CURRENT THERAPY
in Thoracic and Cardiovascular Surgery

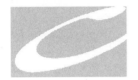

Stephen C. Yang, MD, FACS, FCCP
Associate Professor of Surgery and Medical Oncology
Chief, Division of Thoracic Surgery
Department of Surgery
The Johns Hopkins University School of Medicine
Chief of Thoracic Surgery
The Johns Hopkins Bayview Medical Center
Baltimore, Maryland

Duke E. Cameron, MD, FACS
The James T. Dresher, Sr. Professor of Surgery and Pediatrics
Division of Cardiac Surgery
Department of Surgery
Department of Pediatrics
The Johns Hopkins University School of Medicine
Chief of Pediatric Cardiac Surgery
The Johns Hopkins Hospital
Baltimore, Maryland

CURRENT THERAPY in Thoracic and Cardiovascular Surgery

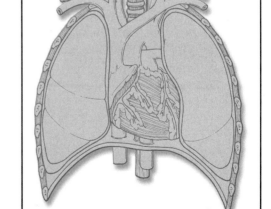

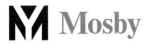
Mosby

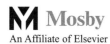
Mosby
An Affiliate of Elsevier

The Curtis Center
170 S Independence Mall W 300E
Philadelphia, Pennsylvania 19106

**WF
970
C976
2004**

Current Therapy in Thoracic and Cardiovascular Surgery   ISBN 0-323-01457-7
Copyright © 2004, Mosby, Inc. All rights reserved.

Library of Congress Cataloging-in-Publication Data

Yang, Stephen C.
Current therapy in thoracic and cardiovascular surgery / [edited by] Stephen C. Yang,
  Duke E. Cameron.
     p. ; cm.
  ISBN 0-323-01457-7
   1. Chest--Surgery. 2. Cardiovascular system--Surgery. I. Yang, Stephen C. II.
Cameron, Duke E.
   [DNLM: 1. Thoracic Surgical Procedures. 2. Cardiovascular Surgical Procedures. WF
970 C976 2004]
  RD536.C875 2004
  617.5′4--dc21

                                                                 2003051392

Vice President, Global Surgery: Richard H. Lampert
Developmental Editor: Kimberley Cox
Publishing Services Manager: Tina Rebane
Project Manager: Norm Stellander
Design Coordinator: Ellen Zanolle

Printed in United States of America

Last digit is the print number: 9 8 7 6 5 4 3 2 1

To our loving families, for their patience, sacrifices, strength, and support

Harry and Muriel Yang
Maria Yang, Kristin, Andy and Alex
Edward and Joanne Cameron
Claudia Cameron, Danielle and Nicole

Contributors

David H. Adams, MD
Marie-Josée and Henry R. Kravis Professor
Department of Cardiovascular Surgery
Mount Sinai School of Medicine
Chairman, Department of Cardiothoracic Surgery
Mount Sinai Medical Center
New York, New York, USA
Conventional Coronary Artery Bypass Surgery

Cary W. Akins, MD
Clinical Professor of Surgery, Harvard Medical School
Visiting Surgeon, Massachusetts General Hospital
Boston, Massachusetts, USA
Coronary Artery Bypass Surgery During Hypothermic Ventricular Fibrillation Without Aortic Occlusion

Scott K. Alpard, MD
Surgical Research Fellow
Division of Cardiothoracic Surgery
University of Texas Medical Branch
Galveston, Texas, USA
Extracorporeal Life Support in the Adult

Nasser K. Altorki, MD
Chief, Division of Thoracic Surgery
Department of Cardiothoracic Surgery
Weill Medical College of Cornell University
New York-Presbyterian Hospital
New York, New York, USA
Ivor-Lewis Esophagectomy

Richard J. Andrassy, MD
Denton A. Cooley Professor and Chairman
Department of Surgery
MD Anderson Cancer Center
Executive Vice President of Clinical Affairs
University of Texas Health Science Center
Houston, Texas, USA
Diaphragmatic Eventration and Plication in the Pediatric Patient

Chandrakanth Are, MD
Assistant Chief of Service
Department of Surgery
The Johns Hopkins Hospital
Baltimore, Maryland, USA
Pulmonary Sequestrations; Laparoscopic Techniques for Gastroesophageal Reflux

Juan P. Arnoletti, MD
Assistant Professor, Department of Surgery
Section of Surgical Oncology
University of Alabama at Birmingham
Birmingham, Alabama, USA
Superior Vena Cava Syndrome

Simon K. Ashiku, MD
Instructor in Surgery
Harvard Medical School
Attending Surgeon, Beth Israel Deaconess Medical Center
Boston, Massachusetts, USA
Carinal Resection

Steven Aufderheide, MD
Department of Anesthesiology and Critical Care Medicine
The Johns Hopkins Medical Institutions
Baltimore, Maryland, USA
Anesthesia for the Thoracic Surgical Patient

Ralph W. Aye, MD
Head, Thoracic Oncology
Swedish Cancer Institute
Swedish Medical Center
Clinical Assistant Professor
Department of Surgery
University of Washington
Seattle, Washington, USA
The Hill Procedure for Gastroesophageal Reflux

Carl L. Backer, MD
A.C. Buehler Professor of Surgery
Feinberg School of Medicine, Northwestern University
Director, Pediatric Heart Transplant Program
Division of Cardiovascular-Thoracic Surgery
Children's Memorial Hospital
Chicago, Illinois, USA
Coronary Artery Disease in Children; Vascular Rings and Pulmonary Artery Slings

Vinay Badhwar, MD
Assistant Professor of Surgery and Pediatrics
University of South Florida
Chairman and Medical Director
Northside Heart Institute
Partner, Cardiac Surgical Associates
St. Petersburg, Florida, USA
Mitral Regurgitation and the Ischemic Heart

Charles E. Bagwell, MD
Professor of Surgery and Pediatrics
Chairman, Division of Pediatric Surgery
Department of Pediatric Surgery
Medical College of Virginia
Virginia Commonwealth University
Richmond, Virginia, USA
Hiatal Hernia and Esophageal Reflux in the Pediatric Patient

N. S. Balaji, MBBS, MS, FRCS
Research Fellow, Foregut Surgery
University of Southern California
Los Angeles, California, USA
Preoperative Evaluation of Gastroesophageal Reflux Disease

Farzaneh Banki, MD
Clinical Instructor, Department of Surgery
University of Southern California Keck School
of Medicine
Los Angeles, California, USA
Benign Strictures of the Esophagus

Hendrick B. Barner, MD
Professor of Surgery
Division of Cardiothoracic Surgery
Washington University School of Medicine
Department of Surgery
Christian Hospital Northwest
Department of Surgery
Barnes-Jewish Hospital
St. Louis, Missouri, USA
Conduit Selection for Coronary Artery Bypass Surgery

Hasan F. Batirel, MD
Assistant Professor, Department of Thoracic Surgery
Marmara University Hospital
Istanbul, Turkey
Lung Amebiasis

Erik Bauer, MD
Resident, Department of Otolaryngology
Washington University School of Medicine
Resident Physician, Department of Otolaryngology
Barnes-Jewish Hospital
St. Louis, Missouri, USA
Tracheostomy

William A. Baumgartner, MD
The Vincent L. Gott Professor
Cardiac Surgeon-in-Charge
Division of Cardiac Surgery
The Johns Hopkins Hospital
Baltimore, Maryland, USA
Neuroprotective Strategies During Cardiac Surgery

Joseph E. Bavaria, MD
Associate Professor of Surgery, Division of
Cardiothoracic Surgery
University of Pennsylvania School of Medicine
Director, Thoracic Aortic Surgery Program
Division of Cardiothoracic Surgery
Hospital of the University of Pennsylvania
Philadelphia, Pennsylvania, USA
Ascending Aortic Aneurysm

Brian T. Bethea, MD
Cardiothoracic Surgery Resident
The Johns Hopkins Hospital
Baltimore, Maryland, USA
Occult Lung Cancer

Michael D. Black, MD
Chief, Pediatric Cardiac Surgery
Director, Pediatric and Adult Congenital Heart Program
California Pacific Medical Center
San Francisco, California, USA
Isolated Ventricular Septal Defect

Steven F. Bolling, MD
Professor of Surgery
Section of Cardiac Surgery
University of Michigan
Ann Arbor, Michigan, USA
Mitral Regurgitation and the Ischemic Heart

Michael Bousamra II, MD
Department of Surgery
University of Louisville
Director of Lung Transplant Program
Jewish Hospital
Louisville, Kentucky, USA
Postoperative Care of the General Thoracic Surgical Patient

Julie R. Brahmer, MD
Division of Medical Oncology
The Sidney Kimmel Comprehensive
Cancer Center at The Johns Hopkins University
Medical Center
The Johns Hopkins Medical Institutions
Baltimore, Maryland, USA
Chemotherapy for Lung Cancer

Jeffrey A. Brinker, MD
Professor of Medicine and Radiology
Department of Cardiovascular Medicine
The Johns Hopkins Medical Institutions
Baltimore, Maryland, USA
Cardiac Pacing in Adults

Derek R. Brinster, MD
Fellow in Cardiothoracic Surgery
Brigham and Women's Hospital
Boston, Massachusetts, USA

Ascending Aortic Aneurysm

Malcolm V. Brock, MD
Division of Thoracic Surgery
The Johns Hopkins Hospital
Baltimore, Maryland, USA

Esophageal Duplication Cysts; Pulmonary Sequestrations

Kelli R. Brooks, MD
Resident, Department of Surgery
Duke University Medical Center
Durham, North Carolina, USA

Tracheoinnominate Artery Fistula

John W. Brown, MD
Harris B. Shumacker Professor of Surgery
Indiana University School of Medicine
Staff Physician, James Whitcomb Riley Hospital
for Children
Indianapolis, Indiana, USA

Congenital Aortic Stenosis; Atrial Septal Defects

Redmond P. Burke, MD
Department of Cardiac Surgery
Miami Children's Hospital
Miami, Florida
Arnold Palmer Hospital
Orlando, Florida, USA

*Patent Ductus Arteriosus and
Aortopulmonary Window*

Harold M. Burkhart, MD
Assistant Professor of Surgery
Division of Cardiothoracic Surgery
University of Iowa
Iowa City, Iowa
Division of Cardiovascular Surgery
Mayo Clinic and Mayo Foundation
Rochester, Minnesota, USA

Mitral Valve Replacement

Brian S. Cain, MD
Kaiser Permanente, East Bay
Cardiac Services Program
Oakland, California, USA

Tension Pneumothorax

Janice Shannon-Cain, CRNA
Anesthetist
Kaiser Oakland Hospital
Oakland, California, USA

Tension Pneumothorax

John H. Calhoon, MD
Professor and Head, Division of Thoracic Surgery
University of Texas Health Science Center,
San Antonio
San Antonio, Texas, USA

Pulmonary Injury

Duke E. Cameron, MD
The James T. Dresher, Sr. Professor of Surgery
and Pediatrics
Division of Cardiac Surgery
Department of Surgery
Department of Pediatrics
Chief of Pediatric Cardiac Surgery
The Johns Hopkins Hospital
Baltimore, Maryland, USA

*Aortic Root Replacement; Tricuspid Valve Operations;
Palliative Operations for Congenital Heart Disease;
Tetralogy of Fallot; Aortic Arch Interruption*

Marcia I. Canto, MD, MHS
Assistant Professor of Medicine
Director, Therapeutic Endoscopy and Endoscopic
Ultrasonography
Division of Gastroenterology
The Johns Hopkins Medical Institutions
Baltimore, Maryland, USA

*Lasers, Stents and Photodynamic Therapy in
Esophageal Cancer*

David J. Caparrelli, MD
Resident, Department of Surgery
The Johns Hopkins Medical Institutions
Baltimore, Maryland, USA

Surgical Approach for Small Cell Lung Cancer

Alan G. Casson, MD
Professor and Head, Division of
Thoracic Surgery
Dalhousie University
Halifax, Nova Scotia, Canada

Carcinoma of the Cervical Esophagus

Stephen M. Cattaneo II, MD
Senior Resident, Department of Surgery
The Johns Hopkins Medical Institutions
Baltimore, Maryland, USA

*Benign Tumors of the Esophagus; Neuroprotective
Strategies During Cardiac Surgery*

Robert J. Cerfolio, MD
Associate Professor, Department of Surgery
University of Alabama at Birmingham
Birmingham, Alabama, USA

Complications of Pulmonary Resections

Ibrahim B. Cetindag, MD
Division of Cardiothoracic Surgery
Southern Illinois University School of Medicine
Springfield, Illinois, USA
Complications of Pulmonary Resections; Surgery for Giant Bullous Disease

Bapsi Chak, MD
Assistant Professor
Department of Radiation Oncology
Vanderbilt University School of Medicine
Nashville, Tennessee, USA
Neoadjuvant Therapy for Esophageal Cancer

Andrew C. Chang, MD
Lecturer, Department of Surgery
Section of Thoracic Surgery
University of Michigan Medical Center
Ann Arbor, Michigan, USA
Transhiatal Esophagectomy

Michael F. Chiaramonte, MD
Clinical Instructor, Division of Plastic Surgery
The Johns Hopkins Medical Institutions
Baltimore, Maryland, USA
Treatment of Sternal Wound Infections

Joseph C. Cleveland, Jr., MD
Assistant Professor of Surgery
Surgical Director, Adult Cardiac Transplantation
Division of Cardiothoracic Surgery
University of Colorado Health Sciences Center
Denver, Colorado, USA
Complications Following Lung Transplantation

Andrew D. Cochrane, FRACS, FRCS
Cardiac Surgeon
Department of Cardiac Surgery
Royal Children's Hospital
Melbourne, Australia
Congenitally Corrected Transposition of the Great Arteries

Neri M. Cohen, MD, PhD
Greater Baltimore Thoracic Surgery
Department of Surgery
GBMC Healthcare
Baltimore, Maryland, USA
Bronchogenic Cysts

Rachel H. Cohn, MS
Clinical Research Coordinator
Department of Cardiothoracic Surgery
Evanston Northwestern Healthcare
Evanston, Illinois, USA
Transmyocardial Revascularization

Brendan J. Collins, MD
Surgical Resident
Department of Surgery
The Johns Hopkins School of Medicine
The Johns Hopkins Hospital
Baltimore, Maryland, USA
Posterior Mediastinal Masses

Paul M. Colombani, MD
Professor of Surgery
Division of Pediatric Surgery
The Johns Hopkins University School of Medicine
Children's Surgeon-in-Charge
Department of Pediatric Surgery
The Johns Hopkins Hospital
Baltimore, Maryland, USA
Pectus Excavatum and Carinatum

Stephen B. Colvin, MD
Chief of Cardiothoracic Surgery
New York University School of Medicine
New York, New York, USA
Mitral Valve Reconstruction

John V. Conte, MD
Associate Professor of Surgery
The Johns Hopkins University School of Medicine
Associate Professor & Director of Cardiopulmonary Transplantation
Division of Cardiac Surgery
The Johns Hopkins Hospital
Baltimore, Maryland, USA
Cardiac Transplant

Denton A. Cooley, MD
President and Surgeon-in-Chief
Texas Heart Institute
Clinical Professor of Surgery
University of Texas Health Science Center, Houston
Houston, Texas, USA
Ventricular Aneurysms

Juan A. Cordero, Jr., MD
Attending Cardiothoracic Surgeon
Good Samaritan Regional Medical Center
Attending Cardiothoracic Surgeon
Phoenix Cardiac Surgery, P.C.
Phoenix, Arizona, USA
Morgagni and Bochdalek Hernias in the Adult

Edward E. Cornwell III, MD
Department of General Surgery
The Johns Hopkins Hospital
Associate Professor of Surgery
Chief, Adult Trauma Service

Department of Surgery
The Johns Hopkins School of Medicine
Baltimore, Maryland, USA
Traumatic Hemothorax

Robert M. Cortina, MD
Attending Thoracic Surgeon
New Hanover Regional Medical Center
Wilmington, North Carolina, USA
Chylothorax

Joseph S. Coselli, MD
Professor and Chief, Division of Cardiothoracic Surgery
Michael E. DeBakey Department of Surgery
Baylor College of Medicine
Chief of Service
Department of Cardiothoracic Surgery
Methodist DeBakey Heart Center
Houston, Texas, USA
Descending Thoracic Aortic Aneurysms

Jane E. Crosson, MD
Assistant Professor of Pediatrics, Director of Pediatric Electrophysiology
The Johns Hopkins University School of Medicine
Baltimore, Maryland, USA
Cardiac Pacing in Children

Benedict D.T. Daly, MD
Professor of Cardiothoracic Surgery
Boston University School of Medicine
Director of General Thoracic Surgery
Boston Medical Center
Boston, Massachusetts, USA
Eventration of the Diaphragm

Thomas A. D'Amico, MD
Associate Professor of Surgery
Department of Surgery
Duke University Medical Center
Durham, North Carolina, USA
Tracheoinnominate Artery Fistula

Alan Dardik, MD, PhD
Division of Vascular Surgery, Department of Surgery
The Johns Hopkins Hospital
Baltimore, Maryland, USA
Combined Carotid and Coronary Disease

Philippe G. Darteville, MD
Professor of Surgery
Paris-Sud University
Paris
Chairman, Department of Thoracic and Vascular Surgery and Heart-Lung Transplantation

Marie Lannelongue Hospital
Le Plessis Robinson, France
Superior Sulcus Tumors

Malcolm M. DeCamp, Jr., MD
Director, Lung Transplant Program
Staff Surgeon, Department of Thoracic and Cardiovascular Surgery
The Cleveland Clinic Foundation
Cleveland, Ohio, USA
Video-Assisted Thoracic Surgery and Pericardial Effusive Diseases

Steven R. DeMeester, MD
Assistant Professor of Cardiothoracic Surgery
Keck School of Medicine of
University of Southern California
Norris Comprehensive Cancer Center
Los Angeles, California, USA
Achalasia

Philippe Demers, MD, MSC, FRCS(C)
Assistant Professor of Surgery
University of Montreal
Staff Surgeon
Montreal Heart Institute
Montreal, Quebec, Canada
Postpneumonectomy Empyema and Bronchopleural Fistula

Claude Deschamps, MD
Cardiothoracic Surgery
The Mayo Clinic
Rochester, Minnesota, USA
Esophageal Reconstruction—Colonic Interposition

Jean Deslauriers, MD, FRCS(C)
Professor of Surgery
Laval University
Division of Thoracic Surgery
Centre de Pneumologie de l'Hopital Laval
Sainte-Foy, Quebec, Canada
Postpneumonectomy Empyema and Bronchopleural Fistula

Frank C. Detterbeck, MD
Cardiothoracic Surgery
University of North Carolina
Chapel Hill, North Carolina, USA
Myasthenia Gravis and Thymoma

E. Gene Deune, MD
Assistant Professor, Division of Plastic Surgery
The Johns Hopkins Hospital
Baltimore, Maryland, USA
Treatment of Sternal Wound Infections

Patrick DeValeria, MD
Assistant Professor, Division of Cardiovascular and Thoracic Surgery
Mayo Clinic Scottsdale
Scottsdale, Arizona, USA
Surgical Management of Pericardial Disease

Daniel J. DiBardino, MD
Surgical Resident
Michael E. DeBakey Department of Surgery
Baylor College of Medicine
Research Fellow
Congenital Heart Surgery
Texas Children's Hospital
Houston, Texas, USA
Descending Thoracic Aortic Aneurysms

J. Michael DiMaio, MD
Assistant Professor
Division of Thoracic and Cardiovascular Surgery
The University of Texas Southwestern Medical Center
Dallas, Texas, USA
Human Immunodeficiency Virus and the General Thoracic Surgeon

Dean M. Donahue, MD
Assistant Professor of Surgery
Harvard Medical School
Division of Thoracic Surgery
Massachusetts General Hospital
Boston, Massachusetts, USA
Acquired Tracheal Stenosis

Donald B. Doty, MD
Adjunct Professor of Surgery
Department of Surgery
University of Utah School of Medicine
Staff Surgeon
Division of Cardiovascular and Thoracic Surgery
LDS Hospital
Salt Lake City, Utah, USA
Spiral Saphenous Vein Bypass Graft for Superior Vena Cava Obstruction; The Small Aortic Root

John R. Doty, MD
Staff Surgeon
Division of Cardiovascular and Thoracic Surgery
LDS Hospital
Salt Lake City, Utah, USA
Spiral Saphenous Vein Bypass Graft for Superior Vena Cava Obstruction; Concomitant Cardiac and Thoracic Operations; The Small Aortic Root

Frank D'Ovidio, MD
Clinical Fellow, Thoracic Surgery
Division of Thoracic Surgery

Toronto General Hospital
Toronto, Ontario, Canada
Non-Small Lung Cancer—Stage I and II Disease

Robert J. Downey, MD
Associate Professor of Surgery
Division of Thoracic Surgery, Department of Surgery
Memorial Sloan-Kettering Cancer Center
New York, New York, USA
Non-Small Cell Lung Cancer—Stage III Disease

George Drugas, MD
Associate Professor of Surgery and Pediatrics
Department of Surgery, Section of Pediatric Surgery
University of Rochester Medical Center
Pediatric Surgeon
Golisano Children's Hospital at Strong Surgery
University of Rochester School of Medicine and Dentistry
Rochester, New York, USA
Congenital Tracheoesophageal Fistula

Brian W. Duncan, MD
Surgeon, Department of Pediatric and Congenital Heart Surgery
The Cleveland Clinic Foundation
Cleveland, Ohio, USA
Transposition of Great Arteries

André Duranceau, MD
Professor of Surgery, Universite de Montreal
Centre Hospitalier de l'Universite de Montreal
Montreal, Quebec, Canada
Pharyngoesophageal Dysfunction and Cricopharyngeal Myotomy

Daniel J. Durand, BS
Medical Student
The Johns Hopkins University School of Medicine
Baltimore, Maryland, USA
Lung Transplantation in the Pediatric Patient

Cornelius M. Dyke, MD
The Sanger Clinic, PA
Gastonia, North Carolina, USA
Cardiac Tumors

Harvey L. Edmonds, Jr., PhD
Professor and Director of Research
Department of Anesthesiology
University of Louisville
Director, Cardiovascular Neuromonitoring
Department of Cardiothoracic Surgery
Jewish Hospital Heart and Lung Institute
Louisville, Kentucky, USA
Intraoperative Cerebral Monitoring

David W. Eisele, MD, FACS
Professor and Chairman
Department of Otolaryngology-Head and Neck Surgery
University of California, San Francisco
San Francisco, California, USA
The Difficult Elective Intubation

John A. Elefteriades, MD
Professor and Chief
Cardiothoracic Surgery
Yale University School of Medicine
Attending Surgeon
Department of Cardiothoracic Surgery
Yale-New Haven Hospital
New Haven, Connecticut, USA
Aortic Dissection

Ronald C. Elkins, MD
Professor Emeritus, Section of Thoracic and
Cardiovascular Surgery
The University of Oklahoma Health Sciences Center
Oklahoma City, Oklahoma, USA
The Ross Operation

Armin Ernst, MD
Assistant Professor of Medicine, Harvard Medical School
Director, Interventional Pulmonology
Co-Director, Medical Critical Care
Beth Israel Deaconess Medical Center
Boston, Massachusetts, USA
Stenting of the Airway

David S. Ettinger, MD
The Alex Grass Professor of Oncology
Department of Oncology
The Sidney Kimmel Comprehensive Cancer Center
The Johns Hopkins Medical Insitutions
Baltimore, Maryland, USA
Chemotherapy for Lung Cancer

L. Penfield Faber, MD
Vice-Chairman and Professor
Department of Cardiovascular-Thoracic Surgery
Rush University Medical Center
Senior Attending Physician
Department of Cardiovascular and Thoracic Surgery
Presbyterian-St. Luke's Medical Center
Chicago, Illinois, USA
Limited Resection Procedures for Lung Cancer

James Fackler, MD
Clinical Director for Pediatric Intensive Care
Associate Professor of Anesthesiology
The Johns Hopkins Medical Institutions
Baltimore, Maryland, USA
*Pediatric Extracorporeal Membrane Oxygenation and
Mechanical Circulatory Assist Devices*

Christopher M. Feindel, MD
Deputy Head
Division of Cardiovascular Surgery
Medical Director, Heart & Circulation
Program
Toronto General Hospital
Toronto, Ontario, Canada
Postinfarction Ventricular Septal Defect

Stanley C. Fell, MD
Professor of Cardiothoracic Surgery
Albert Einstein College of Medicine
Director of Thoracic Surgery (1977-1997)
Montefiore Medical Center
New York, New York, USA
*Esophageal Reconstruction—Reversed and Nonreversed
Gastric Tubes*

Robert L. Ferris, MD, PhD
Assistant Professor
Otolaryngology and Immunology
University of Pittsburgh Eye and Ear Institute
University of Pittsburgh Cancer Institute
Pittsburgh, Pennsylvania, USA
The Difficult Elective Intubation

Farzan Filsoufi, MD
Assistant Professor, Department of
Cardiothoracic Surgery
Mount Sinai School of Medicine
Director, Cardiac Valve Center
Mount Sinai Medical Center
New York, New York, USA
Conventional Coronary Artery Bypass Surgery

Anne C. Fischer, MD, PhD
Assistant Professor of Surgery
Division of Pediatric Surgery
The Johns Hopkins University
Baltimore, Maryland, USA
Congenital Pulmonary Disorders

Elliot K. Fishman, MD, FACR
Professor of Radiology and Oncology
Director, Diagnostic Imaging and Body CT
The Russell H. Morgan Department of Radiology and
Radiological Science
The Johns Hopkins University
Baltimore, Maryland, USA
Radiologic Assessment of the Chest

Torin P. Fitton, MD
Fellow, Cardiac Surgery
Johns Hopkins Hospital
Baltimore, Maryland, USA
Pulmonary Arteriovenous Malformation

Arlene A. Forastiere, MD
Professor of Oncology
Sidney Kimmel Cancer Center
The Johns Hopkins University School of Medicine
Baltimore, Maryland, USA

Neoadjuvant Therapy for Esophageal Cancer

Randall S. Fortuna, MD
Clinical Assistant Professor in Pediatrics
University of Illinois College of Medicine at Peoria
Pediatric Cardiovascular Surgeon
Children's Hospital of Illinois at DSF Saint Francis
Medical Center
Peoria, Illinois, USA

Trauma to the Heart and Great Vessels

Charles D. Fraser Jr., MD
Professor of Surgery and Pediatrics
Department of Surgery
Baylor College of Medicine
Chief of Congenital Heart Surgery
Congenital Heart Surgery Services
Texas Children's Hospital
Houston, Texas, USA

Aortic Valve Repair

Willard A. Fry, MD
Professor Emeritus of Surgery
Northwestern University Medical School
Chicago
Former Chief of the Section of Thoracic Surgery
Evanston Northwestern Healthcare
Evanston, Illinois, USA

Spontaneous Pneumothorax

Henning A. Gaissert, MD
Assistant Professor of Surgery
Division of Thoracic Surgery
Massachusetts General Hospital and
Harvard Medical School
Boston, Massachusetts, USA

*Esophageal Reconstruction—Jejunal Segment
Interposition and Free Graft*

Aubrey C. Galloway, MD
Professor of Surgery
Director, Thoracic Surgery Residency Program
New York University Medical Center
New York, New York, USA

Mitral Valve Reconstruction

Ziv Gamliel, MD, FRCSC, FACS
Division of Thoracic Surgery
University of Maryland
Baltimore, Maryland, USA

Video-Assisted Thoracic Surgery and Esophageal Disease

Brian L. Ganzel, MD
Associate Professor, Department of
Cardiothoracic Surgery
University of Louisville School of Medicine
Louisville, Kentucky, USA

Intraoperative Cerebral Monitoring

Susan Garwood, MB, CHB
Associate Professor, Department of Anesthesiology
Yale University School of Medicine
New Haven, Connecticut, USA

Inotropic Support

A. Marc Gillinov, MD
Surgical Director, Center for Atrial Fibrillation
Department of Thoracic and Cardiovascular Surgery
The Cleveland Clinic Foundation
Cleveland, Ohio, USA

*Surgical Treatment of Atrial Fibrillation; Aortic Valve
Replacement*

Robert J. Ginsberg, MD, FRCSC†
Professor of Surgery
Chairman, Division of Thoracic Surgery
University of Toronto
Toronto, Ontario, Canada

Non-Small Lung Cancer—Stage I and II Disease

Thomas G. Gleason, MD
Assistant Professor of Surgery, Division of
Cardiothoracic Surgery
University of Pennsylvania School of Medicine
Hospital of the University of Pennsylvania
Philadelphia, Pennsylvania, USA

Ascending Aortic Aneurysm

Melvyn Goldberg, MD
Vice-Chairman, Department of Surgical Oncology
Chief, Thoracic Surgical Oncology
Fox Chase Cancer Center
Philadelphia, Pennsylvania, USA

Superior Vena Cava Syndrome

Clifford Goldman, BS, MD
Attending Anesthesiologist and Pain Management
Physician
Holy Cross Hospital
Silver Spring, Maryland, USA

Postoperative Pain Control for Thoracic Surgery

**Terry Gourlay, PhD, BSc (Hons), CBiol, MI Biol,
ILTHE, FRSH**
Department of Cardiothoracic Surgery

---

†Deceased.

Imperial College London
London, United Kingdom
Adult Cardiopulmonary Bypass

Geoffrey M. Graeber, MD
Professor of Surgery
Director of Surgical Research
Section of Thoracic and Cardiovascular Surgery
West Virginia University School of Medicine
Morgantown, West Virginia, USA
Muscle Flaps for Chest Wall Reconstruction

Igor D. Gregoric, MD
Associate Chief, Transplant Service
Director, Mechanical Circulatory Support
St. Luke's Episcopal Hospital
Texas Heart Institute
Houston, Texas, USA
Ventricular Aneurysms

Randall Griepp, MD
Professor of Cardiothoracic Surgery
Mount Sinai Medical Center
New York, New York, USA
Reconstruction of Aortic Arch Aneurysms

Sean C. Grondin, MD, MPH, FACS, FRCSC
Associate Professor of Surgery
University of Calgary
Director of Research, Division of thoracic Surgery
Foothills Medical Center
Calgary, Alberta, Canada
*Pleurectomy for Diffuse Mesothelioma; Evaluation of the
Solitary Pulmonary Nodule; Spontaneous Pneumothorax*

Eugene A. Grossi, MD
Professor of Surgery
Division of Cardiothoracic Surgery
Department of Surgery
New York University School of Medicine
Chief Thoracic Surgery
New York Veterans Administration Hospital
New York, New York, USA
Mitral Valve Reconstruction

Frederick L. Grover, MD
Professor and Chair, Department of Surgery
University of Colorado School of Medicine
Denver, Colorado, USA
Complications Following Lung Transplantation

Robert A. Guyton, MD
Charles R. Hatcher, Jr. Professor of Surgery
Chief of the Division of Cardiothoracic Surgery
Emory University School of Medicine
Atlanta, Georgia, USA
Myocardial Protection

Jeffrey A. Hagen, MD, FACS, FCCP
Associate Professor of Clinical Surgery
Keck School of Medicine
University of Southern California
Chief, Section of Thoracic/Foregut Surgery
LAC-USC Medical Center
Los Angeles, California, USA
Benign Strictures of the Esophagus

Robert L. Hannan, MD
Cardiovascular Surgeon
Miami Children's Hospital
Miami, Florida, USA
Patent Ductus Arteriosus and Aortopulmonary Window

David H. Harpole, Jr., MD
Professor of Surgery
Department of Surgery
Duke University Medical Center
Durham Veterans Administration Hospital
Durham, North Carolina, USA
Benign and Low-Grade Malignant Tumors of the Lung

John Hawkins, MD
Professor of Surgery
University of Utah
Chief, Cardiothoracic Surgery
Primary Children's Medical Center
Salt Lake City, Utah, USA
Pulmonary Valve and Infundibular Stenosis

Stephen R. Hazelrigg, MD
Professor and Chairman
Division of Cardiothoracic Surgery
Southern Illinois University School of Medicine
Springfield, Illinois, USA
Surgery for Giant Bullous Disease

Richard F. Heitmiller, MD
Chief of Surgery
Union Memorial Hospital
Baltimore, Maryland, USA
Cancer of the Gastroesophageal Junction

Alan W. Heldman, MD
Assistant Professor of Medicine
The Johns Hopkins University School of Medicine
Director, Multimodality Cardiovascular Intervention
The Johns Hopkins Hospital
Baltimore, Maryland, USA
Cardiac Catheterization

Neal D. Hillman, MD
Assistant Professor of Surgery
Department of Cardiothoracic Surgery
University of Utah
Salt Lake City, Utah, USA
Pulmonary Valve and Infundibular Stenosis

Roberta Hines, MD
Professor of Anesthesiology
Chairman, Department of Anesthesiology
Yale New Haven Hospital
New Haven, Connecticut, USA
Inotropic Support

Jeff C. Hoehner, MD, PhD
Assistant Professor of Surgery
The Johns Hopkins Medical Institutions
Baltimore, Maryland, USA
Congenital Diaphragmatic Hernia

Katherine J. Hoercher, RN
Director of Research
Kaufman Center for Heart Failure
The Cleveland Clinic
Cleveland, Ohio, USA
Left Ventricular Volume Reduction

Wayne Hofstetter, MD
Assistant Professor, Division of Thoracic Surgery
UCLA School of Medicine
Los Angeles, California, USA
Lymph Node Dissection for Esophageal Cancer

Richard A. Hopkins, MD
Karlson Professor and Chief of Cardiothoracic Surgery
Brown University
Providence, Rhode Island, USA
Valve Replacement in Children

John Howington, MD, FACS
Assistant Professor of Surgery
Department of Surgery
University of Cincinnati College of Medicine
Director, Division of Thoracic Surgery
Department of Surgery
University Hospital
Chief, Division of Thoracic Surgery
Department of Surgical Services
Cincinnati Veterans Affairs Medical Center
Cincinnati, Ohio, USA
Thoracic Incisions

Tain-Yen Hsia, MD
Chief Resident
Division of Thoracic Surgery
The Johns Hopkins Hospital
Baltimore, Maryland, USA
Diaphragmatic Injuries

Charles B. Huddleston, MD
Professor of Surgery
Washington University School of Medicine

St. Louis Children's Hospital
Chief, Pediatric Cardiothoracic Surgery
St. Louis Children's Hospital
St. Louis, Missouri, USA
Complete Atrioventricular Canal

Mark Iannettoni, MD
Johann L. Ehrenraft Professor and Chairman
Department of Cardiothoracic Surgery
University of Iowa Hospitals and Clinics
Roy and Lucille Carver College of Medicine
Iowa City, Iowa, USA
Transhiatal Esophagectomy

Riivo Ilves, MD
Chief, Thoracic Surgery
Department of Cardiothoracic Surgery
Albany Medical Center
Chief, Thoracic Surgery
Department of Surgery
Stratton Veterans Affairs Hospital
Albany, New York, USA
Nissen Fundoplication

David M. Jablons, MD
Associate Professor of Surgery
Chief, Section of General Thoracic Surgery
University of California at San Francisco
San Francisco, California, USA
Tension Pneumothorax

Sanjay Jagannath, MD
Assistant Professor of Medicine
Department of Gastroenterology
The Johns Hopkins Hospital
Baltimore, Maryland, USA
Lasers, Stents and Photodynamic Therapy in Esophageal Cancer

Stuart W. Jamieson, MD
Professor and Head
Division of Cardiothoracic Surgery
University of California, San Diego
Medical Center
San Diego, California, USA
Pulmonary Thromboendarterectomy

Scott B. Johnson, MD
Associate Professor, Division of Cardiothoracic Surgery
University of Texas Health Science Center
University Hospital
Audey-Murphy Veterans Affairs Hospital
San Antonio, Texas, USA
Pulmonary Injury

David W. Johnstone, MD
Associate Professor of Surgery and Oncology
Department of Surgery
Strong Memorial Hospital
Rochester, New York, USA

Chylothorax

David R. Jones, MD
Assistant Professor of Surgery
Division of Thoracic and Cardiovascular Surgery
University of Virginia
Charlottesville, Virginia, USA

Anterior Mediastinal Masses

Larry R. Kaiser, MD
The John Rhea Barton Professor and Chair
Department of Surgery
University of Pennsylvania School of Medicine
Chief of Surgery
Hospital of The University of Pennsylvania
Philadelphia, Pennsylvania, USA

Lung Volume Reduction Surgery—Video-Assisted Thoracoscopic Approach

Tom R. Karl, MD
Professor of Surgery and Pediatrics
University of California, San Francisco
Chief of Pediatric Cardiothoracic Surgery
University of California San Francisco Children's Hospital
San Francisco, California, USA

Congenitally Corrected Transposition of the Great Arteries

Riyad Karmy-Jones, MD
Department of Surgery
University of Washington
Seattle, Washington, USA

Mediastinitis

Edmund S. Kassis, MD
Senior Resident, Department of Surgery
The Johns Hopkins Medical Institutions
Baltimore, Maryland, USA

Pulmonary Fungal Infections

Robert J. Keenan, MD
Professor of Cardiothoracic Surgery
Department of Cardiothoracic Surgery
Drexel University College of Medicine
Philadelphia
Director, Division of Thoracic Surgery
Co-Director, Minimally Invasive Surgery
West Penn Allegheny Health Systems
Program Director, West Penn Center for Lung and Cardiothoracic Surgery
West Penn Hospital
Pittsburgh, Pennsylvania, USA

Belsey Mark IV Repair for Gastroesophageal Reflux

Steven M. Keller, MD
Interim Chair, Cardiothoracic Surgery
Montefiore Medical Center
Professor of Cardiothoracic Surgery
Albert Einstein College of Medicine
Bronx, New York, USA

Mediastinal Lymph Node Dissection for Lung Cancer

Kemp H. Kernstine, MD, PhD
Chief, Section of General Thoracic Surgery
Division of Cardiothoracic Surgery
Department of Surgery
University of Iowa Hospitals and Clinics
Iowa City, Iowa, USA

Pneumomediastinum

Kenneth A. Kesler, MD, FACS
Professor of Surgery
Department of Surgery, Section of Cardiothoracic Surgery
Indiana University School of Medicine
Indianapolis, Indiana, USA

Bronchial Adenomas

Paul A. Kirschner, MD, FACS
Professor Emeritus
Department of Cardiothoracic Surgery
Mount Sinai School of Medicine
New York, New York, USA

Localized Fibrous Tumors of the Pleura

Paul M. Kirshbom, MD
Department of Cardiothoracic Surgery
Emory University School of Medicine
Assistant Professor of Surgery
Department of Cardiothoracic Surgery
Emory University Hospital
Atlanta, Georgia, USA

Hypoplastic Left Heart Syndrome

Lawrence R. Kleinberg, MD
Assistant Professor, Department of Radiation Oncology
Sidney Kimmel Comprehensive Cancer Center at The Johns Hopkins University School of Medicine
Baltimore, Maryland, USA

Radiotherapy for Lung Cancer; Radiotherapy for Esophageal Disease

Christopher J. Knott-Craig, MD, FACS
Professor of Surgery
Chief, Pediatric Thoracic and Cardiovascular Surgery

University of Oklahoma Health Sciences Center
Oklahoma City, Oklahoma, USA
Prosthetic Valve Endocarditis

Neal D. Kon, MD
Wake Forest University School of Medicine
Winston-Salem, North Carolina, USA
Selection of a Cardiac Valve Prosthesis

Stephen J. Korkola, MD
Senior Resident, Cardiothoracic Surgery
Division of Cardiothoracic Surgery
The Montreal General Hospital
McGill University Health Center
Montreal, Quebec, Canada
Traumatic Airway Injuries

Mark J. Krasna, MD, FACS
Chief, Division of Thoracic Surgery
Director, Thoracic Oncology Program
University of Maryland School of Medicine
Baltimore, Maryland, USA
Video-Assisted Thoracic Surgery and Esophageal Disease

Jason J. Lamb, MD
Co-Director, West Penn Center for Lung and thoracic
Disease
Western Pennsylvania Hospital
Pittsburgh, Pennsylvania, USA
Belsey Mark IV Repair for Gastroesophageal Reflux

Rodney J. Landreneau, MD
Director, Comprehensive Lung Center
UPMC Shadyside
Division of Thoracic and Foregut Surgery
Shadyside Medical Center
UPMC Presbyterian University Hospital
Jameson Health System
UPMC St. Margaret Hospital
Pittsburgh, Pennsylvania, USA
Complications of Video-Assisted Thoracic Surgery

David A. Lanning, MD, PhD
Fellow in Pediatric Surgery
Children's Hospital of Michigan
Detroit, Michigan, USA
*Hiatal Hernia and Esophageal Reflux in the Pediatric
Patient*

Christine L. Lau, MD
Resident of Surgery
Department of Surgery
Duke University Medical Center
Durham, North Carolina, USA
Benign and Low-Grade Malignant Tumors of the Lung

Richard H. Lee, MD
Chief Resident, Division of Plastic and
Reconstructive Surgery
The Johns Hopkins Medical Institutions
Baltimore, Maryland, USA
Prosthetic Substitutes for Chest Wall Reconstruction

Robert B. Lee, MD, FACS
Associate Professor, Clinical, of Cardiac and
Thoracic Surgery
Department of General Surgery
University of Mississippi Medical Center
Chief of Surgery
Central Mississippi Medical Center
Jackson, Mississippi, USA
Empyema Thoracis

Steven J. Lester, MD, FACC, FRCPC, FASE
Consultant, Cardiovascular Diseases
Assistant Professor, Mayo Clinic College of Medicine
Department of Medicine, Division of Cardiology
Mayo Clinic Scottsdale
Scottsdale, Arizona, USA
Surgical Management of Pericardial Disease

Jerrold H. Levy, MD
Professor of Anesthesiology
Emory University School of Medicine
Cardiothoracic Anesthesiology and Critical Care
Emory Healthcare
Atlanta, Georgia, USA
Blood Conservation Strategies in Cardiac Surgery

Cleveland W. Lewis, Jr., MD
Director, Thoracic Surgery
Orange Regional Medical Center
Middletown, New York, USA
*Actinomycosis and Nocardial Infections
of the Lung*

Amy M. Lightner, MD
Resident in General Surgery
Massachusetts General Hospital
Boston, Massachusetts, USA
Malignant Tracheal Tumors

R. Eric Lilly, MD
Assistant Professor of Surgery
Brown Medical School
Director, Cardiac ICU
Department of Cardiothoracic Surgery
The Miriam Hospital
Providence, Rhode Island, USA
Valve Replacement in Children

João A. Lima, MD
Associate Professor of Medicine
Department of Cardiology
Director of Cardiovascular Imaging in Cardiology
Department of Cardiology
The Johns Hopkins University
Baltimore, Maryland, USA
Intraoperative Transesophageal Echocardiography

Jonathan Limpert, MD
Department of Surgery
St. Louis University Health Sciences Center
St. Louis, Missouri, USA
Paraesophageal Hernia

Michael J. Liptay, MD
Head, Division of Thoracic Oncology and Section of
Thoracic Surgery
Evanston Northwestern Healthcare
Assistant Professor of Surgery
Northwestern University Medical School
Evanston, Illinois, USA
*Evaluation of the Solitary Pulmonary Nodule;
Pleurectomy for Diffuse Mesothelioma*

Virginia R. Litle, MD
Cardiothoracic Surgery Resident
Division of Thoracic Surgery
University of Pittsburgh Medical Center
Pittsburgh, Pennsylvania, USA
Non-Small Cell Lung Cancer—Stage IV Disease

Alex G. Little, MD
Professor of Surgery
Elizabeth Berry Gray Chair of Surgery
Department of Surgery
Wright State University School of Medicine
Dayton, Ohio, USA
The Failed Antireflux Operation

Thom E. Lobe, MD
Professor of Surgery, Pediatrics and Preventive
Medicine
University of Tennessee
Chairman, Section of Pediatric Surgery
LeBonheur Children's Medical Center
Memphis, Tennessee, USA
Pediatric Tracheal Disorders

Joseph LoCicero, III, MD
Professor and Chair, Department of Surgery
University of South Alabama Health System
Mobile, Alabama, USA
Non-Small Cell Lung Cancer—Chest Wall Invasion

Gary K. Lofland, MD
Professor of Surgery
University of Missouri/Kansas City School
of Medicine
Joseph Boon Gregg Section of Thoracic Surgery
Children's Mercy Hospital
Kansas City, Missouri, USA
Pulmonary Atresia with Intact Ventricular Septum

James D. Luketich, MD
Chief, Division of Thoracic and
Foregut Surgery
Department of Surgery
University of Pittsburgh Medical Center
Pittsburgh, Pennsylvania, USA
Non-Small Cell Lung Cancer—Stage IV Disease

Bruce W. Lytle, MD
Staff Surgeon
Department of Thoracic and
Cardiovascular Surgery
The Cleveland Clinic Foundation
Cleveland, Ohio, USA
Reoperation for Coronary Artery Bypass Surgery

Paolo Macchiarini, MD, PhD
Professor of Surgery
Hannover Medical School
Chief, Department of Thoracic and
Vascular Surgery
Heidehaus Hospital
Hannover, Germany
*Acquired Tracheoesophageal Fistula; Superior
Sulcus Tumors*

Michael J. Mack, MD
Medical Director, Cardiovascular Disease and
Transplantation
Medical City Dallas Hospital
Department of Cardiothoracic Surgery
Cardiopulmonary Research Science and
Technology Institute
Dallas, Texas, USA
*Off-Pump Coronary Artery Bypass Surgery;
Eventration of the Diaphragm*

Michael M. Madani, MD
Assistant Clinical Professor of Surgery
Division of Cardiothoracic Surgery
University of California Medical Center
Chief, Division of Cardiothoracic Surgery
Veterans Affairs Medical Center La Jolla
San Diego, California, USA
Pulmonary Thromboendarterectomy

Kamal A. Mansour, MD
Professor of Surgery
Division of Cardiothoracic Surgery
Emory University School of Medicine
Chief, Department of General
Thoracic Surgery
Veterans Affairs Medical Center
Atlanta, Georgia, USA
Diffuse Esophageal Spasm and Scleroderma

Douglas J. Mathisen, MD
Hermes C. Grillo Professor of Thoracic Surgery
Harvard Medical School
Visiting Surgeon and Chief, General Thoracic
Surgery Unit
Massachusetts General Hospital
Boston, Massachusetts, USA
Malignant Tracheal Tumors; Carinal Resection

Kenneth L. Mattox, MD
Professor and Vice Chairman,
Department of Surgery
Baylor College of Medicine
Chief of Staff
Chief of Surgery
Ben Taub General Hospital
Houston, Texas, USA
Chest Wall Injury and Blunt Cardiac Trauma

Constantine Mavroudis, MD
Professor of Surgery
Feinberg School of Medicine
Northwestern University
Surgeon in Chief, Cardiovascular-Thoracic Surgery
Willis J. Potts Professor of Surgery
Children's Memorial Hospital
Chicago, Illinois, USA
*Coronary Artery Disease in Children; Vascular Rings
and Pulmonary Artery Slings*

John C. Mayberry, MD
Associate Professor of Surgery
Trauma/Critical Care Section,
Department of Surgery
Oregon Health and Science University
Portland, Oregon, USA
Flail Chest and Pulmonary Contusion

Patrick M. McCarthy, MD
Surgical Director, Kaufman Center for Heart Failure
Thoracic and Cardiovascular Surgery
The Cleveland Clinic Foundation
Cleveland, Ohio, USA
Surgical Treatment of Atrial Fibrillation

Walter E. McGregor, MD
Staff Cardiothoracic Surgeon
Department of Cardiothoracic Surgery
Riverside Methodist Hospital
Columbus, Ohio, USA
Complications of Video-Assisted Thoracic Surgery

D. Michael McMullan, MD
Chief Resident, Cardiothoracic Surgery
Division of Cardiothoracic Surgery
University of Washington
Seattle, Washington, USA
Pleural Effusions

Roger B. B. Mee, MB, CH.B, FRACS
Chairman, Pediatric and Congenital Heart Surgery
The Cleveland Clinic Foundation
Cleveland, Ohio, USA
Transposition of Great Arteries

David S. Mendelson, MD
Associate Professor of Radiology
Mount Sinai School of Medicine of New York University
Associate Attending
The Mount Sinai Medical Center
New York, New York, USA
Localized Fibrous Tumors of the Pleura

Walter H. Merrill, MD
Professor of Surgery
Section of Cardiothoracic Surgery
University of Cincinnati
Cincinnati, Ohio, USA
Hypertrophic Cardiomyopathy

Bryan F. Meyers, MD
Associate Professor of Surgery
Department of Surgery
Washington University School of Medicine
St. Louis, Missouri, USA
Tracheostomy

Daniel L. Miller, MD
Associate Professor of Surgery
Section of Thoracic Surgery
Emory University Clinic
Atlanta, Georgia, USA
Bronchiectasis

Joseph I. Miller, Jr., MD
Professor and Chief of General Thoracic Surgery
Emory University School of Medicine
Atlanta, Georgia, USA
Video-Assisted Thoracic Surgery for Pleural Disease

Douglas N. Miniati, MD
Chief Resident
Stanford University Medical Center
Stanford, California, USA
Heart-Lung Transplantation

John D. Mitchell, MD
Assistant Professor of Surgery
Chief, Section of General Thoracic Surgery
Division of Cardiothoracic Surgery
University of Colorado School of Medicine
Denver, Colorado, USA
Congenital and Acquired Esophageal Diverticula

Peter J. Mogayzel, Jr., MD, PhD
Assistant Professor of Pediatrics, Anesthesia and
Critical Care Medicine
Director, Cystic Fibrosis Center
Medical Director, Pediatric Lung
Transplantation Program
The Johns Hopkins School of Medicine
Baltimore, Maryland, USA
*Cystic Fibrosis; Lung Transplantation in the
Pediatric Patient*

Darroch W.O. Moores, MD
Associate Professor of Surgery
Albany Medical College
Attending Surgeon
Department of Surgery
St. Peter Hospital
Albany, New York, USA
Morgagni and Bochdalek Hernias in the Adult

Keith D. Mortman, MD
Clinical Fellow, Division of Thoracic Surgery
Cedars-Sinai Medical Center
Los Angeles, California, USA
Mediastinal Lymph Node Dissection for Lung Cancer

David S. Mulder, MD
H. Rocke Robertson Professor of Surgery
Division of Cardiothoracic Surgery
The Montreal General Hospital
McGill University Health Center
Montreal, Quebec, Canada
Traumatic Airway Injuries

Sudish C. Murthy, MD, PhD
Department of Thoracic and
Cardiovascular Surgery
The Cleveland Clinic Foundation
Cleveland, Ohio, USA
Esophageal Perforation

John L. Myers, MD
Professor of Surgery and Pediatrics
Director, Pediatric and Congenital
Cardiovascular Surgery
Penn State Children's Hospital
Hershey, Pennsylvania, USA
Coarctation of the Aorta

Keith S. Naunheim, MD
Professor of Surgery
St. Louis University
The Vallee L. and Melba-Willman Professor and
Chief of Cardiothoracic Surgery
St. Louis University Health Sciences Center
St. Louis, Missouri, USA
Paraesophageal Hernia

Jonathan C. Nesbitt, MD
Clinical Professor
Vanderbilt University Medical Center
Staff Surgeon
Department of Cardiothoracic Surgery
St. Thomas Hospital
Nashville, Tennessee, USA
Middle Mediastinal Masses

Dao M. Nguyen, MD
Principal Investigator, Thoracic Oncology Section
Surgery Branch
National Cancer Institute
Bethesda, Maryland, USA
*Extended Resection of Primary Lung Cancers Involving
Great Vessels or Heart*

Daniel Nyhan, MD
Professor of Anesthesia
Department of Anesthesia
Associate Professor of Surgery
Department of Surgery
The Johns Hopkins University School
of Medicine
Chief, Division of Cardiac Anesthesia
Department of Anesthesiology/Critical
Care Medicine
The Johns Hopkins Hospital
Baltimore, Maryland, USA
Cardiac Anesthesia

John A. Odell, MB ChB, FRCS(Ed), FACS
Head, Section of Cardiothoracic Surgery
Mayo Clinic Jacksonville
Jacksonville, Florida, USA
Esophageal Trauma

John C. Ofenloch, MD
Chief Resident, Division of Cardiothoracic Surgery
Emory University School of Medicine
Atlanta, Georgia, USA
Diffuse Esophageal Spasm and Scleroderma

Dmitry Oleynikov, MD, FACS
Assistant Professor of Surgery
Joseph and Richard Still Fellow in Medicine
Co-Director of Education and Training
The Minimally Invasive and Computer Assisted
Surgery Initiative
The University of Nebraska Medical Center
Omaha, Nebraska, USA
Surgical Therapy for Barrett's Esophagus

Jonathan B. Orens, MD
Associate Professor of Medicine
Medical Director, Lung Transplantation Program
Division of Pulmonary and Critical Care Medicine
The Johns Hopkins Hospital
Baltimore, Maryland, USA
*Preoperative Evaluation of the Lung Transplant
Candidate*

Mehmet C. Oz, MD
Director, Cardiovascular Institute
Department of Cardiothoracic Surgery
New York Presbyterian Hospital, Columbia University
New York, New York, USA
Mechanical Circulatory Assistance

Charles N. Paidas, MD, FACS, FAAP
Associate Professor, Division of Pediatric Surgery
The Johns Hopkins Hospital
Baltimore, Maryland, USA
Caustic Burns of the Esophagus

Octavio E. Pajaro, MD, PhD
Assistant Professor of Surgery
Mayo College of Medicine
Surgical Director, Lung Transplantation
Chair, Surgical Director, Transplant Research
Committee
Department of Cardiothoracic Surgery
The Mayo Clinic
Jacksonville, Florida, USA
Esophagoscopy

K. Gage Parr, MD
Instructor in Anesthesiology and Critical Care Medicine
Department of Anesthesiology and Critical Care
Medicine
The Johns Hopkins University

Staff Anesthesiologist
Union Memorial Hospital
Baltimore, Maryland, USA
Cardiac Anesthesia

Harvey I. Pass, MD
Professor of Surgery and Oncology
Wayne State University
Karmanos Cancer Institute
Detroit, Michigan, USA
Malignant Mesothelioma

G. Alexander Patterson, MD
Division of Cardiothoracic Surgery
Washington University School of Medicine
Attending Physician
Barnes Jewish Hospital
St. Louis, Missouri, USA
*Lung Transplantation—Surgical Options and
Approaches*

Taine T. V. Pechet, MD
Assistant Professor of Surgery
Division of Thoracic Surgery
Thomas Jefferson University
Philadelphia, Pennsylvania, USA
*Lung Transplantation—Surgical Options and
Approaches*

Walter Pegoli, Jr, MD
Pediatric Surgery
University of Rochester Medical Center
Chief, Pediatric Surgery
Galisano Children's Hospital
Rochester, New York, USA
Congenital Tracheoesophageal Fistula

Carlos A. Pellegrini, MD
The Henry N. Harkins Professor and Chairman
Department of Surgery
University of Washington School of Medicine
Seattle, Washington, USA
Surgical Therapy for Barrett's Esophagus

Bruce A. Perler, MD, FACS
Julius H. Jacobson II Professor of Surgery
Department of Surgery
The Johns Hopkins University School
of Medicine
Chief, Division of Vascular Surgery
Department of Surgery
The Johns Hopkins Hospital
Baltimore, Maryland, USA
Combined Carotid and Coronary Disease

Renzo Pessotto, MD
Consultant Cardiothoracic Surgeon
Department of Cardiothoracic Surgery
Lothian University
Department of Cardiothoracic Surgery
Royal Infirmary of Edinburgh
Edinburgh, United Kingdom
Ebstein's Anomaly

Jeffrey H. Peters, MD
Professor of Surgery
Chief, Section of General Surgery
University of Southern California
Los Angeles, California, USA
*Preoperative Evaluation of Gastroesophageal
Reflux Disease*

Duc Thinh Pham, MD
Cardiothoracic Surgery Fellow
Northwestern Memorial Hospital
Chicago, Illinois, USA
Myasthenia Gravis and Thymoma

Albert J. Polito, MD
Assistant Professor of Medicine
Director, Interstitial Lung Disease Program
The Johns Hopkins University School
of Medicine
Baltimore, Maryland, USA
Diffuse Lung Diseases

Marvin Pomerantz, MD
Professor of Surgery
Section of General Throacic Surgery
Division of Cardiothoracic Surgery
University of Colorado Health
Sciences Center
University of Colorado Hospital
Denver, Colorado, USA
Tuberculous Diseases of the Chest

Ronald B. Ponn, MD
Assistant Clinical Professor
Yale University School of Medicine
New Haven, Connecticut, USA
Mediastinoscopy and Mediastinotomy

Jeffrey L. Port, MD
Assistant Professor of Cardiothoracic Surgery
Department of Cardiothoracic Surgery
Weill Medical College of Cornell University
New York-Presbyterian Hospital
New York, New York, USA
Ivor-Lewis Esophagectomy

W. Thomas Purcell, MD
Chairman, Department of Oncology/
Hematology
Director, Deaconess Billings Cancer Center
Deaconess Billings Cancer Center
Billings, Montana, USA
Chemotherapy for Lung Cancer

Joe B. Putnam, Jr., MD
Chairman and Professor
Department of Thoracic Surgery
Vanderbilt University Medical Center,
Nashville, Tennessee
Pulmonary Metastases

Mohammed A. Quader, MD
Cardiothoracic Surgeon
Nebraska Heart Institute and Nebraska
Medical Center
Omaha, Nebraska, USA
Left Ventricular Volume Reduction

Jan Quaegebeur, MD
Children's Hospital of New York
New York, New York, USA
Pediatric Mitral Valve Disease

Vivek Rao, MD, PhD, FRCS(C)
Staff Surgeon and Surgical Director
Cardiac Transplant and Mechanical Assist
University Health Network
Assistant Professor of Surgery
University of Toronto
Toronto, Ontario, Canada
Mechanical Circulatory Assistance

William J. Ravich, MD
Associate Professor
Division of Gastroenterology
The Johns Hopkins University School
of Medicine
Full-time Staff, Division of
Gastroenterology
The Johns Hopkins Hospital
Baltimore, Maryland, USA
Medical Treatment for Barrett's Esophagus

Anees J. Razzouk, MD, FACC, FACS
Professor of Surgery
Department of Surgery
Chief, Division of Cardiothoracic Surgery
Loma Linda University and Medical Center
Loma Linda, California, USA
Trauma to the Heart and Great Vessels

Ivan M. Rebeyka, MD
Clinical Professor of Surgery and Pediatrics
University of Alberta
Edmonton, Alberta, Canada
Myocardial Protection in Children

V. Seenu Reddy, MD, MBA
Cardiothoracic Surgery Resident
Division of Cardiothoracic Surgery
Emory University Medical Center
Atlanta, Georgia, USA
Substernal Goiter

Carolyn E. Reed, MD
Professor of Surgery
Director, Hollings Cancer Center
Medical University of South Carolina
Charleston, South Carolina, USA
Upper Thoracic Esophageal Cancer

Thomas W. Rice, MD
Department of Thoracic and Cardiovascular Surgery
The Cleveland Clinic Foundation
Cleveland, Ohio, USA
Esophageal Perforation

Robert D. Riley, MD
Assistant Professor of Cardiothoracic Surgery
Wake Forest University
Winston-Salem, North Carolina, USA
Selection of a Cardiac Valve Prosthesis

Richard E. Ringel, MD
Associate Professor of Pediatrics
The Johns Hopkins University School of Medicine
Associate Professor
The Johns Hopkins Hospital
Baltimore, Maryland, USA
Cardiac Pacing in Children

Robert C. Robbins, MD
Associate Professor
Department of Cardiothoracic Surgery
Stanford University School of Medicine
Stanford Hospital
Stanford
Associate Professor
Lucille Salter Packard Children's Hospital
Palo Alto, California, USA
Heart-Lung Transplantation

John R. Roberts, MD, MBA, FACS
Department of Thoracic Surgery
The Sarah Cannon Cancer Center
Centennial Medical Center
Baptist Hospital
Nashville, Tennessee, USA
Substernal Goiter

Mark D. Rodefeld, MD
Assistant Professor of Surgery
Indiana University School of Medicine
Staff Physician, James Whitcomb Riley Hospital
for Children
Indianapolis, Indiana, USA
Congenital Aortic Stenosis; Atrial Septal Defects

Jonathan J. Rome, MD
Associate Professor of Pediatrics
University of Pennsylvania School of Medicine
Director, Cardiac Catheterization Laboratory
Department of Pediatrics
Children's Hospital of Philadelphia
Philadelphia, Pennsylvania, USA
*Percutaneous Catheter Interventions in
Congenital Heart Disease*

Russel S. Ronson, MD
Director of Cardiovascular and thoracic
Surgery Research
Brookwood Hospital
Birmingham, Alabama, USA
Video-Assisted Thoracic Surgery for Pleural Disease

Todd T. Rosengart, MD
Professor of Surgery
Northwestern University Medical School
Owen L. Coow Chair
Division of Cardiothoracic Surgery
Evanston Northwestern Hospital
Chicago, Illinois, USA
Transmyocardial Revascularization

Christopher T. Salerno, MD
Assistant Professor, Division of Cardiothoracic Surgery
University of Washington
Seattle, Washington, USA
*Congenital and Acquired Esophageal
Diverticula*

Piya Samankatiwat, MD, MSc, FRCS (Thailand)
Assistant Professor
Division of Cardiothoracic Surgery
Department of Surgery
Faculty of Medicine, Ramathibodi Hospital
Mahidol University
Bangkok, Thailand
Double Outlet Right Ventricle

Michal Savcenko, MD
Cardiopulmonary Research Science and
Technology Institute
Dallas, Texas, USA
*Video-Assisted Thoracic Surgery and
Mediastinal Disease*

John C. Scatarige, MD
Assistant Professor of Radiology
Department of Radiology
The Johns Hopkins Hospital
Baltimore, Maryland, USA
Radiologic Assessment of the Chest

Hans H. Scheld, MD
Professor and Director, Department of Thoracic and
Cardiovascular Surgery
University Hospital
Muenster, Germany
Intraaortic Balloon Pump

Christof Schmid, MD
Professor and Senior Surgeon
Department of Thoracic and Cardiovascular
Surgery
University Hospital
Muenster, Germany
Intraaortic Balloon Pump

Frank E. Schmidt, MD
Professor of Clinical Surgery
Louisiana State University Health Science Center
Chief, Cardiothoracic Surgery
Veterans Affairs Medical Center
Professor of Clinical Surgery
Medical Center of Louisiana, Charity/University
Campuses
New Orleans, Louisiana, USA

Thoracoplasty

Frank G. Scholl, MD
Assistant Professor
Department of Cardiac Surgery
Vanderbilt University Medical Center
Nashville, Tennessee, USA
Hypertrophic Cardiomyopathy

David S. Schrump, MD
Senior Investigator and Head, Thoracic Oncology
Section, Surgery Branch
National Cancer Institute
Bethesda, Maryland, USA

*Extended Resection of Primary Lung Cancers
Involving Great Vessels or Heart*

Charles F. Schwartz, MD
Assistant Professor of Surgery
Division of Cardiothoracic Surgery
Department of Surgery
New York University School of Medicine
New York, New York, USA
Mitral Valve Reconstruction

Walter J. Scott, MD
Member, Thoracic Surgical Oncology
Fox Chase Cancer Center
Philadelphia, Pennsylvania, USA
Broncholithiasis

Janice Shannon-Cain, CRNA
Anesthesia Instructor
Samuel Merrit College of Nursing
Staff Anesthetist
Kaiser Oakland Hospital
Oakland, California, USA
Tension Pneumothorax

Irving Shen, MD
Assistant Professor
Cardiothoracic Division
Oregon Health Sciences University
Portland, Oregon, USA
*Cardiopulmonary Bypass and Hypothermic
Circulatory Arrest*

Joseph B. Shrager, MD
Associate Professor of Surgery
Department of Surgery
University of Pennsylvania School of Medicine
Chief, Section of General Thoracic Surgery
University of Pennsylvania Health System
Philadelphia, Pennsylvania, USA
*Lung Volume Reduction Surgery—Video-Assisted
Thoracoscopic Approach*

Brett A. Simon, MD, PhD
Associate Professor
Department of Anesthesiology and
Critical Care Medicine
The Johns Hopkins Medical Institutions
Baltimore, Maryland, USA
Anesthesia for the Thoracic Surgical Patient

Sunil Singhal, MD
Resident in Surgery
Department of Surgery
The Johns Hopkins Medical Institutions
Baltimore, Maryland, USA
*Lung Volume Reduction Surgery—Median Sternotomy
Approach*

Arun K. Singhal, MD, PhD
Assistant Professor of Surgery and Physiology
Temple University School of Medicine
Attending Physician
Temple University Hospital
Philadelphia, Pennsylvania, USA
Coronary Endarterectomy

Eric R. Skipper, MD
Surgical Director of Clinical Research
Surgical Director of Cardiac Transplantation
Department of Thoracic Surgery
Carolinas Heart Institute
Carolinas Medical Center
Charlotte, North Carolina, USA
Cardiac Tumors

W. Roy Smythe, MD
Chairman, Department of Surgery
Texas A&M Health Science Center
College of Medicine
Temple, Texas, USA
Chest Wall Neoplasms

Joshua Robert Sonett, MD
Associate Professor of Surgery
Division of Cardiothoracic Surgery;
Director, Lung Transplant Program
Columbia University College of Physicians and
Surgeons
New York, New York, USA
Bronchoscopy

David Spielvogel, MD
Assistant Professor, Department of
Cardiothoracic Surgery
Mount Sinai Hospital
New York, New York, USA
Reconstruction of Aortic Arch Aneurysms

Thomas L. Spray, MD
Professor of Surgery
University of Pennsylvania
Chief, Division of Cardiothoracic Surgery
Alice Langdon Warner Chair in Pediatric
Cardiothoracic Surgery
Children's Hospital of Philadelphia
Philadelphia, Pennsylvania, USA
Hypoplastic Left Heart Syndrome

James D. St. Louis, MD
Brown University
Providence, Rhode Island, USA
Valve Replacement in Children

Peter S. Staats, MD
Associate Professor of Anesthesiology and Critical
Care Medicine and of Oncology
Director, Division of Pain Medicine
Department of Anesthesiology and Critical Care
The Johns Hopkins University School of Medicine
Baltimore, Maryland, USA
Postoperative Pain Control for Thoracic Surgery

Vaughn A. Starnes, MD
Hastings Professor and Chairman
Department of Cardiothoracic Surgery
Keck School of Medicine
University of Southern California
Los Angeles, California, USA
Ebstein's Anomaly

Edward R. Stephenson, MD
Assistant Professor of Surgery
Department of Cardiothoracic Surgery
The Milton S. Hershey Medical Center
Hershey, Pennsylvania, USA
Coarctation of the Aorta

Ken C. Stewart, MD, FRCSC
Assistant Professor
Department of Surgery
University of Alberta
Edmonton, Alberta, Canada
Lung Transplantation—Surgical Options and Approaches

Sean M. Studer, MD
Medical Chief, Lung Transplantation
The Recanati Miller Transplantation Institute
Mount Sinai School of Medicine
New York, New York, USA
*Preoperative Evaluation of the Lung Transplant
Candidate*

David J. Sugarbaker, MD
Richard E. Wilson Professor of Surgical Oncology
Harvard Medical School
Chief, Division of Thoracic Surgery
Brigham and Women's Hospital
Philip L. Lowe Senior Surgeon and Chief of the
Department of Surgical Services
Dana-Farber Cancer Institute
Boston, Massachusetts, USA
*Extrapleural Pneumonectomy for Diffuse Malignant
Pleural Mesothelioma*

Sudhir R. Sundaresan, MD
Associate Professor of Surgery
University of Ottawa

Active Staff, Division of Thoracic Surgery
The Ottowa Hospital General Campus
Ottowa, Ontario, Canada
Acute Airway Obstruction

Thoralf M. Sundt, MD, FACS
Cardiovascular Surgery
Mayo Medical School
Senior Associate Consultant
Mayo Clinic
Rochester, Minnesota, USA
Coronary Endarterectomy

Scott J. Swanson, MD
Chief of Thoracic Surgery
Mount Sinai Medical Center
New York, New York, USA
Lung Amebiasis

Stephen G. Swisher, MD, FACS
Associate Professor of Surgery
Thoracic and Cardiovascular Surgery
MD Anderson Cancer Center
Houston, Texas, USA
Lymph Node Dissection for Esophageal Cancer

Mark A. Talamini, MD
Professor of Surgery
The Johns Hopkins University School of Medicine
Director of Minimally Invasive Surgery
The Johns Hopkins Hospital
Baltimore, Maryland, USA
Laparoscopic Techniques for Gastroesophageal Reflux

Vincent K. Tam, MD
Medical Director
Cardiothoracic Surgery
Cook Children's Hospital
Ft. Worth, Texas, USA
Total Anomalous Pulmonary Venous Connection

Paul C.Y. Tang, MD
Research Fellow, Cardiothoracic Surgery
Yale University School of Medicine
New Haven, Connecticut, USA
Aortic Dissection

Kenneth Taylor, MD, FRCS, FRCSC, FESC, FETCS, FSA
British Heart Foundation Professor of Cardiac Surgery
University of London
Professor and Chief of Cardiothoracic Surgery
Hammersmith Hospital
London, United Kingdom
Adult Cardiopulmonary Bypass

Pierre R. Theodore, MD
Chief Resident, Cardiothoracic Surgery
Department of Surgery
The Johns Hopkins Hospital
Baltimore, Maryland, USA
Sleeve Lobectomy

Vinod H. Thourani, MD
Clinical Fellow (Cardiothoracic)
Emory University School of Medicine
Emory Healthcare
Atlanta, Georgia, USA
Myocardial Protection

Betty C. Tong, MS, MD
Senior Resident, Department of Surgery
The Johns Hopkins Medical Institutions
Baltimore, Maryland, USA
Massive Hemoptysis

Thomas A. Traill, MD
Professor of Medicine
Department of Cardiology
The Johns Hopkins University School of Medicine
Baltimore, Maryland, USA
Evaluating Patients before Coronary Artery Bypass Surgery

Victor F. Trastek, MD
Professor of Surgery
Chair, Board of Governors
Mayo Clinic
Scottsdale, Arizona
The Collis Gastroplasty for Gastroesophageal Reflux

Jonathan Trites, BSc, MD, FRCSC
Assistant Professor, Division of Otolaryngology
Department of Surgery
Dalhousie University
Attending Staff, Otolaryngology–
Head and Neck Surgery
Queen Elizabeth II Health Sciences Centre
Halifax, Nova Scotia, Canada
Carcinoma of the Cervical Esophagus

Timothy H. Trotter, MD, FACS
Assistant Professor, Section of Thoracic and
Cardiovascular Surgery
University of Oklahoma
Oklahoma City, Oklahoma, USA
Prosthetic Valve Endocarditis

Donald D. Trunkey, MD
Professor of Surgery
Department of Surgery

Oregon Health and Science University
Portland, Oregon, USA

Flail Chest and Pulmonary Contusion

Victor T. Tsang, MS, MSc, FRCS
Consultant Cardiothoracic Surgeon
Great Ormond Street Hospital
London, United Kingdom

Truncus Arteriosus

Elaine E. Tseng, MD
Assistant Professor of Surgery
Division of Cardiothoracic Surgery
UCSF Medical Center
San Francisco, California, USA

Cancer of the Gastroesophageal Junction

Anthony P. Tufaro, DDS, MD
Divisions of Plastic and Reconstructive Surgery and
Surgical Oncology
The Johns Hopkins Medical Institutions
Baltimore, Maryland, USA

*Prosthetic Substitutes for Chest
Wall Reconstruction*

Mark W. Turrentine, MD
Professor of Surgery
Division of Cardiothoracic Surgery, Department
of Surgery
Indiana University School of Medicine
Staff Physician, James Whitcomb Riley Hospital
for Children
Indianapolis, Indiana, USA

*Atrial Septal Defects; Congenital
Aortic Stenosis*

Ozuru Ukoha, MD
Assistant Professor of Cardiothoracic
Surgery
Rush University
Senior Attending Physician
John H. Stroger Jr. Hospital of Cook County
Chicago, Illinois, USA

*Palliative Surgical Procedures for
Esophageal Carcinoma*

Ross M. Ungerleider, MD
Professor of Surgery
Chief, Pediatric Cardiac Surgery
Oregon Health Sciences University
Portland, Oregon, USA

*Cardiopulmonary Bypass and Hypothermic
Circulatory Arrest*

Harold C. Urschel, Jr., MD
Professor of Thoracic and Cardiovascular Surgery
University of Texas Southwestern Medical School
Chair of Cardiovascular and Thoracic Surgical Research,
Education and Clinical Excellence
Baylor University Medical Center
Dallas, Texas, USA

Thoracic Outlet Syndrome

John D. Urschel, MD, FRCSC, FRCSEd
Associate Professor, Department of Surgery
McMaster University
Surgeon-in-Chief
St. Joseph's Healthcare
East Hamilton, Ontario, Canada

Infections of the Chest Wall

Eric Valliéres, MD
Surgical Director of the Lung Cancer Program
Swedish Cancer Institute
Surgical Practices
Seattle, Washington, USA

Mediastinitis

Craig A. Vander Kolk, MD
Professor, Division of Plastic Surgery
The Johns Hopkins Hospital
Baltimore, MD

Treatment of Sternal Wound Infections

Ara A. Vaporciyan, MD
Associate Professor of Surgery
Department of Thoracic and Cardiovascular
Surgery
M.D. Anderson Cancer Center
Houston, Texas, USA

Unusual Primary Malignant Neoplasms of the Lung

Wickii T. Vigneswaran, MD, FACS
Associate Professor and Chief of Thoracic Surgery
Director of Lung Transplant, Co-Director of Thoracic
Oncology
Department of Thoracic and Cardiovascular Surgery
Loyola University Chicago, Stritch School of Medicine
Loyola University Medical Center
Maywood, Illinois, USA

Lung Abscess

Antonio L. Visbal, MD
Resident in Cardiovascular and Thoracic Surgery
Mayo Clinic
Scottsdale, Arizona, USA

The Collis Gastroplasty for Gastroesophageal Reflux

Luca A. Vricella, MD
Assistant Professor, Division of Cardiac Surgery
The Johns Hopkins Hospital
Baltimore, Maryland, USA

*Truncus Arteriosus; Aortic Root Replacement; Tricuspid
Valve Operations; Palliative Operations for Congenital
Heart Disease; Tetralogy of Fallot; Aortic Arch
Interruption; Double Outlet Right Ventricle*

Jon-Cecil M. Walkes, MD
Department of Surgery
Baylor College of Medicine
Department of Cardiovascular and Thoracic Surgery
The Methodist Hospital
Houston, Texas, USA

Chest Wall Injury and Blunt Cardiac Trauma

Garrett L. Walsh, MD
Professor of Surgery
Department of Thoracic and Cardiovascular Surgery
The University of Texas M.D. Anderson Cancer Center
Houston, Texas, USA

Pleural Effusions

Sandra M. Wanek, MD
Surgical Critical Care Fellow
Trauma/Critical Care Section, Department
of Surgery
Oregon Health and Science University
Portland, Oregon, USA

Flail Chest and Pulmonary Contusion

Ko-Pen Wang, MD
Director, Lung Cancer Center
Harbor Hospital Center
Director, Interventional Pulmonology
The Johns Hopkins Medical Center
Baltimore, Maryland, USA

Stenting of the Airway

William H. Warren, MD
Thoracic Surgical Associates
Rush University
Chicago, Illinois, USA

Palliative Surgical Procedures for Esophageal Carcinoma

Thomas J. Watson, MD
Associate Professor of Surgery
Division of Cardiothoracic Surgery
University of Rochester School of Medicine and Dentistry
Attending Physician, Strong Memorial Hospital
Rochester, New York, USA

Fibrothorax and Decortication of the Lung

Watts R. Webb, BA, MD
Clinical Professor of Surgery
Louisiana State University School of Medicine
Attending Staff
Charity Hospital of Louisiana
Memorial Hospital
University Hospital
New Orleans, Louisiana, USA

Thoracoplasty

Rick White, MD, FACC, FAHA
Clinical Director, Center for Integrated Non-Invasive
Cardiovascular Imaging
Department of Thoracic and Cardiovascular Surgery
Cleveland Clinic Foundation
Cleveland, Ohio, USA

Left Ventricular Volume Reduction

Richard I. Whyte, MD
Professor, Department of Cardiothoracic Surgery
Stanford University
Head, Division of Thoracic Surgery
Stanford University Medical Center
Stanford, California, USA

Congenital and Acquired Esophageal Diverticula

Earle W. Wilkins, Jr., MD
Clinical Professor of Surgery, Emeritus
Harvard Medical School
Senior Surgeon
Massachusetts General Hospital
Boston, Massachusetts, USA

Left Thoracoabdominal Esophagectomy

Walter G. Wolfe, MD
Professor of Surgery
Department of Surgery
Duke University Medical Center
Durham, North Carolina, USA

Actinomycosis and Nocardial Infections of the Lung

Douglas E. Wood, MD
Chief, General Thoracic Surgery
Endowed Chair in Lung Cancer Research
Department of Surgery, Division of
Cardiothoracic Surgery
University of Washington
Seattle, Washington, USA

Tracheal Release Maneuvers

Kenneth J. Woodside, MD
General Surgery Resident
Department of Surgery
The University of Texas Medical Branch

Galveston, Texas, USA

Extracorporeal Life Support in the Adult

Cameron D. Wright, MD
Associate Professor of Surgery
Harvard Medical School
Associate Visiting Surgeon
Department of Thoracic Surgery
Massachusetts General Hospital
Boston, Massachusetts, USA

Benign Tracheal Tumors; Left Thoracoabdominal Esophagectomy

Alene Wright, MD
Chief Resident, Department of Surgery
Creighton University
Omaha, Nebraska, USA

Broncholithiasis

Manoel Ximenes-Netto, MD, PhD
Professor and Head, Thoracic Surgery Unit
Hospital de Base of the Distrito Federal
Brasilia, Brazil

Esophageal Reconstruction—Reversed and Nonreversed Gastric Tubes; Esophageal Infections

Stephen C. Yang, MD, FACS, FCCP
Associate Professor of Surgery and
Medical Oncology
Chief, Division of Thoracic Surgery
Department of Surgery
The Johns Hopkins University School of Medicine
Chief of Thoracic Surgery
The Johns Hopkins Bayview Medical Center
Baltimore, Maryland, USA

Massive Hemoptysis; Diaphragmatic Injuries; Pulmonary Arteriovenous Malformation; Surgical Approach for Small Cell Lung Cancer; Occult Lung Cancer; Sleeve Lobectomy; Pulmonary Fungal Infections; Lung Volume Reduction Surgery—Median Sternotomy Approach; Posterior Mediastinal Masses; Benign Tumors of the Esophagus; Complications of Esophageal Resection; Concomitant Cardiac and Thoracic Operations

Anthony P. C. Yim, MD
Professor of Surgery and Chief of Cardiothoracic
Surgery
Department of Surgery
Prince of Wales Hospital
Hong Kong, China

General Principles of Video-Assisted Thoracic Surgery

David D. Yuh, MD
Assistant Professor
Division of Cardiac Surgery
Director of Cardiac Surgical Research

The Johns Hopkins Hospital
Baltimore, Maryland, USA

Lung Transplantation in the Pediatric Patient; Cardiac Transplant; Surgical Management of Endocarditis; Pediatric Cardiac Transplantation

Rex C. Yung, MD, FCCP
Assistant Professor of Medicine and Oncology
Director of Pulmonary Oncology
Director of Bronchoscopy
The Johns Hopkins University School of Medicine
Baltimore, Maryland, USA

Assessment of the Patient Undergoing Pulmonary Resection

Martin R. Zamora, MD
Associate Professor of Medicine
Division of Pulmonary Sciences and Critical Care
Medicine
Medical Director, Lung Transplantation Program
University of Colorado Health Sciences Center
Denver, Colorado, USA

Complications Following Lung Transplantation

Kenton J. Zehr, MD
Associate Professor of Surgery
Mayo Medical School
Consultant, Division of Cardiovascular Surgery
Mayo Clinic
Rochester, Minnesota, USA

Mitral Valve Replacement

Lambros S. Zellos, MD, MPH
Fellow, Division of Thoracic Surgery
Brigham and Women's Hospital
Harvard Medical School
Boston, Massachusetts, USA

Extrapleural Pneumonectomy for Diffuse Malignant Pleural Mesothelioma

Harry Zemon, MD
Research Fellow/Senior Surgical Resident
George Washington University Hospital
The John Hopkins University
Baltimore, Maryland, USA

Pediatric Cardiac Transplantaion

George L. Zorn, III, MD
Chief Resident, Department of Thoracic Surgery
University of Virginia
Charlottesville, Virginia, USA

Middle Mediastinal Masses

Joseph B. Zwischenberger, MD
Department of Surgery
University of Texas Medical Branch
Galveston, Texas, USA

Extracorporeal Life Support in the Adult

Foreword

The *Current Therapy* series has been an important addition to the medical and surgical literature over the past several decades. The need for periodic, frequent updates regarding therapy has become essential as the pace of discoveries and the introduction of new concepts and therapies have escalated. This is especially true in the surgical disciplines. *Current Surgical Therapy* is now in its seventh edition, being reissued every 3 years with an entirely new set of contributors. One edition of *Current Therapy in Cardiothoracic Surgery* was issued many years ago and was successful, but no subsequent editions emerged. The present volume is a renewal and, it is hoped, the first of many successful editions of *Current Therapy in Thoracic and Cardiovascular Surgery*.

A superb line-up of experts covering all aspects of thoracic and cardiac surgery has been assembled to participate in this edition. Even though most are from the United States, authors from elsewhere in the world are included, which adds a definite international flavor. All topics in thoracic and cardiac surgery are covered, as well as surgery on the thoracic aorta. This text is of interest to students, residents, fellows, practitioners in private practice, and academicians; however, it will be of most use to private practitioners and academicians. This text provides a quick review of current therapy, only briefly addressing etiology, pathogenesis, and other items that are important but are treated adequately in larger texts. *Current Therapy in Thoracic and Cardiovascular Surgery* is aimed primarily at providing information on up-to-date therapy.

Ultimately, the success of a text such as this depends on its editors. Dr. Stephen C. Yang and Dr. Duke E. Cameron are young but very experienced surgeons. Both are excellent clinicians, superb technical surgeons, and dedicated educators. They provide expertise in the two broad areas covered in this text. They are dedicated to the concept of periodically updating *Current Therapy in Thoracic and Cardiovascular Surgery* with new editions and new contributors.

Many superb textbooks exist in the field of thoracic and cardiac surgery. For these large texts, several years are dedicated to picking appropriate authors, waiting for complete and detailed chapters to be written, extensive editing, and finally the publishing of an edition that is expected to be used for many years. Today, with the pace of new contributions to thoracic and cardiac surgery, therapy is in a constant state of flux and cannot await updating every 6 or 7 years. That makes a text such as this, which is expected to come out every 3 years, essential for the practitioner. I am confident that this edition is the first in a long series that will provide the cardiothoracic surgeon with a current update in this rapidly changing field. I congratulate the two editors, both close colleagues of mine, on a superb job well done.

John L. Cameron, MD, FACS
The Alfred Blalock Distinguished
Senior Professor of Surgery
The Johns Hopkins University School of Medicine
Baltimore, Maryland, USA

Foreword

This follow-up edition to the 1986 book, *Current Therapy in Cardiothoracic Surgery,* is significantly different to warrant a change in its title—*Current Therapy in Thoracic and Cardiovascular Surgery.* Although the change is subtle, this new book significantly expands previously published chapters with updates and new developments while adding a number of new sections covering both thoracic and cardiovascular disease. This edition retains the philosophy of the original book by providing a practical synopsis of the current care of many surgical conditions. In addition to emphasizing surgical techniques, the editors have continued to stress "additional pointers on work-up, postoperative management, and avoidance of pitfalls."

This book is divided into several chapters, allowing the reader easy access to a particular area of interest and providing a succinct but quick read with valuable take-home points. The orientation is primarily centered on diseases with associated operative procedures. The editors have assembled a talented array of authors that reads like a "who's who" in thoracic and cardiovascular surgery.

In the area of thoracic surgery, the editors have added chapters dealing with HIV infection, pulmonary metastases, complications of pulmonary and esophageal resection, the use of muscle flaps for chest wall reconstruction, and lung volume reduction surgery. They have expanded the sections on lung transplantation and video-assisted thoracic surgery as well as introducing a new section entitled "Thoracic Emergencies."

In the area of cardiovascular surgery, the editors have significantly expanded the content dealing with a variety of new procedures and operative techniques. New chapters discuss inotropic support, intraoperative transesophageal echocardiography, concomitant cardiac and thoracic operations, pulmonary thromboendarterectomy, surgical treatment of atrial fibrillation, the Ross procedure, and left ventricular volume reduction. The authors have significantly expanded the section on mechanical circulatory support and that dealing with the thoracic aorta. Within the chapters on pediatric and congenital heart disease, the editors have added chapters dealing with percutaneous catheter interventions, extracorporeal membrane oxygenation, and mechanical circulatory assistance.

I believe that this newest edition of *Current Therapy* provides the cardiothoracic surgical resident and the practicing surgeon with a comprehensive yet succinct reference work on thoracic and cardiovascular diseases. The editors and authors are to be commended for providing the reader with an excellent textbook that is both easy to read and comprehensive in scope.

William A. Baumgartner, MD
The Vincent L. Gott Professor
Cardiac Surgeon-in-Charge
Division of Cardiac Surgery
The Johns Hopkins Hospital
Baltimore, Maryland, USA

Preface

Never before has the young cardiothoracic surgeon been inundated with so much information relevant to our specialty. Our desks overflow with journals, monographs, books, meeting programs, and advertisements, and our computers serve as portals to a seemingly limitless ocean of Web sites, online journals, discussion groups, and product literature. For many cardiothoracic surgeons, access to information is no longer the problem; rather, the problem is access to the wisdom and perspective necessary to digest and interpret that information. This is particularly true for the younger surgeon, whether in training, beginning a practice, or studying for board examinations, but it is also true for the senior surgeon exploring new areas of interest. For both, the challenge of patient care demands a practical perspective and efficient use of time in review of the subject. It is our hope that this new edition of *Current Therapy in Thoracic and Cardiovascular Surgery* meets those needs.

In a real sense, this is the second edition of *Current Therapy* in the area of cardiothoracic surgery. The first, entitled *Current Therapy in Cardiothoracic Surgery* and edited by Hermes Grillo and associates from the Massachusetts General Hospital in Boston, set the bar high for our effort, and we are grateful for the inspiration they provided. In the 15 years since that edition, new therapies and treatment modalities have arisen; some have even come and gone. It is a challenge to decide whether to include novel and experimental treatments in a book such as this, and we have erred toward the side of established therapy, with apologies to the pioneers of our proud specialty. Similarly, use of graphics is limited in a book that aims to be both concise and comprehensive.

Our gratitude to the nearly 300 authors is immense. It is on their shoulders that we stand, and, of course, to them the credit belongs. The experience shared in their chapters probably represents thousands of years of personal hands-on clinical practice.

Our surgical chiefs, John Cameron and William Baumgartner, provided invaluable advice, encouragement, and support for this book and, in no small sense, made it possible.

We are also indebted to many others: close family and friends for their words of wisdom; our residents and students for providing a constant source of learning and a daily reminder of why we love our profession; and our administrative staff—Trisha Arbella, Marvin Borja, and Lori Garrison—who have kept us in line and provided invaluable leg work for this book.

Finally, Richard Lampert, Kimberly Cox, Norman Stellander, and the team at Elsevier have shown admirable patience with our busy clinical schedules, have shepherded us through a bewildering process, and, in our eyes, have earned sainthood.

Stephen C. Yang, MD
Duke E. Cameron, MD

Contents

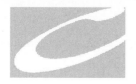

THORACIC SURGERY

RADIOLOGIC ASSESSMENT OF THE CHEST

John C. Scatarige

Elliot K. Fishman

Diagnostic imaging plays a pivotal role in the work-up and management of patients with surgically treatable thoracic disease. To render informed care to these patients, thoracic surgeons should be familiar with the impressive array of imaging options now available to them. In particular, the strengths, limitations, and appropriate clinical use of each of these methods should be understood.

This chapter has two parts. The first part is a review of important technologic advances in the radiologic armamentarium. The second part discusses the application of imaging techniques to specific clinical situations of interest to thoracic and cardiovascular surgeons. This discussion is not exhaustive; it is hoped that interested readers will be stimulated to seek more detailed sources of particular interest.

■ TECHNOLOGIC PROGRESS

Improvements in equipment engineering, detector design, data processing, and radiopharmaceuticals have altered the radiologic landscape drastically. These advances have facilitated the development of noninvasive angiography with computed tomography (CT) and magnetic resonance imaging (MRI), three-dimensional imaging, and metabolic imaging in oncology. Advanced imaging technology has been disseminated rapidly and is now available in most communities.

Filmless Radiography: Digital Radiology and PACS

For decades, chest radiography has involved exposing a 14-inch×17-inch cassette containing film and intensifying screens. After exposure, the film is removed from the cassette and processed in photographic chemicals. The resulting "hard copy" image is embedded on the film and is immutable. Conventional radiographs must be transported, displayed on view boxes, stored, and periodically retrieved and sometimes are lost. Still an area of active investigation, newer digital radiographic technology has been developed as an alternative. The digital radiographic image is collected either on a portable cassette–based system or on a fixed flat panel digital detector. The digitized image that results can be viewed as "soft copy" on a workstation screen where image brightness and contrast can be manipulated by the radiologist. This flexibility is particularly advantageous in the chest, where the lungs and mediastinum can be viewed at different settings, similar to in CT. The study can be stored, retrieved, and transmitted to remote workstations for viewing by the clinician. Other digitized examinations, such as CT, MRI, and scintigraphic studies, can be viewed and stored on the same system.

Picture archiving and communications systems (PACS) increasingly are being adopted by imaging departments as a cost-containment strategy. Their implementation requires considerable initial capital outlay. Still, PACS holds the promise of reducing or eliminating the need to purchase, handle, and store film and offers the prospect of reducing the frustration of lost or misplaced films.

Helical CT

Older CT scanners acquired data sequentially, one image (slice) at a time. This process was time-consuming and often resulted in images degraded by respiratory motion in critically ill or uncooperative patients. Helical CT scanners acquire data continuously while the patient is moved gradually through the scanning aperture. A large volume of data can be collected during a brief interval, even a single breath hold, reducing motion artifacts. The newest generation of helical scanner, called a *multidetector,* permits even more rapid scan data acquisition. When coupled with the timed delivery of intravenous contrast material by power injector, CT angiography

(CTA) and multiphasic (arterial, venous) protocols become feasible. These enormous sets of volumetric data can be transferred to specialized workstations, which allow real-time three-dimensional display in any plane. Volume rendering is the most sophisticated three-dimensional technique. It is particularly useful for depicting thoracoabdominal aortic aneurysms, aortic dissections, and the tracheobronchial tree.

MRI

Similar to helical CT, MRI provides noninvasive multiplanar imaging of the thorax. In contrast to CT, MRI does not require x-rays to detect attenuation differences. MRI depends on differences in the concentration of mobile hydrogen in tissues. These differences become evident when a patient is placed in an external magnetic field and radiofrequency pulses energize the hydrogen nuclei. Many different imaging sequences can be employed in MRI. The complex MRI signal that results can be modified further by the administration of gadolinium, an intravenous contrast agent.

MRI examination times can be long. More recent technical improvements have shortened the procedure greatly, however. Magnetic resonance angiography (MRA) is now possible during a single breath hold. Additional advantages are that follow-up MRI examinations can be performed without concern of radiation dose to the patient or of exposure to radiographic contrast agent. The presence of a cardiac pacemaker and certain vascular clips are contraindications to MRI.

Metabolic Imaging with FDG-PET

Although positron emission tomography (PET) has existed since the 1960s, its serious clinical application did not begin until the 1990s. In contrast to conventional chest x-ray and helical CT, PET is a biochemical and physiologic rather than a morphologic technique. It employs intravenously administered radiopharmaceuticals, which resemble endogenous biologic compounds.

The most frequently employed radiotracer is a glucose analogue, 2-[F-18] fluoro-2-deoxy-D-glucose (FDG). FDG preferentially accumulates in malignant cells because they have a higher rate of glycolysis than most normal tissues. FDG has been shown to be effective in detecting tumor foci in cancers of the lung, head and neck, esophagus, and breast and in lymphoma. In addition, quantitative FDG-PET methods seem to be useful in the early assessment of tumor response to therapy.

When FDG is distributed in the patient, a state-of-the-art PET scanner acquires volumetric whole body data sets, which can be displayed in axial, coronal, and sagittal planes. These images do not provide the spatial resolution of modern helical CT; clinical PET scans usually are viewed and correlated with a CT scan.

■ APPLICATION OF RADIOLOGIC TECHNIQUES IN THORACIC DISEASE

Solitary Pulmonary Nodule

The detection of a solitary pulmonary nodule (SPN) less than 3 cm in diameter on a chest radiograph is a common clinical occurrence. Imaging studies are important in differentiating a benign from a malignant cause and should be undertaken in a methodical manner.

There are two plain film criteria by which an SPN can be declared benign. The first is a lack of change over at least 2 years of observation. In this regard, attempts to locate and obtain prior chest films are frequently rewarding and spare the patient the expense, risk, and anxiety of additional imaging or invasive procedures. Second, one of four patterns of calcification within a well-marginated nodule indicate benignity: diffuse, central, laminar, and popcorn-like.

An SPN not fulfilling these criteria or containing eccentric calcification should be studied with helical CT. CT scan of the entire thorax confirms the nodule in question, precisely localizes it to a lobe and segment, and excludes additional unsuspected nodules. Thinly collimated scans of the nodule in question provide additional morphologic and density criteria. A nodule with a spiculated or irregular border or that is cavitated with a thick, nodular wall is likely malignant. Calcification is exquisitely displayed on CT, facilitating search for one of the benign patterns. A feeding artery and draining vein indicate an arteriovenous malformation. Fat within the nodule indicates a hamartoma or lipoid pneumonia.

Targeted, Enhanced CT

Indeterminate nodules fulfilling neither benign nor malignant criteria can be evaluated further with a rigorous contrast enhancement protocol. The procedure is based on the fact that malignant nodules are more vascular than benign lesions. Unenhanced scans and timed contrast-enhanced helical CT of the nodule are performed. If the SPN of interest measures an increase of 15 Hounsfield units or less during the first 4 minutes after injection, the lesion is likely to be benign and can be followed. Preliminary data suggest that this technique has a sensitivity of 98% for detecting malignancy in nodules 5 mm or larger.

Metabolic Imaging

FDG-PET also can help to classify further an indeterminate SPN. The accumulation of FDG radiotracer in the suspect nodule strongly suggests malignancy. Early data suggest a sensitivity of 90% to 100% for cancer. False-negative examinations have been reported in bronchoalveolar cell carcinoma and carcinoid tumors. In addition, false-positive PET scans have been noted in active granulomatous disease, pneumonia, and abscess. State-of-the-art PET equipment can reliably evaluate nodules 8 mm in diameter. Improvements in the coming years surely will lower this threshold.

Image-Guided Lung Biopsy

Image-guided transthoracic needle biopsy is an accepted technique for the evaluation of an SPN and a variety of focal pulmonary, pleural, and mediastinal processes not accessible to bronchoscopy. In experienced hands, aspiration and core biopsy leads to a definitive histologic diagnosis in greater than 90% of cases. The choice of guidance modality varies with equipment availability, training, and personal preference. In most U.S. centers, fluoroscopic and CT guidance are preferred. Ultrasound is gaining acceptance as a versatile and less cumbersome alternative for sampling masses close to or abutting the chest wall. In a series from the authors' institution, 40% of thoracic biopsies were guided by ultrasound.

Pneumothorax, the most frequent complication, occurs in 8% to 64% of patients. Higher pneumothorax rates are associated with small lesions, masses far from the pleura, biopsies performed under CT guidance, and the use of a shallow pleural puncture angle. Obstructive lung disease is itself an important risk factor for postbiopsy pneumothorax requiring placement of a chest tube.

Preoperative Staging of Lung Cancer

The goal of radiologic staging in non–small cell lung cancer is the accurate separation of patients who have potentially resectable tumors from patients with unresectable primary tumors, unresectable mediastinal nodal metastases, or distant metastases. Chest radiography is not sufficient for this task. The contributions of helical CT and, more recently, FDG-PET have been well studied.

Mediastinal Nodal Metastasis

Accurate detection of metastases to ipsilateral mediastinal and subcarinal nodes (N2) and to the contralateral hilum, mediastinum, and bilateral scalene and supraclavicular lymph nodes (N3) has been the hope of noninvasive imaging. Contrast-enhanced helical CT uses size criteria to predict nodal metastasis: A short-axis diameter of a lymph node that exceeds 1 cm is considered abnormal. These morphologic criteria have fallen short in the face of reactive lymphadenopathy in lung cancer patients and microscopic metastases to lymph nodes normal in size. The sensitivity and specificity of helical CT for staging mediastinal nodes are approximately 75% and 65% respectively.

Evidence has accumulated indicating that FDG-PET is superior to CT in detecting N2 and N3 metastases. A sensitivity of 91% and specificity of 86% have been reported. Thoracic FDG-PET seems to be particularly useful when negative; its high negative predictive value of 95% suggests that these patients could proceed directly to surgery without mediastinoscopy.

Chest Wall, Mediastinal Invasion

CT and MRI have been used to evaluate primary cancers invading the chest wall or diaphragm (T3) and the mediastinum (T4). CT is only about 50% sensitive for diagnosing direct mediastinal invasion and is less accurate for chest wall invasion. MRI has had comparable success. Because of its multiplanar capability, however, MRI generally is preferred for evaluating vascular and brachial plexus involvement by superior sulcus tumors and cancers close to the major vessels, diaphragm, and chest wall.

Distant Metastasis

FDG-PET whole body imaging seems to be more accurate than CT in the detection of distant metastases. MRI classically has been used to evaluate adrenal masses; early experience indicates that PET can differentiate precisely adrenal metastasis from common, incidental adrenal adenomas just as well as MRI. PET is relatively insensitive, however, in the detection of small brain metastases.

Overall Impact of PET

FDG-PET already is having an impact on lung cancer staging. In one study of 102 lung cancer patients clinically staged by conventional means, PET caused 61% to be restaged; the stage was lowered in 20% and raised in 41%.

Preoperative Staging of Esophageal Cancer

The incidence of adenocarcinoma of the esophagus continues to increase. When detected on barium esophagography or endoscopy, early esophageal cancer is managed best surgically. Preoperative staging is necessary for selection of appropriate surgical candidates and for assessment of prognosis. Endoscopic ultrasound at 7.5 or at 12 MHz is unsurpassed at depicting the depth of tumor invasion and spread to locoregional lymph nodes. Laparoscopic staging and video-assisted thoracic surgical (VATS) staging also are accurate for detecting regional and distant metastasis, but these methods are expensive and not without risk.

Contrast-enhanced helical CT of the thorax and abdomen has been the noninvasive procedure of choice for detecting distant disease (M1, stage IV disease). Demonstration of metastases to liver, lung, or mediastinal or retroperitoneal lymph nodes is an indication for a palliative approach to management. The anatomic criteria of CT for lymphadenopathy impose limitations on accuracy, however, similar to the limitations discussed for lung cancer.

Reports indicate that FDG-PET is more accurate than CT in establishing M1 disease in esophageal cancer. In one study with surgery as the gold standard, FDG-PET and helical CT correctly predicted thoracoabdominal lymph node metastases in 83% and 60% of patients. FDG-PET whole body imaging undoubtedly will assume a greater role in the future in evaluating patients with esophageal cancer.

Pulmonary Embolism

In the past, the diagnosis of suspected pulmonary embolism was based on radionuclide ventilation-perfusion imaging (V/Q scan) and catheter pulmonary angiography. V/Q scans provided indirect evidence of emboli, ventilation-perfusion mismatches. Because a substantial percentage of V/Q scans are not diagnostic, catheter angiography often has been needed for a definitive diagnosis, particularly in patients in whom anticoagulation was contraindicated.

Noninvasive CT pulmonary angiography (CTPA) has become a reality, thanks to advances in helical CT technology. Requiring only the intravenous administration of contrast material by power injector, CTPA has replaced V/Q scintigraphy at many institutions. Pulmonary emboli appear as filling defects in the main pulmonary arteries or in the lobar or segmental pulmonary artery branches. Visualization of subsegmental branches has improved with the more narrow collimation, more rapid acquisition times of multidetector scanners, and single breath-hold imaging, which reduces motion artifacts.

CTPA has a sensitivity of 85% to 90% and a specificity of greater than 90% for pulmonary embolism. In patients without demonstrable emboli, CTPA often detects other unsuspected thoracic pathology contributing to the patient's symptoms. Questions have been raised about the safety of withholding anticoagulants in symptomatic patients with CTPA that is negative for emboli. Outcomes data indicate that CTPA has a negative clinical predictive value of 0.99: it is a reliable tool for excluding clinically significant pulmonary embolus.

CT Before Bronchoscopic and Surgical Lung Biopsy
Bronchoscopy in Suspected Lung Cancer

Fiberoptic bronchoscopy (FOB) is an extremely useful procedure for evaluating patients with suspected lung cancer and a host of other focal pulmonary processes. By virtue of its superb anatomic delineation of the tracheobronchial tree, thoracic CT is an efficacious complement to FOB. Preprocedure review of the CT scan by the bronchoscopist has been shown to increase the diagnostic yield of FOB and to reduce the number of subsequent invasive procedures. As a general rule, when the focal abnormality is situated close to a fourth-order bronchus or located more proximally, FOB is likely to yield a definitive diagnosis.

HRCT in Diffuse Lung Disease

High-resolution CT (HRCT) involves the acquisition of narrowly collimated axial images of the lungs, which are reconstructed using a high-resolution algorithm. The resulting images depict the bronchopulmonary anatomy with remarkable clarity. Secondary pulmonary lobules and interlobular septa can be discerned routinely. HRCT is more sensitive than chest radiography in detecting diffuse lung diseases, such as interstitial pneumonia, interstitial fibrosis, sarcoidosis, and lymphangitic carcinomatosis. Frequently the abnormalities shown on HRCT are sufficiently characteristic to suggest a specific diagnosis and potentially to obviate the need for biopsy.

When surgical or VATS biopsy is required to establish a definitive diagnosis, a representative site for biopsy must be selected. Sampling error is a potential problem. HRCT can delineate the lung zones most affected by the process in question and can help the surgeon avoid areas of extensive fibrosis and subpleural honeycombing.

Radiology of the Postoperative Chest

The upright bedside (portable) anteroposterior chest x-ray is the principal means of radiologic surveillance immediately after thoracic surgery. Pneumothorax, atelectasis, pleural effusion, and postoperative pneumonia are readily detected. Radiography easily confirms satisfactory placement of endotracheal, thoracostomy, and nasogastric tubes and vascular catheters. Upright lateral and lateral decubitus radiographs can assess the size and mobility of pleural effusions. When an infected pleural collection is suspected, contrast-enhanced helical CT can localize precisely the extent of the process, assess the thickness of the pleural peel, and assist the surgeon in choosing percutaneous guided or surgical drainage. In critically ill patients, ultrasound equipment can be brought to the bedside to guide diagnostic or therapeutic thoracentesis.

Conventional radiography and helical CT generally are employed for longer term surveillance after curative resection of non–small cell lung cancer. Mediastinal, pleural, or pulmonary recurrences are demonstrable by either method but are discerned more easily on CT. FDG-PET is proving to be more sensitive than CT in this patient group as well. In detecting residual or recurrent lung cancer, the sensitivity and specificity of FDG-PET are 100% and 92% compared with 71% and 95% for helical CT.

Thoracic Aorta

CTA and MRA are replacing invasive catheter angiography in the evaluation of diseases of the thoracic aorta. Beyond imaging the aortic lumen, MRA and CTA allow assessment of the aortic wall, mural thrombus and calcification, and adjacent extraaortic structures. CTA with volume rendering and contrast-enhanced MRA are 100% sensitive and nearly 100% specific in diagnosing type A and B aortic dissections. They permit noninvasive assessment of the extent of the intimal flap, the presence of intramural hematoma, and involvement of ascending aorta and pericardium.

Fusiform and saccular aneurysms are equally well shown by CTA and MRA. Multiplanar contrast-enhanced MRA can show the Adamkiewicz artery in about two thirds of cases. This information potentially could aid the thoracic surgeon in preserving the associated intercostal artery and preventing ischemic spinal cord injury. CTA provides an accessible and quick noninvasive alternative to catheter angiography in cases of suspected aortic injury after high-speed deceleration. CTA is sensitive and reasonably specific in detecting aortic rupture, intimal injury, and traumatic pseudoaneurysm.

Radiologic Screening for Lung Cancer

Many clinical trials employing chest radiography to screen regularly patients at high risk for lung cancer have been conducted. Although early, resectable cancers were detected, none of these trials succeeded in lowering lung cancer–specific mortality, a key outcome measure. Helical CT is much more sensitive than chest radiography in detecting and characterizing small lung nodules. Screening enthusiasts now have shifted attention to CT as a potential screening tool. At this writing, many screening trials are under way or planned, all using a low radiation dose CT imaging protocol.

Results from the initial prevalence screenings indicate that more than 20% of enrolled high-risk patients had one or more lung nodules detected, most of which later were determined to be benign. Follow-up CT protocols will have to triage these patients accurately, minimizing unnecessary intervention for benign nodules, while identifying all cancers. Time will be required to determine whether low-dose CT can detect lung cancer accurately at a resectable stage and at an acceptable cost, while reducing lung cancer–specific mortality.

SUGGESTED READING

Flamen P, et al: Utility of positron emission tomography for the staging of patients with potentially operable esophageal carcinoma, *J Clin Oncol* 18:3202, 2000.

Goodman LR, et al: Subsequent pulmonary embolism: risk after a negative helical CT pulmonary angiogram-prospective comparison with scintigraphy, *Radiology* 215:535, 2000.

Pieterman RM, et al: Preoperative staging of non-small-cell lung cancer with positron-emission tomography, *N Engl J Med* 343:254, 2000.

Sheth S, et al: US guidance for thoracic biopsy: a valuable alternative to CT, *Radiology* 210:721, 1999.

Urban BA, et al: Imaging of thoracic aortic disease, *Cardiol Clin N Am* 17:659, 1999.

ASSESSMENT OF THE PATIENT UNDERGOING PULMONARY RESECTION

Rex C. Yung

In 2001, an estimated 169,500 new cases of lung cancers were expected to be diagnosed in the United States. The current stage distribution of the cases places about 30% in stages I (A and B) and II (A and B), the groups that are potentially resectable for cure. Another 30% to 35% are found to have regional nodal involvement (N1, N2, and N3), previously considered unresectable for cure. With the advent of innovative induction or neoadjuvant chemoradiotherapies, however, a subset of these initial stage IIIA and to a lesser extent stage IIIB patients with nonbulky nodal involvement and good functional status may have good cytoreduction and can be considered for surgical cure as well. If the current multicenter trials of spiral computed tomography (CT) scan as a screening tool for early lung cancer prove CT to be efficacious, 80% to 85% of CT-detected lung cancers may present as stage I small peripheral nodules. There may be a burgeoning expansion of the number of potentially resectable lung cancers.

Most lung cancer cases are found in current smokers and ex-smokers, and the pulmonary reserves of many of these patients with chronic obstructive pulmonary disease (COPD) of varying severity are less than ideal. In addition, many of these patients are elderly, and they may have other severe comorbidities related to tobacco use and cardiovascular, renal, and other organ dysfunction. As a result, currently only about two thirds of the patients with "early stage" lung cancers are offered surgery with curative intent. The following discussion on the assessment of the patient undergoing planned pulmonary resection focuses on the evaluation of pulmonary function as a predictor of perioperative complications and postoperative morbidity and mortality. Based on prospective studies published in the early 1990s by the Lung Cancer Study Group, the standard lobectomy of cancerous tissue and lymph nodes draining a lung lesion is recommended as the minimum ideal resection. The present algorithm also may be adapted to calculate lung function lost from the resection of benign diseases of the lung, although in these cases a lesser resection may be considered.

Many parameters historically have been shown to affect patient outcome after thoracic surgery and pulmonary resection. Advanced patient chronologic age (i.e., patients >70 years) or increased biologic age (i.e., poor functional status, such as Karnofsky Functional Score <70 or Eastern Cooperative Oncology Group score >2) is associated with higher morbidity and mortality. Aside from higher pathologic stage of lung cancer, poor functional status is the main predictor of patient response to therapy and of long-term prognosis in lung cancer. Extent of planned surgical resection,

lobectomy versus pneumonectomy, also affects operative risks. The initial assessment of the patient referred for pulmonary resection consists of a complete careful history taking and physical examination, which affords the surgeon a careful review of the patient's risk factors and the important opportunity to size up the patient's functional status in a way a written summary may not. The value of the experienced physician's clinical "gestalt" should not be minimized.

Many tests, performed in a sequential manner as indicated by the individual case, also are paramount in providing a reasonable prediction of the risks a patient may face for a given planned procedure. These studies include simple assessments, such as observation of the time a subject takes to cover a fixed distance on level ground, how many steps a patient can climb, and measurement of pulse oximetry at rest or at varying levels of exercises. At the other end of the spectrum are invasive studies, such as cardiac catheter measurements of pulmonary arterial pressure at rest and at exercise, pulmonary arterial pressure during transient occlusion of the planned resected vasculature, and serial arterial blood gas analysis during cardiopulmonary exercise testing (CPET). The standard complete pulmonary function tests (PFTs) form the minimal objective test for the assessment of whether an individual can tolerate lung resection.

■ PULMONARY FUNCTION TESTS

PFTs can encompass a range of measurements, derived from several standard maneuvers that are repeated to ensure reproducibility. Repeated measurements are necessary because PFTs are effort-related tests. Good technician instructions to and coaching of the patient are essential, as is good patient understanding, to obtain an accurate and true "best" performance. Spirometry, lung volumes, and the diffusing capacity or gas transfer factor (D_{LCO}) are the measurements included in a "complete" set of PFTs. Spirometry measures airflow over time with volume calculated from the integration of the abovementioned measurements. Spirometry can be presented in the familiar flow-volume loop, which gives a helpful but limited first impression as to whether the patient may have airflow limitations characteristic of an obstructive or restrictive lung disease pattern. The data from spirometry also are presented as the forced vital capacity (FVC) and forced expiratory volume in 1 second (FEV_1) in absolute values (liters) and as a percentage of the "normal" value predicted based on the patient's age, height, and sex and the ratio of the two (FEV_1/FVC) as a percentage. Various other parameters, such as forced expiratory flow, midexpiratory phase ($FEF_{25\%-75\%}$), "midflow," and peak expiratory flow, may be in the report, but these are not discussed further because they contribute little to the reliable prediction of perioperative morbidity and mortality.

Lung volumes can be measured by one of several techniques (helium dilution, nitrogen washout, and body-box plethysmography), and the values are presented in absolute values (liters) and as a percent of the predicted normal. There is much debate among pulmonary physiologists as to the pros and cons of each technique. It generally is accepted that accurate thoracic lung volume and the degree of gas-trapping in patients with severe emphysema and patients with other bullous lung diseases is measured best by body-box plethysmography, but for the practical purpose of assessing the average patient for lung resection, the method of measuring lung volume is less important than careful calibration of the machinery and the patient's performance. The D_{LCO} or the synonymous gas transfer factor is a surrogate measurement of oxygen uptake capacity of the lungs. Deviations from the normal value may represent a complex integration of defects in the pulmonary alveoli epithelium, the pulmonary vasculature, the interface (interstitium) where gas exchange occurs, and even concomitant cardiac diseases. Chronic diseases affecting the pulmonary parenchyma and epithelium (severe emphysema or pulmonary fibrosis) almost always involve the microvasculature to a similar degree; there are, however, conditions that affect the vasculature without obvious impairment of the epithelium or interstitium. These conditions include primary pulmonary hypertension and secondary pulmonary hypertension such as that due to scleroderma and chronic thromboembolism. It cannot be assumed from normal spirometry and lung volumes that a patient has normal gas-exchange capacity.

When assessing a patient for pulmonary resection, how does the surgeon interpret the slew of numbers that usually are included in the standard full PFTs report? The FEV_1 and D_{LCO} are the two parameters that are reliable predictors of postoperative morbidity and mortality. Publications from the 1960s warned against thoracic surgical interventions (often in tuberculosis patients and less often in cancer patients) with FVC less than 60% predicted and in patients with thoracic hyperinflation and "gas-trapping" (total lung capacity and residual volume >120% predicted). The vital capacity has less correlation with airflow obstruction and ventilatory limitation. Based on the ground-breaking work of Cooper, McKenna, Gelb, and others who have revived the study of lung volume reduction surgery (LVRS) for advanced emphysema, clinicians now recognize the unusual opportunity for aggressive curative surgery in the occasional patient with severely limited pulmonary reserve and hyperinflation, with an otherwise potentially resectable lesion located in particularly emphysematous lung. The special cases of lung cancer resection combined with LVRS are addressed briefly later in this chapter.

The acceptable lower limit of FEV_1 associated with an unacceptable risk with lung resection also has evolved over the decades. Although it is true that in the absence of significant preexisting comorbidities, FEV_1 thresholds of greater than 1.5 liters and greater than 2.0 liters indicate adequate pulmonary reserve for lobectomy and pneumonectomy, conversely, these cutoffs are unnecessarily strict and exclude some patients who can undergo lung resections safely. Instead of an absolute value in liters, it is preferable to evaluate the lung functions as a percent of the predicted normal because shorter, older, and female subjects have lower ventilatory and oxygen delivery requirements than do taller, younger, and male subjects. A baseline FEV_1 of equal to or greater than 60% predicted is believed to be a safe cutoff for pulmonary resection not requiring complete pneumonectomy. Normal PFT values do not take into account, however, body weight. In a later section that discusses CPET, which is a more detailed metabolic study dealing with anaerobic thresholds and oxygen consumption, the results are normalized further to body weight to take into account the higher metabolic and ventilatory requirements of a heavier person.

■ PREDICTED POSTOPERATIVE PULMONARY FUNCTION

The limits of surgery depend on the starting pulmonary function and the extent of planned resection for the individual patient. As such, an accurate prediction of the residual postoperative pulmonary functions (FEV_1-ppo and D_{LCO}-ppo) would provide a better measure of a patient's functional reserve after surgery. Several simple arithmetic formulas can be applied to estimate the FEV_1-ppo and D_{LCO}-ppo. The simplest formula assumes equal distribution of lung function between 19 lobar segments (10 on the right and 9 on the left) and approximately 5% function for each segment. The FEV_1-ppo or D_{LCO}-ppo is estimated as follows:

$$\text{Predicted postoperative FEV1-ppo} = \text{preoperative FEV1} \times (\text{no. residual segments})/(\text{no. initial segments})$$

or FEV_1-ppo = $FEV_1 \times (1 - [5.26\% \times$ no. resected bronchopulmonary segments/100]) if the patient starts off with two complete lungs (i.e., no prior lung resections). A slightly more complex formula would exclude from the calculation any lung segments that are not aerated or perfused because they should not contribute to the preoperative baseline lung function.

■ SPLIT-LUNG FUNCTION STUDIES

Although the previous formulas may be easy to use, the accuracy may be affected by the nonhomogeneous distribution of lung function, which applies to many patients with chronic lung conditions, such as emphysema and interstitial lung diseases. Selective bronchospirometry in awake subjects is uncomfortable for patients and challenging to do. In the 1980s and 1990s, work by Olsen, Bollinger, and others refined the technique and validated the benefit of using pulmonary perfusion to estimate quantitatively the amount of functioning lung that may be lost. The "quantitative selective" or "split-lung" function study using radionuclide scanning quantitates the regional lung distribution of the injected technetium-99m-labeled macroaggregates and facilitates a more accurate prediction of the residual percent of preoperative lung function after a planned lung resection.

The current lower thresholds of acceptable FEV_1-ppo and D_{LCO}-ppo have been decreased to a minimum 35% to 40% for FEV_1-ppo and 40% for D_{LCO}-ppo. In general, FEV_1-ppo generally underestimates the residual PFTs and the functional status after resection; this is especially true in patients with severe hyperinflation and nonhomogeneous distribution of emphysematous lung disease who have resection of these dysfunctional lung units.

■ EXERCISE TESTING

Although adopting a simplified estimate of a patient's predicted postoperative residual FEV_1 and D_{LCO} with the aforementioned minimum thresholds can classify most patients into low-risk and high-risk groups, there are many individuals who fall into a gray intermediate zone or whose functional status does not seem to correlate with their PFT measurements. Exercise testing provides an extra measure of fitness or identifies heretofore missed comorbidities, such as occult ischemic heart disease, which may increase postoperative complications.

Different methods of exercise testing have been studied and published. Stair climbing is a convenient, rapid, and essentially free way to estimate exercise capacity and cardiopulmonary reserve, with studies by Pollock and Olsen showing good correlation between number of flights climbed with maximal oxygen consumption ($\dot{V}O_2$max). The drawback has been a lack of standardization, including number and height of the steps and the pace of ascent. Submaximal, level-ground walking timed to cover a certain distance or by graded treadmill exercise may not provide sufficient stress or provide a measurement of the $\dot{V}O_2$max. The recommendation for the best method to obtain an integrated estimate of cardiopulmonary fitness, reserve, and potential for surgical complications is to perform a maximal effort CPET with measurement of $\dot{V}O_2$max.

Protocols exist for CPET with treadmill or with bicycle ergometer, with timed stepped-up or continuous ramp increase in workload until exhaustion. Concomitant cardiac monitoring accompanies the collection and analysis of exhaled gas and arterial blood gas measurement as indicated. Based on the measured $\dot{V}O_2$max expressed as milliliters of oxygen consumed per kilograms of actual body weight per minute (ml/kg/min), patients with $\dot{V}O_2$max equal to or greater than 20 ml/kg/min without cardiac instabilities are candidates for lobectomy and pneumonectomy without further testing. Patients with $\dot{V}O_2$max between 12 and 15 ml/kg/min are at risk for more postoperative cardiopulmonary complications, and an estimate of postoperative residual $\dot{V}O_2$-ppo should be calculated, based preferably on a corresponding quantitative split-lung perfusion study. Patients with $\dot{V}O_2$-ppo less than 10 ml/kg/min are not surgical resection candidates because their rates of postoperative complications, especially of respiratory insufficiency, are prohibitively high. This minimum $\dot{V}O_2$ threshold applies also to patients with severe, heterogeneously distributed emphysema with a lung cancer located in particularly emphysematous lungs who otherwise could be considered for combined LVRS. Although LVRS has benefited selected patients with improvement in postoperative respiratory mechanics and FEV_1, they could not gain pulmonary vascular bed needed for gas exchange, and these patients may die as a result of further increase in pulmonary artery pressure.

■ MISCELLANEOUS ASSESSMENT AND INTERVENTIONS

Arterial blood gas demonstrations of hypercarbia of $PaCO_2$ greater than 45 torr and hypoxemia of PaO_2 less than 55 torr had been regarded in the past as indices of high risk of postoperative complications and contraindications for thoracic surgery. These values now are recognized to be only relative contraindications, and patients undergoing a combined lung cancer/LVRS resection may have at least transient improvement in oxygenation in parallel to improvement in

airflow obstruction. Historically, emphysema patients who have chronic sputum production ("chronic bronchitics" or "blue bloaters") have fared worse prognostically than patients who are "pink puffers" or non–carbon dioxide retainers. The data from LVRS and interim analysis of the National Emphysema Treatment Trial offer similar cautions about thoracic resection of chronic bronchitics with severe airflow obstruction. The finding of hypercarbia should be coupled with an assessment of the patient's bronchitic status.

Other parallel lessons between COPD, major thoracic surgery, and LVRS include in particular attention to nutritional assessment, standard cardiac evaluation, and psychosocial assessment. Malnutrition and weight loss in particular are negative prognostic factors in COPD and cancer. Proinflammatory cytokines, such as tumor necrosis factor-α, interleukin-1, and interleukin-6, are increased in COPD patients in the lower quartile weight group, and these cytokines are increased further in patients with cancer cachexia. Malnourished patients are at increased risk for postoperative respiratory insufficiency and ventilator dependency and a myriad of other complications, such as poor wound healing, sepsis, and other nosocomial infections, which in turn delays healing and recovery.

Cardiac assessment ranges from careful history taking, physical examination, and electrocardiogram integrated into clinical criteria, such as Goldman's, to incorporation with pulmonary risk factors into certain cardiopulmonary risk indices, such as Epstein's. High-risk cardiac patients should be referred for appropriate cardiac stress testing.

Standard interventions carried out during the initial pulmonary assessment include firm recommendation for smoking cessation among active smokers and prescription of tobacco-cessation aids. Bronchodilators are prescribed for patients with obstructive airways disease. Antibiotics are considered for management of airways infections. Emphasis on nutrition includes laboratory assessment; suggestions for nutritional supplements; and, for selected patients, appetite stimulants, such as medroxyprogesterone. Pulmonary and cardiac rehabilitation may warrant a delay in surgery for potential cure of a lung cancer. Lessons from LVRS show the importance of a mandatory and intensive course of rehabilitation in the marginal surgical candidate. Concerns that a delay in surgery would allow a cancer to metastasize during the 6 to 8 weeks of rehabilitation miss the reality that surgeries on lung cancer all too often are performed on understaged tumors, which already may have unrecognized regional nodal or distant metastases. A course of cardiopulmonary rehabilitation and nutritional enhancement may complement the current 2- to 3-month trials of neoadjuvant or induction chemotherapy given to stage II and selected stage III newly diagnosed lung cancer patients, in the hope of reducing the high incidence of postoperative relapses.

■ SUMMARY

Assessment of the pulmonary status of patients undergoing lung resection has become a multidisciplinary process. High-quality PFTs, including spirometric measurement of FEV_1 and gas transfer (D_{LCO}), remain the mainstay initial diagnostic studies. Patients with baseline FEV_1 and D_{LCO}

greater than 60% of predicted should tolerate standard lobectomy. More extensive resections by bilobectomies or pneumonectomy require a careful estimate of the predicted residual lung function. FEV_1-ppo greater than 35% to 40% predicted normal and D_{LCO}-ppo greater than 40% predicted normal are the current thresholds for safe resection. There is some controversy as to whether a quantitative split-lung perfusion study or a maximal CPET should be the next study used to quantify an estimated functional reserve after the proposed surgery. The two tests are complementary, and the sequence in which they are ordered and performed depends on their availability, reliability of the study at the local institution, and costs.

An absolute $\dot{V}O_2max$ of equal to or greater than 20 ml O_2/kg/min consumption provides clearance for a pneumonectomy, whereas a $\dot{V}O_2max$-ppo of less than 10 ml O_2/kg/min is an absolute contraindication for surgery. $\dot{V}O_2max$ of 12 to 15 ml O_2/kg/min or discordant results of the FEV_1-ppo and D_{LCO}-ppo require a more judicious approach, with considerations for therapeutic interventions briefly listed earlier, which may improve the pulmonary and overall functional status of the patient. Until we succeed in better primary and secondary prevention of lung cancer, the goal is to identify all lung cancer patients who potentially may be resected for cure or are candidates for aggressive multimodality therapy that would prolong good-quality survival.

SUGGESTED READING

Armstrong P, et al: Guidelines on the selection of patients with lung cancer for surgery (British Thoracic Society and Society of Cardiothoracic Surgeons of Great Britain and Ireland Working Party), *Thorax* 56:89, 2001.

Pretreatment evaluation of non-small-cell lung cancer: official statement of the American Thoracic Society and European Respiratory Society, with endorsement by the American College of Chest Physicians, *Am J Respir Crit Care Med* 156:320, 1997.

Weisman IM: Cardiopulmonary exercise testing in the preoperative assessment for lung resection surgery, *Semin Thorac Cardiovasc Surg* 13:116, 2001.

Wyser C, et al: Prospective evaluation of an algorithm for the functional assessment of lung resection candidates, *Am J Respir Crit Care Med* 159:1450, 1999.

POSTOPERATIVE CARE OF THE GENERAL THORACIC SURGICAL PATIENT

Michael Bousamra II

Major thoracic surgical resections are attended by significant perioperative morbidity and mortality. Thoracic malignancies are the most commonly encountered surgical problem, and these often occur in elderly patients or patients in a compromised physiologic state. The loss of respiratory function related to lung resection proportionally diminishes pulmonary reserve. Given this adverse environment, perioperative care of thoracic surgical patients hinges on several factors. First is a clinical and quantitative evaluation of the patient before surgery, particularly patients with limited reserve or existing comorbidity. A careful yet expeditious surgery with avoidance of excessive fluid administration is needed because many postoperative complications either are created or are avoided in the operating room. After surgery, frequent, focused patient assessment with anticipation of potential problems is the key to preventing complications or resolving them before they become life-threatening. This chapter emphasizes a pragmatic and reasoned approach to optimize operative results and specifically addresses a variety of common or serious problems that the surgeon encounters in general thoracic surgery.

■ PREOPERATIVE ASSESSMENT: GENERAL COMMENTS

Patient selection always skews surgical results. Inclusion of patients with greater operative risk increases operative morbidity and mortality, yet exclusion of these patients may force them into therapies that are less effective. Patients with lung cancer confront the thoracic practitioner with this problem most frequently. The relative benefits of surgical resection over radiation therapy have never been defined clearly, but surgical cure rates generally are assumed to be twice as high for stage I and II disease. The anticipated relative benefit of surgical resection must be weighed against estimates of operative morbidity and mortality based on patient comorbidity and pulmonary function. It follows that a cogent informed consent and mutual decision to proceed with surgical resection can be one of the first steps toward optimal patient care and the establishment of a trusted patient/physician relationship. Perioperative assessment serves to identify specific problems, assess their severity, and, most importantly, estimate their impact on surgical outcome. Pulmonary function most often is the "hinge of fate." Spirometry and diffusion capacity are static measures of pulmonary function. Exercise oximetry and maximal oxygen consumption studies are dynamic assessments of cardiopulmonary reserve. Exercise desaturation less than 88% is significant, and a myocardial oxygen consumption of less than 12 ml/kg/min may pose a prohibitive risk to surgical resection (provided that body mass index is near normal). Radionuclide split-lung function is particularly helpful in marginal patients in whom lung function is nonuniform (e.g., in cases in which tumors obstruct the airway or in which bullous disease is unilaterally more prominent).

Cardiac function is of penultimate concern. Investigation for coronary artery disease and decreased left ventricular function is necessary. Symptoms of angina and heart failure should be sought. Older patients and diabetics or patients with evidence of prior myocardial damage on electrocardiogram (ECG) should undergo a noninvasive stress test. Cardiac catheterization may be necessary in selected individuals to clarify their preoperative risk and to offer strategies for preoperative intervention, either catheter based or surgical.

Less commonly, patients present with significant alterations in renal, hepatic, and gastrointestinal function or other significant comorbidity. Aside from assessing the immediate effect these problems pose on the postoperative recovery, one also must contemplate the significant effect they may have on long-term survival and the relative merits of surgery.

The preoperative assessment also may dictate surgical strategy. Patients with limited pulmonary reserve may undergo surgical treatment of lung cancer but with a more limited resection. In cases of esophageal cancer, transhiatal resection may be tolerated better than a more radical resection in patients with limited pulmonary reserve or other comorbidity.

■ GENERAL PRINCIPLES OF POSTOPERATIVE CARE

After postsurgical extubation, patients are often semiconscious. Airway protective mechanisms are blunted, and bronchial mucociliary clearance is reduced. Aspiration and atelectasis are prone to occur. Elevation of the head of the bed improves diaphragm position and reduces aspiration risk. Continuous monitoring of cardiac and respiratory systems is a standard of care after major thoracic resections. Pulse oximetry provides a reliable noninvasive assessment of arterial oxygen saturation. Ventilation-perfusion mismatch is readily identified. Intraarterial lines allow systemic pressure monitoring and serial blood gas determinations in patients who may require reintubation. Most patients, as they recover from anesthesia, have carbon dioxide retention, particularly patients with emphysema. In the absence of respiratory distress, most patients can be managed supportively by arousal, bronchodilator treatment, and mild chest physiotherapy.

Continuous ECG recording should be available and is employed routinely in the first 24 to 48 hours after major resections. Cardiac arrhythmias are encountered frequently after pulmonary resections. Increased adrenergic tone, electrolyte imbalance, and mediastinal shift are probable causes of supraventricular tachycardia. Hypoxia and atrial distention from fluid overload are other common causes. Myocardial ischemia may be precipitated by the increased oxygen demand associated with a rapid heart rate or because of hypotension induced by the arrhythmia. Treatment of supraventricular tachycardia with intravenous calcium channel blockers and eventual conversion to oral medication is one standard. Selective β_1-antagonists also may be used while monitoring the patient for secondary effects of bronchospasm and hypotension. Intravenous magnesium sulfate has been shown to be effective in preventing supraventricular tachycardia after pulmonary resection when given within the first 12 hours.

Postoperative care of the thoracic surgical patient can be standardized according to the type of surgery performed. Care pathways and postoperative orders should be formulated for limited pulmonary resection, lobectomy, pneumonectomy, esophageal resection, and nonresectional surgery of the esophagus. These formulas serve as a template for thoracic team members to follow and as a means to recognize problems as deviations from the expected norm. They also ensure that all aspects of patient care are covered. Retrospective comparison studies have shown enhanced outcomes and shortened hospital stay when care pathways are employed. Standard orders should not be implemented without tailoring them to the individual patient's needs. Care pathways routinely encompass patient monitoring, supplemental oxygen needs, intravenous fluids, medications, chest tube management principles, activity, chest physiotherapy, and diet progression.

■ PAIN RELIEF

Intercostal thoracotomy incisions rank at the top of painful exposures. Chest wall splinting and elevation of the diaphragm cause a restrictive ventilatory pattern. All lung volumes are reduced, particularly the expiratory reserve volume, which predisposes the lung to atelectasis. Postthoracotomy pain also inhibits the forceful cough needed to expel retained secretions. Analgesics are essential to improve respiratory mechanics, yet they must be titrated to avoid secondary complications. Narcotic administration by patient-controlled analgesia systems has proved safe and effective, provided that maximal doses are not excessive. Intrathecal narcotic administration provides effective pain relief with a single preoperative injection. It may be attended by mild hypotension, however, inducing a sequence of unwanted volume administration or central line access with short-term vasopressor administration. Epidural analgesic strategies are common. Insertion of the catheter at the lumbar or thoracic level is effective, although more cephalad levels require lower initial infusion rates to avoid an ascending spinal effect and diaphragm paralysis. Usually a local anesthetic is combined with a narcotic. Hypotension can occur but is minimal if the local anesthetic is reduced or avoided. In the older patient, urinary bladder catheterization is necessary. Patient mobility is reduced by all the paraphernalia associated with the epidural and the patient-controlled analgesia systems. This encumbrance detracts from their benefit.

Infusion of local anesthetic through intercostal subpleural catheters can provide effective pain relief with avoidance of the side effects associated with intravenous and epidural narcotic administration. The development of a compact self-contained delivery system has improved patient convenience without impairing patient mobility. Subpleural placement of the catheter can be cumbersome, however, and care must be taken to avoid intercostal vessel puncture. Leakage through the subpleural access site also can diminish the anesthetic effect.

Complications associated with analgesic strategies must be considered. Narcotics produce respiratory depression at high doses. They also contribute to gastrointestinal dysfunction, most significantly postoperative ileus and colonic distention. Vagal irritation during surgery also may play a role in this phenomenon. The problem can be life-threatening due to the risk of bowel ischemia and perforation. Tense abdominal distention also has deleterious effects on ventilation. The best approach is avoidance by restricting oral intake to clear liquids until the patient is passing either flatus or stool. This cautious resumption of diet has no significant effect on overall nutrition, yet spares the occasional patient from significant morbidity. Patients receiving epidural or intrathecal agents should have blood pressure and respirations monitored at frequent intervals. Management optimally is supervised through a pain management team responsible for analgesic administration. Nonsteroidal antiinflammatory drugs are effective adjuncts to postoperative pain relief. Because pulmonary resection patients are fluid restricted, renal dysfunction is more likely to occur with administration of nonsteroidal antiinflammatory drugs, and serum creatinine should be monitored accordingly. Ketorolac has been noted to be particularly effective, but in addition to renal side effects, it is associated with gastric bleeding and perforation. These risks are ameliorated by concomitant administration of misoprostol (Cytotec), a mucosal protective agent, and by limiting therapy to fewer than 6 days.

Postoperative fluid administration generally is limited to approximately 2 liters/24 hr to minimize the tendency to develop pulmonary edema after lung manipulation. This restriction is particularly important after pneumonectomy, when the consequences of pulmonary edema are more grave. Occasionally, patients are struck by a profound thirst and may drink several liters. To avoid fluid overload, an oral fluid restriction should be kept in place for the first 48 to 72 hours. Esophageal resections are not confined by strict intravenous fluid limits because adequate perfusion of the esophageal substitute is of primary importance. With the two-field and three-field dissections inherent in esophageal resection, intraoperative fluid losses are more profound. Systemic perfusion pressures should be supported by liberal volume resuscitation. Dopamine, 1 to 4 µg/kg/min, also may be administered to improve splanchnic perfusion.

Pulmonary toilet measures are crucial in postthoracotomy recovery. Early and frequent ambulation, incentive spirometry, and voluntary coughing to clear secretions all have salutary effects on patient recovery. Chest percussion is indicated in patients with rhonchi and other signs of retained secretions, particularly after major pulmonary resections. Adequate pain control is essential for percussion techniques to be tolerated and beneficial.

Management of intrapleural drainage tubes has long been a matter of individual preference, but several concepts are generally applicable. Patency and function are assessed by tidal movement of fluid within the tube during the respiratory cycle. While tubes are on suction, an air leak may be continuous but usually is more prominent during exhalation. A break in the system is indicated by a new large continuous air leak or one that worsens during inspiration. Evidence suggests that air leaks resolve more quickly when pleural tubes are placed to water seal within 24 to 48 hours of resection rather than remaining on suction until the air leak stops. After any pulmonary resection, a small pneumothorax can be expected. The pneumothorax may increase when the chest tube is placed on water seal. If the pneumothorax is not large and is not associated with respiratory distress or worsening subcutaneous emphysema, it can be observed in hopes of more rapid resolution of the air leak. On chest tube removal, the lung can be reexpanded by placing the chest tube to suction. Approximately 5% to 10% of patients have air leaks beyond postoperative day 5. Increasingly, patients are discharged with a Heimlich valve attached to the chest tube with subsequent removal at an office visit. Observation for worsening pneumothorax and subcutaneous emphysema should be carried out.

■ VENTILATORY SUPPORT

Only a few patients require mechanical ventilation after pulmonary resection. Early extubation generally is favored to reduce the ill effects of positive airway pressure on bronchial closure and minor bronchopleural fistulas. Prolonged intubation also increases the potential for contamination of the bronchial tree. Exceptions to the rule of early extubation include cases with prolonged anesthesia or operations incurring extensive blood loss and fluid administration in which pulmonary edema and temporary deterioration in lung function can be anticipated. Moderate levels of positive endexpiratory pressure (5 to 10 mm Hg), tidal volumes of 8 to 10 ml/kg, and mild hypoventilation reduce airway pressure, minimize alveolar damage, and lower stress on the bronchial closure.

In some patients with marginal pulmonary reserve, particularly patients with emphysema undergoing lung volume reduction, early extubation specifically is advocated. Effective pain relief via an epidural catheter, bronchodilators, and immediate pulmonary toilet measures is essential for success. Part of the rationale for early extubation is to avoid the sudden asynchronous straining of the patient against the mechanically delivered tidal volume. The production of high airway pressures can disrupt parenchymal staple lines and nonsurgical sites, creating a massive air leak. Other patients with diminished pulmonary function who undergo thoracic procedures without bleb resection do not share this pressing need for early extubation.

Significant postoperative bleeding should be uncommon. Most thoracic resections do not require transfusion. Assiduous intraoperative hemostasis can keep blood loss at less than 300 ml for most standard pulmonary resections. Careful inspection of the intercostal space, divided bronchial vessels, and all vascular ligatures before closure is routine. Thoracic cavity irrigation with water readily identifies smaller bleeding points through the clear fluid. If increased bloody chest tube output is noted, serial chest radiographs are needed to assess for retained hemothorax. This is particularly true if the chest tube output suddenly decreases, which may indicate only an obstructed or clotted tube lumen rather than cessation of bleeding. Although no single output value should serve as an absolute mandate for reexploration, hemodynamic instability requires resuscitation and urgent surgical intervention.

■ POSTOPERATIVE CARE OF ESOPHAGECTOMY PATIENTS

Patients undergoing esophageal resection incur a different set of postoperative problems. Respiratory complications head the list of difficulties but for different reasons. Surgery is generally 4 to 8 hours in duration, and abdominal and thoracic cavities are violated. Tissue dissection is extensive, and fluid losses are greater. Pulmonary edema due to fluid resuscitation is more likely.

Airway protective mechanisms are compromised by a cervical esophagogastric anastomosis. Division of the strap muscles and laryngeal retraction result in decreased laryngeal elevation and exposure of the vocal cords during swallowing. The nasogastric tube promotes aspiration, and the intrathoracic stomach is a local reservoir of caustic fluid that can reflux easily into the hypopharynx. Counteractive measures include delaying extubation until the patient is alert and has regained somatic muscle strength. We generally wait 24 hours, particularly if an extended or radical esophagectomy was performed. Fowler's position limits passive reflux. Incentive spirometry and voluntary coughing help clear airway secretions. Feeding is initiated only after a swallow study is reviewed for evidence of aspiration. Initially, thickened liquids are swallowed more safely. Double swallowing improves clearance of the hypopharynx. Chin lowering and dry swallowing exercises improve epiglottic coverage of the glottis.

Unrecognized anastomotic leakage can be life-threatening whether in the cervical or thoracic region. Cervical anastomotic leaks occur more frequently, but usually can be handled effectively by opening the neck for drainage. Anastomotic dilation promotes antegrade flow of swallowed material and more rapid closure of the fistula. On some occasions, the cervical esophagogastric leak drains into the upper mediastinum, and a septic course results. Formal drainage in the operating room is recommended for these cases.

Intrathoracic anastomotic leaks carry a higher mortality. Early recognition and drainage usually are needed for survival. Small radiographically identified outpouchings at the anastomosis that readily drain back into the bowel may be treated conservatively. The common scenario is that of a patient who has not yet been studied or who had a negative esophagogram recently who presents with respiratory distress, fever, and agitation. This syndrome is a manifestation of a leak until proved otherwise. Turbid fluid recovered from the chest tube or radiographic signs such as pneumomediastinum and hydropneumothorax prompt rapid resuscitation and reexploration. Otherwise, an esophagogram should be performed with barium (not diatrizoate [Gastrografin] if there

is a risk for aspiration). Several barium swallows or nasogastric infusion of barium is needed to delineate the anastomosis and fill the stomach. Multiple positions should be used to distend the anastomosis and the gastric staple line along the lesser curve. Delayed films are obtained if no leak is evident initially. Operative drainage, débridement, and decortication are standard therapy. Reanastomosis is usually possible. Buttressed closure with a vascularized pedicle flap of diaphragm or pericardial fat is recommended. Large defects may be treated by T-tube drainage with establishment of an esophagopleurocutaneous fistula. Occasionally, local tissue destruction makes complete débridement and reconstruction untenable. Cervical esophagostomy, gastrostomy, and feeding jejunostomy are recommended for this circumstance, with bowel interposition performed at a later date.

Conduit necrosis is a dreaded complication after esophagectomy. It usually occurs within the first 48 to 72 hours after resection. Hemodynamic instability and anion gap acidosis are hallmarks. Endoscopy reveals a black, necrotic mucosa of the transposed stomach or colon. Torsion of the mesentery or simple vascular insufficiency from the process of conduit mobilization is responsible. Cervical esophagostomy and gastrostomy are recommended with later reconstruction because these patients are usually unstable.

Chylous effusion from thoracic duct transection can have serious consequences. If the main duct has been divided, fluid output may approach 2 liters/day. Lymph loss leads to rapid protein depletion and immunosuppression. Chest drainage in the patient with NPO (nothing per mouth) status is clear, not milky. Few if any other causes explain persistent high chest tube output, but confirmation can be obtained with a fatty meal, usually cream per nasogastric tube. Routine ligation of the thoracic duct during esophagectomy prevents this problem. All lymphatic tissue between the aorta and azygous vein is encompassed by the ligature. If a major duct leak is recognized postoperatively, prompt intervention with duct ligation is the best option because major thoracic duct injuries are unlikely to close with nonoperative measures, and continuing protein losses jeopardize patient recovery.

■ POSTPNEUMONECTOMY EMPYEMA AND BRONCHOPLEURAL FISTULA

Postpneumonectomy empyema and bronchopleural fistula occur in approximately 1% to 5% of pneumonectomy patients. They may become manifest at any time within the first several months after resection, and most occur within 3 to 4 weeks. Fever, malaise, and rising white blood cell count all are signs consistent with an infected pleural space. Patients also may have positive blood cultures. If a postpneumonectomy bronchopleural fistula is present, patients have increased sputum production, which, especially early on, is watery or may have clotted material. Chest x-ray often reveals a contralateral infiltrate in conjunction with a falling air-fluid level on the side of the pneumonectomy. Sepsis, respiratory failure, and mechanical ventilation result from delayed recognition of the problem and greatly complicate treatment.

Management of postpneumonectomy empyema and bronchopleural fistula is challenging under any circumstances.

When diagnosed, a large-bore chest tube is placed to evacuate the pleural space, with care taken to keep the infected pleural space dependent. Bronchoscopy may be needed to assess the bronchial stump for dehiscence. The time-honored procedure described by Clagett and Eloesser involves creation of a transthoracic window by rib resection and marsupialization of the skin to the parietal pleura. The mediastinum must be in a fixed position to prevent any ill effect of the open pneumothorax. The window should be large enough to accommodate the surgeon's hand for easy wound packing. It gradually constricts, but packing continues with ring forceps. Dilute povidone-iodine (Betadine) (10:1 to 20:1) packing is effective at rendering the pleural space culture negative. Each removal of gauze from the chest effectively débrides necrotic material and detritus. When the chest is culture negative, the wound is closed by mobilization of the myocutaneous flaps and filling the pleural cavity with antibiotic solution. Success is achieved in most patients, but reinfection is common. The presence of a bronchopleural fistula complicates matters. It may have been the primary event that caused the empyema. Alternatively the bronchial stump may have broken down because of the empyema. Often the patient develops a contralateral pneumonia or acute respiratory distress syndrome due to aspiration of infected pleural fluid. Mechanical ventilation is inefficient due to loss of a significant fraction of the tidal volume through the bronchopleural fistula. Packing the chest tightly through the Clagett window and sealing it with an airtight drape can limit volume loss. This situation is frequently unstable with continued aspiration of intrapleural contents. Muscle flap coverage of the bronchial stump is needed to prevent continued contamination of the airway and lung. Continued mechanical ventilation increases the risk, however, of reformation of the bronchopleural fistula through the muscle flap. A keen sense of the patient's clinical direction dictates the timing of surgical intervention. Ideally the patient can be recovered and muscle flap coverage performed with the patient off mechanical ventilation in a relatively clean pleural space. When the bronchial stump is closed, management continues as described for postpneumonectomy empyema.

A technique of closed intrapleural irrigation with 0.1% povidone iodine, 40 ml/hr, has been described for treatment of early postpneumonectomy empyema with a small bronchopleural fistula. Irrigation and drainage tubes are placed after débridement of the thorax and muscle flap closure of the bronchus. Irrigation with povidone iodine is continued for 7 days followed by 24 hours of saline irrigation. Chest tubes are removed on obtaining a negative Gram stain for organisms and white blood cells. Tube removal without recurrence of bronchopleural fistula or empyema was reported in all 22 patients studied.

SUGGESTED READING

Bousamra M II: Optimizing results of esophageal resection for benign and malignant disease, *J KY Med Assoc* 99:12, 2001.

Cerfolio RJ, et al: A prospective algorithm for the management of air leaks after pulmonary resection, *Ann Thorac Surg* 66:1726, 1998.

Easterling CS, et al: Pharyngeal dysphagia in postesophagectomy patients: correlation with deglutitive biomechanics, *Ann Thorac Surg* 69:989, 2000.

Graham RJ, et al: Postoperative portable chest radiographs: optimum use in thoracic surgery, *J Thorac Cardiovasc Surg* 115:45, 1998.

Richardson JD, Tobin GR: Closure of esophageal defects with muscle flaps, *Arch Surg* 129:541, 1994.

THORACIC INCISIONS

John Howington

The bony thorax of the chest provides a challenge for adequate exposure in thoracic surgical procedures. Many approaches have evolved for specific pathologic processes in the chest to optimize exposure, while attempting to reduce the morbidity of the procedure. No one approach is best for all thoracic surgical procedures.

Most thoracic operations are facilitated by isolation of the ipsilateral lung with placement of a double-lumen endotracheal tube or a bronchial blocker. All open thoracic approaches cause significant pain for the patient. This pain is best controlled with a well-placed and well-dosed thoracic epidural catheter. Although intercostal blocks, pleural catheters, and patient-controlled analgesia are effective tools, the gold standard for postoperative pain control remains thoracic epidural analgesia.

■ POSTEROLATERAL THORACOTOMY

The posterolateral thoracotomy is the most commonly used approach. It provides excellent exposure of the thoracic spine, esophagus, descending thoracic aorta, and hilum of the lung. It is well suited for decortication of the lung and as an alternative to the median sternotomy for many cardiac procedures.

The procedure begins with the patient in the supine position on a beanbag and with sequential compression devices on the lower extremities. After general anesthesia and proper placement of a double-lumen endotracheal tube (or bronchial blocker) and appropriate monitoring lines, the patient is turned into the lateral decubitus position. The neck should be maintained in a neutral position, and a roll is placed in the axilla to protect the dependent brachial plexus. Pillows are placed between the legs, and adequate padding is provided for the down leg at the level of the knee and ankle. The arms are padded and folded superiorly in a praying position. The table is flexed to open the interspaces on the operative side, and the bed is placed in slight reverse Trendelenburg position to level the chest. Wide adhesive tape is placed across the hip and lower leg to secure the patient and to avoid body rotation during the procedure.

The incision begins at the anterior border of the latissimus dorsi muscle usually at the level of the inframammary crease. The incision curves posteriorly, passes 2 cm below the scapular tip, and ends in the auscultatory triangle inferior to the border of the trapezius muscle at a point midway between the posterior border of the scapula and the thoracic spine. The latissimus dorsi muscle is divided with cautery in line with the skin incision. Alternatively, if sparing of the muscle is desired, flaps can be developed superficial to the latissimus fascia, and the muscle can be retracted posteriorly after the anterior border is released from its attachments. Reflecting the serratus muscle from posterior to anterior by dividing its posterior and inferior fascial attachments provides excellent exposure, while preserving the muscle.

The incision may begin lower if access to the diaphragm, lower thoracic spine, or distal esophagus is needed. In these cases, a more oblique incision that follows the desired interspace is chosen. When performing a thoracotomy for anterior exposure of the spine, the use of fluoroscopy in the anterior-posterior and lateral projections to confirm the desired spine levels facilitates determination of the proper interspace for entering the chest. For tumors that involve the chest wall or superior sulcus, the incision also can be extended cephalad to provide more exposure.

The scapula is retracted superiorly and away from the chest wall, and the ribs are palpated posteriorly along the erector spinae muscles. The second intercostal space is deeper and wider and is readily identified. Insertion of the posterior scalene muscle along the anterior border of the second rib also defines it. The first rib has a broader and more flat feel than the lower ribs but can be difficult to locate in large or obese patients. When the first or second rib is identified, counting down from above can identify the proper intercostal space for the procedure.

The intercostal space chosen varies with the surgical procedure. The fourth interspace provides the best exposure for upper lobe resections and on the left for the aortic arch and proximal descending thoracic aorta. The fifth intercostal space is chosen most often for other pulmonary resections and decortication of the lung. The seventh or eighth intercostal space is chosen for distal esophageal and diaphragm procedures.

Adequate exposure most often can be obtained without routinely taking or dividing (shingling) a rib. The intercostal muscles are divided immediately above the lower rib of the desired interspace with electrocautery. The intercostal muscles may be divided posteriorly to within 2 cm of the

sympathetic chain and anteriorly to within 1 cm of the internal thoracic vessels. With thoracic spine procedures, a rib may be taken to provide wider exposure, and the bony rib may be used for the spinal fusion. Entering the chest through the bed of a resected rib is the preferred approach with extrapleural pneumonectomy and in reoperative thoracic procedures.

The standard wound closure begins with approximation of the intercostal space. The author prefers to place four drill holes with a $1/16$ drill bit in the inferior rib. Four interrupted no. 5 polyester (Ethibond) sutures are placed through the inferior rib and on top of the superior rib. This approach avoids entrapment or injury of the intervening intercostal bundle. This approach was shown to reduce postoperative pain in a randomized trial performed by Cerfolio. The lung always is reinflated before closure. The muscle layers are closed with running no. 1 polyglactin 910 (Vicryl) suture. The subcutaneous tissue is closed with a running 2-0 Vicryl suture. The skin may be approximated with a 4-0 Monocryl (poliglecaprone) subcuticular stitch or skin staples.

When a rib needs to be resected, the periosteum is scored in the middle of the rib with cautery from the level of the erector spinae muscles to the anterior extent of the incision. The periosteum is elevated off the superior portion of the rib from posterior to anterior, and the inferior periosteum is elevated from anterior to posterior. Having elevated the periosteum circumferentially, the rib is cut posteriorly at the level of the erector spinae muscles and anteriorly at the level of the skin incision. The intercostal muscle may be divided on top of the rib anteriorly to within 2 cm of the internal thoracic vessels and posteriorly to within 2 cm of the sympathetic chain. For wound closure, the bed of the resected rib is closed in two layers with running 0 Vicryl sutures. This closure provides a watertight seal of the chest at the completion of the resection. Often the periosteal bed closure is facilitated by placing pericostal sutures through drill holes in the next lower rib and above the superior rib to take tension off the periosteal closure.

■ ANTERIOR THORACOTOMY

The anterior thoracotomy is the preferred approach in an emergency setting, allowing fast access to the left chest, pericardium, and aorta. The incision can be extended across the sternum (clamshell) into the right chest, providing good exposure to the right and left heart and both pleural spaces.

A more limited anterior thoracotomy also is used in an elective setting for surgical lung biopsy in patients unable to tolerate single-lung ventilation. In addition, this incision is appropriate for cardiac surgical procedures and may be more cosmetically appealing in women. The heart and upper and middle lobes of the lung can be accessed from this approach.

After intubation, the patient is left in the supine position, and a rolled blanket is placed under the operative side vertically from the shoulder to the hip. The ipsilateral arm is padded and tucked to the side. The skin incision begins just lateral to the sternal border and follows the inframammary crease to the anterior axillary line. It is best to mark the incision preoperatively in the holding area with the patient sitting up or better still in the standing position. A superior flap is developed, raising skin and adipose and breast tissue off the pectoralis fascia to the fourth or fifth interspace depending on the desired exposure. The pectoralis muscle fibers are divided over the desired interspace, and the pleura is entered on top of the fifth or sixth rib. Care is taken to avoid injury to the internal thoracic vessels when medial exposure is required for pericardial and cardiac procedures. The closure is similar to that described earlier.

■ LATERAL (AXILLARY) THORACOTOMY

The lateral thoracotomy is the author's preferred approach for uncomplicated upper and middle lobe resections by providing excellent exposure of the upper hilum of the lung. This incision along with the anterior thoracotomy is the typical utility incision for video-assisted thoracic surgical lobectomy procedures. The wider interspace through these areas allows for visualization and specimen removal without the use of a rib spreader.

Patient preparation and positioning is the same as that described earlier for the posterolateral thoracotomy. The incision begins in the anterior axillary line over the fourth or fifth intercostal space and is carried posteriorly to the anterior border of the latissimus dorsi muscle. Care is taken to avoid entering the breast tissue in women. The serratus anterior muscle is split in the direction of the muscle fibers. The latissimus dorsi muscle is spared and reflected posteriorly. The fourth intercostal space is chosen for upper lobe resections; however, complete node sampling and division of the inferior pulmonary ligament are difficult from this high anterior approach. Access through the fifth intercostal space provides excellent exposure of the superior hilum, the major and minor fissures, and the paratracheal lymph nodes on right and level 5 and 6 lymph nodes on the left. In addition, adequate exposure is obtained for dividing the inferior pulmonary ligament and removing inferior mediastinal lymph nodes. The wider intercostal spaces anteriorly allow for better exposure with less rib spreading. Closure is the same as for the aforementioned thoracotomy.

■ VERTICAL AXILLARY THORACOTOMY

Vertical axillary thoracotomy is a muscle-sparing approach popularized by Ginsberg and others that provides excellent exposure for middle and lower lobe lung resections. Access to the more superior interspaces and the upper chest can be problematic with this approach, however.

Patient preparation and positioning are the same as that described earlier for the lateral approaches. The incision begins high in the axilla along the anterior border of the latissimus dorsi muscle and is carried down vertically along the posterior axillary line. No skin flaps are developed. The latissimus dorsi muscle is reflected posteriorly, and the posterior border of the serratus anterior muscle is identified. The serratus anterior muscle is reflected anteriorly by dividing the posterior and inferior fascial attachments. Dividing the lower muscle strips of the serratus as they insert on the lower ribs can increase exposure.

The scapula is retracted superiorly and off the chest wall. The sixth intercostal space is used because it provides excellent exposure of the lower hilum. The intercostal muscles are divided anteriorly just short of the internal thoracic artery and posteriorly to the angle of the rib. A Touffier chest retractor is used to separate the ribs, and a second Touffier retractor is used to retract the serratus anteriorly and the latissimus posteriorly. Closure is the same as described earlier.

■ ANTERIOR MEDIASTINOTOMY (CHAMBERLAIN PROCEDURE)

Chamberlain and McNeill introduced the anterior (parasternal) mediastinotomy in 1966. This approach was designed to assist in the diagnosis and staging of left upper lobe lung tumors and to determine resectability when there was concern for mediastinal invasion. This approach is complementary to the standard cervical mediastinoscopy in staging left upper lobe lung cancers.

Left parasternal mediastinotomy allows the surgeon to obtain biopsy specimens of level 6 (preaortic) and level 5 (aortopulmonary window) lymph nodes and anterior mediastinal masses. Right parasternal mediastinotomy allows the surgeon to obtain biopsy specimens of mediastinal masses, along with right-sided mediastinal lymph nodes, including level 3 (prevascular), level 4 (lower paratracheal), and level 10 (tracheobronchial).

The patient is placed in supine position on the operating table. After induction of general anesthesia, a shoulder roll is placed transversely beneath both scapulae, and the bed is placed in reverse Trendelenburg position to reduce central venous pressure. The patient is prepared and draped from the low neck to the epigastrium and from anterior axillary line to anterior axillary line to allow for conversion to an anterior thoracotomy or median sternotomy in the unlikely event that uncontrolled bleeding occurs during the procedure.

The second costal cartilage is identified at the sternomanubrial junction. A 5-cm incision is made over the second or third costal cartilage depending on the location of the mass or lymph nodes in question. The muscle fibers of the pectoralis muscle are retracted with a self-retaining retractor. The cartilaginous portion of the rib may be removed and the mediastinal space entered through the perichondrial bed, or the intercostal muscle above the rib can be divided to provide access. In most cases of mediastinal node biopsy, the internal thoracic vessels can be retracted and spared. Biopsy of mediastinal lymph nodes is assisted by use of a standard mediastinoscope and biopsy forceps. When greater exposure is required or when there is significant concern for injury to the internal thoracic vessels, proximal and distal suture ligation of the internal thoracic vessels is performed, and the vessels are divided.

If the pleural space is not entered, no drainage tube is required. When the pleural space has been entered, a small chest tube or red rubber catheter may be placed to evacuate air from the pleural cavity. If there is no air leak, the tube may be removed in the operating room after suction has been applied to the chest tube and the lung inflated with continuous positive airway pressure to evacuate all pleural air.

The pectoralis major fascia is closed with a running 0 Vicryl suture. The subcutaneous layer is closed with a running 2-0 Vicryl suture. The skin is approximated with a 4-0 Monocryl subcuticular stitch. After closure of the wound, the chest cavity is aspirated by placing the chest tube to 20 cm of suction, and the lung is expanded with a Valsalva maneuver. The tube may be removed in the operating room if no air leak is noted on positive-pressure ventilation and the lung was not biopsied or injured during the dissection. This allows complete reexpansion of the lung and patient discharge from the recovery room on the same day.

■ THORACOABDOMINAL INCISION

The left thoracoabdominal incision offers excellent exposure for thoracoabdominal aneurysms and cancer of the gastro-esophageal junction. This approach provides wide exposure of the lower thorax, upper abdomen, and retroperitoneal space. The patient is positioned similar to the lateral approaches; however, the hips are rotated slightly posteriorly and secured with wide adhesive tape, and the table is tilted slightly to the left.

The incision begins in the upper midline of the abdomen midway between the umbilicus and xiphoid process. It is carried superiorly in a diagonal fashion to the level of the sixth, seventh, or eighth intercostal space. The latissimus dorsi and serratus anterior muscles are divided with electro-cautery. The scapula is retracted superiorly and away from the chest wall, and the ribs are palpated posteriorly along the erector spinae muscles, identifying the proper intercostal space for the procedure.

The level for chest wall opening is determined by the specific operative procedure and the extent of superior exposure required. A seventh intercostal space approach is most commonly used. The intercostal muscles are divided immediately above the lower rib with electrocautery. The muscle division is carried posteriorly to within 2 cm of the sympathetic chain. The intercostal muscle is divided anteriorly to the level of the internal thoracic vessels, which are suture ligated and divided. The costal margin is opened, and a short segment of cartilage is removed to facilitate reapproximation at the time of closure.

The abdomen is opened in layers with electrocautery. The left hemidiaphragm can be opened radially to the esophageal hiatus or circumferentially, leaving a 2- to 3-cm rim of diaphragm attached to the chest wall for later closure. Care is taken to avoid injury to the main left phrenic nerve and its larger branches. Chest and abdominal retractors are placed and opened slowly.

Closure of the incision begins with placement of standard chest drains. The abdomen or retroperitoneum is not drained routinely. The diaphragm is closed with interrupted no. 2 silk horizontal mattress sutures. The costal margin is closed with one or two figure-of-eight no. 2 Vicryl sutures that incorporate the upper edge of the diaphragm to prevent postoperative hernia formation. The rest of the chest is closed as described previously.

■ THORACOABDOMINAL SPINE EXPOSURE

The thoracoabdominal spine exposure approach is used most often for lower thoracic and upper lumbar spine

pathology. The left side is preferred because retraction and mobilization of the liver and inferior vena cava on the right are more problematic than the spleen and aorta on the left. The patient is prepared and positioned similar to the left thoracoabdominal approach described earlier. The table is left level, however, for optimal alignment of the spine. Wide adhesive tape is placed across the hip and lower leg to secure the patient and to avoid body rotation during the procedure.

Care is taken to keep the beanbag below the midline to allow improved visualization of the spine on fluoroscopy. Typically the spinal levels to be exposed and proper spinal alignment are confirmed with anteroposterior and lateral projection fluoroscopy before preparation and draping of the patient. The involved spinal levels are identified under fluoroscopy and marked on the skin. This allows the surgeon to center the thoracotomy incision over the area of spinal pathology.

For spine exposure cases, this approach typically begins with a low posterolateral thoracotomy. The 10th or 11th rib is resected subperiosteally, and the left pleural space is entered through the bed of the resected rib. Chest retractors are placed, and the lung may be packed out of the way with laparotomy sponges or collapsed when lung isolation can be accomplished. Fluoroscopy is used to confirm levels of interest and exposure for fusion. The diaphragm is divided along the posterior and lateral margin, leaving a 2-cm rim of muscle to sew for closure. The peritoneum is left intact and swept from lateral to medial, exposing the lower diaphragm and psoas muscle. Care is taken to avoid injuring the aorta at the hiatus. The segmental vessels over the involved vertebral bodies are ligated and divided.

After completion of the spinal fusion, the diaphragm is repaired with interrupted horizontal mattress no. 2 silk sutures. The bed of the resected rib is closed in two layers with running 0 Vicryl sutures. This closure often is facilitated by placing pericostal sutures through drill holes in the next lower rib and above the superior rib to take tension off the periosteal closure. The remaining layers are closed as previously described.

■ CLAMSHELL THORACOTOMY

Also called *bilateral sternothoracotomy,* the clamshell thoracotomy approach provides excellent exposure for resection of multiple bilateral lung metastases, bulky anterior mediastinal masses with thoracic cavity extension, bilateral lung transplantation, and cardiac procedures in which a median sternotomy is deemed unsafe. In cases of emergent left anterior thoracotomy, extension of the incision to a clamshell approach provides improved access to the heart, mediastinum, hilum, and great vessels for repair of traumatic injuries and exploration and evacuation of both pleural spaces.

After intubation, the patient is left in a supine position. The arms may be placed flexed above the face and secured to an ether screen, or bilateral blanket rolls may be placed vertically behind each posterior axillary line and the arms slightly flexed at the elbow, well padded, and secured at the side with the assistance of sleds. The torso can be elevated off the operating table with sheets.

The inframammary crease is traced with a marking pen from anterior axillary line to anterior axillary line. This is best performed in the preoperative area with the patient in a sitting or preferably standing position. Skin and subcutaneous flaps are developed above the level of the pectoralis major fascia and carried superiorly to the third or fourth intercostal space similar to a mastectomy. The pectoralis muscle fibers are split at the chosen interspace, and bilateral anterior thoracotomies are performed. The right and left internal thoracic vessels are suture ligated proximally and distally and divided. A transverse sternotomy is performed at the level of the two thoracotomies with a sternal saw. A chest retractor is placed in each anterior thoracotomy opening and opened slowly. Care is taken not to open the chest too wide to prevent traction injury of the phrenic nerves. The parietal pleura is divided superiorly to the level to the innominate vein, avoiding injury to the phrenic nerve and the internal thoracic vein as it turns posteriorly to empty into the innominate vein.

Closure begins after adequate bilateral pleural drainage. It is not necessary to drain the mediastinum if the pericardium was not entered. A figure-of-eight heavy stainless steel wire suture is used to approximate the sternum. Three interrupted pericostal sutures are placed on each side with the lower sutures placed through the superior rib and drilled holes in the lower rib. These sutures are crossed and the interspaces pulled together by an assistant while the sternal wire is tightened to provide optimal sternal apposition. The remaining layers are closed as previously described.

■ HEMI–CLAMSHELL THORACOTOMY

The hemi–clamshell thoracotomy approach combines a partial upper sternal split and anterior thoracotomy. It is used most often for anterior Pancoast lung cancers, thymoma with significant extension into the aortopulmonary window, neurogenic tumors involving the proximal brachial plexus, and great vessel pathology.

After induction of anesthesia, a rolled blanket is placed beneath the operative side from the shoulder to the hip. The incision begins at the midsternum and continues to the anterior axillary line in the inframammary crease. The skin and adipose and breast tissue are raised at the level of the pectoralis major fascia to the level of the fourth intercostal space. The pectoralis muscle is divided in the direction of the fibers over the fourth intercostal space. The pleural space is entered at the top of the fifth rib. When this approach is used for lung cancer resection, the pleural space is explored to determine resectability before upper sternal division. The internal thoracic vessels are suture ligated proximally and distally and divided.

Next the skin incision is extended in the midline to the sternal notch, and the deep tissue is divided down to the periosteum of the sternum. The sternum is divided in the midline to the level of the fourth intercostal space. A partial transverse sternotomy is performed from the fourth intercostal space connecting with the midline sternotomy. Retractors are placed in the interspace and between the sternal edges and opened slowly. Care should be taken to avoid undue traction on the brachial plexus by excessive spreading of the sternal retractor.

The closure again begins with placement of the intercostal sutures through drilled holes placed in the inferior rib. Three or four drill holes with a 1/16 bit are placed in the fifth rib. The anterior interspace does not approximate as close as more posterior approaches, making attempts to close the intercostal space unsatisfactory. Using no. 5 polyester (Ethibond) pericostal suture to bring the ribs back to the normal spacing avoids postoperative lung herniation in most cases. When the intercostal space has been returned to the normal space, the sternal edges are reapproximated with no. 6 stainless steel wires. Typically two wires are placed in the manubrium, and two wires are placed around the upper sternum. Placing the lower sternal wire at the top of the fourth rib on the operative side and on top of the fifth rib on the contralateral side provides good apposition of the cut edges of the transverse sternotomy.

■ MEDIAN STERNOTOMY

The median sternotomy is the most common approach for open cardiac procedures. It also provides excellent exposure for thymectomy, anterior mediastinal tumor resection, bilateral lung volume reduction, and bilateral lung metastases resection when the lower lobes (particularly the left lower lobe) are not involved. The median sternotomy has been used for lower tracheal and carinal resections. The median sternotomy approach is advocated for control of a chronic postpneumonectomy bronchial stump fistula. This approach allows access, division, and closure of the bronchus through a clean, uncontaminated field.

This approach begins with the patient in the supine position, with both arms padded and tucked to the side. A double-lumen tube generally is used for pulmonary resections and some mediastinal resections. A single-lumen tube is satisfactory for the other procedures. The skin incision typically begins at the base of the suprasternal notch (or may begin at the sternomanubrial junction for better cosmesis when significant cervical exposure is not required) and ends at the tip of the xyphoid or a few centimeters below. The incision is carried down to the anterior sternal plate in the midline with electrocautery. Following the decussating fibers of the subcutaneous tissues and palpating the lateral margins of the sternum facilitate identification of the midline. The upper rectus fascia is divided along the linea alba with care taken to avoid entry into the peritoneum. Dissection is performed in the midline above the sternal notch. A bridging vein often is encountered and is dealt with best by isolation, ligation, and division. Care should be taken in the retrosternal dissection superiorly to avoid injuring the innominate vein, which lies immediately posterior to this dissection. The xyphoid may be resected or divided in the midline with electrocautery. The inferior retrosternal space is bluntly dissected with the surgeon's index finger. The sternum is divided in the vertical midline with a saw. Bone wax may be used to control marrow bleeding, and electrocautery is used to control bleeding along the cut periosteal edges. A sternal retractor is placed and adjusted to provide evenly distributed pressure on the cut sternal edges. The retractor should not be placed too high on the sternum because this can lead to injury to the brachial plexus. The retractor is opened slowly, with the superior and inferior fascial attachments divided with electrocautery to avoid tearing of the tissues along the innominate vein and the diaphragm.

A partial sternal split of the manubrium is recommended when exposure of the upper mediastinum only is needed. An adequate thymectomy can be performed with this incision; it also is used in conjunction with head and neck procedures for extended tissue dissection or large thyroid tumors.

Closure of both incisions begins after placement of mediastinal drains. The sternal edges are approximated with no. 6 stainless steel wire. Typically, two wires are placed through the manubrium, and four wires are placed immediately around the sternum. Care should be taken to hug the lateral edge of the sternum at the top edge of the corresponding costal cartilage to avoid the internal thoracic vessels and their branches. If bleeding from an internal thoracic vessel occurs, it is controlled best with a figure-of-eight 2-0 silk suture ligature because use of electrocautery often results in ongoing or worsened bleeding. The pectoralis and upper rectus fasciae are closed with a running no. 1 Vicryl suture. The author waits until after sternal approximation and fascial closure to secure the anterior mediastinal chest tube. The chest tube is withdrawn and advanced a few centimeters to ensure the drain was not caught in the wound closure, then secured at the skin with a no. 2 silk suture.

SUGGESTED READING

Bains MS, et al: The clamshell incision: an improved approach to bilateral pulmonary and mediastinal tumor, *Ann Thorac Surg* 58:30, 1994.

Fry WA: Thoracic incisions, *Chest Surg Clin N Am* 5:177, 1995.

Ginsberg RJ: Alternative (muscle-sparing) incisions in thoracic surgery, *Ann Thorac Surg* 56:752, 1993.

Lumsden AB, et al: The surgical anatomy and technique of the thoracoabdominal incision, *Surg Clin North Am* 73:633, 1993.

HUMAN IMMUNODEFICIENCY VIRUS AND THE GENERAL THORACIC SURGEON

J. Michael DiMaio

Since the first reported case of acquired immunodeficiency syndrome (AIDS) in 1981, an estimated 13.9 million people have died as a result of this severe immunosuppression associated with human immunodeficiency virus (HIV) infection. An RNA retrovirus, HIV results in the destruction of immune mediating cells, especially the CD4 subset of human lymphocytes. The resulting absolute neutropenia allows a spectrum of opportunistic infections and malignancies to occur, which, among other criteria, define AIDS.

Despite the decrease in AIDS deaths as a result of highly active antiretroviral therapy, infections and neoplastic complications continue to affect patients with HIV. Specifically the thoracic surgeon is called on to assist in the diagnosis and treatment of a diverse group of common and unusual disorders of the cardiopulmonary system and the esophagus. This chapter outlines the more frequent pulmonary and esophageal complications associated with HIV that require surgical intervention. Disease processes familiar to the thoracic surgeon, such as lung cancer and esophagitis, are reviewed in the setting of HIV infection and AIDS.

■ PULMONARY INFECTION

Patients with HIV/AIDS can be affected by a wide spectrum of pulmonary infections. The thoracic surgeon often becomes the final hope of securing a diagnosis in these patients when less invasive diagnostic procedures, such as sputum studies, bronchoalveolar lavage, pleural biopsies, and transthoracic fine needle aspiration, have been unrevealing. As in all of thoracic surgery, the approach is dictated by the location of the pathology. Cervical mediastinal exploration or left anterior mediastinotomy often provides a tissue diagnosis in patients with mediastinal adenopathy with little morbidity. Patients without mediastinal adenopathy who have peripheral or diffuse lung lesions are candidates for video-assisted thoracic surgery (VATS) even if they may not tolerate single-lung ventilation. VATS allows tissue to be obtained from several areas of the lung and pleura as well as the sampling of associated pleural effusions; this technique can be performed using intermittent apnea if required. Lesions not believed to be accessible by VATS are approached via standard anterior or posterolateral thoracotomy.

Pneumocystis carinii pneumonia (PCP) is an opportunistic pulmonary infection that can be devastating to patients with HIV/AIDS. The thoracic surgeon is frequently asked to assist with the care of these patients because of the association between PCP and spontaneous pneumothoraces. The incidence of pneumothorax in patients with PCP has been reported to approach 5%, and the incidence significantly increases with the use of aerosolized pentamidine and cigarette smoking. Spontaneous pneumothoraces in patients with PCP occur most commonly after the rupture of emphysematous pleural blebs and parenchymal cysts—the result of subpleural necrosis. Histologically, this condition appears as extensive parenchymal necrosis with the complete loss of normal tissue architecture. Clinically, this is manifest as diffuse fibrocystic parenchymal disease with a predilection for the upper lobes of the lung.

The unique effects of PCP infection on the lungs produces pneumothoraces that are often recurrent, are persistent, are associated with significant morbidity and, frequently, are associated with hospital mortalities. Sepkowitz in 1991 found that patients with PCP and a pneumothorax had a 65% ipsilateral and a 65% contralateral recurrence and occurrence rate of pneumothoraces. Similarly, 85% of patients with PCP and a pneumothorax develop a bronchopleural fistula that persists greater than 7 days. Despite improvements in medical and surgical therapy, in patients with PCP who experience a spontaneous pneumothorax, hospital mortality rates of 29% to 50% have been reported.

The treatment of pneumothoraces associated with PCP is a challenge to the thoracic surgeon. Nonoperative therapy using tube thoracostomy with or without a pleural sclerosing agent has been shown to be successful in a few of these patients. Trachiotis in 1996 treated 25 patients in this manner. Of patients, 9 resolved their pneumothorax and bronchopleural fistula, 13 patients were discharged from the hospital with a chest tube and Heimlich valve in place, and 9 patients died in the hospital.

When one considers the cause of a spontaneous pneumothorax in patients with PCP, it is not surprising that lung reexpansion and pleural sclerosis are often ineffective. At the University of Texas Southwestern Medical Center, the initial approach to patients with a history of PCP and a spontaneous pneumothorax has evolved to VATS wedge resection of the area of lung associated with the bronchopleural fistula accompanied by pleural sclerosis, initially with talc poudrage but more recently using mechanical pleurodesis. Use of this technique early in the case of these patients is based on a report comparing 46 patients with PCP and unilateral pneumothorax treated with tube thoracostomy and chemical pleurodesis, VATS wedge resection and pleurodesis, or wedge resection via thoracotomy and pleurodesis. Tube thoracostomy and pleurodesis was successful in only 26% of patients, with 10 hospital deaths, a mean hospital stay of 18 days, and 12 patients who required further therapy. Two thirds of patients treated with wedge resection and pleurodesis via thoracotomy resolved their pneumothorax and bronchopleural fistula with a mean hospital length of stay of 10.3 days. Patients undergoing VATS treatment of pneumothorax experienced an 88% success rate; mean hospital length of stay was 3.6 days.

■ PLEURAL EFFUSION

The incidence of pleural effusion in patients with HIV/AIDS varies widely as does the etiology. Pleural effusions have been reported to occur in 1.7% to 18% of patients with HIV/AIDS. The treatment of these effusions differs from the general population in the need to sample these fluid collections aggressively early in their course. Similarly, chronic and refractory effusions and pleural fluid collections that change

in character must be sampled serially to identify changes in microbiology or the development of malignant effusions.

The exception to this strategy is a pleural effusion resulting from Kaposi's sarcoma (KS). Approximately 50% of patients with KS have either a unilateral or a bilateral pleural effusion. Fluid cytology and pleural biopsy are usually not capable of providing a diagnosis because KS pleural effusions do not contain pathopneumonic cells, and they do not produce parietal pleural changes. Consequently, patients suspected of having a pleural effusion from KS require a lung biopsy for diagnosis. The biopsy specimen is obtained most easily using VATS, and the procedure should be combined with mechanical pleurodesis because of the refractory nature of these pleural effusions.

The diagnosis of tuberculous pleural effusions in HIV/AIDS patients is approached as in non–HIV/AIDS patients. The demonstration of acid-fast bacilli by staining or eventual sputum culture, bronchoalveolar lavage, pleural fluid, or pleural biopsy is confirmatory. Treatment, as in the general population, consists of multidrug antimicrobial therapy. Drainage of the pleural space by tube thoracostomy usually can and should be avoided.

Pleural effusions resulting from malignancies in HIV/AIDS patients, as in the general population, portend a mean survival of less than 90 days. Our approach to these patients has been directed at relieving their symptoms, while minimizing their procedure-associated morbidity and hospital stay. It has been our practice to use the Pleurx (Surgimedics, Denver Biomaterials, Denver, CO) pleural drainage catheter in HIV/AIDS patients with malignant pleural effusion. As previously reported in non–HIV/AIDS patients, this device allows the intermittent drainage of recurring malignant pleural effusions by a patient or caregiver in the home. Inserted using a Seldinger technique, this catheter does not require general anesthesia for insertion and usually is scheduled as an outpatient procedure.

■ THORACIC EMPYEMA

Thoracic empyema does not seem to occur more frequently in patients with HIV/AIDS than in the general population. Similarly an empyema in HIV/AIDS patients usually results from a community-acquired bronchopulmonary infection. When diagnosed by thoracentesis, the optimal treatment for an empyema depends on its phase of development. Repeated thoracentesis or, preferably, drainage of the pleural space by tube thoracostomy combined with appropriate antimicrobial therapy adequately treats most free-flowing exudative pleural effusions. Likewise, the treatment for a well-organized complex empyema is not controversial—thoracotomy, decortication, and prolonged pleural drainage.

The treatment of a loculated fibrinopurulent empyema continues to be a source of debate between advocates of pleural drainage combined with fibrinolytic therapy and advocates of operative drainage. In an attempt to ascertain the optimal therapy for these patients, we previously reported a series of 20 patients randomized to either VATS decortication or tube thoracostomy with pleural streptokinase therapy. This investigation found that patients treated with VATS had a significantly shorter mean hospital stay

($p = .009$), required fewer mean days of chest tube drainage ($p = .03$), and experienced fewer treatment failures ($p = .05$) than patients treated without surgery. Patients who failed nonoperative therapy all were treated successfully using VATS. Our current approach to an HIV/AIDS patient with a fibrinopurulent empyema is VATS decortication, appropriate antimicrobial therapy, and postoperative pleural drainage.

■ ESOPHAGUS

The thoracic surgeon occasionally is asked to participate in the care of HIV/AIDS patients experiencing complications from a diverse group of esophageal infections. Several guiding principles are helpful when evaluating these patients. First, HIV/AIDS patients with symptoms attributable to the esophagus should undergo esophagogastroduodenoscopy (EGD) early in their evaluation. It is unlikely that any other readily available study would identify what is most commonly a complication of an infectious esophagitis as rapidly and accurately as EGD. Direct inspection of the esophageal mucosa allows the experienced endoscopist to identify candida esophagitis and herpetic esophagitis quickly. Other less common infections can be confirmed through biopsy specimens taken during the procedure. Esophageal strictures and fistulas also can be treated at the time of EGD with dilation and covered stent placement.

The thoracic surgeon also should bear in mind that the mainstay of therapy for HIV/AIDS patients with complications of infectious esophagitis is often medical. Strictures, fistulas, ulcers, and their associated symptoms can be temporized with the aforementioned methods of local control. These measures generally fail, however, unless the underlying tuberculosis, *Candida,* cytomegalovirus, herpes, or other infection is treated in a systemic fashion.

■ LUNG CANCER

Bronchogenic carcinoma has been identified as a significant health concern among patients with HIV/AIDS. First reported in 1984, many investigators believed the two diseases were coincidental in light of the prevalence of tobacco use in what was initially a relatively homogeneous population of HIV/AIDS patients. Cottle in 1993 and Barchielli in 1995 were the first investigators to show convincing evidence of an association between lung cancer and HIV/AIDS.

Parker subsequently reported compelling evidence linking HIV/AIDS and lung cancer in 1998. Based on an epidemiologic comparison of the Texas State HIV/AIDS and Lung Cancer registries, Parker found an observed-to-expected lung cancer ratio of 6.5 among patients with HIV/AIDS. It was concluded that there was a significantly increased incidence of bronchogenic carcinoma in HIV/AIDS patients, that these patients were predominantly male and presented at a younger age, and that the tumor histology in these patients followed the trend of the general population.

Whether or not a link between HIV/AIDS and lung cancer is borne out in subsequent investigations, the potential association is clinically relevant for thoracic surgeons. Thurer in 1995 emphasized the need for maintaining a high index of suspicion for malignancy when evaluating pulmonary nodules in HIV/AIDS patients. Thurer's review found that 22% of 37 patients with HIV/AIDS undergoing fine needle aspiration of a solitary pulmonary nodule had bronchogenic carcinoma despite a mean age of only 41 years.

When a diagnosis of bronchogenic carcinoma has been made in a patient with HIV/AIDS, the thoracic surgeon may be asked to evaluate these patients for resection. This decision, as in other patients with lung cancer, should be based on whether a survival or palliation advantage for the patient would be realized over other forms of therapy. Because of the relatively small number of these patients and their brief periods of follow-up, however, few series of HIV/AIDS patients with lung cancer exist from which to draw information.

We have developed treatment algorithms for patients with HIV/AIDS and lung cancer based on our experiences and those reported in the literature. Physicians evaluating these patients should begin by "staging" the HIV/AIDS and the lung cancer. Assessment of a patient's date of seroconversion with HIV, response to therapy and prophylaxis, CD4 count and viral load trends, and the presence of AIDS-defining illnesses or malignancies determines which form of therapy is most appropriate. [Recommendation of CD4 count and viral load not to operate is less than 200].

The assessment of the HIV/AIDS patient is at least as important as the stage of the cancer to the thoracic surgeon. In contrast to patients with HIV, patients who meet the criteria of the Centers for Disease Control for AIDS to have a mean survival of only 3 months with or without therapy for lung cancer. Alshafire in 1997 found that patients with AIDS and lung cancer did not tolerate chemotherapy or external beam radiation therapy. Of the patients in their series, 97% could not complete their scheduled treatment because of debilitating opportunistic infections. Similarly, Thurer found a mean survival of only 4 to 5 months in patients with AIDS who underwent pulmonary resection for stage IA bronchogenic carcinoma. All patients appeared to be cancer free when they died of complications related to AIDS. It has been our practice to recommend only palliative/hospice care for the patient with AIDS and carcinoma of the lung.

For patients with HIV and lung cancer, it is appropriate for the thoracic surgeon to stage the cancer in these patients in the manner to which they are accustomed. After a history, physical examination, and computed tomography scan of the chest, we perform bronchoscopy and cervical mediastinal exploration in patients without evidence of metastatic disease. In addition, because of the association of pulmonary hypertension and HIV, we perform a right heart catheterization and pulmonary spirometry and a diffusion capacity in patients otherwise believed to be candidates for lung resection.

Our experience suggests that patients with HIV found to have "early" stage lung cancer (T1-3, N0-1), without evidence of pulmonary hypertension, tolerate anatomic resection of the tumor without significant morbidity or mortality. We have not resected tumors requiring pneumonectomy in these patients, however. Patients with HIV and advanced stage carcinoma of the lung (stage IIIA and IIIB) generally have not been offered resection. We have found that in contrast to patients with AIDS, some HIV patients with lung cancer have tolerated external beam radiation therapy as palliation for hemoptysis and obstructive symptoms.

SUGGESTED READING

Abolhoda A, Keller SM: Thoracic surgical spectrum of HIV infection, *Semin Respir Infect* 14:359, 1999.

DiMaio JM, Wait MA: The thoracic surgeon's role in the management of patients with HIV infection and AIDS, *Chest Surg Clin N Am* 9:97, 1999.

Thurer RJ, et al: Surgical treatment of lung cancer in patients with human immunodeficiency virus, *Ann Thorac Surg* 60:599, 1995.

Walsh FW, et al: The initial pulmonary evaluation of the immunocompromised patient, *Chest Surg Clin N Am* 9:19, 1999.

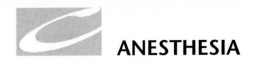

ANESTHESIA

ANESTHESIA FOR THE THORACIC SURGICAL PATIENT

Stephen Aufderheide
Brett A. Simon

This chapter explores each of the components that make up the practice of thoracic anesthesia, beginning with preoperative evaluation, followed by general concepts of intraoperative monitoring, lung isolation, anesthetic techniques, and anesthetic considerations for specific surgeries. A separate chapter discusses in detail postoperative pain management in thoracic surgical patients.

■ PREOPERATIVE EVALUATION

All patients undergoing thoracic surgery should receive evaluation by the anesthesiologist before surgery. The goal is to define the nature and functional status of the patient's relevant primary and coexisting medical conditions so that they may be optimized for surgery, their individual risk may be assessed, and appropriate plans for intraoperative and postoperative care may be made. This anesthetic care plan can be formulated only after consideration of two broad specific areas.

The first consideration is the patient and his or her comorbidities. Because each patient is different, these traits inevitably modify the anesthetic plan, monitoring, postoperative disposition, and postoperative pain management. In general, exercise tolerance is a simple first-pass screening tool—the patient who can walk two to three flights of stairs without pause and has no symptoms of shortness of breath or chest pain may need no further workup. In addition to a standard detailed history and physical examination, specific attention should be paid to the cardiovascular system, including any history of arrhythmias, ischemic disease, valvular pathology, and ventricular dysfunction because the stresses of surgery, volume shifts, and potential hypoxemia may decompensate previously well-controlled disease. Defining the nature and severity of pulmonary dysfunction with appropriate pulmonary function tests may be indicated to optimize the patient's condition with bronchodilators, steroids, or antibiotic therapy and to predict postoperative pulmonary function after resection.

The second consideration is the surgery itself. Different surgical procedures impose different physiologic stresses, which present widely varying management requirements, and it is important to communicate the specifics of the procedure to the anesthesia team so that appropriate plans for intraoperative and postoperative care may be made. Some of these specific issues are covered in the last section of this chapter. Finally, the unique interaction of the specific patient with his or her comorbidities and the specific surgery dictates the anesthetic plan.

■ PREMEDICATION

The choice of preoperative medication to relieve anxiety, alleviate pain, and dry secretions deserves more thoughtful consideration in thoracic surgical patients. Many of these patients have little pulmonary reserve or have thickened pulmonary secretions. Narcotic premedication or antisialagogues are rarely used. More commonly, if any sedation is used, it is given intravenously after monitors are applied. H_2-blockers or equivalent drugs to reduce gastric acid secretion may be given the night before and morning of surgery to reduce aspiration risks, especially in patients who will require repeated airway manipulations. Bronchodilators should be continued through the morning of surgery, with a final treatment given immediately before transfer to the operating room, especially for patients with severe reactive airways disease. A short course of steroids, if not contraindicated for surgical considerations, also may be useful in reducing bronchospasm in certain patients. β-Blockers and most cardiac medications should be continued through the morning of surgery, with the exception of angiotensin-converting enzyme inhibitors, which typically are held because of their persistent vasodilation. Diuretics and oral hypoglycemic agents also typically are held the day of surgery.

■ MONITORING

The American Society of Anesthesiology has determined minimal acceptable standards for intraoperative monitoring, as follows: electrocardiogram, end-tidal carbon dioxide (capnography), pulse oximetry, inspiratory oxygen concentration, and temperature. End-tidal agent analyzers are standard of care in most institutions. Peripheral arterial catheters for continuous monitoring of blood pressure are indicated routinely in many thoracic procedures because of the potential for hemodynamic instability from compression of the heart or major vasculature, effects of anesthesia, and bleeding and for repeated measurement of arterial blood gases to assess gas exchange and oxygenation. Insertion of central venous access with or without a pulmonary artery catheter usually is determined by the patient's comorbidities as much as by the surgery itself. Although intrathoracic intravascular pressure measurements (central venous pressure, pulmonary artery pressure, pulmonary capillary wedge pressure) may be difficult to interpret in a patient with an open chest or in the lateral position, the functional information (cardiac output, stroke volume) obtained from a pulmonary artery catheter remains accurate. Thus, for intraoperative monitoring of patients undergoing lateral thoracotomy with significant cardiac dysfunction or major fluid issues, a pulmonary artery catheter is preferred. For postoperative assessment of fluid status or if the use of vasoactive infusions is anticipated, a central line suffices. Use of transesophageal echocardiography is determined mostly by the patient's comorbidities. Transesophageal echocardiography may be affected adversely by positioning. A subset of patients have substandard windows in a lateral decubitus position.

■ LUNG ISOLATION

The need for single-lung ventilation is unique to thoracic anesthesia and deserves special attention.

Indications

"Absolute" indications for single-lung ventilation, in which single-lung ventilation is required for patient safety or to make surgery possible, typically include isolation of one lung from the other (infection, massive hemorrhage) and ventilation when a major airway has been breached (severe bronchopleural fistula or surgery on a major conducting airway). "Relative" indications, in which lung isolation is not needed for survival but significantly improves the surgeon's operative conditions, are more common reasons for using single-lung ventilation. These situations include thoracotomy or thoracoscopy for lung resection or to facilitate exposure of other intrathoracic structures for surgery of the thoracic aorta, esophagus, heart, and thoracic spine. Contraindications to single-lung ventilation are few and include primarily the inability of a patient to tolerate single-lung ventilation because of hypoxia, hypercarbia, or pulmonary hypertension or the presence of an airway tumor or other abnormality that would prevent lung isolation.

Techniques

Single-lung isolation usually is accomplished by one of two methods: bronchial blocker or double-lumen endobronchial tube. On rare occasions and in pediatric patients, lung isolation also may be achieved by advancing a conventional endotracheal tube (ETT) into a main stem bronchus.

Bronchial Blockers

A bronchial blocker is simply a catheter with a balloon at its tip that is passed through or placed alongside a standard single-lumen ETT and inflated in the main stem bronchus of the operative lung. A fiberoptic bronchoscope is required to position the blocker properly. Historically the original bronchial blocker was a Fogarty embolectomy catheter, which could be difficult to maneuver and was displaced easily because of its low stiffness. The Univent tube (Fuji Systems, Tokyo, Japan) incorporated the blocker catheter into a channel in the wall of a silicon ETT so that it could be advanced or withdrawn as needed. Although more convenient than a Fogarty catheter, it can be difficult to maneuver the blocker toward the left side, and its use must be planned in advance. An endobronchial blocker that can be placed though any adequately sized ETT and guided to the correct position using a small nylon loop that slips over the bronchoscope has been introduced (Arndt Endobronchial Blocker, Cook Critical Care, Bloomington, IN). A special three-port ETT connector allows simultaneous ventilation, bronchoscopy, and introduction of the blocker, greatly facilitating positioning and adjusting of the blocker.

The main advantage of the bronchial blocker is that the single-lumen ETT may be left in place and used for long-term ventilation. The outside diameters of these ETTs are significantly smaller than the double-lumen tubes (DLTs) and may be easier to place in patients with difficult airways, tracheostomies, or other anatomic abnormalities. For patients with limited pulmonary reserve, the balloon may be advanced into a lobar bronchus, and selective lobar blockade may be achieved. Bronchial blockers are ideal for long cases in which lung isolation may be required only for a short period, such as an anterior-posterior thoracic spine stabilization.

There are several disadvantages. Blockers may be difficult to place into the left side, lung deflation is slow because it primarily relies on absorption of trapped oxygen, and suctioning and administration of continuous positive airway pressure (CPAP) to the deflated lung to improve oxygenation may be difficult. Finally, it may be impossible to achieve right lung isolation in the 5% or so of patients with tracheal or proximal right upper lobe bronchial takeoff.

Double-Lumen Endobronchial Tubes

Historically, many DLT choices have been available. Currently, most institutions use a disposable Robertshaw-type tube made of clear, nontoxic plastic and with low-pressure cuffs that position in the trachea and proximal main stem bronchus. These tubes are available in left-sided (endobronchial lumen placed in left main stem bronchus) and right-sided (endobronchial lumen placed in right main stem bronchus) versions over a range of sizes (41 Fr, 39 Fr, 37 Fr, 35 Fr, and 28 Fr). The right-sided DLT has a large lateral Murphy eye and slanted endobronchial balloon designed to decrease the incidence of right upper lobe occlusion.

Choosing the appropriate DLT size is related loosely to patient height, with most men requiring 39 Fr to 41 Fr and most women requiring 37 Fr to 39 Fr. Ultimately, size has to be checked at the time of insertion with backup sizes immediately available. The largest tube that appropriately fits should be used to facilitate suctioning and bronchoscopy and to minimize resistance and permit spontaneous ventilation before extubation in patients with compromised pulmonary function. Positioning of the DLT should be confirmed by fiberoptic bronchoscopy, although if clinical lung isolation is achieved, this can be postponed until after patient positioning. The most common problem is difficulty in passing the endobronchial tube into the left main stem bronchus because of the asymmetry of the right and left bronchi. When this occurs, the tube should be withdrawn well into the trachea, rotated such that the bronchial tube is facing left, and then advanced avoiding further twisting. If further difficulty is encountered, the bronchoscope should be advanced to the tip of the bronchial lumen, the tube pulled back above the carina, the scope advanced into the left side, and the tube advanced over the scope. If this fails, it usually indicates that the tube is too large and should be downsized. Finally, if all else fails, particularly for left-sided tubes, the right main stem bronchus could be occluded gently with the chest open to allow passage into the left bronchus. Position should be confirmed by visualizing the proximal edge of the bronchial cuff alongside the carina by viewing through the tracheal lumen. Tracheal and bronchial cuffs should be inflated with the minimum volumes required to prevent air leaks during ventilation.

When patients need to remain intubated at the end of the surgery and a DLT has been used, it should be exchanged for a conventional ETT if at all possible. After placing an airway exchange catheter in each lumen of the DLT, it is removed under direct laryngoscopy, and the new ETT is placed over both tube exchangers and advanced into the trachea. There are several reasons why the DLT should be exchanged. First, the endobronchial portion can injure the bronchus if left in place for long periods. The internal diameter of the two lumens is small and prone to obstruction by secretions. The longer tube causes more tracheobronchial irritation and may be more uncomfortable for the patient. Finally, a special adapter is used to connect both lumens of the DLT to the ventilator. If this adapter is broken or misplaced, it becomes impossible to ventilate the patient. Most intensive care unit (ICU) personnel do not use DLTs routinely and are not familiar with their use, increasing the risk of problems.

The advantages of using a DLT over a bronchial blocker are many. True lung isolation, in which the lung contents are sealed in or out with access for suctioning, bronchoscopy, or ventilation, can be obtained only with a DLT. The isolated lung is inflated quickly and easily and deflated. CPAP or positive end-expiratory pressure (PEEP) can be applied easily to the appropriate lung to prevent desaturation. Lastly, DLTs are relatively easy to place. The disadvantages are not significant. The large outer diameter of the tube may make insertion difficult and, as stated previously, should be changed if postoperative ventilation is required. Right-sided tubes are slightly more difficult to position because of the need to ensure ventilation of the right upper lobe.

Practical Considerations

To prevent atelectasis and allow time for exhalation, tidal volumes of around 10 ml/kg and rates of 8 to 10 breaths/min should be used. When the lung is isolated, the minute ventilation needs to be maintained, or else a rise in carbon dioxide occurs. Most commonly, the tidal volumes are maintained on single-lung ventilation, allowing a rise in peak inspiratory pressures up to 50%. If peak inspiratory pressures are greater than this and after ruling out other problems (i.e., tube position, bronchospasm, secretions), a decrease in tidal volume may be needed with an increase in respiratory rate to match the original minute ventilation. Care must be taken to ensure adequate time for lung emptying and prevent auto-PEEP. Moderate increases in P_{CO_2} are generally well tolerated and resolve when dual-lung ventilation is resumed.

Oxygen desaturation is not a rare occurrence during single-lung ventilation due to shunting through the nonventilated lung. Whenever severe desaturations occur, inflation of the deflated lung always should be the first strategy. For desaturations that are more modest, optimal function of the ventilated lung first should be ensured. DLT position and function should be verified and secretions and bronchospasm treated. Hand ventilation with sustained inflation recruits atelectatic regions, and if the saturation responds to this maneuver, 4 to 6 cm H_2O PEEP generally maintains recruitment. Intermittent oxygen insufflation via a suction catheter placed into the DLT port of the operative lung frequently helps. Meanwhile, from the surgeon's standpoint, if an anatomic lung resection is being performed, the pulmonary artery branches to that area could be compressed temporarily or ligated expeditiously. If these simple maneuvers fail, a small amount of CPAP may be added to the deflated lung. CPAP is increased slowly from 2 to 10 cm H_2O until desaturation stops or the lung starts to inflate. Although there is a theoretical risk that PEEP to the dependent lung would redistribute blood flow to the nonventilated lung and worsen shunt, in practice this is rarely a problem and PEEP avoids inflating the operative lung and compromising surgical conditions.

Complications

There are two rare but potentially serious complications of lung isolation techniques for which one must be vigilant: airway rupture and dependent lung pneumothorax. Most bronchial injuries occur with insertion of a DLT that is too large for the patient, by overinflation of the endobronchial cuff, or with blind insertion into the distal airway. These complications can be minimized with direct vision of the endobronchial lumen and balloon with the bronchoscope. The endobronchial cuff should be checked throughout the procedure, and the minimum amount of air that eliminates the leak around the bronchial cuff should be used. Dependent lung pneumothorax may be due to overventilation or air trapping in the ventilated lung, with the risk increased with underlying emphysema or bullous disease. Although unusual, pneumothorax must be included in the differential diagnosis if unexplained hypotension and increased airway pressures occur because prompt treatment is required to prevent disaster. Finally, there is some association between DLTs and vocal cord dysfunction, most likely from the large outer diameter of the DLT. Although little can be done to stop this problem, this complication should be kept in mind when discussing risks with patients.

■ CHOICE OF ANESTHETIC

General anesthesia is required for most major thoracic procedures; however, the addition of regional techniques for intraoperative and postoperative pain control allows minimization of sedation and respiratory depression associated with narcotic analgesia. Thoracotomy is one of the most painful incisions in surgery. It has been well documented that thoracic incisions have immediate and intermediate lasting adverse effects on respiratory mechanics. Although these effects are not mediated solely by pain, they can be reduced by certain postoperative pain approaches. The following is a brief discussion of some regional options for pain relief.

A more thorough discussion can be found in the chapter on "Postoperative Pain Control for Thoracic Surgery."

Epidural

Thoracic epidurals often are viewed as the ideal choice for postoperative pain relief. This technique provides little to no systemic narcotic with no shift in the carbon dioxide response curve and excellent pain relief for deep breathing and movement. Catheters may be left in place for several days and titrated to effect. When dosed with continuous infusions of dilute local anesthetic with or without low-dose narcotics, ambulation is possible and hemodynamic effects are minimized. Disadvantages include time added to the procedure, inability to insert the catheter, migration of the catheter after insertion, and hypotension from sympathectomy, particularly when more concentrated local anesthetics are used. Lumbar catheters also may be effective, but the incidence of hypotension and leg weakness is higher than with thoracic catheters. Epidurals are not inserted in patients who will require cardiopulmonary bypass, patients with coagulopathy or thrombocytopenia, or patients taking low-molecular-weight heparins because of the risk of epidural hematoma (although aspirin use or subcutaneous heparin is generally not a contraindication).

Intrathecal Narcotics

Intrathecal administration of narcotics, typically 0.3 to 0.8 mg of preservative-free morphine, can provide good pain relief for 12 to 24 hours postoperatively, generally enough time for most more robust patients to transition smoothly to intravenous patient-controlled analgesia. Advantages include the speed and ease of administration of the narcotic into the intrathecal space. Disadvantages include the slow (1 to 2 hours) onset of analgesia; inability to titrate; and potential side effects of pruritus, urinary retention, and respiratory depression (usually treatable by low-dose naloxone infusion without reversal of analgesia). As with epidurals, this procedure should not be used in patients who are anticoagulated or thrombocytopenic.

Intrapleural Catheter

There has been some controversy as to the efficacy of the intrapleural catheter for pain relief. Although there are studies showing this technique as being inferior, equal to, and superior to epidural catheters, most of the data suggest that intrapleural catheters are inferior to epidural techniques. The advantage to using an intrapleural catheter is that it is inserted under direct visualization by the surgeon so that the local anesthetic is delivered to the desired location nearly 100% of the time. The distribution of the anesthetic is gravity dependent, probably accounting for the variability in effectiveness; the incidence of sympathectomy and hypotension is relatively high; and the absorption of local anesthetic is potentially significant.

Intercostal Nerve Blocks

Intercostal nerve blocks are an effective method of postoperative pain relief for the thoracotomy incision and chest tube sites. Blocks may be performed under direct vision before closure or percutaneously, and the onset of analgesia is immediate. The main disadvantage is the limited duration (3 to 6 hours) of pain relief obtained. The local anesthetic in this area has a high rate of absorption, second only to intravenous administration. This high rate of absorption is responsible for the short duration of action, and it is possible to achieve toxic systemic doses of local anesthetic.

■ ANESTHETIC CONSIDERATIONS FOR SPECIFIC SURGERIES

Bronchoscopy

Flexible bronchoscopy usually is performed outside the operating room with only minimal sedation. In situations in which deeper sedation or prevention of movement is required or rigid bronchoscopy is planned, general anesthesia is necessary. For flexible bronchoscopy, the airway may be secured with an ETT, a laryngeal mask airway, or rarely, intermittent mask ventilation. Using a laryngeal mask airway works well because the device delivers the fiberoptic scope right to the larynx and allows easy ventilation with minimal airway stimulation, but it does not protect the airway from aspiration of gastric contents. Local anesthetic (topical lidocaine solution) should be administered to the larynx and trachea via the scope to decrease stimulation and coughing. Rigid bronchoscopy requires deep muscle relaxation because the risk of airway injury with sudden patient movement is significant. Intravenous anesthetic techniques are preferred because delivery of inhaled anesthetics may be intermittent while sharing the airway with the bronchoscope operator.

Mediastinoscopy

Mediastinoscopy is a relatively short procedure with rare but potentially catastrophic consequences. An important anesthetic concern is to ensure adequate muscle relaxation so that the patient will not move while the scope is in the mediastinum but still be able to reverse the paralysis quickly. A second concern is the potential for injury to mediastinal structures. Vascular structures may be injured or compressed, resulting in bleeding, arrhythmias, and hypotension. Because these are potential hazards and both arms are typically tucked for this procedure, adequate vascular access for acute volume resuscitation is required. The use of an arterial line is not required but is indicated for patients who might not tolerate brief periods of hypotension or swings in blood pressure. Because the innominate artery often can become compressed during the procedure, reducing the ability to measure blood pressure in the right arm when it is most needed, it is our practice to measure blood pressure in the left arm during these procedures. Compromised perfusion to the right side may be monitored by placing the pulse oximeter on the right hand.

Anterior Mediastinal Mass

Patients with large anterior mediastinal masses undergoing mediastinotomy for tissue diagnosis deserve special anesthetic consideration. These tumors may compress the trachea, the main bronchi, or both, making ventilation or passage of an ETT impossible. Airway obstruction may not occur until there is deepening of general anesthesia or muscle relaxation due to reduction in the distending pressure on the intrathoracic airways. Factors that should alert the surgeon and anesthesiologist to this potential but avoidable complication include symptoms of positional (supine) stridor or dyspnea, evidence of intrathoracic variable obstruction on flow-volume loops, and radiographic evidence of tracheobronchial compression. Importantly, it may be possible to get gas into the lung with positive-pressure ventilation, but it may not egress freely, resulting in air trapping, overdistention, reduction of venous return, and hypotension.

When airway compression is at risk, it is reasonable to follow a more conservative approach. Inhaled spontaneous induction should be performed, frequently beginning with the head of the bed elevated 45 degrees. Anesthetic depth should be increased slowly, the table flattened, and assisted ventilation attempted gradually. If assisted ventilation is easy, including complete exhalation, the anesthetic is deepened rapidly, and muscle relaxation is achieved with a short-acting agent.

If at any stage ventilation becomes difficult, this approach permits backing up a step by allowing the anesthetic effects to wear off. In an emergency or if it is impossible to pass an ETT past the obstruction, a backup airway may be provided by passing a rigid bronchoscope past the compression and providing ventilation through it. If a patient with a large, symptomatic anterior mediastinal mass is anesthetized for diagnostic purposes before initiation of definitive treatment, one should consider leaving the patient intubated and sedated until after administration of chemotherapy or radiation therapy because these tumors frequently shrink rapidly, reducing greatly the risk of postextubation airway obstruction.

Tracheal Resection and Reconstruction

Because the airway needs to be shared, communication and planning between the anesthesia and surgical teams is essential for the smooth conduct of these cases. The goal of the anesthetic is to have the patient wide awake and extubated at the conclusion of the case, so short-acting agents with little to no muscle relaxation or narcotic effects are used. An arterial line should be placed, preferably in the left arm. Management considerations for induction of anesthesia and securing the airway for patients with critical tracheal stenosis or tracheomalacia are similar to the considerations discussed previously for large anterior mediastinal masses. These patients likewise are at risk for airway obstruction due to coughing, secretions, or loss of muscle tone and should undergo a gentle inhalation induction with spontaneous respiration until adequate airflow with assisted ventilation is confirmed. When anesthesia is deep enough, either a small ETT is placed and pushed through the obstruction, or a rigid bronchoscope is used to dilate the airway so that an ETT may be passed.

After the trachea is divided following surgical exposure, a sterile wire-reinforced ETT is placed into the distal trachea by the surgeon and connected to sterile tubing passed off the field to the anesthesia circuit. To maintain constant anesthetic depth during the intermittent periods of apnea while the sutures are being placed between the resected ends of the trachea, it is useful to convert to a total intravenous anesthetic, such as propofol, during this portion and usually for the remainder of the procedure. After all the sutures are in place, the neck is flexed, the oral ETT is advanced with surgical guidance into the distal trachea, and the tracheal ends are approximated with the tied sutures. After closure, the chin frequently is tied to the upper sternum with heavy suture to minimize tension on the anastomosis. The patient should be extubated in the operating room wide awake because reintubation is difficult with the neck flexed, and positive-pressure mask ventilation puts the anastomosis at risk. Prophylactic nebulized racemic epinephrine given immediately on extubation may be useful to minimize edema of the larynx or stridor and reduce bronchospasm. If the patient requires reintubation at any time postoperatively, it should be performed over a fiberoptic bronchoscope with the surgeons present, allowing inspection of the anastomosis and precise placement of the ETT cuff.

Thoracotomy

Anesthesia for thoracotomy commonly requires single-lung ventilation. Although single-lung ventilation may not be mandatory for most of the operative procedure, it greatly facilitates surgical exposure. Choice of postoperative pain relief, monitors, and lung isolation techniques already has been discussed. The anesthetic technique should be matched to the intended postoperative pain method chosen. Arterial monitoring of blood pressure is performed frequently because of the possibility of significant bleeding, cardiac irritation, hypoxemia, or hypoventilation requiring blood gas analysis and due to the advanced age and comorbidities of the typical patient. Intraoperative fluid usually is held to a minimum, particularly for pneumonectomies, with the goal of maintaining the patient on the "dry" side of euvolemia. Placement in the lateral decubitus posture requires careful attention to the usual positioning risks.

Thoracoscopy

Thoracoscopy is similar to thoracotomy except that single-lung ventilation is required almost routinely to permit operative exposure in the closed chest. In addition, because this is a minimally invasive technique, postoperative discomfort is also low, and neuraxial pain management is usually not necessary.

Esophagectomy or Esophagogastrectomy

Esophagectomy or esophagogastrectomy may be performed via thoracic, thoracoabdominal (three-incision), or transhiatal approaches. The primary concerns for the anesthesiologist in these surgeries are basically the same. First, there is the risk of hemodynamic compromise. The esophagus lies directly behind the heart, and during dissection of this structure there may be compression of the heart, compromise of venous return, or arrhythmias. This situation is more prominent in transhiatal resections because the surgeon blindly dissects the esophagus with his or her hand in the closed chest cavity. Arterial blood pressure monitoring is mandatory in these surgeries. The second area of concern is the patient's airway after the surgery is complete. Because aspiration is a significant risk with resection of the esophagogastric junction, and reintubation may be more difficult after a long surgery with major fluid resuscitation, our practice is to leave these patients intubated and sedated overnight. If a cervical anastomosis is present, it may be disrupted by aggressive mask ventilation or a failed intubation attempt in an emergency situation. Finally, these cases typically have large third space losses and fluid requirements (although less so for the transhiatal approach), making a central line helpful to guide management. Some thoracic approaches are facilitated by single-lung ventilation to improve surgical exposure and may benefit from postoperative epidural analgesia.

Thymectomy

The most important anesthetic consideration for thymectomy relates to the indication for the procedure rather than the procedure itself. Substernal thymectomy is performed frequently for the neuromuscular disorder myasthenia gravis, a disease characterized by voluntary muscle weakness because of reduced numbers of acetylcholine receptors at the neuromuscular junction. Depending on the severity of the disease, as indicated by the progression from ocular to proximal muscles to bulbar symptoms and the cumulative dose of anticholinesterase, these patients may require a period of mechanical ventilation postoperatively. The anesthetic technique should minimize or eliminate the use of muscle relaxants and, optionally, use neuraxial analgesia techniques to reduce systemic narcotic use and potential respiratory depression. A neostigmine infusion should be started in the operating room and continued to the ICU until the patient can resume his or her oral medication regimen. As with other anterior mediastinal masses, airway compression and compromise may require special management if present.

Lung Volume Reduction

Lung volume reduction surgery for advanced emphysema is a procedure with a true team approach, with close communication between the pulmonologists, surgeons, anesthesiologists, and critical care physicians. With typical forced expiratory volume in 1 second (FEV_1) values in the 600- to 800-ml range, these patients do not meet classic criteria for extubation even before they have surgery, and it is imperative that their preoperative condition and hospital course be optimized. At many institutions, patients undergo a preoperative course of pulmonary rehabilitation, exercising with supplemental oxygen to improve their conditioning, strength, psychological state, and nutritional status. All respiratory infections and reactive airway diseases must be treated. Because these patients have marginal pulmonary mechanics, it is essential that effective postoperative pain control be provided to reduce splinting and permit slow, deep breathing and clearance of secretions.

From an anesthetic point of view, at our institution, patients undergoing lung volume reduction surgery receive no narcotics or benzodiazepines so to reduce the risk of respiratory depression, and all pain relief is provided by an epidural catheter. High thoracic epidurals are placed with minimal or no sedation so that a segmental sensory block can be confirmed before induction of general anesthesia. If the epidural cannot be established in the operating room, it is started in radiology under fluoroscopy guidance. General anesthesia proceeds with propofol, muscle relaxants, and epidural analgesia. An arterial line, central line, and double-lumen ETT are placed. Nebulized bronchodilators

are given if needed. Mechanical ventilator settings using low rates (6 to 8 breaths/min) and long expiratory times keep peak pressures low, particularly when operating on the second side (and ventilating the newly reduced lung). For sternotomy approaches, the DLT is changed to a large single-lumen tube before sternal closure to facilitate spontaneous breathing on emergence from anesthesia. When awake, these patients undergo β_2-agonist treatments, with the head of the bed elevated to maximize pulmonary function. Blood gases are obtained serially over the next 15 minutes to 2 hours, while providing bronchodilators, pain control with epidural dosing, and verbal encouragement to maximize pulmonary function. When the P_{CO_2} is found to be decreasing or at least constant, the ETT is removed, and the patient is observed until the condition remains stable. Only at this time is the patient transferred out of the operating room to the ICU.

Many potential problems are encountered in these challenging cases. Air trapping and auto-PEEP are common and may result in reduced venous return and hypotension. In addition, these patients usually are managed "dry," increasing the risk of hypotension from air trapping, anesthetic side effects, and sympathectomy from epidural dosing. Due to the potential for hemodynamic instability, the arterial line should be placed before induction. For the same reasons, central access is helpful to assist fluid management, particularly in the postoperative period. Although unilateral and bilateral thoracoscopic approaches sometimes are performed, we still place and confirm thoracic epidural catheters to reduce pain and postoperative pulmonary dysfunction in the event that it becomes necessary to convert to a thoracotomy (muscle-sparing) incision. Air leaks should be identified and estimated quantitatively by the amount lost per breath of tidal volume. Larger leaks (>50% tidal volume lost) may need to be addressed surgically. Otherwise, low tidal volumes and minimization of chest tube suction (none usually used) should be instituted. Finally, it is crucial that postoperative care include meticulous attention to pain control, secretions, bronchospasm, patient encouragement, and early ambulation. Epidural analgesia should not be reduced for hypotension; rather a vasoconstrictor infusion should be added. It is not unusual for the first P_{CO_2} in the ICU to be 60 to 70 torr. As long as the patient has good pain control, air leaks are manageable, and the patient is breathing in a reasonably organized manner without bronchospasm, this value should improve steadily over the first few hours.

SUGGESTED READING

Brodsky JB, Fitzmaurice B: Modern anesthetic techniques for thoracic operations, *World J Surg* 25:162, 2001.

Seigne PW, et al: Anesthetic considerations for patients with severe emphysematous lung disease, *Int Anesthesiol Clin* 38:1, 2000.

Shah JS, Bready LL: Anesthesia for thoracoscopy, *Anesthesiol Clin N Am* 19:153, 2001

Slinger PD, Johnston MR: Preoperative assessment for pulmonary resection, *Anesthesiol Clin N Am* 19:411, 2001.

Wilson RS: Lung isolation: tube design and technical approaches, *Chest Surg Clin N Am* 7:735, 1997.

THE DIFFICULT ELECTIVE INTUBATION

Robert L. Ferris
David W. Eisele

◼ DEFINITION

Airway obstruction can occur during the induction of general anesthesia. A *difficult airway* is defined as a clinical situation in which a conventionally trained anesthesiologist experiences difficulty with mask ventilation, tracheal intubation, or both. This situation is approached best by anticipating a potentially difficult airway and paying careful attention to the management of the patient. Particular modifications to the standard algorithmic approach to the difficult intubation, as devised by the American Society of Anesthesiologists (Figure 1), may be necessary in patients undergoing thoracic and cardiovascular surgery. This chapter addresses the approach to the expected difficult airway, a diagnosis made after a thorough history, physical examination, and consideration of the patient's prior experiences with general anesthesia.

◼ PATIENTS AT RISK

Identification of the patient with a difficult airway requires a careful airway history to detect medical, surgical, and anesthesia-related factors that could indicate the presence of a difficult airway. A history of dyspnea, stridor, or noisy breathing should be noted. Tracheal narrowing may be secondary to external compression from an anterior mediastinal mass or a substernal goiter. Compression of the airway may be insidious when it is at the intrathoracic level and at the bronchial level. In these situations, a patient may be asymptomatic with airway compression and manifest difficulty only after induction of anesthesia when voluntary control of the airway is lost. Other conditions associated with the presence of a difficult airway include prior difficult intubation, obesity/obstructive sleep apnea, prior radiation therapy, pregnancy, congenital or acquired deformities, trauma, infections, and neoplasms. Certain classification systems have been developed to rate the anticipated difficulty of intubation, including the Mallampati criteria, thyromental distance measurement, and the degree of neck extension. Briefly, these systems correlate upper airway anatomic measurements and relationships with the probability of difficulty during endotracheal intubation.

Specific conditions related to thoracic and cardiovascular surgery may contribute to the development or exacerbation of a difficult airway during endotracheal intubation or extubation. A well-planned approach to the intubation of these patients, including appropriate preoperative discussion with the anesthesiologist, in most cases avoids the need for urgent decision making and potential complications.

◼ EVALUATION OF THE ANTICIPATED DIFFICULT AIRWAY PATIENT

All patients with a suspected difficult airway should undergo systematic airway evaluations, including examination of the anterior neck, specifically as an entry point for cricothyroid membrane puncture, cricothyroidotomy, or tracheostomy. Anatomic factors, such as obesity or tumor; previous surgery (head and neck, cervical spine); radiation; or tracheal deviation may make cricothyroidotomy or tracheotomy difficult.

Preoperative information regarding the likelihood of encountering a difficult airway should be obtained. Chest and neck computed tomography scans provide airway anatomic information in addition to the presence and location of extrinsic or intrinsic masses that may interfere with the placement of an endotracheal tube (ETT). An anterior mediastinal mass may cause tracheal compression to the degree that passage of an ETT is problematic. Additional airway information may be gained from flow volume loops. This test can help distinguish between fixed or variable intrathoracic and extrathoracic airway obstruction. The latter information may help to guide the expected needs of the patient in securing a safe airway in the operating room.

To plan accordingly, an anticipated difficult airway may be visualized preoperatively using the fiberoptic scope before attempted intubation is undertaken. Fiberoptic bronchoscopy also frequently is necessary to position double-lumen ETTs in thoracic surgery, and evaluation of the upper airway should be performed before placement of the ETT. Other scenarios may predispose a cardiothoracic surgical patient to airway difficulty during intubation or extubation, including tracheomalacia, tracheal stenosis (after prior tracheal surgery or intubation injury), laryngospasm, and tracheoesophageal fistula. The relative influence of these conditions should be evaluated thoroughly before attempted endotracheal intubation.

◼ MANAGEMENT OF THE DIFFICULT AIRWAY

It may be difficult to predict which patients will develop near or total airway obstruction. Appropriate equipment and personnel should be available for this scenario. Having an emergency airway cart available in the operating room is invaluable (Table 1). In addition, having identifiable experts in airway management, especially anesthesiologists and head and neck surgeons who can be summoned for assistance, is extremely beneficial for the management for the unanticipated difficult airway. Basic requirements include a thorough knowledge of upper airway anatomy, a planned team approach, and facility with several different methods of instrumentation.

Useful techniques to secure the airway after failed endotracheal intubation include continued mask ventilation, rigid endoscopic intubation, flexible fiberoptic nasotracheal intubation, the laryngeal mask airway (LMA), and transtracheal jet ventilation. If these methods fail and mask ventilation

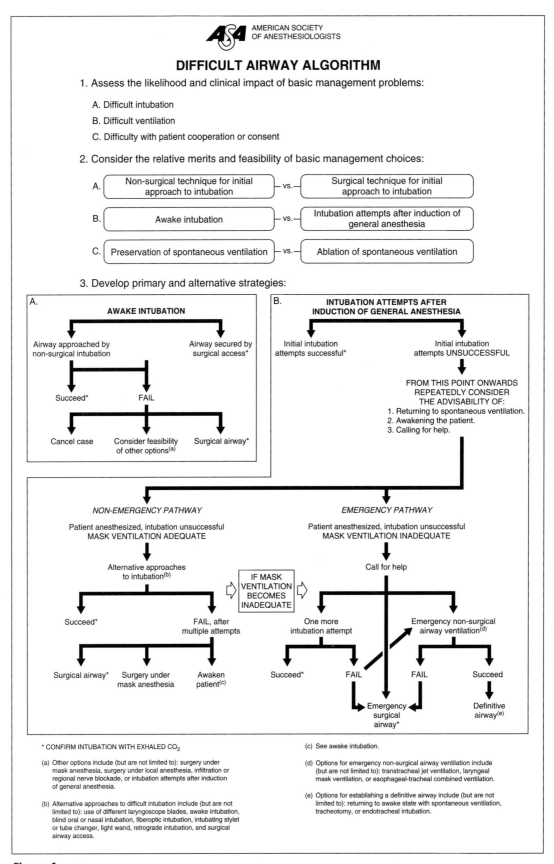

Figure 1
Algorithmic approach to the difficult airway, as developed by the American Society of Anesthesiologists.

Table 1 Adult Emergency Airway Cart

Dedo laryngoscope, Hollinger laryngoscope
Laryngeal suction tips
Rigid bronchoscope (6 × 35) with adapter
Bronchoscope suction tips
Fiberoptic bronchoscope
Jet ventilation setup
Eschmann stylet
Light source and fiberoptic cables
Tracheotomy set
Local anesthetic set (lidocaine with 1/100,000 epinephrine)
Jolly tube
Alligator forceps
Tooth guard
Scalpel handle, no. 15 scalpel blade
Cup forceps, straight and up-biting
Assorted laryngeal mask airways
Assorted endotracheal tubes
Assorted tracheostomy tubes
Mayo scissors
Kelly clamp
Towels, towel clip

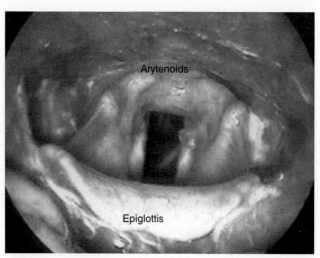

Figure 2
Fiberoptic endoscopic view of the larynx from above. The epiglottis, supraglottic structures, and true vocal folds are visible. Careful advancement of the bronchoscope toward the vocal folds enables injection of local anesthetic before placement of the bronchoscope, then the endotracheal tube into the trachea.

is not possible, a surgical airway should be created. The latter option may include either a cricothyroidotomy or a tracheostomy. Some surgeons suggest cannulation of the femoral vessels for cardiopulmonary bypass if tracheal compression reduces airway size to less than 50% of normal; patients with lesser degrees of obstruction may benefit from sterile preparation of the groin for access to the femoral vessels for cannulation and cardiopulmonary bypass should the need arise. The American Society of Anesthesiologists has developed an algorithm for the management of the difficult airway (see Figure 1). Modifications to this algorithm may be appropriate depending on the specific needs relating to a particular patient's condition.

■ TECHNIQUES FOR MANAGEMENT OF THE DIFFICULT AIRWAY

The following techniques may be employed depending on the equipment available and on the experience and proficiency of the surgeon and anesthesia team.

Fiberoptic Nasotracheal Intubation
Intubation under the guidance of a flexible bronchoscope is a safe method for intubating the awake patient with a difficult airway. An indication for fiberoptic intubation is impaired access to the larynx via the oral cavity. This difficulty may be related to trismus, oral cavity obstruction due to tumor, edema or hematoma, upper airway neoplasms, infections, cervical spine trauma, and morbid obesity.

To perform fiberoptic intubation, the patient's nose is topically decongested and anesthetized. The pharynx also is anesthetized with lidocaine or benzocaine spray. Having the patient sit rather than lie supine facilitates visualization of the larynx by the intubator, who faces the patient. Passage of successively larger, lubricated (2% lidocaine jelly) nasopharyngeal airways through the larger nasal cavity helps dilate

the nasal passage. A nasotracheal tube (≥7-mm I.D.), softened by soaking in warm saline, is passed through the nose and nasopharynx into the oropharynx. Care must be taken to avoid passage of the tip of the ETT too far into the pharynx, which may elicit gagging.

A lubricated fiberoptic bronchoscope is passed through the ETT, taking care not to pass it through the Murphy eye of the tube. Secretions are suctioned away. The glottis is visualized (Figure 2), and the larynx is anesthetized with 2 to 3 ml of 1% lidocaine delivered through the bronchoscope side port. The suction port is occluded temporarily during lidocaine instillation. The fiberoptic bronchoscope is advanced through the glottis and into the trachea. The ETT is advanced over the fiberoptic bronchoscope into the trachea. The position of the ETT above the carina is confirmed visually. If there is difficulty in advancing the ETT into the larynx, the tube should be rotated and gently readvanced. Continued inability to advance the tube may necessitate the use of a smaller ETT.

Oral fiberoptic intubation is a good alternative to nasotracheal fiberoptic intubation if the nasal cavity or nasopharynx is obstructed or if there is active nasal hemorrhage. This method requires good oropharyngeal anesthesia and cooperation because gagging may make this technique difficult. An oral airway guide for fiberoptic intubation facilitates orotracheal fiberoptic intubation. The use of an Ovassapian airway guide is preferable because it can be removed easily when the ETT has been placed adequately, without disconnecting or removing the ETT.

Fiberoptic intubation requires skill, time, and the patient's cooperation. Complications include hemorrhage, esophageal intubation, laryngospasm, and other potential complications of intubation. Failure to intubate by this method is uncommon.

Laryngeal Mask Airway

The LMA is a ventilation device consisting of a tube with an inflatable silicone mask. The deflated mask is placed into the pharynx and positioned above the larynx. The mask cuff is inflated without holding the device. This creates an air seal in the pharynx above the larynx. Although most commonly used for nonemergency airway control during general anesthesia, the LMA is an alternative for temporary emergency airway control if standard mask ventilation is adequate and endotracheal intubation is unsuccessful. After the airway is stabilized with the LMA, an ETT can be placed. Intubation with a small (<6.0 mm I.D.) ETT directly through the LMA can be performed. Alternatively an Eschmann stylet (gum elastic bougie) can be placed through the LMA into the trachea, and the LMA can be exchanged for an ETT over the stylet.

Fiberoptic visualization of the airway can be performed through the LMA, alongside an Eschmann stylet, and this may facilitate passage of the stylet into the trachea. The appropriate size ETT and fiberoptic bronchoscope needs to be selected for use with each LMA size. The compatibility of the tube and its adapter should be tested before insertion because the outside diameter of ETTs may vary. In addition, the ETT can be bronchoscopically guided into the airway after an appropriately sized ETT is loaded onto the bronchoscope.

The LMA is not as effective as an ETT in preventing pulmonary aspiration of gastric contents. The contraindications to using the LMA are similar to those for facemask ventilation and include patients with hiatal hernias and patients who are at risk for aspiration. Other contraindications for an LMA include severe trismus, obstruction of the glottic or subglottic larynx, pharyngeal or supraglottic mass, and laryngospasm.

Light Wand

The light wand (Trachlight; Laerdal Medical, Wappinger Falls, NY), also called the *lighted stylet,* is an intubating stylet with a handle and a malleable, fiberoptic light source at its tip. An ETT is placed on the lubricated light wand, and the tip of the ETT is placed blindly into the hypopharynx and directed toward the glottis. The light on the stylet transilluminates the neck and directs placement of the ETT into the larynx. Then the ETT is advanced into the larynx.

Overall, the advantages of the light wand are that it is easy to learn, is simple to operate, is lightweight, is portable, works well in settings of poor ambient lighting, is applicable in situations in which cervical spine mobility is limited, and is not hampered significantly by blood or secretions. Situations in which the light wand may not be applicable include obese patients with thick necks or other patients with anterior cervical pathology, in which it may be difficult to visualize the cervical illumination, and patients with upper airway pathology, such as neoplasms, which may preclude the use of blind intubation techniques.

Bullard Laryngoscope

The Bullard laryngoscope (Circon, Stamford, CT) is a rigid, curved fiberoptic laryngoscope with an attachable ETT stylet designed to allow direct visualization of the glottis. The blade of the laryngoscope is placed in the oropharynx, the tongue and epiglottis are lifted, and the glottis is visualized. The ETT is advanced over the stylet into the trachea.

Compared with flexible fiberoptic laryngoscopes, the Bullard laryngoscope is more portable and rugged. The illumination characteristics of the Bullard device, although adequate, may be inferior to the flexible fiberoptic laryngoscope, however. In some patients, the Bullard laryngoscope may not be long enough to expose the glottis, although an attachable blade extender is available. Also, the Bullard scope blade and ETT combination is bulkier than the flexible intubating fiberscope and requires a greater degree of mouth opening. As with any fiberoptic instrument, blood, secretions, or vomitus may interfere with visualization.

Rigid Endoscopic Intubation

This technique relies on the use of a closed laryngoscope, which is commonly used for diagnostic and therapeutic direct laryngoscopy. These instruments facilitate intubation or the use of a rigid bronchoscope to allow for direct airway intubation and ventilation. In contrast to the standard Macintosh and Miller blade laryngoscopes used commonly by anesthesiologists, a closed-tube laryngoscope displaces tissues circumferentially, improving visualization of the larynx and suctioning. A closed-tube laryngoscope is useful in several situations, including the presence of obstructing oropharyngeal or supraglottic laryngeal masses or tumors; the inability to visualize the glottis due to anatomic distortions from tumor; friable or bleeding tumors; or fixed glottic, subglottic, or tracheal lesions. The rigid bronchoscope can be used in the same situations and is the preferred method for airway management in situations of tracheal or bronchial foreign bodies and selected obstructing tracheal tumors.

When the glottis is visualized with the laryngoscope, there are two options for intubation. The first option is to intubate through the laryngoscope. The trachea can be intubated directly through the laryngoscope, and the patient can be ventilated. Certain rigid laryngoscopes (i.e., the Hollinger or anterior-commissure scope) accommodate only a 5-mm I.D. or smaller uncuffed ETT. The second option is to place an Eschmann stylet (gum elastic bougie) through the laryngoscope into the trachea. Using the Seldinger technique, the laryngoscope is removed, leaving the Eschmann stylet in place, and the patient is intubated over the Eschmann stylet. The Eschmann stylet accommodates ETTs of 6 mm I.D. and larger. Using the larger diameter Dedo rigid laryngoscope, direct placement of a wider ETT is possible (≤7.5 mm I.D. cuffed tube); this enables the patient to be ventilated and stabilized with the endotracheal cuff inflated. The laryngoscope can be removed by detaching the proximal ventilator adapter from the ETT and grasping the tube with a long alligator forceps. The forceps hold the tube in place while the laryngoscope is removed, and the ETT adapter is replaced, allowing mechanical or bag ventilation through the tube as desired. Another alternative for ventilation, when the glottis is exposed with the closed laryngoscope or rigid bronchoscope, is jet ventilation. A jet ventilator adapter can be attached to the end of the laryngoscope and used to ventilate the patient. Alternatively a flexible-tube jet ventilator can be passed into the trachea through the laryngoscope, and jet ventilation can be performed.

A rigid bronchoscope can be used to intubate the trachea directly. This method may be beneficial for the bypass of tracheal obstructions and for the management of foreign bodies in the airway. When the bronchoscope has been placed through the glottis and into the trachea under direct vision, the end of the bronchoscope is occluded with an eyepiece, and the respiratory circuit is attached to the ventilation side port of the bronchoscope. An Eschmann stylet also can be passed through the bronchoscope and used to facilitate the placement of an ETT after the bronchoscope has been withdrawn, as described earlier.

Cricothyroidotomy

Cricothyroidotomy refers to the surgical opening of the cricothyroid membrane, which is identified by palpating the cricothyroid space between the thyroid and cricoid cartilages. The skin over the cricoid cartilage is injected with local anesthetic if the patient is conscious. The neck is prepared with antiseptic solution. The thyroid cartilage is stabilized with the nondominant hand, and an incision is made with a scalpel through the skin, subcutaneous tissue, and cricothyroid membrane. An ETT or tracheotomy tube is inserted through the cricothyroid incision and passed caudally into the trachea. Small-diameter tubes (e.g., a no. 4 tracheotomy tube) are necessary because the cricothyroid space is approximately 9 mm wide.

In general, direct laryngoscopy should be performed after emergency cricothyroidotomy to assess internal laryngeal injury. Any laryngeal cartilage injury should be repaired. Conversion to a formal tracheotomy should be performed if long-term ventilation (>7 days) or upper airway bypass is anticipated. Cricothyroidotomy should not be performed in children because of the small size of the pediatric cricothyroid space; instead a tracheotomy is preferred.

Tracheotomy

Tracheotomy can be performed under local anesthesia as an option for management of the anticipated difficult airway. Also, tracheotomy serves as an alternative to cricothyroidotomy for emergency surgical airway access. It is the procedure of choice in a child, in a patient with an unidentifiable cricothyroid membrane, and in a patient with subglottic stenosis or obstruction. A vertical midline incision is made through the skin and subcutaneous tissue, while stabilizing the larynx with the nondominant hand. An extended neck provides better anatomic identification, assuming this is not otherwise contraindicated. The tracheal rings are divided vertically in the midline and opened with a finger or instrument. After the ETT has been directed caudally through the

tracheotomy, care must be taken to avoid main stem bronchus intubation by maintaining the tip of the ETT in the trachea.

■ PATIENT EXTUBATION

Extubation of a patient with a difficult airway must be considered carefully. If upper airway edema is suspected from multiple attempts at endotracheal intubation, steroids may be given and the head of the bed elevated to reduce swelling. As is necessary for intubation, a plan for airway management during emergence from anesthesia and extubation must be in place. Emergency airway equipment should remain available during a patient's emergence from anesthesia. The operating room team must be vigilant after extubation and during recovery from anesthesia so as to prevent postanesthetic airway obstruction. A careful airway history should be obtained to detect medical, surgical, and anesthesia-related factors that could indicate the presence of a difficult airway from prior extubations. Deflation of the ETT cuff should be performed to see if the patient can breathe around the tube, indicating that upper airway swelling might have gone down. Planning should include the consideration of extubation when the patient is awake and options for management if airway obstruction occurs after extubation.

■ SUMMARY

Although particular scenarios unique to thoracic and cardiovascular surgery may contribute to difficulty with elective endotracheal intubation, the anticipated difficult airway should be approached using an algorithm guided by standard principles of airway control. Preoperative planning and discussions between the surgeon, anesthesiologist, and patient facilitate the establishment of a plan of action and enable the necessary equipment and experienced personnel to be assembled.

SUGGESTED READING

Eisele DW: Airway emergencies. In Eisele DW, McQuone S, editors: *Emergencies in head and neck surgery,* St Louis, 2000, Mosby, p 111.

Langeron O, et al: Prediction of difficult mask ventilation, *Anesthesiology* 92:1229, 2000.

Weymuller EA: Acute airway management. In Cummings CW, et al, editors: *Otolaryngology/head and neck surgery,* ed 3, St Louis, 1998, Mosby-Year Book, p 2368.

POSTOPERATIVE PAIN CONTROL FOR THORACIC SURGERY

Clifford Goldman

Peter S. Staats

Pain is our silent, internal alarm system. Without this system, humans would not recognize and respond appropriately to life-threatening diseases and injuries. A person incapable of feeling pain would be unlikely to enjoy longevity. When creating the pain response, however, nature did not anticipate our ability to perform pain-inducing surgical procedures during which we inflict pain as a by-product of rehabilitative and life-supporting operations. Postoperative pain can be especially problematic when it interferes with activities that promote healing (e.g., breathing or walking) and when it is allowed to dredge such deep pathways that the "pain alarm" becomes stuck, transforming what should have been short-term discomfort into chronic pain that continues despite removal of the pain-invoking noxious stimuli. When this happens, pain becomes a threat to health.

The chain of events that triggers postoperative pain begins when tissue damaged by surgical manipulation becomes inflamed and activates the terminals of the sympathetic nerves. This process releases the chemicals and mediators (histamines, bradykinins, and prostaglandins) that cause peripheral sensitization of nociceptors, lowering their threshold to the point where ordinarily nonpainful stimuli invoke pain. A concurrent central nervous system effect causes Aδ and C nerve fibers to transmit information that creates a condition of hyperexcitability at the synapses in the dorsal horn. The heightened intensity and duration of response of the dorsal horn neurons to stimuli (primary hyperalgesia) also broaden the scope of this response, expanding the perception of pain in response to stimuli originating beyond the ordinary receptive field (secondary hyperalgesia). This heightened responsiveness in the dorsal horn is known as *wind-up phenomenon* or *central sensitization*. Finally, central sensitization activates *N*-methyl-D-aspartate (NMDA) receptors at the spinal cord level, creating new connections among neurons. The changes invoked by central sensitization may create conditions that lead to the postoperative development of chronic neuropathic pain.

Postoperative pain delivers an unnecessary message and can be pathologic (inhibiting the mobility that enhances recovery, inducing stress-related damage to the cardiovascular system, and creating chronic pain states), so it is important to optimize pain management interventions. Because postoperative pain occurs in a chain reaction, there are multiple options for the timing and nature of these interventions. Administration of nonsteroidal antiinflammatory drugs (NSAIDs) can decrease the impact of peripheral sensitization by inhibiting the production of prostaglandins. Initiating analgesia before surgery using regional anesthetic and neuraxial techniques may preempt development of central sensitization by blocking transmission through the C fibers. This preemptive analgesia may prove to be a powerful means of controlling postoperative pain, decreasing morbidity, and preventing the development of chronic pain.

In the case of thoracic surgery, postoperative analgesia is not only important for patient satisfaction, but also it is a paramount factor affecting patient outcomes because decreasing pain decreases cardiovascular and respiratory morbidity, shortens hospital stays, and reduces the incidence of chronic postthoracotomy pain. During the postoperative period, patients must breathe deeply and cough sufficiently to clear secretions. Intense postthoracic pain may reduce postoperative pulmonary function, however, by causing diaphragmatic dysfunction (as the natural tendency toward pain avoidance leads postthoracic patients to limit painful chest wall motion). This diminished function results in an inability to clear secretions and in a decreased functional residual capacity, both of which may last for 7 to 14 days postoperatively. Decreased functional residual capacity leads to atelectasis and to ventilation-perfusion mismatching, resulting in postoperative hypoxemia, pneumonia, and prolonged mechanical ventilation.

By using epidural local anesthetics or opiates to control pain, pulmonary function improves, and postoperative pulmonary complications can be avoided. In addition, many patients undergoing thoracic surgery have cardiovascular disease and have a significantly increased risk of developing perioperative myocardial ischemia. Administration of epidural local anesthetics or opioids to control pain results in improved regional blood flow to poststenotic regions of the myocardium. By preventing pain-related postoperative complications, it is possible to shorten hospital stays and decrease associated costs.

Because anesthetic decisions made preoperatively and during the operation can have an impact on postoperative analgesic requirements, postoperative analgesia may be more appropriately considered *perioperative* analgesia. The multiple modalities for pain control include administration of parenteral narcotics and adjunct analgesics (e.g., NSAIDs), regional techniques (e.g., intercostal blocks and drug delivery via intrapleural catheter), and neuraxial techniques (e.g., epidural administration of opiates and local anesthetics). Properly implemented, these analgesic techniques, alone or in combination, can have a significant impact on postoperative outcomes.

■ SYSTEMIC ANALGESICS

The intravenous (IV) administration of opioids has long been the method of choice for controlling postoperative pain. The adjunctive use of newer medications, such as NSAIDs, cyclooxygenase type II antagonists, and NMDA receptor antagonists, reduces dose requirements and side effects while increasing efficacy.

Development of patient-controlled analgesia (PCA) has improved the postoperative administration of IV opioids by making consistent pain relief readily available (when patients recover from sedation) through an easily adjusted method of administration associated with reduced toxicity. The most commonly used medications for PCA are morphine, fentanyl, and hydromorphone. Although PCA reduces the incidence of respiratory depression in patients, this method of delivery does not reduce the incidence of other side effects of opioids, including pruritus, nausea, vomiting, biliary spasm, constipation, and urinary retention. If pain is well controlled with PCA, this technique can improve postoperative respiratory function.

The ability of patients to escalate the dosage of opioids with PCA is limited to avoid sedation and the respiratory depression that compromises pulmonary function. To avoid subjecting patients to pain that cannot be controlled with PCA and to avoid opioid-produced respiratory depression, some physicians use combined techniques, such as continuous epidural local anesthetic infusion with demand dosing of opioids via PCA.

■ REGIONAL ANESTHETIC TECHNIQUES

Regional anesthetic techniques, such as paravertebral or intercostal nerve blocks, can be performed preoperatively to use the benefits of preemptive analgesia and achieve 6 to 12 hours of good postoperative pain relief. The first step in performing paravertebral blocks for thoracotomy is identifying and marking a position 2.5 cm lateral to the superior borders of the T6-8 spinous processes. A 22-gauge spinal needle is advanced at the skin to the transverse process. After contacting bone, the needle is walked off the superior aspect of the transverse process and advanced approximately 1 cm. After negative aspiration of blood or air, 5 ml of local anesthetic is injected. Prolonged relief has been produced by placing a catheter in the paravertebral space and providing a continuous infusion of local anesthetic. The benefits of this procedure include ease of technique and preservation of pulmonary function. Possible complications include pneumothorax, intravascular injection of local anesthetic causing seizure, increased plasma levels of local anesthetic, nerve damage, and spinal anesthesia.

Intercostal nerve blocks for thoracotomy are performed by first identifying the sixth through eighth ribs ipsilateral to the incision site. Then a 22-gauge spinal needle is advanced to bone at a point proximal to the incision site along the rib. When it contacts the rib, the needle is walked off the inferior aspect of the rib and advanced 0.5 cm. After negative aspiration of blood or air, 3 to 5 ml of local anesthetic is injected. The risks and benefits of this procedure are similar to those associated with paravertebral nerve blocks except that the incidence of spinal anesthesia is extremely rare with intercostal nerve blocks. Contraindications for both of these procedures include bleeding diathesis, local infection, and sepsis.

Newer techniques, such as cryoablation of the intercostal nerve, can provide 1 to 3 months of good analgesia. When a cryoprobe ($-60°$ C) touches a nerve, the extreme cold degenerates the nerve axons but does not damage the surrounding connective tissue (perineurium). This procedure is performed before closing the thoracotomy incision. Using a nerve hook, the intercostal nerve is removed from the subcostal groove, and the cryoprobe is placed on the nerve for at least 30 seconds. If the cryoprobe misses direct application by 2 to 3 mm, cryoablation may fail. It is important to pierce the parietal pleura before applying the probe to the intercostal nerve.

By reducing pain, cryoanalgesia diminishes the need for postoperative opioid administration and improves pulmonary function. Patients generally experience moderate shoulder pain on the first postoperative day, which usually is attributed to the chest tube and abates when the tube is removed on the second or third postoperative day. Sensation begins to return in the dermatomal distribution of the intercostal nerve within 2 to 3 weeks after cryoablation. At 6-month follow-up, cryoanalgesia patients report a significant incidence of intercostal paralysis and dysesthesias, but this is virtually indistinguishable from nerve injury caused by the surgical manipulation. Cryoanalgesia has proved to be a reliable and effective means of achieving postoperative pain control; considering the long duration of analgesia it provides, this modality may be the treatment of choice for patients with increased risk of developing chronic chest wall pain.

Many thoracic surgeons employ interpleural regional analgesia for postoperative pain control. This technique may allow the local anesthetic to block the intercostal nerves, the thoracic sympathetic nerves, and the nerve endings within the pleura itself. Interpleural analgesia involves inserting a catheter (usually intraoperatively) into the thoracic cage between the parietal and visceral pleura, generally in the eighth intercostal space over the superior border of the rib. Alternatively, it may be placed through the same insertion site of an indwelling chest tube. When these techniques are performed percutaneously, a Touhy needle is walked off the superior border of the rib, and the pleural cavity is entered using a loss-of-resistance technique. The usual dosing is an initial bolus of 10 to 20 ml of 0.25% bupivacaine with 1:200,000 epinephrine followed by an infusion through the catheter of the same concentration at 5 ml/hr. An alternative is to administer a bolus dose of 20 to 30 ml of 0.25% bupivacaine with epinephrine every 4 to 6 hours, increasing the concentration of bupivacaine to 0.50% if necessary.

To avoid failure, the chest tube must be clamped before administration of the local anesthetic and stay clamped for 5 to 15 minutes. Posterior placement of the catheter, dilution of the local anesthetic secondary to pleural effusion, loculation of the local anesthetic by adhesions, and the presence of a bronchopleural fistula also can impede pain relief.

This technique is not appropriate for postoperative analgesia after an anterior thoracotomy incision, but it is indicated for cases of multiple rib fractures, postherpetic neuralgia, and chronic pancreatitis. Interpleural regional analgesia is contraindicated in patients with coagulopathy, local infection, sepsis, and conditions affecting distribution of the local anesthetic within the pleural space (e.g., pleural adhesions). Reported complications secondary to interpleural administration of local anesthetic include pneumothorax, systemic toxicity from the local anesthetic, pleural effusion, Horner's syndrome, phrenic nerve paralysis, bleeding, infection, and catheter breakage. Results with use of interpleural analgesia for thoracotomy are equivocal, possibly because some physicians employ a less than optimal technique. Further study and physician education is required to determine the efficacy of this technique for postoperative pain control.

■ NEURAXIAL OPIOIDS AND LOCAL ANESTHETICS

Neuraxial techniques for postoperative analgesia include intrathecal and epidural administration of opioids in combination with local anesthetics. Neuraxial opioids act as agonists at the μ and κ receptors located in Rexed's laminae I, II, and V in the dorsal horn gray matter. Binding these receptors inhibits afferent transmission. Local anesthetics act by blocking sodium channels in the axons of the Aδ and C fibers returning to the dorsal horn, inhibiting the afferent transmission of painful stimulus from the periphery.

There are fewer side effects associated with neuraxial opioids than seen with systemic administration because neuraxial doses are significantly smaller than doses required by systemic administration. Intrathecal dosing requires 100 times less medication than systemic administration and 10 times less than epidural administration. Common side effects of neuraxial opioid administration include respiratory depression, pruritus, nausea, vomiting, constipation, and urinary retention. Respiratory depression depends on the lipophilicity of the drug and can occur 2 hours or 6 to 12 hours after injection. The relative contraindications of neuraxial techniques include coagulopathy, sepsis, and local infection.

Intrathecal opioids provide 12 to16 hours of analgesia with an onset time of approximately 1 to 2 hours. A single intrathecal injection of opiates, most commonly morphine, may be used alone or in combination with an epidural infusion. Because it is hydrophilic, morphine achieves greater dermatomal spread than other opioids. A typical dose for intrathecal morphine is 0.3 mg, and the solution generally is administered into the L3-4 intervertebral space with a 25-gauge spinal needle to decrease the risk of postdural puncture headache. This technique obviates the need to insert an epidural catheter (which can be difficult and can increase risk of infection) and reduces the occurrence of hemodynamic changes or the motor blockade that may occur with the epidural administration of local anesthetics. The main disadvantage is that this technique, which carries similar risks as placement of an epidural catheter, does not provide analgesia past the first postoperative day.

Continuous epidural catheter infusion is the technique most often used for postoperative analgesia because it provides prolonged pain control compared with a single intrathecal administration. Also, epidural administration of opioids and local anesthetics decreases the incidence of pulmonary complications after thoracotomy compared with systemic opioid administration. Epidural opioids may be administered alone or, more commonly, in combination with local anesthetics. When using local anesthetics, the epidural catheter should be placed at T7 to block the T6-8 dermatomes and ensure good analgesia for thoracotomy. Epidural catheters are placed by introducing a 17-gauge Touhy needle through the ligamentum flavum into the epidural space using a loss-of-resistance technique. After injecting 5 ml of saline to expand the space, an epidural catheter is inserted through the Touhy needle. Injection of a test dose of lidocaine with epinephrine ensures that the catheter is not intravascular or intrathecal.

Opioids that have been administered alone in the epidural space include fentanyl, hydromorphone (Dilaudid), methadone, and meperidine, but morphine generally is used because of its hydrophilicity. Morphine is administered as a single 4 to 6-mg bolus in a 10- to 15-ml volume, with a continuous infusion rate of 0.1 to 0.8 mg/hr. The onset of analgesia occurs in 30 to 60 minutes, and the duration of effect is approximately 12 to18 hours.

The main benefit of infusing epidural opioids without local anesthetics is to avoid hypotension secondary to sympathectomy and motor blockade. Systemic side effects are more frequent with opioids alone, however, than with the combination epidural/local anesthetic therapy due to the higher dose of opioids when administered alone and the faster systemic absorption through the epidural fat and venous plexus. Local anesthetics generally are administered epidurally in combination with opioids to limit the dosage and decrease the side effects of both agents. A bolus of 6 to 8 ml of 0.25% bupivacaine is administered via the catheter to obtain anesthesia of the T6-8 dermatomes for preemptive analgesia, then a continuous infusion is employed for postoperative analgesia. A commonly used regimen is 0.125% bupivacaine with 5 μg/ml of fentanyl administered at a continuous rate of 4 to 6 ml/hr. If epidural PCA is available at the hospital, boluses of 2 to 4 ml can be self-administered by the patient every 10 minutes in conjunction with the continuous infusion.

The main disadvantages of neuraxial local anesthetics are postoperative hypotension, weakness, and urinary retention. The incidence of complications from thoracic epidural placement is low, however, and some can be avoided by proper positioning. These complications include postdural puncture headache, postoperative radicular pain, nerve palsies secondary to positioning, nerve injuries, and epidural hematoma. Epidural hematoma is the most devastating complication of epidural catheter placement; fortunately, its incidence is low and usually associated with coagulopathy.

■ SUMMARY

Many of the multiple modalities of treatment for postthoracotomy pain are not readily available to all physicians because of limited institutional resources. Currently, most hospitals in the United States use continuous epidural infusion of opioids with the adjunct of epidural or IV PCA for postoperative analgesia because these are the most widely studied techniques. Although new techniques, such as cryoablation, are not yet widely available, further study may prove the efficacy of these modalities.

SUGGESTED READING

Benumof JL, Alfery DD: Anesthesia for thoracic surgery. In Miller RD, editor: *Anesthesia*, ed 5, New York, 2000, Churchill Livingstone, p 1722.

Conacher ID: Post-thoracotomy analgesia, *Anesthesiol Clin N Am* 19:66, 2001.

Liu S, et al: Epidural anesthesia and analgesia, *Anesthesiology* 82:1474, 1995.

Peeters-Asdourian C, Gupta S: Choices in pain management following thoracotomy, *Chest* 115:122S, 1999.

Richardson J, et al: A prospective, randomized comparison of preoperative and continuous balanced epidural or paravertebral bupivacaine on post-thoracotomy pain, pulmonary function and stress responses, *Br J Anaesth* 83:387, 1999.

Staats PS, Panchal SJ: Pro: the anesthesiologist should provide epidural anesthesia in the coronary care unit for patients with severe angina, *J Cardiovasc Thorac Anesth* 11:105, 1997.

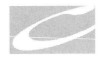

BRONCHOSCOPY: DIAGNOSTIC AND THERAPEUTIC APPLICATIONS

Joshua Robert Sonett

The comfortable and facile use of flexible and rigid bronchoscopy enables the thoracic surgeon to diagnose pathologic lesions and to perform direct interventions to relieve obstructed airways. Current techniques in the endobronchial treatment of lung and airway diseases continue to evolve but are already essential in the complete care of patients with benign and malignant problems and patients with airway complications related to lung transplantation. The ability to triage open surgical techniques with flexible and rigid endobronchial techniques empowers the thoracic surgeon to apply best specific diagnostic and therapeutic interventions based primarily on the needs and pathology of the patient.

■ INDICATIONS

The indications for awake flexible bronchoscopy are numerous and primarily can be considered diagnostic or therapeutic (Table 1). *All patients undergoing open lung resection should have a diagnostic flexible bronchoscopy performed by the operating surgeon.* This procedure can be performed at the time of resection through the endotracheal tube. Direct visualization of the airway by the surgeon helps secure operative intentions as to the type and extent of resection needed and to suction secretions and to rule out anatomic anomalies and other synchronous or endobronchial lesions (less common). Postoperatively the use of awake flexible bronchoscopy can offer crucial support to the patient with marginal pulmonary function who is having difficulty clearing secretions. Bedside bronchoscopy may be performed primarily with topical anesthesia and should be invoked liberally for patients who clear secretions poorly or have clinical or radiologic evidence of atelectasis. Rigid bronchoscopy is a crucial element in the care of any patient with proximal airway obstruction, compression, or life-threatening hemoptysis. Indications for the use of rigid bronchoscopy

and its need to be readily available are listed in Table 1. The ability to attain and maintain a safe airway with rigid bronchoscopy is an invaluable and necessary technique. Additionally, routine tumor débridement may be facilitated greatly when using a rigid bronchoscope even when combined with a flexible bronchoscope.

■ TECHNIQUES

Techniques in flexible bronchoscopy are well described, and the practicing thoracic surgeon should be comfortable with awake bronchoscopy in and out of the operating room. Supplemental intravenous sedation may be used as needed or as tolerated; however, proper local anesthetic preparation and techniques are perhaps the most important component of performing an awake evaluation of the airway and vocal cords. Pretreatment with 10 ml of 1% lidocaine (Xylocaine) delivered by nebulizer may be helpful but is not essential. The nares and posterior pharynx are anesthetized by application of 2% to 4% lidocaine jelly swabbed into the nares and posterior pharynx with a cotton-tipped applicator. Supplemental oxygen may be applied easily by a nasal cannula placed in the patient's mouth. Bronchoscopy is begun via the nares; when the vocal cords are visualized, 1% lidocaine is applied directly in two to three 5-ml aliquots. This maneuver allows the vocal cords time to become anesthetized before instrumentation and prevents coughing. Then the examination and procedure for the rest of the tracheobronchial tree may be performed.

Rigid bronchoscopy is performed in the operating room with general anesthesia. Adequate patient relaxation, optimal oxygenation, and clearance of the hypopharynx of secretions are important steps before attempts at insertion of the bronchoscope. The teeth are protected with a mouth guard, then the rigid bronchoscope is inserted by the surgeon under direct vision. The tip of the epiglottis is visualized through the bronchoscope, then the tip of the rigid bronchoscope is used to elevate the epiglottis, and the vocal cords are visualized. Helpful techniques after insertion include packing the hypopharynx with a moist large gauze roll to provide an airway seal at the level of the cords. After insertion and direct inspection, a flexible bronchoscope introduced through the rigid bronchoscope should be used to gain better visualization of the distal airway or to deliver adjuvant laser ablation to lesions that were directly débrided. *When laser ablation is performed under general anesthesia, supplemental oxygen must be reduced to the lowest levels to avoid combustion in the airway.*

Table 1 Indications for Flexible and Rigid Bronchoscopy

INDICATION	BRONCHOSCOPY
Diagnostic	
Infiltrate	Flexible
Tumor	Flexible
Carcinoid	Flexible with rigid standby
Tracheal stenosis	Flexible with rigid standby
Intervention/Therapeutic	
Clearance of secretions	Flexible (bedside)
Removal of foreign objects	Rigid
Hemoptysis	Flexible and rigid
Tumor removal	
Direct débridement	Flexible and rigid
Laser	Flexible with rigid standby
Photodynamic therapy	Flexible
Brachytherapy	Flexible
Relief of endoluminal extrinsic compression/obstruction (±) stent	Flexible and rigid

■ THERAPEUTIC APPLICATIONS

Débridement

Patients with persistent symptoms of airway obstruction after maximal treatment may be considered for endobronchial palliation. Evaluation of patients with pulmonary insufficiency and malignant airway obstruction should begin with a chest x-ray and a computed tomography scan of the chest. An initial treatment of external beam radiotherapy for patients with malignant airway disease not only avoids invasive endobronchial manipulations, but also devascularizes tumor bulk, making débridement safer. Debulking of airway lesions may be performed with a variety of techniques, including direct manual débridement and coring, laser ablation, and photodynamic therapy.

The modality or combination of techniques used may depend on the lesion, the preferences of the patient, and the experience of the surgeon. In general, the most efficient debulking method is by direct manual débridement and "core out." The use of laser to ablate remaining luminal irregularities or bleeding can be helpful. Primary laser débridement, with flexible bronchoscopy alone, is best reserved only for smaller, minimally obstructive lesions. The use of photodynamic therapy or brachytherapy is even more selective. Photodynamic therapy may have its best application for endobronchial lesions that are completely occluding an airway with total opacification of the lung. Indirect tissue destruction may occur with less concern of airway perforation.

Stents

Endobronchial stents can afford excellent palliation for patients with intrinsic and compressive lesions of the airway. The major selection of stent choices is between rigid Silastic stents and expandable metal or Silastic covered expandable metal stents. Silastic stents offer the advantages of significantly less reactive endobronchial granulation tissue and the ability to remove the stents easily. These attributes make Silastic stents an excellent choice for nonmalignant disease, such as bronchial stenosis after lung transplant or tracheal stenosis. Insertion requires the use of rigid bronchoscopy as depicted in Figure 1.

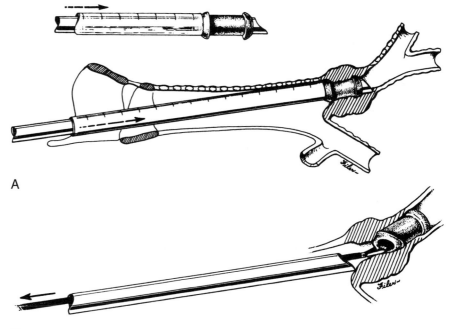

Figure 1
A and **B**, Rigid bronchoscopy placement and repositioning of a Silastic endobronchial stent. (*Reprinted with permission from Sonett JR, et al: Ann Thorac Surg 59:1417, 1995.*)

A

B

Silastic stents have the disadvantages of frequent migration and a mucous impaction due to small internal diameter-to-external diameter ratio.

Expandable metal stents have improved markedly the ease of insertion of endobronchial stents. The expandable nature of the stents has made them less prone to migration and mucous plugging (improved diameter-to-external diameter ratio), and a wide variety of sizes has enabled placement in secondary bronchi and in the trachea. These stents can be placed in an awake patient with fiberoptic bronchoscopy or in the operating room with the patient under general anesthesia. Placement of the stents under general anesthesia is preferred so that simultaneous dilation, débridement, and adjustments to the stent location may be performed. Expandable metal stents should be used with great caution in benign disease and only as a last resort. In patients with benign airway disease, granulation tissue, and subsequent stricture in response to the stent may be as debilitating as the original pathologic condition.

■ RESULTS OF TREATMENT

The palliative and therapeutic benefits of interventional bronchoscopy and endobronchial therapy are an essential component in the care of the thoracic surgical patient. The use of the varying techniques and modalities should be tailored to each patient and his or her pathology. In malignant disease, immediate palliation of debilitating airway symptoms may be attained with little potential morbidity, making the use of these techniques valuable even in patients with terminal cancer. Palliation of airway symptoms for even a few months may offer valuable quality time to patients in their greatest time of need. A general algorithm for the use of endobronchial therapy in malignant disease is provided in Figure 2, and an algorithm for lung transplant patients is provided in Figure 3. The use of endobronchial stents in nonmalignant disease carries higher morbidity in regards to long-term complications; permanent metal stents in this population should be used only in carefully selected patients

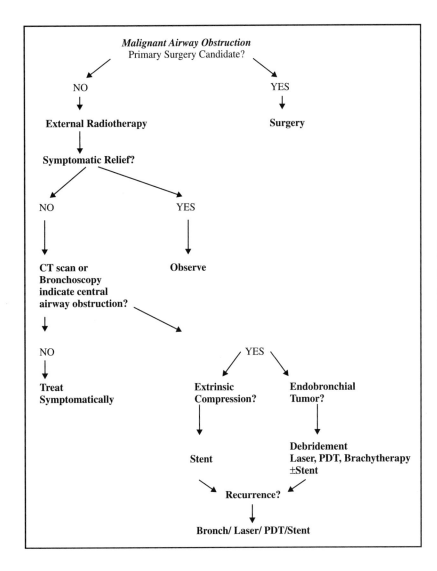

Figure 2
Treatment algorithm for patients with symptomatic malignant airway obstruction. CT, computed tomography; PDT, photodynamic therapy. (*From Sonett J:* Md Med J *47:260, 1998.*)

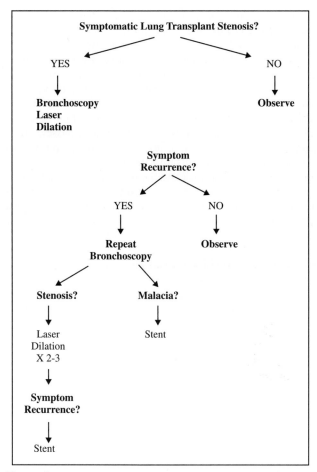

Figure 3
Algorithm for treatment of lung transplant stenosis/malacia.
(*From Sonett J:* Md Med J *47:260, 1998.*)

who have failed all other therapies, including dilation and the possible use of Silastic stents.

SELECTED READING

Golden AJ, et al: Bronchoscopy, lung biopsy, and other diagnostic procedures. In Murray JF, Nadel JA, editors: *Respiratory medicine,* Philadelphia, 1994, WB Saunders, p 711.

Keshavjee S, Ginsberg RJ: Rigid bronchoscopy. In Pearson FG, et al (eds): *Thoracic surgery,* New York, 1995, Churchill Livingstone, p 190.

Sonett JR: Endobronchial stents: primary and adjuvant therapy for endobronchial airway obstruction, *Md Med J* 47:260, 1998.

Sonett JR, et al: Endobronchial management of benign, malignant, and lung transplantation airway stenosis, *Ann Thorac Surg* 59:1417, 1995.

Sonett JR, et al: Removal and repositioning of "permanent" expandable wire stents in bronchial airway stenosis after lung transplantation, *J Heart Lung Transplant* 17:328, 1998.

ESOPHAGOSCOPY

Octavio E. Pajaro

Esophagoscopy is a diagnostic and therapeutic modality for the general and thoracic surgeon. Although endoscopy is performed most frequently by the gastroenterologist, the general surgeon needs to understand the indications, contraindications, risks, and therapeutic potential of the rigid and flexible procedures. Esophagoscopy is invaluable in the evaluation of esophageal pathology. Coupled with ultrasound guidance, esophagoscopy is required for the proper staging of esophageal cancer and has proved helpful in lung cancer staging and in evaluating some mediastinal tumors.

◼ ESOPHAGEAL ANATOMY

The esophagus is a muscular tube that begins at the distal margin of the cricopharyngeus muscle. This location corresponds to the level of the cricoid cartilage anteriorly and the space between the sixth and seventh cervical vertebrae posteriorly. The esophagus provides continuity of the posterior oropharynx with the stomach. Its inner circular and outer longitudinal muscle layers characterize the esophagus throughout its course. The average length of the esophagus is 25 cm from the cricopharyngeus muscle to the stomach.

The approximate distance from the upper incisors to the cricopharyngeus muscle is approximately 16 cm; to the aortic constriction, approximately 23 cm; and to the gastroesophageal junction, 40 cm.

■ INDICATIONS

The use of esophagoscopy should be considered every time one is evaluating abnormal esophageal symptoms, pathology, or radiographic findings; this includes dysphagia, reflux symptoms, gastrointestinal bleeding, odynophagia, upper abdominal pain, and persistent vomiting of unknown etiology. Pertinent radiographic abnormalities that should be evaluated with endoscopy include suspected neoplasm, esophageal or gastric ulcer, and upper gastrointestinal tract strictures or obstruction. Other less common findings that require endoscopy are chemical burns, thoracic trauma, esophageal perforation, fistulization with the airway, and Barrett's esophagus.

Flexible endoscopy also should be done at the beginning of every surgical esophageal procedure, not only as a powerful teaching tool, but also to verify pathologic findings or equivocal results if performed by another physician. In addition, it can help to plan alternative approaches and access response to preoperative therapy (e.g., induction chemoradiation therapy for cancer). It is useful to leave the endoscope in the esophagus during the operative procedure to help locate difficult lesions or when minimally invasive approaches are performed to avoid penetration of the mucosal layer (e.g., myotomy). In these latter cases, the esophagus can be insufflated under irrigation at the end of the procedure to check for mucosal defects.

Therapeutic indications for esophagoscopy include the dilation of strictures, the treatment of gastroesophageal varices, and the palliation of malignant esophageal obstruction using stents and laser therapy. The therapy of esophageal cancer with photodynamic therapy is actively being investigated.

The coupling of esophagoscopy with ultrasound (EUS) has widened the indications for esophagoscopy. The use of ultrasound allows for further characterization of tumors and paraesophageal lymph nodes. Leiomyomas, extramucosal tumors, and cysts can be differentiated with ultrasound techniques. Depth of invasion of esophageal cancers can be assessed accurately with EUS. Assessment of tumor depth, size of paraesophageal lymph nodes, and biopsy specimens of the mass itself and of the paraesophageal lymph nodes is required for preoperative staging of esophageal cancers. Biopsy specimens of precarinal lymph nodes and aortopulmonary window lymph nodes can be obtained in the evaluation of lung cancer. Other mediastinal tumors not originating from the lung or esophagus have been evaluated using EUS.

■ CHOICE OF INSTRUMENTS

The rigid esophagoscope compared with a flexible scope allows for larger biopsy specimens, better visibility in the event of any bleeding, and easier removal of foreign objects.

Rigid endoscopy does not allow for evaluation of the whole length of the esophagus. It is technically more difficult, has poorer visualization, and requires more anesthesia to perform.

Flexible esophagoscopy not only allows for better visualization and evaluation of the entire length of the esophagus, but also enables one to visualize the stomach and duodenum. The flexible esophagoscope is by far the most widely used technique and most commonly required for the evaluation of symptoms consistent with obstruction (masses, strictures) or gastroesophageal reflux. Esophagoscopy is essential for the evaluation of the total length of Barrett's esophagus because this may dictate the operative approach when planning a resection. After inspection of a mass or mucosal abnormality, biopsy specimens generally can be obtained if appropriate.

■ CONTRAINDICATIONS

Contraindications to performing esophagoscopy are rare. The main concern when performing an esophagoscopy is preventing a complication, such as causing a perforation or injuring the patient from the maneuvers required to pass the endoscope. Patients who have evidence of cervical instability, either from trauma or from degenerative diseases, would be at high risk during esophagoscopy. The presence of a perforation may dissuade one from endoscopy for fear of worsening the defect. Clinically unstable patients—from a hemodynamic standpoint or bleeding—and patients who cannot cooperate even with sedation should not undergo the procedure. Early esophagoscopy after a surgical anastomosis (<4 weeks) also would be considered high risk.

■ TECHNIQUE

In most cases for flexible esophagoscopy, topical and light intravenous sedation is required, generally not as deep as that used for bronchoscopy. Continuous monitoring of electrocardiogram, blood pressure, and oximetry is mandatory. In addition to supplemental oxygen, intubation and defibrillation should be readily available. Patients are placed in the left lateral decubitus position. The scope is inserted with the greatest bend aimed toward the anterior position, to allow for proper orientation while doing the procedure. Extreme care is taken to cannulate the esophagus and not to force the end to avoid accidental perforation. Semiconscious patients are asked to swallow. If the vocal cords are seen, gentle insufflation is performed to help visualize the cricopharyngeus orifice. As the scope is passed into the esophagus, one should be cognizant of the distance marker at the incisors so that standard intraluminal landmarks or abnormal pathology can be noted. After briefly inspecting the stomach and duodenum, the end of the scope is retroflexed to visualize adequately the distal side of the esophagogastric junction and the cardia. Then the scope is gently withdrawn, the stomach is suctioned to aspirate as much air as possible, and the esophagus is inspected carefully again verifying the distance from the incisors of any abnormalities.

For rigid endoscopy, general anesthesia usually is required, sometimes in the operating room. In the supine position, a roll is placed behind the shoulders to help hyperextend the neck. Care is taken during the entire procedure to protect the teeth, especially incisors, from injury; rubber guards for the upper teeth should be placed. With the dominant hand inserting the scope, the index finger on the other should be between the scope and upper incisors at all times, while the thumb pushes the scope upward (anterior) to avoid trauma. As with the flexible scope approach, the esophagus is cannulated carefully, but in this instance, the cricopharyngeus always is visualized directly before advancing the scope. Because insufflation of the esophagus is not possible, the scope should be advanced more slowly than with the flexible approach. Long-tipped suction and grasping devices should be readily available. If the scope is being used for dilation, a wire or other long passer should be used to identify the true orifice.

■ COMPLICATIONS

The risk of esophageal perforation from esophagoscopy has become low (0.1% to 0.2%) with the use of flexible scopes, but perforation still is encountered more commonly with the rigid technique. The site of perforation is at the most narrow regions—in the normal esophagus at the cricopharyngeus, at the aortic knob, or above the esophagogastric junction—or at benign or malignant strictures.

Repeated esophagoscopies can be performed even in irradiated patients with a low incidence of complications. Early diagnosis and prompt appropriate treatment need to be instituted the moment a perforation occurs. Early on, symptoms of this highly dreaded complication can be mild and nonspecific, but they can progress rapidly to obvious signs, including pain, fever, cardiovascular collapse, sepsis, pleural effusions, pneumothorax, pneumomediastinum, and palpable subcutaneous emphysema.

■ SUMMARY

The diagnostic role of esophagoscopy lies in its ability to visualize the entire length of the esophageal mucosa, stomach, and duodenum and in its ability as EUS to evaluate the depth and character of esophageal masses, allowing accurate biopsy of mediastinal and esophageal masses and lymph nodes. The therapeutic role of esophagoscopy rests on the ability to address strictures and obstructions with dilations, stents, and lasers. Coupled with photodynamic therapy, there is hope potentially to treat esophageal cancers. Complications are rare. Esophagoscopy plays no role in the evaluation of esophageal function.

SUGGESTED READING

Ackroyd R, et al: Photodynamic therapy for dysplastic Barrett's oesophagus: a prospective, double blind, randomised, placebo controlled trial, *Gut* 47:612, 2000.

Barr H, et al: Review article: the potential role for photodynamic therapy in the management of upper gastrointestinal disease, *Aliment Pharmacol Ther* 15:311, 2001.

McGarrity TJ, et al: Apoptosis associated with esophageal adenocarcinoma: influence of photodynamic therapy, *Cancer Lett* 163:33, 2001.

Wax MK, et al: Safety of esophagoscopy in the irradiated esophagus, *Ann Otol Rhinol Laryngol* 106:297, 1997.

MEDIASTINOSCOPY AND MEDIASTINOTOMY

Ronald B. Ponn

Surgical assessment of the mediastinum is probably the most common operating room procedure performed by general thoracic surgeons. Although the usual indication for mediastinoscopy and mediastinotomy derives from the importance of nodal status on lung cancer prognosis and treatment, the procedures also are useful for diagnosing other neoplastic, granulomatous, and miscellaneous causes of lymphadenopathy or anterior mediastinal mass. In addition to its use as a diagnostic modality, mediastinoscopy can be used to assess tracheal or mediastinal invasion by the neoplastic processes. Endoscopic examination of the upper mediastinum was described about 50 years ago, originally via a scalene incision and later by a midline low cervical approach. The mediastinoscopes commonly used today are hollow, beveled metal tubes with distal illumination and lateral slits for instrumentation.

■ MEDIASTINOSCOPY

Cervical mediastinoscopy provides access to the superior mediastinum in the region of the trachea, including the left and right paratracheal and subcarinal lymph nodes. Assessment of neoplastic invasion or encasement of the airway and blood vessels also is possible.

Indications and Contraindications

Although mediastinoscopy may be useful for diagnosing any superior mediastinal adenopathy or mass, whether neoplastic, granulomatous, infectious, or inflammatory, it is applied most commonly for staging the N (node) factor in cases of known or suspected lung cancer. Pulmonary resection after documentation of mediastinal (N2) disease is associated with poor long-term survival. Most surgeons do not recommend resection as primary therapy in patients with clinical N2 disease. The role of resection after induction therapy in this group is under investigation. With a negative predictive value of greater than 90%, mediastinoscopy is more reliable than current noninvasive means for identifying patients who are likely to benefit from thoracotomy as the next step in their treatment.

The reported accuracy of computed tomography (CT) varies widely. As the threshold for defining radiographic adenopathy has been lowered over time to 1 cm, sensitivity has increased at the cost of specificity. Of enlarged nodes on CT, 20% to 40% are benign, due to reaction to postobstructive pneumonia or an unrelated process. The role of positron emission tomography (PET) using glucose analogues to assess metabolic activity as a marker of neoplasm seems promising but has not yet achieved sufficient accuracy that positive mediastinal foci reliably can be considered malignant in all cases. There is general agreement that biopsy of nodes that are enlarged by CT criteria or are positive on PET is indicated in otherwise resectable cases. In contrast, surgeons vary in their application of mediastinoscopy in patients with nodes of normal size. Proponents of routine mediastinoscopy stress that tumor metastases often are found in nodes that are not enlarged and that even in cases of peripheral cancers with a normal mediastinum by CT scan the yield of surgical biopsy can be 10%. Others use mediastinoscopy selectively. Common indications include the presence of a central primary tumor, a peripheral tumor with chest wall invasion, the potential need for a pneumonectomy, and the presence of enlarged N1 nodes.

In general, the safety and potential yield of mediastinoscopy make it prudent to have a low threshold for including it as part of the evaluation of the lung cancer patient. If a decision is made to bypass mediastinal biopsy, it must be based on a high-quality CT scan, interpreted in collaboration with an experienced thoracic radiologist, and a negative PET scan, if available. At the extreme positive end of the radiographic spectrum, it is often reasonable to accept clinical N2 staging without tissue in the presence of obvious massive, confluent adenopathy or invasion that is not consistent with any benign process.

Contraindications are few. Patients who have permanent tracheostomies after laryngectomy are not candidates for cervical mediastinoscopy. A large goiter or extensive calcification or aneurysm of the aortic arch or innominate artery may make the procedure hazardous. Previous sternotomy also mistakenly is considered a contraindication, unless significant mediastinitis occurred during the initial operation. Prior thyroidectomy may obscure the midline but is not associated with any particular hazards because the pretracheal fascia was not entered. In cases of prior mediastinoscopy, adhesions are usually present, most importantly between the trachea and the innominate artery. Nonetheless, redo mediastinoscopy has been shown to be safe. Superior vena cava obstruction is another situation in which mediastinoscopy requires extra care but remains feasible. In this setting, the most troublesome bleeding is usually from superficial veins rather than the vertically oriented deeper veins that can be avoided by keeping to the midline. In addition, with superior vena cava syndrome cases, diagnostic tissue often can be obtained from a high paratracheal site, obviating the need for significant dissection.

Technique

In most instances, mediastinoscopy is performed as an outpatient procedure. Because of the small but real potential for bleeding, it is prudent to limit the venue to hospital-based units rather than free-standing ambulatory facilities. Alternatively, some surgeons prefer to proceed directly to thoracotomy at the same session when mediastinal evaluation is negative. Mediastinoscopy is performed under general anesthesia. The patient is positioned with the occiput of the head at the top of the operating table, the neck is extended with an interscapular roll, and the back of the table is elevated 20 to 30 degrees. Care should be taken to position the endotracheal tube so that it is not in the way of the scope. Preparation and draping include the anterior chest for possible sternotomy, but this area is not shaved. Circulation to the right arm is monitored with a radial artery cannula or a pulse oximeter because a dampened waveform may indicate innominate artery compression and decreased right carotid perfusion.

A 3- to 4-cm incision is made between the sternocleidomastoid muscles about 2 cm above the sternal notch and carried through the platysma. The midline is opened vertically between the two layers of strap muscles down to the trachea. Occasionally the thyroid isthmus must be retracted cephalad to provide access to the trachea and in rare instances divided and oversewn. The thyroidea ima artery or branches of the inferior thyroid vein rarely must be ligated. It is essential to assess the area just above the sternal notch during this dissection because the innominate artery may be drawn up into the neck by cervical extension (especially in young persons) and be subject to injury.

When an adequate area of trachea is exposed, the pretracheal fascia is incised and elevated. A pretracheal tunnel is fashioned by blunt dissection with the index finger. During palpation and later visualization, mediastinoscopy should be thought of as a "tracheocentric" procedure (i.e., anatomic location is defined at all times by the relationship of the finger, the endoscope, and the dissecting instruments to the trachea). Fibrous bands sometimes are encountered between the trachea and fascia, especially at the level of the innominate artery. Thereafter a gentle side-to-side sweeping motion during digital advancement suffices to clear the pretracheal and paratracheal spaces. The dorsal aspect of the finger senses the tracheal rings during passage, while the volar aspect identifies the innominate artery anteriorly. More distally, one palpates the aortic arch, the lymph node–bearing areas, and often the carina and proximal main stem bronchi (Figure 1). During this dissection, the surgeon forms a mental image of any lymphadenopathy, mass, or invasion in relation to the normal structures of the upper mediastinum.

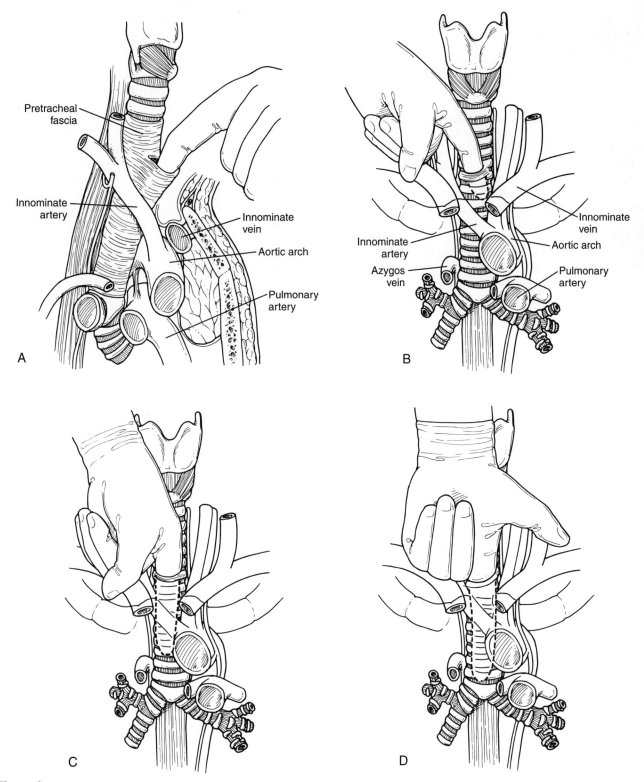

Figure 1

Development of the pretracheal tunnel and identification of landmarks and pathologic involvement. Oblique **(A)** and anterior **(B)** views of the dissecting finger entering the pretracheal space and palpating the innominate artery. **C,** Beyond the artery, the tunnel is extended by distal progression and lateral sweeping. **D,** Finger fully inserted and palpating the aortic arch, nodes, and sometimes the carina and proximal bronchi. (*From Ponn RB, Federico JA: Mediastinoscopy and staging. In Kaiser LR, et al, editors:* Mastery of cardiothoracic surgery, *Philadelphia, 1998, Lippincott-Williams & Wilkins, p 18; with permission.*)

To access the nodes, the pretracheal fascia must be penetrated. This can be done digitally now or later via the mediastinoscope. Enlarged right paratracheal nodes are often subject to easy freeing by looping the finger around the innominate artery and bluntly dissecting the nodes against the chest wall.

The mediastinoscope is introduced into the pretracheal tunnel. The scope should be advanced only if a tunnel is visible and the device passes easily. Blunt dissection is performed using a metal or disposable plastic suction-cautery device. If the extrafascial space has not been entered by finger dissection, it is opened using the sucker. This is accomplished best in the mid to low pretracheal region by angling the end of the scope anteriorly to tent up the pretracheal fascia (Figure 2). The mediastinum is inspected before any biopsy specimens are taken. One should try to identify the azygos vein, the tracheal bifurcation, the proximal main stem bronchi, and the pulmonary artery. When these landmarks are noted, lymph nodes in the right and left paratracheal and subcarinal regions are sought. Nodes are identified by color and consistency, location with respect to anatomic structures, and the map generated by palpation. All target nodes are partially dissected free before any biopsy specimens are taken to prevent minor bleeding from obscuring the field. Because the color of vascular structures can be similar to lymph nodes, aspiration with a long needle is carried out before biopsy if there is any doubt. Nodes are dissected with the suction-cautery. When sufficiently separated from surrounding tissue, the node is grasped with a large cupped laryngeal forceps or similar instrument, and traction is applied under direct vision. If the sample cannot be delivered by gentle pulling and twisting, further dissection is indicated. It may be helpful to introduce a second dissector or forceps to divide tethering attachments while traction is maintained on the node by the first forceps. Alternatively, further dissection may be achieved by removing

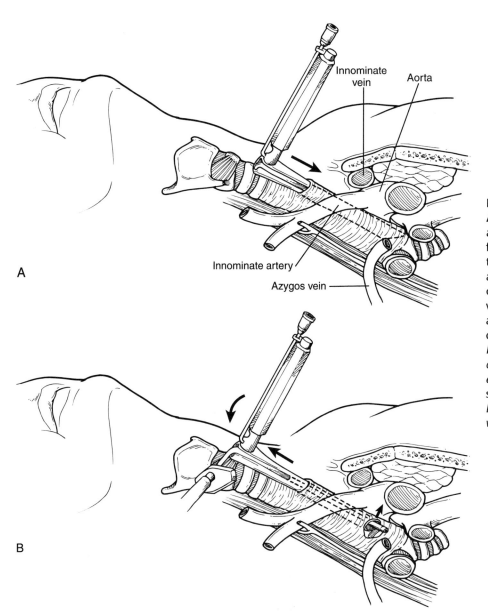

Innominate vein

Aorta

Innominate artery

Azygos vein

A

B

Figure 2
A, The passive angle of the mediastinoscope within the pretracheal fascia aims the bevel directly at the trachea. **B**, The scope must be angled anteriorly to tense the fascia so that it can be penetrated with the sucker. The innominate artery is subject to compression during this maneuver. (*From Ponn RB, Federico JA: Mediastinoscopy and staging. In Kaiser LR, et al, editors:* Mastery of cardiothoracic surgery, *Philadelphia, 1998, Lippincott-Williams & Wilkins, p 20; with permission.*)

the scope and reintroducing the index finger. The actual biopsy specimen is always taken through the scope under direct vision. Although it is preferable to remove an entire lymph node, large size, friability, or adherence often limits the biopsy to an incisional sample taken with the laryngeal forceps.

The extent of biopsy specimens depends on the clinical situation and operative findings. In rare instances of a completely solidified mediastinum that makes anatomic definition impossible, needle aspiration for cytology or a core biopsy taken by cutting needle may provide a diagnosis. In most cases, however, it is possible to obtain substantial lymph node samples. In sarcoidosis, lymphoma, or mediastinal mass, all that is needed is diagnostic tissue from a single site. For staging lung cancer, in contrast, it is preferable to sample more than one level. Nodes are taken from the high and low right paratracheal, subcarinal, and left paratracheal areas (levels 2R, 4R, 7L, and 4L). Level 4L nodes are sometimes difficult to find, and in some cases it is prudent not to dissect aggressively to avoid injury to the left recurrent laryngeal nerve. Also, if there is obvious tumor at a high level or a site contralateral to the primary tumor, other nodes need not be accessed because staging would not be affected. In general, however, it is more expedient to sample all levels rather than to wait for frozen section confirmation.

The operative sites are inspected for bleeding. The mediastinoscope is withdrawn slowly because its presence can perpetuate bleeding by keeping the tunnel open, preventing tissue coaptation, or can tamponade lateral bleeders. Most bleeding is minor and can be controlled by packing with oxidized cellulose. If there is bleeding from a visible small vessel, metal clips can be applied, most often for bronchial artery branches in the subcarinal space. When cautery is used at any point during mediastinoscopy, it should be applied directly to the bleeding site and at low wattage to prevent thermal injury to vital structures. For closure, the strap muscles are reapproximated to the midline with a single absorbable suture, and the skin is closed with a subcuticular suture. Ridge formation is lessened if the platysma is not closed separately. The patient usually is discharged after a period of standard postoperative observation. Unless there is suspicion or indication of a problem, routine chest film and laboratory studies are unnecessary, although pneumothorax is a rare complication.

Variations of cervical mediastinoscopy allow access to areas not reached by the standard pretracheal procedure. *Extended cervical mediastinoscopy* adds the subaortic and anterior mediastinal regions (levels 5 and 6). Digital dissection is carried out anterior to the aortic arch in the space between the innominate and left common carotid arteries. After palpation, the mediastinoscope is passed, and samples of lymph nodes or mass are taken as in the standard operation. This approach is used mostly in conjunction with pretracheal mediastinoscopy for the assessment of left upper lobe lung cancers. In *mediastinopleuroscopy*, the pleural space is entered intentionally—posterior to the innominate artery on the right or between the carotid and subclavian arteries on the left. This approach allows assessment of the upper pleural space, pleural fluid sampling, and sometimes lung biopsy in addition to the usual access to the upper mediastinum and is used most commonly for lung cancer diagnosis and staging.

Complications

In experienced hands, mediastinoscopy is associated with a low operative risk. Mortality varies from none to 0.08% in large series, whereas complications are noted in about 3%, but only 0.5% are major. The most feared problem and the source of most deaths is bleeding from one of the large vessels subject to injury in the upper mediastinum—the aorta and its branches, the azygos vein, superior vena cava, and pulmonary artery. Tight packing of the tunnel with gauze sponges or oxidized cellulose controls most bleeding, at least temporarily. If open repair is needed, the approach—sternotomy or thoracotomy—is based on the location of the injury, the resectability and location of the tumor, and the patient's hemodynamic status. Although a sternotomy is faster and does not require repositioning, thoracotomy is acceptable if the surgeon believes that rapid vascular control and tumor resection can be achieved. In either case, placement of a double-lumen endotracheal tube facilitates the operation greatly.

Nonvascular major structures that can be injured include the tracheobronchial tree, the esophagus, and important nerves. Treatment of airway or esophageal perforation depends largely on whether the diagnosis is made early or only after complications have appeared. Recurrent nerve paralysis may be permanent or temporary. Pneumothorax can occur from pleural puncture but is under tension only if there is a pulmonary parenchymal injury and insufficient pleural venting. Rare complications include phrenic nerve injury, thoracic duct injury, mediastinitis, venous air embolism, stroke, tumor implantation, and mediastinal lymph node necrosis.

■ ANTERIOR MEDIASTINOTOMY

Anterior or parasternal mediastinotomy provides access to the subaortic and anterior mediastinal nodes (levels 5 and 6) on the left and to anterior mediastinal masses, the upper anterior hilar structures, and portions of the upper lobes and pleura on both sides. The standard Chamberlain procedure often is replaced by anterior mediastinoscopy, an examination using a mediastinoscope passed through a small parasternal intercostal incision.

Indications and Contraindications

Cancer of the left upper lobe is the most common indication. Tumors in this location can drain to the superior mediastinal stations and levels 5 and 6. Anterior mediastinotomy often is planned in combination with cervical mediastinoscopy and performed if findings are negative in the superior mediastinum. There is evidence that fully resected left upper lobe cancers with N2 disease confined to the subaortic region have a surgical 5-year survival of 25% to 30%—more than three times that of other N2. Most surgeons perform surgical biopsy of these nodes only when there is radiographic lymphadenopathy. If one practices routine mediastinoscopy, however, the pattern of drainage noted indicates that cervical mediastinoscopy be performed for left upper lobe tumors. In addition to nodal staging, anterior mediastinotomy is useful for assessment of direct neoplastic invasion of the mediastinum and upper anterior hilum, including the proximal left pulmonary artery and superior vein. It also is an ideal procedure for biopsy of many anterior mediastinal masses, such as lymphoma, thymoma, and germ cell tumors. In some cases, hilar masses and upper lobe pulmonary lesions can be approached via this route.

Prior sternotomy, usually for cardiac procedures, is not a contraindication but warrants caution. The presence of an internal mammary artery bypass graft may make deep biopsy of subaortic nodes hazardous because the course of the graft is usually anterior to the hilum. Biopsy of large masses that abut the anterior parasternal chest wall does not endanger the graft, however.

Technique

Mediastinotomy generally is performed as an outpatient procedure. A double-lumen endotracheal tube is not essential but may be helpful, especially for examination of pathology that does not reach the chest wall. A transverse incision is made lateral to the sternum at the second or third costal level, and the pectoralis fibers are split to expose the cartilage. In the classic Chamberlain procedure, the cartilage is resected subperichondrially. The internal mammary vessels are best avoided but may be ligated. The pleura is dissected away from the mediastinum. Large anterior tumors are identified and biopsy specimens are obtained at this point. For deeper assessment of the subaortic and anterior hilar areas, combined digital dissection and direct vision extend access inward until the aorta, pulmonary artery, and intervening space are identified. As in cervical mediastinoscopy, a mental image of the anatomy and pathology is formulated. Enlarged nodes or areas of tumor invasion are sampled by incisional or excisional biopsy as in cervical mediastinoscopy, with prior needle aspiration used if needed to differentiate a vascular from a solid structure. It is often helpful to open the pleura and obtain specimens from either or both the mediastinal or pleural sides. When anterior mediastinotomy is performed in conjunction with cervical mediastinoscopy, the neck incision usually is left open during the latter procedure to allow bidigital palpation of the upper hilar and subaortic regions to assess for fixation and invasion. Drainage usually is not needed. If the pleura was entered, air is evacuated during a Valsalva inspiration through a small tube that is then withdrawn. If the lung has been biopsied, a small tube can be left in place and connected to standard pleural suction or a Heimlich valve.

In most cases, the standard Chamberlain procedure described previously can be modified by eliminating costal cartilage resection and proceeding via a second interspace incision. This approach is especially easy with large mediastinal masses. For deeper evaluation, a small intercostal incision followed by placement of a short mediastinoscope is currently the favored approach.

Complications

Mortality is rare. Bleeding from major local vessels is possible and should be handled in a manner similar to that described for mediastinoscopy—initial packing and open control if needed. Pneumothorax is treated according to its severity. Diaphragmatic paralysis or hoarseness occurs rarely from damage to the phrenic or recurrent laryngeal nerve. Chylothorax has been reported. Tumor implantation in the incision can occur, more commonly with large lymphomas or germ cell tumors than with lung cancers.

■ NOTE ON ALTERNATIVE PROCEDURES

Although surgical biopsy of the mediastinum is a safe and valuable means of diagnosing abnormalities and staging lung cancer, other approaches may be equally useful and indicated in some cases. These include transcarinal/transbronchial needle aspiration during bronchoscopy, transthoracic mediastinal or hilar aspiration or core biopsy, endoscopic (transbronchial or transesophageal) ultrasound–guided needle aspiration, and videothoracoscopic evaluation. Although the scope of this chapter precludes discussion of these modalities, thoracic surgeons should be familiar with the advantages and limitations of these techniques and apply them as indicated by the nature of individual cases and the availability of local expertise.

SUGGESTED READING

Ginsberg RJ: The role of preoperative surgical staging in left upper lobe tumors, *Ann Thorac Surg* 57:526, 1994.

Ponn RB, Federico JA: Mediastinoscopy and staging. In Kaiser LR, et al, editors: *Mastery of cardiothoracic surgery*, Philadelphia, Lippincott-Williams & Wilkins, 1998, p 11.

Puhakka HJ: Complications of mediastinoscopy, *J Laryngol Otol* 103:312, 1989.

Shields T: The significance of ipsilateral mediastinal lymph node metastasis (N2 disease) in non-small cell carcinoma of the lung, *J Thorac Cardiovasc Surg* 99:48, 1990.

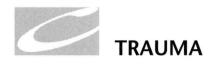

TRAUMA

PNEUMOMEDIASTINUM

Kemp Kernstine

The presence of pneumomediastinum implies that there is or has been a breech of an air-containing mediastinal structure. Air, saliva, gastric secretions, bile, ingested food, and drink all are noxious agents that can contaminate the mediastinum. To maintain hemostasis, the mediastinum is replete with lymphatics that drain and contain acute perforations. Inflammation that results from the perforation, especially the edema, may contain a perforation. The rate of the inflammatory process varies significantly and depends on the age of the patient; the patient's immune and nutritional status; and associated comorbid factors, such as cancer, steroids, diabetes, and other chronic illnesses. Pneumomediastinum may be a stable incidental finding on a radiographic study or may be a progressively worsening clinical finding resulting in hemodynamic collapse. In either case, there must be a positive pressure source of air through a defect in the mediastinal structure, peritoneal cavity, neck or head, and face for it to occur. If the finding continues to worsen, either a "ball-valve" mechanism or continuous positive airflow source is present that produces sufficient air pressure into the mediastinum that overcomes the normal adherence of the mediastinal planes. Clinical suspicion gained from clinical data and invasive and noninvasive tests may help to determine the location and size of the perforation and help determine the manner of treatment. Time is crucial because as the edema worsens, healthy tissues are destroyed by the inflammation and violaceous material.

Air in the mediastinal tissues may originate from the respiratory tract, such as after trauma to the facial bones, larynx, hypopharynx, trachea, and main stem bronchi. Dental procedures that use compressed air to clear surgical debris may result in facial and neck subcutaneous emphysema and pneumomediastinum; similar situations may occur using compressed-air surgical machinery even when performing peripheral extremity surgery. Rigid bronchoscopy, especially endobronchial tumor "coring" procedures and laser bronchoscopy, may cause airway perforation. Severe straining or Valsalva maneuver, such as with weight lifting, or sudden impact to the chest from trauma or sports may cause severe damage to the alveolus, main bronchi, and airway subdivisions; this also can result in complete bronchial disruption.

This disruption has been described in children with severe croup. Airway obstruction from foreign body, tumor, or extrinsic compression from inflamed peribronchial nodal tissue may result in air trapping and eventual alveolar rupture. Barotrauma may occur with scuba diving and flying in nonpressurized planes. Alveolar trauma also may occur from mechanical ventilation with excessive airway peak and mean airway pressure and excessive lung volumes. Air released from the ruptured alveolus dissects toward the mediastinum along the vascular structures and planes surrounding them.

Mediastinal air also may originate from the esophagus. Iatrogenic injury accounts for 65% to 70% of perforation cases. Other causes include Boerhaave's syndrome, esophageal apoplexy or effort-induced esophageal damage, and spontaneous rupture of esophageal tumors. Effort-induced esophageal perforations may occur with straining during defecation, childbirth, and seizures. Pneumomediastinum more frequently occurs after cervical esophageal perforations than after thoracic or abdominal esophageal damage. The stomach and small and large bowel that herniate into the mediastinum may strangulate and leak their contents into the mediastinum.

Peritoneal air may enter the mediastinum through the esophageal hiatus and the foramen of Morgagni. Carbon dioxide insufflation used during laparoscopic surgery may result in mediastinal emphysema but rarely has any untoward effects. Forced air entering the vagina or through a rectal perforation also may enter the mediastinum.

Gas-forming bacteria resulting in descending necrotizing or acute bacterial mediastinitis may cause pneumomediastinum. Frequently, patients have had prior surgery, trauma, or infections of the oropharynx, mediastinum, or chest. Nonpathologic mediastinal emphysema may be present on the chest radiograph after surgery or trauma but usually resolves in 2 to 7 days. Nonpathologic mediastinal air is seen in more than 10% of patients after tracheostomy.

Diagnostic testing may misdirect the clinician or delay therapy, putting the patient at greater risk for complications and death. What are the appropriate means to evaluate patients given the different situations? What tests should be performed and when? Finally, what surgical means are necessary to repair the damage?

■ HISTORY

Spontaneous or effort-induced pneumomediastinum (Hamman's syndrome) usually occurs in young males, frequently adolescents. Rarely, it may occur in infants with respiratory distress, children with asthma, or children after strenuous play. Nearly half of all childhood pneumothoraces, pneumomediastinum, and pneumopericardium are associated with asthma, and one quarter of patients will have or have had pneumonia. In adults, straining against a closed glottis, such as during weight lifting, mountain climbing, contact sports, and blunt chest trauma, may result in pneumomediastinum. Mediastinal air may occur with sudden increases in lung volume with inhaled recreational drug use, such as smoking marijuana or crack cocaine. It also has been reported in cases after use of ecstasy, "speed," and heroin, although the mechanism is unclear. Patients who have interstitial lung disease such as that associated with pulmonary fibrosis, bleomycin-induced lung disease, and dermatomyositis may be more prone to development of mediastinal air. Mediastinal emphysema after paraquat ingestion is almost universally fatal.

Mediastinal emphysema can result in substernal pleuritic chest pain that may radiate to the neck or to the back, dyspnea, or cough. Patients with diabetic ketoacidosis may develop pneumomediastinum of respiratory or, less frequently, esophageal origin. It may be associated with a low-grade fever and a mildly elevated white blood count. The patients are rarely severely ill but can have hemodynamic instability. In children and especially infants, the immaturity of the fascial planes allows dissection into the pericardium, resulting in pneumopericardium, and into the anterior mediastinum, elevating the thymus on the lateral chest radiograph, the "sail" sign.

More severe injuries worthy of rapid diagnostic evaluation usually are associated with a severe antecedent event. Severe straining with emesis, dysphagia, chills, odynophagia, pain in the floor of the mouth after dental or head and neck surgery, recently aspirated food, recent pneumonia, or recent asthmatic attack may result in acute mediastinal emphysema. Ventilator-dependent patients with higher airway pressures with possibly a prior history of emphysema or increased peak and mean airway pressure may develop pneumomediastinum. The pyriform sinus, trachea, or proximal bronchia may be perforated after trauma or instrumentation (e.g., from intubation) and may develop mediastinal and subcutaneous emphysema. Other iatrogenic causes include esophageal instrumentation with rigid esophagoscopy and dilation (especially pneumatic); sclerosing varices; stent placement; nasogastric, Cantor, and Sengstaken-Blakemore tubes; salivary bypass tubes; and esophagoscopy, especially in patients with cervical osteoarthritis.

■ PHYSICAL EXAMINATION

Physical findings may help to identify the location of and response to the mediastinal violation. Possible findings include anxiety, somnolence, and confusion; elevated or significantly depressed body temperature; hypotension; tachycardia; tachypnea; and palpable or visible subcutaneous air in the neck, chest, and face that may progress across the torso, pubis, and extremities. The pitch of the voice may be a high, nasal quality from air dissecting into the paranasal sinuses and posterior mediastinal fascial planes. Pneumothorax and hydrothorax may result in deviation of the mediastinal structures and the trachea. Asthma has been associated with pneumomediastinum, but wheezing may occur as a result of the inflammatory response as well. Breath sounds may be absent owing to the presence of a pneumothorax or pleural fluid collections, from a perforated viscus, hemothorax, or empyema. Along with wheezing, rales, and rhonchi may be a sign of severe inflammation, which implies that a delay has occurred to the time of presentation. "Hamman's crunch" (crepitant sound heard at auscultation that varies with heartbeat) results from air/inflammation within or outside the pericardium. Ecchymosis, masses, and erythema may be present on the face, neck, or torso. There may be peritoneal signs in cases in which there is peritoneal contamination or abdominal distention of intraperitoneal air. Typically the history and physical examination are sufficient to determine the mechanism and timing of the injury and the patient's physiologic response.

■ DIAGNOSTIC TESTS

The best tests to evaluate pneumomediastinum are tests that rapidly help to determine the location and size of the perforation, estimate the degree of contamination, and help the clinician to develop a plan of treatment. A chest radiograph defines the findings and may identify a pneumothorax, degree of pneumomediastinum, presence of air-fluid levels in the mediastinum, and fluid, and potentially loculations in the pleural space. Air frequently is seen streaking along the left heart border and in some cases free peritoneal air. Air at the junction of the diaphragm and left heart "V" sign frequently is associated with Boerhaave's syndrome. Patients who present with spontaneous pneumothorax should have repeated chest radiographs to follow the course and potential development of pneumothorax that might be unrecognized initially and potentially progress toward tension. Repeated chest radiographs may be necessary to follow the course of the mediastinal emphysema, especially in a patient who is mechanically ventilated or who has severe pulmonary compromise.

Computed tomography (CT) of the neck, chest, and as necessary the abdomen may verify the presence of air and fluid contamination and help to identify the source of mediastinal air. CT contrast with oral dilute barium should be used judiciously. Barium in the mediastinum does not appear to increase the mortality or morbidity, but it can cause a chronic granulomatous reaction and may reduce the radiologic visibility for later contrast studies.

When oropharyngeal, tracheal, or upper esophageal perforation is suspected, triple endoscopy (laryngoscopy, bronchoscopy, and esophagoscopy) is used to evaluate and characterize the damage and to plan therapy. Laryngopharyngoscopy is safe to perform in suspected injuries of the head and neck region. Bronchoscopy is mandatory. The area of airway damage may be hemorrhagic, ecchymotic, or edematous. Esophageal endoscopy to visualize adequately a potential perforation requires air insufflation that may worsen the air-fluid contamination of the mediastinum and potentially may increase the size of the perforation. The sensitivity of esophagogastroscopy is poor compared with other potential tests. In trauma cases, esophagoscopy misses 15% to 30% of the perforations. We use esophagoscopy intraoperatively to identify better the injury and its relationship to the inflamed mediastinal tissues. Usually the scope can be palpated even through the most inflamed mediastinal tissue, with the lighted tip helping to identify the location of the perforation. Using it in this fashion, esophagoscopy does not delay the treatment or worsen the injury.

Contrast-enhanced fluoroscopy of the pharynx, esophagogastric region, or airways may help to define the injury better. This is our modality of choice for identifying the source of mediastinal air when the pharynx, esophagus, or stomach is thought to be the source. Diatrizoate meglumine (Gastrografin) is water-soluble and may be diluted by enteric contents and may not identify the perforation, especially in more distal locations, such as the stomach and duodenum. One disadvantage of diatrizoate meglumine is that if it is aspirated, acute respiratory distress syndrome may result. To avoid this, we introduce diatrizoate meglumine in relatively small amounts through a fluoroscopically placed nasoenteric tube to evaluate for and locate the perforation. If no leak is identified under gravity filling of the enteric tube, forceful infusion and esophageal distention may help to identify the damage better. If no leak is found, the nasoenteric tube is removed, and the patient is given thin barium to swallow. If no leak is found with thin barium study, thicker consistency barium is used. Thick barium better delineates small mucosal tears. If no leak is found on the barium study, there is still a 5% to 10% risk that a perforation is present. When the clinical suspicion remains high, to allow for potential esophageal spasm to subside, a repeat thin barium study is performed in 12 to 24 hours. The repeat study should reduce the likelihood of a missed perforation to less than 1% to 2%.

■ TREATMENT

Spontaneous pneumomediastinum usually resolves promptly. If wheezing or pneumonia is present, it should be treated. The patient should rest, be provided with adequate analgesics, and be monitored clinically. Patients without a history of emesis or straining may be observed as an outpatient, depending on the degree of their chronic illness and potential debility associated with the pneumomediastinum. Supplemental oxygen to speed the resolution of the pneumomediastinum has been used, but there is no proven benefit. There is no evidence that prophylactic antibiotics are of any benefit. If there is any question of esophageal perforation, however, an esophagogram should be performed. On repeated chest radiographs, if the pneumomediastinum worsens or pneumothorax develops, chest tube thoracostomy may be necessary. CT or bronchoscopy may be necessary to identify the presence and location of damage. Especially in children, the occurrence of pneumomediastinum may identify patients with asthma and warrant pulmonary function testing at a later time.

Pneumomediastinum in a mechanically ventilated patient may result in tension pneumothorax and severe hemodynamic compromise. When found, repeated chest radiographs should be performed to follow the process. Equipment for emergent chest tube placement should be immediately available. If a pneumothorax is present, even if small, a chest tube should be placed. The airway pressure (peak and mean) should be minimized and the tidal volume reduced. The patient should be sedated and treated for bronchospasm. Auto-positive end-expiratory pressure should be avoided and routinely evaluated. The patient should be weaned from positive pressure and extubated as soon as medically possible.

When patients are undergoing evaluation for pneumomediastinum, they should remain NPO (take nothing by mouth), antibiotics should be initiated to treat potential pathogens, and the patient should be intravenously hydrated. Nasogastric drainage may be necessary to reduce ongoing soilage while the evaluation is being performed. If there is suspicion of a pharyngoesophageal or gastric perforation, the nasogastric tube should be placed fluoroscopically to reduce the likelihood of further damage from tube placement. If a clinically significant perforation is found and appropriate testing is completed, the patient should be hemodynamically stabilized and prepared for the operating room. The following principles should guide the operating surgeon: (1) Stop ongoing contamination by closure of the perforation or, in the case of severe or chronic esophageal perforation, diversion of the enteric contents. (2) Drain the contamination and any inflammatory fluid. (3) Débride the devitalized tissues surgically or by forceful irrigation. We combine antibiotics and forceful irrigation to assist in treating the local bacterial contamination. (4) Correct any distal obstruction. (5) Plan for postoperative nutritional support.

Results of preoperative testing should help determine the operative approach. For the posterior and middle mediastinal structures, those more likely to cause a pneumomediastinum, a right-sided thoracotomy would be performed. The upper two thirds of the esophagus, the entire thoracic trachea, and the proximal 3 to 4 cm of the left main stem bronchus are approached most easily through a fourth to fifth intercostal space incision. Injuries to the distal third of the esophagus and to the distal left main stem bronchus are approached most easily through the left chest. In adjacent tracheoesophageal or bronchoesophageal injuries, fistulas may be avoided by interposing a vascular pedicle. Long-term drains should be avoided near suture lines.

Pharyngeal or cervical esophageal leaks, if small, may be treated with systemic antibiotics for 5 to 7 days. The patient should remain NPO and the esophageal study repeated in 3 to 5 days to follow the course of healing. Afterwards, oral antibiotics should be continued for 2 weeks or until the patient has responded clinically. Nonoperative management of thoracic esophageal leaks may be performed when there is minimal to no signs of sepsis, there is good nutritional status, the leak is contained within the mediastinal pleura, the fluoroscopically evaluated contrast material drains back out of the perforation into the esophagus without any significant pooling, and there is no distal obstruction or malignancy. For patients with thoracic esophageal perforations, the resultant inflammation may make the repair much more difficult, from the surgeon's standpoint in performing it and in the patient's ability to tolerate it. Surgical judgment is necessary to determine how best to repair an esophageal perforation. The use of a primary closure versus a diversion technique depends on the patient's health status, the time from the perforation, and the degree of mediastinal inflammation. If the esophageal perforation has occurred less than 24 hours from time of repair, the 30-day mortality has been found to be approximately 10%; however, if operative treatment is delayed more than 24 hours, the mortality is 40%.

In neonates, the immature mediastinal fascial planes, especially those around the pulmonary veins and arteries, may allow for pneumopericardium. These infants may develop severe hemodynamic compromise or death. A subxiphoid drain may be necessary to decompress the pericardium. Pneumopericardium also may occur in adults, but the utility of a mediastinal tube may not be as effective.

For patients with tracheobronchial rupture or perforation, the mediastinal and fascial tissues may contain the tear while limiting the bacterial contamination and soilage of the mediastinum. When tracheal or bronchial disruption is greater than one third of the circumference of the airway, or if the pneumomediastinum is progressively worsening, or if a pneumothorax has developed or is unresolved after closed chest tube thoracostomy, surgical repair is indicated. Repair of a bronchial rupture after closed chest trauma has a mortality rate of 30%. Of these tears, 80% are located within 2 to 3 cm of the carina. These repairs typically are performed through a right thoracotomy, but higher laryngeal-tracheal injuries are approached with a low "collar" incision. The same surgical principles should be followed—débride devitalized tissues, perform all anastomoses to healthy tissue, and adequately drain the area. In some blast-type injuries, the lobe or the lung may need to be resected.

Pneumomediastinum after laparoscopic surgery is not associated with any morbidity or mortality and may be safely observed. When associated with pneumothorax, there is significant risk, however, and the pneumomediastinum should be treated with chest tube thoracostomy.

After dental and head and neck surgery, a paratonsillar, retropharyngeal, or submental infection or abscess may occur. Infections typically are from mixed aerobic and anaerobic organisms. They may result in a synergistic, necrotizing cellulitis. This infection travels along the natural planes of the face, nasal sinuses, neck, and mediastinum. The patient may present with acute respiratory stridor, altered phonation, Ludwig's angina, Lemierre's syndrome, dyspnea, and hemodynamic compromise. CT helps determine the extent and degree of the inflammatory process and direct the course of therapy. Antibiotics should be administered to treat mixed infections. Cultures should be taken of any purulent material. Any inflamed and necrotic areas found on CT or at surgical exploration should be surgically débrided and drained. For patients with processes extending below the thoracic inlet, a cervical mediastinal scope, video-assisted approach, and possible thoracotomy may be necessary to achieve access for débridement and drain placement. Tracheostomy may be necessary in cases of severe dyspnea, hemorrhage, or posterior pharyngeal/laryngeal edema. Despite early recognition and aggressive treatment, the mortality has been reported to be 40% to 50%.

SUGGESTED READING

Abolnik I, et al: Spontaneous pneumomediastinum: a report of 25 cases, *Chest* 100:93, 1991.

Chalumeau M, et al: Spontaneous pneumomediastinum in children, *Pediatr Pulmonol* 31:67, 2001.

Liptay MJ, et al: Acute and chronic mediastinal infections. In Shields TW, et al: *General thoracic surgery*, ed 3, New York, 2000, Lippincott, Williams & Wilkins.

Wright CD, et al: Nonneoplastic disorders of the mediastinum. In Fishman AP: *Fishman's pulmonary diseases and disorders*, ed 3, New York, 1998, McGraw-Hill.

FLAIL CHEST AND PULMONARY CONTUSION

Sandra M. Wanek

John C. Mayberry

Donald D. Trunkey

Chest trauma in a civilian population accounts for 10% to 15% of all trauma admissions and is associated with 25% of deaths due to trauma. Injury to the chest wall is the most common thoracic injury, and the presence of rib fractures is associated with 12% mortality. Fractures involving the upper six ribs are associated with life-threatening intrathoracic injuries, whereas fractures involving the lower six ribs are related to spleen, liver, or kidney damage. The trauma patient with multiple rib fractures resulting in a flail segment has significantly higher morbidity predominantly due to an underlying pulmonary contusion. Elderly patients with preexisting comorbidities and age-related physiologic changes also tend to fare worse.

■ DIAGNOSIS AND TREATMENT OF FLAIL CHEST

Flail chest is the most serious chest wall injury encountered. Mechanically, it is a complete disruption of a portion of the chest wall by segmental fractures of two or more adjacent ribs. It also may result from disruption of the ribs from the sternum at the costochondral cartilage and a fracture in the rib. Aside from the deleterious effects on chest wall mechanics, the force required to cause a flail chest places the patient at significant risk for other intrathoracic injuries.

Noting the paradoxical wall movement in a spontaneously breathing patient is the best way to make the diagnosis. If the patient is intubated, the positive-pressure ventilation may prevent the altered chest wall movement. In this situation, diagnosis may be overlooked unless sought by palpation of the chest wall, compression over the sternum, and bilateral compression on the rib cage to note fractures or crepitation. The specific fracture pattern described previously also may be seen on chest radiograph or computed tomography scan.

Pain management is a significant component to treating the patient with a flail chest. The disruption of chest wall mechanics may decrease tidal volume and impair the ability to generate an effective cough. This situation leads to the development of hypoventilation and places the patient at great risk for subsequent atelectasis and pneumonia. If there is an associated pulmonary contusion, lack of an effective cough impairs the ability to clear the associated hemoptysis, and this further contributes to the development of obstruction, intrapulmonary shunting, and pneumonia. Unless the segment is large, these alterations generally can be managed without intubation in 65% to 75% of patients by use of incentive spirometry and aggressive pulmonary toilet. This approach requires active participation on the part of the patient, which can be achieved only with adequate pain control.

Oral narcotics are rarely effective for pain control during the acute treatment phase of a flail chest. Intravenous narcotics are able to provide adequate pain relief, but the degree of sedation as a side effect may impair the patient's ability to participate with pulmonary toilet. If the flail segment is small, however, intravenous narcotics may be sufficient without oversedation. For patients who are in extreme pain or in whom the flail segment is large, the preferred option for pain management is thoracic epidural. An extradural combination of a low-dose narcotic and local anesthetic acts synergistically to provide excellent pain control without sedation. The patient now can deep breathe, can cough, and has increased mobility. This helps to prevent hypoventilation, increases clearance of secretions, and improves the patient's chance of avoiding intubation.

Treatment of a flail chest is centered on adequacy of oxygenation and ventilation and pain control. Patients who are able to maintain oxygen saturation greater than 90% on 6 liters of oxygen with a normal respiratory rate and normocarbia can avoid intubation. Intravenous narcotics are given for pain control with frequent assessment. We recommend an analogue pain scale of 1 to 10 be done along with other vital signs. If pain control is inadequate and there are no contraindications, such as spine fractures or coagulopathy, a thoracic epidural is placed. Deterioration in respiratory function at any time prompts intubation to maintain normal chest wall movement for pain control and to normalize respiratory functions.

Patients with severe flail chest expected to require prolonged ventilatory support should be considered for early tracheostomy. This procedure is useful for clearance of secretions and blood in patients with an underlying pulmonary contusion. Because these patients are prone to have prolonged weaning, tracheostomy also allows for intermittent bilevel ventilation in the later stages of weaning from full-support mechanical ventilation.

Selected patients with flail chest with or without chest wall deformity may be considered for operative stabilization. Indications for flail chest fixation include pain control and failure to wean from mechanical ventilation. Several methods have been described using Kirschner wires, wire cerclage, and Judet staples (Figure 1). Our experience has been predominantly with 3.5-mm acetabular reconstruction plates secured with wire suture. More recently, we have been using smaller titanium mandible reconstruction plates secured with self-tapping screws. Stabilizing every other fractured rib is adequate to provide normalization of chest wall movement, decreasing pain and improving respiratory mechanics. Absorbable plates and screws are available and may be considered for use in children and adolescents. Our experience with these devices is still limited, however.

■ DIAGNOSIS AND TREATMENT OF PULMONARY CONTUSION

Pulmonary contusion is a diffuse hemorrhage into the parenchyma resulting from blunt and penetrating trauma. The latter is associated with medium-velocity and high-velocity gunshot wounds and shotgun blasts. It commonly appears within several hours as a patchy opacity on the chest radiograph. This opacity tends to progress or "blossom" over the next several days, and this distinguishes it from an infiltrate initially presenting 2 to 3 days later due to gastric aspiration, atelectasis, or pneumonia.

Hemoptysis is a common consequence of pulmonary contusion. Small peripheral lesions may produce only blood-tinged sputum. Injuries near the hilum may develop massive bleeding, however, into the tracheobronchial tree. Rarely the pulmonary contusion may be so extensive and destructive to the pulmonary tissue that the hemoptysis contributes to life-threatening airway obstruction. For these lesions, immediate resection of the damaged lung tissue is required.

Treatment of a pulmonary contusion as an isolated injury is conservative in nature. Attention to pulmonary toilet, the use of incentive spirometry, and surveillance for pneumonia are paramount. The historical admonition to avoid fluid resuscitation in patients with pulmonary contusion is not valid, and the use of diuretics as an initial treatment modality is of unproven benefit and may be deleterious. Overresuscitation also should be avoided because this contributes to pulmonary edema and hypoxia. Strict attention to volume status is crucial; monitoring of central venous pressure and urine output is mandatory. The use of a pulmonary artery catheter also may be necessary in selected patients for tight control of their fluid status. Drainage of effusions, pneumothorax, or hemothorax is important to promote lung expansion and maintain minute volume. Prophylactic antibiotics are not currently recommended. Although young healthy patients are likely to have enough pulmonary reserve to tolerate a pulmonary contusion without intubation, smokers, the elderly, and patients with underlying pulmonary disease often require temporary ventilatory support.

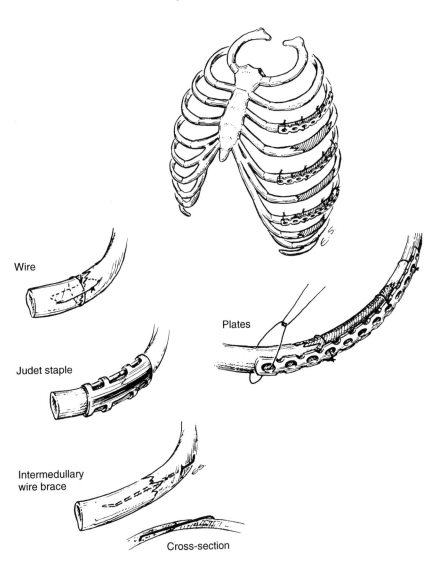

Wire

Plates

Judet staple

Intermedullary
wire brace

Cross-section

Figure 1
Techniques for surgical repair of flail chest:
simple wire fixation, Judet staple wrap,
intermedullary Kirschner wire, and metal
plating with wire cerclage.

SUGGESTED READING

Ahmed Z, Mohyuddin Z: Management of flail chest injury: internal fixation versus endotracheal intubation and ventilation, *J Thorac Cardiovasc Surg* 110:1676, 1995.

Cohn SM: Pulmonary contusion: review of the clinical entity, *J Trauma* 42:973, 1997.

Hoff SJ, et al: Outcome of isolated pulmonary contusion in blunt trauma patients, *Am Surg* 60:138, 1994.

Richardson JD, et al: Selective management of flail chest and pulmonary contusion, *Ann Surg* 196:481, 1982.

Voggenreiter G, et al: Operative chest wall stabilization in flail chest: outcomes of patients with or without pulmonary contusion, *J Am Coll Surg* 187:130, 1998.

CHEST WALL INJURY AND BLUNT CARDIAC TRAUMA

Kenneth L. Mattox
Jon-Cecil M. Walkes

Blunt chest injury is the predominant mode of intrathoracic trauma. Injury may occur to the chest wall, to one of the three thoracic visceral cavities, or to both areas combined. This chapter focuses on chest wall and blunt cardiac injuries.

■ CHEST WALL FRACTURES

Blunt chest wall trauma can produce various direct injuries to the chest wall, such as sternal, clavicular, and scapular fractures and muscle hemorrhage. The internal consequences of blunt chest wall trauma include blunt cardiac injury, pericardial tamponade, pericardial rupture, pulmonary contusion, tracheobronchial tears, great vessel injury, and diaphragmatic tears. Secondary iatrogenic injuries, such as pulmonary insufficiency and cardiac depression, may be the result of employing long-established therapeutic modalities, such as the choice and volume of resuscitative fluids. Iatrogenic perforation by various catheters and tubes also is common.

Fracture of the sternum or disruption of the costal chondral junction is usually secondary to anterior energy forces, such as the chest impacting the steering wheel, prolonged external cardiac massage during cardiopulmonary resuscitation, and severe blows to the anterior chest (i.e., athletic events). A sternal fracture is usually horizontal and may be nondisplaced and unrecognized. Displaced fractures create an overlap and pose pain control and cosmetic challenges. Overlapping fractures to the sternum usually are repaired operatively with simple wire closure. Separation of the costochondral junction usually does not require surgery.

Blunt injuries to the heart are associated with sternal fractures in less than 25% of cases. In most of these cases, a diagnosis of "mild cardiac contusion" is based on nonspecific criteria, such as an elevation of cardiac enzymes or a variety of abnormal electrocardiogram (ECG) findings. Virtually all patients with this "diagnosis" are admitted to the hospital for observation only and rarely require any further cardiac evaluation or therapy.

■ BLUNT CARDIAC TRAUMA

Since the 1970s, *cardiac contusion* has referred to everything from minor conditions resulting in a slight elevation of cardiac enzymes to complex injuries, such as septal defect or frank cardiac rupture. Because of its nondescript nature and inconsistent clinical spectrum, the term *cardiac contusion* should be omitted from the surgical vernacular. Its use to describe a patient's condition provides no clinical insight or specific indication for treatment.

■ NEW TERMINOLOGY FOR BLUNT CARDIAC INJURY

The term *myocardial contusion* has been used for decades and is the subject of hundreds of published articles. A fatal complication or surgical intervention rarely is described in patients with "myocardial contusion," although many authors propose a complex algorithm of evaluation and monitoring of these patients. In the long-standing trauma scoring system, myocardial contusion carries a trauma score of 3, undoubtedly a much higher score than such a minor injury should command. Conversely, a rupture of the free wall of the heart, an acute septal defect, a fracture or occlusion of a coronary artery, and a cardiac valve tear all could be assigned a theoretical trauma score of 3 (for a diagnosis of myocardial contusion), rather than a more appropriate score of 4 or 5. With this significant dichotomy and confusion relating to the terminology, a new classification of blunt cardiac injury has been suggested (Table 1).

■ ETIOLOGY AND DIAGNOSIS

The associated morbidity and mortality seen in patients with sternal fractures often are due to severe concomitant injuries. In 1962, Gibson reported an 11-year series of 80 patients with sternal fractures. He reported 19 deaths, with the leading cause of death being severe head injury. Although it seems obvious that the heart would suffer a significant amount of injury due to its intimate association with the sternum, there does not seem to be a consistent, demonstrable association between sternal fractures and blunt myocardial contusion and dysfunction.

Although it is relatively easy to diagnose a sternal fracture clinically and radiologically, the diagnosis of blunt cardiac injury is more elusive. Diagnosing a sternal fracture typically can be made on physical examination and on the lateral chest x-ray. Patients typically present with ecchymosis or skin defect over the sternum in association with an appropriate deceleration mechanism. The diagnosis is confirmed on supine chest x-ray with an additional lateral view. The diagnosis of blunt myocardial injury is usually nebulous. As a result of the confusing and nebulous association of the relationship between sternal fracture and heart injury, the use of the term *myocardial contusion* (in association with sternal fracture) varies in the literature from 1.3% to 62% depending on the precise definition of myocardial contusion used.

Of significant interest is the paucity of blunt cardiac injuries reported in professional athletes, especially American football players. Despite the tremendous blows to the midsternum week after week, blunt cardiac injury is virtually never diagnosed in this group. Sternal fracture is reported frequently, however, after external cardiac massage for cardiopulmonary resuscitation (CPR). With this lesser "impact" (with CPR), sternal fractures and rupture of a heart chamber are recognized complications from CPR. The exact incidence of free wall cardiac rupture, especially right ventricular wall rupture, or even "cardiac contusion" after external cardiac compression has not been established.

The surgeon treating a patient with anterior chest trauma, sternal fractures, anterior rib fractures, or possible blunt cardiac trauma is seeking answers to a list of questions. The initial examinations, tests, and imaging should answer the following:

Is the patient hemodynamically stable?
Are there any associated injuries?
Is there need for hospitalization or just extended cardiac monitoring for arrhythmias?
Is there an osseous injury requiring immobilization?
What is the timing of any fracture fusion operation?
Is there cardiac muscle dyskinesis, coronary artery insufficiency, hemopericardium, cardiac valvular insufficiency, ventricular septal hematoma or dyskinesis, or evidence of a traumatic septal defect or a left-to-right shunt?
What tests would answer these questions in the hemodynamically stable patient and in the unstable patient?

PHYSICAL EXAMINATION

The recommended anatomic injury scores for physiologic or anatomic abnormalities addressed in this chapter are cited in Table 1. The patient with blunt cardiac injury may present with a wide range of symptoms from obvious sternal ecchymosis and associated fracture to no notable chest wall abnormality. The most consistent finding in a patient with blunt cardiac injury is a rib fracture; this in and of itself is not indicative of blunt cardiac injury. A patient with a significant blunt cardiac injury may present with elevated central venous pressure or hypotension or both, especially if the injury has an accompanying hemopericardium. Septal and valvular defects have an associated murmur. In our experience, patients with clinically significant blunt cardiac injury often do not present with associated murmurs. Physical examination must be coupled with laboratory and imaging studies, such as ECG and transesophageal echocardiography (TEE), to aid in diagnosis. Patients with sternal fractures complain

of significant pain and often describe a "click" in the midsternum with movement or coughing.

LABORATORY AND ANCILLARY EVALUATIONS

The initial diagnostic approach to the patient suspected of having a blunt cardiac injury does not differ from that of the "standard" trauma patient. The first priority is the primary and secondary survey, as recommended by the American College of Surgeons Advanced Trauma Life Support Course. The chest x-ray, particularly the lateral view, is part of the secondary survey and diagnoses horizontal displaced sternal fractures. The baseline ECG is obtained, recognizing that this alone lacks the sensitivity and specificity to diagnose blunt cardiac injury. Helling showed a 54% incidence of abnormal ECGs in 64 patients evaluated for blunt cardiac injury. Of the ECG abnormalities, 49% were nonspecific ST-segment depression and T-wave changes. Maenza noted in a meta-analysis that abnormal ECGs and myocardial injury were not consistent. Patients with free wall rupture, subtle wall defects, and cardiac valvular disruption have been known to present without any ECG abnormalities. In a "stable" patient with a high index of suspicion for blunt cardiac injury, however, an initial "abnormal" ECG warrants admission to a telemetered bed for 8 to 24 hours.

Laboratory tests often are used as an adjunct in the diagnosis of blunt cardiac injury, but similar to the ECG, the use of these markers is limited by the lack of a precise definition of blunt cardiac trauma. Even among authors who have reported some utility for these tests, the ideal timing of the test after injury is controversial. The most frequently used markers are creatinine kinase–myocardial bands (CK-MB) and troponins. Troponins, even those elevated for post–myocardial infarction, are unreliable to pinpoint specifically serious cardiac injury after blunt trauma. One confounding variable is the fact that CK-MB also is found in skeletal muscle. Consequently the relevance of an elevated CK-MB level in a patient with multiple long bone fractures and chest wall trauma is questionable. Adams found in 44 patients studied that there was a direct correlation between elevated troponin levels and blunt cardiac injury as defined by ECG in patients having myocardial infarction, but the exact relationship between troponin levels and clinically significant myocardial injury is variable. These enzymes have not been shown to affect therapeutic options, decisions, timing of operation, or extent of hospitalization. Use of CK-MB and troponin levels has not been shown to affect outcome after blunt cardiac injury.

IMAGING

During the patient evaluation process, the surgeon seeks data determining the need for hospitalization, operation, and surgical intensive care. If surgery is required, a precise definition of the area of injury must be determined. The focused abdominal sonography for trauma (FAST), transthoracic echocardiography or TEE, and cardiac catheterization are the diagnostic imaging options.

Table 1 New Terminology and Scoring System for Blunt Cardiac Injury	
BLUNT CARDIAC INJURY WITH	**TRAUMA SCORE**
No ECG, physiologic, or anatomic abnormality	1
Minor ECG abnormality	1
Major ECG abnormality	1
Cardiac enzyme elevation	1
Free wall hematoma	2
Septal hematoma	2
Septal defect	4
Valvular insufficiency	4
Free wall rupture	5
Cardiac herniation	5
Coronary artery injury	5

From Adams JE, et al: *Am Heart J* 131:308, 1996.
ECG, electrocardiogram.

FAST

The FAST has been standardized with four ports to look for blood in the abdomen or the pericardial sac. Hemopericardium can be shown 30 minutes before the development of pericardial tamponade syndrome. This rapid test is performed by surgeons in the emergency department, operating room, and intensive care unit.

TEE

Transthoracic echocardiography or TEE can be performed. TEE is used often by surgeons, anesthesiologists, and cardiologists to show septal defects, abnormal cardiac wall motion, hemopericardium, valvular insufficiency, and dyskinesis. TEE might provide enough information for the surgeon to proceed with an operation or may be followed by cardiac catheterization if necessary.

■ TREATMENT

Sternal Fracture

Sternal fractures, in the absence of cardiac injury, are repaired for two reasons: to control pain and for cosmesis. A transverse or vertical incision at the area of the fracture usually is sufficient to expose the deformity. The overriding edges of the fracture must be reduced. Wire sutures are placed and secured, as is done for any median sternotomy closure. Patients resume normal activity (excluding contact sports) when discharged from the hospital. Results are extremely good, and complications are rare.

Anterior Rib Fractures

Anterior rib fractures, similar to all rib fractures, usually are treated nonoperatively. If painful, the patient might require intercostal nerve blocks. Commercially available circumferential binders should be avoided because they restrict respiratory movement and are associated with an increased rate of pneumonia. Operative fixation of rib fractures rarely is required and usually is reserved for patients with a "flail chest" and ventilator dependency. Operative fixation might have some theoretical advantage in decreasing the length of time the patient has pain from this injury.

Sternal Chondral Separation

Separation of the sternal chondral junction may occur in the absence of rib or sternal fracture and may be caused by anterior blunt force trauma. This condition may be very painful and takes several weeks to heal. Operative fixation is not required. Long-term pain in the region of the separation is not unusual. There is no specific treatment other than pain management.

Blunt Cardiac Trauma with Mild ECG Abnormalities

Patients with blunt cardiac injury as indicated by ECG or enzyme abnormalities are treated with simple observation, usually in the emergency department or "chest pain" monitored unit. In these cases, operation has virtually never been reported. In rare instances, a cardiac arrhythmia might develop, and medical treatment of the arrhythmia might be indicated.

Cardiac Rupture

Hemopericardium detected by the FAST usually is treated with anterolateral thoracotomy. Subxyphoid pericardiotomy and needle pericardiocentesis have less utility than was perceived formerly. Hemopericardium from blunt cardiac trauma may not be clinically manifest for several days, or the patient may present with full-blown pericardial tamponade. Blunt cardiac injuries requiring surgery are usually single case reports. The most commonly ruptured chamber is the right atrium, followed by the right ventricle. Simple cardiorrhaphy is accomplished with a running suture, usually 4-0 polypropylene. Pledgets are rarely, if ever, necessary in repair of a cardiac injury, with the possible exception of the right ventricle. Thoracotomy on a right ventricular free wall rupture might be required in the emergency department at the time of presentation.

Traumatic Ventricular Septal Defect

Similar to cardiac free wall rupture, blunt injury to the ventricular septum with development of a ventricular septal defect might be immediately manifest by acute congestive heart failure or could be delayed for several days. Some delayed cases are associated with a left ventricular aneurysm. Operative repair is required for hemodynamically significant ventricular septal defects and is performed on cardiopulmonary bypass.

Traumatic Valvular Insufficiency

Traumatic valvular tears have been described for the aortic, mitral, and pulmonary valves, resulting in valvular insufficiency. Repair for left-sided hemodynamically significant lesions is performed on cardiopulmonary bypass. Although an occasional cardiac valve repair by resuspension or chordae reattachment has been reported, most single case reports have cited valvular replacement.

Pericardial Tear with Cardiac Herniation

Cardiac herniation through a pericardial tear is rare. Pericardial tears secondary to blunt chest trauma have been described at the right, left, and midline diaphragmatic locations. Herniation through a relatively small rent in the pericardium can result in almost immediate death. Herniation through a larger tear can result in intermittent hypotension due to positional changes with spontaneous reduction of the herniation and sometimes recurrent herniation and hypotension. Often the exact pathology is not "discovered" until the time of operation, when closure of the rent is accomplished along with repair of other associated injuries.

■ RESULTS

The mortality and complications after simple blunt chest injury with blunt cardiac manifestations of ECG or enzymatic elevations are extremely low. Patients with septal, free wall, valvular, and pericardial tears have mortality rates greater than 50%. Delayed repair of septal or valvular rupture may be performed several days, weeks, or months after the initial injury.

SUGGESTED READING

Adams JE, et al: Improved detection of cardiac contusion with cardiac troponin I, *Am Heart J* 131:308, 1996.

Helling TS, et al: A prospective evaluation of 68 patients suffering blunt chest trauma for evidence of cardiac injury, *J Trauma* 29:916, 1989.

Maselli D, et al: Posttraumatic left ventricular pseudoaneurysm due to intramyocardial dissecting hematoma, *Ann Thorac Surg* 64:830, 1997.

Pretre R, Chilcott M: Blunt trauma to the heart and the great vessels, *N Engl J Med* 336:626, 1997.

Reginato E, et al: Post-traumatic mitral regurgitation and ventricular septal defect in absence of left pericardium, *Thorac Cardiovasc Surg* 28:213, 1980.

TRAUMATIC AIRWAY INJURIES

Stephen J. Korkola

David S. Mulder

Hospital personnel dealing with trauma see acute airway injuries relatively infrequently. This observation may be explained by the fact that major trauma to the upper airway is often fatal at the scene, and patients do not survive to the hospital secondary to aspiration of blood, secretions, and debris causing airway obstruction. Ongoing advances in prehospital care and regionalization of trauma centers will increase the number of patients surviving to hospital attention, however. The subset that does survive requires the treating team to be capable of rapidly diagnosing and treating these injuries.

Blunt airway trauma may involve the larynx, the cervical and mediastinal trachea, or the intrathoracic bronchi. Injuries can range from mild insignificant mucosal edema to airway transection, or complete obstruction from aspirated blood, or extrinsic compression from hematoma or subcutaneous emphysema, with ensuing cardiorespiratory collapse.

■ CAUSES OF INJURY

The upper airway is relatively protected against blunt trauma by the sternocleidomastoid muscles laterally, the cervical spine posteriorly, and the mandible anteriorly. The anterior protection afforded by the mandible becomes ineffective, however, with the neck in extension, leaving the larynx and trachea vulnerable and exposed. Sudden deceleration characterizing motor vehicle accidents allows the hyperextended neck to strike the dashboard or steering wheel. Other relatively common mechanisms include "clothesline" injuries, whereby the anterior neck is injured by a fixed rope or wire making contact while riding a motorcycle,

snowmobile, or all-terrain vehicle. Similarly, sports involving pucks, balls, or other missiles traveling at high velocity may strike the anterior neck, resulting in traumatic injury to the airway.

Mechanisms of blunt injury include direct and indirect causes. The upper airway may experience direct compressive forces against the anterior vertebral bodies of the cervical spine. The larynx and trachea respond to this compressive force by absorbing some of the energy or by fracturing. In general, as the patient ages, the cartilage becomes less resilient and unable to absorb energy, making the likelihood of fracture greater. Injury to the cricoid cartilage carries a particularly high risk of airway compromise because the circumferential ring provides little room for the expansion of hematomas or mucosal edema.

In addition to the direct compression type of injury, indirect mechanisms may play a contributing role in airway injury after blunt trauma. A sudden increase in intratracheal pressure against a closed glottis may induce linear tears in the membranous trachea. Anterior-posterior compression of the thoracic cage results in lateral movement of the lung hila with possible tearing of the relatively fixed trachea and main stem bronchi. Sudden acceleration-deceleration induces shearing forces in the trachea around its fixed points at the cricoid cartilage and carina.

Penetrating injuries to the airway depend on the instrument inflicting the damage. The type, length, and angle of insertion of a knife or other sharp instrument are important determinants of injured structures. The trajectory and muzzle velocity of the bullet are important in gunshot wounds. Associated injuries to the esophagus and great vessels are relatively common in these cases.

■ EVALUATION

The diagnosis of an acute airway injury may be obvious and recognized immediately or occult and go unrecognized for weeks. Injuries to the larynx are characterized by varying degrees of hoarseness, stridor, dyspnea, cough, hemoptysis, cervical and facial subcutaneous emphysema, loss of laryngeal prominence, cervical hematoma, and ecchymosis. More distal injuries to the tracheobronchial tree inside the chest present with dyspnea, cough, and hemoptysis, with varying degrees of subcutaneous emphysema. Pneumomediastinum may be characterized by crepitations on auscultation of the heart (Hamman's crunch), whereas intrapleural bronchial disruption may lead to pneumothorax with loss of breath sounds, tympany, mediastinal shift, or tension pneumothorax, resulting in cardiovascular collapse. After placement of a chest tube for pneumothorax, continued air leak and failure of the lung to reexpand with suction may suggest bronchial disruption. Patients may deteriorate after intubation and positive pressure ventilation; with a large tear, the ventilated air takes the path of least resistance out the defect and into the chest tube system (compounded with suction), resulting in inadequate ventilation of both lungs. Total disruption or obstruction of the airway presents not with stridor or hoarseness, but rather cyanosis, loss of consciousness, bradycardia, hypotension, and inevitable cardiorespiratory arrest. More recently, fiberoptic laryngoscopy and bronchoscopy has taken on an important role in the trauma room for diagnosing and managing acute airway injuries.

Radiographic investigations play little role in the diagnosis of airway injury during the initial assessment, especially in the unstable patient in whom the airway has not yet been secured. A portable chest x-ray and lateral cervical spine films may prove useful, however, after the primary survey to aid in the diagnosis of subtler injuries. The cervical spine film not only detects bony injuries, but also is useful in assessing for deep cervical air not detected on physical examination. The portable chest x-ray is always readily available and allows one to diagnose pneumothoraces, pleural effusions, pneumomediastinum, and subcutaneous air not appreciated on physical examination. Other findings, such as fractured ribs or a widened or deviated mediastinum, may provide clues to other important injuries. Computed tomography may play a role in diagnosing and characterizing laryngeal injuries in the stable patient, allowing better preparation for surgical repair.

■ INITIAL TREATMENT

Acute management of the airway should follow the guidelines proposed and updated regularly by the American College of Surgeons Committee on Trauma for Advanced Trauma Life Support. The approach should be well organized with numerous backup plans should things not go as expected. Orotracheal intubation with appropriate cervical spine precautions and direct laryngoscopy may be an appropriate first step in trying to secure the airway. Caution is advised, however, in the presence of maxillofacial trauma or suspicion of laryngeal trauma. Flexible bronchoscopy plays an adjuvant role in diagnosing and managing the injured airway. It is usually available and relatively easy to perform even in the most difficult airway, while maintaining cervical spine immobilization. It also allows the accurate placement of distal tubes in the airway that can act as a stent for the disrupted trachea or main stem bronchi. It does take some time to perform in the acute situation, however, even in experienced hands. The status of the larynx can be assessed and a decision made to continue with tube insertion over the bronchoscope versus aborting the intubation and proceeding with surgical airway management.

■ SURGICAL MANAGEMENT

The use of cricothyrotomy in the patient with traumatic airway injuries may play a lifesaving role in carefully selected patients. It is particularly useful when orotracheal intubation is not possible or contraindicated. It is contraindicated, however, in the setting of laryngeal or cricoid cartilage injury. Although often thought of as a quick and reliable method of obtaining control of the airway, it may not be straightforward in the presence of neck hematomas and significant subcutaneous emphysema.

There are few indications to perform tracheostomy in the acute setting. The trachea is deep within the neck, and it is surrounded by a range of thyroid sizes and many large veins that are often dilated in the face of respiratory distress. This makes tracheostomy in the emergency department a challenging undertaking. In the presence of significant laryngeal injury precluding orotracheal intubation and cricothyrotomy, however, it should be the appropriate alternative. It also may be indicated in cases of partial disruption of the cervical trachea when the tube can be inserted directly through the injured area. This maneuver helps minimize the amount of viable trachea that later facilitates repair. When complete transection of the cervical trachea has occurred, the distal portion often retracts into the mediastinum. It is located by finger palpation, pulled out into the neck with a nontraumatic instrument, and intubated to secure the airway.

Rarely a patient may require cardiopulmonary bypass or extracorporeal membrane oxygenation for cardiorespiratory support while awaiting definitive repair of severe airway trauma. These maneuvers require specialized personnel, are time-consuming to instigate, and require systemic heparinization that usually is contraindicated in the trauma patient with other associated injuries.

A patient who deteriorates after intubation, ventilation, and appropriate chest tube placement and subsequently develops a massive air leak requires immediate flexible bronchoscopy with selective positioning of the endotracheal tube depending on the findings. The timing and type of definitive surgical repair depend on the site and extent of the injury to the airway and on the location and severity of associated injuries. Surgical exploration for laryngeal trauma usually is indicated for injuries causing obstruction sufficient to require surgical control of the airway, uncontrolled subcutaneous emphysema after airway management, extensive mucosal lacerations/disruption with exposure of cartilage, and displaced fractures. There is no advantage in delaying definitive repair unless other, more life-threatening, injuries take priority. Steroids may be beneficial if administered early to help limit laryngeal edema. In addition, patients should receive broad-spectrum antibiotic coverage to prevent chondritis and perichondritis resulting from contact of exposed cartilage with the contaminated airway lumen. These complications contribute to delayed healing and the formation of excessive granulation tissue and fibrous scar that leads to increased risk of stricture formation.

Laryngeal injuries requiring surgical reconstruction should be undertaken with the help of an otolaryngologist. Fractures of the thyroid cartilage can be reduced with titanium miniplates, plates, or fine wires. Dislocated arytenoids should be repositioned onto their cricoarytenoid facet, preferably from inside, under direct vision with the laryngoscope. The completely avulsed arytenoids should be repositioned to provide bulk to the posterior glottis and reduce the risk of future aspiration. Cricoid fractures are reapproximated with fine wire or nonabsorbable suture. Most injuries to the larynx are associated with mucosal disruptions that may be exposed through a midline incision in the thyroid cartilage and repaired directly with fine chromic catgut sutures, tying the knots outside the lumen if possible. Local mucosal flaps from the piriform sinus or free buccal grafts may be required for larger areas of devitalized tissue.

Recurrent laryngeal nerve injury may be secondary to complete disruption, contusion, or edema. Exploration of the nerves generally is not indicated for two reasons. First, the results of repair have been disappointing, and, second, the contused nerve with potentially recoverable function may be irreversibly damaged during exploration. Months may be required for spontaneous recovery of nerve function.

The indications for stent placement after laryngeal reconstruction are controversial. In general, injuries involving the anterior commissure, comminuted fractures of the thyroid cartilage in which the fixation technique does not afford rigid immobilization, and injuries with extensive mucosal edema or tissue grafting should have a stent placed. A variety of homemade and commercially available prostheses are available and are generally left in place for 2 weeks. Extensive reconstruction of the larynx may require the placement of a tracheostomy (if not present already) to allow the repair to heal and edema to resolve. The tracheostomy should be placed at least two tracheal rings below the repair, using strap muscles and the thyroid gland to isolate the suture line from the tracheostomy site. Tracheostomy placement also may be required for airway protection when the recurrent nerve is injured.

In general, injuries to the trachea involving greater than one third of the circumference should be repaired surgically to prevent late stenosis formation. Similar to laryngeal injuries, operative intervention usually is required when there is increasing subcutaneous emphysema, persistent pneumothorax, or clinical deterioration despite chest tube placement and mechanical ventilation.

Injuries involving the cervical trachea are approached best through a collar incision with or without median sternotomy as the need arises. The patient is placed supine with a sandbag under the shoulders and a doughnut ring pillow under the occiput. The head of the bed may be elevated to decrease venous pressure and bleeding. The incision is made 1 to 2 cm above the sternal notch and extended laterally to the medial border of each sternocleidomastoid muscle. Flaps are developed superiorly and inferiorly under the platysmal layer to expose the larynx, entire cervical trachea, esophagus, and associated great vessels. Both groins and the chest are prepared routinely should the need for cardiopulmonary bypass arise or a segment of greater saphenous vein is needed. Injuries to the mediastinal trachea and bronchus are approached best through a posterolateral thoracotomy. Exposure to the trachea, carina, right main stem, and proximal left main stem bronchi are approached best through the right chest. This approach also affords excellent exposure of the proximal esophagus. More distal injuries on the left

should be exposed through a left thoracotomy, generously mobilizing the aorta. Repair of simple lacerations of the trachea and bronchi are repaired primarily using interrupted sutures of 3-0 polyglactin 910 (Vicryl) to reestablish mucosal-to-mucosal continuity. Débridement of devitalized tissue should be performed with caution to leave the greatest amount of viable trachea for repair. Suture lines performed through the chest are reinforced with pedicled flaps of pleura or pericardium wrapped around the anastomosis. Alternatively a pedicle of intercostal muscle may be used. Repairs in the neck are reinforced with mobilized strap muscles. More complex injuries involving complete transection of the trachea with large amounts of devitalized tissue are repaired with interrupted sutures of 3-0 Vicryl after careful débridement. Pericartilaginous sutures are placed on the rigid portion of the trachea, and simple interrupted sutures placed on the membranous portion. To help create a tension-free anastomosis, length may be gained by mobilizing the trachea distally to free up both hila, allowing the structures to shift superiorly. The trachea is mobilized in the anteroposterior plane to avoid damage to the vascular supply, which enters on the lateral aspects.

At the end of the procedure, the patient's chin may be sutured to the anterior chest to prevent the patient from extending the neck and stressing the suture line. This suture is left in place for approximately 1 week and removed after flexible bronchoscopy is performed to assess the integrity of the anastomosis.

■ POSTOPERATIVE CARE

Careful attention is paid to tracheobronchial toilet, by removing any blood, secretions, and debris with regular bronchoscopic examinations and suctioning as necessary over the first 2 to 3 days. Nasotracheal suctioning should be used cautiously when there is a tracheal or bronchial suture line. If possible, patients should be kept with the head of bed elevated to reduce edema and encourage healing. There is a relatively high incidence of associated chest wall injury, which necessitates adequate pain control for optimal respiratory function. Intercostal nerve blocks and epidural anesthesia have proved useful in the early postoperative period. The endotracheal tube is removed after secretions are manageable, and the patient is able to ventilate adequately on his or her own.

■ COMPLICATIONS

Patients surviving acute trauma to the airway and their associated injuries may be subject to many delayed complications. This is especially true if the injuries went unrecognized at the time of the initial assessment. Frequent repeat examinations of the airway with fiberoptic laryngoscopy and bronchoscopy are useful to detect problems early. Stenosis of the airway and glottic scarring may become evident if stridor presents weeks to months after the initial injury. This may be treated by carbon dioxide laser radial incision and dilation. Stenoses secondary to loss of cartilaginous support may be managed with free grafts of rib cartilage. In selected cases, resection of the stenosis and end-to-end anastomosis may be necessary.

Dysphonia and vocal fatigue may result from scarring of the vibrating surface of the vocal cords or deficient glottic closure from vocal cord paralysis. Collagen or fat implants and medialization thyroplasty may prove useful in restoring vocal function with ongoing rehabilitation and the help of a speech-language pathologist. Interventions for vocal dysfunction should be delayed for at least 6 to 12 months to ensure that spontaneous recovery of function will not occur.

■ CONCLUSION

Traumatic injuries to the airway constitute a relatively small percentage of patients presenting to the emergency department. Medical personnel dealing with these patients must be comfortable with all the options of acute airway management because patient survival depends on the ability to secure the airway at the initial assessment. Surgical techniques for definitive repair and reconstruction of the proximal airway have yielded good results, although late stenoses and voice dysfunction remain significant problems.

SUGGESTED READING

Bertelsen S, Howitz P: Injuries of the trachea and bronchi, *Thorax* 27:188, 1972.

Cassada DC, et al: Acute injuries of the trachea and major bronchi: importance of early diagnosis, *Ann Thorac Surg* 69:1563, 2000.

Mathisen DJ, Grillo HC: Laryngotracheal trauma, *Ann Thorac Surg* 43:254, 1987.

Ogura J: Management of traumatic injuries of the larynx and trachea including stenosis, *J Laryngol Otol* 85:1259, 1971.

Rossbach MM, et al: Management of major tracheobronchial injuries: a 28-year experience, *Ann Thorac Surg* 65:182, 1998.

TRAUMATIC HEMOTHORAX

Edward E. Cornwell III

Thoracic trauma is a major contributor to death due to injury, accounting for approximately 25% of all trauma deaths in the United States. Thoracic trauma by its nature implies potential lethality occurring due to (1) major hemorrhage from the heart, great vessels, pulmonary parenchyma, and chest wall vasculature and (2) respiratory failure as a result of acute traumatic lung injury. Consequently, major thoracic trauma results in mortality in nearly 10% of cases.

Traumatic hemothorax presents a broad spectrum of clinical challenges. On the one hand, nearly 90% of patients are treated successfully with appropriate chest tube placement and management. On the other hand, a small subset of patients require operative intervention for hemorrhage control and are saved by attention being paid to special surgical considerations. This chapter addresses traumatic hemothorax with special attention paid to (1) the particulars of tube thoracostomy, (2) the management of residual hemothorax, and (3) special considerations in patients requiring surgical intervention.

■ TUBE THORACOSTOMY

Posttraumatic hemothorax of sufficient size to be apparent on chest x-ray is most commonly due to laceration of the lung parenchyma or chest wall vessels (intercostal or internal mammary). Standard treatment is a large-caliber (32 to 40 Fr) chest tube that allows for evacuation of blood, reduces the risk of clotted hemothorax, and provides for ongoing determination of the extent of thoracic bleeding. In more than 90% of patients with blunt trauma and more than 80% of patients with penetrating trauma, bleeding is self-limited, and operative intervention is unnecessary.

Beyond the standard principles of chest tube placement (i.e., incision in fifth intercostal space at the mid axillary line, finger exploration of thoracic cavity before tube placement, and placement of the tube overlying the superior border of the rib), two practical maneuvers deserve special emphasis. First, the importance of the follow-up x-ray after tube placement cannot be overemphasized. This x-ray helps to confirm that minimal chest tube output is due to cessation of bleeding rather than accumulation of a large clotted hemothorax. Second, the rotation (or "spinning") of the tube before securing it to the chest wall with a nonabsorbable suture is of importance. This rotation should avoid the bending or "kinking" of the tube sometimes seen on follow-up x-ray, which may have the consequence of impeding adequate evacuation of blood.

■ ROLE OF ANTIBIOTICS

A major complication of thoracic trauma and chest tube placement for traumatic hemothorax is empyema. There is some suggestion in the literature that the site and setting of tube placement (i.e., prehospital, emergency department, intensive care unit, operating room) and the physician performing the procedure (surgeon versus nonsurgeon) may affect the incidence of posttraumatic empyema.

Considerable attention has been paid to the question of prophylactic antibiotic use in injured patients requiring tube thoracostomy to reduce the incidence of empyema. Because bacterial contamination occurs before antibiotics are administered, antibiotic use constitutes early presumptive therapy rather than true prophylaxis. An evidence-based review performed by the Practice Management Guidelines Workgroup of the Eastern Association for the Surgery of Trauma has addressed the topic of antibiotic use in tube thoracostomy for traumatic hemopneumothorax. On the basis of 11 prospective trials and 2 meta-analyses, the following statement was generated:

> There are sufficient class 1 and 2 data to recommend prophylactic antibiotic use in patients receiving tube thoracostomy following chest trauma. A first-generation cephalosporin should be used for no longer than 24 hours. The data suggest there may be a reduction in the incidence of pneumonia but not empyema in trauma patients receiving prophylactic antibiotics when a tube thoracostomy is placed.

It remains poorly explained and perhaps even counterintuitive that reduction of pneumonia rather than empyema is the reasonable expectation with the use of a short course of periprocedural antibiotics for chest tube placement in the injured patient.

■ RESIDUAL HEMOTHORAX

After placement of a chest tube for a traumatic hemothorax, current guidelines recommend immediate surgery if 1500 ml of blood is evacuated initially or if drainage of more than 200 ml an hour for the ensuing 2 to 4 hours occurs. These guidelines roughly coincide with the amount of bleeding that would produce hemorrhagic shock in a previously healthy 70-kg patient (class 3 hemorrhage). Occasionally, despite the aforementioned safeguards, thoracic blood collections are drained only partially. This residual blood, which already is contaminated, may serve as the nidus for the development of an empyema or fibrothorax. The uncommon but frustrating scenario of chest tube placement, incomplete evacuation, tube adjustment, and perhaps tube replacement, followed by numerous x-rays and computed tomography (CT) scans is a memorable one for any physician caring for large numbers of trauma patients. This scenario ultimately may lead to thoracotomy and decortication to liberate trapped lung parenchyma.

Advances in video-assisted thoracic surgery (VATS) have allowed for development of a minimally invasive method for draining retained traumatic hemothorax and have decreased the risk of development of empyema or fibrothorax. Several considerations regarding VATS evacuation of clotted hemothorax deserve emphasis: (1) Progressive clot organization and adhesion formation presents about a 3- to 5-day "window" when semisolid clot and residual serum can be evacuated via VATS with a high degree of success. (2) Because the procedure is done with single-lung ventilation, with collapse of an already injured and contused lung, complete reevacuation is a challenge and may take several days following the procedure. (3) The local response to the lung injury may promote local vasodilation and perfusion of nonventilated lung. The resultant increase in the alveolar-arterial gradient may

exacerbate relative hypoxemia around the time of the VATS evacuation of the hemothorax. The result of the latter two considerations produces a scenario that may alarm the uninitiated but should be met with patience and persistence—that is, the clinical and radiographic picture (progressive hypoxemia and a markedly abnormal chest x-ray postoperatively) initially will leave one to conclude that the operation has made the patient worse. A critical care bed should be available after the procedure, but the usual pattern over the ensuing 24 hours is one of clinical and radiographic clearance.

Until more recently, the standard chest x-ray was used most frequently to identify cases in which evacuation of residual hemothorax is appropriate. Clinical experience suggests that the chest radiograph is insufficient to distinguish between retained hemothorax and other conditions (e.g., contusion, atelectasis, intraparenchymal hemorrhage) that are not amenable to VATS removal. In one series in which plain x-rays were compared with thoracic CT scans, the surgeons' and the radiologists' interpretations of chest x-rays were incorrect in nearly half of the cases. A recommendation was made to use chest CT scan on or about the third postinjury day in patients in whom chest x-ray would suggest the possibility of residual traumatic hemothorax.

■ SURGICAL CONSIDERATIONS

One of the underappreciated and potentially devastating consequences of thoracotomy for ongoing thoracic bleeding is systemic air embolism. When one considers the clinical circumstances, perhaps it is surprising this complication does not happen more frequently: (1) The patient typically has major ongoing hemorrhage that leads to depressed intravascular volumes and pressures. (2) The most common scenario is that of a bullet injury that has destroyed much of the pulmonary parenchymal architecture. (3) Shortly after intubation, the patients have a high positive airway pressure combined with low intravascular pressure in the face of abnormal communication between these two components of the pulmonary anatomy. The resulting scenario of air escaping the small airways and entering the bronchial veins and ultimately the pulmonary vein becomes understandable, producing a systemic air embolism. Because the above-mentioned contributing factors are all unavoidable, the one modification that might be offered is a heightened sense of urgency and rapid transport to the operating room of these patients before intubation, where possible. At this point, positioning, rapid preparation, and draping of the patient should occur first, reserving intubation for a point as close in time as possible to the actual incision. This practice decreases the length of time when increased airway pressures are present in combination with ongoing pulmonary bleeding. If the injury is to the left chest, advancing the tube down into the right main stem bronchus and keeping the left lung collapsed also may be of benefit if the collapse can be tolerated by the patient. When the thorax is entered, occluding the pulmonary hilum with a vascular clamp or with the surgeon's fingers can impede the continuous passage of air into the coronary, cerebral, and other systemic arteries. In this regard, one of the major advances in trauma surgery in the 1990s was the advanced use of the stapling device to facilitate

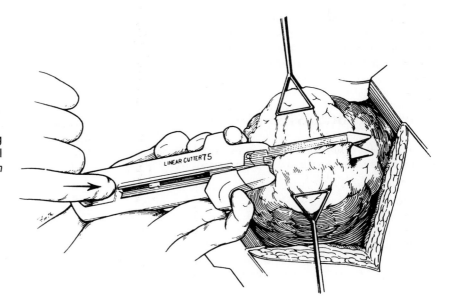

Figure 1
Pulmonary tractotomy using linear cutting stapler. (*From Asensio JA, et al:* J Am Coll Surg *185:486, 1997; with permission from the American College of Surgeons.*)

pulmonary tractotomy for hemorrhage control and to minimize introduction of systemic air.

■ PULMONARY TRACTOTOMY

Injury to the lung parenchyma is the most common cause of traumatic hemothorax requiring lifesaving thoracotomy for hemorrhage control. Until more recently, these patients typically were managed with simple oversewing, wedge resection, or anatomic resection. The aforementioned concerns of systemic air embolism have led to the practice of early hilar cross-clamping by some surgeons. Whatever technique is used, early hemorrhage control is the hallmark of this lifesaving procedure.

With the common use of staplers in surgery, pulmonary tractotomy for hemorrhage control has become one of the major advances in thoracic trauma surgery. The technique can be performed with either single-lumen or double-lumen endotracheal intubation. With a Duval lung clamp placed parallel to the track of the bullet, the stapling device is positioned so that one of the arms is placed through the entrance and exit wound of the lung (Figure 1). When the stapler is fired, the bullet track is exposed fully allowing the surgeon to suture directly bleeding vessels and transected bronchi (Figure 2). Among the patients in the author's experience is a 14-year-old whose vascular injury from a proximal branch of the pulmonary artery was managed with staple tractotomy through the central portion of the left upper lobe. The tractotomy facilitated lifesaving control of brisk hemorrhage, without any resection of pulmonary tissue. The suture that was crucial to create cessation of bleeding subsequently was found to be so centrally placed as to catch a tiny corner of pericardium, yet pneumonectomy or even wedge resection or lobectomy was avoided. Staple pulmonary tractotomy has been shown in several series to provide rapid, effective exposure to bleeding pulmonary parenchymal vessels and transected bronchi.

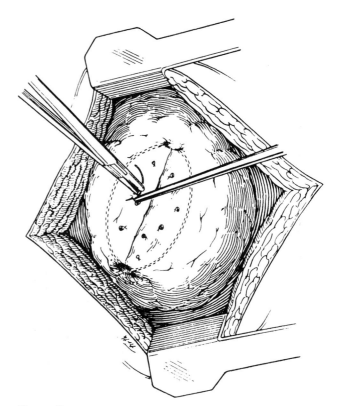

Figure 2
Suture ligation of bleeding vessels and transected bronchi after pulmonary tractotomy. (*From Asensio JA, et al:* J Am Coll Surg *185:486, 1997; with permission from the American College of Surgeons.*)

■ SUMMARY

Although most patients experiencing traumatic hemothorax can be managed by appropriate placement of a large-bore chest tube, the principles of periprocedural antibiotic coverage, attention to complete evacuation of accumulated blood, and attention to newer surgical considerations facilitate optimal outcome for patients with a wide variety of injury severity.

SUGGESTED READING

American College of Surgeons Committee on Trauma: *Advanced trauma life support for doctors,* ed 6, Chicago, 1997, First Impression.

Asensio JA, et al: Stapled pulmonary tractotomy: a rapid way to control hemorrhage in penetrating pulmonary injuries, *J Am Coll Surg* 185:486, 1997.

Ho AM: Is emergency thoracotomy always the most appropriate immediate intervention for systemic air embolism after lung trauma? *Chest* 116:234,1999.

Luchette FA, et al: Practice management guidelines for prophylactic antibiotic use in tube thoracostomy for traumatic hemopneumothorax: the EAST practice management guidelines work group. Eastern Association for Trauma, *J Trauma* 48:753, 2000.

Velmahos GC, et al: Predicting the need for thoracoscopic evacuation of residual traumatic hemothorax: chest radiograph is insufficient, *J Trauma* 46:65, 1999.

ESOPHAGEAL TRAUMA

John A. Odell

The most common cause of esophageal trauma is that which follows an endoluminal procedure, such as endoscopy, dilation, or transesophageal ultrasound (Table 1). Considering the frequency of these procedures, the risk of perforation or damage is small. In addition, because perforation is a well-recognized complication of these procedures, a high index of suspicion for these injuries exists, and when they occur, treatment usually can be instituted early. This situation does not exist with other traumatic causes of esophageal injury. Blunt traumatic rupture of the esophagus is extremely rare. Barometric trauma to the esophagus is seen commonly in Boerhaave's syndrome associated with forceful vomiting. Another variant may occur when air or gas is forced into the esophagus, such as when a tire is bitten and pressurized gas is forced into the mouth or a pressurized soda bottle cap is opened with teeth. With respect to penetrating trauma, the cervical portion of the esophagus is relatively unprotected, whereas the intrathoracic portion of the esophagus has a protected posterior relationship lying on the vertebral column: In the neck, it is vulnerable to penetrating injury; in the chest, it is infrequently damaged. The esophagus also is surrounded by other major structures, such as the trachea, aorta, and heart. Penetrating injuries commonly also damage these structures, resulting in death with the esophageal injury not being recognized or distracting the clinician away from the esophageal injury because of more obvious dramatic signs.

■ RECOGNITION OF THE INJURY

If one considers what one eats, drinks, and refluxes up and down the esophagus, it is apparent that the normal esophageal mucosa is extremely resilient. When the mucosa is breached and penetration beyond the esophagus occurs, contamination, representing the varied bacterial flora of the mouth present in swallowed saliva or food, is initiated. These organisms acting together cause a virulent form of necrotizing infection that resembles aspiration-associated lung abscess or human bites. The resulting infection may be contained in the mediastinum, may spread widely through the loose areolar tissue surrounding the esophagus within the mediastinum and neck, or rupture into the pleural space causing an empyema. Morbidity and mortality increase proportionally to the delay in diagnosis. It is important that the injury be recognized early. The clinician should understand the full spectrum of presentation and the nuances of infrequent, but well-described traumatic scenarios (e.g., intramural esophageal dissection).

The classic symptoms are dysphagia or odynophagia, but many patients do not have these symptoms. When mediastinitis is established, signs of local and systemic sepsis may be present. There may be pain with neck movement. Classic signs are subcutaneous emphysema and cervical hematoma, but these presentations also are variable. A large intrathoracic perforation may allow direct pleural fistulization with little

---

Table 1 Types of Esophageal Injury

Endoscopic trauma—esophagoscopy, dilation, transesophageal echocardiography

Blunt traumatic injury—rupture, traumatic tracheoesophageal fistula

Barometric trauma—Boerhaave's syndrome, intramural esophageal dissection, intramural esophageal hematoma, air-pressure injuries

Penetrating trauma

Caustic injury

Foreign body in the esophagus

or no evidence of subcutaneous emphysema. A presentation in which food contents are noted in the chest tube after drainage of empyema is a frequent occurrence. With lower perforation of the esophagus, pain and symptoms of upper abdominal rigidity may be present.

The plain radiograph may show mediastinal widening with or without air-fluid loculi, subcutaneous emphysema, and a pleural fluid collection, which also may have an air-fluid level. Occasionally, computed tomography may identify loculations of fluid. When a leak is suspected, a contrast study usually is performed. Thin barium rather than diatrizoate sodium (Gastrografin) is favored: Extraluminal contrast with Gastrografin is poorly seen sometimes and if there is communication with the airway may cause pulmonary edema. Barium was one of the early contrast agents used for bronchograms, so it is reasonably well tolerated if aspiration occurs. The disadvantage with barium is that it tends to remain visible in the injury tract or mediastinum and may cause a foreign body–like reaction. Follow-up barium swallows to assess the continued presence of a leak or the size of the leak may require preswallow radiographs and careful interpretation because of preexisting barium from a previous study.

In some injuries, the likelihood of esophageal injury is high and definitely should be considered, such as transmediastinal injuries. A common scenario is one in which a stab wound by a right-handed assailant enters the left side of the neck, which causes a right pneumothorax or empyema. The trachea or esophagus or both invariably are damaged. Similarly, patients with bullet wounds that traverse the mediastinum should have the esophagus checked.

Esophagoscopy, either with a rigid or a flexible instrument, is not done for diagnostic purposes. Rather, it is useful in patients who require immediate exploration for concomitant injuries in whom contrast studies cannot be performed. The site of trauma is often difficult to see, and reliance on hematoma, blood clot, air leak, and other indirect evidence is sometimes necessary. If traumatic injury to the esophagus is a strong possibility and exposure of the neck or chest has been performed for concomitant injuries, careful inspection of the esophagus should take place. Insufflating air into the esophagus through a nasogastric tube and looking for bubbles in the dissected operative site submerged with saline may sometimes reveal the leak. In some patients, a contrast study may need to be done after these surgical procedures or completion of resuscitation to look for other injuries.

■ MANAGEMENT

A broad clinical spectrum of esophageal trauma ranges from contained small leaks that are recognized early to large leaks with severe mediastinal infection. Factors that are believed to influence management include site of the leak (cervical, thoracic, or intraabdominal), severity of sepsis, length of time from perforation to diagnosis, patients with preexisting esophageal disease in whom the esophageal injury occurred while undergoing endoscopy or dilation, and other comorbidities.

Despite the underlying cause of the esophageal injury, the main consequences are perforation and leakage. Generally, efforts should be directed toward limiting soilage, encouraging healing of the perforation by suture or drainage, and maintaining nutrition of the patient. In some patients, healing is unlikely to occur because of severe sepsis or extensive damage, and other forms of management need to be considered. A basic schema for the management of esophageal trauma is shown in Figure 1.

A reasonable starting point for the discussion of esophageal trauma is to separate patients with preexisting esophageal disease from patients with a normal esophagus. This distinction is important because if preexisting disease is present, it may need to be dealt with at the same time as management of the leak or perforation. An additional consideration is that healing is unlikely to occur in the presence

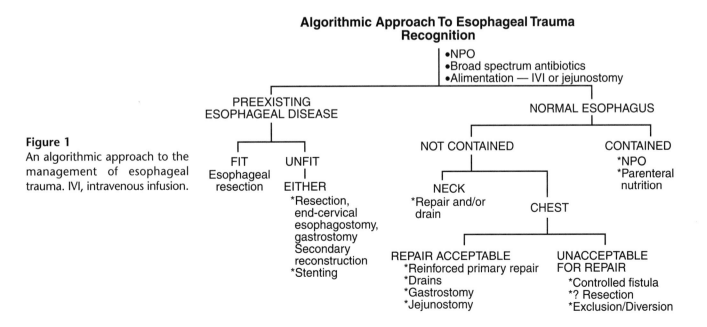

Algorithmic Approach To Esophageal Trauma Recognition

Figure 1
An algorithmic approach to the management of esophageal trauma. IVI, intravenous infusion.

of distal obstructing carcinoma. If the patient's general condition is good, primary resection and reconstruction with stomach should be considered. Usually these patients are seen early after the injury has occurred (usually from endoscopy), and the consequences of infection are often less. Some patients with a stricture may be managed in the same manner as patients with a normal esophagus if the stricture can be dilated. In patients with achalasia, a myotomy should be performed at the same time as repair, commonly on the side opposite the site of repair. If the patient's condition is unstable, resection and drainage with end-cervical esophagostomy and gastrostomy with delayed reconstruction should be pursued. Decisions are difficult in patients in whom comorbidities and metastases exist. Often there is pressure on the surgeon to perform some sort of intervention because of an iatrogenically produced perforation. Occasionally a stent may be passed across the site of disruption to seal the leak, but it often fails to achieve complete exclusion.

Rarely, in some patients with a normal esophagus, there are few or no symptoms and no signs of sepsis, with a leak well contained within the mediastinum. In these instances, the patient is observed carefully, given broad-spectrum antibiotics, and fed intravenously; the barium swallow is repeated at regular weekly intervals.

If the leak is not contained, the site of the perforation dictates further management. Esophageal injury in the neck, if seen early, is managed by exploration and repair with a soft drain placed to the area. This repair may be reinforced by adjacent tissue or muscle. If a leak is not apparent after 5 days, the drain is removed; if present, the drain remains until the leak closes. If the leak in the neck is seen late, only the abscess is drained, and no attempt is made to repair the site of disruption.

Esophageal leaks in the chest, unless in the rare instance in which the leak is contained without symptoms, are managed by thoracotomy and repair in virtually every patient no matter the length of time that has passed since the injury. This is a change from the more traditional approach, in which, if presentation was late, it was believed that suture closure invariably broke down. Excellent results of late repair have been reported by many groups, particularly from Massachusetts General Hospital. In many of these patients, thoracotomy would be necessary in any event, for management of the empyema and wide drainage of the mediastinum. Repair adds little to the morbidity of the procedure. The operative side is dictated by the injury. Upper thoracic leaks are approached best through the right side; lower esophageal leaks (below the aortic arch) may be approached from either side, or the approach may be dictated by the side the tract drains toward or the side that has the larger pleural fluid collection. I tend to approach lower leaks from the left because a gastrostomy and feeding jejunostomy can be performed fairly easily without redraping.

At operation, the lung is decorticated, and the pleural space is evacuated of debris. The extent of reaction involving the pleura is often dramatic; even in patients with leakage for a few hours, the pleura is reddened and edematous. The mediastinum is widely opened and all necrotic tissue removed. Externally the leak in the esophagus often appears smaller than the mucosal tear. It is important that the esophageal muscle is opened and removed if necrotic, until

the full extent of the mucosal tear is exposed. If a penetrating injury was the cause of leakage, through-and-through leaks should be excluded with esophagostomy. The repair is closed with interrupted absorbable sutures. If possible, the esophageal muscle is reapproximated over the repair; in some instances in which necrotic muscle has been excised, this is not possible. All repairs are buttressed by additional tissue. The pleura is often thickened and edematous and is commonly used, but other tissue, such as intercostal muscle (without periosteum, as bone can form and cause external narrowing), pericardial fat, diaphragm, stomach, or omentum, can be used. The tissue buttress provides an extra layer of reinforcement to prevent and contain any leak. The repair is tested by instilling air into the esophagus via a nasogastric tube, while the operative site is flooded with saline. The chest is washed out thoroughly and cleaned of debris. If the opposite pleural space was opened during débridement, that side also needs tube thoracostomy drainage. Chest tubes are placed close to the site of repair. When the chest is closed, a draining gastrostomy and feeding jejunostomy are performed. A nasoesophageal tube is positioned in the esophagus close to the repair and placed on intermittent suction and limits to some degree soiling by saliva in the acute phase. Enteral feeding is started as soon as bowel function returns.

Further management is directed toward reducing infection and preventing breakdown of the repair. Approximately 15% to 50% of repairs break down. Effort on reducing leakage is time well spent. Broad-spectrum antibiotics are administered particularly to deal with organisms commonly found in the mouth. The stomach is kept well drained to prevent reflux of gastric contents through the repair. An H_2-blocker is given to reduce stomach acidity. The chest tubes are kept in place until a barium swallow is performed on postoperative day 6 or 7 and shows no leak. The rationale is that if a leak develops, it is better to have it controlled by localization along the tube tract. Patients with residual but contained leaks (no leakage via the chest tubes) have chest drains removed because they no longer serve a purpose. Conservative management is continued, and contrast studies are repeated weekly. Mucus in the chest tube, the development of a new pneumothorax or air-fluid levels, or the development of an air leak at any stage indicates a breakdown of the repair. The chest tubes allow conversion of the repair to that of a controlled fistula: The pleural contamination causes an effective pleurodesis around the chest tubes. At this later stage after repair, I am not obsessive about keeping the patient strictly nothing per mouth (NPO) because a nasoesophageal tube is difficult to keep in place for a long time, especially if the patient's morale is declining. In addition, saliva is swallowed continually, and contamination does occur. Water is allowed to be taken by mouth. If a late leak develops but has good drainage, patients are encouraged to take water. The rationale is that water washes out debris, dilutes organisms, and does not seem to delay healing. If a leak is apparent through the chest tube, this is confirmed and followed, usually without contrast studies by observing the presence or absence of swallowed methylene blue egressing through the chest tube. When methylene fluid no longer is seen, contrast studies are used. Methylene blue is not used intraoperatively to localize the site of perforation—it widely stains tissues, making visualization difficult. Generally over time (a few weeks), the leak slowly diminishes and closes. After the acute phase has passed, the chest tube can be converted to an open system and withdrawn. Although a general pessimistic attitude exists toward esophageal leaks, largely due to the accompanying severe mediastinitis and pleural infection, it sometimes is gratifying and surprising that extensive esophageal injuries heal with simple adherence to basic principles of effective drainage.

Numerous other approaches to a perforation that are "not readily reparable" are advocated, which remains undefined. Esophageal exclusion and diversion has been used by some authors for most esophageal perforations. Most authors reserve it for the patient in whom there is extensive tearing and soiling of the mediastinum. Side- or end-cervical esophagostomy can be performed. If necessary, the stomach is excluded from the esophagus by various methods, including staples and ligatures of absorbable or nonabsorbable sutures, passed through a Rumel tourniquet, either around the esophagogastric junction or across the lower end of the esophagus. The disadvantage of these approaches is that an additional procedure is necessary when healing of the perforation has occurred; this may include repair of the cervical esophagus and bougienage of the occluding staples. These additional procedures have an added morbidity and may be unsuccessful in that a further leak or stricture may be produced. This is why the aggressive approach of repair and drainage previously described is advocated.

Another form of management that has been effective for the "not readily reparable" injury is the use of an esophageal T-tube to convert the leak into a controlled fistula. The T-tube (and chest tube) should not be placed against the aorta because erosion occurs. It is extremely difficult to justify the effectiveness of these exclusion procedures. Is a lateral cervical esophagostomy more diverting than a sump nasoesophageal tube? Is banding or stapling the distal esophagus more efficient than a gastrostomy tube placed on suction?

In a review of 13 collected series totaling 589 patients, Jones and Ginsberg reported an overall mortality of 22% for esophageal perforation. Primary repair was associated with the lowest mortality. Patients treated nonoperatively also had a 22% mortality. Exclusion and diversion was associated with a mortality of 39%. Selection bias may be responsible for the different results and choice of therapy. Cause, location, delay in treatment, underlying disease, and type of treatment identified significant risk factors for death from esophageal trauma.

■ CORROSIVE INJURY

There are two scenarios in which corrosive injuries commonly occur. The first scenario is usually a child, occasionally an adult, who inadvertently swallows the caustic agent. In these patients, the volumes are usually small, and the noxious taste makes the patient immediately spit out the agent. This often results in damage localized mainly to the oropharynx or larnyx or both, with usually, but not always, limited involvement of the esophagus. The other scenario is in adults who attempt suicide and who swallow larger volumes of the caustic agent and have more severe injuries. The injury may be severe enough to cause perforation of the esophagus and stomach, and in some instances necrosis may extend to involve the liver, spleen, pancreas, and duodenum. There also can be extensive damage to the larynx, and tracheostomy may be necessary to maintain an airway.

The list of agents may include sulfuric acid, hydrochloric acid, sodium hydroxide, and potassium hydroxide (e.g., oven cleaners, toilet bowl cleaners, drain cleaners). Dishwasher detergents, Clinitest tablets, and small batteries may contain strong alkaline elements. Ammonia and hypochlorite solutions are less caustic. Acids produce injury by coagulation necrosis, whereas alkaline agents produce injury by liquefaction necrosis.

Treatment is usually supportive, unless perforation or fullthickness necrosis is present. Laparotomy or thoracotomy with resection of necrotic stomach or esophagus is necessary if there is full-thickness esophageal necrosis or perforation, peritoneal signs, or a persistent alkaline pH reading on the nasogastric tube aspirate (this indicates destruction of acidproducing gastric glands). Restoration of gastrointestinal continuity is not pursued until recovery has occurred. Endoscopy, usually done cautiously with minimal insufflation under general anesthesia, is useful to assess the depth and extent of injury and involvement of the stomach. It also is useful to exclude patients with minimal injury who do not require hospital admission. The degree of injury has been classified as follows: erythema and edema, first-degree burns; noncircumferential ulceration and white plaques, seconddegree burns; and circumferential ulceration, white plaques and sloughing, third-degree burns. Steroids have serious side effects with little benefit. Any oral diet is withheld until patients are swallowing their saliva without pain. Then patients are started on a liquid diet and advanced slowly to a soft diet over several days. Repeat barium swallows may be necessary to determine the presence of perforation or stricture. Strictures usually occur 2 to 4 weeks after caustic insult.

Esophageal stricture is to be anticipated and needs to be managed by dilation. Some authors recommend immediate gastrostomy for passage of a string through the esophagus and out the nasopharynx to facilitate retrograde dilation or placement of an endoesophageal stent.

■ ESOPHAGEAL FOREIGN BODIES

Similar to corrosive injuries, children and adults present with two distinct patterns of esophageal foreign body lodgment. Children swallow a large variety of objects, predominantly toys and coins. In adults, food boluses, bone splinters, and fish bones are common. Safety pins, hairpins, and defective dentures have become less common and replaced by more "modern" foreign bodies, such as buttons, batteries, beverage can openers, and cocaine packages.

Adults with esophageal foreign bodies usually know what has become stuck. Many patients have strictures of the esophagus and have had episodes of food "sticking" previously. The common site of lodgment is the cervical portion at the cricopharyngeus muscle. In an adult, a foreign body in the distal esophagus or repeated episodes of food impaction always should prompt suspicion for an underlying esophageal disorder.

When the history is suspicious for a retained esophageal foreign body, chest and lateral cervical radiographs should be obtained. The foreign body may be obvious; subcutaneous emphysema would indicate that a perforation has occurred. A barium swallow is not usually performed because it may radiographically mask the foreign body. Esophagoscopy is performed if there is any suspicion of a foreign body even if physical examination and radiographic interpretation are normal. Soda drinks (in the belief that the bubbles can dislodge the food bolus) have no proven benefit and may induce regurgitation, vomiting, and aspiration. Papain should not be used to dissolve a meat bolus because perforation has been described. Usually the foreign body is extracted best under general anesthesia using rigid esophagoscopy. If the object is larger than the esophagoscope, it is grasped under direct visualization and brought into the opening of the scope. With a firm grasp of the object, the scope, forceps, and foreign body are withdrawn as a unit. Particular care is necessary in the removal of sharp objects. The sharp points may need to be covered with suction tubes or withdrawn with the sharp end trailing. Occasionally a fiberoptic extraction may be useful by gently insufflating the esophagus and providing a wider esophageal aperture to retract the object.

After the foreign body is removed, it is advisable to reinspect the impaction site to exclude a mucosal tear or esophageal pathology. In some instances, a contrast study also may be necessary.

■ INTRAMURAL HEMATOMA/DISSECTION

Intramural hematoma/dissection is an uncommon condition, which should be recognized specifically because it is managed conservatively. The condition variously has been termed *intramural hematoma*, *submucosal hematoma*, and *intramural esophageal dissection*. Two theories of pathogenesis have been proposed. Bleeding may occur spontaneously beneath the submucosal layer, resulting in a hematoma, which may track over a considerable distance and obstruct the esophageal lumen by varying degrees. It may rupture into the esophagus, resulting in hematemesis as the presenting symptom. The other theory suggests that the mucosa tears first with secondary dissection of the submucosal layer. Approximately one third of patients either have a medical condition predisposing to coagulopathy or are on anticoagulants. Apart from symptoms of bleeding and obstruction, some patients have chest or back pain, odynophagia, nausea, or vomiting. Women are affected more commonly than men, and this condition occurs more often in the elderly.

The diagnosis is made best by oral contrast studies. Occasionally the hematoma and mucosal tear may be visible at endoscopy, but invasive procedures usually are not recommended because of concern about extending or perforating a contained process.

Management is nonoperative, including analgesics, antibiotics, and intravenous alimentation while healing occurs. If stability or healing is shown by repeat esophagram after a week, a soft diet can be instituted and the patient discharged.

SUGGESTED READING

Barros JL, et al: Foreign body ingestion: management of 167 cases, *World J Surg* 15:783, 1991.

Bufkin BL, et al: Esophageal perforation: emphasis on management, *Ann Thorac Surg* 61:1447, 1996.

Cameron JL, et al: Selective nonoperative management of contained intrathoracic esophageal disruptions, *Ann Thorac Surg* 27:404, 1979.

Jones WG, Ginsberg RJ: Esophageal perforation: a continuing challenge, *Ann Thorac Surg* 53:534, 1992.

Shama DM, Odell JA: Penetrating neck trauma with tracheal and oesophageal injuries, *Br J Surg* 71:534, 1985.

Wright CD, et al: Reinforced primary repair of thoracic esophageal perforation, *Ann Thorac Surg* 60:245, 1995.

PULMONARY INJURY

Scott B. Johnson
John H. Calhoon

Injury to the lungs can cause significant morbidity and mortality in patients who have sustained thoracic trauma. Traumatic lung injury is commonly blunt or penetrating. Motor vehicle accidents, shootings, and stabbings account for most injuries seen at trauma centers. Iatrogenic injuries to lung parenchyma also can be a significant source of in-hospital morbidity given that life-sustaining supportive care is not without risk. Examples include barotrauma or air embolism secondary to high-pressure ventilation, pneumothoraces from central venous line placements, and pulmonary injury caused by inadvertent placement of feeding catheters or nasogastric tubes into the airway. In the 20th century, during World War I, mortality from chest wounds was greater than 50%, which decreased to less than 10% in World War II and even less in the Korean and Vietnam wars. In civilian practice, supportive measures and tube thoracostomy are sufficient treatment for nearly 85% of patients with pulmonary trauma.

■ PREOPERATIVE EVALUATION AND TREATMENT

Pulmonary injury frequently is associated with injuries to other major organ systems. The basics of airway, breathing, and circulation continue to be important in the treatment of patients who have sustained significant pulmonary injury. Patients who are comatose, moribund, or in respiratory distress usually require intubation and mechanical ventilation. Cardiopulmonary resuscitation remains the mainstay of initial treatment in patients who experience cardiorespiratory collapse. Vital signs should be assessed early while performing the primary survey because they may signal the need for immediate lifesaving therapy. In a patient who has sustained a gunshot wound to the chest who is tachycardic, tachypneic, and hypotensive with no breath sounds on the side of injury, an ipsilateral tube thoracostomy should be placed before performing any further diagnostic studies. In a patient who likewise has sustained a gunshot wound to the chest but is in no distress with normal vital signs, a more leisurely workup and evaluation is possible. When a major pulmonary injury is suspected, two large-caliber intravenous lines should be inserted, one centrally if possible. A blood sample should be obtained simultaneously for a type and crossmatch. A pulse oximeter is a useful, noninvasive method of continuously monitoring trends in oxygenation, whereas insertion of an arterial catheter can provide instantaneous measurement of blood pressure and allows for frequent blood gas measurements that may help guide resuscitation.

When the patient is stabilized, a more careful, thoughtful, yet rapid history should be obtained whenever possible. This history should include facts such as the circumstances of the accident and mode of injury (e.g., speed of vehicles involved, location of the patient with respect to the vehicle, restraints used, time to extrication, fatalities at the scene, problems encountered by emergency medical services in the field, caliber of the weapon, distance from the assailant, or type of knife used). In addition, a past medical history should be obtained to include as a minimum a list of current medications and allergies. A past medical history is particularly important when dealing with elderly patients who may be on anticoagulants or who have chronic conditions such as renal insufficiency, cardiac disease, or chronic obstructive pulmonary disease. In performing the secondary survey, the trauma victim should be completely disrobed for evaluation of all wounds and injuries. This evaluation should include the patient's entire back and skin, which often can indicate or give subtle clues to the injury of other structures. Entrance and exit wounds can be less than obvious—often this is the case with ice pick wounds or low-velocity gunshot wounds. When the patient is hemodynamically stable, an upright posteroanterior and lateral chest radiograph should be obtained in full inspiration. A hematocrit, electrocardiogram, urinalysis, and other routine laboratory work should be obtained. When indicated, special studies, such as sonography, can be obtained later to rule out cardiac injuries and to determine whether or not a diaphragm laceration or disruption is present.

If the patient has a penetrating missile injury and there is suspicion of injury to mediastinal structures, evaluation of the esophagus and great vessels should be performed. Contrast esophagography, esophageal endoscopy, angiography, and bronchoscopy all are useful in diagnosing mediastinal visceral injury. Ongoing significant air leaks or an air leak coupled with hemoptysis is an indication to perform bronchoscopy to rule out major tracheobronchial injury. This may be done at the bedside or in the operating room depending on the patient's hemodynamic stability and acuity of other injuries. In addition, computed tomography of the chest can be helpful in diagnosing pulmonary contusions, pleural fluid collections, thoracic aortic injuries, and diaphragmatic disruptions. Transesophageal echocardiography, if available and performed by experienced personnel, can be an invaluable diagnostic tool and help guide inotropic supportive measures when necessary. The clinician must remember, however, that special studies are time-consuming, often are falsely negative or positive, and can impose risk while delaying appropriate and indicated therapy. Special studies should be obtained only when specifically indicated in a hemodynamically stable patient.

■ SURGICAL INDICATIONS

Absolute indications for surgery are exsanguination and uncontrollable air leak from a chest cavity. Either of these usually becomes evident after the placement of a thoracostomy tube. Simple tube thoracostomy is done best with rolled sheets under the affected side, with placement into the fourth or fifth intercostal space mid to anterior axillary line, with the tube directed posteriorly. Initial drainage from chest tubes should be noted. Frequently, tube thoracostomy results in a large initial blood loss that rapidly subsides with full expansion of the lung and approximation of the two pleural surfaces. Nonetheless, immediate surgery should be considered in patients who initially have greater than 1200 ml of drainage from chest tubes. In addition, urgent surgery should be considered in patients who continue to bleed greater than 400 ml after the first hour, or 200 ml after the second hour, or who continue to bleed greater than 100 ml/hr without indications of slowing because this usually suggests an injury to either a major pulmonary vessel or systemic artery that requires surgical ligation or repair. These guidelines are not absolute, however. One may decide to continue to observe a stable patient who is continuing to bleed if he or she is coagulopathic, in which case transfusion of appropriate clotting factors rather than immediate operation may be more appropriate; likewise, one may decide to explore a patient who has had less blood loss if his or her vital signs are deteriorating, or if the bleeding is increasing rather than decreasing, or if a significant intrathoracic hematoma is seen on chest radiograph despite appropriately placed thoracostomy tubes. The surgeon should proceed to surgery only if the overall clinical situation warrants. Rarely, if the patient with massive bleeding has vital signs that are deteriorating rapidly, the patient may require an emergency department thoracotomy as a lifesaving maneuver.

A tracheobronchial injury should be suspected in any patient with a massive air leak. Tracheobronchial injury also should be suspected in trauma patients who present with or subsequently develop subcutaneous emphysema.

Bronchoscopy is indicated when tracheobronchial injury is suspected. It can give important information regarding the presence and location of specific injuries and be useful in planning surgical approach. It also can aid in securing the airway. It is common for patients who have sustained significant pulmonary trauma with an air leak to require ventilatory assistance for associated pulmonary contusion. Mechanical ventilation often worsens air leaks secondary to positive pressure forces. Most *parenchymal* lung injuries associated with air leaks respond to low ventilatory pressures, chest tube drainage, and patience. In patients who are unstable secondary to large ventilatory volume loss, the surgeon can attempt under bronchoscopic guidance to place the endotracheal tube down past the injury (if in the trachea) or down into the contralateral main stem bronchus if immediate control of the airway or more effective ventilation becomes necessary. In these cases, the chest tube should be placed to water seal rather than to suction to minimize pressure gradients and subsequent ventilatory volume loss. In patients with massive, uncontrollable air leaks or confirmed major tracheobronchial disruption, immediate surgical exploration may be the patient's only chance for survival.

Relative indications for surgery include retained foreign body, undrained large hemothoraces, sucking chest wounds or defects, and, on rare occasions, flail segment. Other relative late indications for surgery include persistent air leaks, entrapped lung, persistent hemoptysis, empyema, and (late recognized) bronchial disruption. Well-placed chest drains, good pulmonary toilet, aggressive use of diagnostic and therapeutic bronchoscopy, and occasionally the skill of the invasive radiologist often can treat or avoid these complications altogether.

■ SURGICAL CONSIDERATIONS

Good anesthetic technique is crucial to a successful surgical outcome. A well-functioning peripheral arterial line, a central venous pressure/volume line, and multiple large-bore peripheral intravenous access lines are helpful to have and be secured *before* positioning. Transesophageal echocardiography can be useful in assessing volume status and detecting air emboli to the left side of the heart and can help direct inotropic support. The time that it takes to place either a double-lumen endotracheal tube or a balloon-tipped, single-lumen tube is invariably worth the effort. Single-lung ventilation often can be crucial in allowing the surgeon exposure of important structures. Intraoperative bronchoscopy, in addition to diagnosing tracheobronchial injury, can be used to confirm endotracheal tube placement. When indicated, the judicial use of intravenous nitroglycerin, dopamine, milrinone, or inhaled nitric oxide can augment ventilation and perfusion significantly in patients requiring single-lung ventilation or patients who have sustained significant pulmonary injury.

■ POSITIONING AND OPERATIVE APPROACH

Positioning of patients undergoing surgery to repair pulmonary injuries requires consideration of not only exposure to the injured lung parenchyma and tracheobronchial tree, but also other injuries the patient may have sustained. In planning the operative approach, the surgeon must consider all structures that may need repair, such as the brachiocephalic vessels, diaphragm, esophagus, heart, and chest wall. In most cases, priority should be given first, however, to obtaining adequate intravenous access, obtaining control of the airway, and evaluating adequately and working up other injuries the patient may have sustained.

Bilateral injuries or injuries involving the heart are approached best through either a median sternotomy with both arms tucked or a bilateral "clamshell" anterolateral thoracotomy with both arms out. If a median sternotomy is used to explore the lungs, the incision should be generous and the pleura opened widely. Dividing the pericardial hilar attachments can provide additional exposure and allow delivery of most of the lung into the wound, while helping to preserve cardiac output. An indication to use this approach includes large air leaks from both chest cavities in which one suspects either a major proximal tracheal injury or major bilateral parenchymal injuries that may require resection or other operative intervention. It must be kept in mind, however, that exposure of the pulmonary hilum is suboptimal with this approach, especially to the left side. Unilateral thoracic injury is approached best through a posterolateral thoracotomy because this provides optimal exposure to the lung apices, the diaphragm, the pulmonary hilum, and the esophagus. If the injury appears to be located inferiorly within the chest, a sixth or seventh interspace incision should be made. Conversely, if the injury is in the clavicular, cervical, or apical area, exploration is made best in the third or fourth interspace. An anterolateral thoracotomy provides less exposure to the posterior mediastinal structures and hilum but can be done with the patient in the supine position with the arms out, allowing for emergent entrance into the pleural space. This incision can be extended across the sternum (hemi-clamshell) to gain access to cardiac structures when necessary. In the stable patient in whom a major cardiac or pulmonary hilar injury is not likely present, a thoracoscopic exploration sometimes can suffice. This approach also is performed best in a full lateral decubitus position.

■ TECHNIQUES

When the pleural space is entered, a systematic exploration should be done with evacuation of fresh blood, clot, and any foreign material. Severe bleeding usually can be controlled with digital pressure until its source can be identified accurately and controlled more precisely with a clamp or stitch. Bleeding from lung parenchyma can be profound, and occasionally temporary manual occlusion of the hilum is necessary for control. Profound air leaks caused by major tracheobronchial injury often can be controlled temporarily by having the anesthesiologist advance the endotracheal tube distal to a tracheal injury or down into the opposite bronchus while the surgeon guides it with manual palpation. In the rare patient with a large tracheal defect, this maneuver sometimes can be done directly through the wound using forceps. Under difficult circumstances, a sterile catheter can be brought directly through the operative field and ventilation performed using high-frequency, low tidal volume techniques directly through the injured segment. Using the above-mentioned techniques, one usually can obtain adequate ventilation, arrest life-threatening hemorrhage, and begin to assess the injury more carefully to plan definitive repair.

Repair of pulmonary injuries presents unique technical challenges and considerations. Parenchymal air leaks tend to close with reexpansion alone, although large leaks can lead to poor oxygenation and inadequate ventilation. Air leaks may require increased ventilatory support, usually at the expense of higher airway pressures. This situation can lead to perpetuation of the air leak and a self-defeating situation. In addition, higher ventilatory pressures can lead to an increased host systemic inflammatory response, mediating further pulmonary damage distant to the site of injury. For these reasons, air leaks should be sought at the time of exploration and repaired if possible. Isolated, peripheral air leaks sometimes can be sutured primarily and closed; however, the visceral pleura supports suture ligatures poorly, and attempting simple suture repair often leads to more air leaks. Because of this, we prefer to use stapled pneumorrhaphy for these types of peripheral injuries. Occasionally in the stable patient, available tissue sealants can be used to cover a wide or deep area when sutures or staples are ineffective, particularly in the fissure.

The trachea and bronchus have a relatively poor blood supply that often can lead to a tenuous repair. Tracheal injuries usually can be fixed using straightforward surgical techniques. Stellate injuries can be repaired by débridement followed by primary closure with or without a pericardial patch or resection with primary anastomosis. Methods to reduce tension on a tracheal anastomosis include mobilization of the pretracheal space, chin flexion, division of pericardial and pulmonary attachments, release of suprahyoid structures, and reimplantation of the left main stem bronchus. We prefer to use a monofilament, long-term absorbable suture in a figure-of-eight technique anteriorly (around the cartilage) and a running technique posteriorly (for the membranous portion). Primary repair should be buttressed with intercostal muscle, pleural, pericardial, or omental flaps. Bronchial injuries can be treated similarly or resected based on the location and extent of the injury. In cases that require formal resection, we prefer to use a stapler for the bronchial stump. The stump can be buttressed with appropriate flaps when indicated.

Bleeding parenchyma usually responds to simple cauterization so long as large vessels are not involved. In the case of deeper parenchymal injuries with active bleeding, tractotomy may be a useful approach. Coined by Mattox, *tractotomy* involves the unroofing of pulmonary bleeders by dividing (usually with the aid of a stapling device) the lung parenchyma overlying a missile tract, allowing direct suture ligature of bleeding vessels. When doing this, care should be taken, however, to ensure large portions of lung are not devitalized, which could lead to further sepsis. If large areas of lung parenchyma are involved and bleeding is centrally located or massive, anatomic resection, such as lobectomy, may be required. When peripheral areas of parenchyma have been injured and are bleeding (which is commonly the case), simple pneumorrhaphy using a stapling device is an excellent method of controlling the hemorrhage. As a last resort, in the patient in whom bleeding is so massive that control is impossible, pneumonectomy may be required. Mortality in these cases is high.

■ NONOPERATIVE THERAPY

Occasionally a gunshot wound to the thorax is associated with little or no hemopneumothorax. In addition, bullets rarely cause complications while stationary. As a result, the presence of a bullet within the parenchyma is in itself not an indication for tube thoracostomy or surgery. Surgery should be reserved for patients who have ongoing hemorrhage or who have significant respiratory compromise secondary to air leaks. Most patients with parenchymal lung injury can be managed with simple tube thoracostomy or ventilatory support alone. In addition, with the increasing use of specialized imaging studies, such as sonography, computed tomography, and magnetic resonance imaging, and other diagnostic tests whose high sensitivity often leads to false-positive results, one must be cautious of overtreatment. The presence of a small hemothorax or small pneumothorax within the chest cavity seen on computed tomography scan associated with a bullet is not by itself an indication for surgery, unless the patient has appropriate clinical findings to suggest an operation is otherwise necessary.

■ CRITICAL CARE ISSUES

Good critical care management is important in treating patients who have sustained pulmonary injury. Traumatic pulmonary injury can lead to release of immune mediators that can cause a systemic inflammatory response, further injuring lung parenchyma distant to the site of the traumatic injury. This situation can lead eventually to fulminate respiratory failure and an acute respiratory distress syndrome–type pattern commonly seen in multiply-injured patients. The thoracic surgeon should be competent in the use of ventilator support strategies to limit hypoventilation, hypoxemia, and barotrauma that may contribute further to injury. Ventilatory principles include avoiding high peak pressures, minimizing the need for prolonged high inspiratory oxygen concentrations, and maintaining normal carbon dioxide levels and acid-base status. These strategies may include using prolonged inspiratory times and short (but adequate) expiratory times (i.e., reverse inspiratory/expiratory ratios) and changing from a volume control mode to a pressure control mode of ventilation. Positive end-expiratory pressure may be necessary to improve oxygenation but may worsen shunt fractions and increase mean airway pressures. This situation may lead to increased intravascular fluid volume requirements. In this case, pulmonary arterial catheterization may be indicated to gauge fluid volumes and shifts better. Vigilance at the patient's bedside may be necessary to maximize ventilatory support, limit additional parenchymal lung injury, and maintain adequate ventilation and cardiac output.

■ MORBIDITY AND MORTALITY

Complications of pulmonary injury are common and range from simple atelectasis and hematoma to retained hemothoraces, severe pulmonary contusion, pneumonia, and empyema. Early bronchoscopy and aggressive pulmonary toilet along with adequate pain relief should be employed liberally. Retained hemothorax frequently may lead to entrapped lung (fibrothorax) and the subsequent development of an empyema. Intrathoracic fluid collections, fever, and leukocytosis all are suggestive of empyema. Most small intraparenchymal hematomas and contusions eventually heal with supportive therapy alone.

Death from isolated pulmonary injury requiring simple pneumorrhaphy or tractotomy is rare (<1%) in the absence of significant comorbidities or other injuries. When a major resection is required or when pulmonary injury is associated with other body organ injuries (especially in patients who have sustained severe blunt trauma), mortality may exceed 25%. Patients with a documented systemic air embolism secondary to a penetrating pulmonary injury have a mortality rate exceeding 90%, as do patients who have required an emergent pneumonectomy for exsanguinating hemorrhage in the setting of hypotensive shock.

■ LEGAL IMPLICATIONS

Historically, little attention is given to the legal aspect of penetrating wounds. A careful history should be obtained to include all circumstances of the injury. All physical evidence should be preserved. The weapon, the missile, and any product of the weapons discharged should be marked and noted. Clothing should be retained for examination of any entrance or exit sites or traces of gunpowder. The surgeon should describe as specifically as possible findings such as garment orientation, location of any burned or débrided tissue, or unburned powder fragments that possibly could trace the missile to a weapon. The operative report should include a detailed description of the entrance and exit wounds. An estimate of the proximity of the firearm should be made by the appearance of the wound. Contact wounds have a flash burn and bruises. Wounds inflicted from further away, but still relatively close, may be "tattooed" with burnt powder, whereas more distant wounds lack this. Well described are the differences in kinetic energy that result by using the formula K is proportional to $1/2\ MV^2$ (where K is the kinetic energy, M is the mass of the missile, and V is muzzle velocity.) For example, a 22-caliber weapon has only 75 foot-lb of kinetic energy at the muzzle, whereas a 38 special has 350 foot-lb.

Many police weapons now carry greater than 1000 foot-lb of kinetic energy. Hunting rifles can have even greater kinetic energy at the muzzle, ranging from 2000 to 3000 foot-lb. The type of the missile also is important with respect to injury of the lung and chest wall. Missiles that are hollow or soft point expand and dissipate their energy internally, potentially creating a tremendous amount of parenchymal injury. As with all penetrating pulmonary injuries, injuries to other organ systems, such as to the abdominal viscera, must be considered. A careful catalogue of all the injuries not only is medically indicated, but also has important legal implications.

■ CONCLUSION

Blunt chest injuries tend to have a much higher mortality than penetrating injuries because of the propensity for multiple system damage, particularly head trauma. They are responsible for 50,000 deaths and 1.5 million disabling injuries every year. Improvements in motor vehicle seat belts and air bags have helped to decrease this morbidity and mortality. Many automobile accidents involve the indiscriminate use of mind-altering drugs. It is important to document clinical findings of inebriation, laboratory blood alcohol levels, and results of blood and urine toxicology screens for the medical record.

SUGGESTED READING

Cryer HG, et al: Shock, transfusion, and pneumonectomy: death is due to right heart failure and increased pulmonary vascular resistance, *Ann Surg* 212:197, 1990.

Gillette MA, Hess DR: Ventilator-induced lung injury and the evolution of lung-protective strategies in acute respiratory distress syndrome, *Resp Care Rev* 46:130, 2001.

Hoff SJ, et al: Outcome of isolated pulmonary contusion in blunt trauma patients, *Am Surg* 60:138, 1994.

Richardson JD, et al: Management of transmediastinal gunshot wounds, *Surgery* 90:671, 1981.

Wall MJ Jr, et al: Pulmonary tractotomy with selective vascular ligation for penetrating injuries to the lung, *Am J Surg* 168:665, 1994.

DIAPHRAGMATIC INJURIES

T. Y. Hsia

Stephen C. Yang

Senertus described the first traumatic diaphragmatic injury in 1541. Today, our understanding of the pathophysiology and management of diaphragmatic injury and rupture continues to come from the trauma literature. With the advent of modern high-speed transportation and increased firearm violence in society, traumatic diaphragmatic injury appears to be a disease in evolution. Injury to or rupture of the diaphragm due to penetrating and blunt truncal trauma is seen with increasing frequency. In North American series, the prevalence of diaphragmatic rupture among blunt trauma victims ranges from 0.8% to 8%, whereas 10% to 42% of all penetrating left thoracoabdominal trauma victims sustained diaphragmatic injury. As a result of a greater awareness, routine use of chest radiographs in the initial evaluation of trauma patients, availability of minimally invasive techniques, and improved access to modern trauma care systems, surgeons increasingly are facing the diagnosis and management of diaphragmatic injuries.

■ CLASSIFICATION

Diaphragmatic injuries can be classified according to the mechanism of injury, side involved, unilateral or bilateral location, clinical sequelae after the onset of injury, and severity of the anatomic disruption. The last-mentioned has an important practical application in predicting outcome and associated visceral injury because these patients with diaphragmatic injuries are at risk for severe multisystem trauma. Likewise, greater than 95% of all injuries to the diaphragm occur from either penetrating or blunt trauma. Other causes include inadvertent operative tears, spontaneous or effort-related ruptures, and erosions by chest tubes or subphrenic abscesses. Blunt diaphragmatic rupture occurs mainly from high-speed motor vehicle crashes when the rapid deceleration results in a nonuniform pressure load on the inflexible central tendon. In particular, lateral impact to the torso is three times more likely to rupture the diaphragm than from a frontal direction. The diaphragm is buffered by the liver on the right, so 95% of injuries occur on the left; bilateral injuries occur in less than 3% of all cases. Compared with the left, patients with right hemidiaphragm ruptures tend to have worse increased multiorgan involvement, more hypovolemic shock, lower Glasgow Coma Scale score, and higher mortality. Bilateral ruptures, including ruptures involving the pericardium, are rare in patients who reach the hospital alive.

Injuries to the diaphragm due to stab or gunshot wounds should be suspect if the skin entry site lies between the fourth intercostal space to the umbilicus. There is no predisposition for either hemidiaphragm; however, injury to the left is more frequent because of the greater number of right-handed assailants. Defects from penetrating injures are usually smaller than defects caused by blunt trauma and potentially more dangerous in terms of delayed abdominal organ obstruction and strangulation. Many trauma surgeons believe, however, that penetrating injuries to the right diaphragm rarely become symptomatic.

Diaphragmatic injury or rupture also can be classified by the time of presentation. Three clinical phases follow the onset of traumatic diaphragmatic injury: acute, latent, and obstructive phases. The acute phase begins with the original trauma and ends with the apparent recovery from other injuries and may mask the diaphragm injury. Most patients (60%) have nonspecific left upper quadrant, lower thoracic, or shoulder pain. About one third have only a chest wall laceration and no herniation through a small diaphragm tear. The rest have, however, severe acute symptoms of dyspnea, hypotension, or cyanosis due to compression of the lung and mediastinal shift from the herniated organs.

In the latent or interval phase, symptoms are variable and nonspecific as the patient compensates for having intrathoracic abdominal contents. The symptoms suggest other disorders, such as peptic ulcer disease, gallbladder disorder, partial bowel obstruction, and chronic obstructive pulmonary disease. Symptoms of intermittent bowel obstruction aggravated by eating or lying on the left side are relieved by belching, vomiting, or flatus.

Finally, the obstructive phase may occur at anytime when bowel obstruction occurs after incarceration of herniated viscera, leading to necrosis if diagnosis and treatment are delayed further. In one series, the onset of the obstructive phase ranged from 20 days to 28 years; however, 90% usually present with strangulation by 3 years. These patients present with symptoms consistent with slow progressive herniation of stomach and bowel contents into the chest cavity, including nausea, vomiting, abdominal pain, and obstipation, finally leading to respiratory distress, shock, obstruction, strangulation, and signs of viscus perforation.

Although diaphragmatic injury is rarely a direct cause of posttraumatic death, it is a marker of severe injury and is associated with significant mortality and morbidity. The American Association for the Surgery of Trauma has developed a diaphragm organ injury scale (Table 1). The grading scheme is an anatomic description and assists in the assessment of severity score.

Table 1 Diaphragm Organ Injury Scale	
GRADE*	**INJURY DESCRIPTION**
I	Contusion
II	Laceration ≤2 cm
III	Laceration 2-10 cm
IV	Laceration >10 cm with tissue loss ≤25 cm^2
V	Laceration with >25 cm^2 tissue loss

*Advance one grade for bilateral injuries.

Adapted from Moore EE, *J Trauma* 36:300, 1994.

■ DIAGNOSIS

The diagnosis of acute diaphragm injury or rupture is a clinical challenge, especially in patients who do not have obvious indications for emergent exploration. Because diaphragmatic defects do not heal and eventually can lead to a latent visceral herniation, delayed diagnosis can be catastrophic. Review of the literature shows that missed diagnosis of diaphragmatic injury or rupture approaches 66%.

Previous clinical history from patients or care providers often can provide specific clues. Knowledge of the mode of injury is key, particularly if there was a previous stab wound. With previous blunt trauma, intermittent bowel obstruction without a previous abdominal incision should raise the possibility of diaphragm disruption. Findings on physical examination should raise suspicion. Inspection of the involved hemithorax may reveal ipsilateral prominence and decreased intercostal retraction or paradoxical motion of the left upper abdominal quadrant on respiration. There may be tympany or dullness on percussion. Auscultation may reveal decreased breath sounds, bowel sounds, or shifting of the cardiac sounds to the contralateral side.

Plain chest films are the initial screening test of choice, but 75% are nondiagnostic. Findings suggestive of a diaphragm defect include an indistinct costophrenic angle, elevated or indistinct hemidiaphragm, air-fluid levels in the chest, and abnormal pleural densities. Right diaphragm injuries rarely are detected, with higher false-negative rates in cases in which penetrating injuries result in a smaller defect compared with defects seen in blunt rupture. Computed tomography and ultrasonography are often positive when there is frank visceral protrusion into the chest. Diagnostic peritoneal lavage may be helpful in the acute setting but carries a 25% to 34% false-negative rate.

For left-sided ruptures, the diagnosis usually is made if a nasogastric tube passed into the stomach is seen in the hemithorax, or an upper gastrointestinal contrast series reveals a narrowing of the obstructed stomach or bowel segment above the diaphragm. If an aortogram is performed for other reasons, the splenic or gastric vessels may be seen above the diaphragm. Although the use of radionuclide scanning, fluoroscopy, or magnetic resonance imaging has shown relative accuracy in the diagnosis of blunt diaphragmatic rupture in stable patients treated conservatively, their use in unstable patients with multiple injuries is impractical. The efficacy of these more advanced imaging studies remains unknown without large prospective series. Right-sided ruptures may show a total or partial ("mushroom" projection) liver herniation with or without associated bowel contents.

Owing to the difficulty in diagnosis and the high mortality associated with missed diaphragmatic injuries, some surgeons have supported mandatory laparotomy for all patients with penetrating injury to the lower chest or abdomen. With the advent of endoscopic techniques, however, evaluation of the diaphragm and other structures can be performed effectively, while avoiding the morbidity of an open procedure. In two prospective series from the University of Southern California, diaphragmatic injuries were present in 42% of all patients who presented with penetrating trauma to the left thoracoabdominal region. This region was defined as the area enclosed by the nipple line superiorly and costal margin inferiorly over the anterior and posterior chest to the sternum and spine medially. Although 60% of patients who met the indication for an emergent open operation had a diaphragmatic injury on exploration, laparoscopy also was diagnostic for a diaphragmatic injury in 26% of patients who were stable and asymptomatic. As a result, routine laparoscopy is recommended to evaluate occult diaphragmatic injuries in stable patients with a left thoracoabdominal penetrating injury who otherwise have no other indication for an open operation. Tension pneumothorax, which should be diagnosed clinically, must be relieved first with a thoracostomy tube before abdominal insufflation in the presence of a diaphragmatic defect. In patients with previous abdominal surgery, a video-assisted thoracic surgical approach may be preferred to evaluate the diaphragm when intraabdominal injuries have been ruled out.

Diagnosis in the latent phase can be difficult. This is particularly true in patients with right-sided hernias due to the vague symptoms. Often, patients may not recall any previous history of trauma, and physical examination may reveal bowel sounds over the chest. In one series of patients with late posttraumatic diaphragmatic hernia, 4 of 10 were diagnosed by chest films, and 5 were diagnosed by diatrizoate meglumine (Gastrografin) contrast studies.

■ MANAGEMENT

The surgical approach to repair acute diaphragmatic injury or rupture depends on the mechanism of injury, condition of the patient, and time of presentation. Shock should be corrected, and a nasogastric tube should be in place to decompress the stomach. During induction of anesthesia, the surgeon must be present in case a rapid thoracotomy is required. In hemodynamically stable patients who sustain thoracic trauma, immediate life-threatening injuries should be addressed first, with emergent anterolateral thoracotomy or median sternotomy required to control active intrathoracic bleeding and relieve pericardial tamponade, if present. When these injuries are controlled, the diaphragm can be inspected thoroughly for defects. Even the smallest of defects should be closed. Subsequent laparotomy can be performed to explore the abdomen for other injuries, but diaphragmatic defects can be repaired from either approach. When both cavities need to be explored, separate incisions are favored over a continuous one because of the higher morbidity.

In patients who require emergent laparotomy for suspected intraabdominal injuries, thorough inspection of both hemidiaphragms is mandatory, regardless of the track of the penetrating missile or direction of the blunt impact. Diaphragmatic rupture resulting from blunt trauma should be approached through a laparotomy because of the high incidence of simultaneous intraabdominal solid organ injuries. Similarly, hemodynamically stable patients whose diaphragm injury is confirmed by noninvasive imaging or by laparoscopy, laparotomy should be performed to rule out occult intraabdominal injuries.

In contrast to the acute presentation, many authors prefer a thoracotomy approach for injuries and hernias that present in a delayed fashion. Although this approach provides excellent exposure to divide the adhesions between the trapped viscera and lung parenchyma, a transabdominal approach may be preferable for left hemidiaphragmatic hernias in which segments of small or large bowel may have to be resected and anastomosed. A thoracotomy approach should be used, however, for all right-sided diaphragmatic defects, regardless of the timing after initial injury.

The herniated viscera first is reduced carefully and returned to the abdominal cavity. The preferred method of closure of the diaphragmatic defect is by interrupted full-thickness nonabsorbable 0 or no. 1 sutures. Other methods include a continuous running two-layered simple horizontal mattress and figure-of-eight interrupted sutures. None of these methods has been proved more efficacious than the other. Adhesions should be taken down, the lung decorticated, and, if necessary, the diaphragm loosened from the lower rib to take tension off the repair. In instances in which the pericardium is involved, the heart should be put back into its anatomic position and the pericardial defect closed loosely with running absorbable sutures. If there is a lack of lateral diaphragm tissue to approximate when the injury is at the periphery, the diaphragm may be advanced upward by placing pledgeted horizontal sutures through the edge of the defect and then through the intercostal muscles on either side of a higher rib. A limited thoracoplasty of the angle of ribs 8 through 10 may be needed to approximate the diaphragm edges. For the chronic rupture, a splenectomy may need to be performed, followed by enlargement of the defect to facilitate repair. Finally, on the rare occasion when the tissue loss is extensive, closure of the defect can be achieved with fascia lata, biologic material such as bovine pericardium, or synthetic material such as Gore-Tex or Marlex. Because postoperative atelectasis and pleural effusions are common, tube thoracostomy is recommended; however, some surgeons prefer aspirating the pleural cavity at the completion of the repair.

■ OUTCOME

Mortality and morbidity in patients with acute diaphragmatic injuries differ considerably from patients with a delayed presentation. In the former, multiorgan trauma is usually present, and irreversible shock and head injury are cited most often as the causes of early death (approaching 40%). With strangulated bowel, the mortality rate increases to 80%. When these injuries are isolated and repaired adequately, complications are rare and usually pulmonary in nature. With the chronic type, sepsis and multisystem organ failure are the usual causes of mortality. In the presence of bowel strangulation and gangrene, a much higher postoperative mortality (66%) and morbidity (80%) are encountered compared with patients with an uncomplicated operative approach.

SUGGESTED READING

Boulanger BR, et al: A comparison of right and left blunt traumatic diaphragmatic rupture, *J Trauma* 35:255, 1993.

Murray JA, et al: Penetrating left thoracoabdominal trauma: the incidence and clinical presentation of diaphragm injuries, *J Trauma* 43:624, 1997.

Reber PU, et al: Missed diaphragmatic injuries and their long-term sequelae, *J Trauma* 44:183, 1998.

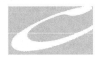

ACUTE AIRWAY OBSTRUCTION

Sudhir Sundaresan

Acute airway obstruction is a life-threatening emergency and, when recognized, must be dealt with expeditiously and effectively. The patient typically presents with shortness of breath, noisy respiration, and intolerance of the recumbent position. Stridor signifies an advanced degree of fixed mechanical upper airway obstruction. Cough and hemoptysis may be present and are usually features of airway tumors. Often, these patients have experienced gradually worsening airflow limitation before their acute presentation; frequently, they have been misdiagnosed as having asthma or chronic obstructive pulmonary disease, with resultant prescription of inhalers or corticosteroids, with no benefit.

■ EVALUATION

The evaluation begins with a careful history, if this can be obtained. Any history of recent or remote endotracheal intubation or tracheostomy raises the possibility of a fibrous tracheal stricture complicating either of these interventions. Cough and hemoptysis may signify the presence of a primary benign or malignant airway tumor. Prior history of treatment for thoracic malignancies (e.g., lung, esophageal, thyroid carcinomas) points to a local airway recurrence as a potential cause of symptoms. Certain distal malignancies (particularly renal cell cancers) are known to metastasize to the airway and can cause acute airway obstruction, so having knowledge of these lesions is important.

The posteroanterior and lateral chest radiograph is the most basic radiologic investigation and should be obtained initially in all patients. The plain chest radiograph may be helpful if there is a bulky intrathoracic mass causing extrinsic airway compression. Otherwise, plain radiographs are not particularly helpful for assessment of intrinsic airway pathology. Helical computed tomography with multiplanar (three-dimensional) reconstruction generates excellent anatomic detail with respect to location, length, and severity of airway narrowing. This technique has effectively replaced plain airway tomography and has become the imaging study

of choice for airway assessment. The only drawback of helical computed tomography is the significantly longer breath-hold necessary to complete it (15 to 45 seconds), making it unsuitable for some patients with critical airway obstruction.

Flow volume loops from patients with fixed upper airway obstruction have characteristic features. These studies are used more for academic purposes, however, than for any practical benefit for the patient and can be omitted. Ultimately, bronchoscopy is the crucial modality for assessment of the nature and severity of the airway pathology. This examination should be performed in the operating room after gathering as much information about the patient and the airway as possible. This strategy facilitates the assessment of the cause of the problem and implementation of measures to secure a satisfactory airway until more definitive therapy can be administered.

■ TREATMENT

General Measures

Before any diagnostic or therapeutic interventions can be started, the patient must be stabilized. The following are general measures that can be applied to any patient with critical upper airway obstruction. They can be used alone or in combination, depending on the clinical situation. Several of these measures (in particular, the use of diuretics, steroids, and racemic epinephrine) are applicable more to the postoperative setting, where edema of the glottis or subglottic structures plays a major role in airflow obstruction. These measures still may be valuable, however, in the emergency stabilization of patients with upper airway obstruction if edema (superimposed on the underlying airway pathology) is considered to be a significant factor.

1. Elevation of the head of the bed
2. Humidified oxygen delivered by high-humidity facemask
3. Diuretics (furosemide, 20 mg intravenously immediately and every 6 to 8 hours for 24 hours)
4. Steroids (usually dexamethasone, 4 to 6 mg intravenously every 6 hours for 24 to 48 hours)
5. Racemic epinephrine, administered by nebulizer (can be repeated every 4 to 6 hours)
6. Heliox, a helium-oxygen mixture

Airway narrowing results in airway turbulence and resistance. Because the resistance to the flow of turbulent gases is proportional to the density of the gas, heliox (only one third as dense as room air) decreases airflow turbulence and resistance.

Anesthetic Management

Careful anesthetic management of the patient before and during bronchoscopy is crucial. The fundamental principle is the avoidance of any paralytic agents until the secure status of the airway has been verified. Satisfactory topical anesthesia of the upper airway should be achieved before the patient enters the operating room. This is achieved by having the patient gargle a dilute solution of viscous lidocaine, then inhale nebulized 1% lidocaine (20 ml).

Fiberoptic bronchoscopy is performed to visualize the pathology, assess the distance from the vocal cords to the lesion, and verify that a secure airway (rigid bronchoscope or endotracheal tube) can be passed distal to the lesion, if necessary. In this setting, I prefer to use a laryngeal mask airway, which can be well seated into position using a combination of intravenous anesthesia (continuous propofol infusion) and inhalational anesthesia, but with meticulous avoidance of any paralytic agents. The prior administration of topical anesthesia facilitates the procedure, in that the laryngeal mask airway can be positioned in the hypopharynx and the bronchoscope passed beyond the vocal cords into the airway, with minimal coughing and stressful reaction by the patient. During the conduct of the bronchoscopy, the patient is asleep but breathing spontaneously, receiving gentle assisted manual ventilation by the anesthesiologist. More lidocaine can be used (sparingly) to irrigate the epiglottis, vocal cords, and upper airway as the bronchoscope is advanced under direct vision.

When the pathology has been identified, judgment is required to decide on the overall security of the airway. Ideally the fiberoptic bronchoscope is passed beyond the offending pathology into the distal trachea. Care is necessary to avoid direct trauma to the lesion because this may result in swelling or bleeding, both of which may worsen an already tenuous situation. Biopsy specimens of any suspected tumor are obtained best after placement of a more secure airway. When these considerations have been addressed, the appropriate-size rigid bronchoscope is selected and prepared. The patient can be paralyzed, the laryngeal mask airway removed, and the rigid scope advanced carefully into the distal trachea beyond the lesion. Further bronchoscopic maneuvers are described in the next section. The objective is to achieve an airway of satisfactory caliber so that on completion of the entire procedure, the patient is breathing spontaneously and extubated, awaiting definitive therapy at another procedure. After extubation, the general measures described earlier are implemented in the postanesthesia care unit. The patient subsequently is observed in the intensive care unit until more definitive management is given.

Surgical Management

The use of a rigid bronchoscope in this situation offers many advantages: excellent visualization, secure ability to ventilate and suction, and the ability to biopsy and core-out tumors adequately or dilate tight strictures. Strictures resulting from prior endotracheal intubation or tracheostomy are treated best by dilation as a temporizing measure until definitive treatment (usually resection) is performed. Dilation usually can be done using a graduated series of rigid bronchoscopes, starting with a pediatric scope (if necessary) and progressing through 7-mm and 8-mm sizes. The ability to pass an 8-mm rigid bronchoscope beyond the stricture ensures an adequate-caliber airway; if the stricture initially was noted to be tight, it may not be prudent to attempt to pass larger (e.g., 9-mm) rigid scopes because of the potential for creating a linear split of the airway. Occasionally, tight strictures have a shallow "neck," making it difficult to engage a rigid bronchoscope at that level. In this circumstance, I have found the use of esophageal dilation balloons useful (Boston Scientific Corporation, Natick, MA). The yttrium aluminum garnet (YAG) laser plays virtually no role in the acute or definitive management of postintubational strictures of the airway.

The acute management of airway tumors consists of rigid bronchoscopy and core-out of the obstructing intraluminal component of the tumor. This particular maneuver is best done using the Wolf rigid bronchoscopes (Richard Wolf Medical Instrument Corporation, Vernon Hills, IL). The Wolf bronchoscopes feature a sharp "chisel-tip," which facilitates fracturing large loose pieces of the protruding tumor, allowing them to be extracted using a foreign body forceps. All tissue extracted in this manner is sent for pathologic evaluation. If troublesome bleeding ensues, it can be managed readily by irrigation with dilute epinephrine solution or gentle tamponade using epinephrine-soaked pledgets. Electrocautery also can be applied to focal bleeding sites, although the fraction of inspired oxygen must be reduced deliberately first.

Definitive Management

As indicated earlier, the definitive management of the different lesions causing acute airway obstruction is highly variable, depending on circumstances related to the lesion itself and the general status of the patient. These options are discussed in greater detail elsewhere in this book. Tracheal resection and primary anastomosis constitute the ideal treatment for strictures, benign tumors, and localized primary airway malignancies. More extensive primary airway cancers and secondary airway involvement from other malignancies are treated using various approaches, centered mainly on external beam radiation. Other palliative options may be used alone or in combination, including brachytherapy, stent placement, periodic use of the YAG laser, and, more recently, photodynamic therapy. Tracheostomy, which traditionally was used for palliation in this setting, essentially has been supplanted by the various aforementioned techniques.

SUGGESTED READING

Courey MS: Airway obstruction: the problem and its causes, *Otolaryngol Clin N Am* 28:673, 1995.

DeLaurier GA, et al: Acute airway management: role of cricothyroidotomy, *Am Surg* 56:12, 1990.

Horak J, Weiss S: Emergent management of the airway: new pharmacology and the control of comorbidities in cardiac disease, ischemia, and valvular heart disease, *Crit Care Clin* 16:411, 2000.

Stanopoulos IT, et al: Laser bronchoscopy in respiratory failure from malignant airway obstruction, *Crit Care Med* 21:386, 1993.

TENSION PNEUMOTHORAX

Janice Shannon Cain
Brian S. Cain
David M. Jablons

■ BACKGROUND

The most common cause of tension pneumothorax is mechanical ventilation with positive-pressure ventilation in patients with visceral pleural injury. A tension pneumothorax can complicate a simple pneumothorax, however, after penetrating or blunt chest trauma in which a parenchyma lung injury has failed to seal. Similarly, traumatic defects in the chest wall may cause a tension pneumothorax if incorrectly covered with occlusive dressings or if the defect itself constitutes a flap-valve mechanism. Tension pneumothorax also may occur after a misguided attempt at subclavian or internal jugular venous catheter insertion or from markedly displaced thoracic spine fractures.

Tension pneumothorax complicates less than 2% of patients experiencing an idiopathic spontaneous pneumothorax, but it is a common manifestation of rib fractures or barotrauma in patients requiring mechanical ventilation. In a tension pneumothorax, this expanding intrapleural air may occur quickly or gradually, depending on the extent of lung injury and respiratory status of the patient.

■ PHYSIOLOGY

Tension pneumothorax develops secondary to a bronchopleural fistula (BPF), which typically acts as a one-way valve that allows air to enter the pleural space from a defect in the lung parenchyma or airway. A BPF develops secondary to barotrauma caused by episodes of markedly elevated airway pressure, such as during a violent cough or Valsalva maneuver or instances of increased airway pressures due to positive end-expiratory pressure (PEEP) causing intrapleural pressure to rise precipitously. As a result of air in the pleural space under pressure (especially if the patient is on positive-pressure ventilation), the ipsilateral lung collapses, and the mediastinum shifts to the opposite chest, interfering with expansion of the contralateral lung and compromising venous return to the heart. Although it is debated which of these factors plays a more critical role in tension physiology, the accompanying hypotension is due to impaired filling pressures. Tension pneumothorax, especially in a patient being ventilated, is life-threatening and demands acute diagnosis and immediate intervention.

■ DIAGNOSIS

The symptoms of tension pneumothorax can be divided into early and late symptoms. Early symptoms include tachypnea or air hunger, tachycardia or bradycardia, and distended neck veins. Late symptoms are chest pain, severe dyspnea and respiratory distress, hypoxemia, hypercarbia, hypotension, and a depressed level of consciousness.

Physical findings (signs) also can be divided into early and late findings. Early signs are absent breath sounds, hyperresonance to percussion, distended neck veins, and asymmetric chest movement. Late signs include contralateral tracheal and mediastinal deviation (on chest x-ray) acidosis, cyanosis, and, if centrally monitored, equalization of filling pressures and depressed cardiac output.

In the unusual situation in which an x-ray has been performed in the setting of tension pneumothorax, one might visualize contralateral mediastinal shift and relative lucency of the hemithorax due to intrathoracic air accumulation. Subcutaneous emphysema may be observed on plain films or clinical examination. Computed tomography reveals the same findings but adds little to plain chest x-ray. Tension pneumothorax is a clinical emergency that often does not allow for radiologic verification (portable chest x-ray) before intervention. When a "tension" pneumothorax is diagnosed by computed tomography, it is usually an incidental finding in a patient with severe chronic obstructive pulmonary disease and subtle clinical findings (e.g., elevated mean airway pressures, progressive but slowly wavering hypoxia).

It is crucial that the possibility of acute occult tension pneumothorax be entertained in any critically ill patient being mechanically ventilated who has high peak airway pressures (>30 to 35 cm H_2O), is requiring high PEEP (>15 cm), has severe chronic obstructive pulmonary disease, or decompensates immediately after an intervention (e.g., central line placement, bronchoscopy, deep endotracheal suctioning). In these settings, the combination of clinical suspicion and physical signs warrants intervention (needle decompression, tube thoracostomy) before radiologic confirmation. Bilaterally well-placed chest tubes are typically well tolerated barring complications (e.g., coagulopathy) and often are lifesaving.

■ TREATMENT

Emergency Needle Decompression and Aspiration

A standard large-bore intravenous catheter is inserted into the thorax allowing pressured intrapleural air to escape and the lung to reexpand. This maneuver converts the tension pneumothorax into a simple pneumothorax. One should not wait for a chest x-ray for confirmation of the diagnosis because needle decompression has a relatively good risk-to-benefit ratio when the clinical findings support tension pneumothorax and because the treatment is lifesaving.

The needle thoracentesis procedure is as follows: The second intercostal space is identified in the mid clavicular line on the side of the tension pneumothorax. The chest is surgically prepared. The area is anesthetized locally if the patient is conscious or if time permits. The patient is placed in a semiupright position if a cervical spine injury has been excluded and the patient is hemodynamically stable. Keeping the Luer-Lok in the distal end of the catheter, the surgeon inserts an over-the-needle 14- to 18-gauge (2 inches or 5 cm long) catheter into the skin and directs the needle just over (superior to) the rib into the intercostal space. The surgeon punctures the parietal pleura, then removes the Luer-Lok from the catheter and listens for a sudden escape of air when the needle enters the parietal pleura, indicating that the tension pneumothorax has been relieved. The needle is removed, and the Luer-Lok is replaced in the distal end of the catheter. The plastic catheter is left in place, and a bandage or small dressing is applied over the insertion site. When the immediate tension has been relieved, the clinical situation should improve quickly (i.e., increased blood pressure and cardiac output, decreased airway pressures, improved oxygenation), and any pressors may need to be adjusted quickly. When needle decompression has improved the immediate crisis, formal tube thoracostomy needs to be performed.

Tube Thoracostomy Drainage

Subsequent definitive treatment usually requires only simple insertion of a chest tube. Chest tube insertion may be performed as follows: The insertion site is planned as the fifth intercostal space, just below the nipple level, between the anterior and mid axillary line. The chest is surgically prepared and draped at the predetermined site of insertion. The skin and rib periosteum are locally anesthetized. The surgeon makes a 2- to 3-cm transverse (horizontal) incision at the predetermined site and bluntly dissects through the subcutaneous tissues and intercostal muscles, just over the top of the rib. The surgeon punctures the parietal pleura with the tip of a clamp and spreads the jaws of the clamp before putting a sterile gloved finger into the incision and into the pleural cavity. This maneuver helps to avoid injury to the lung and to clear any nearby intrapleural adhesions. The proximal end of the thoracostomy tube is clamped, and the thoracostomy tube is advanced into the pleural space to the desired length. The surgeon looks for "fogging" of the chest tube with expiration or listens for air movement. The end of the thoracostomy tube is connected to an underwater seal apparatus. The tube is sutured in place. A dressing is applied, and the tube is taped to the chest with a mesentery. The surgeon obtains a chest x-ray and arterial blood gas values or institutes pulse oximetry monitoring as indicated by the clinical scenario.

Pigtail Catheter-Combination Therapy

The practitioner should have shown facility with drainage of pleural effusions before treatment of emergency situations with pigtail catheters. These catheters typically are inserted using the Seldinger technique, and the larger bore needle, which allows placement of a wire, permits release of entrained air from the pleural space. This temporizes the situation, then the catheter can be placed over the wire in a calm manner, sewn into place, and connected to suction. Perhaps due to the resistance from the length of the catheter, 40 cm H_2O suction seems to work best with these catheters.

One caveat is that should the catheter become kinked, a tension pneumothorax could recur. Padding the skin exit site usually prevents this complication. Pigtail catheters have little role in a patient critically ill in the intensive care unit. Formal tube thoracostomy with a minimum of a 28 Fr chest tube remains the gold standard. Small soft catheters often kink or plug with fibrin, creating a more ominous emergency because

tension pneumothorax is not considered, as there is a "tube" in place. Clinical suspicion and judgment must prevail, and formal 28 Fr or larger tube should be placed. Pigtail catheter treatment has a role in patients with sufficient reserve, minimal symptoms, and reasonable performance status only. In critically ill patients with borderline hemodynamics or significant comorbidities (e.g., acute respiratory distress syndrome, stiff lungs), formal tube thoracostomy is the standard of care.

■ MANAGEMENT

While performing one of the aforementioned treatments electively, the patient should be in a monitored setting. Adjuncts include the ability to assess the patient's respiratory status (pulse oximetry), high flow oxygen, and ventilator or intensive care support. After the procedure, one may choose to monitor blood gases, obtain an electrocardiogram, and confirm lung reexpansion on chest x-ray. In patients who resolve their tension physiology but have a persistent BPF, operative intervention may be required. If the patient is well enough to tolerate single-lung ventilation, thoracoscopy may be appropriate.

■ COMPLICATIONS

Untreated tension pneumothoraces are associated with high mortality and are surgical emergencies. This chapter has outlined simple, lifesaving treatment strategies. The most common complications are secondary to tube placement and include further parenchymal lung injury; inappropriate tube placement (e.g., in the lung fissure, extrapleural or subdiaphragmatic); bleeding due to intercostal vessel injury or lung injury, especially if the patient is coagulopathic; and creation of an additional BPF, especially in a patient with severe bullous emphysema. The last-mentioned is the most ominous iatrogenic complication. Almost all these complications can be controlled or minimized with the correct clinical acumen and skill training.

■ CONCLUSION

Tension pneumothorax is a simple yet life-threatening problem when it occurs, especially in critically ill, positive-pressure–ventilated patients. Typical presenting signs and symptoms and immediate and definitive therapies have been described. Understanding the basic physiologic derangements prepares the clinician to diagnose and treat this uncommon yet critical clinical situation.

SUGGESTED READING

American College of Surgeons: *Advanced trauma life support for doctors*, ed 6, Chicago, 1997, First Impression.

Barton E: Tension pneumothorax, *Curr Opin Pulm Med* 5:269, 1999.

Sabiston DC: *Sabiston textbook of surgery: the biological basis of modern surgical practice*, ed 16. Philadelphia, 1997, WB Saunders.

MASSIVE HEMOPTYSIS

Betty C. Tong

Stephen C. Yang

■ BACKGROUND

Massive hemoptysis is an unusual but life-threatening condition, with reported mortality of up to 80% when treated conservatively. At present, there is no established definition for this diagnosis; however, most agree that a volume of blood greater than 600 ml expectorated within 24 hours qualifies as massive hemoptysis. Appropriately, major hemoptysis is defined as 100 ml of blood within 24 hours, and exsanguinating hemoptysis is defined as more than 1000 ml/24 hr, or a rate greater than 150 ml/hr.

Massive hemoptysis may result from many disease states. Historically the presentation of hemoptysis was pathognomonic of tuberculosis. Currently, tuberculosis remains the most common etiology, followed by other inflammatory states such as bronchiectasis and chronic bronchitis. Malignancy is another common cause of massive hemoptysis, with occurrence of 36% in some series. Approximately 3% of patients with primary lung cancer experience massive terminal hemoptysis; this is associated most commonly with cavitating squamous cell carcinoma. Other less common causes include mitral stenosis, arteriovenous fistula, and trauma to pulmonary vasculature (Table 1).

During episodes of massive hemoptysis, bleeding can arise from the bronchial, pulmonary, or systemic circulation. Bleeding from the bronchial artery system accounts for 95% of cases of massive hemoptysis. Tuberculosis alone is responsible for 70% of these cases, followed by aspergilloma (especially in an old tuberculous cavity), histoplasmosis, bronchiectasis, and lung abscess.

Approximately 5% of cases arise from the pulmonary circulation. Common causes include pulmonary hypertension; true and false aneurysms of the pulmonary artery; and iatrogenic causes such as overanticoagulation, bronchoscopy, or pulmonary artery injury secondary to placement of pulmonary artery catheters. Hemoptysis is often the first clinical manifestation of pulmonary artery dissection, pseudoaneurysm formation, or rupture resulting from overinflation of a pulmonary artery catheter balloon. Arteriovenous malformations are associated most often with Osler-Weber-Rendu disease and result in a left-to-right shunt of the pulmonary arterial vasculature. As the disease progresses, the vessel wall becomes thinner and more prone to rupture. Pulmonary venous hypertension resulting from mitral stenosis, pulmonary vein stenosis, fibrosing mediastinitis, and pulmonary embolus also may result in hemoptysis caused by bleeding from the pulmonary circulation.

The nonbronchial systemic circulation accounts for the remaining 1% of massive hemoptysis. Inflammatory and

Table 1 Common Causes of Hemoptysis
Inflammatory
Tuberculosis
Aspergillosis
Bronchiectasis
Chronic bronchitis
Necrotizing pneumonitis
Cystic fibrosis
Lung abscess
Neoplastic
Bronchogenic carcinoma
Bronchial adenoma
Primary tracheal tumors
Vascular
Pulmonary embolism/infarction
Arteriovenous fistula
Traumatic
Lung contusion or laceration
Bronchial rupture
Foreign body
Iatrogenic
Invasive monitoring (pulmonary artery catheter)
Bronchoscopy
Pulmonary vein manipulation (ablation, stenting)
Cardiac
Mitral stenosis
Acute pulmonary edema
Coagulation disorders

neoplastic states induce neovascularization from collateral arteries, as shown by injection studies. Other systemic sources of bleeding include trauma, tracheoinnominate fistulas, and thoracic aortic aneurysms communicating with the bronchial artery system.

■ EVALUATION AND INITIAL MANAGEMENT

Evaluation of the patient presenting with massive hemoptysis should begin with maneuvers to secure a patent airway and quickly localize the bleeding site. It is important to verify the lungs as the source of blood versus other potential sources, such as the nose, mouth, pharynx, or gastrointestinal tract. A few key elements elicited from the patient's history should provide useful information in this regard, including duration of bleeding, appearance and amount of blood or clot, and associated activity that may induce or is causally related to the bleeding. Associated chest pain, presence of wheezing or bubbling of secretions, prior history of cardiac or pulmonary disease, and history of smoking suggest the lungs as a potential bleeding source.

Initial management of the patient who presents with massive hemoptysis includes admission to an intensive care unit or monitored setting with strict bed rest. In the acute setting, airway protection must be a priority. The anesthesia team should be notified early in the event that intubation becomes necessary, potentially with a double-lumen endotracheal tube. The patient should be positioned in a semi-upright manner or with the bleeding side dependent to minimize the risk of contamination into the contralateral side. Humidified oxygen should be administered via facemask. For cases arising from pulmonary artery catheter placement, proximal reinflation of the balloon may provide temporary control of bleeding, yet potentially may worsen the injury.

Large-bore intravenous access should be obtained. Pertinent laboratory studies include complete blood count, serum chemistry, coagulation studies, and arterial blood gas. Also, blood must be sent for type and crossmatch, and blood products should be available for possible transfusion or to reverse coagulopathy. Sputum samples should be sent for Gram stain and acid-fast bacilli and for culture, particularly for *Mycobacterium tuberculosis*. Intramuscular codeine may be used for cough suppression, as variations in thoracic pressure produced by violent coughing may exacerbate the hemoptysis. Anxiolytics also may be administered for light sedation. These agents must be used with caution to avoid oversedation and aspiration from suppression of the cough reflex.

A chest radiograph is crucial on initial examination. Often the chest radiograph is sufficient to determine whether the bleeding originates from the left or right side by revealing the presence of a mass, cavity, or other lesion and localized infiltrate or atelectasis. In some states, such as bronchitis, bronchiectasis, pulmonary embolism, bronchogenic carcinoma, and pulmonary artery dissection or rupture, the chest radiograph may be normal. In these cases, chest computed tomography may offer additional information. Other studies that may be helpful include pulmonary angiography, selective bronchial arteriography, and ventilation-perfusion scans. In the acute situation, stabilizing the patient must be a priority and may preclude a complete radiologic workup.

The patient's medical status should be optimized with control of hypertension and, if not contraindicated, reversal of anticoagulation. Broad-spectrum antibiotic therapy has been advocated in cases when the patient's sputum is purulent. Bedside evaluation of pulmonary function is helpful in determining whether the patient may tolerate future operation. Other therapeutic agents, such as intravenous vasopressin, conjugated estrogens, and protamine, have been used in the past but are of little clinical benefit.

■ BRONCHOSCOPY

After initial stabilization, every patient should undergo bronchoscopy. Most authors recommend that bronchoscopy be performed either during the acute bleeding episode or within 24 hours of initial presentation. Bronchoscopy is useful not only as a means of clearing the airway of blood, but also for identifying the bleeding site and source. Rigid bronchoscopy offers advantages including superior visualization, control of the airway, and suctioning of clot and debris. It also provides a means for instrumentation, especially for patients presenting with exsanguinating hemoptysis or patients who are not operative candidates. Flexible fiberoptic bronchoscopy is often more readily available, can be done at the bedside, and is easier to perform, especially in the intubated patient. Regardless of the method used, it is helpful to have two separate suction devices while performing this procedure.

Many therapeutic interventions may be applied during bronchoscopy. Bronchial lavage with iced saline or topical epinephrine may be used to induce bronchial artery constriction and hypothermic vasospasm in areas of neovascularization. For cases of severe bleeding in which immediate pulmonary resection is indicated, bleeding can be localized and controlled during bronchoscopic examination. This is useful in isolating the bleeding side and preventing contamination into the contralateral side until the resection can be performed.

■ MECHANICAL VENTILATION

When it is determined from which side the bleeding originates, a double-lumen endotracheal tube may be used for intubation. Alternatively, a no. 8/14 Fr Fogarty catheter may be passed through the rigid bronchoscope and used to isolate the bleeding lung. Before use, the Fogarty catheter is modified with a 30- to 40-cm segment of plastic tubing interposed between the proximal end of the hub and the Luer-Lok fitting of the catheter. This modification enables the physician to remove the bronchoscope without disrupting the catheter already in place. Isolation of the bleeding side allows for single-lung ventilation and decreases the risk of aspiration during pulmonary resection. When the bleeding bronchus has been isolated and cross-clamped, the catheter may be removed, and bilateral ventilation may be safely resumed.

Because the tracheobronchial tree is asymmetric, the established method for controlling the hemorrhage differs for each side. For bleeding on the left side, the modified Fogarty catheter is passed through the rigid bronchoscope into the left main stem bronchus, just distal to the carina. The catheter balloon is inflated (with radiopaque dye if fluoroscopy is available), which subsequently isolates the left lung. A single-lumen endotracheal tube is inserted into the trachea approximately 2 cm above the carina to provide single-lung ventilation via the right lung. Alternatively, a commercially available bronchial blocker may be placed directly through an endotracheal tube under direct vision with a flexible bronchoscope. After catheter placement, a chest x-ray should be obtained to ensure that the catheter balloon is not obstructing the left upper lobe bronchus.

The right main stem bronchus is significantly shorter than that on the left, and the right upper lobe bronchus originates from a more proximal location. Bleeding on the right side is isolated by intubation of the left main stem bronchus with a single-lumen endotracheal tube. The cuff of the endotracheal tube is inflated, providing selective ventilation of the left lung via the endotracheal tube.

■ BRONCHIAL ARTERY EMBOLIZATION

Because most cases of massive hemoptysis arise from the bronchial arterial circulation, embolization of bleeding bronchial arteries has been shown to play a major role in the successful management of this problem. Bronchial artery embolization (BAE) first was described by Remy in 1974. Since then, many studies have validated its role in the management of massive hemoptysis.

The procedure usually is performed by the vascular interventional radiologist using a transfemoral approach with the patient under local anesthesia. Embolization of selected bronchial arteries is achieved using absorbable gelatin sponge material (e.g., Gelfoam), nonabsorbable particles, or Hilal coils. An absolute contraindication to BAE is visualization of an anterior spinal artery arising from cervicointercostal or intercostobronchial trunks, or from the intercostal artery.

BAE should be considered for patients in whom a bleeding site has been localized. For patients undergoing pulmonary angiography with intent to identify a source of hemoptysis, BAE is a useful therapeutic procedure. There are many advantages to BAE in the management of massive hemoptysis. It is a minimally invasive technique that may be performed on patients who might not otherwise tolerate surgical management. Also the relatively high success rate of this procedure may facilitate a delay of surgery so that an operation can be performed on a nonemergent basis. One must consider, however, that BAE is an invasive procedure with associated potential complications, and its use may adversely delay surgical intervention.

Reported success rates for BAE and the immediate cessation of bleeding range from 77% to 95%. Long-term follow-up reveals bleeding recurrence rates of 42%, however, which may be due in part to the underlying pathology. The rate of recurrence in patients presenting with aspergilloma is higher than that for patients with active tuberculosis. Also, patients with numerous systemic collateral vessels have a higher likelihood of recurrent bleeding because not all vessels are accessible for embolization. Finally, degradation of agents used in embolization results in recanalization of bleeding vessels. Complications associated with BAE are relatively uncommon, with rates ranging from 4% to 11%. Reported complications include subintimal blood vessel dissection from catheter manipulation; distal arterial occlusion, including that of the cerebral vessels; and spinal cord complications, such as Brown-Séquard syndrome and transient or permanent paraparesis.

BAE is an important adjunct in the treatment of massive hemoptysis. It is highly successful in the immediate control of bleeding and should be considered for every patient in whom a bleeding source can be identified. It is the primary treatment of choice for all patients with massive hemoptysis, especially patients considered to be nonoperative candidates. The risk of recurrence is significant, however, and semielective surgical resection of the underlying pathology should be considered when the patient is stabilized.

■ SURGICAL MANAGEMENT

Surgery provides definitive management for the problem of massive hemoptysis with lower recurrence rates compared with BAE. Surgical morbidity and mortality rates rise, however, with increasing amounts of preoperative blood loss and in cases performed under emergent conditions. Bleeding greater than 600 ml in a 24-hour period or at a rate greater than 150 ml/hr, tracheoinnominate fistula, aortobronchial fistula, and rupture of the pulmonary vasculature secondary to chest trauma or iatrogenic injury all are indications for immediate operation (Table 2). Surgery may be performed

Table 2 Surgical Indications for Massive Hemoptysis
INDICATIONS FOR IMMEDIATE SURGERY
Total amount of bleeding >600 ml/24 hr
Bleeding rate >150 ml/hr
Tracheoinnominate fistula
Aortobronchial fistula
Trauma
INDICATIONS FOR URGENT SURGERY (24-28 HR AFTER INITIAL EVENT)
Fungal mass
Lung abscess
Persistent radiodense lesion
Irretrievable endoluminal obstructing clot

on an urgent basis (delayed 24 to 48 hours after initial presentation) for cases due to the presence of fungal mass, lung abscess, persistent radiodense lesion, or irretrievable endoluminal obstructing clot.

Patient selection is crucial in the operative management of massive hemoptysis. First, the patient must be able to tolerate a thoracotomy and possible lung resection. Second, enough lung parenchyma should remain after resection to preserve pulmonary function and avoid the use of supplemental oxygen. Finally the bleeding source must be amenable to surgical control. Contraindications for surgery include inability to localize the site of bleeding, the presence of disseminated carcinoma with distant metastasis, involvement of the mediastinum and great vessels, poor pulmonary function as shown by forced vital capacity less than 40% or forced expiratory volume in 1 second less than 40%, and severe advanced cardiopulmonary disease.

Objectives of surgical management include control of the bleeding source and excision of the pathologic lesion while preserving as much normal lung parenchyma as possible. Operative procedures for the control of massive hemoptysis include selective vessel ligation, wedge resection, segmentectomy, lobectomy, bilobectomy, and pneumonectomy. Early dissection and division of the offending bronchus and extrapleural dissection are recommended. Endoluminal catheters employed for isolation of bleeding bronchi may be removed and double-lung ventilation resumed when the bleeding bronchus has been ligated and the lung tissue resected. For patients who may not tolerate extensive lung resection, cavernostomy or thoracoplasty may be considered. In certain instances, intrapericardial control of the pulmonary artery may be necessary.

Overall surgical mortality has been reported to be 7% to 25%, with lower rates reported in more recent years. The main predictor of surgical outcome is the patient's preoperative rate of bleeding. Because of this strong association, some advocate delaying surgery until 5 to 10 days after the acute episode of hemoptysis. This delay allows for clearing of the bronchial tree of residual blood and partial recovery of the lung parenchyma. Although the extent of pulmonary resection usually is related to the degree of morbidity and mortality, it remains an independent predictor of outcome. Other factors that influence surgical morbidity and mortality include the mechanism of bleeding, aspiration into the contralateral lung, baseline pulmonary function, and preoperative functional status. Common postoperative complications include aspiration, need for tracheostomy, respiratory failure, bronchopleural fistula, and empyema.

■ CONCLUSION

Massive hemoptysis is a relatively uncommon yet life-threatening condition with significant associated morbidity and mortality. Early diagnosis using bronchoscopy and therapeutic intervention are the current accepted methods for initial cessation of bleeding. Surgery provides definitive

management, but the timing of operation is critical. Ideally, surgery should be reserved for highly selected patients who can tolerate thoracotomy and possible lung resection and in whom active bleeding has been well controlled.

SUGGESTED READING

Fernando HC, et al: Role of bronchial artery embolization in the management of hemoptysis, *Arch Surg* 133:862, 1998.

Garzon AA, et al: Exsanguinating hemoptysis, *J Thorac Cardiovasc Surg* 84:829, 1982.

Knott-Craig CJ, et al: Management and prognosis of massive hemoptysis, *J Thorac Cardiovasc Surg* 105:394, 1993.

ESOPHAGEAL PERFORATION

S. C. Murthy
T. W. Rice

Although no absolute consensus regarding the management of esophageal perforation exists, clinicians universally agree that it presents a daunting challenge. With rare exception, the diagnosis portends an ominous prognosis if left untreated. The consequences of esophageal perforation are related to extravasation of oral and gastric secretions (including bacteria) into the mediastinum, which precipitates an intense inflammatory process that rapidly overwhelms local defenses and ultimately culminates in septic shock. The infection results in descending mediastinitis for cervical perforation, in empyema for thoracic perforation, and in peritonitis for abdominal perforation.

Review of the literature documents almost 1500 cases of esophageal perforation between 1935 and 2000. Data from these reports are summarized in Figure 1. Greater than 80% of perforations occur within the thoracic esophagus, and abdominal perforation is rare (Figure 1A). Overall, the most common etiology for perforation is esophageal instrumentation (e.g., endoscopy, dilation) (Figure 1B). In early reports, barogenic (Boerhaave's syndrome) and traumatic perforation were predominant. As techniques for endoluminal management of esophageal diseases were developed and disseminated, however, iatrogenic causes superseded spontaneous perforations. Four major treatments for esophageal perforation are described. These therapies and their respective frequencies are shown in Figure 1C. Mortality of the entire cohort was 25%.

The symptom complex of esophageal perforation depends greatly on the anatomic location, extent, and duration of the injury. A small, contained perforation noted shortly after endoscopy may be of academic interest only. Patients with Boerhaave's syndrome can present to a local emergency department in extremis, however. Cervical perforation frequently is accompanied by neck pain. Distal esophageal injury produces a low chest pain similar to pain associated with myocardial infarction, pancreatitis, perforated peptic ulcer, or acute aortic dissection. Neck crepitus often accompanies cervical perforation; Hamman's crunch is more commonly a sign of thoracic perforation. Dysphagia is invariably present regardless of location of the perforation. Fever, odynophagia, tachycardia, and tachypnea suggest advanced illness.

A diagnosis of esophageal perforation should be suspected in any patient who develops signs or symptoms after esophageal instrumentation. Perforation should be considered if a young patient (<50 years old) experiences low chest pain and evidence of a systemic inflammatory response. An elderly patient may have a more insidious onset of signs and symptoms making early diagnosis more difficult. Depending on its acuity, patients with barogenic perforation may present with Mackler's triad (chest pain, subcutaneous emphysema, history of emesis). A chest radiograph may show pneumomediastinum, cervical subcutaneous emphysema, or hydropneumothorax.

A contrast study with barium sulfate is the test of choice to confirm perforation. We prefer the barium esophagogram because of its higher sensitivity and lower toxicity if aspirated. Cervical perforations are more difficult to identify due to the rapid passage of contrast material through the cervical esophagus. Chest computed tomography scan may show extraluminal gas or extravasation of oral contrast material. If an esophagogram is not possible (e.g., intubated patient), esophagoscopy is a useful adjunct.

Early diagnosis and contained perforation are favorable predictors for recovery. In sick individuals, immediate

A

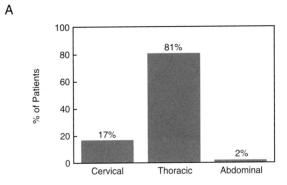

B

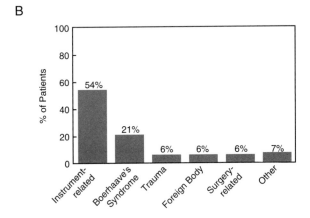

C

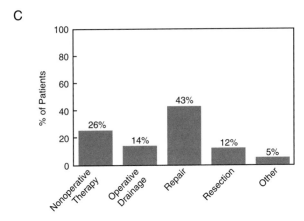

Figure 1
Summary of data collected from 1484 patients with esophageal perforation. **A,** Location. **B,** Etiology. **C,** Therapy.

management entails débridement and drainage of necrotic tissue, control of tissue soilage, and expert critical care. Whenever possible, a secondary objective of restoring alimentary tract continuity should be considered.

Management can be either nonoperative or operative. To tailor therapy appropriately, knowledge of the etiology, location, duration, and underlying esophageal pathology is essential. Age, comorbid disease, and response to injury also help to define the illness score. Together, these data should stratify patients into appropriate treatment algorithms.

■ NONOPERATIVE THERAPY

Nonoperative therapy classically is reserved for elderly patients with multiple comorbid illnesses who present acutely ill after an iatrogenic or spontaneous perforation. Management includes nasogastric decompression, percutaneous drainage (usually tube thoracostomy), and broad-spectrum antibiotics. The antibiotic regimen must include coverage for oral flora (penicillin, clindamycin). Parenteral nutrition begins if the patient shows early survival. Surgical intervention (e.g., diversion, drainage, enteral feeding access) generally is reserved for patients with recovery potential (i.e., sepsis resolution). Despite this conservative approach, the observed mortality of 36% for patients treated is far less than would be expected. Only more recently has it become clear which patients survive with nonoperative management.

Guidelines now exist for nonoperative management of esophageal perforation. Cameron et al successfully managed a cohort of eight patients (all operative candidates) without surgical intervention. Patient criteria were disruption of the esophagus contained within the mediastinum or between the mediastinum and the visceral pleura, free drainage of the cavity back into the esophagus, minimal symptoms, and minimal signs of sepsis. Treatment of these patients should include broad-spectrum antibiotics, parenteral alimentation, possible nasogastric tube decompression, and, most importantly, immediate consideration for operative intervention should symptoms worsen or early sepsis develop. In Cameron's series, oral intake was reinstituted after an esophagogram showed contraction of the mediastinal cavity and closure of the esophageal disruption (7 to 38 days). Length of hospitalization averaged 1 month.

Another condition that responds well to nonoperative therapy is microperforation. This subtle full-thickness disruption is a frequent complication of aggressive esophageal dilation. The patient usually complains of greater than expected chest discomfort after the dilation. An esophagogram may be normal (or show mucosal irregularity), but a chest computed tomography scan shows a small amount of extraluminal gas. It is prudent to observe these patients in the hospital for 24 hours. During this time, patients should be given broad-spectrum antibiotics and kept on nothing-per-mouth status (NPO). A repeat contrast study should be obtained the following day to document healing.

Although still in its infancy, the development of covered esophageal stents has the potential to impact greatly management of malignant esophageal perforation. Patients with advanced, obstructing esophageal cancer who sustain perforations during stricture dilation are ideal candidates for the application of this technology. In general, these patients are poor surgical candidates; the less invasive approach of endoluminal stenting is a reasonable compromise to surgical intervention. Stents are best considered palliative therapy and should be avoided in operative candidates.

■ OPERATIVE THERAPY

When operative therapy is indicated, possible approaches include operative drainage, perforation repair, esophageal resection, and esophageal exclusion/diversion. The choice of therapy varies with the presentation of the illness.

Operative Drainage

Operative drainage is useful for cervical perforation. For iatrogenic cervical injuries, the location of the perforation commonly is found within Killian's triangle. Defined superiorly by the inferior constrictors and inferiorly by the cricopharyngeus muscle, the area is susceptible to disruption because of the absence of an organized muscularis layer. Neck hyperextension and anterior cervical osteophyte formation may compromise the region further. Narrowing of the esophagus at the upper esophageal sphincter serves as the first major impediment to the passage of ingested foreign bodies.

Operative drainage for cervical esophageal perforation is conducted through an oblique left neck incision placed over the sternocleidomastoid muscle. The muscle and carotid sheath are displaced laterally, and the airway, thyroid, and strap muscles are retracted medially. Division of the omohyoid muscle and middle thyroid vein improves exposure. Blunt mobilization of the cervical esophagus is usually sufficient for proper drainage of the infected space. Even for early perforations, the cephalad aspect of the posterior mediastinum is contaminated and requires drainage. For advanced cases, a mediastinoscope can be inserted alongside the esophagus to enable débridement and drainage of the posterior mediastinum. Repair of the associated mucosal interruption is not essential, provided that adequate drainage is achieved. To reduce the incidence of stricture or persistent esophagocutaneous fistula, repair is recommended for perforations with limited soilage and inflammation. Nasogastric decompression, parenteral nutrition, and broad-spectrum antibiotics are important adjuncts.

When patients with cervical perforation present with signs of descending mediastinitis (sepsis, Hamman's crunch, right pleural effusion), cervical drainage alone is usually insufficient. A collar incision may be necessary to débride the anterior and the posterior mediastinum; a right thoracotomy often is required to drain the descending infection completely. Wound complications are reduced by avoiding sternotomy. Left thoracotomy provides inadequate exposure to the superior mediastinum. Mediastinal irrigation catheters have no proven benefit.

Drainage alone rarely suffices for intrathoracic perforation. An uncommon clinical scenario arises when a patient with a suspected intrathoracic perforation is explored, and evidence of tissue soilage and mediastinal emphysema is found, but the perforation is not. In these cases, even intraoperative endoscopy (and esophageal insufflation) may fail to locate the perforation site. Wide drainage is the only recourse. Before abandoning a repair attempt, the muscularis mucosa layer over the area of the suspected perforation should be dissected gently to ensure that a subtle mucosal defect is not hidden under reannealed muscle.

It is crucial that all contaminated spaces be drained. This entails examination of both chest cavities for thoracic perforation. Because most distal esophageal perforations are approached through the left chest, right-sided thoracoscopy is a useful therapeutic adjunct.

Esophageal Repair

Operative repair should be considered the mainstay of surgical therapy for esophageal perforation. Unless significant tissue necrosis and inflammation exist, repair should be attempted for most thoracic and abdominal perforations. Primary repair is usually safe for perforations diagnosed within 24 to 48 hours of the injury, and there are reports of successful repair for chronic perforation. Advantages of repair are control of tissue soilage and prompt restoration of alimentary tract continuity. Primary repair should not be considered if either cancer or end-stage achalasia (i.e., megaesophagus) is present. Resection is the preferred option for these conditions.

The abscess resulting from perforation usually necessitates access into the left pleural space, and consequently a posterolateral left thoracotomy through interspace 6 or 7 is preferred. Single-lung ventilation is necessary, and a lung decortication usually is required to treat the associated empyema. The distal esophagus should be mobilized circumferentially and examined thoroughly. A small muscle defect often conceals a large linear mucosal disruption. The muscle must be incised and frequently débrided to expose the ends of the tear. The mucosa and submucosa appear viable in most cases. Precise reapproximation of the mucosa and submucosa is crucial to the success of the repair. A continuous 3-0 polydioxanone suture works well (Figure 2). As an alternative, a linear stapler may be used to coapt these layers.

The muscularis mucosa is closed over the mucosal repair when possible. Continuous or interrupted suture technique is employed. More importantly, buttressing of the repair with transposed, healthy tissue always should be undertaken.

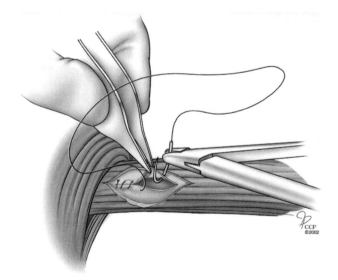

Figure 2

During exploration of the thoracic esophagus for perforation, a small muscle defect often hides a large mucosal disruption. The muscle must be dissected to reveal the entire defect. Meticulous suture technique is used to coapt the mucosal edges. Alternatively a linear stapler may be used for mucosal reapproximation.

To this end, several techniques have been described. Rotation of the pleura (Grillo flap) is quick, easy, and the most commonly practiced technique (Figure 3). As a result of the local inflammatory response, the pleura is markedly thickened and vascularized. It is simple to manipulate and mobilize. From the standard left chest approach, the pleura can be dissected easily from the chest wall and off the aorta. Care must be taken to prevent inadvertent dissection of the aortic adventitia as the flap is elevated posteriorly. The flap is usually receptive to interrupted absorbable sutures and is tacked over the repair. A 360-degree wrap of the distal esophagus is not advocated.

Another technique employs an intercostal muscle flap. The muscle flap should be harvested before placement of the rib spreader to prevent injury to the intercostal vascular pedicle. A subperiosteal dissection is used to elevate the vascular pedicle and attached muscle from the underside of the rib above the thoracotomy. The muscle flap is mobilized posteriorly until the desired length is obtained. Because of the attached periosteum, the flap may calcify over time. This muscle flap should not be used to encircle the esophagus because ossification of the flap can entrap the esophagus.

Although less commonly employed, a rotation flap of diaphragm is an option if neither pleura nor intercostal flaps are satisfactory. Being mindful of the phrenic neurovascular bundle, a paddle of diaphragm based on a branch of the arborizing phrenic artery can be rotated over the repair. The muscle flap should be dissected carefully off the peritoneum inferiorly and the central tendon of the diaphragm avoided. The resulting defect in the diaphragm must be closed meticulously with large-gauge suture.

The gastric fundus also has been used as a repair buttress. Because reflux and obligate postoperative hiatal hernia are concerns with this technique, it should be avoided. Epicardial fat pad, extrathoracic muscles (e.g., latissimus dorsi or serratus anterior) and omentum are other options for repair coverage. Experience with these tissues is limited, as are their indications.

A perforation sustained during dilation of a benign stricture poses an additional problem. In these cases, the perforation frequently is just proximal to the stricture. Repair of the perforation is destined to fail, unless the distal obstruction can be alleviated as well. For peptic strictures, intraoperative endoscopy and dilation is warranted. If the obstruction is relieved, the question of adding an antireflux procedure to the operation remains. Some surgeons have argued that a fundoplication be added. This could serve to buttress the primary closure suitably and provide an effective reflux deterrent. In patients with severe reflux disease, however, because the esophagus is foreshortened, any antireflux surgery should include a lengthening procedure (Collis gastroplasty). Adding a simple fundoplication to the repair must be questioned. The addition of a gastroplasty to the operation further complicates the surgery and can be justified only in early perforations. A more prudent course might be to manage the reflux disease medically and reserve reflux surgery for recurrence.

If a perforation is sustained during esophageal dilation for achalasia, the myotomy must be completed surgically. After the perforation is repaired, a Heller myotomy should be performed 180 degrees from the repair. This must be

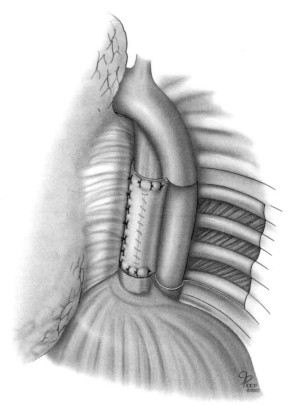

Figure 3
Pleural flap buttressing of a repaired perforation.

carried onto the proximal fundus, and the submucosa must be liberated completely.

Repair is usually the best option for nonmalignant perforation. In cases of delayed diagnosis (>48 hours), significant tissue necrosis or septic shock makes failure of the repair more likely. Some clinicians advocate resection; however, others have added an exclusion/diversion procedure to protect a high-risk repair. The esophagus can be excluded functionally by a loop cervical esophagostomy that may be reversed when the repair heals. Cervical esophageal stricture and recurrent laryngeal nerve injury may complicate this approach. A noncutting linear stapler (with absorbable or titanium staples) can be applied to the distal esophagus to prevent reflux of gastric secretions over the repair site. If there has been no damage to the mucosa, the esophageal lumen spontaneously reconstitutes within 2 to 4 weeks, and little evidence of the stapling is noted on follow-up endoscopy. Little evidence supports routine use of adjunctive exclusion/diversion procedures.

A primary repair should be accompanied by wide mediastinal drainage, esophageal decompression (nasogastric tube with or without gastric tube), and a parenteral feeding route (central venous line). For more involved cases, enteral feeding access (J-tube) is prudent. Patients should be kept NPO, and arrangements for long-term antibiotics (2 to 4 weeks) should be made. In an uncomplicated case, it is reasonable to expect healing within 7 to 10 days. An esophagogram should be obtained before any decision regarding reinstitution of oral feeding is made. As shown by

Cameron et al, in the absence of illness, a contained leak after repair is seldom problematic and resolves with nonoperative measures.

Esophageal Resection

As intensive care and surgical techniques improve, esophageal resection can be performed with limited mortality. This limited mortality promotes the incorporation of esophagectomy into the treatment algorithm for esophageal perforation. Although the specific indications for resection are guided largely by clinical judgment and anecdotal experience, esophagectomy is the procedure of choice for malignant perforation (iatrogenic or spontaneous) in a fit patient with resectable disease.

Iatrogenic perforation of a cancer in the distal esophagus commonly is diagnosed early enough to permit a transhiatal approach to the resection. When there is any question of left (or right) pleural space involvement, a limited thoracotomy is warranted. A decision to delay or to reconstruct the alimentary tract immediately is made intraoperatively based on many of the variables previously discussed. If immediate reconstruction is appropriate, a gastric conduit can be placed in either orthotopic or heterotopic (substernal) positions. A substernal colon conduit usually is employed for delayed reconstruction. This procedure can be undertaken safely 3 to 6 months after recovery from the initial operation. Esophagectomy is also the treatment of choice to manage perforation in end-stage achalasia (megaesophagus) because there is little reason to spare the esophagus in these patients.

Finally, esophageal resection (and end-cervical esophagostomy) may be a better option than operative drainage, diversion/exclusion, or high-risk repair for the critically ill patient with an intrathoracic perforation. This solution abrogates the possibility of persistent tissue soilage and perpetuation of sepsis that frequently accompanies other therapies. Current data establish the safety of esophagectomy as primary treatment for esophageal perforation.

Esophageal Diversion/Exclusion and T-Tube Drainage

Although numerous case reports have been written on esophageal diversion/exclusion and T-tube drainage, their use as primary therapy for perforation is not warranted. When diversion/exclusion of the esophagus was introduced in the 1960s, suture material was less refined, and breakdown of primary repair occurred frequently. Because mortality of elective esophagectomy was greater than 25% at the time, it was reasonable to consider alternatives for management of the disease. Our analysis suggests, however, that diversion/exclusion or T-tube drainage should be avoided in most circumstances.

Percutaneous drainage (T-tube) of the esophagus should not be considered equivalent to drainage of the biliary system. Bile is sterile, whereas oral and gastric secretions are not. Experience with this approach for high-risk cases or to salvage a failed repair has been disappointing. In addition to an unacceptably high mortality rate, protracted hospitalization, frequent displacement of the T-tube, and persistent fistula have been observed. Salvage esophagectomy with end-cervical esophagostomy is preferred for these difficult cases.

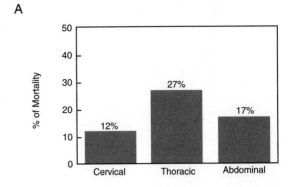

A

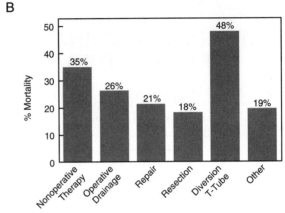

B

Figure 4
Summary of the hospital mortality of 1484 patients treated for esophageal perforation. **A**, Location. **B**, Therapy.

■ RESULTS

Approximately one quarter of patients studied over 65 years died of perforation. A summary of mortality by location of perforation (Figure 4A) and therapy (Figure 4B) is shown. As expected, mortality from thoracic perforation is greater than that from other locations. Resection and repair are the best treatment options with mortality rates in the 20% range. In more current series, mortality rates of less than 10% for these options have been shown.

■ CONCLUSION

Despite remarkable advances in the surgical sciences, esophageal perforation continues to present a difficult clinical challenge. When diagnosed early, survival should be expected. Surgical therapy must include wide débridement and drainage of infected tissue, interruption of the chemical and bacterial insult, and skilled postoperative management. A buttressed primary repair should be considered for most patients, and little hesitation should be given toward proceeding to esophagectomy if indicated.

SUGGESTED READING

Cameron JL, et al: Selective nonoperative management of contained intrathoracic esophageal disruptions, *Ann Thorac Surg* 27:404, 1979.

Dipierro FV, et al: Esophagectomy and staged reconstruction, *Eur J Cardiothorac Surg* 17:702, 2000.

Grillo HC, Wilkins EW Jr: Esophageal repair following late diagnosis of intrathoracic perforation, *Ann Thorac Surg* 20:387, 1975.

Iannettoni MD, et al: Functional outcome after surgical treatment of esophageal perforation, *Ann Thorac Surg* 64:1606, 1997.

Jones WG II, Ginsberg RJ: Esophageal perforation: a continuing challenge, *Ann Thorac Surg* 53:534, 1992.

TRACHEOINNOMINATE ARTERY FISTULA

Kelli R. Brooks
Thomas A. D'Amico

With an incidence of less than 1%, tracheoinnominate artery fistula (TIF) is an infrequent, albeit devastating, complication of tracheostomy or tracheal reconstruction. Approximately 10% of all posttracheotomy bleeding episodes are due to TIF, with peak occurrence in the first 3 weeks postoperatively. Incidence is greatest in patients with head injuries that result in irritability and ceaseless patient movement. Other predisposing conditions include steroid administration, stomal infection, sepsis, hypotension, malnutrition, abnormal neck positioning due to neurologic disorders, and the need for high-pressure ventilation requiring high cuff pressures to prevent air leaks. TIF also has been shown in patients with tracheal malignancy after radiation therapy to the mediastinum.

■ PATHOGENESIS

TIF most commonly develops after tracheostomy or tracheal resection. Three scenarios for the development of TIF after tracheostomy have been proposed. First, the elbow of the tracheostomy tube may abut the posterosuperior innominate artery and with time cause mechanical erosion into the artery in a tracheostomy placed below the fourth tracheal ring or with a tracheostomy placed in the standard position (between the second and third tracheal ring), if the innominate artery is in an unusually high position (Figure 1). Alternatively, when the cuff pressure exceeds the capillary perfusion pressure of the tracheal wall, tracheal necrosis eventually may occur and extend through the anterior wall of the trachea into the posterior innominate artery, resulting in TIF (Figure 2). Finally, the tracheostomy tube may be misfitted or the tip misplaced, applying direct anterior pressure onto the tracheal wall next to the innominate artery and resulting in subsequent erosion into the artery; this is particularly common in tubes with a 90-degree angle (Figure 3).

■ DIAGNOSIS

Early recognition and prompt management are the keys to long-term survival in patients who develop TIF. One must have a high index of suspicion when incisional or tracheal bleeding occurs more than 48 hours after tracheostomy. Early posttracheotomy bleeding (<48 hours after the procedure) most likely originates from the skin, subcutaneous tissue, or thyroid. After this time, significant tracheostomal or tracheal bleeding should be presumed secondary to TIF until proved otherwise.

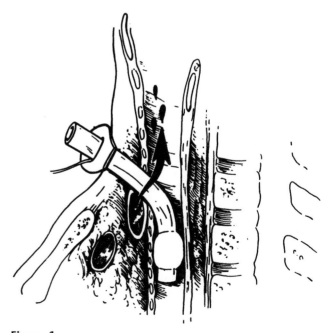

Figure 1
Tracheoinnominate fistula due to erosion of the elbow of a low-lying tracheostomy tube into the innominate artery. (*From Dyer RK, Fisher SR: In Wolfe WG, editor:* Complications in thoracic surgery, *St. Louis, 1992, Mosby-Year Book, p 296.*)

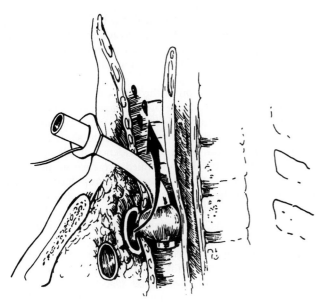

Figure 2
Tracheoinnominate fistula due to an overinflated tracheostomy cuff. (*From Dyer RK, Fisher SR: In Wolfe WG, editor:* Complications in thoracic surgery, *St. Louis, 1992, Mosby-Year Book, p 296.*)

The diagnosis of TIF usually is made on the basis of clinical events; however, radiologic confirmation sometimes is required. A sentinel bleeding episode occurs in approximately 40% to 50% of patients before the development of massive hemorrhage. The blood may appear less saturated than expected for an arterial source, owing to associated hypoxia.

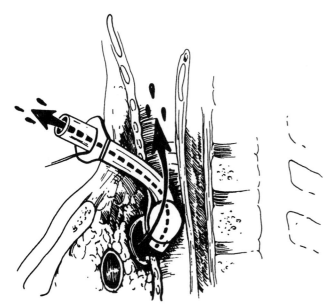

Figure 3
Tracheoinnominate fistula due to acute angulation of the tracheostomy tube. (*From Dyer RK, Fisher SR: In Wolfe WG, editor:* Complications in thoracic surgery, *St. Louis, 1992, Mosby-Year Book, p 297.*)

Rigid bronchoscopy, performed in the operating room, is the most effective diagnostic procedure. The rigid bronchoscope allows identification of the sources and access to remove blood and clot from the airway. The rigid scope can be used to compress the artery against the posterior sternum to control the bleeding temporarily, while providing ventilation.

Flexible bronchoscopy through the partially withdrawn tracheostomy tube may identify the fistula, but is useful neither in removing blood from the airway nor in compressing the fistula. Occasionally, in a stable patient with only minimal to moderate tracheal bleeding from an undetermined source, arteriography may be performed to confirm the presence of a TIF; however, the sensitivity of arteriography is only 20%. The most effective arteriographic view is a lateral projection of a direct injection into the innominate artery showing an irregularity of the posterior arterial wall.

■ PREOPERATIVE MANAGEMENT

In the case of massive hemorrhage, immediate preoperative control of bleeding is necessary for patient survival. If the fistula is discovered during rigid bronchoscopy, the scope may be used for temporary occlusion. Alternatively the cuff of the tracheostomy tube may be hyperinflated to produce occlusion and compression of the fistula, which is successful in approximately 85% of cases. The ideal method involves orotracheal intubation and simultaneous removal of the tracheostomy tube. Hyperinflation of the cuff of the endotracheal tube is usually successful, and the removal of the tracheostomy catheter provides superior operative exposure.

If endotracheal occlusion of the TIF is unsuccessful, the tracheostomy incision should be enlarged, and blunt finger dissection should be performed in the anterior paratracheal plane, as with performing cervical mediastinoscopy. Using this technique, the innominate artery may be mobilized away from the trachea, allowing digital compression of the vessel against the posterior table of the sternum to control the hemorrhage (Utley maneuver).

While the surgeon accomplishes control of the hemorrhage, additional personnel should be ensuring adequate intravenous access, beginning resuscitative measures, and securing an adequate supply of blood products in preparation for emergent surgical repair. Most importantly, an adequate airway must be maintained, which may require aggressive, albeit careful, suctioning of blood and clot from the airways. Unless the patient has undergone prior median sternotomy, cardiopulmonary bypass should not be required in the repair of a TIF. If the development of TIF is associated with tracheal dehiscence after extensive resection, however, with loss of control of the distal airway, the emergent establishment of cardiopulmonary bypass may be the only possible lifesaving measure.

■ SURGICAL MANAGEMENT

When the diagnosis of TIF is established, surgical repair must be performed expeditiously yet judiciously. Every effort should be made to control the fistula before undertaking the extensive surgical dissection required to complete this difficult repair successfully. The chance of survival if attempting repair on an actively bleeding patient or hemodynamically unstable patient is dismal. Attention to correct patient positioning, the placement of a bladder catheter and electrocautery pads, and the administration of perioperative antibiotics is advantageous.

The chest and neck should be prepared and draped in sterile fashion from the mandible to the knees, allowing bilateral access to the cervical, thoracic, and femoral regions. If desired, the tracheostomy site may be excluded with biodraping. Femoral arterial access for blood pressure monitoring and arterial blood gas sampling may be obtained at this point, if a left radial arterial catheter has not been placed already. Access to the right radial artery usually is avoided because division of the innominate artery precludes accurate assessment at this source.

There are two approaches that may be employed for adequate exposure in the repair of the fistula. A "trapdoor" incision may be used, by extending the tracheostomy incision laterally into the right cervical region and inferiorly to the midsternum. After dividing the manubrium and upper sternum, the approach is completed with horizontal extension into the right third or fourth intercostal space. This approach is advocated to reduce the incidence of postoperative mediastinitis and sternal dehiscence.

The preferred approach is through a standard median sternotomy, which provides superior exposure, especially for the identification and management of anomalous anatomic variations. After sternotomy, the thymus is divided, and the innominate vein is retracted superiorly to expose the innominate artery. No attempt should be made to identify the fistula at this point.

Proximal and distal control of the innominate artery is obtained subsequently. Before repair, the anatomy of the left common carotid artery must be ascertained; anomalous origin of the left carotid from the trunk of the innominate is present in approximately 20% of whites and 30% of African Americans. In this case, proximal control of the innominate trunk should be obtained distal to the origin of the left carotid, preserving cerebral blood flow. If this cannot be performed due to the presence of inflammation, a bypass to the left carotid must be performed before ligation.

The distal innominate artery may be visualized by applying gentle caudad traction to the trunk. Distal control of the vessel should be obtained proximal to the bifurcation of the right carotid and right subclavian arteries, to preserve perfusion to the right upper extremity; at present, no cases of subclavian steal have been reported. If this control is not possible because of fistula location and vessel inflammation, the confluence must be resected; if significant upper extremity ischemia is present postoperatively, femoral-to-axillary bypass may be performed.

After proximal and distal control of the innominate artery has been achieved, it is safe to proceed with identification of the fistula tract by dissecting the inflamed innominate artery away from the trachea. The involved segment of the innominate artery is resected, and the proximal and distal stumps are oversewn with monofilament suture. Care should be taken to resect all inflamed and diseased artery. No segment of artery or the arterial stumps should

be left adjacent to the inflamed trachea. This situation may be avoided by allowing retraction of the proximal stump and by performing dissection of the distal stump so that it can be covered with surrounding soft tissues.

Unilateral interruption of the right carotid artery is well tolerated, and the incidence of neurologic sequelae due to division of the innominate is extremely rare. Carotid stump pressure may be checked before ligation to show adequate collateral circulation. Additional evidence of adequate collaterals is shown by the continued presence of the right superficial temporal artery pulse, equal pupillary response under light anesthesia, and pulsatile back bleeding from the transected vessel. Adequate resuscitation before clamping and division of the innominate is necessary for adequate collateral circulation to be present.

Bypass grafting of the right carotid is not recommended at the time of operation; not only is grafting usually unnecessary, but also grafts would be placed in a contaminated field. If it becomes apparent after division of the innominate artery that cerebral perfusion is inadequate, however, a bypass to the carotid may be performed from the contralateral carotid, subclavian, or axillary artery, using saphenous vein.

Attention then is turned to the tracheal defect. After débridement, closure with simple interrupted absorbable sutures (preferably in a longitudinal fashion) is performed. Extensive resection and reconstruction of the trachea is prone to fail in this setting, owing to the amount of inflammation and subsequent foreshortening of the trachea. Further resection must not be performed if it would result in an anastomosis under tension. Alternatively, any residual defect may be managed with vascularized soft tissue, which covers the defect and minimizes dead space, to decrease incidence of infection. Suitable sources for soft tissue coverage include the sternocleidomastoid muscle, thymus, pericardium, and omentum (mobilized with right gastroepiploic artery).

The wound should be irrigated and mediastinal drains placed before sternal closure. The neck wound is left open with packing and frequent dressing changes. At the conclusion of the procedure, a neurologic examination should be performed as soon as is feasible. Postoperative care includes appropriately directed intravenous antibiotics, dressing changes, and aggressive pulmonary toilet. If the patient is still ventilator dependent after 7 to 10 days, replacement of the tracheostomy may be considered if the wound is granulating well, and there are no signs of infection.

■ CRITICAL ISSUES

The development of TIF is associated with a mortality approaching 75%; prevention cannot be excessively stressed. Tracheostomy and tracheal resection should be performed by experienced surgeons and under optimal conditions. When creating a tracheostomy, it is essential to use tracheostomy tubes limited to 60-degree angulation, with large-volume, low-pressure cuffs, and to ensure that the tracheotomy is created between the second and third tracheal rings. When performing mediastinal tracheostomy, the innominate artery should be ligated and divided electively. During tracheal resection and reconstruction, the tracheal suture line should not be performed under tension and must be covered with soft tissue. Caregivers must perform sterile, gentle, and adequate endotracheal suctioning and ensure that the ventilator tubing does not cause traction on the tracheostomy cannula.

When TIF occurs, early recognition and prompt control of hemorrhage are paramount because one third of patients exsanguinate preoperatively. Resection without reconstruction of the involved segment of the innominate artery is associated with a significant reduction in postoperative rebleeding (60% versus 7%) and death (64% versus 10%) compared with repair or reconstruction. Appropriate antibiotics and careful attention to wound care postoperatively help prevent the additional complications of wound infection and sternal breakdown resulting from operating in this contaminated field.

SUGGESTED READING

Cooper JD: Trachea-innominate artery fistula: successful management of 3 consecutive patients, *Ann Thorac Surg* 24:439, 1977.

Deslauriers J, et al: Innominate artery rupture: a major complication of tracheal surgery, *Ann Thorac Surg* 20:671, 1975.

Dyer RK, Fisher SR: Tracheal-innominate and tracheal-esophageal fistulas. In Wolfe WG, editor: *Complications in thoracic surgery,* St. Louis, 1992, Mosby-Year Book, p 294.

Jones JW, et al: Tracheo-innominate artery erosion: successful surgical management of a devastating complication, *Ann Surg* 184:194, 1976.

Wright CD: Management of tracheoinnominate artery fistula, *Chest Surg Clin N Am* 6:865, 1996.

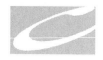
CONGENITAL DIAPHRAGMATIC HERNIA

Jeff C. Hoehner

The management of congenital diaphragmatic hernia (CDH) is controversial and challenging. It is now clear that the diaphragmatic defect develops early in gestation and disallows normal early branching of the tracheo-bronchial tree and the pulmonary vascular bed. This process involves not only the lung on the affected side, but also on the contralateral side. The resulting pulmonary hypoplasia leads to a pathophysiologic condition termed *persistent pulmonary hypertension* or *persistent fetal circulation*. Because of high pulmonary vascular resistance, desaturated blood is shunted through the patent ductus arteriosus and foramen ovale, bypassing the lungs. This persistent right-to-left shunting results in a vicious cycle of hypoxia, hypercarbia, and acidosis, causing death in some infants. Nevertheless, with the recognition and improved treatment of this physiologic process, the overall mortality of newborns with CDH presenting with respiratory distress has improved to 65% to 80%.

Surgical correction no longer is considered an emergency, and immediate repair probably is contraindicated in most infants. Early respiratory stabilization has become the mainstay of therapy. It is believed that the existing high pulmonary vascular resistance results from a combination of spasm in the distal pulmonary arteries and a fixed reduction in the total cross-sectional area of the pulmonary arterial bed due to hypoplasia. A relative surfactant deficiency also may be involved. Management is aimed at decreasing the severity and the frequency of pulmonary arterial spasm, allowing improved compliance by remodeling. The pattern/mode of ventilatory support is designed to minimize the undesirable effects on pulmonary blood flow and pulmonary parenchyma (i.e., barotrauma). Differing pharmacologic agents have been useful, as has the introduction of extracorporeal membrane oxygenation (ECMO) in some infants. Ultimate success in the most severely affected patients hinges on remodeling of the pulmonary vasculature and true pulmonary growth.

■ PRENATAL CARE

Currently, most infants born with CDH are diagnosed after a prenatal ultrasound examination. The diagnosis should be complemented by a careful search for other congenital anomalies, particularly anomalies of the cardiovascular and nervous systems. The current standard of care is to ensure the health of the mother and fetus, while bringing the neonate to delivery as close to term as possible. The greatest advantage of prenatal diagnosis is that it allows parental education about possible treatments and outcomes before delivery. It also allows the fetus and mother to be referred safely to an appropriate perinatal center where the full array of respiratory care expertise and strategies are immediately available, including inhaled nitric oxide, oscillating ventilators, and possibly ECMO. A spontaneous vaginal delivery is preferred unless obstetric issues supervene. Because no reliable prenatal predictors of disease severity currently exist, appropriate patient selection for fetal intervention is unclear.

■ PERIOPERATIVE CARE

When an infant with CDH is born, efforts should be directed toward stabilizing the tenuous cardiopulmonary system, while provoking the least iatrogenic injury. It is essential to consider CDH as a physiologic, not a surgical emergency.

Resuscitation begins with endotracheal and nasogastric intubation to facilitate ventilation and gastrointestinal decompression. Mask ventilation is contraindicated because it worsens bowel distention. Arterial and venous access can be acquired through the umbilicus. If the umbilical venous catheter can be passed into the right atrium, it is useful for mixed venous blood gas analysis. Although the postductal umbilical artery is appropriate for blood pressure monitoring, it is essential to monitor arterial oxygen saturation in a preductal location as well. An important part of the treatment decision algorithm requires an estimation of whether the infant has sufficient pulmonary parenchyma to allow for adequate gas exchange and survival. Although controversial, an infant unable to saturate fully the preductal hemoglobin with oxygen and achieve a P_{CO_2} level less than 50 mm Hg in the face of maximal conventional therapy probably possesses pulmonary hypoplasia incompatible with life.

What embodies standard or conventional treatment is controversial. Although a strategy based on muscle paralysis and induced alkalosis with hyperventilation is traditional and widespread, many currently advocate strict avoidance of all paralyzing agents. More recent treatment algorithms take advantage of native respiratory effort, with respiratory support only to achieve adequate chest wall movement. For this strategy, sufficient supplemental oxygen is administered to maintain preductal oxygen saturation greater than 80%. The postductal values are virtually disregarded other than as an index of right-to-left shunting. Because oxygen delivery, not oxygen saturation, is the goal, this approach requires adequate circulating hemoglobin levels and arterial perfusion pressure. "Permissive hypercapnia" is allowed to avoid iatrogenic barotrauma. Blood, crystalloid, and cardiotonic drugs typically are employed. Evidence suggests that an infant born with CDH possesses a surfactant deficiency, and early surfactant administration may improve outcome. Agents directed toward ameliorating pulmonary hypertension, such as the α-adrenergic antagonist tolazoline, although sometimes effective, often precipitate systemic hypotension with predictable tachyphylaxis. If there is an improvement in the postductal oxygen saturation with an intravenous bolus of 1 to 2 mg/kg, a continuous infusion is initiated. Newer agents, such as inhaled nitric oxide (iNO), acting to relax smooth muscle in the pulmonary arteriole, also may be useful. Because iNO is rapidly bound to and inactivated by hemoglobin, systemic effects are virtually absent when inhaled. iNO is delivered by the respirator in the 25 ppm range. Although theoretically appealing, the clinical efficacy of iNO in CDH patients has been difficult to show in initial limited trials.

If the above-mentioned measures remain ineffective in maintaining adequate oxygen delivery and achieving an acceptable serum pH, ECMO may be employed. The first CDH patients to receive support in this fashion underwent venoarterial ECMO with drainage of the right heart via the jugular vein and infusion into the aortic arch via the carotid artery. The right neck is the preferred site, via either a transverse or a longitudinal (carotid endarterectomy) incision. The vessels are controlled, and appropriate-size cannulae (i.e., 8 to 10 Fr arterial, 10 to 14 Fr venous) are inserted. Care is taken to avoid air embolus. Systemic heparinization is employed. Dedicated experienced perfusionists are mandatory. The neck wound is closed, and the cannulae are secured well within the vessels and along the neck and skull. Alternatively, venovenous ECMO employing either two-vein cannulation or cannulation of a single vessel with a dual staged lumen cannula remain options. Duration of an ECMO "run" may last days to several weeks, and repair of the diaphragmatic defect may take place concomitantly. Although many institutions rely heavily on this technology and applaud its liberal use, there are no well-controlled studies to support strongly the contention that ECMO improves survival. Comparative reports from two centers using different management strategies, one using ECMO and the other not, revealed virtually identical survival rates.

■ TIMING OF SURGERY

Historically, CDH has been considered a surgical emergency. Infants were rushed to the operating room as soon as possible after birth, believing that reducing the viscera from the chest would relieve the compression of the lungs. It now seems clear that emergency surgery only adds surgical and anesthetic morbidity to an unstable patient without reversing the underlying physiologic problem. Immediate repair of the hernia does not increase the surface area available for gas exchange in hypoplastic lungs. Atelectasis does not exist, and alveoli do not expand on decompression of the chest. If adequate gas exchange is achieved perinatally, it is possible that anesthesia or surgery may induce recurrent, refractory, or unstable pulmonary vasospasm. An ill-timed operation can initiate this process and may lead to the demise of the infant. Current data suggest that prolonged preoperative stabilization with delayed repair may improve outcome.

It is a popular belief that surgery should be performed when pulmonary vascular tone is maximally stabilized, as determined through preductal-postductal oximetry and serial cardiac echocardiography with Doppler. More recent reports have shown that minute ventilation improves over the first several days of life, necessitating reduced mechanical support with concomitant improvement in blood gas parameters. A timely operation often can be performed after several days with minimal supplemental oxygen and airway support. It is speculated that the hypertrophied muscle in the intraascinar arterioles is undergoing remodeling, and preoperative stabilization allows improvement in vessel cross-sectional area and reactive vasospasm.

Although most patients with CDH experience respiratory distress at birth, approximately 5% to 20% of children with diaphragmatic hernias are diagnosed after the neonatal period. Their presentation is extremely varied and may be associated with misleading clinical and radiologic assessments. They rarely present with severe respiratory distress and accordingly the above-mentioned supportive measures are not applicable. Nevertheless, elective surgical repair is indicated in these patients as well to treat and prevent worsening respiratory symptoms and to prevent incarceration/ strangulation.

■ SURGICAL REPAIR

Based on clinical stability, repair of CDH can be performed either in the operating room or in the intensive care unit (ICU). Advantages of the operating room include improved lighting and a thermally controlled and isolated environment with immediate access to all required materials. For infants in whom repair is to take place while on ECMO, however, issues involving intravenous access, heat loss, oxygenation, and, to some extent, hemodynamics are solved. Because transportation of a precarious infant requiring an oscillating ventilator, nitric oxide, or ECMO may add prohibitive risk, these infants may be better served having a surgical repair in the ICU.

Although left-sided and right-sided defects require different approaches, certain operative elements remain common. In my opinion, most defects should be repaired transabdominally, although a thoracic approach can be used and is preferred by a few clinicians. One advantage of a thoracic approach may be improved exposure and easier reduction of the right lobe of the liver through a right-sided defect when concerns of hepatic venous kinking arise. The advantages of an abdominal exposure include (1) simpler, easier, and more expeditious reduction of viscera from the chest; (2) accurate visualization of the defect; (3) precise reconstruction of a normal, dome-shaped diaphragm; (4) the ability to gain abdominal domain through abdominal wall stretching or the use of prosthetics, allowing replacement of the viscera within the abdominal cavity without further restricting ventilation; and (5) the ability to perform a Ladd procedure or correct any additional intestinal anomalies in the patient deemed stable to undergo such a procedure. Visualization of the lung, an associated sac, or the occasional extralobar sequestration is equivalent from either an abdominal or a thoracic approach.

Surgical preparation should include the abdomen and the chest on the side of the defect. A subcostal incision performed 2 cm below the rib margin is preferred by most surgeons. This incision also allows the development of an internal oblique/transversalis muscle flap if required. Gentle reduction of the viscera, which may include the entire alimentary canal, spleen, liver, kidney, and adrenal, should proceed in an orderly fashion, with removal of the spleen and the liver last. Extreme caution avoids injury to either the spleen or the liver, as hemorrhage from these organs can be difficult to control in a newborn. With relocation of the liver, kinking of the hepatic veins must be prevented.

On either side, the diaphragmatic defect, typically posterolateral, is seen best after visceral reduction is complete. When a true hernia sac exists, it should be resected. The anterior rim of the diaphragm usually is better developed than the posterior component. The posterior rim, which is always present to some degree, is unrolled as it is dissected free from the posterior chest wall just cephalad to the adrenal. When adequate diaphragmatic tissue exists, a primary repair approximating anterior and posterior elements is accomplished with nonabsorbable suture material. Sutures may be placed in a horizontal mattress fashion, preferably with pledgets, to prevent the sutures from pulling through the thin diaphragmatic muscle. Although it is possible to anchor some of the anterior diaphragm to the tissue overlying a posterior rib, inordinate effort to achieve a primary repair under tension is not suggested. A successful repair would be jeopardized in such circumstances, and diaphragmatic closure using a muscle flap or prosthetic material is a better alternative. Current series report a 35% to 55% incidence of CDH repair using either a flap or a prosthesis. If a prosthetic patch is deemed necessary, lyophilized dura, Marlex, or most frequently Gore-Tex, can be used. A template slightly overestimating the defect is created and transferred to the Gore-Tex sheet. Unused Gore-Tex can be used to assist in subsequent abdominal wall closure. The posterior attachment of the patch is started medial-to-lateral with nonabsorbable suture material and completed in a circumferential fashion. Although prosthetic patches are employed frequently, more recent studies indicate that the recurrence rate is high, almost 50%, and suggest this is not an acceptable long-term solution for the child with CDH. Techniques that involve intercostal, rectus abdominis, and reversed latissimus dorsi muscle flaps also have been used. My preference for closure of a large defect incorporates an internal oblique/transversus abdominis flap, as originally described by Simpson. Briefly, a pedicle muscle flap, including the transversus and internal oblique muscles, is fashioned from the anterior abdominal wall after separation from the external oblique muscle. The flap is swung posteriorly, hinged along the anterior leaf of the diaphragm, and sutured to the posterior muscular rim of the diaphragm. The inferior cut margin of the subcostal laparotomy incision becomes the most dorsally located portion of the flap approximated to the posterior diaphragmatic lip. It is imperative that adequate distance be maintained between the subcostal incision and the costal margin if a muscle flap is to be fashioned and provide adequate length.

After the defect is closed, the viscera must be returned to the abdominal cavity and abdominal wall closure attempted. This is not always accomplished easily, and systematic stretching of the abdominal wall often creates much-needed intraabdominal domain. The use of a chest tube provides no added benefit, and its use is discouraged. The abdominal wall is closed in layers, preferably with interrupted 2-0 or 3-0 absorbable suture material. Interrupted sutures are preferred if the closure is under tension. If the abdominal wall closure is tight and there is a risk of restricting ventilation or creating an abdominal compartment syndrome, a prosthetic sheet is used to bridge the fascial defect in a fashion similar to ventral hernia repair. Alternatively a temporary prosthetic pouch or "silo" may be created in a fashion similar to that employed for repair of omphalocele or gastroschisis. Development of skin flaps with skin closure alone, allowing an incisional hernia to remain, is also an option.

■ RESULTS OF TREATMENT

Reported survival statistics for CDH patients are affected by small series size, referral patterns, exclusion criteria, and variations in treatment. Improvements in prenatal diagnosis, acute medical support, and transport have allowed sicker infants to reach referral centers and be included in survivorship data, partially offsetting potential achievements in improved care. A review of 18 series including nearly 900 patients treated between 1989 and 1998 yielded an overall survival rate nearing 65%, replacing the historically quoted 50% survival rate based on older series.

Beyond survival itself, studies addressing the long-term morbidity after treatment of CDH using current technology are lacking. Complications in patients treated for CDH fall into two broad categories: pulmonary and nonpulmonary. Nonpulmonary complications include foregut dysmotility, chylothorax, scoliosis, pectus excavatum, adhesive intestinal obstruction, diaphragmatic hernia recurrence, and abdominal wall hernias. Thrombosis, bleeding, stroke, intracranial bleeding, and neurocognitive consequences also must be included as complications for patients who were maintained on ECMO. Clinically apparent gastroesophageal reflux is prevalent (80% at discharge, 30% at 1 year) and is presumably secondary to small stomach size and to the loss of normal anatomic relationships that oppose reflux. Although near-uniform success is achieved with medical therapy, surgical correction is sometimes necessary. Growth failure and neurodevelopmental abnormalities (including hearing and visual problems) are also significant (30% to 50%), particularly during the first 2 years.

Given the severe respiratory distress apparent in these infants at birth, it is truly remarkable that near-normal to normal respiratory function is experienced in most survivors as they reach adulthood. Tremendous potential for alveolar growth with concomitant pulmonary capillary growth exists after birth. Respiratory function is believed to normalize after alveolar growth. Detailed studies testing lung function 6 to 18 years after CDH repair revealed either normal or near-normal formal pulmonary function parameters. This is based on studies in the pre-ECMO era, however, and does not apply to infants salvaged with the more advanced technology currently available. Most surgeons have witnessed, with increasing frequency, infants with severe chronic pulmonary disease requiring tracheostomy and long-term mechanical ventilation. One justification for the development of therapy through fetal intervention is to avoid these debilitating forms of morbidity and have an impact on quality of life in addition to survival.

SUGGESTED READING

Azarow K, et al: Congenital diaphragmatic hernia—a tale of two cities: the Toronto experience, *J Pediatr Surg* 32:395, 1997.

Grosfeld JL, Klein MD, editors. Congenital diaphragmatic hernia. In: *Seminars in pediatric surgery*, vol 5, Philadelphia, 1996, WB Saunders.

Langer JC, et al: Timing of surgery for congenital diaphragmatic hernia: is emergency operation necessary? *J Pediatr Surg* 23:731, 1988.

Moss RL, et al: Prosthetic patch durability in congenital diaphragmatic hernia: a long-term follow-up study, *J Pediatr Surg* 36:152, 2001.

Simpson JS, Gossage JD: Use of abdominal wall muscle flaps in repair of large congenital diaphragmatic hernia, *J Pediatr Surg* 6:42, 1971.

Wilson JM, et al: Congenital diaphragmatic hernia—a tale of two cities: the Boston experience, *J Pediatr Surg* 32:401, 1997.

DIAPHRAGMATIC EVENTRATION AND PLICATION IN THE PEDIATRIC PATIENT

Richard J. Andrassy

Diaphragmatic eventration may be caused by phrenic nerve injury or congenital muscular deficiency of the diaphragm. This results in an abnormal elevation of the diaphragm that causes paradoxical motion of the affected diaphragm during inspiration and expiration. In addition, frequently there is a shift of the mediastinum and decreased intrathoracic space for pulmonary expansion. The congenital form generally results from incomplete development of the muscular portion or central tendon. This condition has been reported to be more common on the left side, although it has been seen on either side and occasionally can be bilateral. Congenital eventration can be seen in association with other congenital anomalies, including pulmonary sequestration, congenital heart disease, tracheomalacia, cerebral agenesis, and trisomic chromosomal abnormalities. Phrenic nerve palsy is seen secondary to phrenic nerve injury in the newborn. This condition occasionally has been seen in association with Erb's palsy as a result of birth injury or iatrogenic damage. Phrenic nerve injury is a well-known complication of pediatric cardiac surgery and has been reported in 1% to 2% of cases. Most phrenic nerve palsies recover spontaneously, generally within 2 to 3 weeks. Surgical procedures on the neck, mediastinal tumors, or resection of thoracic masses may lead to injury as well.

Eventration secondary to muscular hypoplasia may be difficult to distinguish from paralysis, which is a consequence of traction injury to the nerve roots of the phrenic nerve during traumatic delivery. Newborns with diaphragmatic eventration may be asymptomatic or present with respiratory distress, tachypnea, or pallor. These neonates may suck poorly and tire easily during feeding, resulting in failure to thrive. Patients on a ventilator with positive-pressure ventilation may be difficult to diagnose because paralysis may obscure the diagnosis. Difficulty with weaning may lead one to consider the diagnosis, however. Older children may present with recurrent pneumonias or gastrointestinal symptoms, including vomiting, pain, and gastric volvulus.

■ DIAGNOSIS

Chest x-ray showing a unilateral or bilateral elevated diaphragm may lead to suspicion of the diagnosis. This suspicion can be confirmed by ultrasonography or fluoroscopy showing paradoxical motion of the diaphragm and mediastinal shift. Many of these children may have evidence of pneumonia, atelectasis, or decreased lung volume. Occasionally, older children first may have a diagnosis made during evaluation for gastrointestinal complications.

■ INDICATIONS FOR SURGERY

Indications for surgery in patients with diaphragmatic eventration include respiratory distress that requires continued ventilation, failure to wean effectively, recurrent pulmonary infections, and failure to thrive secondary to poor intake. Newborns and young patients should be considered for surgical intervention early to prevent pulmonary damage or persistent pulmonary dysfunction. Evidence of permanent phrenic nerve injury should lead to early consideration of primary phrenic nerve repair or diaphragmatic plication. If the cause is uncertain, failure to wean from positive-pressure ventilation after 2 to 3 weeks would indicate the need for plication. Diaphragmatic plication may be performed transthoracically or transabdominally. It has been suggested to approach the right side through the chest and the left side through the abdomen. It has been my personal preference to perform all diaphragmatic plications through the chest because the branches of the phrenic nerve are identified more easily and can be preserved and avoided via the thoracic approach. The abdominal approach, particularly on the left, is also easy and has been used more frequently when associated intraabdominal surgical procedures are performed. Diaphragmatic plication is an easy surgical procedure, generally performed by thoracotomy through the sixth or seventh interspace. Multiple nonabsorbable large-caliber sutures are placed by staggered bites across the diaphragm. Multiple parallel sutures are placed, then pulled up to ascertain adequate flattening and plication of the diaphragm. Additional imbricating sutures can be placed in the diaphragm to plicate further or flatten the diaphragm to maximize the intrathoracic space. Generally the chest tube can be removed within 1 or 2 days, and the patient is weaned successfully from ventilatory support within several days. Marked improvement in pulmonary function and decreased gastrointestinal symptoms are seen. Complications generally are related to associated anomalies. It is rare to need synthetic material to reinforce the diaphragmatic plication; however, in instances of severe attenuation of the medical diaphragm, synthetic reinforcing material can be placed.

Bilateral congenital eventration in the diaphragm has been reported and is exceedingly rare. These patients generally have severe respiratory insufficiency and a high mortality rate if not treated aggressively. Bilateral diaphragmatic plication may result in early weaning from the ventilator and return to normal pulmonary function. Patients with known phrenic nerve transection should be considered for primary microsurgical repair. Diaphragmatic electrical pacing has been used infrequently in pediatric patients. Long-term results have suggested that the plicated diaphragm maintains adequate growth in proportion to the contralateral side. Normal values of pulmonary function tests are obtained, and diaphragmatic plication does not interfere with further overall development of the diaphragm or chest wall.

■ CONCLUSION

Diagnosis of congenital or acquired diaphragmatic eventration should lead to early consideration of surgical plication when spontaneous recovery does not appear to occur within 2 to 3 weeks of diagnosis. The surgical repair is relatively easy, complications are generally minor, and the long-term results are excellent.

SUGGESTED READING

Kizilcan F, et al: The long-term results of diaphragmatic plication, *J Pediatr Surg* 28:42, 1993.

Langer JC, et al: Plication of the diaphragm for infants and young children with phrenic nerve palsy, *J Pediatr Surg* 23:749, 1988.

Rodgers BM, Hawks P: Bilateral congenital eventration of the diaphragms: successful surgical management, *J Pediatr Surg* 21:858, 1986.

Smith CD, et al: Diaphragmatic paralysis and eventration in infants, *J Thorac Cardiovasc Surg* 91:490, 1996.

Tsugawa C, et al: Diaphragmatic eventration in infants and children: is conservative treatment justified, *J Pediatr Surg* 32:1643, 1997.

CONGENITAL TRACHEO-ESOPHAGEAL FISTULA

Walter Pegoli
George Drugas

Congenital malformations of the trachea and esophagus may occur separately or in combination. The reported incidence of tracheoesophageal malformations is 2.4 per 10,000 live births. Population studies have found a slight but statistically significant male preponderance. The etiology of tracheoesophageal anomalies is not known.

■ ANATOMY AND CLASSIFICATION

The most useful and practical classification of tracheoesophageal anomaly is based on simple anatomic description:

1. Esophageal atresia with distal tracheoesophageal fistula—86%
2. Esophageal atresia without tracheoesophageal fistula—8%
3. Tracheoesophageal fistula without esophageal atresia—4%
4. Esophageal atresia with fistulas to upper and lower pouch—1%

5. Esophageal atresia with proximal tracheoesophageal fistula—1%

Esophageal atresia with a distal tracheoesophageal fistula is
the most common anomaly. The upper esophagus ends
blindly usually at the level of the third thoracic vertebra. The
fistula usually originates near the carina off the posterior
membranous wall of the trachea. The blood supply to the
upper esophageal pouch is axial arising from the thyrocervical trunk. The blood supply to the lower esophagus is
segmental from the aorta.

Isolated esophageal atresia usually is associated with a
long gap between the two ends of the esophagus. The length
of the upper pouch is similar in all of the anomalies. The
lower pouch is short, however, measuring only 1 to 2 cm
above the level of the diaphragm. Isolated tracheoesophageal
fistula is usually cervical in location with a fistula inserting
more cephalad on the posterior membranous trachea than
on the anterior aspect of the esophagus.

Esophageal atresia with proximal tracheoesophageal fistula has a fistula arising proximal to the tip of the upper
esophageal pouch. The distal esophageal pouch is markedly
shortened. Esophageal atresia with proximal and distal fistulas usually is associated with a normal gap between the
esophageal segments.

■ ASSOCIATED ANOMALIES

At least 50% of infants with esophageal atresia have one or
more associated anomalies. Most common are major cardiac
malformations (15% to 30% incidence), particularly patent
ductus arteriosus, ventriculoseptal defects, atrial septal
defects, right aortic arch, and tetralogy of Fallot. These cardiac problems are responsible for most deaths. The spectrum
of anomalies most often associated with esophageal atresia
may be arranged into the acronym, *VACTERL* (*V* = vertebral,
A = anorectal, *C* = cardiac, *T* = tracheo, *E* = esophageal,
R = renal, *L* = limb). Infants with esophageal atresia and the
VACTERL association have a higher mortality rate.

In 1962, Waterston developed a risk factor classification
that grouped patients with tracheoesophageal malformations according to birth weight, pneumonia, and associated
congenital anomalies. With advances in neonatal critical care
and anesthesia, however, this classification is of historical
interest only. Modern predictors of survival in cases of
esophageal atresia are based on birth weight and the presence or absence of structural congenital heart disease.
Low-birth-weight infants with major congenital heart disease have a significant survival disadvantage.

■ DIAGNOSIS AND CLINICAL FINDINGS

The prenatal diagnosis of esophageal atresia by ultrasonography is based on the presence of maternal polyhydramnios
and the finding of an absent or small stomach bubble.
Sonographic visualization of a blind upper esophageal
pouch has been reported but is an inconsistent finding.

Most infants with esophageal atresia are symptomatic
within the first hours of life. The earliest sign is excessive

salivation. If feeding is initiated, coughing, choking, and
cyanosis ensue. The diagnosis of esophageal atresia can be
confirmed by attempting to pass a 10 Fr Replogle tube
through the mouth and into the esophagus. Failure to
advance the tube beyond 10 cm from the nose or mouth is
pathognomonic for esophageal atresia. Injection of contrast
material into the upper pouch is unnecessary and can precipitate aspiration.

Radiographs are valuable to determine the presence or
absence of a distal esophageal fistula. Air in the stomach
and bowel confirms the presence of a distal tracheoesophageal fistula. Absence of air in the abdomen typically
represents an isolated esophageal atresia without a distal
tracheoesophageal fistula. The diagnosis of tracheoesophageal fistula without esophageal atresia is considerably
more difficult and requires a high index of suspicion based
on clinical symptoms. The diagnosis can be made by barium
esophagography in the prone position, but bronchoscopy or
esophagoscopy may be required to confirm the diagnosis.

The incidence of recognizable congenital defects associated with esophageal atresia ranges from 50% to 70%.
Physical examination focused on seeking associated anomalies, echocardiography, renal ultrasonography, and chromosomal analysis is important in evaluating infants with
tracheoesophageal anomalies.

■ PREOPERATIVE MANAGEMENT

Pneumonitis is the result of aspiration of pharyngeal secretions or reflux of gastric acid through the tracheoesophageal
fistula. Aspiration pneumonia is the most significant preoperative problem facing infants with tracheoesophageal
anomalies. The cornerstones of management consist of
measures that prevent aspiration and treat pneumonitis. A
Replogle tube (sump catheter) should be positioned in the
upper pouch. The catheter should be maintained on low continuous suction. The infant should be positioned in a semi-
upright position to minimize reflux of gastric acid through
the tracheoesophageal fistula. Broad-spectrum antibiotics
are indicated in the presence of pneumonitis. Routine endotracheal intubation should be avoided because of the risk of
gastric perforation and worsening abdominal distention
secondary to positive-pressure ventilation. This is especially
of concern in patients with associated duodenal atresia.
Vitamin K is administered preoperatively in all surgical newborns to decrease the likelihood of bleeding complications.

■ OPERATIVE MANAGEMENT

The operative approach to infants with tracheoesophageal
malformations depends on the anatomic anomalies present.
Infants with birth weight less than 1500 g and major congenital anomalies are poor candidates for extensive primary
reconstruction. These infants are served better with gastrostomy decompression and placement of a central venous
catheter for nutritional support to allow for the stabilization
and treatment of associated medical or surgical problems.
Healthy infants with minor or no associated anomalies are
treated best with prompt primary repair.

Esophageal Atresia with Distal Tracheoesophageal Fistula

Immediate operative intervention for infants with esophageal atresia and distal tracheoesophageal fistula is unnecessary. A period of 24 to 48 hours for resuscitation and delineation of associated anomalies is current standard therapy.

Repair of the anomaly is undertaken under general endotracheal anesthesia. It is imperative that the endotracheal tube be placed carefully to avoid intubation of the fistula. Some anesthesiologists intubate under bronchoscopic guidance to avoid inadvertent fistula cannulation. Additionally, to avoid positive-pressure ventilation, some anesthesiologists favor initiating the procedure under continuous spinal anesthesia to allow for spontaneous ventilation. General anesthesia with positive-pressure ventilation can be initiated when the fistula has been operatively controlled.

The operative approach is through a posterolateral thoracotomy incision opposite the aortic arch as defined by preoperative echocardiography. In 95% of infants, the procedure is performed through the right chest. The latissimus dorsi and serratus muscles may be divided, or they can be retracted using a muscle-sparing technique to expose the chest wall. The chest is entered through the fourth intercostal space. Most pediatric surgeons proceed using a retropleural dissection. In this extrapleural approach, parietal pleura is dissected gently away from the chest wall using moistened cotton-tip applicators or gauze to dissect the pleura anteromedially as the rib spreader is sequentially opened. Proponents of this technique cite a diminished risk of empyema secondary to anastomotic leak. Other surgeons prefer, however, a transpleural approach, citing shorter operative times and low rates of empyema formation secondary to an anastomotic leak with current antibiotic therapy.

Along the posterior mediastinum, the azygos vein is isolated, ligated, and divided. The lung and pleura are retracted gently medially exposing the upper pouch, distal tracheoesophageal fistula, trachea, and vagus nerve. The upper pouch is dissected circumferentially. This dissection is aided by placement of a large-bore Foley catheter transorally into the proximal pouch. A traction suture can be placed through the apex of the pouch and catheter to assist in immobilization. Because the blood supply of the proximal pouch originates from the thyrocervical trunk and ramifies through the submucosal plexus, extensive dissection does not pose a risk of ischemic injury. During the dissection, care must be taken to avoid injury to the posterior membranous wall of the trachea.

The lower esophagus is dissected circumferentially at the level of the fistula. After circumferential dissection, the fistula is controlled with a vessel loop passed around the distal esophagus to allow for further exposure and to impede the flow of anesthetic gases into the distal esophagus. The esophagus is transected several millimeters away from the origin of the fistula to avoid narrowing the tracheal lumen. The fistula is closed using interrupted absorbable sutures. The integrity of the closure can be tested by filling the thoracic cavity with saline and watching for bubbles on ventilation. The distal esophagus is thin-walled and depends on segmental blood supply. Extensive dissection of the lower segment should be avoided. Injury to the segmental vessels may result in ischemia of the lower esophagus and predispose to anastomotic complications.

The most dependent portion of the lower pouch is incised transversely. Traction sutures are placed laterally. An end-to-end, full-thickness anastomosis is performed using interrupted absorbable sutures. The back wall of the anastomosis is performed first using 5-0 sutures with the knots tied on the inside of the lumen. Thereafter, a 10 Fr catheter is placed transnasally into the esophagus by the anesthesiologist and advanced under direct visualization into the stomach. The anterior layer of the anastomosis is completed over the catheter. The tube ensures esophageal patency and may be used for early postoperative enteral feedings. The tracheal suture line may be reinforced using adjacent tissue, preferably intercostal musculature or pleura. This maneuver decreases the likelihood of recurrent fistula formation.

When the anastomosis is complete, a chest tube is placed and secured to the lateral chest wall adjacent to the esophagus. This tube drains the retropleural space in the event of an anastomotic leak.

Occasionally the distance between the upper and lower esophageal segments limits the ability to perform a tension-free anastomosis easily. Extensive mobilization of the distal esophagus may damage the segmental blood supply and result in an ischemic injury. Blood supply to the proximal pouch is nonsegmental, however. To lengthen the upper esophageal segment, Livaditis reported the use of a circular myotomy on the proximal pouch. One or more myotomies can be performed to increase the length of the upper pouch. If the gap cannot be bridged to achieve a primary anastomosis, the lower pouch is tacked to the chest wall using permanent sutures, and a gastrostomy is performed. Esophageal reconstruction is deferred until a later date.

In cases of long gap esophageal atresia when a delayed primary anastomosis cannot be performed, esophageal replacement is indicated. The choice of esophageal substitutes includes colonic interposition, gastric transposition, or reversed gastric tube interposition.

Tracheoesophageal Fistula without Esophageal Atresia (H Type)

The diagnosis of congenital H-type tracheal esophageal fistula requires a high index of suspicion. This anomaly usually presents within the first few days of life when the infant manifests feeding difficulties or has unexplained oxygen desaturation episodes during feeding. Older infants and children may present with recurrent episodes of aspiration pneumonia or excessive flatulence.

If the diagnosis is suspected, real-time esophagography may establish the diagnosis. A small nasogastric tube is placed in the distal esophagus, and contrast medium is injected gradually under fluoroscopic guidance. As the tube is withdrawn slowly into the cervical esophagus, the fistula may be identified. Bronchoscopy with esophagoscopy, using blue dye technique, can confirm the diagnosis. Methylene blue is injected gently into the upper trachea via an endotracheal tube during esophagoscopy. The fistula orifice may be identified. If this procedure is performed immediately before operative fistula ligation, a Fogarty catheter may be passed through the fistula to aid in identification at exploration.

Most H-type fistulas may be closed successfully using a cervical collar incision. A right-sided approach is advocated to avoid injury to the thoracic duct. The sternocleidomastoid muscle is retracted posteriorly, and the dissection proceeds to the carotid sheath. Identification of the trachea and esophagus is facilitated by the placement of endotracheal and nasogastric tubes. The recurrent laryngeal nerve, lying in the tracheoesophageal groove, must be identified and preserved. Identification of the fistula is facilitated by the presence of a previously placed Fogarty catheter or feeding tube through the fistula. The proximal esophagus is encircled with a vessel loop. The fistula is divided and closed sequentially using absorbable sutures. It is important to leave extra tissue on the tracheal side to avoid narrowing the tracheal lumen during closure. Most surgeons interpose adjacent strap muscle tissue between the opposing suture lines to reduce the likelihood of fistula recurrence.

Isolated Esophageal Atresia without Fistula

Infants with pure esophageal atresia manifest near-complete absence of an intraabdominal esophagus. The proximal and distal ends of the esophagus are rudimentary and separated by a long gap. Clinically, these patients mimic patients with esophageal atresia and a distal tracheal esophageal fistula. The abdomen is scaphoid, however, and a plain abdominal radiograph is gasless. Classically, patients with pure esophageal atresia are managed by creating a cervical esophagostomy and placement of a gastrostomy tube. Subsequently the esophagus is replaced with either stomach or interposed colon. Some authors describe delaying primary repair, however, for 6 to 8 weeks to allow for differential esophageal growth. Bougie dilation of the upper and lower pouches may be performed during this time. Suction on the upper pouch and gastrostomy feedings are maintained until the pouches are less than 1 cm apart. A primary anastomosis can be performed via a right thoracotomy with high likelihood for success.

■ COMPLICATIONS

Hospital survival rates range from 85% to 95%. Death results most frequently from congenital or chromosomal defects. The most significant postoperative complication is an anastomotic leak. Leaks are apparent when saliva is seen in the chest tube placed at the time of surgery. Leaks usually are well tolerated, and most close spontaneously. During the time interval before closure, central hyperalimentation is required. Ultimately a barium contrast esophagram is required to evaluate for the presence of a stricture and to confirm resolution of a leak. Complete disruption of the anastomosis requires cervical esophagostomy and gastrostomy. After an adequate time interval, esophageal substitution is required.

Stricture

Esophageal anastomotic strictures are common. Conditions predisposing to stricture include anastomotic tension, leak, and gastroesophageal reflux. Stricture is manifested by choking, dysphagia, and aspiration pneumonitis. The diagnosis is made by contrast esophagography. Primary treatment is dilation. Dilation is repeated until the stricture is resolved. If there is no resolution of the stricture in 6 months to 1 year, resection of the stricture should be considered.

Gastroesophageal Reflux

Gastroesophageal reflux is present in most infants with esophageal atresia. Conditions for reflux are enhanced by poor motility of the lower esophageal pouch and an altered angle of His secondary to surgical manipulation at the time of anastomosis. Most infants with reflux respond well to conservative measures consisting of upright feedings, thickening of feeds, H_2 blockers, and promotility agents. Antireflux procedures are reserved for patients refractory to maximal medical management.

Recurrent Tracheoesophageal Fistula

Recurrent tracheoesophageal fistula is an uncommon complication after esophagoesophagostomy; incidence ranges from 5% to 10%. The etiology has been attributed to an anastomotic leak with local inflammation and erosion through the previous site of a tracheoesophageal fistula repair. Recurrent respiratory infections, abdominal distention, and choking spells may indicate recurrence. Esophagoscopy performed in the prone position is the most reliable method of establishing the diagnosis. Recurrent fistulas in the neck may be repaired from a cervical approach. Fistulas in the thorax require thoracotomy. In either setting, bronchoscopy with cannulation of the fistula is a reliable diagnostic method and is invaluable in treating the fistula during the operative procedure. The fistula is approached transpleurally, with division and closure of the fistula being the operation of choice. To prevent fistulization, pleura, intercostal musculature, or pericardium should be interposed between the esophagus and the trachea.

SUGGESTED READING

Beasley SW, Myers NA: Diagnosis of congenital tracheoesophageal fistula, *J Pediatr Surg* 23:415, 1988.

Benjamin B, Pham T: Diagnosis of H-type tracheoesophageal fistula, *J Pediatr Surg* 26:667, 1991.

Holman WL, et al: Surgical treatment of H-type tracheoesophageal fistula diagnosed in an adult, *Ann Thorac Surg* 41:453, 1986.

Vos A, Ekkelkamp S: Congenital tracheoesophageal fistula: preventing recurrence, *J Pediatr Surg* 31:936, 1996.

CAUSTIC BURNS OF THE ESOPHAGUS

Charles N. Paidas

Prevention programs, consumer products safety commissions, lobbying by the medical profession, and heightened consumer awareness all have contributed to diminishing significantly the devastating effects of caustic ingestions. Socioeconomic factors, such as parental job absenteeism, job relocation, and overall rising hospital costs, are a few of the seldom spoken about family consequences, however, of this entirely preventable injury. Higher crime rates and attempted suicide among the patient population are hidden psychological aspects of caustic burns.

The incidence of severe ingestion (requiring hospitalization or esophageal replacement) has been reduced dramatically. Despite the observed reduction, accidental ingestions in children younger than 5 years old and suicide attempts in individuals 15 to 40 years old remain the two most common types of ingestions. Regardless of the cause, the most common agent is an alkaline household liquid cleaner. Compared with ingestion of solids, injuries resulting from ingestion of liquids are much more severe.

■ PATHOLOGY

The extent and severity of the esophageal injury depend on the amount and the nature of the ingested material. Strong acid or alkali ingestions constitute the two most common types of caustic ingestions. These substances can be sold in liquid or solid/particulate forms. Strong acid substances are found in industrial and swimming pool cleaning solutions, battery fluids, and a variety of antirust compounds. Strong alkaline-containing substances include household cleaning products, such as toilet bowel and oven cleaners and bleach used for clothes washing; Clinitest tablets; and personal hygiene products. The common weak alkali is ammonia hydroxide found in most bleach solutions. The clinical significance of weak alkalis is the fact that they cause much less injury and require far less therapy.

Acid burns cause a coagulative necrosis and a superficial eschar that protects the deeper layers from damage. In liquid form, transit of ingested acid is rapid, and acid burns tend to spare the oropharynx, produce skip injuries to the esophagus, and frequently cause injury to the stomach and duodenum. Acids tend to taste bitter and cause immediate pain, however, which leads to spitting the acid out usually well before it reaches the esophagus and stomach.

The alkaline burn is characterized by liquefactive necrosis, meaning there is far greater penetration at the level of the oropharynx and esophagus. There is frequently penetration of all layers of the esophagus causing substantial secondary edema. In addition, the pathology of the strong alkali is exacerbated by the fact that these substances are odorless and tasteless, escaping many of the oropharyngeal protective mechanisms associated with an acid burn. In general, the potential for perforation and circumferential scar formation is greatest with an alkaline ingestion.

A special case of caustic alkali occurs with the ingestion of batteries used for hearing aids, watches, and computer games. These batteries should pass through the colon within 4 days. Batteries larger than 15 mm are not likely to pass beyond the pylorus in children younger than 6 years old. These situations require radiographic localization and more than likely endoscopic retrieval from the stomach because this is the likely point of failure to pass.

Most caustic ingestions involve the oropharynx, lips, and gums. As is the case for most foreign body ingestions, the most common sites for pathology within the esophagus are its three areas of narrowing: the cricopharyngeus, the level of the aortic arch, and the gastroesophageal junction.

■ CLINICAL FINDINGS AND EMERGENCY DEPARTMENT MANAGEMENT

The initial clinical presentation comprises oropharyngeal pain; irritability; and, in severe cases, excessive salivation, dysphagia, and eventually airway compromise. Hoarseness and stridor are signs of serious airway injury that mandate intubation. Retrosternal pain, neck crepitus, and sudden onset of epigastric pain imply full-thickness esophageal damage. In contrast, 20% of children present with no symptoms at all. At least half this asymptomatic group have on admission or insidiously develop esophageal injury requiring treatment. A 24-hour period of observation is reasonable, even for asymptomatic patients, especially if there is any question about the circumstances of the event.

Emergency department management should begin with the standard assessment of the ABCs (airway, breathing, and circulation) (Figure 1). When the patient is stable, posteroanterior and lateral upright chest and abdominal radiographs should be obtained looking for pleural effusion or free air. Children with no visible signs or only lip swelling or redness can be observed in the hospital or a short-stay unit for 24 hours to ensure they can tolerate oral feedings. All children with oral lesions require esophagoscopy (preferably rigid) and if necessary bronchoscopy. Ingestion of particulate caustic substances results in signs of contact readily visible in the oropharynx. Particulate matter rarely gets beyond the oropharynx because the child usually spits it out. Liquid caustic agents (acid or alkali) contribute to more pathology down the length of the esophagus. Children who have ingested liquids more frequently require esophagoscopy. Under no circumstances should there be blind passage of a nasogastric or orogastric tube.

The keystone of emergency management is rigid or flexible esophagoscopy, which should be performed within 24 hours of the injury because the risk of mechanical perforation 2 to 3 days later is significant. The indications for esophagoscopy include all patients with stridor, vomiting, drooling, or intended ingestion. The procedure always should stop at the first sign of pathology below the cricopharyngeus.

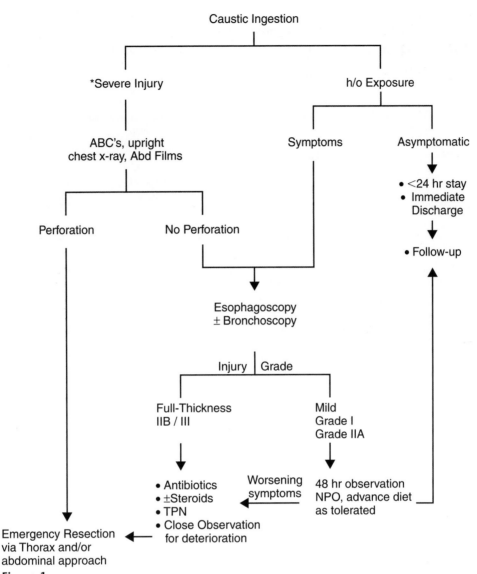

Figure 1
Algorithm for acute management of caustic ingestion. *Severe Injury = respiratory compromise, neck crepitus, severe epigastric or retrosternal pain, unknown corrosive, or intentional ingestion.

Distance from the upper incisors to the pathology should be recorded. If there are respiratory signs and symptoms, laryngoscopy and bronchoscopy should be performed. Grading of the esophageal burn should be performed during esophagoscopy (Table 1).

Patients with grade 1 injuries have superficial burns causing edema and hyperemia. These patients can be observed, a normal diet can be advanced, and the patient ultimately can be followed in an outpatient clinic. These superficial injuries cause mucosal sloughing and should heal without a stricture. Grade II injuries penetrate into the muscular layer of the esophagus and can result in either patchy (IIA) or circumferential (IIB) injury. Ulcerations (superficial and deep) and pseudomembranes are found during endoscopy. Grade III injuries are full-thickness injuries, and mediastinitis or peritonitis occurs by 48 hours. All grade III and more

than 75% of circumferential grade IIB burns cause esophageal stricture and, as expected, are associated with a higher incidence of infection. In contrast, no stricture formation is observed with grade I or grade IIA burns. Circumferential ulceration is usually easy to recognize. Grade III endoscopic findings classically are characterized by a gray mucosal slough, thrombosed submucosal vessels, and black eschar.

Acute management of caustic ingestion should be dictated by the endoscopic grading of the esophagus and the status of the patient (see Figure 1). Patients with mild exposure with symptoms and severe injury (including intentional ingestion or ingestion of an unknown substance) should be evaluated for perforation using endoscopy. If there is no evidence of perforation, patients with mild exposure (e.g., bleach and detergent) can be observed and possibly discharged from the

DEGREE OF INJURY	DEPTH	ENDOSCOPY
Grade I	Mucosal	Superficial hyperemia and edema
Grade II	Partial Thickness	Mucosal sloughing, friable,
A	Patchy	superficial ulcers,
		pseudomembranes
B	Circumferential	Circumferential
		deep
		ulceration
Grade III	Full Thickness	Eschar,
		gray
		black
		Ulcers
		transmural
		necrosis

Table 1 Classification of Esophageal & Gastric Burns

emergency department with follow-up instructions or observed for 24 hours. In contrast, signs of respiratory distress (hoarseness or stridor), mediastinal air, and pneumoperitoneum all require a different treatment algorithm. Patients may require intravenous antibiotics, mechanical ventilation, possible esophagogram, and drainage of the mediastinum if free contrast material into the pleural space is shown or esophageal resection if there is obvious necrosis. A contained mediastinal leak that returns contrast material back into the esophagus may be observed without the need for immediate drainage. Pneumoperitoneum is an absolute indication for laparotomy and resection of all dead tissue. Laparoscopic evaluation of the pneumoperitoneum is not indicated but may be useful to evaluate the abdomen if there is isolated mediastinal pathology.

All grade IIB or III pathologies require antibiotics for oropharyngeal flora. A penicillin derivative or clindamycin is appropriate. Corticosteroids (2 to 2.5 mg/kg/day) have not been shown to improve outcome or avoid stricture formation. Some centers continue to add them to their treatment algorithm, however. If steroids are used, they should be instituted within the first 24 hours of ingestion and for 3 weeks thereafter. Early introduction of parenteral nutrition is essential for all patients with perforations and for patients with poor gastric motility. Alternatively, enteral feedings should be introduced within 48 hours for all grade I and IIA patients. Open gastrostomy is helpful for grade IIB and III patients.

■ OPERATIVE CONSIDERATIONS

The two most important lessons learned about esophageal perforations are as follows: (1) Delay in diagnosis of a perforation is uniformly fatal, and (2) there is no optimal substitute for the native esophagus. All things being equal, the radical approach to the possibility of perforation is observation.

One should have a high index of suspicion for grade IIB and III esophageal burns and use contrast studies to disprove a leak. Peritoneal signs, pneumoperitoneum, and clinical deterioration (altered mental status, persistent acidosis, coagulopathy) mandate operation. Necrotic tissue must be

removed, holes closed, and mediastinum adequately drained. Laparoscopic evaluation of the abdomen also may be included in the treatment algorithm if there is a question of periesophageal or gastric pathology. Despite these precepts, individualization of care is appropriate for all grade IIB or III burns.

Circumferential grade IIB burns can be managed with an open gastrostomy and insertion of a string through the gastrostomy that exits in a transnasal route. Beginning at 4 weeks postburn, serial dilations using progressive antegrade bougienage from the oropharynx or retrograde stringing bougienage through the gastrostomy are effective. Retrograde string bougienage or antegrade dilations should be performed at 2- to 3-week intervals for three consecutive dilations. Optimal caliber bougienage is 48 to 50 for adults and 34 to 36 for children. The circumferential burn is associated with a high incidence of stricture formation that is usually unresponsive to steroids but amenable to dilation. Injection of the stricture with triamcinolone (30 mg/ml) also may be effective. Failure of the stricture to resolve with any of the above-mentioned measures after a maximum of 12 months requires esophageal replacement. Malignant degeneration is possible at the area of the stricture but it takes 40 or more years to manifest. Frequent surveillance for squamous cell carcinoma of the esophagus is warranted if the stricture appears to respond to dilations beyond the 1-year interval.

Operative intervention should begin with direct visualization of the distal esophagus and the entire stomach via the abdomen if there is pneumoperitoneum or signs of peritonitis. Isolated mediastinal air can be managed with direct inspection of the thorax, open débridement of necrotic tissue, and drainage of the mediastinum. A combined approach (chest and abdomen) is occasionally necessary; laparoscopy can be used. Removal of the entire esophagus is possible through a transhiatal approach followed by a cervical esophagostomy. Evidence of stomach necrosis (black eschar or submucosal vessel thrombosis) mandates a total gastrectomy, cervical esophagostomy, and jejunal feeding tube. Isolated stomach injury is uncommon, and if gastric necrosis is found, a thorough transhiatal look at the esophagus is necessary.

The possibility of the need for esophageal replacement usually is considered after 1 year of dilations, stricture injections, and antacid therapy. Options for esophageal replacement include reverse gastric tube, gastric pull-up, and colon or jejunal interposition. For the colon interposition, options include retrosternal isoperistaltic right colon based on the middle colic artery or use of the left colon, vascularized by the left colic artery. All types of replacements are roughly equivalent in technical difficulty and outcome. Most centers today use the gastric pull-up or colon interposition, however. Retrosternal or native esophageal bed position of the replacement is surgeon dependent. Microvascularized free jejunal grafts can be used for repairing residual defects. Short-term complications of replacement include leak, devascularization, and stricture formation. Long-term complications depend on the type of replacement. Stomach conduits have the problem of continued gastric acid secretion and the possibility of reflux (acid or alkaline bile) and

dysplasia. The colon and the jejunum can become redundant and require revision. Overall, there is no real optimal substitute for native esophagus. At all costs, therapy should attempt to save the patient's esophagus.

SUGGESTED READING

Anderson KD, et al: A controlled trial of corticosteroids in children with corrosive injury of the esophagus, *N Engl J Med* 323:367, 1990.

De Jong AL, et al: Corrosive esophagitis in children: a 30-year review, *Int J Pediatr Otorhinolaryngol* 57:203, 2001.

Hugh TB, Kelly MD: Corrosive ingestion and the surgeon, *J Am Coll Surg* 189:508, 1999.

Karnak I, et al: Esophageal perforations encountered during the dilation of caustic esophageal strictures, *J Cardiovasc Surg (Torino)* 39:373, 1998.

Trowers E, et al: Chemical and radiation-induced esophageal injury, *Gastroenterol Clin N Am* 4:657, 1994.

HIATAL HERNIA AND ESOPHAGEAL REFLUX IN THE PEDIATRIC PATIENT

David A. Lanning
Charles E. Bagwell

Normal gastroesophageal function is a complex process of events coordinated in the esophagus, stomach, and duodenum. Continued research has improved understanding of the physiology of this process and the pathophysiology of gastroesophageal reflux disease (GERD) and has identified the patients who will most likely benefit from a gastric fundoplication procedure. With more long-term data and outcomes analysis demonstrating excellent results from operative treatment for GERD, surgical intervention is being instituted more often and earlier, especially in patients who do not respond favorably to medical therapy. Gastric fundoplication is the third most common operation performed by pediatric surgeons.

■ CLINICAL PRESENTATION

During the first several months of life, infants' lower esophageal sphincters are physiologically incompetent, and

emesis ("spitting up") of small amounts of feeds is common. However, severe gastroesophageal reflux (GER) can have a number of pathologic gastrointestinal and respiratory manifestations (Table 1). Failure to thrive is one of the more common effects of recurrent vomiting and, when severe, caloric deprivation can develop, as well as severe dental decay or chronic laryngeal inflammation in the older child. Furthermore, the effects of chronic exposure to gastric acid in the esophagus can result in esophagitis, Barrett's esophagus, or esophageal stricture. Diagnosis of esophagitis generally requires biopsy confirmation because ulceration may not be visible endoscopically in children with this process, even in severe cases.

Repeated emesis with periodic aspiration can also lead to pulmonary disorders, including recurrent pneumonia, bronchitis, and bronchiectasis. Also, multiple studies have shown that vagal reflexes triggered from small amounts of acid reflux into the mid or upper esophagus may produce laryngospasm and/or bronchospasm. This may explain the

---

Table 1 Gastrointestinal and Respiratory Manifestations of GERD

1. Failure to thrive
2. Severe and chronic emesis
3. Malnutrition
4. Esophageal stricture
5. Apneic or asthmatic episodes
6. Chronic stridor
7. Sudden infant death syndrome
8. Recurrent pneumonia, bronchitis, and bronchiectasis

increased incidence of asthma in patients with GERD, as well as the reduced frequency of asthma symptoms after antireflux surgery. Reflux-induced laryngospasm may also be responsible for obstructive apnea, recurrent stridor, acute hypoxia, and even sudden infant death syndrome.

Many patients with central nervous system disorders such as mental retardation, brain injury, cerebral palsy, and Down's syndrome have GERD. Whether the reflux is due to chronic supine positioning, abdominal spasticity, diaphragmatic flaccidity, scoliosis, or a neurologic motility disorder remains unclear, but the degree of reflux generally correlates with the severity of the central nervous system deficit. Cystic fibrosis is also associated with an increased incidence of GERD, possibly secondary to chest physiotherapy, postural drainage, or esophageal dysfunction. GERD may also play a role in patients with chronic laryngitis and otitis media.

■ DIAGNOSIS

There are a variety of diagnostic tests available to diagnose GERD, including barium esophagography, 24-hour pH monitoring, and esophagogastric scintigraphy. The diagnostic modality used can vary according to the physician's preference and the patient's presentation. Diagnostic work-up for GERD should be undertaken if a patient presents with episodic, forceful vomiting; symptoms after age 6 months; prior treatment with acid-reducing or prokinetic medications; or evidence of pathologic reflux (see Table 1).

An upper gastrointestinal study is a moderately sensitive test that can also document an unsuspected congenital or anatomic lesion, such as a gastric (or duodenal) web, stenosis, or malrotation. The false-positive rate with this study can be reduced by assessing the number of reflux episodes after instilling an amount of contrast (in the mouth or stomach) similar to a normal feeding. The upper gastrointestinal study may also identify motility disorders (such as those seen after repair of esophageal atresia) and provide information on gastric emptying.

Intraesophageal pH monitoring (generally 12 to 24 hours) is the most sensitive and specific test for diagnosing GERD and provides precise quantification of esophageal exposure to gastric juice. In addition, one can assess ability of the esophagus to clear refluxed acid as well as to correlate reflux episodes to the patient's symptoms. Data are compiled using several parameters to generate a reflux "profile," which can be analyzed by a computer program to determine severity of the disease based on variance from normal values of spontaneous reflux at various ages. Despite technical improvements in performing intraesophageal pH monitoring that have resulted in less patient discomfort, this technique has not gained general acceptance.

While having a lower sensitivity and specificity for the detection of reflux than pH monitoring, technetium 99m sulfur colloid scan also allows quantification of gastric emptying. This information may be critical to determine which patients require a gastric emptying procedure in addition to fundoplication. This study uses a "mixed meal" to assess emptying rates for both liquids and solids. Normally, 70% of a test meal leaves the stomach within 1 hour of oral feeding.

Those that retain greater than 50% of a radiolabeled meal after 90 minutes in the absence of mechanical obstruction are considered to have delayed gastric emptying.

Esophageal manometry is accurate for determining lower esophageal sphincter pressure and the potential for reflux, but it is not often used for diagnosing reflux in children. However, the test may be helpful in identifying patients with esophageal dysmotility states such as achalasia. Such patients generally do not do well with fundoplication alone and may benefit from motility-stimulating agents or other surgical intervention (myotomy) in addition to fundoplication.

■ INDICATIONS FOR SURGERY

Patients with history of an acute life-threatening event and reflux should be monitored in a hospital setting until they can undergo an antireflux procedure. Patients with other conditions that are unlikely to respond to medical treatment, such as esophageal stricture or Barrett's esophagus, or children with symptoms from a demonstrated hiatal hernia should also be offered an antireflux procedure. Neurologically impaired (NI) patients referred for gastrostomy (for feeding alone) may not require an extensive workup beyond an upper gastrointestinal series and gastric emptying studies; the majority of patients benefit from fundoplication with or without pyloroplasty (depending on gastric emptying study results). Medical therapy for GERD is generally undertaken initially for patients with non–life-threatening gastrointestinal or pulmonary symptoms such as failure to thrive, esophagitis, asthma, or pneumonia. Treatment includes smaller but more frequent meals and prone positioning with elevation of the head of the crib; some advocate thickening of feeds with cereal. Children for whom conservative measures fail may also be placed on antacids, H_2 blockers, and/or prokinetic agents. However, after a trial period of 6 to 8 weeks, the effectiveness of conservative and medical treatment should be reevaluated; generally surgery is recommended if symptoms persist. For patients with esophagitis, a similar trial of medical treatment may be initiated, but surgical therapy is recommended for those who do not demonstrate histologic improvement on repeat biopsy. The decision for surgical intervention is often difficult and may require repeated evaluation of the patient's clinical course and discussions with the child's primary pediatrician and family.

■ SURGICAL TREATMENT

Patients considered for an antireflux procedure should be studied with an upper gastrointestinal series to rule out esophageal stricture, assess gastric/duodenal anatomy, and assess gastric motility and emptying. Any question of abnormal gastric motility should be quantified by technetium scan, and a pyloroplasty considered if more than 50% of the radiolabeled material remains in the stomach at 90 minutes. Increasing the high-pressure zone in the lower esophagus and the length of abdominal esophagus, as well as accentuating the angle of His, involves major objectives of surgical treatment.

The fundoplication should prevent reflux of gastric juice into the esophagus yet allow for normal swallowing. Although the ability to "burp" gas from the stomach is desired, it is difficult to construct a wrap that allows this to occur in a predictable fashion. Also, the surgical repair should minimize the risk of paraesophageal hernia and not significantly slow esophageal, gastric, or intestinal motility.

The standard surgical treatment for GERD with which all techniques are compared is the Nissen fundoplication. The 360-degree posterior fundic wrap has a number of subtle variations, but the principles are the same. The approach can be transabdominal or through the left chest. Most are performed through an upper midline incision, reserving the thoracic approach to patients with a tight stricture or severe esophageal shortening or for complex operations, including those on patients with severe kyphoscoliosis. After the left triangular ligament is taken down and the left lobe of the liver is retracted to the right, the phrenoesophageal ligament is divided and a right angle is used to encircle the esophagus, taking care not to injure the esophageal wall or vagus nerves. A Penrose drain is placed around the esophagus for traction, allowing the distal thoracic esophagus to be freed up into the mediastinum. The crura are then reapproximated with interrupted silk sutures. The short gastric vessels are ligated with silk ties to obtain a redundant portion of fundus that can be easily passed behind the esophagus to form a "floppy" wrap. With an esophageal bougie in place, the edges of the wrap are approximated using silk sutures to include a portion of the underlying esophageal muscularis, which lessens the frequency of a "slipped" wrap postoperatively. The superior edge of the wrap is secured to the diaphragm as another step to avoid the "slipped" wrap. Most patients have a gastrostomy tube placed in the anterior wall of the stomach using a Stamm technique of double concentric purse-string sutures. A gastrostomy tube is brought out through the left upper quadrant of the abdominal wall, and the stomach is secured to the parietal peritoneum and fascia with interrupted sutures. A standard Heineke-Mikulicz pyloroplasty may be constructed in patients with delayed gastric emptying. Also, an appendectomy is generally performed, especially in NI patients.

A multicenter, retrospective review of 7,467 patients who underwent surgical treatment for GERD demonstrated good to excellent results in 95% of neurologically normal (NN) and 85% of NI patients. Sixty-four percent of the patients underwent a standard Nissen fundoplication, 34% a Thal fundoplication, and fewer than 2% received a Toupet fundoplication, with similar reoperative and complication rates. Major complications occurred in 4.2% of NN and 12.8% of NI patients, including recurrent reflux secondary to wrap disruption (7.1%), respiratory events (4.4%), gas bloat syndrome (3.6%), and intestinal obstruction (2.6%). The reoperative rate was 3.6% in NN and 11.8% of NI patients. The authors concluded that surgery should be recommended for patients with persistently symptomatic GERD after receiving maximal medical therapy. The Nissen and Thal fundoplications have similar results and are both effective techniques. Similar to previous studies, the authors demonstrated that NI patients have lower success rates and higher complication rates than NN children, but the majority still benefit from operative treatment.

An alternative procedure to a Nissen fundoplication is the modified Thal anterior fundoplication. This technique is characterized by reconstruction of the angle of His using an anterior fundoplication consisting of a 180-degree wrap. Initially, the distal esophagus is circumferentially mobilized and the posterior crural defect is reapproximated. With an esophageal dilator in place, the upper gastric cardia is sutured to the anterior two thirds of the esophagus and diaphragm at the level of the hiatus. One reported benefit is that more patients are able to burp in the postoperative period; in addition, this technique is useful in patients with a large liver, a short esophagus, or a tiny stomach (i.e., those with pure esophageal atresia) and in patients who undergo an extended myotomy for achalasia. Bliss et al retrospectively reviewed 46 patients who had undergone a Thal fundoplication. Of the 22 patients who consented to follow-up evaluation, 83% were clinically asymptomatic at 2 years and 66% were reflux free on physiologic testing. Despite the low number of patients in this study, these results concur with those presented in the multicenter study of Fonkalsrud et al and suggest that the Thal procedure compares favorably with the Nissen fundoplication.

The Toupet is a third antireflux procedure advocated by some pediatric surgeons; its distinction is the creation of a valve from the gastric fundus passed behind the esophagus. Once the distal esophagus is mobilized and the crura are reopposed, a large bougie is placed in the esophagus, and the gastric fundus is brought behind the esophagus and sutured to the right crus. A second row of sutures is placed on the right between the fundus and the esophagus with a final row of sutures placed on the left side between fundus and esophagus. As a result, the fundus encircles the esophagus approximately 270 degrees to create an obturator effect at the hiatus. Bensoussan reported on 112 patients with medically refractory GERD over a 10-year period who underwent a Toupet partial fundoplication. The mean follow-up period for 95 of the patients was 3.5 years for NI children and 4.9 for NN children. Although 6 patients had temporary dysphagia and 2 with food impaction, more than 90% of patients were free of symptoms. The authors concluded that the Toupet partial posterior fundoplication is as easy to perform and equally effective as the Nissen wrap. In addition, the ability to belch is retained, postoperative dysphagia is less common, and gas bloat syndrome is avoided. However, although the procedure is associated with a significant number of early complications (24% in NI patients and 18% in NN patients), the long-term outcome of the Toupet antireflux procedure was excellent in 90% of patients.

Laparoscopic Nissen fundoplication is another surgical option to treat GERD. Although multiple studies have shown comparable long-term outcome and earlier recovery than with open fundoplication in adults, the data for children are less clear. In a 4-year series, Rothenberg evaluated laparoscopic Nissen fundoplication in 220 consecutive patients. With only 18 patients lost to follow-up after the first year, there were 7 patients with recurrence of their reflux symptoms and documented breakdown of their fundoplication or development of a hiatal hernia. However, all 7 underwent a successful second laparoscopic repair (with 2 receiving a pyloroplasty). Two of the three late failures were thought to result from the development of large hiatal hernias. The intraoperative and postoperative complication rates were 2.6% and 7.3%, respectively, and the average time to discharge was 1.6 days. The operative time in the last 30 cases was considerably shorter than at the beginning of the experience (average of 55 minutes compared with 109 minutes in the first 30 cases). The author concludes that despite a steep learning curve, laparoscopic Nissen fundoplication has clinical results comparable to the open approach with significantly less morbidity and a shorter period of hospitalization.

In a retrospective review, Levy et al compared 171 pediatric patients with Nissen fundoplication to 236 patients with a modified Rossetti fundoplication, an open procedure characterized by liver retraction without mobilization, no crural repair, no ligation of short gastric vessels, and a 2-cm floppy fundic wrap. The incidence of dysphagia, postoperative hiatal hernia, need for esophageal dilation, revision of fundoplication, time to discharge, and operative time were reviewed. There was no difference in any of these parameters between the techniques; however, the mean operative time and the incidence of recurrent reflux were lower in the modified Rossetti group compared with the Nissen group. The authors concluded that the modified Rossetti fundoplication requires less operative time, has a low complication rate, and is their procedure of choice for patients who require an open fundoplication for treatment of gastroesophageal reflux.

Cameron et al reviewed 79 patients over a 5-year period who underwent an uncut Collis-Nissen fundoplication for the select group of patients with shortened esophagus from chronic esophagitis. After esophageal mobilization and division of short gastrics, the intraabdominal esophagus is lengthened by stapling parallel to the lesser curve with an esophageal bougie in place. The crura are closed followed by a 360-degree posterior wrap. The anterior stomach is then sutured to the lesser curve to cover the staple line and the wrap

is secured to the diaphragm and crura. Despite 77% of the patients being NI, the authors demonstrated a 97% control rate for GERD with a median follow-up of 1.8 years. Only 2 of the children had documented recurrent GERD and only 1 required repeat fundoplication. Postoperative complications were noted in 26% (minor 23%, major 3%) with one postoperative mortality. The authors conclude that the uncut Collis-Nissen fundoplication has acceptable morbidity and mortality in this select population and should be considered in children with neurologic impairment or chronic lung disease.

■ CONCLUSIONS

Operative treatment for GERD provides excellent results with minimal morbidity and mortality. Future studies will further delineate which procedure is optimal for a given patient based on their anatomy, physiology, and clinical presentation. Finally, further investigation will also determine the role of more minimally invasive procedures in the treatment of pediatric patients with GERD.

SUGGESTED READING

Bagwell CE: Gastroesophageal reflux in children. In Nyhus LM, editor: *Surgery annual*, Norwalk, CT, 1995, Appleton & Lange, p 133.

Fonkalsrud EW and Ament ME: Gastroesophageal reflux in childhood, *Curr Probl Surg* 31:1, 1996.

Fonkalsrud EW, et al: Surgical treatment of gastroesophageal reflux in children: a combined hospital study of 7467 patients, *Pediatrics* 101:419, 1998.

Johnson DG: The past and present of antireflux surgery in children, *Am J Surg* 180:377, 2000.

CYSTIC FIBROSIS

Peter J. Mogayzel, Jr.

Cystic fibrosis (CF) is the most common life-shortening autosomal recessive disorder in whites, affecting approximately 1 in 3200 live births. CF is a multisystem disease that affects the lungs, sinuses, gastrointestinal tract, pancreas, hepatobiliary system, sweat glands, and reproductive tract. The production of sputum with abnormal viscoelastic properties leads to airway obstruction, bacterial infections and subsequent bronchiectasis, chronic obstructive pulmonary

disease, and eventually respiratory failure. However, there is a wide phenotypic spectrum of disease presentation and severity.

Advances in medical therapies have led to a substantial improvement in survival for patients with CF. Today most patients live into adulthood with an excellent quality of life (Figure 1). However, many patients experience pulmonary complications that potentially require surgical intervention. The approach to pulmonary disease in CF is constantly changing, and the advent of successful lung transplantation has altered traditional approaches to surgical treatments of CF pulmonary complications.

■ PATHOPHYSIOLOGY

CF is caused by mutations in the cystic fibrosis transmembrane conductance regulator gene *(CFTR)*. *CFTR* functions as a

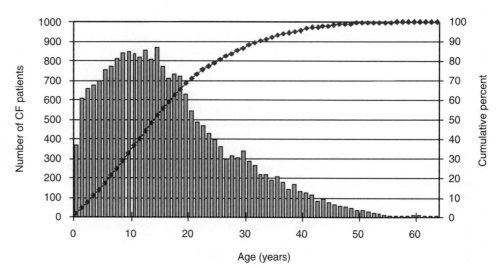

Figure 1
Age distribution of the CF patient population in the United States. (Data from the *1999 Cystic Fibrosis Foundation patient registry annual data report.*)

chloride channel on the apical surface of epithelial cells in several tissues, including the lung. Affected cells also have defects in sodium, bicarbonate, and water transport, leading to the production of highly viscous secretions that are difficult to clear from the airway. Over time, the airways of patients with CF become colonized with various types of bacteria. The presence of these organisms and the resulting purulent sputum leads to a cycle of bacterial overgrowth, inflammation, and lung damage. Also over time, parenchymal lung destruction occurs, leading to bronchiectasis, obstructive lung disease, and respiratory failure.

The onset of lung disease in patients with CF is variable. Lung growth and development in utero are thought to be normal. Lung damage in patients with CF has traditionally been ascribed to chronic infections and subsequent neutrophil-mediated inflammatory response. Recent studies have demonstrated inflammatory cytokines in the lungs of infants with CF before acquiring any bacterial pathogens. These and other findings suggest that patients with CF have a proinflammatory milieu in their lungs predisposing to lung damage.

Bacterial colonization in the airways of patients with CF becomes increasingly common over time. *Haemophilus influenzae* and *Staphylococcus aureus* are frequently found in the sputum of children with CF, and eventually about 80% of patients become colonized with *Pseudomonas aeruginosa.* Other potential pathogens, including *Stenotrophomonas maltophilia, Burkholderia cepacia,* and *Aspergillus* species, are commonly found in the sputum of patients with CF. Overgrowth of bacteria leads to "CF or pulmonary exacerbations" characterized by increased coughing, dyspnea, fatigue, weight loss, and occasionally fevers. These symptoms can arise acutely or can develop subtly over an extended period of time. Pulmonary exacerbations are treated with oral or intravenous antibiotics.

Ultimately, patients with CF develop bronchiectasis, and the frequency of pulmonary exacerbations increases as pulmonary function declines. Patients with advanced CF lung disease can develop several pulmonary complications, including pneumothorax, hemoptysis, and infections with bacteria, that are resistant to multiple antibiotics.

■ MEDICAL THERAPY

The mainstay of therapy for CF has been nutritional support with pancreatic enzyme replacement therapy, chest physiotherapy to clear airway secretions, and antibiotics to treat pulmonary infections. The use of the mucolytic agent recombinant human deoxyribonuclease I (rhDNase), inhaled antibiotics, and devices to aid in chest physiotherapy have become widespread. Additionally, patients with CF require treatment for multiple nonpulmonary problems, including malabsorption due to pancreatic insufficiency, distal intestinal obstruction syndrome, sinus disease, diabetes, osteoporosis, and infertility.

■ SURGICAL CONSIDERATIONS

As the pulmonary function of patients with CF declines, they develop more pulmonary complications that may require surgical intervention. Traditional approaches to the problems of severe bronchiectasis, hemoptysis, and pneumothorax are evolving due to the introduction of minimally invasive thoracic procedures and the advent of lung transplantation as a viable option for patients with end-stage CF.

■ SURGICAL RESECTION

In some patients, localized disease can be a source for recurrent infections and pulmonary exacerbations. When patients are selected appropriately, lobectomy can lead to a dramatic decline in the number and severity of pulmonary exacerbations. Resection works best for patients with one region that is clearly much more diseased than the rest of the lungs. The upper lobes are usually affected first in patients with CF and typically have more disease than the remainder of the lung. Several published reports confirm that the right upper and middle lobes are the most likely to require resection. Although lobectomy, and even pneumonectomy, has been advocated for patients with advanced lung disease, these patients are less likely to have a sustained benefit from lung resection. In these cases, lobectomy should be considered a temporizing measure that will probably not slow rapidly progressive loss of lung function.

Lobectomy can be contemplated for patients who have a localized region of bronchiectasis or atelectasis serving as a nidus of infection. Surgical resection should only be considered in patients who have not responded to aggressive medical therapy, including several extended courses of intravenous antibiotics lasting 3 to 4 weeks. Before it has been decided that medical therapy failed, patients should also be treated with rhDNase, inhaled antibiotics, and aggressive chest physiotherapy for an extended period. Flexible fiberoptic bronchoscopy can also be performed to remove mucus plugs and identify atypical organisms that have not been recovered in expectorated sputum.

Preoperative evaluation should include pulmonary function tests, thoracic computed tomography, and ventilation/perfusion scans to identify lung regions with a disproportional amount of disease. Although the upper lobes are usually the most severely affected in CF, any lobe can require resection. Lung function of patients undergoing lobectomy should be optimized before surgery; therefore, patients should be treated with intravenous antibiotics based on sputum cultures, and aggressive chest physiotherapy for an extended period before surgery.

At the time of surgery, airway secretions should be aggressively cleared by bronchoscopy after intubation to avoid intraoperative mucus plugging and to limit postoperative atelectasis. Significant bleeding can occur during lobectomy in patients with CF for a number of reasons. Bronchial artery enlargement and collateralization with pulmonary arteries create a very vascular pulmonary parenchyma. Adhesions of the visceral and parietal pleurae are common findings. In addition, patients with CF typically have very large hyperplastic peribronchial lymph nodes that can be quite vascular.

Postoperatively, patients should be extubated as quickly as possible and encouraged to perform maneuvers that improve clearance of airway secretions. Adequate pain management is essential to allow patients to perform adequate chest physiotherapy and incentive spirometry to prevent atelectasis. Placement of an epidural catheter preoperatively should be encouraged. Antibiotics should be continued postoperatively for a total of 2 to 3 weeks.

Improvement in postoperative pulmonary function testing is a good prognostic indicator that suggests a sustained improvement in lung function is likely. However, changes in pulmonary function testing after lobectomy can be quite variable. Lobectomy may not influence gas exchange because the resected tissue was not involved in gas exchange. Ultimately, the goal of surgery is to decrease infections, thereby preventing parenchymal damage and slowing the inevitable loss of lung function.

■ PNEUMOTHORAX

Pneumothorax is a poor prognostic indicator in CF. Approximately 1.5% of adult patients have a pneumothorax requiring a chest tube each year. Traditionally, the high likelihood of recurrence has led many centers to advocate early pleurodesis in the management of pneumothorax. However, pleurodesis typically leads to dense pleural adhesions that complicate lung transplantation. Therefore, a more conservative approach is now advocated in the management of pneumothorax. Chest tube drainage with a small-bore catheter with expectant management is recommended for patients experiencing an initial pneumothorax. Pleural adhesions usually prevent complete collapse of the lung in these patients, and chest tube drainage successfully treats an initial pneumothorax in a majority of patients.

Management of patients with a persistent air leak or recurrent pneumothoraces is more problematic. Pleurodesis via the instillation of doxycycline, quinacrine, or talc has been used effectively to treat pneumothorax in patients with CF for some time. Instillation of sclerosing agents has two advantages: it can be performed without surgical intervention and critically ill patients can be managed without general anesthesia. However, there are significant disadvantages to this approach, including the formation of lung adhesions to the parietal pleura, affecting diaphragm function and potentially complicating or even excluding transplantation. These issues have encouraged most centers to pursue a more directed approach to pneumothorax management. Thoracoscopy with resection or laser ablation of blebs and local pleural abrasion leads to the resolution of almost all pneumothoraces. Some authors have also advocated a local application of talc poudrage by thoracoscopy. These procedures should minimize pleural adhesions in anticipation of lung transplantation. Thoracotomy with surgical pleurodesis, partial pleurectomy, oversewing, or stapling of subpleural blebs should be reserved for the most severe cases. If lung transplantation is considered, talc pleurodesis and pleurectomy should be avoided.

■ MASSIVE HEMOPTYSIS

Hemoptysis is a common problem for patients with advanced CF lung disease. Many patients produce blood-streaked sputum on a regular basis. Bleeding arises from enlarged and tortuous bronchial arteries and can be eroded by bacterial overgrowth. Massive hemoptysis occurs in 1% to 2% of adults with CF and can be life-threatening. Massive hemoptysis is often defined as expectoration of more than 240 ml of blood within 24 hours, or recurrent bleeding of more than 100 ml of blood/day for several days over a short period of time. Initial evaluation should include physical examination, chest radiograph, complete blood count with platelet count, prothrombin time, and partial thromboplastin time.

Hemoptysis usually responds to medical therapy, including intravenous antibiotics and discontinuation of rhDNase and nonsteroidal antiinflammatory agents. However, massive or recurrent hemoptysis often requires bronchial artery embolization. If possible, localizing the source of bleeding before angiography is preferable. Chest radiographs and physical examination are occasionally helpful in localizing the source of bleeding. Patients sometimes have a warm or bubbling sensation that localizes the involved region. However, bronchoscopy is the best method of identifying a site of active bleeding and should be performed once the hemoptysis has improved, but while the patient is still bleeding.

Hemoptysis often arises from more than one vessel, necessitating embolization of all the vessels supplying the affected area. Recurrent hemoptysis is not uncommon, and it can be difficult to treat because each episode may be due to bleeding from a different region. Small vessels are difficult to embolize, and recently formed arteriovenous communications may also complicate treatment. Recently, several case reports have described the successful use of oral tranexamic acid to treat recurrent hemoptysis.

Life-threatening hemoptysis is rare. Before embolization, bronchoscopy can be used to tamponade the airway with a balloon catheter or gel foam pledgets. To prevent asphyxiation in life-threatening episodes of hemoptysis, selective or double-lumen intubation can be performed. Iced saline lavage or topical therapy with α-adrenergic receptor agonists or thrombin and intravenous vasopressin has also been used successfully to control hemorrhage. Lung resection may be necessary in cases of uncontrollable or recurrent hemoptysis that is unresponsive to embolization.

■ LUNG TRANSPLANTATION

Respiratory failure is the predominant cause of death in patients with CF. As lung transplantation has evolved over the past decade, it has become an option for many children and adults with end-stage CF. To avoid potentially catastrophic infections, both lungs need to be replaced with or without concomitant heart transplantation. In the United States, bilateral, sequential lung transplantation is the preferred operation; however, many European centers do the "domino" procedure, and perform heart-lung transplants in patients with CF. A limited number of centers have performed simultaneous lung and liver transplants to treat both CF pulmonary and liver disease.

Patient selection and the timing of referral are vitally important in achieving good transplant outcomes. Because priority is not given to sicker patients on the lung transplant waiting list, referral timing is an important issue. Unfortunately, mortality in CF cannot be predicted unequivocally by objective testing. Traditionally, a forced expiratory volume in 1 second (FEV_1) of less than 30% of predicted has been used as a guide for transplant referral because it is associated with a 2-year survival rate of about 50%. However, it is clear that the rate of decline in pulmonary function is also an important prognostic indicator of mortality, and should be taken into account when evaluating patients for transplantation. For example, relatively stable patients can develop a rapid decline in pulmonary function during adolescence that may be a harbinger of early mortality.

The difficulty in predicting mortality and obtaining suitable organs has led to the development of living donor lobar transplantation (LDLT). This technique uses the lower lobes from two adult donors to replace the lungs of a child or small adult. Although this technique was developed for patients who most likely would not survive to transplantation due to the severity of their disease, LDLT has been advocated by some centers as a primary therapy for patients who are less ill.

Evaluation for lung transplantation is similar for patients with and without CF (see "Lung Transplantation"). Important relative contraindications to transplantation for patients with CF include malnutrition, liver disease, previous thoracic procedures (lobectomy, severe pleural symphysis), uncontrolled diabetes, osteoporosis, poor compliance with previous medical therapy, and colonization with resistant organisms, particularly *B. cepacia*. The upper airway and residual tracheobronchial tree serve as potential reservoirs for postoperative infections. For this reason, some centers advocate aggressive treatment of potential sinus disease in transplant candidates with endoscopic surgery and antibiotic irrigation. Preoperative sputum colonization can also influence postoperative infections. For example, *Aspergillus* infections are more common in patients with CF who are colonized with this organism. Patients colonized with *B. cepacia* have increased mortality rates within the immediate postoperative period due to infectious complications and poorer longterm survival. However, recent studies suggest that this increased mortality may be limited to those patients who are colonized with *B. cepacia* genomovar III.

Adults with CF typically do not have more complications after transplantation than do other recipients. However, children with CF have been shown to have more episodes of rejection and a higher rate of posttransplant lymphoproliferative disease than children with other diagnoses. In 2002, 171 bilateral lung transplants were performed in adults with CF in the United States according to the United Organization for Organ Sharing (UNOS). The survival rates at 1 and 5 years after transplantation for patients with CF are 83% and 51%, respectively. Overall, patients with CF have survival that is as good as, or better than, lung transplant recipients with other diseases.

■ SUMMARY

The treatment of pulmonary complications in patients with CF is constantly changing. The advent of lung transplantation as a viable option for patients with end-stage CF and the introduction of minimally invasive thoracic procedures have altered traditional approaches to the problems of bronchiectasis, hemoptysis, and pneumothorax. Lung transplantation has given many patients with end-stage CF hope for not only a longer life, but also a better quality of life. However, successful lung transplantation can be achieved only through the timely evaluation of appropriate patients.

SUGGESTED READING

Schidlow DV, et al: Cystic Fibrosis Foundation consensus conference report on pulmonary complications of cystic fibrosis, *Pediatr Pulmonol* 15:187, 1993.

Mendeloff EN, et al: Pediatric and adult lung transplantation for cystic fibrosis, *J Thorac Cardiovasc Surg* 115:404, 1998; discussion 413, 1998.

Yankaskas JR, Mallory GB Jr. Lung transplantation in cystic fibrosis: consensus conference statement, *Chest* 113:217, 1998.

CONGENITAL PULMONARY DISORDERS

Anne C. Fischer

Congenital lung malformations represent a diverse spectrum of developmental defects. A high index of suspicion for these relatively rare malformations is essential in evaluating a thoracic lesion in a child. Congenital lung malformations have variable clinical presentations, may involve other associated congenital anomalies, and may present early in infancy with respiratory distress or remain asymptomatic until adolescence or adulthood (Table 1). The revolution in prenatal imaging has enabled earlier detection of pulmonary anomalies. Prenatal characteristics, such as the echogenicity of lung parenchyma, cystic components, and associated physiologic features such as hydrops and intrathoracic mass effects, accurately identify a fetal lung lesion. Definitive diagnosis may be elusive, however, because the spectrum of these characteristics may overlap. Prenatal imaging has led to a greater understanding of the natural history and the underlying pathophysiology of these lesions. These advances have been quintessential in defining criteria for early therapeutic intervention in lesions adversely affecting fetal development as opposed to expectant management with postnatal resection in most cases.

Identifying the developmental defects of these malformations requires a brief review of normal lung development. A highly orchestrated interaction occurs during development between the endoderm of the foregut and the invaginated mesenchyme. The primitive foregut is the anlage of pulmonary and gastrointestinal systems, which clarifies a persistent connection in some anomalies. Lung development is initiated at 3 weeks' gestation during the *embryonic* stage, when the tracheal diverticulum diverges from the primitive foregut. Maturation of the conducting airways from trachea to terminal bronchioles is completed by the end of the *pseudoglandular* stage (16 weeks' gestation). The development of the gas exchange system, a highly differentiated respiratory unit, occurs in the remaining 24 weeks *in utero* during the *canalicular* and *terminal sac* stages to add the respiratory bronchioles and alveoli to the pulmonary matrix. The final 4 weeks represent an exponential increase in the lung's surface area through alveolar growth, which continues postnatally until 8 years of age.

■ BRONCHOGENIC CYSTS

Bronchogenic cysts arise from abnormal budding of the tracheobronchial tree to form a cystic mass of nonfunctioning tissue. The cysts are lined with bronchial epithelium and mucous glands. Their anatomic location correlates with their time of appearance in development. Two thirds of these cysts separate early in development and are mediastinal, centrally located, and attached firmly to the trachea and carina. These solitary cysts are well-encapsulated spherical lesions, filled with fluid from the entrapped mucus-secreting cells. The cysts remain asymptomatic until superimposing infection occurs. In comparison, peripheral cysts occur later in development, are typically multiple, and are located in the periphery of the lower lobes. Because they occur during rapid bronchial division, a bronchial communication is more common and may contain an air-fluid level in the presence of a residual communication to the tracheobronchial tree. Rapid enlargement of the cyst leading to a pneumothorax can occur, especially in the setting of a large coexistent bronchial communication.

Mediastinal and peripheral types present usually as asymptomatic lesions, unless the cyst enlarges causing respiratory compromise in the neonate or until secondary infection intercedes later in life. In the former case, the mass effect of the cyst causes compression of the airway and distal pulmonary hyperinflation, worsening the respiratory compromise. A chest radiograph is diagnostic in greater than 77% of cases. Radiographs after a respiratory exacerbation in an infant need to be obtained sequentially to detect a subtle underlying bronchogenic cyst. Routine thin-section computed tomography with contrast material to delineate

Table 1 Characteristics of Congenital Malformations

TYPE	TYPICAL PRESENTATION	COMMUNICATION TO TRACHEOBRONCHIAL TREE	ASSOCIATED ANOMALIES
Bronchogenic Cyst	Asymptomatic*		−
Mediastinal Cyst	Asymptomatic central cyst	+/−	
Peripheral Pulmonary Cyst	Respiratory distress in infants	+	
CCAM	Antenatally diagnosed	+	20% Anomalies Overall
I (50%)	Asymptomatic		−
II (42%)	Symptomatic in newborn		Majority of Anomalies
III (3%)	Symptomatic in newborn		−
CLE	Majority diagnosed as neonate (LUL, RML)	+	20% Cardiac Anomalies
Pulmonary sequestration	Incidentally detected (lower lobes)	−	Anomalous systemic blood supply
Extralobar (25%)	Neonate-dyspnea or difficulty feeding	−	Potential GI tract connection
Intralobar (75%)	Later in childhood—recurrent pneumonia	−	−

*Later presentations with infection.

CCAM, congenital cystic adenomatoid malformation; CLE, congenital lobar emphysema; LUL, left upper lobe; RML, right middle lobe.

mediastinal structures is highly accurate and superior in showing these lesions. Prenatal diagnosis typically detects a simple cyst, but the differential diagnosis includes esophageal duplication cysts, a type I congenital cystic adenomatoid malformation (CCAM), and a congenital diaphragmatic hernia. Intrauterine cyst aspiration to alleviate a mediastinal shift can be performed; reaccumulation may necessitate repeated aspirations.

Regardless of location, the therapy is surgical resection; an urgent resection is indicated in the symptomatic patient. Mediastinal lesions can be enucleated thoracoscopically or via a thoracotomy. Segmental or lobar resection is curative for peripheral lesions. Asymptomatic lesions require resection because they can become acutely symptomatic or undergo malignant degeneration, as has been reported with rhabdomyosarcoma.

■ CYSTIC ADENOMATOID MALFORMATIONS

CCAMs are multicystic or mixed intrapulmonary masses from bronchiolar proliferation without alveoli. These cystic structures may interconnect and often communicate with the tracheobronchial tree. They usually are localized to one lobe with the following distribution: left lower lobe, 25%; left upper lobe, 20%; right lower lobe, 19%; and right upper lobe, 10%. Stocker subclassified CCAMs based on the cyst size and number. All lack cartilage and have a predominance of elastin. Type I malformations are the most common (>50%) and typically have a dominant large cyst (usually >2 cm). Type II malformations are multiple smaller cysts (<1 cm), occur 42% of the time, and are a mixture of cystic and adenomatous areas. There is a high incidence of associated congenital anomalies (26%), including renal dysgenesis, cardiac anomalies, imperforate anus, and congenital heart disease. Type III malformations are a solid-appearing adenomatous variant with tiny cysts (<0.5 cm). Poor prognostic indicators often are associated with type III cysts because these lesions tend to be large and capable of producing fetal hydrops and pulmonary hypoplasia.

Prenatally the presentation of a CCAM is highly variable, with detection at 12 to 14 weeks' gestation. The typical ultrasound appearance is macrocystic (type I) or echogenic (type II or III) depending on the underlying histology. Doppler ultrasonography prenatally can confirm the diagnosis and detect an anomalous blood supply consistent with a sequestration. An echogenic lung mass, such as a type III CCAM, can be confused with a congenital diaphragmatic hernia due to the heterogeneity of the mass. Fetuses with large CCAMs may be associated with severe hydrops and intrathoracic mediastinal compression causing pulmonary hypoplasia of the normal lung. Large masses may result in caval obstruction, impaired cardiac filling, and subsequently nonimmune hydrops. The presence of hydrops correlates with a higher mortality rate of greater than 65%; polyhydramnios also is associated with higher mortality. CCAMs may grow progressively or regress by unclear mechanisms; 25% resolve spontaneously (Figure 1). The potential for spontaneous involution limits a clear-cut prognosis. Treatment is dictated by the degree of the secondary effects of the CCAM. Needle aspirations are problematic with reaccumulation, whereas

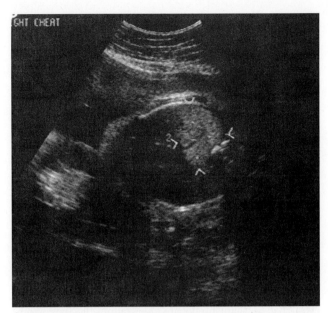

A

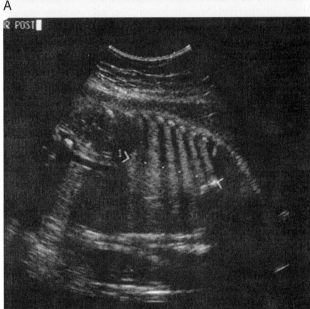

B

Figure 1
Ultrasound of thoracic mass. **A,** Transverse view. **B,** Coronal view. This congenital cystic adenomatoid malformation was visible at 18 weeks' gestation and resolved by 35 weeks' gestation.

thoracoamniotic shunts have decompressed type I cysts successfully but may migrate. Large masses causing fetal hydrops and fetal demise require *in utero* intervention to reverse the hydrops.

Postnatally the size of the lesion dictates the degree of respiratory distress. Large cysts can produce symptoms with compression of the contralateral lung. Typically, type I cysts may remain asymptomatic, discovered incidentally or when infectious complications intervene, such as recurrent pneumonias localized to the same lobe or a lung abscess.

Type II and III microcytic lesions are associated more frequently with distress in the newborn period. A radiograph or computed tomography scan can show in severe cases the hyperexpanded lung with contralateral herniation and mediastinal shift. Definitive therapy necessitates surgical resection. CCAMs have been associated with embryonal rhabdomyosarcomas and bronchoalveolar carcinoma. An elective anatomic lobectomy and a partial segmental resection are the standard options. Postoperatively, respiratory compromise may worsen acutely in neonates with coincident pulmonary hypoplasia and pulmonary hypertension, requiring extracorporeal membrane oxygenation.

■ PULMONARY SEQUESTRATION

A pulmonary sequestration is an ectopic mass of nonfunctioning lung tissue with an anomalous systemic blood supply that lacks an anatomic communication to the tracheobronchial tree. Sequestrations are classified as either intralobar or extralobar. Most are intralobar sequestrations that have anomalous intraparenchymal tissue without an investing pleura. Extralobar sequestrations have a separate visceral pleura and are extrinsic to the normal lobe. Both types have the same histology and primarily are considered vascular anomalies, reflecting the anomalous systemic blood supply. Multiple variations of systemic and pulmonary arterial supply with pulmonary venous drainage have been described. The typical blood supply is from the systemic circulation arising from the descending or abdominal aorta (75%) or other thoracic vessels (25%). Multiple theories attempt to postulate the derivation of sequestrations. Most theories propose the sequestrations as accessory lung buds developing off an anomalous aortic branch that separate due to traction on growth. Others propose that sequestrations are acquired as a postinfectious malformation; however, these sequestrations are detected congenitally without an associated inflammatory or infected component. Extralobar sequestrations are thought to occur later in gestation; any anomalous growth in the distal lung bud develops in an extrapulmonary fashion.

Most sequestrations are in the left lower lobes. Of sequestrations, 5% are located below the diaphragm, however, or are detected as an abdominal or retroperitoneal mass, called an *abdominal accessory lobe*. The systemic feeding arteries often are multiple and branch off the aorta; 15% are infradiaphragmatic. The most common type is the "Rokitansky lobe," which occurs on the left with a feeding vessel from the aorta. Sequestrations often have a patent communication with the gastrointestinal tract. Extralobar types are associated with congenital anomalies (40%), which include congenital diaphragmatic hernia, bronchial atresia, colonic duplication, pulmonary hypoplasia, absent pulmonary artery, vertebral anomalies, and esophageal communication. As a result of the associated diaphragmatic defects, radioisotope scanning of right lower lobe lesions can distinguish a herniated liver from a right lower lobe sequestration.

Typically the extralobar sequestration is asymptomatic and found incidentally due to the associated congenital anomalies. Despite no communication with the tracheobronchial tree or adjacent lung, the sequestration may become infected by hematogenous spread, causing respiratory distress.

Symptoms are primarily respiratory; however, the coincident large venous shunts to the systemic circulation create secondary cardiac manifestations. Typical venous drainage is to the systemic circulation (inferior vena cava, azygos vein, or portal vein), creating a left-to-right shunt. Large shunts potentially create high-output cardiac failure. The *scimitar syndrome* is due to anomalous venous return to the vena cava, creating a left-to-right shunt, and the venous drainage appears as a sickle-shaped shadow in the right lower lobe. Intralobar lesions remain asymptomatic until hemoptysis or recurrent infections occur. Plain radiographs show a cystic or atelectatic mass and are not diagnostically accurate. Definitive diagnosis requires documenting a systemic arterial supply by Doppler ultrasound or nuclear magnetic resonance angiography: both techniques are used more frequently than angiography, the prior gold standard. All sequestrations should be excised to avoid future complications with infection and fatal hemoptysis. Intrapulmonary lesions may require a lobectomy, whereas extrapulmonary lesions simply are excised.

■ CONGENITAL LOBAR EMPHYSEMA

Congenital lobar emphysema is a rare cause of respiratory distress and is characterized by overexpansion of a pulmonary lobe and alveolar overdistention resulting from a one-way valve of inflation. The upper lobes are involved most commonly with the following incidence: left upper lobe, 42%; right middle lobe, 35%; right upper lobe, 21%; and bilaterally, 20%. The etiology is not clear in most cases. Bronchial cartilaginous dysplasia and polyalveolar lobes are the intrinsic pathologies, shown in a quarter of cases each. Extrinsic compression can occur from an intrathoracic mass, such as a vascular or cardiac anomaly, teratoma, vascular ring, or patent ductus arteriosus. Of associated malformations, 20% are cardiac anomalies (patent ductus arteriosus, ventricular septal defect, tetralogy of Fallot). More than half are diagnosed by 1 month of age; presentation after 6 months is unusual. The presentation is moderate distress initially until the lobe gradually enlarges causing cyanosis. Severe life-threatening distress is rare but may require immediate surgical intervention and immediate thoracotomy to allow the overinflated lobe to herniate, to relieve the intrathoracic compression followed by a lobectomy. A chest radiograph is sufficient to diagnose a large emphysematous lobe with atelectasis in the ipsilateral lobe. Bronchoscopy can exacerbate the underlying pathophysiology of congenital lobar emphysema, creating a life-threatening situation. Bronchoscopy should be employed in the scenario of an inhaled foreign object or mucous plugging.

■ SUMMARY

The various congenital lung malformations are relatively unusual individually. Early diagnosis requires a familiarity with the presentations and a compulsive evaluation because the malformations are difficult to detect. Early diagnosis is amenable to an uncomplicated surgical resection, whereas a delay in diagnosis can be associated with substantial morbidity.

SUGGESTED READING

Coran AG, Drongowski R: Congenital cystic disease of the tracheobronchial tree in infants and children: experience with 44 consecutive cases, *Arch Surg* 129:521, 1994.

Hebra A, et al: Bronchopulmonary malformations. In Ashcraft KW, et al, editors: *Pediatric surgery,* Philadelphia, 2000, WB Saunders, p 273.

Kravitz RM: Congenital malformations of the lung, *Pediatr Clin North Am* 41:453, 1994.

Nuchtern JG, Harberg FJ: Congenital lung cysts, *Semin Pediatr Surg* 3:233, 1994.

Puvabanditsin S, et al: Congenital lobar emphysema, *J Cardiovasc Surg* 41:953, 2000.

PEDIATRIC TRACHEAL DISORDERS

Thom E Lobe

Tracheal problems in children encompass a wide variety of conditions, including congenital obstructing lesions, tumors, trauma, tracheomalacia, and congenital tracheal stenosis.

■ UPPER AIRWAY

Laryngeal lesions include atresia, webs, laryngomalacia, redundant mucosal folds, cysts, subglottic stenosis, and vocal cord paralysis. Other common examples of obstructing lesions of the upper airway include intraglossal enteric cysts, cervical cystic hygroma, subglottic cysts, duplications, and glottic webs. Symptoms include prolonged expiration, voice alterations, and stridor, and the diagnosis can be made best by endoscopy. Emergency treatment may require cricothyroidotomy or tracheostomy, but definitive therapy for these conditions is usually delayed.

Laryngotracheal/esophageal clefts present with intermittent symptoms, usually a hoarse or whispered cry. Endoscopy is essential for accurate diagnosis, and intubation of the bronchi may be required to sustain the patient until a definitive procedure is performed.

A "pig bronchus" to the right upper lobe (bronchial take-off from the distal trachea) often is associated with other congenital anomalies and presents with chronic atelectasis, recurrent infections, bronchiectasis, or cyst formation. Resection rarely is required in the presence of obstruction or chronic infection.

The hallmark of tracheal agenesis is when an infant can be ventilated satisfactorily using a bag and mask but not using endotracheal tube intubation, when it is impossible to intubate the infant, or when the esophagus repeatedly gets intubated.

This diagnosis is based on a high index of suspicion. Bronchoscopy is usually necessary and should be performed in the operating room with the intention of carrying out the transesophageal intubation. Most of these cases are associated with a variety of lethal anomalies.

Vascular rings also are associated with tracheal abnormalities. These infants usually present with noisy breathing, and about half present with recurrent infections. Of patients, 20% have what is labeled a "dying spell," 14% present with dysphagia or cough or both, 11% have failure to thrive, and approximately 6% present with aspiration. In most cases, an accurate diagnosis can be made with a barium swallow that can be supplemented with bronchoscopy if necessary. Arteriography rarely is necessary. One of the less common vascular rings, the pulmonary artery sling, usually presents with a high degree of tracheal or bronchial stenosis. This lesion has a characteristic appearance on bronchoscopy, on which the trachea appears flattened in the anterior-posterior diameter. Vascular rings require a high degree of suspicion to make the diagnosis, after which all these lesions can be addressed using either open or thoracoscopic techniques.

■ TUMORS

Common tumors of the larynx and upper trachea include neurofibromatosis and vascular lesions such as hemangiomas and lymphangiomas. True tumors of the tracheobronchial tree are infrequent in children and are rarely malignant. Tumors of the trachea usually present with wheezing, stridor, or cough and only occasionally present with hemoptysis or pneumonia. Benign tumors more often present in the cervical trachea, whereas the opposite is true of malignant tumors. Complete resection usually is indicated, and only rarely is a lesser procedure appropriate.

■ TRAUMA

Although tracheal trauma is rare in children, it can be dramatic in its presentation. Often, there are visible contusions to the chest wall. The primary indication of trauma is when, in the course of the initial resuscitation, a nasogastric tube is placed, and a radiograph is taken that shows a pneumothorax with a nasogastric tube located in the chest cavity.

Bronchoscopy is diagnostic, and most injuries can be repaired successfully.

CAUSTIC INJURY

Although caustic ingestion occurs much less frequently today, severe caustic injury can damage the airway and the more commonly injured esophagus. In suspected cases, the airway should be inspected with an endoscope at the time of diagnostic esophagoscopy. When injury to the trachea is suspected, careful surveillance for pneumothorax or pneumomediastinum should be carried out. Repair in these cases can be difficult.

LARYNGOMALACIA

Laryngomalacia nearly always presents with stridor. Feeding difficulties also predominate along with failure to thrive and obstructive apnea. Cyanosis can be seen in nearly 40% of infants with laryngomalacia. Gastroesophageal reflux disease (GERD) occurs in about one fourth of cases; rarely a patient presents with cor pulmonale.

Endoscopy may show inspiratory collapse of prominent cuneiform cartilages, anterior collapse of the cuneiforms and arytenoids, or a posteriorly displaced epiglottis. Supraglottoplasty is proposed as an effective treatment by some. This involves trimming the supraglottic larynx with a carbon dioxide laser.

TRACHEOMALACIA

Tracheomalacia is seen in a variety of clinical situations, and making an accurate diagnosis and planning effective management can be problematic. For patients whose airway is floppy and for whom continuous positive airway pressure maintains a patent airway, continuous positive airway pressure delivered either by mask or by nasal prongs can provide relief until the trachea grows. In our experience, tracheostomy rarely is needed, and when it is, special tracheostomy cannulae are required to prop open the malacic trachea.

When tracheomalacia is seen after tracheostomy, an anterior cricoid suspension or simple trachea stomal closure can eliminate the problem. Some authors use synthetic splints of Marlex or Vicryl to build a scaffold around the malacic airway to give it external support.

The primary surgery of choice for severe tracheomalacia is aortopexy. We usually use computed tomography (CT) to assess the anatomy. When the thymus is interposed between the underside of the sternum and the aortic arch so as to suggest that there is room to displace the trachea anteriorly, an aortic suspension seems to be of some use. We resect the thymus and suture the anterior fascia of the transverse aortic arch or a reflected flap of pericardium to the sternum under bronchoscopic guidance using either open or thoracoscopic technique. Another option is to place a Palmaz stent bronchoscopically to prop open the airway. This is effective not only for tracheomalacia, but also for patients whose heart or a tumor compresses the airway.

ACQUIRED PROBLEMS

Among acquired problems are papillomas, granulation tissue, and scar. Subglottic papillomas and scar causing obstruction of the airway can be dealt with effectively with laser ablation. Although many surgeons prefer the carbon dioxide laser, we prefer to use the KTP/532 laser, which requires less energy to achieve the same surgical goal and, in theory at least, results in less tissue damage and subsequent scarring. Tracheobronchial stenoses should be considered as a cause of persistent pulmonary problems in infants with bronchopulmonary dysplasia.

TRACHEAL STENOSIS

Short segment tracheal stenosis can be dealt with either by simple resection or by laser release with balloon dilation. The resection is usually straightforward, and we believe that any lesion of less than or equal to 1 to 1.5 cm is treated best with a simple resection and reanastomosis. This approach usually is reserved for segments no longer than four to six tracheal rings. Longer segments, up to a maximum of 50% of the length of the trachea, need a concomitant laryngeal or bronchial release to relieve tension on the anastomosis. Sometimes, these cases need a polytetrafluoroethylene (Teflon) or Silastic stent to prevent anastomotic narrowing, and these patients may benefit by a postoperative splint to hold the neck in flexion until the anastomosis heals. Cardiopulmonary bypass should be considered for these procedures.

Rarely, simple wedge tracheoplasty may play a role, particularly in the cervical tracheal stenosis. Use of anterior cricoid resection has been described in the successful management of short segment subglottic stenosis.

There are a variety of proposed tracheoplasties that have varying utility. The use of castellated incisions is appealing because it results in minimal disruption of the mucosa, but prolonged intraluminal stenting is mandatory. A slide tracheoplasty is another option; the stenosis is transected obliquely at its midpoint from posterior to anterior. The distal end is slit anteriorly, the proximal end is slit posteriorly, and a "fish-mouth" type of anastomosis is carried out by "sliding" the segments toward each other and sewing them together.

Other approaches use pericardial or other biomaterial patches, much as one uses a patch for repair of a vascular stenosis. More recently, some success has been reported using free tracheal allografts, auricular cartilage as a tracheal graft, thyroid alar cartilage, or aortic homograft. Approaches in development include the concept of tissue engineering a new trachea or tracheal cartilages for replacement. When all else fails, a segmental lung transplant can work. Although this approach does not deal with the trachea directly, the bronchial segment can be anastomosed directly to a short, proximal tracheal segment to achieve a satisfactory result.

CONGENITAL TRACHEAL STENOSIS

Congenital tracheal stenosis is a challenging problem in pediatric thoracic surgical practice. These infants often present in extremis with multiple congenital anomalies. Although the operations for repair are technically straightforward, the postoperative care can make the difference between a successful outcome and death.

Sometimes the diagnosis becomes obvious when an infant is in respiratory distress and an endotracheal tube cannot be passed. Other patients may present with more subtle symptoms, such as when a significant tracheal narrowing goes unnoticed for months or years until an acute event precipitates a life-threatening emergency. When the diagnosis of tracheal stenosis is suspected, the proper sequence of diagnostic studies avoids unnecessary delay or disaster.

The cause of most congenital obstructions of the tracheobronchial tree is unknown. Presumably, some vascular accident or disruption of organogenesis occurs at a critical time during the formation of the airway. Associated anomalies of the respiratory tract and esophagus are found frequently; these anomalies are listed in Table 1.

■ DIAGNOSTIC CONSIDERATIONS

In our experience, diagnostic imaging alone is capable of determining the precise diagnosis in nearly every case. Because instrumentation of the airway may precipitate disaster, we prefer (assuming the patient's condition would allow it) a carefully planned workup consisting of radiographs before considering endoscopic instrumentation of the airway.

The first study should be the chest radiograph, on which either a unilateral or a generalized aeration problem usually is noted. When a unilateral problem is present, there usually is an obvious discrepancy between aeration and lung size between sides. If bronchial atresia is present, the ipsilateral lung usually is atretic, small, and opaque, and there is contralateral overexpansion of the other lung. In addition, the vascularity in the contralateral lung is increased because blood that normally would be directed to the atretic lung is added to the blood going to the remaining, normal lung.

If bronchial stenosis occurs, aeration of the involved lung still can occur, but the lung, even though it contains air, remains small and hypoplastic. The pulmonary artery also is hypoplastic; the lung is small, radiolucent, and hypovascular. Rarely, bronchial stenosis may lead to air trapping; in this case, the involved lung or lobe is large and hyperlucent.

With tracheal stenosis, inhibition of the flow of air into the lungs can result in small, clear lungs. In other cases, air trapping, on expiration, results in large, hyperlucent lungs. Specific areas of stenosis, either in the trachea or in the bronchi, often can be seen on plain films. When this is not possible, one can use regular tomography, CT, or magnetic resonance imaging.

If detailed information regarding the specific underlying anatomy is required, it often is best to use contrast bronchography. This study produces the most detailed images of the underlying tracheobronchial abnormality, but it is not required in every case. Some advocate high kilovoltage with added filtration and magnification techniques for evaluation of the airway on plain films.

When a symptomatic infant first is recognized, we begin with standard imaging of the chest in anticipation of visualization of the column of air in the tracheobronchial tree from the larynx to the hila of the lungs. This usually can be accomplished so that the entire airway is sufficiently well visualized to verify or to exclude the presence of an obstruction or a stenotic lesion. When tracheomalacia also is suspected, lateral views under fluoroscopy with or without contrast material in the esophagus usually suggest the diagnosis. The esophagogram may be helpful to identify gastroesophageal reflux and any vascular ring that coexists. For completeness, we prefer contrast-enhanced CT of the chest. CT allows us to visualize any vascular abnormalities that we may have missed otherwise, and it can assist in evaluating the costal cartilages as potential graft material.

When the radiographic findings are not conclusive in an infant, we perform a bedside inspection with a small (1.3-mm) flexible endoscope. This technique is safe and accurate, and

---

Table 1 Anomalies Associated with Congenital Tracheal Stenosis

MORE COMMON ANOMALIES	LESS COMMON ANOMALIES
Airway	Airway
Bronchial stenosis	Laryngomalacia
Tracheal bronchus	Cardiovascular
Tracheomalacia	Triventricular communis
Tracheal web	Coarctation of the aorta
Congenital subglottic stenosis	Dextrocardia with patent ductus arteriosus
Laryngeal hypoplasia with complete absence of the	Ventricular septal defect
glottic and subglottic airways	Skeleton
Pulmonary	Hemivertebrae in the cervical, thoracic, or lumbar
Hypoplasia of one or both lungs	regions
Unilateral pulmonary agenesis	Hypoplasia or absence of the thumb
Congenital lobar emphysema	Proximal radioulnar synostosis
Esophageal	Widened pedicles of vertebrae L2 to L4
H-type tracheoesophageal fistula	Hypoplastic mandible
Congenital stenosis of the upper esophagus	Genitourinary
Gastroesophageal reflux	Imperforate anus with rectovaginal fistula
Diaphragm	Gastrointestinal
Accessory diaphragm	Extrahepatic portal hypertension
Diaphragmatic hernia	

it enables the clinician to assess the nature of the problem and to plan for operative intervention. We reserve more definitive operative bronchoscopy to be performed (if needed) under anesthesia at the time that operative reconstruction is planned. The approaches to the congenitally stenotic tracheobronchial tree range from careful observation with intensive respiratory supportive therapy using either the placement of long-term endotracheal stents or the forceful dilation of the stenosis (with or without concomitant injection of corticosteroids) to the operative placement of prosthetic devices or, more definitively, tracheal grafts of pericardium, myoosseous flaps, periosteum, or cartilage.

■ NONOPERATIVE MANAGEMENT

Nonoperative management consists of regular chest physiotherapy, which is intensified when there is an intercurrent respiratory infection; humidification of the inspired air; and administration of antibiotics, when appropriate. Endotracheal intubation or suctioning is kept to a minimum. Although this therapeutic rationale may play a role in selected cases with minimal stenosis, its major value is that it serves as a reasonable guideline for the perioperative management of these patients.

The use of steroids, with or without balloon dilation, in the primary management of tracheobronchial stenoses is controversial. Forceful dilation of the airway usually leads to acquired stenosis, the healing of which is accompanied by epithelial growth and by various degrees of subepithelial fibrosis and granulation tissue.

Every infant with stenosis of the airway does not require operative intervention. It is the clinician's responsibility to determine which infants would respond poorly to nonoperative management and which infants would require a more invasive approach. In our opinion, the indications for operation include severe life-threatening obstruction, recurrent admissions to the hospital, persistent symptoms that suggest small airway obstructive disease, and failure to thrive, all of which can be caused entirely by the airway stenosis. Nonoperative maintenance and observation in anticipation of growth of the airway with the child may lead to complications or death, which could be avoided with early operative intervention.

■ OPERATIVE THERAPY

Some authors advocate endoscopic management as the initial approach to the stenotic trachea, especially for acquired lesions, such as subglottic stenosis. The role of endoscopic procedures in congenital stenoses, particularly the long segment variety, is probably limited.

A reversed bronchial segment for total tracheal reconstruction of the trachea may be useful in selected cases. Bronchoplasty with an adjacent segmental bronchus or a free cartilage graft also is appealing; however, for isolated bronchial stenosis, occasionally the best option is to perform a pulmonary resection.

In 1982, Kimura et al described a split-thickness costal cartilage graft for the management of tracheal stenosis.

Because cartilage is a semirigid, living, autologous tissue, which derives its nutrients via diffusion, and because it is not dependent on a direct vascular supply, it is an ideal material for use as a tracheal graft. Tension does not seem to be a problem with the Kimura type of cartilage graft because it becomes incorporated into the tracheal wall. It allows for adequate ventilation, while natural growth enlarges the tracheal lumen with time.

Because of the high incidence of unrecognized associated anomalies, we advise waiting for a karyotype and assessing the central nervous system as part of the preoperative assessment when the clinical condition of the patient allows this luxury. Expectant management and dilation of the congenital stricture (with or without the concomitant use of steroids) have proved disappointing in our experience. Bronchoscopy can be useful, particularly to assess the airway beyond the stenosis. Often, there is only enough room for insertion of the telescope alone. This procedure can be performed conveniently at the time of operative repair.

Operative reconstruction using an autologous cartilage graft or processed dura (as opposed to resection in every case) has proved successful for the management of tracheal stenosis in our experience. Complex lesions that involve the carina and extend onto one or both of the main stem bronchi can be managed successfully by suturing multiple pieces of cartilage together and by using a postoperative endotracheal stent. Also described are the use of vascularized sternohyoid myocutaneous flap, omental pedicle flap, construction of a sliding flap tracheoplasty for upper tracheal stenosis, and esophageal tracheoplasty for long segment stenosis.

■ OPERATIVE TECHNIQUE

In the absence of a pulmonary arterial sling, we prefer to approach intrathoracic tracheal, carinal, and right bronchial stenoses via a right anterolateral thoracotomy through the fourth intercostal space, using a retropleural dissection. This approach always provides adequate exposure, and cardiopulmonary bypass does not seem to offer any particular advantage. Although the retropleural approach may not be necessary, it is familiar to anyone who has ever repaired a tracheoesophageal fistula, and it provides excellent exposure of the anatomy. The lungs are retracted anteriorly and inferiorly, exposing the mediastinum. Division of the azygos vein is usually necessary. Taking care not to injure the esophagus or vagus nerve, the trachea is exposed. By carefully retracting the pulmonary hilum inferiorly, adequate exposure of the carina and both main stem bronchi to their pulmonary hila can be gained. With this exposure, the narrowed segment or segments can be identified easily. When the length of the narrowed segment has been determined, the graft can be harvested. We use the sixth costal cartilage, split lengthwise along its broad axis, as the graft. This choice has two distinct advantages. First, no additional incision is necessary. Second, this is a long piece of cartilage with a gentle curve at one end. Accordingly, it can be applied easily to the area of the carina and can extend distally onto the main stem bronchus in instances in which the stenosis involves that part of the airway. We dissect the cartilage from its bed, leaving the underlying pleura intact.

When the graft has been harvested, the trachea is incised lengthwise through the stenosis. The endotracheal tube can be advanced beyond the incision into the left main stem bronchus and secured there until the anastomosis is completed. Alternatively the distal airway can be intubated from the operative field, using a sterile endotracheal tube and a sterile ventilator circuit. After the airway is established, the anastomosis can be accomplished easily.

We prefer to use a running, absorbable suture, placed through the full thickness of the cut edge of the trachea and the graft. The edge of the graft is seated on the cut edge of the trachea, and the perichondrial surface is positioned toward the lumen. In some instances, it may be necessary to sew multiple pieces of cartilage together to provide additional width or length or to reconstruct the carina. When the anastomosis is completed and appears to be airtight, with or without fibrin glue, a stent (if used) can be placed so that its tip is beyond the suture line.

GERD is a frequently overlooked condition. It is believed that the failure rate for laryngotracheal reconstruction is higher for patients with uncontrolled GERD. These patients require more postoperative procedures, especially if a stent is present. When GERD occurs with a stent in place, prime conditions exist for formation of excessive granulation tissue and scarring; this may have an important effect on successful decannulation. Infants who fail decannulation after an apparently successful laryngotracheal reconstruction and who are discovered to have GERD are able to be decannulated after control of the GERD. For postoperative care, two key points include the use of an endotracheal tube as a stent positioned past the most distal suture line in the best (largest and most stable) bronchus (cutting additional holes for air exchange as necessary) and the use of paralysis or sedation.

■ RESULTS

Results from tracheobronchoplasty are generally good. Most of the failures are due to either associated anomalies or complex lesions for which the repair crosses the carina.

SUGGESTED READING

Desai D, et al: Tracheal neoplasms in children, *Ann Otol Rhinol Laryngol* 107:790, 1998.

Jacobs JP, et al: Tracheal allograft reconstruction: the total North American and worldwide pediatric experiences, *Ann Thorac Surg* 68:1043, 1999.

Kimura K, et al: Tracheoplasty for congenital stenosis of the entire trachea, *J Pediatr Surg* 17:869, 1982.

Lobe TE, et al: Successful management of congenital tracheal stenosis in infancy, *J Pediatr Surg* 22:1137, 1987.

Slimane MA, et al: Tracheobronchial ruptures from blunt thoracic trauma in children, *J Pediatr Surg* 34:1847, 1999.

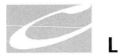

LARYNX AND TRACHEA

TRACHEOSTOMY

Erik Bauer

Bryan F. Meyers

■ TERMINOLOGY

Confusion exists regarding the use of the terms *tracheotomy* (from Greek *trachea arteria* [rough artery] and *tome* [cut]) and *tracheostomy* (from *stoma* [opening or mouth]). Although the terms often are used interchangeably, most practitioners recognize a difference. *Tracheotomy* refers to the procedure creating an opening designed to be temporary, whereas *tracheostomy* refers to creation of a permanent, mature opening, such as that required after total laryngectomy. The opening itself is a *stoma* or *tracheostoma*, and the tube traversing the opening is a *tracheostomy tube*.

■ INDICATIONS FOR TRACHEOSTOMY

There are four major reasons to secure a surgical airway. Although none are absolute indications for tracheostomy, any of them could serve as justification given the appropriate clinical setting. The indications include bypassing upper airway, providing support for prolonged mechanical ventilation, assisting in clearance of lower respiratory tract secretions, and protecting the airway against aspiration of oral or gastric secretions.

Relief of upper airway obstruction historically has been the primary indication for tracheostomy. Endotracheal intubation, when possible, should be the first-line treatment for acute airway obstruction in the emergent setting. In cases of mechanical or anatomic obstruction, however, attempts at translaryngeal intubation may carry an unacceptable risk of further airway compromise. These cases include congenital anomalies, maxillofacial trauma resulting in deformation or instability of the airway, upper airway foreign bodies, infectious or postoperative swelling of the soft tissues of the upper airway, or tumor masses of the upper aerodigestive tract or surrounding soft tissues. Care should be taken to identify impending airway obstruction so that tracheostomy can be performed in an appropriately controlled setting.

Prolonged ventilatory support exposes patients to a variety of complications related to pressure and friction of the endotracheal tube against the tissues of the upper airway and glottis. These include mucosal lesions, posterior glottic and subglottic stenosis, tracheal stenosis, and cricoid abscess. Patient comfort is an additional consideration in awake patients requiring mechanical ventilatory support. If support for longer than 10 to 14 days is anticipated, a timely tracheostomy may be performed to avoid the associated risks of prolonged translaryngeal intubation.

Pulmonary toilet is rarely the sole reason for tracheostomy. Selected patients with pneumonia, bronchiectasis, chronic aspiration, neurologic compromise, or laryngeal disorders may be unable to clear pulmonary secretions or protect their airway from orogastric contents. A tracheostomy tube can combat these problems by providing a direct passage for suctioning and an inflated cuff to separate the digestive and respiratory tracts. Patients with chronic aspiration also may benefit from the placement of a gastrostomy tube.

■ TECHNIQUES OF TRACHEOSTOMY

A surgical airway may be created by four techniques: cricothyrotomy, minitracheostomy, percutaneous dilational tracheostomy, and conventional tracheostomy. All four techniques have merits and drawbacks that are important to the practicing surgeon performing tracheostomy procedures.

Cricothyrotomy

Cricothyrotomy (also called *cricothyroidotomy*) is an emergency procedure recommended for urgent, short-term airway control. It is a simple and effective way to secure an emergency airway in patients with facial trauma, airway obstruction, or other conditions precluding orotracheal or nasotracheal intubation. Although the complication rate is many times that of elective tracheostomy, it can be lifesaving in skilled hands. Cricothyrotomy is preferable to emergency tracheostomy because the cricothyroid membrane is closer to the skin surface, and less dissection is required to reach the airway. In the elective setting, however, tracheostomy is preferred because long-term intubation through the cricothyroid membrane carries an unacceptably high risk of subglottic stenosis and other damage to the subglottic larynx. An emergency cricothyrotomy should be converted to a formal tracheostomy soon after the patient is stabilized.

For this procedure, the patient is positioned supine with the neck in a neutral position, an adequate sterile field is prepared, and local anesthetic is infiltrated. The thyroid cartilage is retracted superiorly, and a horizontal skin incision is made just below, entering the cricothyroid membrane with a short, stabbing motion. A blunt scalpel handle or a tracheal spreader is inserted into the incision and twisted vertically to open the airway. A small cuffed endotracheal or tracheostomy tube is inserted and secured.

Minitracheostomy

Minitracheostomy originally was described as a means of securing either an emergent or an elective airway and providing pulmonary toilet and temporary ventilation through a small incision. In this rapid technique, local anesthetic is infiltrated, a 1-cm stab incision is made in the cricothyroid membrane, and a 4- to 6-mm inner diameter cannula is inserted into the trachea. The cannula is secured to the neck by sutures or soft ties.

The stoma provided by this method is likely to be inadequate to support mechanical ventilation. It has potential value for the management of postoperative bronchial secretions and atelectasis but is not an alternative to conventional tracheostomy for patients requiring mechanical ventilatory support. Available devices include Seldinger style "over-the-wire" kits and simple trocar-based catheters. In the authors' experience, the Seldinger design minimizes the risk of false passage into the pretracheal plane or the membranous trachea. More recently introduced minitracheostomy products include large and small sizes, and with the larger sizes, the distinction between a minitracheostomy and a percutaneous dilational tracheostomy has blurred. Generally a minitracheostomy kit includes only a single obturator that serves as a dilator. The larger the size of the device, the more difficult it would be to place in an awake patient with local anesthetic. If a large size lumen is desired, a percutaneous or open tracheostomy should be considered.

Percutaneous Dilational Tracheostomy

Percutaneous dilational tracheostomy was adapted from the technique of percutaneous nephrostomy tube insertion and was described by Toye and Weinstein in 1969 and 1985. This method has the advantage of being quick, efficient, cost-effective, and safe when performed on properly selected patients. Widespread adoption of this technique by practitioners unfamiliar with open tracheostomy has shown a potential for numerous complications, however. It is recommended that surgeons performing percutaneous tracheostomy be skilled in conventional tracheostomy as well, given that conversion to an open technique may be required. Relative contraindications to percutaneous tracheostomy include young age, obesity or deformity resulting in loss of normal landmarks or anatomic relationships of the cartilages, calcified tracheal rings, thyromegaly, and coagulopathy. Percutaneous tracheostomy is absolutely contraindicated in emergency situations.

Percutaneous tracheostomy is performed most commonly in the intensive care setting for patients requiring prolonged mechanical ventilation with an endotracheal tube already in place. The patient is positioned, prepared, and draped similarly to a conventional tracheostomy. Percutaneous introducer sets contain an introducer needle, a guidewire, and either serial dilators or a single graduated dilator. A tracheostomy tray and standard intubation equipment also should be readily available should the need arise, and a long endotracheal tube ventilation catheter may be left in place as a guide for rapid reintubation.

The procedure may be performed "blindly," with the introducer needle passed through the skin using palpable landmarks, or preferably with bronchoscopic surveillance to guide passage of the device more safely. In the latter method, the endotracheal tube is withdrawn to the level of the cords, and a bronchoscope is passed to monitor the entry of the introducer and dilators into the trachea. A prospective study by Berrouschot compared outcomes in 41 patients who underwent blind percutaneous dilational tracheostomy versus 35 patients who underwent the same procedure with bronchoscopic monitoring. Although the complication rate overall was similar, the severity of complications was greater in the blind passage group. Bronchoscopic monitoring is recommended to minimize the risk of complications resulting from improper placement of the introducer.

A qualified person should monitor the patient and provide sedation with benzodiazepines or propofol. Lidocaine with 1:100,000 epinephrine is infiltrated into the skin overlying the second and third tracheal rings. After careful palpation of the landmarks, a 1-cm vertical incision is placed extending inferiorly from the cricoid cartilage. The introducer needle is advanced through the anterior tracheal wall, aspirating constantly, and the position of the needle tip in the trachea is confirmed when air is withdrawn. In a modified Seldinger technique, a J-wire is passed through the introducer to maintain a position within the trachea, then serial dilators (12 to 36 Fr) are threaded to enlarge the stoma to a diameter sufficient for the tracheostomy tube (Figure 1). The tube is passed over the appropriate-sized dilator and advanced into the trachea over the guidewire assembly (Figure 2). Finally, the dilator and guidewire are removed, and the tracheostomy tube is sutured to the skin. Subsequent care and monitoring is similar to that for conventional tracheostomy.

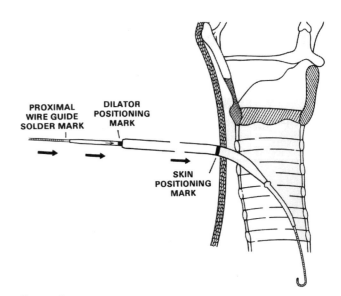

Figure 1

A guidewire has been placed through the anterior tracheal wall in the desired location of the tracheostomy. One of a series of dilators is being passed over the guidewire to create an appropriately sized opening for tube placement. (Diagram reproduced from package insert of Ciaglia percutaneous tracheostomy introducer set, with permission granted courtesy of Cook Critical Care, Bloomington, IN.)

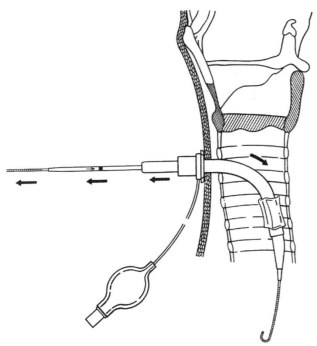

Figure 2

When the tube path has been dilated appropriately, a tracheostomy tube is inserted by loading it onto a dilator. The dilator and tube are advanced into position, and the dilator subsequently is removed. (Diagram reproduced from package insert of Ciaglia percutaneous tracheostomy introducer set, with permission granted courtesy of Cook Critical Care, Bloomington, IN.)

Conventional Elective Tracheostomy

Elective open tracheostomy ideally is carried out in the operating room with adequate instrumentation, lighting, and assistance. The patient is positioned supine, with a shoulder roll to extend the neck and provide optimal access to the trachea. Lidocaine with 1:100,000 epinephrine is infiltrated locally. A horizontal incision is made halfway between the sternal notch and the cricoid cartilage, preferably in a skin crease. The skin, subcutaneous tissue, and platysma are serially incised, revealing the strap muscles. The fascia separating the right and left sternohyoid and sternothyroid muscles is incised vertically, and the muscles are retracted laterally from the midline. The thyroid isthmus typically is retracted superiorly without division. If necessary, the isthmus may be divided between two clamps, and the cut ends may be oversewn. A cricoid hook is placed between the cricoid cartilage and the first tracheal ring to retract the trachea superiorly, and a Kitner dissector is used to release the fine fascia from the anterior tracheal wall. The trachea is entered through a horizontal incision between the second and third or third and fourth tracheal rings. Wide division between the two rings generally makes it unnecessary to resect or divide any of the rings, minimizing damage to the trachea.

In cases in which a long-term tracheostomy is desired, a Bjork flap may be developed by isolating the anterior segment of the tracheal ring below the incision, leaving an inferiorly based flap that may be sutured to the inferior skin margin. Due to the risk of a late, persistent tracheocutaneous fistula, this technique should be avoided if only a temporary stoma is desired. In obese patients or patients with short necks in whom reinforcement is needed to prevent collapse of the stoma, sutures may be placed around the tracheal rings lateral to the opening and secured to the subcutaneous tissues to facilitate changing of the tracheostomy tube.

Placement of the tube is confirmed by direct communication with the anesthesiologist regarding carbon dioxide return, airway pressures, and patient oxygen saturation values. Ventilation is initiated through the tracheostomy tube as the translaryngeal endotracheal tube is withdrawn. Any concerns regarding inappropriate placement or malfunction of the balloon cuff should result in removal of the tracheostomy appliance and advancement of the endotracheal tube to allow safe ventilation during troubleshooting. When adequate placement is ensured, the tube flange is sutured to the skin in four quadrants to prevent displacement of the tube before the stoma is mature. Postoperatively a chest x-ray is obtained to confirm placement of the tube and exclude pneumothorax.

■ COMPLICATIONS OF TRACHEOSTOMY

Complications of tracheostomy can be divided conveniently into those occurring in the intraoperative, early postoperative, and late postoperative periods. Intraoperative complications include bleeding, which is typically minor and easily controlled by cautery or ligation of small bleeding vessels. A high-riding innominate artery may be the source of more serious bleeding, however. Incorrect placement of the tracheostomy device should be a rare occurrence in an elective tracheostomy procedure in which an airway is secured first by endotracheal intubation and the tube is placed directly into the trachea. Malpositioning of the device occasionally may occur in blind percutaneous tracheostomy, and care must be taken to verify the intratracheal position before continuing on with the completion of the procedure. Cardiopulmonary arrest may occur as a result of failure to obtain an airway or as a consequence of tension pneumothorax. Finally, pneumothorax or pneumomediastinum may result from damage to the apex of the pleural space in the lower lateral limits of the tracheostomy incision. A postoperative chest radiograph is important to exclude pneumothorax and confirm placement of the tracheostomy appliance.

Early postoperative complications may include tube obstruction from inspissated mucus or clotted blood. These obstructions can be prevented by humidified air by tracheostomy mask and by meticulous postoperative nursing care. Suturing the tube flange to the skin at the time of the operation may prevent displacement of the tube. If positive-pressure ventilation is used, however, care should be taken not to pack or suture the wound tightly because this can lead to the development of subcutaneous emphysema.

Among late complications is the most feared adverse sequela of tracheostomy, the rare and life-threatening tracheo–innominate artery fistula (discussed in a separate chapter). The risk of tracheo–innominate artery fistula is increased by low placement of the stoma (below the third tracheal ring), an aberrantly high innominate artery, erosion of the tracheal wall resulting from excessive cuff pressure, tube torsion, and local tissue effects such as wound infection or previous radiation treatment. Treatment involves control of the hemorrhage by overinflation of the tracheostomy tube cuff or by using a gloved finger to hold pressure at the bleeding site. Orotracheal intubation with a second endotracheal tube placed with its cuff below the hemorrhage may help buy time and stability while the patient is transported emergently to the operating room. Definitive treatment involves division of the innominate artery, which, if done without extraanatomic bypass, carries the risk of cerebral infarction and upper extremity ischemia. The damaged segment of trachea also may be resected, and an end-to-end anastomosis may be performed with vascularized tissue interposed between the vascular and the tracheal suture lines.

Tracheal stenosis, another late complication related to local pressure effects, may arise at either the level of the cuff or the location of the tube tip. Incidence has decreased significantly since the advent of high-volume, low-pressure cuffs. The classic work by Cooper and Grillo showed that stenosis was caused by pressure leading to local ischemia, followed by local infection and fibrosis. Maintaining cuff pressure less than 25 cmH_2O, the pressure at which submucosal capillaries are occluded, can prevent the complication. Stenosis also can occur at the tracheal stoma, from softening and displacement of the anterior tracheal wall or from formation of granulation tissue. If necessary, these nodules of granulation tissue can be removed surgically.

■ SUMMARY

Current techniques for the placement of tracheostomy appliances range from urgent cricothyrotomy to formal and conventional open tracheostomy. The selection of a single technique depends on the specific clinical problem creating the need for the tracheostomy and the practitioner's skill and comfort with each type of procedure. It is likely that demand will increase for the less invasive, percutaneous placement of tracheostomy devices because this strategy avoids the transport of ventilated patients from the intensive care unit to the operating room. It will be important for surgeons to become familiar with these newer techniques and to lead the efforts in validating the safety and efficacy of such alternatives.

SUGGESTED READING

Barba CA, et al: Bronchoscopic guidance makes percutaneous tracheostomy a safe, cost-effective, and easy-to-teach procedure, *Surgery* 118:879, 1995.

Berrouschot J, et al: Perioperative complications of percutaneous dilational tracheostomy, *Laryngoscope* 107:1538, 1997.

Cooper JD, Grillo HC: Experimental production and prevention of injury due to cuffed tracheal tubes, *Surg Gynecol Obstet* 129:1235, 1969.

Esses BA, Jafek BW: Cricothyroidotomy: a decade of experience in Denver, *Ann Otol Rhinol Laryngol* 96:519, 1987.

Freeman BD, et al: A prospective, randomized study comparing percutaneous with surgical tracheostomy in critically ill patients, *Crit Care Med* 29:926, 2001.

Gysin C, et al: Percutaneous versus surgical tracheostomy: a double-blind randomized trial, *Ann Surg* 230:708, 1999.

BENIGN TRACHEAL TUMORS

Cameron D. Wright

Benign tracheal tumors are very rare and are often misdiagnosed for years. Hemoptysis is less common than it is in malignant tumors. Cough and airway obstructive symptoms predominate. Adult-onset asthma is often misdiagnosed, and steroids are given for "unresponsive" wheezing. Various types of tumors can develop in the epithelium, blood vessels, nerves, and supporting structures of the trachea (Table 1). Papillomas are the most common benign tumors in the pediatric population. The most common benign mesenchymal tumor is a chondroma, whereas fibromas account for 20% of all benign tumors.

■ RADIOLOGIC EVALUATION

Plain chest radiographs frequently miss tracheal tumors. Computed tomography (CT) is currently the radiologic procedure of choice for defining tracheal tumors. The shape and origin characteristics can suggest a benign tracheal tumor (i.e., a rounded, pedunculated lesion). Encasement or invasion of adjacent structures suggests a malignant tracheal tumor. The effective tracheal luminal diameter can be estimated. The location of the tumor dictates the surgical approach to the tumor. Multiplanar and three-dimensional reconstruction can be performed but rarely add any significant useful information. Magnetic resonance imaging likewise adds little to an axial CT scan of the trachea and is rarely useful.

■ BRONCHOSCOPIC EVALUATION

Bronchoscopy should be performed on all patients with suspected tracheal tumors. Information about the tumor itself (location in trachea, distance in centimeters from the cricoid

Table 1 Benign Tracheal Tumors

Glomus tumors	Chondroblastoma
Papilloma	Schwannoma
Pleomorphic adenoma	Paraganglioma
Granular cell tumor	Hemangioendothelioma
Chondroma	Vascular malformation
Leiomyoma	Carcinoid tumors
Fibrous histiocytoma	Mucoepidermoid tumor
Amyloidoma	

or carina, site of origin [pedicle, cartilaginous wall, membranous wall], mobility, status of overlying mucosa, length of involved trachea, and degree of tracheal obstruction), any associated lesions, and possible obstructed secretions can be obtained. In rare cases of severe airway obstruction, an airway can be obtained by rigid bronchoscopy and cored out or laser débridement. In general, rigid bronchoscopy should be used to evaluate tracheal tumors because the optics are superior to flexible bronchoscopes, large biopsy samples can be obtained, bleeding can be controlled, and, most important, the airway can be controlled if necessary. Flexible bronchoscopy can be carried out through the rigid bronchoscope to assess the more distal airway. Small, readily removable benign-appearing tumors do not always need to undergo biopsy as long as a frozen section is performed at the time of resection to confirm their benign nature. Sessile, indeterminate tumors should always be biopsied first to help guide the proposed resection margins of the tumors. Flexible bronchoscopy is very helpful in placing the endotracheal tube in the correct location at the time of operation. For small tumors in the mid or distal trachea, the tube is left in the usual subglottic position. Proximal small tumors are typically bypassed with the aide of a bronchoscope directing the endotracheal tube well past the tumor. Large distal tumors are typically bypassed by guiding a wire-wound armored endotracheal tube with a flexible bronchoscope. Often the cuff does not need to be inflated due to the severity of obstruction of the combination of the tumor and endotracheal tube.

■ INDICATION FOR OPERATION

Essentially, all benign tracheal tumors should be removed because of their potential for airway obstruction. The rare truly pedunculated tumor may be removed endoscopically and closely observed thereafter to monitor for local recurrence. Multiple papillomas are typically treated by YAG laser débridement, and interferon therapy is often used for recurrent papillomas.

■ OPERATIVE APPROACH

The three common operative approaches to tracheal resection are cervical, cervicomediastinal, and transthoracic. The body habitus of the patient greatly influences the operative approach at the border zones of the trachea. The ideal patient is tall and thin and has a narrow anteroposterior diameter of the chest. A benign tumor of the distal third of the trachea in such an ideal patient can almost always be resected through the anterior (cervicomediastinal) approach. In general, tumors in the upper third of the trachea are resected through a cervical collar incision. Anterior approaches (cervical and cervicomediastinal) involve placing the patient supine with the neck extended by means of a roll or an inflatable bag under the shoulder. Subplatysmal flaps are elevated to the top of the thyroid cartilage and to the clavicles. The strap muscles are separated in the midline and mobilized off the thyroid and trachea. The thyroid isthmus is dissected out and divided to fully expose the upper trachea and anterior cricoid. Fibrofatty tissue over the trachea is divided down to the sternal notch to fully expose the anterior surface of the trachea. A cervicomediastinal exposure starts with a collar incision exactly as described earlier.

Once the trachea is exposed from cricoid to the sternal notch, the upper mediastinum is opened. The incision is taken down onto the manubrium, which is cut with a sternal saw or Lebsche knife. A small spreader is inserted after hemostasis of the sternum is obtained. The innominate vessels are mobilized as much as possible to assist retraction but not bared on their undersurfaces to avoid contact with the airway (and possible anastomosis) postoperatively. The innominate vessels can be gently retracted inferiorly and a long tunnel created in the pretracheal plane of the deep cervical fascia down to the carina. This potential space is bluntly mobilized with a finger and is all loose areolar tissue.

Tumors in the distal third of the trachea, especially in obese or elderly kyphotic patients, are usually approached transthoracically. To facilitate the intrathoracic exposure, the flexible armored endotracheal tube is bronchoscopically directed down the left main bronchus and the cuff is inflated to allow the right lung to collapse. A right posterolateral thoracotomy is made through the fourth or fifth interspace. The azygous vein is ligated and divided. The distal trachea is dissected out on the anterior surface after division of the mediastinal pleura and a "reverse mediastinoscopy" is accomplished by dissecting the loose areolar tissue from the anterior wall of the trachea up into the neck to allow greater tracheal mobility.

■ INTRAOPERATIVE VENTILATION

Cardiopulmonary bypass is never necessary to resect a benign tracheal tumor. Once the airway is opened and transected, ventilation is easily carried out by a separate flexible armored endotracheal tube that is also connected to the anesthesia machine. This tube can be passed in and out of the divided trachea as necessary to ventilate the patient. The cuff can usually be partially inflated to such a level that it promotes sufficient sealing to allow positive pressure ventilation as it is inserted into and removed from the trachea. High-frequency jet ventilation is almost never necessary for simple trachea resections. When all of the sutures in the tracheal anastomosis are placed, the regular indwelling endotracheal tube is carefully advanced into the distal airway (avoiding entanglement with the anastomotic sutures) to resume normal ventilation.

■ TRACHEAL RESECTION AND RECONSTRUCTION

The principles and techniques of tracheal resection are the same regardless of the approach to the airway. The segment of trachea to be resected is dissected circumferentially, staying immediately adjacent to the trachea to avoid injury to the recurrent laryngeal nerves. Although malignant tumors and benign stenoses often have transmural changes that allow ready identification of the abnormal trachea, the external trachea in benign tumors is normal and palpation is an unreliable guide to the exact location of the tumor. Intraoperative bronchoscopy allows precise identification of the limits of the tumor. A 25-gauge needle can be used to pierce the airway where the transilluminated bronchoscopic light suggests the margin should be. If it is not precisely correct, it can be removed with impunity and redone to accurately delineate the lesion. The proximal and distal margins can then be marked with sutures at the appropriate locations to guide the tracheal transection. In general, the distal tracheal margin is transected first to allow easy ventilation of the distal airway. The proximal segment to be removed is then completely dissected free (the membranous wall of the trachea is usually much easier to dissect off the wall of the esophagus once the airway is transected), and the proximal margin is transected. The lateral soft tissue attachments of the trachea where the blood supply enters should not be dissected off more than 7 to 8 mm or so to prevent ischemia.

The margin necessary for benign tumors is quite minimal (usually 1 to 2 mm), so extensive resections are uncalled for. Nonetheless, the proximal and distal margins should be checked by frozen section to ensure they are clear. Tumors with low-grade malignant potential (e.g., mucoepidermoid tumors) should be resected with wider margins. Lateral traction sutures of 2-0 Vicryl are placed at the 3- and 9-o'clock positions on both the proximal and distal trachea. Starting in the midline posteriorly, circumferential interrupted 4-0 Vicryl sutures are placed 3 to 5 mm back from the cut edge, with all of the knots on the outside of the trachea. Each suture is snapped together once the needle is cut off and then snapped again to the surgical drape in an organized fashion to allow the anterior-most sutures to be tied first and the first posterior suture to be tied last. When all of the sutures are placed, the temporary field endotracheal tube is removed and the native endotracheal tube is readvanced across the anastomosis into the distal airway. The elevation of the shoulders is removed, and the head is flexed forward by the anesthesiologist to allow the cervical trachea to devolve into the mediastinum. The lateral traction sutures are first tied, followed by the 4-0 sutures starting anteriorly. The anastomosis is examined bronchoscopically to ensure it is technically correct. It is then checked for air leaks by inflating the lungs to 30 to 35 cm of water pressure while the anastomosis is under saline. If the anastomosis lies under the innominate artery, it is separated from it by a pedicled strap muscle or thymus flap. Patients are extubated in the operating room and a routine tracheostomy is not indicated. A guardian chin stick (from the chin to the chest) of heavy silk or nylon is placed to prevent hyperextension of the head (however, this does not approximate the chin to the chest; rather, it allows the chin to be in a neutral position).

■ RESULTS

The results are usually excellent for tracheal resection for benign tumors. Complications should be rare after tracheal resection for benign tumors as anastomotic problems are usually the result of excessive tension due to lengthy resections. Temporary or permanent vocal cord dysfunction should be infrequent (<5%), as is wound infection (<2%). Anastomotic morbidity (dehiscence or stricture) occurs in less than 1% due to the limited amount of trachea resected. Local recurrence likewise should be rare because these are benign tumors.

SUGGESTED READING

Desai DP, et al: Granular cell tumor of the trachea, *Otolaryngol Head Neck Surg* 120:595, 1999.

Dorfman J, et al: Primary tracheal schwannoma, *Ann Thorac Surg* 69:280, 2000.

Kim KH, et al: Pleomorphic adenoma of the trachea, *Otolaryngol Head Neck Surg* 123:147, 2000.

Lange TH, et al: Tracheobronchial glomus tumor, *Ann Thorac Surg* 70:292, 2000.

Mathisen DJ: Surgery of the trachea, *Curr Probl Surg* 35:453, 1998.

Perelman MI, et al: Primary tracheal tumors, *Semin Thorac Cardiovasc Surg* 8:400, 1996.

MALIGNANT TRACHEAL TUMORS

Amy M. Lightner
Douglas J. Mathisen

Primary malignant tumors of the trachea are uncommon, occurring with an annual incidence of only 2.7 per 1 million persons. Their rarity often leads to delayed diagnosis, which underscores the importance of knowing the tumors' salient characteristics.

Adenoid cystic carcinoma is the most common surgically treated primary malignancy of the trachea, making up 40% of tumors in the Massachusetts General Hospital (MGH) series. Gender incidence is approximately equal, and age incidence is spread throughout adulthood with a small peak in the 50s. This tumor is known for its slow-growing nature, insidious presentation, and its tendency to recur several years after initial treatment. This tendency to recur is likely because of its ability to spread submucosally and perineurally for long distances. Adenoid cystic carcinoma is often large and bulky when diagnosed.

Primary squamous cell carcinoma of the trachea made up 35% of the MGH series but has the highest overall incidence among primary tracheal malignancies. It is more common in men, smokers, and patients in their 60s and 70s. It too may be bulky and compress adjacent structures at presentation, or it may be ulcerative or spreading. Squamous cell lesions can be multiple, extend along a significant length of trachea, and typically grow more rapidly than adenoid cystic tumors. Squamous cell and adenoid cystic tumors spread to regional lymph nodes; adenoid cystic tumors occasionally metastasize to other organs (lungs, bone), whereas squamous cell tumors are more likely to be associated with second primary tumors of the aerodigestive tract.

Other primary malignancies of the trachea are uncommon and usually represent only one or two patients in reported series. These tumor types include carcinoids, adenocarcinomas, small cell carcinoma, and adenosquamous carcinoma. Rarely, metastatic lesions or locally invasive laryngeal, thyroid, esophageal, or lung cancers involve the trachea.

Symptoms of tracheal malignancy usually reflect worsening airway obstruction. Initial shortness of breath can progress rapidly to stridor. Cough and wheezing (sometimes misdiagnosed as asthma) are frequent complaints; hemoptysis and recurrent pneumonitis are occasional signs of tracheal tumors. Dysphagia or hoarseness may signal recurrent nerve or esophageal involvement.

■ TREATMENT OPTIONS

In general, if preoperative evaluation (see later) reveals that a tracheal tumor is not metastatic and can be resected safely with primary tracheal or carinal reconstruction, this course should be pursued. Postoperative, full-dose, mediastinal radiation therapy (5000 cGy), about 1 month after surgery and regardless of nodal status, has been our practice.

Primary radiotherapy is a good treatment option in palliative cases or when surgery does not seem technically feasible. Laser photocoagulation, cryotherapy, or electrocautery sometimes are useful in palliation, treating benign lesions, or helping relieve airway obstruction before definitive surgery. Chemotherapy does not yet play a prominent role in treatment of malignant tracheal tumors.

■ PREOPERATIVE ASSESSMENT

Patients often are misdiagnosed with benign cough or asthma due to an initial plain chest radiograph that is read as "normal." Careful inspection of these films is useful, however, and may show an irregular tracheal air column or extratracheal involvement of tumor. Other radiographic studies also are helpful to the surgeon in delineating location, size, and characteristics of the mass, including plain x-ray with a lateral view of the neck, tracheal tomograms, magnetic resonance imaging with sagittal and coronal views of the trachea, spiral computed tomography scan of the neck and chest with three-dimensional reconstruction, barium swallow to assess for esophageal involvement with tumor; and fluoroscopy to study laryngeal function.

The need for definitive diagnosis and precise measurements of tracheal tumors usually leads to endoscopy as part of the patient's evaluation. Rigid bronchoscopy is preferred in assessing these lesions. The wide scope allows for an ample biopsy specimen and for airway patency should the tumor begin to bleed; this procedure should be approached with great caution and in an appropriate setting. Measurements begin at the incisors and are taken to the carina, distal and proximal tumor margins, and vocal cords. Determining the extent of the tumor along the trachea is important because it enables one to plan how surgery should be approached.

Some patients, who may have been slow to present or misdiagnosed, are found to have a tracheal cancer in an emergent situation in which relief of airway obstruction is required. The airway is best secured in the operating room. An initial "core-out" of the tumor via rigid bronchoscopy may be necessary to allow a small endotracheal tube to pass (some institutions use laser therapy or electrocautery in these circumstances). Attempting to pass a large endotracheal tube before bronchoscopic evaluation may complete a near-total obstruction if the tumor begins to bleed or is sheared off by the tube. When a patent airway is secured and the patient is stabilized, the remainder of the preoperative workup can proceed as noted earlier.

■ SURGERY

Circumferential, segmental resection followed by primary reconstruction is the appropriate operation for tumors of the trachea or carina. The amount of airway that eventually is resected depends on intraoperative frozen section results, but enough trachea must remain after resection to allow for a relatively tension-free anastomosis. In young, thin patients, 50% of the trachea usually can be removed safely, but elderly and overweight patients have much less leeway in this regard.

Placement of an inflatable bag underneath the patient's shoulders is useful for hyperextension of the neck during surgery. Other positioning varies by tumor location, but the surgical field should include the chin, neck, and chest, in case the resection becomes more extensive than initially anticipated.

Anesthesiologists specially trained in thoracic procedures are helpful during these cases, as airway management can be challenging. A slow, inhalational induction with a volatile anesthetic generally is used, and intubating past the tumor sometimes requires a small endotracheal tube or a core-out by the surgeon before the principal procedure. Ideally the patient is extubated at the end of the case to avoid the possibility of the endotracheal tube cuff contacting the fresh anastomosis. Total intravenous anesthesia using short acting agents, such as Remifentanil and Propotol, has become an increasingly popular alternative.

Resection

The approach to the tumor depends on the site of the lesion (Table 1). After a cervical collar incision or right thoracotomy is made, the trachea is freed anteriorly by gentle, blunt dissection of the pretracheal plane. The recurrent laryngeal nerves should be identified if the tumor extends outside the lumen of the trachea. If one nerve is involved by tumor, great care must be taken to preserve the other nerve. Circumferential dissection of the trachea about 1 cm above and below the area of tumor is performed, followed by dissection of the area containing the mass (beginning on the side of the trachea opposite the lesion). Preservation of the lateral blood supply of the remaining trachea is imperative and is achieved best by limited lateral dissection and avoiding extensive lymph node dissection.

Before distal transection of the trachea, lateral traction sutures of 2-0 polyglactin 910 (Vicryl) are placed at the 3- and 9-o'clock positions, full thickness around a tracheal ring, about 1 cm beyond the anticipated line of transection. The trachea is opened gently and inspected, then cleanly transected. Similar sutures are placed above the upper level of transection, and this part of the specimen is transected. Frozen sections should be sent from both margins. If the tumor involves the carina or low trachea, it may be easier to transect the upper margin first. Additional exposure of the distal trachea is achieved by dividing the manubrium and spreading it with a small, pediatric sternal spreader. Ventilation is carried out by a sterile endotracheal tube across the operative field, with sterile connecting tubing passed off to the anesthesiologist.

Partial-thickness or full-thickness esophageal resection also can be performed if the tracheal tumor involves the muscular wall of the esophagus. Tumors of the upper trachea that involve the larynx may require partial or total laryngectomy. One or both thyroid lobes may need to be removed if involved by tumor.

Reconstruction

The individual anastomotic sutures (4-0 Vicryl) are placed full thickness, 3 to 4 mm apart, with the knots to lie on the outside. Intermittently removing the endotracheal tube facilitates placement of the sutures. The first stitch is placed posteriorly at the 6-o'clock position. Each subsequent suture is placed "inside" the prior suture, and all are clipped carefully to the drapes to keep them in proper sequence. All sutures are placed before tying begins. Before tying the anastomotic sutures, the anesthesiologist flexes the neck and advances the oral endotracheal tube across the anastomosis. The lateral traction sutures are tied together (to approximate the tracheal ends) before tying the anastomotic sutures. The anastomotic sutures are tied in reverse order of placement. It is crucial that the anastomotic tension not be excessive because this can lead to either separation or stenosis. A suprahyoid release should be performed if excessive tension exists.

Closure

After reconstruction, a soft suction drain should be placed in the pretracheal plane. We place one heavy "guardian" stitch in the skin, from the area just below the chin to the presternal region. This effectively prevents the patient from suddenly hyperextending the neck and placing excessive tension on the anastomosis. The suture is removed on the seventh postoperative day.

■ MORBIDITY, MORTALITY, AND RESULTS

The most serious complication after tracheal resection is dehiscence or partial separation of the anastomosis. This condition results from devascularization of the trachea or from excessive anastomotic tension and presents with subcutaneous emphysema, stridor, and respiratory distress. It is managed best with a tracheostomy or T-tube. Laryngeal release sometimes results in postoperative aspiration. Hoarseness is related to manipulation of the recurrent laryngeal nerves and can be either temporary or permanent. Airway edema with stridor is treated with diuresis, 24 hours of steroids, and elevation of the head of the bed. If edema does not improve, a small, uncuffed endotracheal tube can be inserted carefully over a flexible bronchoscope. It should be left in place for 48 hours, then the situation should be reassessed.

Operative mortality for the 132 patients who had primary reconstruction was 5% (7 cases). One of the deaths was after a tracheal resection (1 of 83) and reconstruction, and the other 6 were after carinal surgeries (6 of 49).

As a result of the rarity of malignant tracheal tumors, few data exist regarding long-term outcomes of tracheal resection and reconstruction for malignancy. The MGH series, published in 1990, reported on 147 patients who underwent surgery (with or without primary reconstruction) for tracheal and carinal tumors over a 26-year period.

Table 1 Recommended Approaches to Tracheal Tumors	
TUMOR SITE	**APPROACH/INCISION(S)**
Upper trachea	Cervical collar incision ± extension through upper sternum
Midtrachea	Cervical collar incision ± median sternotomy
Lower trachea/ carina	High, right posterolateral thoracotomy

In general, the results were excellent. Of these patients, 70% were alive and tumor-free at the time of publication, although the cases were spread over many years so that follow-up time was variable. Survival was longer with adenoid cystic tumors than with squamous cell carcinoma: Median survival for patients with adenoid cystic tumors treated with resection (with or without irradiation) was 118 months compared with only 34 months for squamous cell carcinoma treated in similar fashion. The presence of positive lymph nodes at surgery or of invasive cancer at a resection margin were negative prognostic factors in squamous cell carcinoma but seemed to have little relationship to survival in adenoid cystic carcinoma.

SUGGESTED READING

Grillo HC, Mathisen DJ: Primary tracheal tumors: treatment and results, *Ann Thorac Surg* 49:69, 1990.
Mathisen DJ: Primary tracheal tumor management, *Surg Oncol Clin N Am* 8:307, 1999.
Mathisen DJ: Surgery of the trachea, *Curr Probl Surg* 35:453, 1998.

TRACHEAL RELEASE MANEUVERS

Douglas E. Wood

Disorders involving the airway are relatively uncommon. Most thoracic surgeons see only the occasional patient with tracheal or bronchial pathology. However, both benign and malignant obstructions of the central airway cause significant morbidity and mortality. Successful management may correct or palliate impending suffocation, dyspnea, and obstructive pneumonia. Tracheal resection and reconstruction may preclude the need for a life-long tracheostomy, allow preservation of laryngeal function in patients with benign strictures, and provide treatment with curative intent for airway tumors.

Tracheal reconstructive procedures are frequently regarded as complex operations with high morbidity and mortality. This may prevent their consideration as a viable treatment option for many patients. However, excellent results can be obtained in appropriately selected patients with a combination of well-planned anesthetic airway management, meticulous operative technique, and careful postoperative care. Reconstructive techniques of the airway have developed only recently. Laboratory and clinical experience by Grillo in Boston and Pearson in Toronto resulted in successful tracheal resection and reconstruction in the 1960s. Animal experimentation and clinical experience have led to refinements in surgical technique allowing tracheal and carinal reconstruction to be readily applied to both benign and malignant airway pathology.

The most common indication for tracheal resection and reconstruction is postintubation or posttracheostomy stenosis. Primary tracheal tumors, tumors invading the airway, and idiopathic tracheal or laryngotracheal stenosis are the other indications for tracheal reconstructive surgery. Airway tumors involving the carina or primary lung cancer involving the carina may be managed by carinal resection and reconstruction with many of the same considerations for airway release maneuvers.

Experimental anatomic studies in cadavers allow quantification of anastomotic tension with various degrees of resection. Anastomoses with more than 1200 *g* of tension have a high probability of anastomotic complications in clinical studies. Without specific airway release maneuvers, this allowed only an approximately 2-cm resection of airway with primary reconstruction. Cadaver studies have shown an exponential rise in anastomotic tension with increasing lengths above 2 cm. These pioneering cadaver and animal studies by Grillo and colleagues revealed a variety of techniques that allowed longer lengths of primary airway resection and reconstruction while maintaining a suture line tension of less than 1200 *g*, thereby reducing unacceptable anastomotic complications.

■ BRONCHOSCOPIC EVALUATION

The most important component in evaluating a patient before resection is the bronchoscopic evaluation. The carefully performed bronchoscopy provides clear information on the extent of pathology, the site and approach of planned resection, and the anticipated length of resection, allowing the surgeon to anticipate the potential need for airway release maneuvers. With rigid bronchoscopy, it is possible to identify the anatomic location and diameter of the lesion and to record its position in relation to important landmarks. Although flexible bronchoscopy provides adequate diagnostic information regarding the airway anatomy and extent of the lesion in most cases, rigid bronchoscopy facilitates examination of the airways distal to an obstructing lesion and provides for a more direct and accurate measurement of the length of an airway lesion and its relationship to airway landmarks. Rigid bronchoscopy has the added advantage of being able to simultaneously provide ventilation while traversing a benign stenosis or obstructing tumor. Rigid bronchoscopy can more directly and more reliably stabilize a central obstructed airway while providing ventilation through the bronchoscope. It also has the advantage of larger instrumentation to facilitate mechanical débridement of endoluminal tissue and aspiration of secretions and blood.

The surgeon performing airway resection and reconstruction should be skilled in both flexible and rigid bronchoscopy and have a broad spectrum of bronchoscopes and bronchoscopic instruments, as well as a team that is familiar and comfortable with both endoscopic approaches to airway evaluation. A bronchoscopy report should describe the lesion, including the amount of endoluminal disease and extrinsic compression. The description should include the degree of compromise of the lumen and what portion of the airway circumference is involved. Measurements can be obtained to measure the length of the lesion and its distance from normal landmarks. The simplest technique is to measure the relational distances between the vocal cords, cricoid cartilage, top of lesion, bottom of lesion, carina, and major bronchial bifurcations. A schematic drawing can then be produced in the operating room and in the patient's medical record to quantitatively describe the stricture or tumor so that it can be easily interpreted for surgical planning.

■ TRACHEAL BLOOD SUPPLY

Advances in tracheal reconstructive surgery required a clear understanding of tracheal blood supply (Figure 1). Tracheal release maneuvers have been developed to provide airway mobilization without concomitant devascularization of the trachea. In 1977, Salassa and colleagues described the diverse origin of tracheal blood supply, as well as five routes of collateral arterial blood supply. Arterial flow originates from the inferior thyroid, subclavian, supreme intercostal, internal mammary, innominate, and superior and middle bronchial arteries. The five arterial connections that provide important tracheal collateral circulation are (1) a lateral longitudinal collateral that links the lateral segmental vessels, (2) transverse intercartilaginous arteries that connect the right and left sides, (3) tracheoesophageal vessels that contribute to both structures, (4) connections of the proximal cervical trachea blood supply from the inferior thyroid artery with the segmental lateral tracheal blood supply of the mid portion of the trachea, and (5) connection of the carinal nodal or bronchial arteries with the more proximal segmental tracheal blood supply.

Two important aspects of these findings are that the tracheal blood supply is segmental and that lateral tracheal blood supply must be preserved to maintain airway viability. Interruption of this lateral blood supply and skeletonization of the airway to improve mobility will result in a high incidence of anastomotic complications and the potential for devastating long segment ischemic necrosis of the residual trachea. This knowledge and experience have produced one of the dominant principles in tracheal surgery—skeletonization of the proximal and distal tracheal margins should be performed only to the extent needed to complete the anastomosis, usually 5 to 7 mm. The other two dominant principles of airway reconstructive surgery are resection to a normal

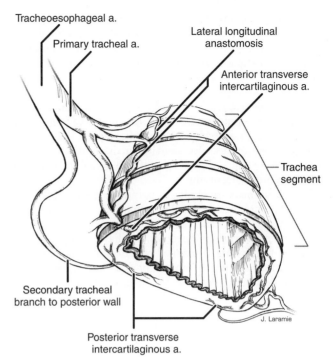

Figure 1
Tracheal blood supply, demonstrating the primary vessels entering the lateral wall of the trachea and showing the lateral longitudinal collaterals and transverse intercartilaginous collaterals. Note the relatively avascular plane along the anterior tracheal wall.

airway and completion of a tension-free anastomosis. Tracheal release maneuvers are fundamental to achieving these goals.

■ STANDARD TRACHEAL RELEASE MANEUVERS

Routine tracheal release maneuvers are the dissection of the avascular pretracheal plane and neck flexion. Both of these procedures are simple and effective and should be performed routinely for all resections of the trachea or carina. These two maneuvers provide assurance of a tension-free anastomosis in nearly all short-segment tracheal resections and are the only airway release maneuvers required in over 90% of patients. At the University of Washington, primary tracheal resection and reconstruction of segments up to 6.5 cm have been performed using these release maneuvers alone.

Early experience with tracheal resection showed that up to 2 cm could be resected and reconstructed without any specific release procedures. It is difficult to quantify the additional length of resection allowed by dissection of the avascular pretracheal plane, but this probably allows an additional 1 to 2 cm of resection. Development of the pretracheal plane is a simple procedure that also helps with surgical exposure. It should be performed routinely early in the dissection for tracheal resection. From a cervical approach, this is similar to development of the plane for mediastinoscopy, directly incising the pretracheal fascia and performing digital blunt dissection over the anterior surface of the trachea down to the carina and mainstem bronchi (Figure 2).

The mediastinoscope and its dissector are sometimes useful in complete dissection of this plane and allow an extension of the dissection over each mainstem bronchus beyond what can be reached with digital dissection alone. For transthoracic tracheal or carinal resection, this plane can be developed in reverse, inserting a finger along the pretracheal plane cephalad and bluntly dissecting up to the level of the thyroid isthmus. Occasionally, mediastinoscopy before the transthoracic approach is helpful to widely develop this plane before thoracotomy.

Previous mediastinoscopy or paratracheal dissection may make this mobilization of the pretracheal plane extremely difficult and less effective. In cases of a proximal lung cancer with potential carinal resection, mediastinoscopy is best deferred to the time of planned resection so as not to compromise this important component of airway mobilization.

Neck flexion and extension have a major impact on tracheal tension. There is wide variability among individuals in the amount of cervical versus intrathoracic trachea with the head in a neutral position. In a young person with a flexible long neck, as much as 60% of the trachea may lie above the thoracic inlet on full neck extension. Conversely, neck flexion devolves the cervical trachea into the mediastinum and, in this same individual, may result in the cricoid cartilage lying at the level of the thoracic inlet with a total intrathoracic trachea. Mulliken and Grillo demonstrated in their human cadaver studies that 15 to 35 degrees of neck flexion would allow a tracheal sleeve resection of just over 7 tracheal rings or 4.5 cm of trachea and still permit end to end anastomosis with tension of less than 1200 g. From this experience we can extrapolate that moderate neck flexion of up to 35 degrees adds approximately 2.5 cm of resectable trachea beyond the known 2 cm that could be resected before the development of airway release maneuvers. This degree of neck flexion is usually comfortable for the patient. If needed, further neck flexion beyond 35 degrees may permit resection of an additional 1 to 1.5 cm of trachea, but this may be more uncomfortable to maintain for the patient in the postoperative period.

During the exposure and resection of a tracheal lesion via a cervical approach, the neck is maximally extended by use of a roll underneath the shoulders. When the anastomotic sutures have been placed, but before being tied, the shoulder roll can be removed and the neck flexed forward by the anesthesiologist, bringing the proximal and distal tracheal ends together for a tension-free anastomosis (Figure 3). The head flexion is not simply an elevation of the head, as for intubation, but is an actual rotation of the head forward, bringing the chin down toward the manubrium.

There are several ways to maintain this position in the postoperative period. Some have developed elaborate neck braces to prevent postoperative neck extension. The simplest, least expensive, and probably most effective technique, however, is to place a guardian suture from the chin to the upper anterior chest. At the completion of the procedure with the neck in the desired position, a heavy suture is placed just posterior to the tip of the chin and deep within the presternal soft tissue at the level of the sternal manubrial junction (Figure 3, inset). It is important to not be overzealous in tightness of the suture, positioning the patient in a more flexed position than is necessary, which may be uncomfortable in the postoperative period. When only a minimal amount of tracheal length is excised, it may be adequate to allow the head to be in a neutral position, using the guardian suture to prevent postoperative neck extension by the patient. These sutures are effective reminders for the patient during sleep or other unconscious movement, to prevent neck extension beyond the degree determined at time of surgery. There is no scientifically established period of time that these guardian sutures stay in place, but the most common practice in major centers is to keep these in place for 7 days postoperatively, at which time the guardian suture is removed. At that time the patient is instructed to consciously avoid neck extension—a restriction that he or she gradually forgets simultaneous with a progressive healing that no longer requires movement restriction.

The process is similar for patients with transthoracic tracheal resections except that in a lateral position, the anesthesiologist will flex the head forward at the appropriate time and place towels or blankets behind the head to maintain

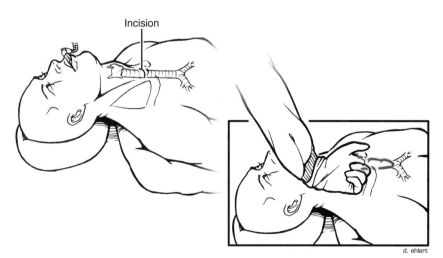

Incision

Figure 2
Development of the avascular pretracheal plane is an essential component of airway mobilization and should be performed routinely.

d. ehlert

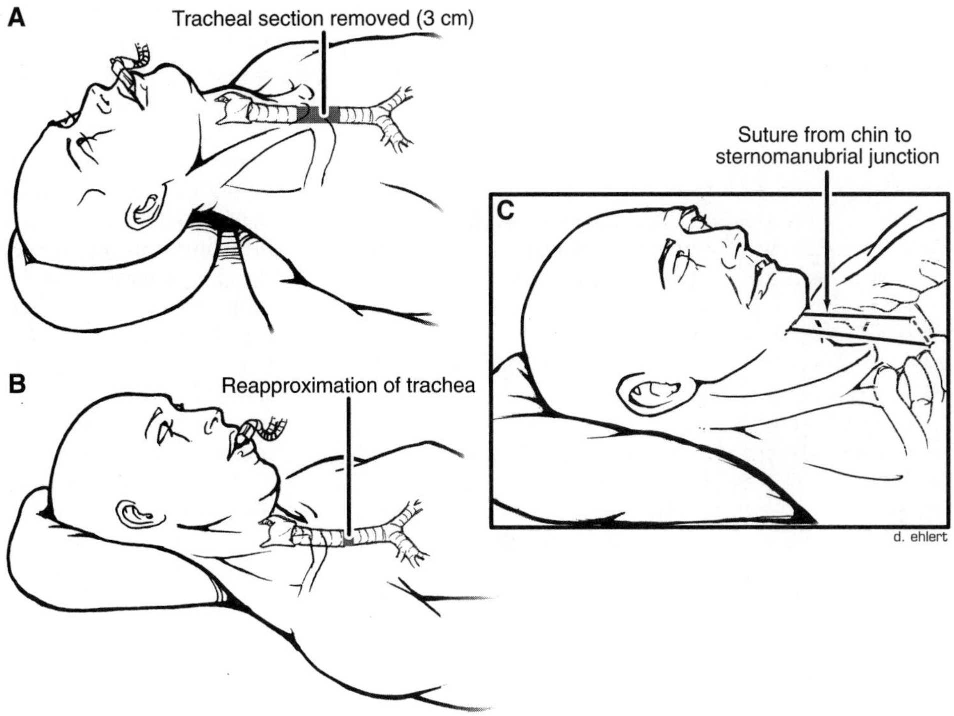

A   Tracheal section removed (3 cm)

B   Reapproximation of trachea

C   Suture from chin to sternomanubrial junction

d. ehlert

Figure 3
Although the routine position of neck extension results in a long gap between proximal and distal tracheal segments **(A)**, neck flexion allows the cervical trachea to descend into the mediastinum, allowing resection of longer segments and maintaining a tension-free anastomosis **(B)**. Placement of a "guardian" suture between the chin and the sternomanubrial junction helps to maintain the neck flexion in the early postoperative period **(C)**.

this position. The most critical time to directly and manually support the flexed position is during emergence from general anesthesia and the early time in the postanesthesia care unit. The guardian suture is an effective reminder when the patient is awake and alert, but before this time he or she may inadvertently pull against the guardian suture without recognizing painful feedback. This requires diligence of the surgical, anesthesia, and nursing team during extubation and the immediate postoperative period.

There is a large degree of variability in the range of neck flexion and overall less cervical mobility with advancing age. Previous cervical spine pathology, kyphosis, and advancing age may all diminish the potential benefit desired from neck flexion alone. However, neck flexion combined with pretracheal dissection is all that is required to reduce anastomotic tension in the vast majority of airway resective procedures.

■ SELECTIVE TRACHEAL RELEASE MANEUVERS

When there is still excessive anastomotic tension despite the maneuvers of pretracheal dissection and neck flexion, two additional selective maneuvers may be used—laryngeal release and/or hilar release. A laryngeal release maneuver is necessary in approximately 8% of patients undergoing tracheal resection for postintubation injuries and approximately 15% of patients undergoing resection for tracheal tumors. A laryngeal release may provide 2 to 3 cm of additional tracheal mobility. However, this transmits only to the proximal trachea and does not have much use in improving mobility for resections in the distal trachea and carina.

Two types of laryngeal release maneuvers have been described: infrahyoid laryngeal release described by Dedo and Fishman and the suprahyoid laryngeal release reported by Montgomery.

The infrahyoid laryngeal release involves division of the thyrohyoid muscle along the superior border of the larynx and bilateral division of the superior cornu of the larynx. Sternohyoid and omohyoid muscles are preserved and the thyrohyoid membrane is divided to allow the larynx to drop away from the hyoid cartilage, providing a total caudal laryngeal mobilization of approximately 2 to 3 cm. Some authors have added division of the inferior constrictor muscles that are attached to the posterior border of the thyroid cartilage to maximize its caudal mobilization. The major complication of this technique is a common occurrence of postoperative odynophagia and aspiration. In the original report of Dedo and Fishman, the return of swallowing function took 3 to 14 days, but other authors have reported a significant incidence of long-term swallowing difficulties after the infrahyoid laryngeal release.

Montgomery developed the suprahyoid release in which the larynx, cricoid, and proximal trachea are released by dividing the suprahyoid laryngeal suspensory attachments. This technique involves division of the stylohyoid, mylohyoid, geniohyoid, and genioglossus muscles along with bilateral division of the hyoid bone anterior to the digastric muscle attachments (Figure 4). This allows the hyoid and laryngeal apparatus to descend 2 to 3 cm caudally for similar mobilization as that achieved by an infrahyoid laryngeal release. The supraglottic approach is generally preferred due to fewer problems with postoperative swallowing dysfunction compared with the infrahyoid approach, while yielding similar degrees of proximal tracheal mobilization. However, even

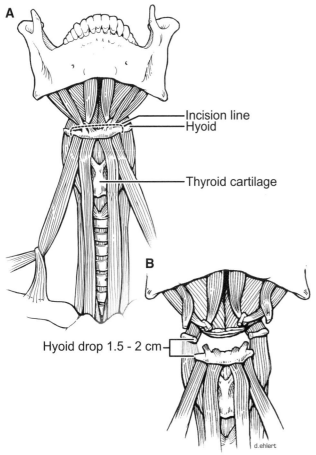

A

Incision line
Hyoid

Thyroid cartilage

B

Hyoid drop 1.5 - 2 cm

d.ehlert

Figure 4
A suprahyoid laryngeal release (of Montgomery) divides the hyoid attachments of the stylohyoid, mylohyoid, geniohyoid, and genioglossus muscles and divides the hyoid bone anterior to the insertions of the digastric muscles.

patients who have the suprahyoid release have a greater problem with postoperative aspiration and swallowing difficulties than do those without a laryngeal release; therefore, this maneuver should be performed only when routine mobilization techniques are inadequate to provide a low tension anastomosis.

The infrahyoid and suprahyoid release maneuvers can be performed through the standard neck incision used for a cervical tracheal resection. Because a laryngeal release adds negligible tracheal mobility to the distal trachea, it is rarely useful to add this maneuver to a transthoracic distal tracheal or carinal resection.

Hilar release maneuvers provide significant mobilization of the mainstem bronchus, allowing the carina and distal trachea to be mobilized more cephalad and release anastomotic tension in the lower trachea. A hilar release provides little mobility to the upper cervical trachea and is not often used for proximal tracheal resections. However, it may be occasionally useful for added mobility in a cervical resection of a long airway lesion that extends into the distal portion of the trachea, requiring a separate thoracotomy or thoracoscopy for distal mobilization.

For most distal tracheal or carinal resections, a right hilar release is performed during a right thoracotomy approach, which is the primary approach for most distal airway procedures. However, a right-sided release can also be accomplished through a median sternotomy and with a thoracoscopy if necessary. A left-sided hilar release can also be performed for additional mobility but is less gratifying than a right-sided hilar release because the left mainstem bronchus and hilum are still restricted by the aortic arch. In an extensive carinal resection with concomitant pneumonectomy, a contralateral thoracotomy or thoracoscopy may be necessary to achieve adequate mobilization of the remaining lung to achieve primary reconstruction. This should be anticipated and performed as the initial step of the operation to avoid an inadequate resection or a difficult or impossible reconstruction.

A hilar release has progressive components depending on the degree of mobilization required. Division of the pulmonary ligament during a right thoracotomy for airway resection should be a routine part of the procedure allowing the hilum to rise in a more cephalad direction. When additional mobilization is required, this can be accomplished with a partial or complete pericardial release. The primary component of this is a U-shaped incision in the pericardium around the anterior, caudal, and posterior aspect of the inferior pulmonary vein (Figure 5). Division of the pericardial reflection attached to the atrium and vena cava completes this maneuver, which allows 2 to 3 cm of cephalad mobilization of the right hilum and right main stem bronchus. An additional 0.5 to 1 cm of mobilization can be obtained by completing a circumferential pericardial division around the hilum. When this is performed, care should be taken to maintain the bronchial artery blood supply and the hilar and subcarinal nodal blood supply, which may provide important collaterals to the distal trachea.

■ CONCLUSION

Tracheal release maneuvers have allowed progressively longer and more aggressive airway resections with primary reconstruction. Until a satisfactory prosthetic conduit is available for tracheal replacement, maneuvers to mobilize the trachea and provide a tension-free anastomosis are critical for the success of tracheal surgery. Optimal results are dependent on careful preoperative planning with bronchoscopy, knowledge of the tracheal blood supply, and the progressive maneuvers for achieving an anastomosis without tension. Pretracheal dissection and neck flexion should be a routine part of every tracheal or carinal resection and provide adequate mobilization in the vast majority of cases. When mobilization is required in the proximal trachea, a suprahyoid laryngeal release can produce 2 to 3 cm of additional tracheal length. For distal tracheal and carinal lesions, a hilar release provides the same degree of mobility to the distal airway. Airway surgery experience, meticulous surgical technique, and attention to the tenets of tracheal surgery—resect to normal airway, maintain tracheal blood supply, and tension-free anastomosis—are critical for the success of tracheal reconstructive procedures.

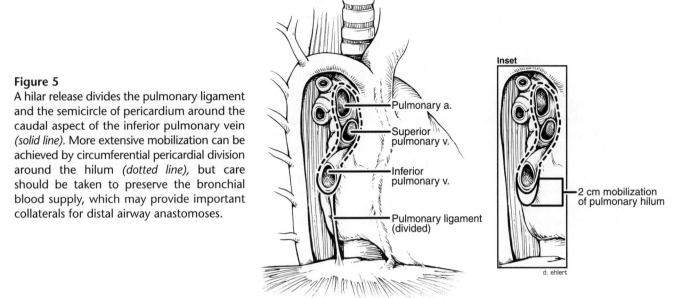

Figure 5
A hilar release divides the pulmonary ligament and the semicircle of pericardium around the caudal aspect of the inferior pulmonary vein *(solid line)*. More extensive mobilization can be achieved by circumferential pericardial division around the hilum *(dotted line),* but care should be taken to preserve the bronchial blood supply, which may provide important collaterals for distal airway anastomoses.

SUGGESTED READING

Grillo HC: Notes on the wind pipe, *Ann Thorac Surg* 47:9, 1989.
Heitmiller RF: Tracheal release maneuvers, *Chest Surg Clin North Am* 6:675, 1996.
Montgomery WW: Suprahyoid release for tracheal anastomosis, *Arch Otolaryngol* 99:255, 1974.
Mulliken JB, Grillo HC: The limits of tracheal resection with primary anastomosis, *J Thorac Cardiovasc Surg* 55:418, 1968.
Salassa JR, et al: Gross and microscopical blood supply of the trachea, *Ann Thorac Surg* 24:100, 1977.

ACQUIRED TRACHEOESOPHAGEAL FISTULA

Paolo Macchiarini

The vast majority of acquired benign tracheoesophageal fistulas (TEFs) are due to pressure necrosis at the site of a cuffed tracheal or tracheostomy tube (Table 1). This injury can progress, in the presence of excessive tube motion or concomitant comorbidity (e.g., infections, hypotension, steroids, diabetes), to a full-thickness perforation of the tracheal and esophageal wall, especially when the inflated cuff compresses a rigid nasogastric tube against the fixed prevertebral plane. This etiology explains why TEFs usually occur at the cervical or, less frequently, at the intrathoracic level near the carina.

■ CLINICAL PRESENTATION AND DIAGNOSTIC INVESTIGATIONS

Timely diagnosis is one of the keys to the successful management of patients with a TEF. In many cases, the history

Table 1 Etiology Other Than Postintubation of Acquired Benign Tracheoesophageal Fistula
Blunt or penetrating neck and thoracic trauma
Granulomatous mediastinal infections
Immunodeficiency syndrome
Foreign bodies
Complications after cervical spine or head and neck surgery
Transhiatal esophagectomy

will be obvious—patients have a history of recent intubation. Often, however, the clinical presentation is not so obvious and varies according to whether the patient is still mechanically ventilated (Table 2). Usually, there is no appreciable abnormality seen in plain chest films and tomograms, except some nonspecific signs like dilation of the distal esophagus and herniation of the sealing cuff outside the tracheal wall. Computed tomography (CT) or three-dimensional spiral CT of the neck may be helpful but lack anatomic details. By contrast, bronchoscopy (1) confirms clinical suspicion; (2) exactly defines the site of the TEF; (3) determines its relationship to the vocal cords, carina, and orifice of the tracheotomy; and (4) establishes the presence of circumferential stenosis, inflammation, or injury of the tracheal wall. Esophagoscopy is usually less informative but important to assess the status of the distal esophagus (e.g., reflux or reactive esophagitis or hiatal hernia). Contrast esophagography may be diagnostic but cannot delineate the exact anatomic extension of esophageal defects.

■ THERAPEUTIC INDICATIONS

Spontaneous closure is very uncommon and observed only in a small minority (<1%) of patients weaned off the ventilator with a very small TEF located at the cervical level and those with minimal symptoms or clinical signs of sepsis, for which an open cervical drainage, draining gastrostomy, and feeding jejunostomy usually are curative. Some other patients (5% to 9%) are never weaned from ventilatory support because the underlying disease has a fatal outcome and the conditions of the tissues surrounding the fistula do not ensure satisfactory healing. In these circumstances, a curative surgical repair is not possible and the therapeutic goals are to place a definitive new tracheostomy tube and, more important, the cuff below the TEF, to remove the nasogastric tube, and to place a gastrostomy and feeding jejunostomy. These maneuvers usually permit adequate ventilatory support and nutrition and prevent pulmonary infection and ongoing soilage. More aggressive surgery, including an esophageal diversion, is usually associated with high mortality and morbidity, and the outcome is almost always fatal.

The vast majority (90%) of patients with an acquired benign TEF are, however, curable with surgical repair, provided that certain preoperative guidelines are fully respected.

■ PREOPERATIVE MANAGEMENT

The following are the cardinal principles on how to preoperatively manage a patient with acquired benign TEF: (1) delay the operative repair until ventilatory support is no longer required, (2) hemodynamically stabilize the patient, (3) prevent pulmonary complications by removing the indwelling nasogastric tube (increases ischemia of the party tracheoesophageal wall and favors gastroesophageal reflux), (4) place a new low-pressure, high-volume (long) tracheostomy tube whose cuff remains below the TEF (minimizes soiling of the tracheobronchial tree, cough-swallow syndrome, and repeated pulmonary infections), and (5) place a draining gastrostomy (prevents gastroesophageal reflux) and feeding jejunostomy (achieves satisfactory nutrition). Fluid resuscitation, systemic antibiotics, respirator support, and nutritional support, although essential, may be totally ineffective if the five cardinal principles are not realized.

These critical principles usually improve the general and local conditions (e.g., catabolic status, bacteremia, aspiration pneumonitis, ischemia of the fistulous tissues) so drastically that surgical repair can then be performed in the majority of cases with excellent results.

■ OPERATIVE TECHNIQUES

A TEF is usually repaired either with direct closure of the tracheal and esophageal defects with or without pedicled muscle flaps or with segmental tracheal resection and anastomosis with esophageal closure. Both procedures usually require a cervical or cervicomediastinal incision only. Only those rare TEFs located just above or near the carina must be accessed via a right posterolateral thoracotomy through the fourth intercostal space, although in my personal experience, a transpericardial approach through a median sternotomy can be safely performed, provided the patient has no active general or local infection.

The ideal candidate for the direct tracheal and esophageal closure is the spontaneously breathing patient who has a small and very well localized fistula with a morphologically normal trachea. Segmental tracheal resection and anastomosis with esophageal closure should be reserved for those patients whose tracheal defect is either too large to allow direct closure or near to totally circumferential. Because the

Table 2 Signs and Symptoms of Acquired Tracheoesophageal Fistula	
MECHANICALLY VENTILATED PATIENTS	**WEANING PATIENTS**
Sudden, massive bloated abdomen	Marked increase of saliva in the trachea
Abnormal secretions in and/or aspiration of liquids from the airway	Airway aspiration of feeding/gastric contents or bile
Suction of gastric contents or tube feedings from the airway	Cough while swallowing (liquids or particulate food in the tracheal aspirate)
Repeated and unexplained pneumonia (RLL)	Repeated gastric juice aspiration in GER patients
Cuff air-tightness cannot be obtained	
Unexplained egress of gases on the machine	

RLL, right lower lobe; GER, gastroesophageal reflux.

diagnosis of TEF is now made earlier, esophageal diversion is becoming rarer.

The anesthetic management differs depending on whether a tracheostomy is present. In patients without a tracheostomy but who have a small TEF, and normal trachea, a small orotracheal tube (<7 mm) can be passed distal to the lesion. In patients with a tracheostomy and more severe damages, ventilation can be best provided through an orotracheal tube placed just proximal to the tracheal defect, while delivering small ventilation volumes to avoid esophageal distention; meanwhile, the tracheostomy orifice is manually obliterated. If the degree of the tracheal stenosis is subocclusive, an endotracheal or long tracheotomy tube is passed through the tracheostomy orifice beyond the diseased tracheoesophageal segment. Once the airway is resected, ventilation is provided through a cross-field sterile tube placed into the distal trachea. For TEFs located just above the carina, the airway can be secured by using the former method or inserting a double-lumen tube into the left main bronchus. An alternative technique would be to insert two high-jet ventilation catheters into both main bronchi, but this method is complicated, risky, and mostly ineffective.

Direct Closure of the Tracheal and Esophageal Defects

A cervical approach is used for all lesions located at least 3 cm above the carina. The patient is placed in the supine position with a small roll beneath the shoulder, with the head hyperextended and resting on a rubber ring turned to the right. The tracheal stoma is first excluded from the operative field. The incision is made on the anteromedial border of the left sternocleidomastoid muscle, covering the lower two-thirds distance between the left ear lobe and sternal notch; if required, this can be eventually extended down the midline over the upper portion of the sternum. The subcutaneous tissues and platysma muscle are divided, sparing the branch of the cervical cutaneous nerve that lies in the upper third of the field, thereby avoiding hypoaesthesia and dysaesthesia in the submandibular skin area. The sternocleidomastoid muscle is dissected away from the underlying muscles, and the omohyoid and prethyroid muscles are divided to expose the jugular vein, carotid artery, and thyroid gland. The middle thyroid vein (if present) and the inferior thyroid artery are ligated and divided; this allows forward and contralateral retraction of the thyroid, pharynx, and larynx, putting the deep cervical fascia under tension (Figure 1). The recurrent laryngeal nerve is then exposed but not dissected in the tracheoesophageal groove. There usually are sequelae of local inflammation, which makes identification of the nerve difficult. It is therefore wiser to identify it, in these situations, at a location remote from the fistula and to protect it from retractor injuries. Unfortunately, identification of the fistulous tract may not be simple and usually requires a more extensive and circumferential dissection than expected. Practically, dissection is relatively simple above the fistula but more difficult below its lower limit. This is because the incision gives a limited operative field, even after partial upper sternotomy and lateral retraction of the trachea (mobilization of the trachea is usually limited by the rigidity of the endotracheal tube).

Once the fistulous tract has been dissected and excluded, it is divided. This process is sometimes more hazardous

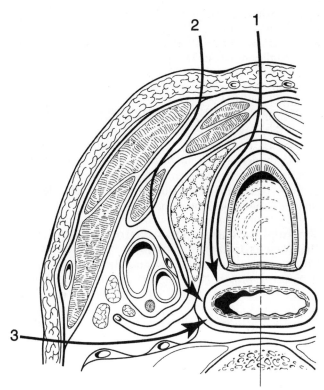

Figure 1
Among the different approaches to the tracheoesophageal groove (1, medial to the thyroid; 2, lateral to the sternocleidomastoid muscle; 3, dorsal to the sternocleidomastoid muscle), the one between the thyroid gland and the carotid-jugular vessels is the less traumatic and ischemic and gives a more anatomic view and safer exposure to the lesion.

at the tracheal than the esophageal level because the tracheal membranous dehiscence is usually longer and larger than that expected from the preoperative endoscopic evaluation and there usually is some mediastinal scar around the tracheal split. A simple means to avoid an excessive and irreversible tracheal division is to keep, in the tracheal division line, a small autologous patch of the surrounding esophagus. Closure of the membranous tracheal defect can then be accomplished directly using interrupted sutures of 4-0 polydioxanone (PDS; Ethicon, Inc., Sommerville, NJ) placed gently to include an esophageal patch, tying the knots outside the lumen. Indirect tracheal closure with the transposition and suture of surrounding strap muscles should be avoided because it is often associated with some degree of late tracheal stenosis or granulation. The esophageal defect is then repaired with a two-layer closure using interrupted 4-0 polyglactin (Vicryl; Ethicon, Inc.), after complete exposure of the mucosal defect and débridement of all devitalized mucosa beyond the fistulous edges.

The need to buttress the repair with a pedicle flap of strap muscle is debatable because it may compress the overlapping suture lines. Alternatively, the esophagus may be mobilized, rotated, and fixated to the prevertebral plane to separate the suture lines. This, however, requires further esophageal dissection and devascularization. Concomitant with the

Table 3 Advantages of the Two-Layer Direct Esophageal Closure With Tracheal Resection And Anastomosis

Fashioned by an anterior incision
No extensive tracheal devascularization
Larger operative field with complete exposure
One-stage tracheal repair
Muscle interpositions or esophageal rotation are unnecessary because anastomoses do not overlap

primary repair, the mediastinum must be débrided and drained to abort the septic process.

Tracheal Resection and Anastomosis With Primary Esophageal Closure

This technique has several advantages over the previously described approach (Table 3). The patient is placed in the supine position with a small inflatable pillow beneath the shoulder and the head hyperextended. An anterior cervical U-shaped incision is used (Figure 2), incorporating the tracheostomy stoma if present. Similar to that used for a tracheal resection, the skin, subcutaneous fat, and platysma are elevated as one layer and the flap is raised to the level of the suprahyoid region. Inferiorly, the incision can be extended vertically just below the manubrial notch, if needed; after an upper sternotomy, the anterior mediastinum can be fully exposed. Although median sternotomy invites the potential for sternal osteomyelitis and mediastinitis, it may be used for those TEFs located near or just above the carina.

The sternohyoid muscles are divided in the midline, and the thyroid isthmus is divided and ligated to expose the anterior surface of the trachea. The trachea is freed circumferentially only above and below the site of the fistula. Care is taken to maintain the dissection as close as possible to the outer tracheal surface to avoid injury to both recurrent laryngeal nerves while preserving the lateral blood supply to the unresected trachea. The trachea is then divided above and below the damaged area, through healthy tissue, placing two lateral traction sutures in the distal tracheal wall. It is of paramount importance to ensure that the cut tracheal end has a normal diameter and mucosal appearance. Once the distal airway is divided, ventilation is usually obtained by inserting a cross-field endotracheal tube into the distal tracheal airway. The original endotracheal tube is withdrawn by the anesthetist, and its tip is secured with silk sutures, so that it may be guided back easily through the glottis when the anastomosis is being completed.

Opening the airway gives a complete exposure to the esophageal defect (Figure 3A). The edges of the esophageal defect are débrided and a two-layer closure, as described earlier, is made over a nasogastric tube, because narrowing of the esophagus to this degree is well tolerated (Figure 3B and 3C). After closure of the esophageal defect, the tracheal ends are reapproximated in an end-to-end manner using a continuous 4-0 PDS suture on the membranous wall and interrupted 3-0 Vicryl on the remaining anterior cartilaginous wall. Before completing the anastomosis, the distal ventilation system is removed and the original endotracheal tube is advanced past the anastomosis line, using the previously placed traction suture for guidance.

Excessive anastomotic tension should be avoided by limiting the length of tracheal resection and by performing a tracheal mobilization or laryngeal release maneuver. Of these, the suprathyroid release is preferred because it does not risk injury to the superior recurrent nerve and, thus, disorders of deglutition. The tracheal stoma can be simply resected or left in place if patients require postoperative mechanical ventilation or when the extent of the tracheal damage does not permit tracheal reconstruction. In these situations, it should be left in place and closed later with a myoplasty.

If the length of the posterior defect of the membranous wall and damaged trachea exceeds the amount of trachea that can be safely resected, one can close the posterior defect longitudinally along the membranous tracheal wall, borrowing some esophageal wall if needed. This limits the amount of trachea to be resected and allows reconstruction that otherwise would be impossible. However, it can be done only if

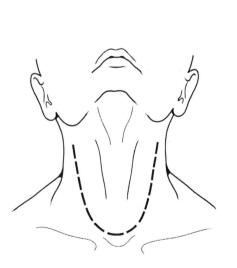 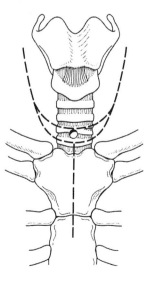

Figure 2
U-shaped cervical incision. The tracheal stoma can be simply resected (right) while performing the collar incision if it does not directly communicate with the fistula.

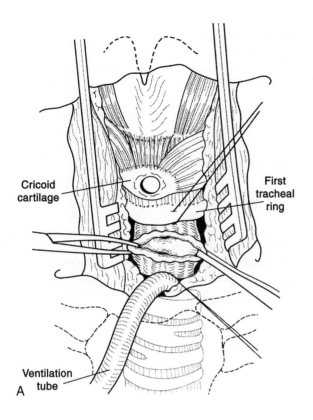

Cricoid cartilage

First tracheal ring

Ventilation tube

A

Figure 3
(A) Exposure and repair of the esophageal defect after tracheal resection. The diseased trachea is divided above and below the damaged area (including the stoma), and ventilation is obtained by inserting a cross-field endotracheal tube into the distal airway. The esophageal defect is held up between forceps to exposure to the muscularis and mucosa. **(B)** Débridement of both esophageal walls is necessary to avoid healing problems. A two-layer closure with interrupted sutures is performed over a nasogastric tube. **(C)** The muscularis is dissected from the mucosa over 180 degrees so that a more solid mucosa plate can be sutured.

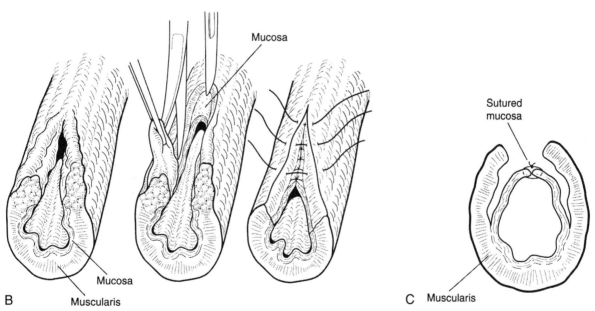

Mucosa

Mucosa

Muscularis

B

Sutured mucosa

C   **Muscularis**

the cartilaginous tracheal wall is healthy. For those situations where the length of the tracheal damage exceeds the limits of reconstruction, closure should still be attempted by buttressing it with strap muscle and maintaining an open airway with a tracheal T tube, thereby permitting definitive oral alimentation and avoiding permanent feeding tubes.

Esophageal Diversion
Esophageal diversion may be useful when the above described techniques are not possible, especially in hemodynamically unstable patients who cannot tolerate a prolonged anesthesia episode or extensive mediastinal manipulation. A combination of cervical esophagostomy (Figure 4), gastrostomy, stapling proximal and distal to the perforation, and T-tube drainage may be used as diversionary techniques. The stapled-off (but not divided) esophagus has a remarkable ability to reestablish its own continuity, regardless of whether absorbable or nonabsorbable staples are used. However, one should keep in mind that (1) continuity should be reestablished at a later date (with stomach or colon), (2) the creation of

Table 4 Results After Surgical Repair of Postintubation Tracheoesophageal Fistulas

| Author (year) | No. of Patients | TYPE OF OPERATION, n | | | TEF Recurrence, n (%) | Mortality, n (%) |
		Simple Closure	TR + EC	ED		
Couraud et al (1989)	16	9	5	2		1 (6)
Mathisen et al (1991)	38	9	29	-	3 (8)	4 (10)
Macchiarini et al (2000)	32	15	14	3	1 (3)	1 (3)
Total	86	33	48	5	4 (5)	6 (7)

EC, esophageal closure; ED, esophageal diversion; TEF, tracheoesophageal fistula; TR, tracheal resection.

a blind esophageal pouch can be a major source of pulmonary sepsis and increases dead space ventilation, and (3) a stricture may occur at the injured site left to heal by scarring.

Esophageal diversion is by far the most complicated, risky, and invariably successful surgical repair of TEFs and therefore should be reserved for (1) large TEFs located just above or near the carina, (2) persistence of tracheobronchial soilage after conservative maneuvers, (3) necrotic and infective neck lesions that are jeopardizing anastomotic healing, and (4) patients who can never be extubated after closure.

■ RESULTS

Table 4 details the worldwide surgical experience with acquired benign TEF. In our experience, esophageal closure

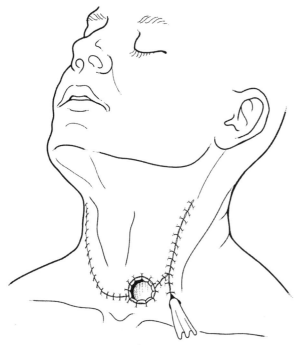

Figure 4
An end esophagostomy for esophageal diversion.

combined with tracheal resection and reconstruction resulted in a significantly lower incidence of tracheal complications (tracheal granulomas or stenosis requiring laser or reoperation) and better long-term results, suggesting that it should be the preferred type of repair for acquired benign TEFs.

■ CONCLUSION

Acquired benign TEFs usually result from erosion of the tracheal and esophageal walls by an endotracheal or a tracheostomy tube cuff, especially when a rigid nasogastric tube is in place. Despite the fact that TEFs have become infrequent with the use of high-volume, low-pressure cuffs, they still represent a life-threatening condition. Most are diagnosed in patients who are mechanically ventilated and, due to the negative effects of positive-pressure ventilation on tracheal suture lines, repair should be delayed until patients are weaned. In the interim, the nasogastric tube should be withdrawn, a tracheostomy tube should be placed so that the balloon rests below the site of the fistula, and draining gastrostomy and feeding jejunostomy tubes suppress gastroesophageal reflux and permit adequate nutrition, respectively. This strategy usually avoids the soilage of the tracheobronchial tree, deterioration of pulmonary function, and need of esophageal diversion. After the patient is weaned from the ventilator, a one-staged anterior approach that includes esophageal two-layer closure and segmental tracheal resection and primary reconstruction definitely corrects the fistula and removes concurrent tracheal disease; this should be regarded as the preferred type of surgical repair.

SUGGESTED READING

Couraud L, et al: Treatment of esophago-tracheal fistulae secondary to respiratory intensive care, *Ann Chir* 43:677, 1989.

Dartevelle P, Macchiarini P: Management of acquired tracheo-esophageal fistula. In Mathisen DJ, editor: *The trachea, Chest Surg Clin North Am*, Philadelphia, 1996, WB Saunders, p 819.

Macchiarini P, et al: Evaluation and outcome of different surgical techniques for postintubation tracheoesophageal fistula, *J Thorac Cardiovasc Surg* 119:268, 2000.

Mathisen DJ, et al: Management of acquired nonmalignant tracheoesophageal fistula, *Ann Thorac Surg* 52:759, 1991.

ACQUIRED TRACHEAL STENOSIS

Dean M. Donahue

Acquired tracheal stenosis results from either intrinsic tracheal pathology (postintubation, inflammatory, idiopathic) or extrinsic compression (goiter, vascular rings, mediastinal masses). Postintubation lesions are the most common cause of acquired tracheal stenosis. These injuries result from pressure necrosis created by the endotracheal tube, a tracheostomy tube, or balloon cuffs. These areas of necrosis heal by scar formation, creating varying degrees of airway obstruction. An understanding of the mechanism of injury may aid in reducing the incidence of these preventable lesions.

■ MECHANISM OF INJURY

Pressure from an endotracheal tube that traverses the larynx may cause mucosal ulceration at contact points, such as the vocal cords, the arytenoids, and the cricoid cartilage. Ischemia and necrosis of the tracheal mucosa can occur from overinflation of a low-pressure cuff of an endotracheal tube. This creates a circumferential injury to the tracheal wall that, if the erosion is deep enough, damages all layers of the trachea. These wounds heal by cicatrization, creating a circumferential stenosis. The full-thickness nature of most clinically significant postintubation lesions is important. Because these lesions are full thickness, they are treated definitively by resection and reconstruction. Most stenotic lesions are not amenable to treatment by modalities aimed at the inside of the tracheal lumen, such as laser ablation.

Stenosis also can occur at the insertion site of a tracheostomy tube. Leverage on the tracheostomy tube from attached ventilator tubing can erode part of the tracheal wall. When the tracheostomy tube is removed, the lateral tracheal walls may collapse, creating a triangular-shaped lesion. The posterior wall of the trachea frequently is uninvolved in a stomal stenosis. An improperly placed tracheal stoma also can result in a stenosis. If the tracheostomy is placed too high on the trachea, the tube can erode into the anterior wall of the cricoid cartilage, resulting in a subglottic stenosis.

■ CLINICAL PRESENTATION

Tracheal stenosis should be considered in any previously intubated patient who manifests signs and symptoms of upper airway obstruction. Symptoms depend on the severity of the stenosis and typically progress from dyspnea on exertion to wheezing and ultimately to stridor. As the stenosis evolves, small amounts of mucus may worsen acutely the obstruction at the level of the stenosis.

■ DIAGNOSTIC STUDIES

Bronchoscopy is mandatory in all patients with tracheal stenosis. If tracheal stenosis is suspected, bronchoscopy is best done in the operating room. This allows for rigid bronchoscopy and tracheal dilation if airway compromise develops. Bronchoscopy allows for precise identification of the location and extent of the stenosis. Because these patients have been intubated previously, it is important to evaluate the laryngeal aperture and function completely before proceeding to tracheal reconstruction. A thorough examination and evaluation of vocal cord function is mandatory.

Radiographic studies of the trachea are helpful in defining the extent of a tracheal lesion. Lateral films of the neck can show most lesions in the upper trachea. Patients with an existing tracheostomy stoma or tracheostomy scar should have a radiopaque marker placed on the skin to identify its relationship to the stenosis. Tomograms of the trachea allow for precise measurement of the length of the lesion and the distance from the vocal cords and carina.

Although computed tomography is valuable in assessing local extent of malignant tracheal pathology, it is of lesser value in assessing benign postintubation stenosis. A computed tomography scan is helpful in airway narrowing caused by compression from a substernal goiter or vascular lesions.

In patients with a tracheostomy tube in place, the tube should be removed during radiographic examination. Tube removal must be done with strict supervision, and emergency equipment must be available for immediate tube reinsertion.

■ INDICATIONS FOR SURGERY

Treatment of stenotic lesions depends on the degree of symptomatic airway obstruction. Minimally symptomatic lesions may be followed with attention paid to the onset of dyspnea on exertion. If a lesion produces symptoms that limit the activity of a patient, surgical correction should be considered. In addition, strictures can recur or respond poorly to repeated dilations, and these should be resected. For causes due to extrinsic narrowing, the primary underlying problem (mediastinal mass or vascular ring) should be addressed.

■ TREATMENT OPTIONS

Resection and reconstruction is the treatment of choice for symptomatic tracheal lesions. Optimal timing of the repair is crucial to its success. There are circumstances when definitive surgical repair should be delayed. These include patients who remain on positive-pressure ventilation, the presence of inflammation in the area of the planned resection, and patients on systemic corticosteroids. Repair in these instances may lead to anastomotic dehiscence and restenosis. Patients with tracheal stenosis who present with acute airway obstruction or have contraindications to surgical repair may be managed temporarily with tracheal dilation using a rigid bronchoscope. If immediate restenosis is a concern, a tracheostomy tube or T-tube can be placed while the patient is prepared for surgical repair. Patients without an existing stoma should have the tube placed directly through the lesion itself to avoid damaging uninvolved trachea. If there is a preexisting stoma located away from the site of stenosis, the tube should be replaced with one through the stenosis allowing the old stoma to heal. This tube may provide additional length of trachea to be used for reconstruction. Some patients are at high risk for recurrence after tracheal resection and are best treated long-term with a tracheal T-tube. This group includes patients with long segment stenosis, patients who cannot be weaned off of high-dose steroids, or patients with lesions resulting from radiation treatment of Hodgkin's disease.

■ SURGICAL TECHNIQUE

The procedure begins with rigid bronchoscopy to evaluate the larynx and trachea. If initial inspection reveals that the tracheal lumen is less than 6 mm in diameter, dilators are passed through the bronchoscope; this is followed by passing progressively larger rigid bronchoscopes beyond the stenosis to complete the dilation. This dilation allows placement of an endotracheal tube for ventilation during the early part of the procedure. Measurements are obtained beginning at the carina and defining the inferior border of the stenosis, the superior border of the stenosis, the cricoid cartilage, and the vocal cords. These measurements are necessary in planning the resection and helpful in deciding if a laryngeal release procedure is needed. The extent of local inflammation also should be determined because the presence of intense inflammation may delay definitive surgical correction. These patients are managed temporarily by dilating the stenosis and possibly inserting a Silastic T-tube.

The patient is positioned with the neck hyperextended. In a young person, this brings more than half of the trachea above the sternal notch. The surgical field extends from the chin to below the sternum. Exposure is obtained through a low collar incision, but occasionally an upper sternotomy is required. The upper and lower skin flaps are elevated deep to the platysma from above the cricoid cartilage to the sternal notch. The strap muscles are separated from the midline. The thyroid isthmus is divided between clamps and suture ligated. The anterior surface of the trachea may be dissected safely from the cricoid cartilage to the carina because the blood supply enters the trachea laterally. Successful repair depends on preservation of the blood supply to the trachea, which comes in segmentally. It becomes important not to devascularize the trachea circumferentially over more than a 1- to 2-cm length on either side of the stenosis.

The area of stenosis is usually clearly visible on the outer surface of the trachea due to its full-thickness nature. If the cartilaginous rings are not destroyed, the patient is bronchoscoped, and a small-gauge needle is inserted into the trachea. Under direct vision through the bronchoscope, this needle is positioned to determine the superior aspect of the stenosis. A fine suture is placed on the outer tracheal wall to mark the area of stenosis, and the patient is reintubated.

Circumferential dissection is carried out along the area of the stenosis, keeping the dissection directly on the tracheal wall to avoid injury to the recurrent laryngeal nerves. Tiny blood vessels are cauterized carefully as they are encountered.

The trachea is encircled with a Penrose drain for traction. No more than 1 to 2 cm of normal trachea should be dissected on either side of the area to be resected. This reduces the risk of devascularizing the portion of the trachea that is to be used for reconstruction.

The trachea is divided at the lower level of the stenosis. The patient is intubated across the operative field. The patient is ventilated while the stenotic segment is retracted upward. The dissection continues close to the tracheal wall to avoid injury to the recurrent laryngeal nerves. A rubber catheter is sutured to the endotracheal tube to facilitate replacement of the tube after the repair sutures are placed. The endotracheal tube is withdrawn upward through the vocal cords. Polyglactin 910 (Vicryl) traction sutures are placed on the lateral walls of each end of the trachea 1 cm from the divided edge of the airway. The patient's head is flexed to reduce tension on the repair. The traction sutures are drawn together to evaluate the degree of tension on the anastomosis. If the amount of tension seems excessive, a laryngeal release maneuver is required. The anastomotic sutures are placed in a manner that keeps the knot outside of the tracheal lumen. Each full-thickness suture is placed approximately 3 mm from the cut edge of the trachea. A 4-0 Vicryl suture is placed into approximately the middle of the membranous wall. This posterior suture is the last suture tied and is held by a hemostat at the upper end of the surgical field. Interrupted 4-0 Vicryl sutures are placed individually toward the operator's side of the field; this is continued to the level of the lateral traction suture. Sutures are placed from the initial midline stitch sewing away from the operator's side to the level of the lateral traction stitch on the opposite side of the field. Each of these sutures is secured individually to the side of the drapes with hemostats. The endotracheal tube can be removed from the distal end of the trachea intermittently to facilitate placement of the sutures. The sutures for the anterior portion of the trachea are placed anterior to the lateral traction sutures. These are all clipped to the drapes below the incision. When all sutures have been placed, the endotracheal tube is advanced through the vocal cords into the distal trachea. The patient's head is positioned to maintain the neck in flexion. The lateral traction sutures on each side are tied, approximating the ends of the trachea. The anastomotic sutures are tied beginning with the anterior tracheal wall sutures. The trachea is rotated slightly by gently pulling each lateral traction suture to facilitate tying of the posterior sutures. If possible, the thyroid isthmus is approximated over the anastomosis. A drain is inserted lateral to the incision and placed in the pretracheal plane. The strap muscles are approximated, and the platysma and skin are closed with subcutaneous sutures. At the conclusion of the procedure, a heavy suture is placed from the submental crease to the presternal skin to maintain the neck in flexion.

■ POSTOPERATIVE MANAGEMENT

Patients wake up and are extubated in the operating room. The surgeon must assess the airway and be certain that the anastomosis is satisfactory. If there is concern that the airway is not satisfactory, a tracheostomy is performed through a small vertical incision away from the anastomosis. The anastomosis should be covered with either mobilized thyroid isthmus or pedicled strap muscle flap. In general, tracheostomy rarely is needed. In our own series, only 27 of 503 patients required a tracheostomy. This typically was due to laryngeal edema or vocal cord paralysis, but some were done routinely early in our experience with laryngotracheal reconstruction. We now find the routine use of tracheostomies in this patient population unnecessary.

The patients are observed overnight in an intensive care unit, watching for signs of tachypnea, dyspnea, or stridor. Oral intake usually is begun under close observation with a thick liquid or soft solid diet. Thin liquids are avoided initially. If a laryngeal reconstruction was performed, or if there is hoarseness, oral intake is delayed further. The surgical drains are managed based on their output, typically being removed by the second postoperative day. Although it is usually not needed, flexible bronchoscopy may be done postoperatively to evaluate the larynx and anastomosis and clear any retained secretions. The guardian chin stitch is cut on the seventh postoperative day.

RESULTS

We reported our series of 503 patients who underwent tracheal resection and reconstruction for postintubation tracheal stenosis. There were 440 patients with a good result categorized by completely normal function and bronchoscopic evaluation. The results were satisfactory in 31 patients who either could perform normal activities but were stressed on exercise or had abnormalities such as a paralyzed or partially paralyzed vocal cord. There were 20 failures treated with tracheostomy ($n = 11$), T-tube ($n = 7$), or dilations ($n = 2$). The average length of follow-up was 3 years.

There were 12 perioperative deaths, with anastomotic dehiscence accounting for 7 deaths. Two patients were on ventilators at the time of resection, and three required postoperative reintubation for retained secretions. One patient required early reintubation and reoperation to stabilize a flail chest. One patient had received mediastinal irradiation for Hodgkin's disease and failed to heal despite omental wrapping. Two patients had a tracheal–innominate artery fistula after dehiscence. One patient had isolated tracheal–innominate artery hemorrhage, probably because of intraoperative trauma. Two patients died of airway obstruction secondary to residual tracheal malacia. There was one postoperative fatal myocardial infarction. One patient died at home with respiratory failure of unknown cause.

There were 53 patients who had previous resection and reconstruction. In 75.5% of these patients, the outcome was good; in comparison, 86% of patients without prior resection and reconstruction had good results. The failure rate of this group was 5.6% with a 3.8% mortality, comparing unfavorably with 3.6% and 2.1% in the group without prior resection. Despite a high proportion of good results (87%), reconstruction after tracheal surgery led to the highest failure rate. Previous T-tube placement, laser therapy, or tracheoesophageal fistula repair did not seem to affect outcome adversely.

Results varied slightly depending on the level of anastomosis. The failure rate progressively increased with a higher level of anastomosis. The failure rates were 2.2% for

a trachea-to-trachea anastomosis, 6.0% for a trachea-to-cricoid anastomosis, and 8.1% for a trachea-to-thyroid anastomosis. Minor complications also became more prevalent with each level, from 16% to 17.1% to 21% with major complication rates of 13.9%, 15.4%, and 12.9%.

Of patients, 49 had a laryngeal release procedure to reduce tension on the anastomosis. The average length of resection in these patients was 4.4 cm. Five patients required laryngeal release with reoperation. The patients who underwent previous laryngeal release had a good outcome. Of the 41 patients requiring laryngeal release with their initial operation, 77% ($n = 31$) had a good result, and 9.1% ($n = 4$) had a satisfactory result. The rate of failure or death was each 6.8%. All five patients who underwent laryngeal release as part of a reoperation had a good outcome.

COMPLICATIONS

Complications of tracheal resection and reconstruction are infrequent. In 49 patients, granulation tissue formed at the site of tracheal anastomosis. Only 5 of 317 (1.6%) patients have had granulation occur since 1978, when the suture material used for anastomosis was changed to an absorbable suture material, in contrast to 44 of 186 (23.6%) patients whose anastomosis was constructed with nonabsorbable suture. Of these 49 patients, 38 were managed by bronchoscopic removal of granulation tissue. Of 11 with more complicated cases, 5 required reoperation for second resection and reconstruction, all with good results. Four patients required tracheostomy, one of which was temporary.

Anastomotic dehiscence or restenosis occurred in 29 patients. Seven patients with this complication died; two also had innominate artery erosion. Eight patients were managed with repeated resection and reconstruction all with either good ($n = 6$) or satisfactory ($n = 2$) results. Four patients required permanent tracheostomy. Five required a T-tube, three of which were temporary. Three patients had dehiscence of a small portion of their anastomosis. Two of these required reexploration and primary closure, and one patient with a minimal leak was managed successfully with drainage of the cervical wound and antibiotics. Two patients required repeated dilations.

A total of 25 patients had varying degrees of laryngeal dysfunction after the operation. Fourteen had minor or temporary dysfunction that required no specific treatment. Eleven patients had more severe dysfunction. Of these, seven required tracheostomy; four were temporary. One patient required a permanent T-tube, another a subglottic stent. Two patients required gastrostomy tube feedings for persistent aspiration secondary to glottic dysfunction. One death occurred in this group. Laryngeal complications—aspiration or vocal cord dysfunction—appeared in 4 of 9 patients undergoing thyrohyoid laryngeal release (44%) and in 8 of 40 (20%) undergoing suprahyoid release. Laryngotracheal resection (trachea-to-thyroid cartilage anastomosis) plus laryngeal release in eight patients led to three minor and four major complications in six of the eight patients. These complications included dysphagia in three, with aspiration also in one, and malacia in one and dehiscence in whole or in part in three. Three of the four patients with major complications ultimately had good results.

Five patients bled from the innominate artery. Three of them died, two of whom had concomitant anastomotic separation. One patient was managed successfully with repair of the artery, and one was managed by division of the innominate artery.

Infectious complications developed in 34 patients. Wound infections accounted for 15 of these. Nineteen patients had bronchitis or pneumonia. Fourteen of these required bedside bronchoscopic treatment and antibiotics. Five more severe cases resulted in one death. Three patients were managed with temporary tracheostomy and two with reintubation.

■ CONCLUSION

The causes of postintubation stenosis have been well documented. Prevention is possible by use of large-volume, low-pressure cuffs and careful management of ventilator tubes attached to a tracheostomy. Only for highly selected lesions are treatments such as repeated dilation, steroid injections, laser treatment, and stenting appropriate. Segmental tracheal resection remains the preferred definitive treatment for postintubation stenosis. In our series, good or satisfactory results were obtained in 93.7% of all resections, with failure in 3.9% and mortality of 2.4%. Our good or satisfactory results of 90.3% after the more complex single-stage resection and reconstruction of subglottic larynx and trachea for stenosis at this difficult level confirm the appropriateness of this approach. In these patients, failure occurred in 8.1% and death in 1.6%. The increased failure rate counsels a continued cautious approach to laryngotracheal reconstruction. A permanent tracheal T-tube may be the best solution for a patient with extensive tracheal damage that would defy reconstruction.

■ SELECTED READING

Donahue DM, et al: Reoperative tracheal resection and reconstruction for unsuccessful repair of postintubation stenosis, *J Thorac Cardiovasc Surg* 114:934, 1997.

Gaissert H, et al: Temporary and permanent restoration of airway continuity with the tracheal T-tube, *J Thorac Cardiovasc Surg* 107:600, 1994.

Grillo HC, et al: Postintubation tracheal stenosis: treatment and results, *Thorac Cardiovasc Surg* 109:486, 1995.

Grillo HC, et al: Idiopathic laryngotracheal stenosis and its management, *Ann Thorac Surg* 56:807, 1993.

Grillo HC, et al: Laryngotracheal resection and reconstruction for subglottic stenosis, *Ann Thorac Surg* 53:54, 1992.

STENTING OF THE AIRWAYS

Armin Ernst
Ko-Pen Wang

Stents are endoprostheses implanted into central airways to alleviate intrinsic or extrinsic airway obstruction. Early reports of stent placement into the airways date back to the beginning of the 20th century. Due to inadequate materials and equipment, however, stent placement has had only limited applications. The first stent that has found widespread use was the T-tube, or Montgomery stent, introduced in 1962 for the treatment of subglottic stenosis. A further advance was the introduction of a dedicated indwelling silicone tube stent in 1989 by Dumon in France. This date indicates the start of the modern era of airway stents, and the Dumon stent to date represents the gold standard for safety and ease of application. Metal stents also have been in use since the mid-1980s. Because the initial designs were laid out for vascular or gastrointestinal purposes, the initial results when placed into the airways were sometimes disastrous. In the 1990s, numerous new designs of metal stents were introduced, and their implantation into the tracheobronchial tree and safety record are vastly improved.

Discussions frequently arise around the question whether metal versus silicone stents are better and safer. This discussion is not helpful because neither stent design is currently optimal for all indications; the stent type should be chosen according to a patient's specific problem. New stent designs combining properties of both types, bioabsorbable stents, and other innovations are in development and may make the discussion and need for choice moot in the future.

■ INDICATIONS FOR STENTING

Indications for consideration of airway stents are listed in Table 1. In general, intrinsic airway obstruction should be relieved and airway patency reestablished as much to the normal lumen size as possible; this can be achieved by dilation, laser resection, or other means. For stents to be effective, airways distal to the obstruction need to be patent. Airway stents are most effective when placed into large central airways. Lobar orifices only rarely are stentable or leave a patient with good results. Airway fistulas often can be treated well with stenting from either airway or esophagus, and this treatment modality has changed significantly the morbidity and mortality for patients with malignant tracheoesophageal fistulas.

Table 1 Indications for Airway Stents

Extrinsic obstruction
Malignant intrinsic obstruction after airway patency has been
   reestablished
Benign intrinsic stenosis after dilation
Airway fistula
Tracheomalacia in select cases

Sizing and choice of the optimal stent dimensions may be difficult. Length and diameter can be measured during bronchoscopy, or an airway computed tomography (CT) scan with reconstruction may be useful (Figure 1). Stents need to be long enough to cover the area in question and should fit snugly in diameter. Stents chosen too small migrate; those too large may exhibit excessive forces on the airway wall. When choosing a particular stent type, several characteristics should be kept in mind.

Silicone stents require rigid bronchoscopy for placement. They are removed easily even after long periods and have a good track record. Silicone stents do not conform to changes in airway diameters in the diseased airway and tend to migrate more frequently than metal stents. Silicone stents can be custom made in different shapes.

Metal stents may be placed with a flexible bronchoscope. They adjust to varying airway diameters and shapes and have a favorable inner-to-outer diameter compared with silicone stents. They rarely migrate but can break and cause significant granulation tissue to form. Removal after 6 to 8 weeks can be difficult or impossible.

Carinal abnormalities or obstructions near the carina may be difficult to treat with tube stents, and frequently a Y-shaped stent is the more satisfactory solution. Alternatively, multiple metal stents can be placed into the proximal end of the right and left main bronchus and distal trachea, formulating a Y-stent *in vivo*.

Patients with benign airway disorders represent a difficult population when stenting is considered. Because of the inherent complications associated with airway stents, the indications have to be strict. It is imperative to document objectively symptomatic improvement with the use of an endoprosthesis. We perform a preprocedural functional assessment, including pulmonary function tests and an exercise assessment such as a 6-minute walk test. After the stent has been placed, we repeat these tests. If there is no objective improvement, the stent is removed. Because metal stents may not be removable after several weeks, experts are divided on their safety in their use for benign disease.

■ SILICONE STENTS

The most commonly used silicone stent is the Dumon stent (Figure 2), but other models are available. The chosen stent is loaded into the distal opening of the rigid introducer tube either by a dedicated device or by folding it and pushing it into the tube. The diameter of the ventilating scope has to be adjusted to the stent size, and some systems are color coded to allow for optimal matching of the introducer tube and bronchoscope diameter. The introducer with the stent is passed to the distal end of the stenotic area. The stent may be pushed out with the introducer plunger or the help of forceps while the scope introducer tube is withdrawn slowly. The stent unfolds in the airway when released. If the stent is too proximal, it may be pushed gently with the tip of the rigid bronchoscope, and if it is deployed too distally, it can be

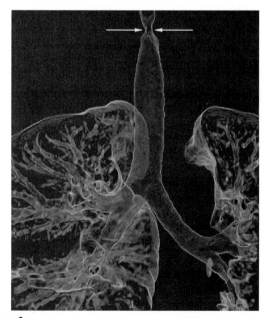

Figure 1
Computed tomography (CT) reconstruction of an airway (external rendering). A stenotic area in the subglottis is shown. Specialized software and multidetector CT scanners are necessary for high-quality images.

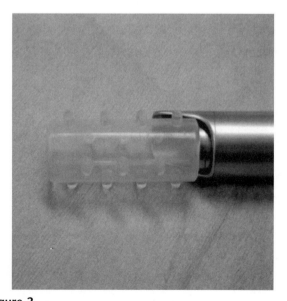

Figure 2
Dumon silicone stent that is deployed through a rigid bronchoscope.

pulled back with the help of forceps. A properly sized stent fits snugly into the airway when completely unfolded. External studs or protrusions on the end are designed to minimize migration risk.

Montgomery T-tubes are designed to be used for subglottic or high tracheal obstructions. They are available in different diameters, and their proximal and distal length can be cut to fit the patient (Figure 3). Care must be taken to leave enough distance to the vocal cords to ensure a good voice. The stent is placed through a tracheal stoma leading with the distal end toward the carina. When the distal and proximal ends are advanced into the trachea, gentle traction is applied to the external limb to allow the stent to straighten out. Minor adjustment may be made with the help of the rigid bronchoscope. The stent is removed easily through the stoma by gentle pulling and generally should be capped to allow for a good voice and minimize secretion buildup. Suctioning and stent care can be performed through the external limb.

Y-stents, such as the Freitag or dynamic stent, require a skilled endoscopist in order to be placed successfully. These stents cannot be loaded into a rigid bronchoscope. Special introduction forceps are available to place the stent through the vocal cords into the trachea with a laryngoscope providing visualization. We often perform direct suspension laryngoscopy to expose the vocal cords and provide ventilation. The stent is advanced with the forceps through the cords and placed into the trachea. This is followed by rigid bronchoscopy to ensure proper placement and to allow for necessary adjustments.

■ METAL STENTS

Most experts agree that older stents, such as the Gianturco stent, have no place anymore in the treatment of airway disorders. This discussion concentrates on newer,

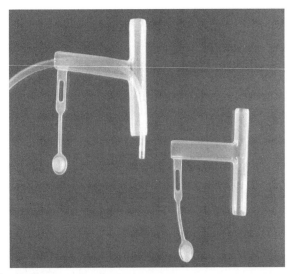

Figure 3
Montgomery T-tubes. The suction catheter may be advanced through the external limb.

second-generation models. An exception is the Palmaz stent. This stent is used rarely in adult airway disorders because its design allows the stent to crush with coughing. It is still in use in the pediatric population, however, as it is currently the only commercially available metal stent in small enough sizes.

In adult applications, most metal stents used now are made from metal alloys (e.g., nickel, titanium, or nitinol). These stents are self-expanding and possess a "shape memory," which allows them to resume their original shape after having been compressed.

Metal stents commonly are placed with a flexible bronchoscope under conscious sedation or with rigid bronchoscopy. In the unstable patient or when working in a single airway, the use of an orotracheal tube or laryngeal mask airway under general anesthesia by flexible bronchoscope or rigid open ventilating scope is the safer choice. Metal stents are generally available covered or uncovered. Membrane-covered stents are intended to be used to prevent tumor ingrowth into the lumen of the stent in malignant stenosis and to block a leakage in patients with airway fistula.

The stent is secured onto an introduction catheter and held in place with either a sheath or other removable system. A guidewire is placed into the airway past the lesion. The catheter is advanced over the guidewire into the airway until the stent is in the desired location. This advancement can be performed easily visually, but especially for the novice, fluoroscopy can be performed to adjust the stent placement. When the location is satisfactory, removing the sheath or pulling a string, which releases the stent to the preset diameter, deploys the stent. It is safe to choose a slightly larger stent, but incomplete expansion results in the stent being longer than it would have been if completely expanded. Metal stents are easier to pull back for adjustment, but pushing them distally is more difficult. In case of uncertainty, it is preferable to deploy the stent too distally and pull the stent back, if needed. Stents usually take 24 to 48 hours to reach their maximum diameter and may be dilated from the inside with balloon dilators.

When a stent has been placed, follow-up needs to be arranged. In the case of metal stents, we perform bronchoscopy within 6 weeks. This allows for necessary adjustments because most stents are not yet embedded. Specific follow-up schedules differ between centers. Airway CT scans are becoming increasingly popular because they are noninvasive.

Preprocedural steroids and antibiotics have no proven value and should be avoided. All patients with airway stents should carry a card identifying the type, size, and location, together with contact numbers for the center that placed the stent. A medical alert bracelet also may be helpful. Patients with tracheal stents need to be informed that there are no contraindications for intubation. Most tracheal stents can be intubated, but it may require flexible bronchoscopic guidance.

■ CONCLUSION

Although there have been significant improvements in stent design, more advances will be seen in the next few years.

Hybrid stents that are made from silicone but are compressible similar to metal stents are already becoming available in Europe. Other concepts include stents made from bioabsorbable materials and materials impregnated with radioactive or chemotherapeutic compounds. As with most complex airway procedures, airway stenting should be performed in a center comfortable with this therapy, which has all the necessary experience and technology available.

SUGGESTED READING

Bolliger CT: Airway stents, *Semin Respir Crit Care Med* 18:563, 1997.

Dumon JF: A dedicated tracheobronchial stent, *Chest* 97:328, 1990.

Freitag L, et al: Management of malignant esophagotracheal fistulas with airway and double stenting, *Chest* 110:1155, 1996.

Wahich M, et al: The Montgomery T-tube tracheal stent, *Clin Chest Med* 24:437, 2003.

Wang KP: Preliminary experiences of self-expandable wire stent or "wall stent" for bronchial obstruction, *J Bronchol* 4:120, 1997.

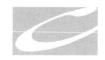

PULMONARY SEQUESTRATIONS

Chandrakanth Are
Malcolm Brock

A pulmonary sequestration is a rare abnormality that constitutes approximately 0.15% to 6.4% of all congenital pulmonary malformations. First described and classified by Pryce in 1946, it is defined as a mass of nonfunctioning, embryonic lung tissue that receives all or most of its arterial blood supply from anomalous systemic arteries. The etiologies proposed include (1) abnormal traction by persistent systemic arteries on the lung bud causing separation from the parent tracheobronchial tree, (2) adhesion of the lung bud to caudally migrating celomic organs, and (3) an insufficient pulmonary arterial supply causing persistence of collateral systemic arteries with subsequent cystic degeneration and fibrosis.

Pulmonary sequestrations commonly present in two forms. Intralobar sequestration (ILS) is characterized by abnormal pulmonary tissue completely invested in normal pleura. Extralobar sequestration (ELS) consists of nonaerated pulmonary tissue with its own visceral pleural investment and is anatomically as well as physiologically distinct from the normal lung. In either type of sequestration, the blood supply is from an abnormal source, usually the descending thoracic or abdominal aorta.

ILS is the more common of the two forms, accounting for about 75% of pulmonary sequestrations, and is located invariably in the posterior basilar regions of the lower lobe (2:1 ratio of left-sided to right-sided lesions). Its blood supply originates in 70% of patients from the thoracic aorta and enters the lung via the inferior pulmonary ligament. Its venous drainage is usually via the appropriate pulmonary veins into the left atrium. A right-sided ILS is more likely to have more frequent anomalies of pulmonary venous drainage, such as the scimitar syndrome. There are bronchial communications in a small subset of patients, and its chief pathologic characteristics are chronic inflammation, cystic change, and fibrosis. ILS occurs equally as frequent in males and females and is usually not associated with other congenital anomalies.

Similar to ILS, the arterial supply for ELS is from the descending thoracic aorta in 70% to 80% of patients. Venous drainage occurs typically via the azygous and hemizygous system, but it can occur via the superior vena cava into the right atrium. Although ELS tissue is most commonly located in the posterior left costodiaphragmatic sulcus between the lower lobe and the hemidiaphragm, it is occasionally found in the mediastinum, pericardium, and abdomen. ELS usually lacks an obvious communication with the tracheobronchial tree. Pathologically, ELS resembles normal parenchyma. There is a male preponderance, and more than 50% of the time it is associated with other congenital anomalies. There is a 30% prevalence with congenital diaphragmatic hernias alone.

■ SYMPTOMS

Most commonly, patients with ILS present with recurrent or persistent pneumonia, lung abscess, low-grade fever, or hemoptysis. Although it is considered to be a congenital pulmonary anomaly, ILS is almost never seen in neonates, and over half of all patients reach 20 years old before the correct diagnosis is made. Only a few patients are asymptomatic on presentation.

ELS, on the other hand, will present in the first few months of life because large sequestered portions of lung cause symptoms such as hemorrhage, respiratory distress, feeding intolerance, and congestive heart failure in infancy. Congestive heart failure, in the absence of congenital cardiac disease, occurs in these infants as a result of massive arteriovenous shunting that leads to high-output cardiac failure. Only 15% of patients are diagnosed based on incidental findings on chest radiographs or have lesions found unexpectedly during surgical repair of a congenital diaphragmatic hernia. Incidental autopsy diagnosis of ELS is rare.

■ DIAGNOSIS

In ILS, physical signs are nonspecific and sporadic. A chest radiograph can demonstrate an infiltrate or abscess involving the posterobasal regions of the left lower lobe. If there is a patent, abnormal communication with the tracheobronchial tree, air-fluid levels may be present. Additional imaging with ultrasonography, computed tomography, and magnetic resonance imaging may be needed for ILS. Ultrasound can help diagnose the source of arterial blood supply. All patients with suspected right-sided ILS should have pulmonary arteriography performed before surgery to define their pulmonary vein anatomy.

In ELS, routine prenatal ultrasonography helps in early diagnosis. Nevertheless, any newborn presenting with respiratory distress should have a chest radiograph taken. Ninety percent of ELS anomalies appear as posterior mediastinal masses or as triangular masses with their apices toward the hilum. In about 10% of patients, the sequestrations communicate with the stomach or esophagus, and these communications must be ruled out preoperatively by an upper gastrointestinal series.

Table 1 Indications for Specific Management of Pulmonary Sequestrations

	INTRALOBAR SEQUESTRATION	EXTRALOBAR SEQUESTRATION
Conservative	Active infection responsive to antibiotics	Uninfected tissue, no associated anomalies. Small asymptomatic, with poor feeding artery
Surgical	Persistent or recurrent pneumonia Hemoptysis	All symptomatic anomalies Undiagnosed posterior basal mediastinal masses Hematemesis/vomiting due to esophageal communication Congestive heart failure (arteriovenous shunting)

■ TREATMENT

In general, resection is recommended for both ILS and ELS. Surgery should be considered only after the size, caliber, and quality of the artery supplying the sequestration have been thoroughly assessed. The principles of treatment include the following: (1) resection of sequestrated segment with as little normal lung as possible, (2) establishment of early vascular control of the aberrant arterial blood supply, and (3) exclusion of foregut communications or other congenital anomalies. The management strategies for both ILS and ELS are listed in Table 1.

For ILS, surgery should be performed with adequate antibiotic coverage during a quiescent phase of the illness when there is minimal inflammation. Surgical resection of the affected area is the most reliable method of eliminating the long-term, recurrent nature of ILS infections. Due to residual chronic inflammation and the difficulty of surgical dissection, a limited segmental resection in the absence of inflammation is possible in only a fourth of patients. Most cases require a formal lobectomy with special attention paid to the source of arterial blood supply.

■ SURGICAL TECHNIQUE

The standard practice has been to approach these lesions through a thoracotomy on the side of the sequestration. The sequestered segment is resected in ELS, whereas in ILS a lobectomy is usually required. In both types, the majority of these lesions are in the basal segments of the lower lobe. Fewer than 15% occur in the upper lobes.

■ SPECIAL CONSIDERATIONS

One of the first objectives of the surgical procedure is to identify the arterial blood supply. In 75% of patients, the anomalous artery arises from the descending thoracic or infradiaphragmatic aorta. If not found in the usual location, other probable vessels of origin include the subclavian, intercostal, phrenic, internal thoracic, celiac trunk, and left gastric arteries. Rarely, coronary and innominate arteries have been the sources of arterial blood supply.

Careful thought should be given in cases involving children, adolescents, and young adults referred for resection of any type of an inflammatory lesion in the lower lobes of the chest because there is a real possibility of ILS in the differential diagnosis. Takedown of the pulmonary ligament and inadvertent transection of a systemic anomalous artery in these patients could be lethal because of retraction of the vessel into the mediastinum or abdomen. In these patients, the anomalous systemic artery in the inferior pulmonary ligament should be approached early in the operation and preferably suture ligated only after appropriate proximal and distal vascular control has been established. Often, the artery can be located by inspection or palpation within the inferior pulmonary ligament itself.

Systemic arterial inflow to the sequestration is multiple in 15% to 20% of the patients. A search for additional feeding vessels is mandatory. When a systemic artery is less than 3 mm in diameter, multiple feeding arteries are the rule rather than the exception.

Other coexisting anomalies may be present. One must be familiar with anatomic variations such as anomalous pulmonary venous return, especially for right-sided ILS lesions. A thorough search preoperatively must be made to rule out abnormal communications to the stomach or esophagus. If a bronchopulmonary foregut communication also exists, the sequestration can have both a pulmonary and an abnormal systemic arterial supply. Finally, in all patients with ELS, a coexisting diaphragmatic hernia must be sought and repaired.

■ OTHER TREATMENT MODALITIES

There are other treatment strategies other than traditional surgery. Prenatal injection of pure alcohol can lead to resolution of ELS. For small lesions, a video-assisted thoracoscopic approach can be used to resect sequestrations reportedly with minimal postoperative pain and better aesthetic results. As with the open approach, identifying the blood supply and safely ligating should be done with care, because it can be challenging to isolate without the advantage of manual palpation. Finally, in patients with major comorbidities for surgery, arterial embolization of the feeding artery can also be performed.

SUGGESTED READING

Stocker JT, Kagan-Hallet K: Extralobar pulmonary sequestration; analysis of 15 cases, *Am J Clin Pathol* 72:917, 1979.

Stocker JT, Makzak HT: A study of pulmonary ligament arteries: relation to intralobar pulmonary sequestration, *Chest* 86:611, 1984.

Zylak CJ, et al: Developmental lung anomalies in the adult: radiologic-pathologic correlation, *Radiographics* 22:S25, 2002.

BRONCHOGENIC CYSTS

Neri M. Cohen

Bronchogenic cysts are rare congenital anomalies of pulmonary development that can present at any time (infant, child, adult). The cyst represents the end result of an independent nest of lung cells that separate from the developing lung bud and proceeds to develop separately from the rest of the lung. This abnormal bud subsequently differentiates into a fluid-filled, blind-ended pouch. They are usually found in the mediastinum (85% to 90%) or in the pulmonary parenchyma (10% to 15%), are usually centrally located, and can be associated with the major airways (trachea, bronchi), esophagus, or cardiac structures. There may exist an identifiable channel between the cyst and the airway. They are the most common benign cysts of the mediastinum and represent 15% to 20% of all mediastinal masses. Up to 70% of patients manifest symptoms directly related to the mass effect of the cyst. Symptoms of compression are more common in the pediatric population (70%) than in adults (60%). In symptomatic patients, the most common complaint is pain (48%), followed by cough (33%), recurrent infections (24%), and dysphagia (10%).

■ DIAGNOSTIC INVESTIGATIONS

The lesion is usually detected on a routine chest radiograph. Intrapulmonary bronchogenic cysts are usually sharply defined, solitary, noncalcified, round opacities confined to a single lobe. They can present as a homogeneous water density, as an air-filled cyst, or with an air-fluid level. Mediastinal bronchogenic cysts are similarly described, presenting in the middle, posterior, or superior mediastinum in close association with the trachea or major bronchi. Because of the central location of the mass, subsequent imaging studies should be obtained to further define the relationship of the cyst to the surrounding mediastinal structures.

Computed tomography (CT) typically shows a sharply marginated mediastinal mass of soft tissue or water attenuation. Most appear cystic, although a minority may appear solid, confounding the diagnosis. Magnetic resonance imaging (MRI), by demonstrating marked increased signal intensity within the lesion on T2-weighted images, is useful for elucidating the true cystic nature of the lesion. In rare circumstances, cardiac gated MRI can define the proximity to and involvement of the tracheobronchial tree, esophagus, pericardium, and heart. Ultrasonography (US) and transesophageal echocardiography (TEE) are useful in distinguishing bronchogenic from pericardial cysts. Bronchoscopy for airway evaluation and esophagoscopy for complete evaluation of the aerodigestive tract usually only reveal evidence of extrinsic compression. If there is an adequate window, image-guided aspiration of the fluid frequently confirms the diagnosis by cytology.

■ INDICATIONS FOR TREATMENT

Treatment is indicated for all cysts that are increasing in size, causing symptoms, or developing complications. All pediatric cysts should be resected. Some authors believe that the possibility of malignancy must also be considered as an indication to resect all cysts. Enlarging cysts have been reported to cause compression of major airways, blood vessels, and the esophagus that can at times be quite dangerous. Life-threatening complications can occur in up to 3% of patients. Other complications—infection, hemorrhage into the cyst, esophagobronchial or pleurocutaneous fistula, malignancy, esophageal compression, arrhythmias, or ventricular outflow tract obstruction—can occur in up to 25% to 30% of patients.

■ THERAPEUTIC ALTERNATIVES

Close Expectant Observation

Small, asymptomatic, bronchogenic cysts (either peripheral or central) can be safely followed with serial interval imaging studies. Once the pathology is defined and the diagnosis is confirmed, chest radiography is usually sufficient for monitoring. Initial frequent studies at short intervals can yield to annual films over time. Cysts that are detected in the pediatric population, and in the adult, cause symptoms, have air-fluid levels, are particularly large, or are in a position to potentially cause life-threatening problems should undergo definitive surgical treatment.

Simple Aspiration

Patients who either refuse surgical resection or are medically unfit for invasive procedures may be treated with image-guided percutaneous needle aspiration of the cyst. This procedure confirms the diagnosis by yielding mucoid material with cytologic examination demonstrating ciliated columnar epithelial cells. If the cyst can be completely aspirated and the epithelial lining destroyed (necrosis, infection), aspiration may result in a durable cure. Unfortunately, the epithelial lining is rarely destroyed with this approach, and thus most cysts treated in this fashion recur.

■ SURGERY

Minimal Invasive Techniques

Superior mediastinal and upper paratracheal cysts can be treated with video-assisted cervical mediastinoscopy techniques. The bronchogenic cyst is identified visually and confirmed with needle aspiration of mucoid fluid. The cyst wall is opened widely with either biopsy forceps, laparoscopic cautery scissors, or ultrasonic scalpel, and the contents are completely evacuated under videoscopic visualization. Definitive treatment to prevent recurrence requires destruction of the secretory epithelial lining of the cyst. Sclerosing agents (e.g., tetracycline, doxycycline, hypertonic saline) have been used to obliterate the lining. Alternatively, the mediastinoscope can be advanced into the cyst cavity and the lining resected or ablated with the cautery or harmonic scalpel. It is usually quite challenging to dissect and resect the cyst from the surrounding tissues through the mediastinoscope. For cysts that are inaccessible through a cervical approach, video-assisted thoracoscopy may be technically feasible for similar endocavitary decompression and ablation of the cyst lining or for complete excision of the cyst. Muscle-sparing minithoracotomy is reserved for those patients who have persistent symptoms and for whom minimally invasive scope-guided therapy fails.

Thoracotomy

Recognition of bronchogenic cysts in the pediatric population should prompt surgical resection to prevent their compression of adjacent structures that may result in growth and development abnormalities. Cysts that have air-fluid levels or clinical evidence of recurrent infection are often in direct communication with the tracheobronchial tree and frequently are within the pulmonary parenchyma. These cysts should be completely dissected free and excised from the surrounding tissues. This allows direct closure of any communication between the cyst and the airway. Pulmonary-sparing procedures should be used (e.g., stapled wedge resection, cautery dissection, segmentectomy) when possible. When the cyst is found to communicate with the esophagus, meticulous dissection with great attention to careful closure of the esophageal wall and buttressing of the suture lines with vascularized tissue is required.

■ PREFERRED APPROACH

Simple, small, uncomplicated, asymptomatic bronchogenic cysts presenting in adulthood can be followed closely by serial chest x-ray films. Other cysts should be treated by the simplest successful method possible. Percutaneous aspiration and drainage can be used for rapid decompression and relief of life-threatening symptoms and to confirm the diagnosis. If this fails to yield a durable result, endocavitary video-assisted scope-guided techniques (using the viewing working mediastinoscope and/or thoracoscope) have a high likelihood of success if the secretory epithelial lining of the cyst can also be destroyed. Thoracotomy is reserved for failures of scope-guided therapy, those presenting in childhood, or complications such as infected cysts. Surgical therapy is directed toward complete resection of the bronchogenic cyst with direct closure of communications to the aerodigestive tract while preserving functioning lung tissue.

SUGGESTED READING

Lin JC, et al: Video-assisted thoracic surgery for diseases within the mediastinum, *Surg Clin North Am* 80:1511, 2000.

Martinod E, et al: Thoracoscopic excision of mediastinal bronchogenic cysts: results of 20 cases, *Ann Thorac Surg* 69:1525, 2000.

Ribert ME, et al: Bronchogenic cysts of the mediastinum, *J Thorac Cardiovasc Surg* 109:1003, 1995.

Schwartz DB, et al: Transbronchial fine needle aspiration of bronchogenic cysts, *Chest* 88:573, 1985.

Urschel JD, Horan TA: Mediastinoscopic treatment of mediastinal cysts, *Ann Thorac Surg* 58:1698, 1994.

PULMONARY ARTERIOVENOUS MALFORMATION

Torin P. Fitton
Stephen C. Yang

Pulmonary arteriovenous malformations (PAVM) are uncommon lesions involving cardiothoracic surgeons and have become even rarer with continued advances in transcutaneous embolotherapy. PAVM describes a direct communication between the pulmonary arterial and venous vasculature, ranging in size from microscopic foci to large, complex, multitributary aneurysms. Grossly, PAVM are oval or spherical, red masses averaging 1 to 5 centimeters in diameter, although the lesions range from 1 millimeter to as large as 10 centimeters. Histologic sectioning demonstrates a plexiform mass of dilated vascular channels supplied and drained by single or multiple afferent and efferent vessels. Approximately 60% of PAVM are associated with the autosomal dominant disorder hereditary hemorrhagic telangiectasia (HHT). This disorder, also known as the Osler-Weber-Rendu syndrome, is characterized by extrapulmonary AVM and PAVM. Isolated lesions have also been described in a variety of acquired conditions, including hepatic cirrhosis, mitral stenosis, thoracic trauma, schistomiasis, actinomycosis, and metastatic thyroid carcinoma. Although initially described in 1897 by Churton, the precise pathogenesis in both congenital and acquired PAVM remains unclear.

■ CLINICAL MANIFESTATIONS

Classically, the triad of dyspnea on exertion, cyanosis and clubbing should alert the clinician to the possibility of a PAVM, although it occurs in only 10% of cases. In fact, the initial presentation is most commonly that of extrapulmonary hemorrhage, including epistaxis, intracranial or gastrointestinal bleeding. This reflects the close association with HHT and its mucocutaneous and cerebral telangiectasias. Pulmonary symptoms of PAVM occur secondary to the anatomic right-to-left shunt and loss of capillary filtering function caused by the direct communication between artery and vein. Physiologically, the right-to-left shunt induces hypoxemia and reactive polycythemia, manifested clinically as dyspnea on exertion, breathlessness and central cyanosis. The absence of the capillary bed in PAVM facilitates paradoxical emboli. Embolization to the central nervous system is the most common complication of PAVM, occurring in 30% of patients, and manifests as a transient ischemic attack, stroke or cerebral abscess. Central nervous system embolic events are associated with significant morbidity and mortality, and are the primary reason for aggressive management. Rare, but potential fatal complications of PAVMs include hemoptysis or hemothorax. Signs suggestive of these complications include pleuritic chest pain with friction rub, decreased lung sounds and percussional dullness.

■ DIAGNOSTIC MODALITIES

Chest roentography is the initial diagnostic exam since 90% of patients with PAVM will demonstrate an abnormality. On chest X-ray, a homogenous, oval mass with an artery radiating from the hilum and vein deviating toward the left atrium is suggestive of a PAVM. The lesions are equally distributed between the right and left lungs, and most commonly found in the lower lobes. Individuals with HHT are more likely to have multiple lesions distributed bilaterally. Additional imaging is needed to evaluate a suspected PAVM, and includes contrast-enhanced computed tomography (CT) and pulmonary angiography. Computed tomography is readily available, noninvasive and has been demonstrated to be more sensitive than conventional angiography in defining PAVM angioarchitecture. Although false positive results occur with vascular tumors, CT is the diagnostic procedure of choice. Hyperselective pulmonary angiography is still routinely performed in most centers to confirm the diagnosis, and used to classify the lesion before therapeutic intervention.

PAVM are classified according to the number and diameter of the afferent vessels supplying the lesion. A simple PAVM has a single artery while complex PAVM have two or more feeding vessels. Most studies have found 80% of PAVM to be simple and 20% complex, although some clinical investigations have concluded the opposite. The diameter of the afferent vessel is important in determining prognosis and timing of embolization. PAVMs with afferent arteries >3 mm in diameter have been implicated in central nervous system complications. Another more detailed classification was described by Anabtawi in 1965 and shown in Table 1. The description is based on a number of anatomic characteristics such as number, size, and location, as well as the presence of a fistula, aneurysm, anomalous venous drainage and other specific criteria.

Other investigative modalities for evaluating PAVM include contrast echocardiography and magnetic resonance angiography. The obvious advantages include ease of performance and avoidance of contrast injection. However, echocardiogram is too sensitive, often diagnosing PAVM of insignificant consequence. It has been abandoned as a modality for either primary evaluation or postembolization follow-up. Magnetic resonance angiography has shown no advantages versus conventional CT.

■ TREATMENT

Observation is indicated in very few patients—those asymptomatic lesions measuring less than 15 mm. These should be monitored with routine CT every 6-12 months. The significant complications associated with PAVM, especially those involving the CNS, mandate aggressive intervention. Prior to widespread availability of transcutaneous embolotherapy, indications for resection included: (1) progressive enlargement on serial radiographic exams, (2) severe hypoxemia, and (3) paradoxical emboli. The advances in transcutaneous interventional procedures have facilitated expansion of the indications to include any asymptomatic PAVM with an afferent artery >3 mm in diameter to prevent possible sequalae. In addition, aggressive therapy is indicated in those patients with Osler-Weber-Rendu disease because complications are highest in this group if left untreated.

Surgery
Surgical intervention was the only available option for the management of PAVMs until embolotherapy was introduced in 1976. Intraoperative management included ligation, local excision, segmentectomy, lobectomy, and even pneumonectomy for large, centrally located lesions. Surgery is associated with excellent long-term outcome, few postoperative complications and minimal mortality. With the availability of embolotherapy, the length of stay and cost associated with a thoracotomy may now be prohibitive. Surgery is still indicated in certain situations when: (1) personnel experienced in embolization are unavailable; (2) acute, hemodynamic instability occurs from hemorrhage; (3) location or angioarchitecture of PAVM makes embolotherapy too hazardous; and (4) severe, life-threatening allergies to intravenous contrast are present.

Parenchyma-sparing procedures are the optimal treatment to maximize available lung and reverse the complications of the anatomic shunt. Recent case reports suggest that lung transplantation is an option in recurrent, debilitating PAVM resistant to repeated embolization. However, determining the timing of transplantation is difficult, since survival data without transplantation is unavailable and the potential for recurrence in the donor lung is unknown.

Embolotherapy
Transcutaneous embolization (TCE) utilizing coils or detachable silicon balloons is now considered the first and most optimal form of treatment for most lesions. Under angiographic guidance, the occlusion device is placed in the proximal neck of the PAVM. Multiple coils or balloons can be placed, facilitating successful embolization of even large PAVM. Post-placement angiography confirms obliteration of the lesions. Repeat CT scans are performed at one

Table 1 Anatomic Classification of Pulmonary Arteriovenous Malformations

TYPE	NUMBER	SIZE	AV FISTULA	AV ANEURYSM	ANOMALOUS VENOUS DRAINAGE	OTHER
I	Multiple	Small	+	−	−	
II	Single	Large	−	+	−	Peripheral
IIIa	Single	Large	−	+	−	Central
IIIb	Single	Large	−	+	+	
IIIc	Multiple	Small	+	−	+	
IVa	Single	Large	−	+	−	Systemic artery communication
IVb	Single	Large	−	−	−	Pulmonary vein varix
V	Single	−	−	−	+	

Adapted from Anabtaw IN, et al. Pulmonary arteriovenous aneurysms and fistulas: anatomic variations, embryology, and classification, *Ann Thorac Surg* 1:277, 1965.
AV, arteriovenous.

month and one year. Patients are continued on antibiotic prophylaxis before all dental and surgical procedures. The efficacy and safety of TCE has been demonstrated in multiple trials. Postprocedural imaging studies have confirmed successful embolization in 96% of cases. The most common complication is post-embolization pleurisy secondary to pulmonary infarction caused by occlusion of the afferent artery side branches supplying normal lung. Other rarer complications include balloon or coil migration, lesion recanalization, air embolism, and deep venous thrombosis at the catheterization site. The incidence of complications is 1.6%, though none have resulted in permanent disability. Recurrence of symptoms after embolization suggests recanalization of embolized lesions or the development of new lesions. The minimal morbidity of TCE facilitates multiple repeat procedures.

◼ CONCLUSION

PAVM are rare lesions with severe multisystem sequalae if left unrecognized and untreated. Aggressive intervention is warranted in all symptomatic lesions, patients with Osler-Weber-Rendu disease, and any asymptomatic PAVM with an afferent artery >3 mm in diameter. TCE is a safe, proven and efficacious therapy with minimal morbidity and negligible mortality. Surgical intervention on the part of the cardiothoracic surgeon is rarely indicated except in highly select instances.

SUGGESTED READING

Gossage JR, Kanj G: Pulmonary arteriovenous malformations: a state of the art review, *Respiratory and Critical Care Medicine* 158:643-61, 1998.

Iqbal M, Rossoff LJ, Steinberg HN, et al: Pulmonary arteriovenous malformations: a clinical review, *Postgraduate Medical Journal* 76:390-94, 2000.

Puskas JD, Allen MS, Moncure AC, et al: Pulmonary arteriovenous malformations: therapeutic options, *The Annals of Thoracic Surgery* 56:253-8, 1993.

Reynaud-Gaubert M, Thomas P, Gaubert JY, et al: Pulmonary arteriovenous malformations: lung transplantation as a therapeutic option, *European Respiratory Journal* 14:1425-28, 1999.

Shields TW, LoCicero III J, Ponn RB, editors: *General thoracic surgery*, 5th ed., Philadelphia, 1995, Lippincott, Williams and Wilkins, Volume 1: 975-84.

LUNG NEOPLASMS

EVALUATION OF THE SOLITARY PULMONARY NODULE

Michael J. Liptay
Sean C. Grondin

Solitary pulmonary nodules (SPNs) are a common problem presented to the thoracic surgeon. With the advent of more efficient radiologic scanners and various lung cancer screening initiatives, an increasing number of smaller sized SPNs are being detected. The primary objective in evaluating the SPN is prompt identification and treatment of early-stage lung cancers. A secondary but important objective is the avoidance of surgical morbidity in the diagnosis of benign lung lesions.

■ DEFINITION

An SPN is a single lesion in the lung less than 3 cm in diameter. It is surrounded on all sides by lung parenchyma with no associated hilar adenopathy or pleural effusions. Most SPNs are asymptomatic on discovery. Lesions greater than 3 cm in size are considered to be lung masses and generally are considered malignant until proved otherwise. Surgical excision is indicated on discovery in most lung masses.

■ INCIDENCE

SPNs are found in approximately 1 in 500 chest radiographs. Annually, this translates into more than 150,000 patients in the United States with newly found pulmonary lesions seeking care. Much of the literature more than 10 years old focuses on SPNs seen on chest x-rays. These lesions tend to be greater than 1 cm in diameter. With a growing number of small SPNs less than 1 cm, algorithms for treatment must be updated. Few data exist on the characteristics of benign versus malignant lesions of 1 cm or less in size and selection criteria for the various available diagnostic and treatment modalities. New approaches are needed to guide further diagnostic and therapeutic maneuvers in patients with small SPNs.

■ FOCUSED HISTORY AND PHYSICAL EXAMINATION

A careful history and physical examination are required to assess the patient-specific malignant potential of the SPN. Patient-specific factors that increase the risk of malignancy in SPNs include advancing age, history of smoking (>10 pack-years), asbestos exposure, chronic obstructive pulmonary disease, and a history of prior malignancy. Questions are asked regarding symptoms such as cough, hemoptysis, and chest pain and systemic signs of infection or inflammation. History of tuberculosis, recent travel to endemic areas of pulmonary mycotic infections, exposure to unusual pets or birds, and previous lung disorders may prove pertinent.

The initial evaluation is accompanied by a frank discussion of the available options for diagnosis and management. These options include further radiologic examinations, such as serial computed tomography (CT) scans and positron emission tomography (PET) scans, and tissue diagnosis using needle biopsy or video-assisted thoracic surgery (VATS) wedge resection.

■ NONINVASIVE EVALUATION

Radiologic characteristics of malignancy include increasing nodular size, spiculated or nonuniform nodular edges, and no evidence of calcifications. Completely calcified nodules categorically can be regarded as benign, whereas lesions with eccentric areas of calcification still may be malignant. A diligent search for previous radiographs that date back 2 years is appropriate in all patients. If stability in size and appearance can be confirmed over that time frame, the lesion safely can be considered benign and may be followed on a more casual basis. The use of statistical models to assign a percentage for chances of malignancy to each patient has not proved superior to the judgment of an experienced physician.

Current Trends in Screening
Based on the results of the large randomized controlled trials evaluating screening chest x-rays and sputum cytologies of the 1970s, screening for lung cancer was concluded to provide little if any benefit to patient survival. Arguments have been waged on both sides of the issue, citing faulty study designs and inappropriate end points. Nonetheless, no recommendations currently are in place for regular radiologic screening of even high-risk populations (i.e., former or current cigarette smokers) for lung cancer. Despite the lack

of irrefutable evidence, several groups nationwide are performing radiologic lung cancer screening examinations. This practice has led to an increasing number of patients seeking diagnostic guidance for asymptomatic small nodules not previously considered significant with conventional chest x-rays. The thoracic surgeon must assess the multifactorial presentation of each patient before recommending a strategy.

Low-Dose CT

Several studies have been published examining the role of CT in early detection of lung cancers. The most widely quoted study by Henschke et al noted 27 of 28 lung cancers found in 1000 smokers were early-stage resectable lesions. This finding is contrasted with the 15% overall survival rate for lung cancers not found on screening techniques. Many of these lesions were in the range of 1 cm in diameter. SPNs of this size often are not visualized on standard chest x-ray. The authors also noted a fourfold increased identification of these small cancers with low radiation dose CT scans compared with chest x-ray.

The negative results of the early randomized trials using chest x-ray may be irrelevant with respect to modern available technology. With chest x-ray performed every 4 months, only 29% of the lung cancers detected in the screened population were found to be resectable. This finding is in contrast to the results of the Henschke group, which detected 96% resectable and 85% stage Ia tumors using low-dose CT scan.

High-Resolution CT

Because intravenous contrast medium typically is necessary and multiple image acquisitions are required, high-resolution CT with measurements of enhancement with contrast blood flow and calculations of Hounsfield units has been advocated by some groups. High-resolution CT has not received the widespread attention of the noncontrast faster studies more amenable to screening techniques, however. As with all noninvasive testing currently available (including PET), the accuracy for these studies is limited in nodules 1 cm or less in size. It is hoped that improvements in the next generation of machines along with more experience in evaluating these tiny nodules will aid in identifying patients who might benefit from early surgical intervention, while sparing patients with benign lesions from invasive procedures (Table 1).

Table 1 Current Algorithm Used by the Authors as Reported by the ELCAP Study Group for Newly Discovered Small Solitary Pulmonary Nodules

SIZE	ACTION
<5 mm	Observe with serial chest CT scan in 4 mo (then 6-mo intervals for 2 yr if stable)
6-10 mm	Case-by-case assessment (serial chest CT follow-up versus VATS resection)
>10 mm	Obtain tissue diagnosis (VATS versus FNA)

CT, computed tomography; ELCAP, Early Lung Cancer Action Project; VATS, video-assisted thoracic surgery; FNA, fine needle aspiration.

PET

PET uses radiolabeled glucose to exploit the increased metabolic rate and glucose uptake of lung tumors compared with normal lung parenchyma. A meta-analysis of 40 studies that comprised 1474 SPNs noted the mean sensitivity and specificity of PET to be 96% (range 83% to 100%) and 74% (range 50% to 100%). For all patients, PET has been shown to have a diagnostic accuracy rate near 90%. False-negative findings occur frequently in association with bronchioalveolar carcinoma, carcinoid tumors, and SPNs less than 1 cm in diameter. The lack of wide availability and the unreliability in the evaluation of SPNs less than 1 cm in diameter has made PET less useful in the ever-growing subset of nodules near 1 cm in size. It is hoped that refinements in equipment and interpretation will continue to add to the utility of this promising new technology in the evaluation of the small SPN.

■ INVASIVE DIAGNOSTIC TECHNIQUES

Bronchoscopy

Although diagnostic bronchoscopy typically is performed immediately before all planned lung resections, the yield of bronchoscopic tissue diagnosis for peripheral SPNs is too low (<20%) to recommend it routinely as the only invasive examination in the workup of the SPN. In patients with other pulmonary symptoms, such as recurrent pneumonias or hemoptysis, a bronchoscopy should be strongly considered.

Fine Needle Aspiration

With the increasing identification of smaller nodules often less than 1 cm in diameter, the utility of transthoracic fine needle aspiration is decreased. The most significant limitation in needle biopsy is the inability to determine definitively a specific benign diagnosis. In only 10% to 20% of cases, a specific benign pathologic diagnosis is conferred. This leaves the remainder of patients to require further investigations or, at a minimum, continued radiologic follow-up.

VATS Wedge Resection

VATS wedge resection for the diagnosis and treatment of SPNs is the most common use of the technique. This minimally invasive surgery allows a complete resection of the nodule (as opposed to the sampling of a needle biopsy) that is tolerated far better than a traditional thoracotomy. Likewise in most cases, if a malignancy is found on VATS, the patient may undergo an anatomic resection with nodal dissection under the same anesthesia. The percentage of indeterminate SPNs found to be malignant on VATS resection has been reported to be 45% to 75% in most series. The most frequent benign diagnoses are granulomas, hamartomas, other inflammatory lesions, and intrapulmonary lymph nodes.

VATS Technical Considerations

Several techniques have been reported that are designed to aid in the VATS localization of the SPN for excision. In our experience, most outer third parenchymal SPNs and interfissural SPNs can be accessed and resected with a review of the chest CT scan to guide placement of thoracoscopy ports.

The access ports are positioned in a triangular fashion to allow for digital palpation and inspection of the lung surface. The positioning of one port site directly over the nodule area aids in the tactile identification of the lesion. Endoscopic stapling devices, especially devices able to roticulate, have made thoracoscopic wedge resections straightforward and routine. We have found little use for needle-wire localization, tattooing, ultrasound, or other localizing procedures.

OPTIONS: FOLLOW, BIOPSY, REMOVE

Balancing the risks of a diagnostic surgical procedure for benign disease versus the ability to resect an early-stage lung cancer is the crux of the issue for treating physicians. Newly detected SPNs must be assumed to be malignant until proved otherwise. The only nodules that may be dismissed without further workup are nodules proved to have not grown over at least a 2-year period by x-ray or nodules with clear-cut benign calcifications radiographically.

Likewise, all lesions that have grown on follow-up or are larger than 3 cm should be removed unless the patient is of prohibitive operative risk. Most patients fall between these two categories and require further diagnostic workup and consideration. In most patients with noncalcified indeterminate SPNs near 1 centimeter in size, the options for diagnosis are observation for growth, radiologic guided needle biopsy, or resection. The prescribed approach is based on the synthesis of radiologic appearance and patient-specific risk factors.

Individual surgeons need to establish their own algorithms for the evaluation and treatment of the SPN. These algorithms must be based on the accepted national guidelines and the availability of local expertise and testing. Likewise, management decisions must be influenced by the perceived surgical risk of the specific patient.

The minimally invasive surgical approach to the peripheral indeterminate SPN offers almost 100% diagnostic accuracy and avoids a delay in the treatment of potentially curable small lung cancers. If a diagnostic VATS wedge resection may be performed with minimal morbidity and a brief hospital stay, perhaps a lower probability of malignancy is acceptable for surgery. In patients with significant comorbidities imposing added risk to the surgical approach, more testing and stringent criteria are warranted before considering resection.

FUTURE CONSIDERATIONS

As with all patient care decisions, the foundation of the evaluation of the SPN is a careful history and physical examination with particular emphasis on the risk factors for malignancy. History and physical examination are supplemented by radiologic testing, including a CT scan and potentially a PET scan. The assessment of malignant potential and individual patient-specific risk factors combine to formulate a strategy of biopsy, resection, or serial observation. The integration of new technologies, such as three-dimensional growth assessment and computer-assisted radiologic diagnosis, will aid in evaluation of numerous small SPNs.

SUGGESTED READING

Gould MK, et al: Accuracy of positron emission tomography for diagnosis of pulmonary nodules and mass lesions: a meta-analysis, *JAMA* 285:914, 2001.

Hazelrigg SR, et al: Video-assisted thoracic surgery for diagnosis of the solitary pulmonary nodule, *Chest Surg Clin N Am* 8:763, 1998.

Henschke CI, et al: Early Lung Cancer Action Project: overall design and findings from baseline screening, *Lancet* 354:99, 1999.

Ost D, Fein A: Evaluation and management of the solitary pulmonary nodule, *Am J Respir Crit Care Med* 162:782, 2000.

Swensen SJ, et al: Lung nodule enhancement at CT: multicenter study, *Radiology* 214:73, 2000.

BRONCHIAL ADENOMAS

Kenneth A. Kesler

Bronchial adenomas are an unusual but interesting group of mainly low-grade but potentially malignant neoplasms, accounting for up to 2% of all pulmonary tumors. The term "bronchial adenoma" has been a collective description for numerous neoplasms, including the more common typical and atypical carcinoid tumors, and the rarer tumors of salivary gland origin, including adenoid cystic carcinoma, mucoepidermoid carcinoma, acinic cell carcinoma, and oncocytoma. Both typical and atypical carcinoids are now included under the category of neuroendocrine lung cancer. Carcinoid tumors constitute the benign end of the neuroendocrine tumor spectrum compared with large cell neuroendocrine and small cell lung carcinomas, which are clearly more malignant. Typical carcinoids, the most common "bronchial adenoma" histology subtype, are categorized as well-differentiated neuroendocrine tumors, arising from Kulchitsky's cells in the bronchial mucosa. These tumors usually present in non-smokers during the fourth to fifth decades of life. From 60% to 70% of these tumors originate in the central airways, with metastases, mainly to regional lymph nodes, present in less than 15% of cases. Approximately one third of pulmonary carcinoids have atypical features. Compared with typical histology, atypical carcinoids normally occur in an older population, more frequently are found in the lung periphery (60% to 70%), and have a higher rate of regional lymph node metastases (30% to 50%).

Tumors of salivary gland origin are most commonly found in the trachea, but they can arise in main stem or lobar bronchi. Although all of these tumors demonstrate different and distinct histology, they have common biologic features, including the tendency to originate and slowly grow in major airways, and if metastases do occur, they are usually limited to regional lymph nodes. As opposed to their more common non–small cell lung cancer counterparts, bronchial adenomas are highly curable with surgical therapy, even in the presence of regional lymph node metastases, which represents the mainstay of therapy.

■ DIAGNOSIS

The presenting signs and symptoms associated with bronchial adenomas depend on tumor location and size. Peripheral tumors most often present as a solitary pulmonary nodule, which are usually asymptomatic and incidental findings on radiographic studies. More commonly, however, these tumors present with clinical and/or radiographic findings consistent with varying degrees of endobronchial obstruction. The vascularity of these tumors is also well known, and hemoptysis is a not infrequent presenting symptom. The symptoms of cough, hemoptysis, and repeatedly localized pulmonary infections, either as a triad collectively or separately, constitute the majority of symptoms in patients with a true bronchial adenoma. Because of the relative slow growth, symptoms frequently persist for many months, or even years, before diagnosis. With subtotal airway obstruction, wheezing may occur, which commonly leads to an erroneous initial diagnosis of asthma. Occasionally, subtotal airway obstruction can create a "ball-valve" effect resulting in lobar or total lung hyperexpansion radiographically. Finally, in approximately 4% of cases, carcinoid tumors are metabolically active with patients manifesting the "carcinoid syndrome," which most commonly occurs in the setting of a large primary tumor or hepatic metastases. Metabolically active carcinoid tumors can also produce ACTH, resulting in Cushing's syndrome.

All patients suspected of having a bronchial adenoma should undergo computed tomography (CT) scanning of the chest and upper abdomen. CT best defines the endobronchial and parenchymal component of these tumors. A CT scan of centrally located tumors can define the degree of airway obstruction and tumor location before bronchoscopic evaluation. Secondary parenchymal abnormalities, such as atelectasis, bronchiectasis, or more severe sequelae of chronic airway obstruction, can also be defined. Finally, CT scanning can demonstrate the presence of enlarged peribronchial and/or mediastinal lymph nodes, which are suspicious for metastatic disease. With respect to nuclear medicine imaging, positron emission tomography scans are frequently false negative; however, many carcinoid tumors are identified on octreotide studies, which can be helpful in select cases. For peripheral tumors, CT-guided fine-needle aspiration biopsy can be diagnostic, but atypical carcinoids occasionally resemble small cell lung carcinoma on cytologic analysis. If a conclusive cytologic diagnosis cannot be made, then wide wedge excision is recommended.

For endobronchial tumors, preoperative fiberoptic bronchoscopy is mandatory for not only diagnostic purposes but also to define surgical anatomy. Fiberoptic bronchoscopy for biopsy of carcinoid tumors has been notoriously difficult or fraught with bleeding complications, as many of these are either submucosal and/or vascular in nature, leading some clinicians to recommend general anesthesia with rigid bronchoscopy for diagnostic biopsy. Injection of dilute epinephrine over the planned biopsy site for vasoconstriction is usually successful in preventing significant hemorrhage. Transbronchoscopic fine-needle aspiration biopsy of endobronchial carcinoid tumors can be more easily obtained; however, again, cytologic results must be interpreted with some degree of caution. Finally, we believe that in the classic clinical setting of an otherwise healthy young to middle-aged patient with a long history of recurring pulmonary infections consistent with airway obstruction, and bronchoscopic evidence of a discrete but vascular endobronchial tumor, direct surgical extirpation with intraoperative frozen section analysis of airway margins as well as the tumor itself is not unreasonable for both diagnostic and therapeutic purposes.

■ SURGICAL TECHNIQUES

Anesthesia preparation is similar to any standard anatomic pulmonary resection that uses a thoracotomy approach including preinduction epidural catheter placement for postoperative pain control, percutaneous radial artery and central venous catheter placements, and an indwelling urinary catheter. For endobronchial tumors, after induction of anesthesia, fiberoptic bronchoscopy is repeated by the surgeon through a single-lumen endotracheal tube to identify the proximal and distal extent of the neoplasm, noting precisely the locations where bronchial transection at the time of thoracotomy will provide a 3- to 5-mm tumor-free margin. Additionally, if the site of tumor attachment to the bronchial wall can be determined, then the bronchotomy should be initiated on the opposite wall. A double-lumen endobronchial tube is then placed for selective lung ventilation. If a left-sided bronchial sleeve resection is anticipated, a right-sided endobronchial tube is preferred, which will greatly facilitate peribronchial dissection and bronchial anastomosis. For all other sleeve and nonsleeve resections, a standard left-sided endobronchial tube is acceptable.

Most surgeons agree that the surgical approach to these tumors, as with other neoplasms, should involve the three following principles: (1) complete excision of the tumor, (2) the sparing of as much uninvolved lung parenchyma as possible, and (3) lymph node sampling or dissection. For a small (<2 cm) peripheral "solitary pulmonary nodule," wide wedge excision using video-assisted thoracoscopic techniques, if anatomically and technically feasible, is performed. If frozen section analysis is able to confirm a typical carcinoid tumor and preoperative CT scan has not demonstrated evidence of peribronchial or mediastinal lymph node enlargement, then this minimally invasive procedure alone usually represents adequate therapy. For larger parenchymal lesions or nodules poorly accessible to wide thoracoscopic excision, we use a total muscle-sparing thoracotomy to accomplish a wedge excision with adequate surgical margins. If a typical carcinoid histology is identified by frozen section analysis, we would then take advantage of the open approach to perform complete peribronchial and mediastinal lymph node dissection before thoracotomy closure. Although controversial, should an atypical carcinoid or other more malignant pathologic subtype of "bronchial adenoma" be identified at the time of frozen section analysis, we believe that in an otherwise healthy patient, lobectomy along with complete lymph node dissection is prudent from an oncologic standpoint given the higher incidence of lymphatic invasion in this setting, without adding significant short- or long-term morbidity.

The majority of typical carcinoids, tumors of salivary gland origin, and some atypical carcinoids originate within the main stem or lobar bronchi. Preserving pulmonary parenchyma in these cases by, for example, avoiding pneumonectomy when possible is recommended. Although formal anatomic resections are still the most commonly performed operations for extirpation of these tumors, given their slow rate of growth and low-grade malignant potential, they are not infrequently amenable to sleeve resection techniques. When smaller tumors arise in the longer left main stem bronchus, occasionally sleeve resection of the airway alone can be accomplished without removing pulmonary parenchyma. When these tumors arise in or near the orifice of a major airway, such as the right upper, left upper, or left lower lobe bronchi, bronchial sleeve resection, including a 3- to 5-mm proximal and distal tumor-free margin, is recommended for parenchymal salvage.

If a lobar sleeve resection is anticipated, we typically use a standard posterolateral thoracotomy approach, dividing the latissimus dorsi muscle, mobilizing without dividing the serratus anterior muscle, and then entering the pleural cavity through the fifth intercostal space after lung deflation.

After pleural cavity and mediastinal inspection, we begin by dividing all segmental pulmonary artery branches supplying the lobe that is to be removed. The pulmonary vein is then doubly ligated, usually with a vascular stapling device, and then divided. At this point, a peribronchial lymph node dissection is performed, which is not only necessary to expose and identify the sites of proximal and distal bronchial division but also potentially therapeutic. At our institution, peribronchial lymph node dissection is accomplished under loop magnification using a standard extended electrocautery blade, to separate the lymph nodes from the airway using judicious blunt and low-level electrocautery dissection while tying to avoid stripping of the bronchial adventitia. Peribronchial lymph nodes are not removed in the rare circumstance of transbronchial tumor extension with direct involvement and adherence of overlying lymph nodes. Larger bronchial arteries, which normally course beneath the carina, as well as on the superior aspect of both main stem bronchi, are ligated with small surgical clips followed by sharp scalpel division without the use of electrocautery to maintain the patency of smaller side branches supplying the residual airways. Similarly, sensory nerves from the vagus to the affected lobe are secured with small vessel clips and then sharply divided, with attempts to spare other branches.

For right upper lobe sleeve resections, a complete peribronchial dissection includes tracheobronchial angle (ATS level 10R), bronchus intermedius (ATS level 11R), and subcarinal lymph node (ATS level 7) lymph node stations. For left-sided sleeve resections, all lymph nodes on the superior aspect of the distal left main stem bronchus (ATS level #10L), peribronchial lymph nodes including nodes commonly found in the minor carina (ATS level 11L), and subcarinal lymph node stations (ATS level 7) are excised. All lymph node stations are usually submitted for permanent, as opposed to frozen section, pathologic analysis. Finally, a mediastinal lymphadenectomy can be performed either at this time or on completion of the procedure.

Using a scalpel, a small bronchotomy is made at the proximal or distal site of planned bronchial division. The airway is retracted upward with a nerve hook, and the bronchial lumen is inspected to ensure a tumor-free margin. Both proximal and distal bronchotomies are then completed, sharply dividing the bronchus at a 90-degree angle. We agree with other authors that spatulation techniques to correct diameter discrepancies before bronchial anastomosis are usually not necessary and may result in poor anastomotic healing. The bronchial segment on the excised lobe is inspected and, if gross proximal and distal margins deemed satisfactory, sent for frozen section analysis. Arguably, the most important aspect to successful bronchial healing is to minimize tension at the anastomosis. Accordingly, before beginning the bronchial anastomosis, complete division of the pleura reflection circumferentially around the superior aspect of the pulmonary hilum and division of the inferior pulmonary ligament is accomplished. In addition, a U-shaped pericardotomy around the inferior pulmonary vein allows an additional 2 to 4 cm of cephalad rotation of the lower lobe and therefore is routinely performed at our institution, particularly for right upper lobe sleeve resections.

The preference of suture material and suture techniques used for bronchial anastomoses varies widely among institutions. Some authors advocate using a running absorbable monofilament closure of the cartilaginous wall with an interrupted suture closure of the membranous wall. We however, have avoided use of absorbable monofilament suture because of the potential for intraluminal granuloma formation, as well as the possibility that the relatively "sharp" edges of this suture material may result in the dreaded complication of pulmonary artery erosion. Another suture technique, perhaps best described as a "closed" interrupted technique, uses absorbable braided sutures, which are sequentially placed and tied, until the anastomosis is complete. We prefer an "open" interrupted technique, using 4-0 absorbable braided suture materials. One or two interrupted sutures are initially placed and tied to secure the deepest aspect of the anastomosis. The remainder of the sutures are placed in an open fashion, without tying, beginning adjacent to the deep sutures and progressing superiorly and inferiorly until both membrane–cartilaginous junctions are approached (Figure 1). Sutures are advanced slightly farther on the proximal cartilaginous wall to correct any discrepancy in lumen diameter, such as advancing 3 mm on the proximal airway while advancing only 2 mm on the distal airway. All sutures, with the exception of the sutures near the membrane–cartilaginous junctions, are then tied in reverse order of placement. Finally, interrupted sutures are placed through the membranous walls, spaced to correct any residual diameter disparity. All remaining sutures are then tied. We have found this open interrupted technique allows more precise suture placement and therefore avoids narrowing of segmental airways, particularly during left-sided lobar sleeve resections. Regardless of the bronchial anastomotic technique used, the surgeon must continually ensure that the cartilaginous and membranous walls of the proximal and distal bronchi are properly aligned to avoid anastomotic twisting and that discrepancies of lumen diameters are being corrected.

After completion of the anastomosis, the remaining lung is judiciously reinflated and the bronchial suture line is inspected under water. As bronchial adenoma patients have rarely undergone preoperative chemotherapy or radiation therapy, we do not routinely wrap these bronchial anastomoses, unless some form of carinal resection was performed. We would, however, wrap large-diameter mediastinal airway anastomoses with a local flap of either pericardium or thymic tissue. After thoracotomy closure, the patient is reintubated with a single-lumen endotracheal tube and bronchoscopy is performed to assess the bronchial

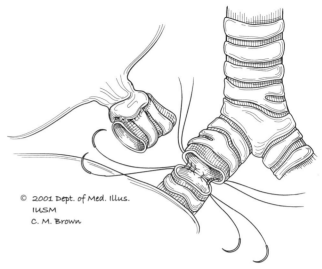

© 2001 Dept. of Med. Illus.
IUSM
C. M. Brown

Figure 1
After placing and tying deep anchoring sutures, we prefer to place the remainder of sutures in an open (untied) fashion. A secure end-to-end anastomosis is established by a "cheating" method or advancing suture bites slightly farther on the larger-diameter proximal bronchus with shorter advancement on the smaller-diameter distal bronchus. (*Courtesy C.M. Brown, IUSM, Department of Medicine, 2001*).

anastomosis as well as aspirate any blood or secretions from the airways. Postoperative pain control is of utmost importance after sleeve resections to optimize pulmonary toilet, because complications stemming from retained endobronchial secretions are common. The patient should be taught respiratory exercises preoperatively that are supervised postoperatively and supplemented with mucolytics and bronchodilators when indicated. If conservative measures fail, then therapeutic bronchoscopy is performed until the patient can sufficiently mobilize his or her own secretions. Diagnostic bronchoscopy is indicated after sleeve resection in patients with persistent fever, leukocytosis, and air leakage to evaluate anastomotic healing. Should significant dehiscence of the anastomosis be demonstrated, then consideration should be given to performing completion pneumonectomy. Minor areas of bronchial dehiscence can be treated conservatively, with most resulting in uncomplicated healing. Urgent completion pneumonectomy should be considered, however, for any patient with delayed bronchial healing and hemoptysis if an underlying pulmonary artery fistula is suspected.

Finally, although it is tempting to endoscopically resect these benign appearing endobronchial tumors, a significant bronchial wall component is usually present that would preclude complete removal. Certainly, endoscopic excision or debulking using an Nd:YAG laser, cryoprobe, or electrocautery for high-risk or elderly patients to relieve the symptoms of endobronchial obstruction can result in prolonged palliation. Compared with most non–small cell lung cancer patients with compromised pulmonary function, patients with bronchial adenomas are typically younger and healthier. Operative mortality rates should therefore be low and range between 1% and 3% for all extirpative operations, including sleeve bronchoplasty, lobectomy, and even pneumonectomy, if a parenchymal sparing procedure is not possible.

■ PROGNOSIS

The anticipated 5- and 10-year survival rates after resection of a typical carcinoid tumor are excellent and estimated to approach 90% and 85%, respectively. Metastases to either parabronchial or mediastinal lymph nodes appear to have only a minor negative prognostic effect, which underscores the importance of removing regional lymph nodes at the time of surgery. In contrast, however, atypical carcinoids have distinctly inferior survival rates ranging from 40% to 76% at 5 years, which decreases to a 18% to 50% 10-year survival rate. The role of adjuvant chemotherapy and/or radiation therapy after resection of an atypical carcinoid tumor is controversial. If regional lymph node metastases are present, we ordinarily recommend a standard small cell chemotherapeutic regimen with cis-platinum and etoposide after recovery. We believe that the benefit of adjuvant chemotherapy in this setting has the potential to be analogous to the benefit of chemotherapy after wedge excision of an undiagnosed pulmonary nodule that proves to be a small cell lung carcinoma. The role of adjuvant chemotherapy and/or radiation therapy for atypical carcinoids with regional lymph node metastasis is clearly deserving of further study, however. Survival statistics after excision of the rare endobronchial salivary gland tumors have been less well established but likely range between the reported survival rates of typical and atypical carcinoids depending on the degree of tumor differentiation and the presence or absence of lymph node metastases.

SUGGESTED READING

Dusmet ME, McKneally MF: Pulmonary and thymic carcinoid tumors, *World J Surg* 20:189, 1996.

Faber LP: Sleeve resections for lung cancer, *Semin Thorac Cardiovasc Surg* 5:238, 1993.

Kulke MH, Mayer RJ: Carcinoid tumors, *N Engl J Med* 340:858, 1999.

Travis WD, et al: Survival analysis of 200 pulmonary neuroendocrine tumors with clarification of criteria for atypical carcinoid and its separation from typical carcinoid, *Am J Surg Pathol* 22:934, 1998.

BENIGN AND LOW-GRADE MALIGNANT TUMORS OF THE LUNG

Christine L. Lau
David H. Harpole, Jr.

■ BENIGN LUNG TUMORS

Oldham summarized benign tumors of the lung and bronchi and reported that most of these lesions initially present as solitary peripheral nodules on routine chest radiographs. Often these tumors are asymptomatic and are diagnosed after being removed for suspicion of cancer. Benign tumors are commonly noted to represent less than 15% of lung neoplasms, but the actual percentage varies based on size, location, age of the patient, growth pattern, and method of detection. Categorization of benign lung tumors is based mostly on modification of Liebow's original scheme based on the embryologic origins. Tumors of epithelial, mesodermal, and mixed types exist. Arrigoni et al reported a review of 130 benign lung tumors from a single institution and found the vast majority were hamartomas (76.9%), followed by localized fibrous mesothelioma (12.3%), with the remainder being a diverse group of lesions that included xanthomatous and inflammatory pseudotumors, lipomas, leiomyomas, hemangiomas, and others.

Hamartoma

Hamartomas are abnormal combinations of normal tissues; in the lung, they are composed mostly of cartilage, gland-like structures, and fat. They are the most common benign tumor, usually are peripherally located, and represent 8% of lung tumors. Hansen et al retrospectively reviewed 89 cases of pulmonary hamartomas and found the majority of lesions were discovered between the ages of 40 and 70 years, with a slightly greater prevalence seen in males. Only 39% of patients had symptoms, with the most common being cough and dyspnea, pneumonia, hemoptysis, and pain. The majority of these lesions are found on routine chest radiographs. On radiologic examination, a lobulated, circumscribed, well-demarcated mass is seen, and classically, "popcorn-like" punctate calcifications are appreciated. When these lesions do grow, they grow slowly. Treatment depends on location, but wedge resection is appropriate when a nodule suspicious for cancer is found at operation to be a hamartoma. Recurrence after resection is not seen.

Mesenchymal Tumors

These uncommon benign tumors include localized fibrous mesothelioma, chrondromas, lipomas, leiomyomas, xanthomas, and granular cell myoblastomas. They are mostly located in the airways and thus have a tendency to be symptomatic. Treatment is complete surgical excision. Typically a sleeve resection with bronchoplastic reconstruction is performed. It is rare to require an anatomic pulmonary resection. Lymph node dissection is unnecessary.

Mucosal Associated Lymphoid Tumors (Pseudolymphoma)

These uncommon tumors are commonly located in the airways and therefore have a tendency to be symptomatic. The diagnosis of pseudolymphoma is controversial. Initially, it was believed that these tumors all represented reactive lymphoid hyperplasia. It is now known, however, that not all of these tumors are inflammatory lesions; at least some are actually low-grade B-cell lymphomas, and therefore, when identified, these lesions should not be included as pseudolymphomas. Radiographically, an air bronchogram is described with pseudolymphomas, apparently resulting from lymphoid aggregates surrounding a normal bronchus. Histologically, mostly mature lymphocytes admixed with plasma cells are found. Well-defined germinal centers are appreciated, and surrounding lymph nodes are negative for the presence of lymphoma. Treatment consists of lobectomy or segmentectomy with hilar lymph node dissection. Negative lymph node involvement provides valuable prognostic information and aids in distinguishing pseudolymphomas from lymphomas. The subsequent local development of lymphoid malignancies has been reported, after resection of apparent pseudolymphomas.

Miscellaneous

Teratomas are very rare in the lung and appear to occur more frequently in females between the ages of 1 and 60 years. Like teratomas found in the mediastinum, these lesions can behave in a benign or malignant fashion. They are more commonly located in the periphery, and although often asymptomatic, hemoptysis and, uncommonly, the expectoration of hair can be seen.

Intrapulmonary thymomas are also rarely reported, mostly as case reports in the literature. The sex ratio appears to be equal, and they occur in a wide age range. Usually these lesions are peripheral, and there may be a trend to occur in the right lung. They may be asymptomatic or present with symptoms from myasthenia gravis (muscle weakness) just as thymomas in the mediastinum. Multiple lung thymomas may also occur. Treatment is resection.

■ LOW-GRADE MALIGNANT TUMORS OF THE LUNG—BRONCHIAL ADENOMAS

Bronchial adenomas are a group of three histologic types of tumors: bronchial carcinoids, adenoid cystic carcinoma, and mucoepidermoid carcinoma. Representing 1% to 2% of all lung tumors, bronchial adenomas were described by Kramer in 1930 as a group of tumors with a prognosis better than that of bronchogenic carcinomas. Although these tumors are less aggressive, they are cancerous lesions with a potential to metastasize to regional lymph nodes as well as distally.

Bronchial Carcinoids

Bronchial carcinoids represent the vast majority of bronchial adenomas (85%), occur equally among men and women, and are seen in all age groups. Bronchial carcinoids are members of the APUD (amine precursor uptake and decarboxylation) family of Kulchitsky's neural crest cells. The cytoplasm of tumor cells of bronchial carcinoids contains neurosecretory granules identified by argyrophilic staining or electron microscopy.

Carcinoids are characterized as typical or atypical based on biologic aggressiveness that is appreciated microscopically. Typical carcinoids are composed of similar-sized clusters of cells in a fibrovascular stroma, whereas atypical carcinoids appear more disorganized, have mitotic figures and display nuclear pleomorphism with granular chromatin. Arrigoni et al described the more aggressive nature of atypical carcinoids compared with typical lesions. Actually, carcinoids are part of a range of neuroendocrine tumors, with small cell lung cancers being the most aggressive. Based on this observation, these tumors have been categorized as Kulchitsky I (typical carcinoid), II (atypical carcinoid), and III (small cell lung cancer).

The clinical presentation of bronchial carcinoids is dependent on whether they are centrally or peripherally located. The majority (60%) are central, and patients present with symptoms of cough (52%), hemoptysis (30%), or dyspnea and wheezing (25%), and usually an abnormal chest radiograph. When located peripherally, bronchial carcinoids are frequently asymptomatic. The carcinoid syndrome with sweating, flushing, and diarrhea is an infrequent presentation, occurring in less than 10% of patients. The diagnosis of a bronchial carcinoid depends on histologic confirmation. Bronchoscopy can often be used to obtain tissue; however, these tumors have a tendency to bleed profusely. Thus, biopsy in the operating room using a rigid bronchoscope is preferred. The typical bronchoscopic appearance has been described as mulberry-like.

The treatment of bronchial carcinoids without mediastinal lymph node involvement is surgical resection. Peripheral tumors commonly are treated with a formal lobectomy to allow assessment of surrounding lymph nodes. The trend is to treat central carcinoids with conservative surgical treatment, with bronchoplastic techniques if possible to allow for pulmonary parenchymal conservation. Various approaches (with limited success) have been used for metastatic spread of pulmonary carcinoids, including multiagent chemotherapy consisting of streptozotocin and 5-fluorouracil. Additionally, the long-acting somatostatin analogue octreotide can be used to treat typical carcinoid syndrome symptoms, although these tend to be uncommon in pulmonary carcinoids. Aggressive atypical carcinoids are often treated as small cell lung cancers, with responses seen similar to chemotherapy and radiation therapy. Survival after surgical resection is excellent, especially for typical carcinoids, where a greater than 90% 5-year survival is seen. Harpole et al identified early pathologic stage (I or II), typical histology, and asymptomatic presentation as favorable factors affecting survival in a multivariate analysis.

Adenoid Cystic Carcinoma (Cylindroma)

Adenoid cystic carcinomas, previously referred to as cylindromas, represent 10% of all bronchial adenomas. These tumors can be seen in all age groups, usually arising in the trachea or main bronchi and thus frequently are symptomatic (cough, hemoptysis, stridor, or respiratory distress) at presentation. Radiographically, a centrally located mass may be evident with the appearance suggestive of bronchogenic carcinoma. Adenoid cystic carcinomas are slow growing but unfortunately show a predilection for perineural, submucosal, and distant metastatic spread. Histologically, adenoid cystic carcinomas have three distinct patterns of growth: cribriform, tubular, and solid. Definitive diagnosis requires tissue confirmation frequently obtainable on bronchoscopic biopsy. Treatment consists of surgical resection, with preoperative radiation frequently given for large tumors. Complete resection is optimal but can only be performed in approximately 60% of cases. Despite the relentless progression of unresectable residual tumor, prolonged survival with minimal morbidity is often obtainable.

Mucoepidermoid Carcinoma

Mucoepidermoid carcinomas represent 1% to 5% of bronchial adenomas and also usually originate in the trachea and proximal bronchi. Because of their central location, these tumors commonly are symptomatic, frequently presenting with cough, hemoptysis, or airway obstruction. Additionally, these tumors are often evident radiographically. Mucoepidermoid carcinomas are derived from minor salivary gland tissue of the proximal tracheobronchial tree and, histologically, are composed of squamous and intermediate elements with intracellular bridges as well as glandular components. Based on mitotic activity, level of necrosis, and nuclear pleomorphism, these tumors are classified as low or high grade. Low-grade tumors prognostically behave in a benign fashion, whereas high-grade mucoepidermoid carcinomas progress rapidly. Bronchoscopic biopsy provides the diagnosis, and treatment is surgical resection when possible. Adjuvant radiation is used for high-grade lesions, but its role remains unclear. Decreased survival is seen with high-grade lesions, incomplete resections, or lymph node or distant metastatic spread at time of diagnosis. Adenosquamous carcinomas are similar pathologically to mucoepidermoid carcinomas but appear in a peripheral location and have an aggressive course.

SUGGESTED READING

Arrigoni MG, et al: Atypical carcinoid tumors of the lung, *J Thorac Cardiovasc Surg* 64:413, 1972.

Arrigoni MG, et al: Benign tumors of the lung: a ten-year experience, *J Thorac Cardiovasc Surg* 60:589, 1970.

Hansen CP, et al: Pulmonary hamartoma, *J Thorac Cardiovasc Surg* 104:674-678, 1992.

Harpole DH: Bronchial adenomas. In Sabiston DC Jr, editor: *Textbook of surgery: the biological basis of modern surgical practice*, Philadelphia, 1997, WB Saunders, p 1860.

Harpole DH, et al: Bronchial carcinoids tumors: a retrospective analysis of 126 patients, *Ann Thorac Surg* 54:50, 1992.

Paladugu RR, et al: Bronchopulmonary Kulchitsky cell carcinoma: a new classification scheme for typical and atypical carcinoids, *Cancer* 55:1303, 1985.

SURGICAL APPROACH TO SMALL CELL LUNG CANCER

David J. Caparrelli
Stephen C. Yang

Small cell lung cancer (SCLC) accounts for approximately 20% to 25% of all bronchogenic cancers and distinguishes itself from non–small cell lung cancer (NSCLC) in biologic behavior as well as in its response to treatment. SCLCs are rapidly growing high-grade malignancies with a propensity for early metastasis to distant organs. Nearly two thirds of all patients with SCLC have *extensive*, disseminated disease at the time of initial diagnosis, whereas one third have *limited* disease. This classification, although introduced when radiotherapy was the primary treatment modality, is still used today in conjunction with the TNM staging system. *Limited* disease is defined as tumor that can be encompassed by a radiotherapy portal. Due to the aggressiveness of SCLC most patients with *limited* disease present in stage IIIa or IIIb. Only a small percentage of patients (approximately 5% of all SCLC) present in clinical stage I with an asymptomatic solitary pulmonary nodule on chest radiography. Due to its aggressive behavior and often late presentation, SCLC remains a therapeutic challenge despite significant advances in medical and surgical oncology.

The optimal treatment regimen for SCLC has been a controversial topic for several decades. After a report by the British Medical Research Council in 1973 randomizing patients to either surgery or radiotherapy for the treatment of SCLC, surgery as the primary therapeutic option for SCLC was abandoned. Subsequently, SCLC has been shown to be highly sensitive to combination chemotherapy, with numerous clinical trials reporting response rates of 80% to 90%. Therefore, it is this treatment modality combined with local radiotherapy that has been the cornerstone of treatment for SCLC during the past 25 years. Despite advances in chemotherapeutics, patients treated with *extensive* stage SCLC still have a median survival of only approximately 9 months. For *limited* disease, treatment with chemotherapy and radiation results in median survival of 15 to 18 months and 5-year survival rates in the 19% to 23% range.

A major drawback to this therapeutic approach is the high rate of local recurrence. After chemoradiotherapy, the primary tumor bed and its associated hilar and mediastinal lymph nodes are the first site of failure in nearly 50% of all recurrences. It is this statistic that has led many to reconsider the role of surgery as the primary component of a multimodality approach to the treatment of *limited* stage SCLC. Further, the use of surgery in an "adjuvant" role, following induction chemotherapy for more advanced, yet still resectable, disease has been gaining favor. Finally, the use of "salvage" surgery has been suggested for both persistent tumor at the primary site after nonsurgical therapy and isolated tumor recurrence at the primary site after a complete response to treatment.

■ PRIMARY SURGERY

Much of what is known regarding the efficacy of surgical resection in *limited* stage SCLC has been derived from an analysis of patients in whom the diagnosis of SCLC was made at the time of thoracotomy. In certain patients at high risk for lung cancer who present with a peripheral mass in clinical stage I disease, many surgeons proceed directly to resection without a pathologic diagnosis. A review of the literature suggests that in this small subset of patients who have stage I SCLC, surgical resection alone will be curative in up to 25%. When combined with postoperative chemotherapy, 5-year survival rates from 40% to 70% have been reported.

Based on these data, when presented with a patient with a solitary peripheral nodule and pathologic diagnosis of SCLC by fine needle aspiration (FNA), it is important to recognize that this patient may be a candidate for surgery and should not be immediately referred for chemotherapy. It is also important to remember that NSCLC, carcinoid tumors, and other neuroendocrine malignancies can be misdiagnosed as SCLC. In addition, up to 15% of SCLC lesions have a mixed histology containing NSCLC components. The surgical workup of these patients starts by evaluating the mediastinum with mediastinoscopy, because the decision to proceed with surgical resection as the primary treatment modality requires the absence of nodal metastases to these areas for any survival benefit. If mediastinal N2 or N3 disease is present, the role of surgery is less clear but still may play a role as "adjuvant" therapy following induction chemotherapy (a topic to be more thoroughly discussed later in this chapter). Although 2-[fluorine-18]fluoro-2-deoxy-D-glucose positron emission tomography is both sensitive and specific (>90%) for mediastinal lymph node metastases in NSCLC, this tool has yet to supplant mediastinoscopy as the diagnostic modality of choice for lymph node staging in SCLC.

Noninvasive staging with nuclear bone scanning and computed tomography of the head, chest, and upper abdomen is also necessary before proceeding to thoracotomy. For those patients whose diagnosis was made at the time of the operation, a noninvasive metastatic workup is carried out postoperatively for the purposes of precise cancer staging and planning of adjuvant therapy.

Whether diagnosed preoperatively or at the time of thoracotomy, complete surgical resection is the key to success for stage I SCLC. Because of a high incidence of intrapulmonary and hilar lymph node metastasis, lobectomy is recommended for complete resection of the primary tumor, as well as for examination of regional lymph nodes. Wedge or segmental resection should only be considered in those patients who are unable to tolerate a more extensive resection due to poor pulmonary function. Further, mediastinal lymph node sampling, or formal dissection, should be undertaken at the time of thoracotomy. Because mediastinoscopy is not as accurate in staging SCLC as is NSCLC and because radiotherapy is recommended when disease has spread to the mediastinum, lymph nodes should be sampled even if a preoperative mediastinoscopy was found to be negative.

The current recommendations for clinical stage I SCLC include mediastinoscopy first and, if negative, complete surgical resection with adequate mediastinal lymph node sampling or dissection, followed by five or six courses of combination chemotherapy. Postoperative radiotherapy is suggested when regional or mediastinal nodal disease is found at the time of operation; the role of prophylactic cranial irradiation in this setting remains controversial.

■ "ADJUVANT" SURGERY AFTER INDUCTION CHEMOTHERAPY

As with stage I SCLC, much has been learned from a retrospective analysis of patients who underwent surgical resection for more advanced disease. Many patients with clinical N1 or minimal N2 disease and resectable primary lesions have undergone surgery before the initiation of adjuvant chemotherapy. In this population, 5-year survival rates of only 20% to 30% have been reported. However, improvement in long-term (5-year) survival has been demonstrated when surgery is used as the "adjuvant" therapy after two or three cycles of induction chemotherapy. In patients who are downstaged to N0 at the time of surgery, 5-year survival rates can reach 60% to 70%. Survival rates drop, however, to 30% to 40% when nodal disease is persistent at the time of surgical resection. In these trials, chemotherapy and radiotherapy were also administered postoperatively as components of the treatment regimen.

Although somewhat encouraging, not all data support the use of surgical resection in node-positive, resectable SCLC. A randomized trial in 1991 by the North American Lung Cancer Study Group showed no difference in survival between patients receiving nonsurgical versus surgical treatment after chemotherapy for *limited* disease. This trial, however, differed from other studies in that chemotherapy was not administered postoperatively. Despite a lack of consensus on the management of node positive (N1, N2) SCLC, there remains support for surgical resection to provide local tumor control, accurately stage the disease, and confirm histology. In fact, there have been reports that after chemotherapy, resected specimens are devoid of SCLC cells yet show evidence of viable, less chemosensitive NSCLC cells.

Surgical resection as a component of a multimodality approach to *limited* stage, node-positive SCLC (including preoperative and postoperative chemotherapy and radiotherapy) should be encouraged based on the currently available literature. However, further prospective randomized trials are needed to definitively define the role of surgical resection in *limited*, node-positive SCLC.

SALVAGE SURGERY

Although SCLC is highly sensitive to chemotherapy and radiotherapy, there are a few patients who have resolution of their nodal disease but have persistent densities at the primary site after completion of these nonsurgical therapies. For these patients, resection may be indicated because continued chemotherapy and maximized radiation doses rarely translate into disease-free and long-term survival. Moreover, histologic analysis of these specimens often reveals a residual component of relatively chemotherapy-resistant NSCLC. Further, patients who develop locally recurrent disease have an extremely poor prognosis, due to limitations in alternative drug and radiation therapies. In a retrospective analysis by Shepherd et al in 1991, the projected 5-year survival after salvage surgery in 28 patients with persistent or recurrent disease following combined modality therapy was 23%. Although there are limited prospective data demonstrating improvement in survival after surgery in locally persistent or recurrent SCLC, resection offers the best chance for local control and may improve the outcome in this subset of patients who otherwise have an extremely poor prognosis. In this subset of patients, mediastinoscopy should always be performed before thoracotomy to assess nodal status for tumor resectability.

SUMMARY

Despite advances in both medical and surgical oncology over the past several decades, the optimal management of *limited* SCLC has yet to be determined. Early results and the advent of chemotherapy caused a shift in the standard of initial care away from surgical resection in the 1970s. However, poor outcomes from recent trials suggest that, in certain patient populations, surgical resection may play a role in a multimodality approach to this high-grade malignancy. Surgical resection as the primary treatment modality, followed by chemotherapy and radiotherapy, has shown promise in stage I SCLC. For *limited* stage, node-positive disease, the role of "adjuvant" surgery needs to be further investigated and should be considered, particularly to provide adequate local control of the disease. Finally, for locally recurrent or persistent disease following nonsurgical therapy, surgical resection should be considered given the limited success of other treatment modalities in this setting. In any of these cases, mediastinoscopy must be performed first to assess mediastinal nodal status.

SUGGESTED READING

Fujimori K, et al: A pilot phase 2 study of surgical treatment after induction chemotherapy for resectable stage I to IIIA small cell lung cancer, *Chest* 111:1089, 1997.

Ginsberg RJ, Shepherd FA: Surgery for small cell lung cancer, *Semin Radiat Oncol* 5:40, 1995.

Inoue M, et al: Surgical results for small cell lung cancer based on the new TNM staging system, *Ann Thorac Surg* 70:1615, 2000.

Inoue M, et al: Results of preoperative mediastinoscopy for small cell lung cancer, *Ann Thorac Surg* 70:1620, 2000.

Urschel JD: Surgical treatment of peripheral small cell lung cancer, *Chest Surg Clin North Am* 7:95, 1997.

NON–SMALL CELL LUNG CANCER—STAGE I AND II DISEASE

Frank D'Ovidio
Robert J. Ginsberg

Lung cancer is the leading cancer-related cause of death in the Western world. About 160,000 new patients are diagnosed each year with this disease in the United States. Non–small cell lung cancer (NSCLC) accounts for about 80% of cases. In North America, the early stages of the disease (stage I and II), when the potential for cure is greater, are diagnosed in less than 25% of patients.

Surgical treatment for early stage NSCLC is the treatment of choice. In general, the following surgical oncologic principles must be applied:

1. The tumor and its draining intrapulmonary lymphatic tributaries and lymph nodes should be resected in their entirety whenever possible.
2. The tumor should be excised completely without spilling or traversing.
3. The surgeon should resect en bloc any structure invaded by tumor to achieve negative margins.
4. At a minimum, multistation lymph node sampling should be performed in all patients. When hilar nodal disease is present, an ipsilateral mediastinal lymph node dissection is required.

Risk factors for cardiopulmonary events should be identified preoperatively. The anticipated resection must be planned carefully after detailed pulmonary evaluation to ensure a reasonable quality of life without chronic respiratory failure.

Smoking cessation, pulmonary rehabilitation, and patient education on how to perform respiratory exercises effectively optimize the postoperative course. All preexisting medical problems should be identified and corrected.

■ STAGE I DISEASE (T1/2N0)

Diagnosis and Staging

Solitary pulmonary nodular lesions with a diameter 3 cm or less often are discovered on routine chest x-ray. Malignancy must be ruled out. A search for previous chest x-rays for comparison is valuable. No change in size over 2 years usually indicates a benign lesion.

High computed tomography (CT) scan Hounsfield units indicating a calcific lesion may allow a benign diagnosis. Positron emission tomography (PET) scans can be used to differentiate benign from malignant nodules, although

bronchoalveolar carcinoma may result in false-negative PET results, whereas active granulomatous nodules are detected as false-positive results. Subcentimeter malignant nodules may escape PET detection, 0.8 cm being the quoted lower diameter limit for PET accuracy. Percutaneous needle biopsy or transbronchial biopsy under fluoroscopy can be performed.

The increasing use of low-dose, high-resolution spiral CT scans for lung cancer screening will identify an increasing number of subcentimeter nodules in the future. Patients with nodules suspected of being malignant that elude tissue diagnosis require surgical intervention for diagnosis, either open surgery or video-assisted thoracic surgery (VATS), to permit needle aspiration, core biopsy, or wedge resection. VATS resection of the subcentimeter, nonsubpleural nodule may require localization methods, such as needle hooking, methylene blue staining, or transthoracic ultrasonography.

Treatment

Trials in patients with T1N0 lesions (>1 cm in diameter) comparing lesser resection, such as segmentectomies or wedge resections, with complete anatomic lobar resections have confirmed the validity of the latter approach because of a significantly higher local recurrence rate after lesser resections. In patients with subcentimeter lesions discovered by CT scan, the role of lesser resections is being investigated. These T1 lesions still may require a pneumonectomy for complete resection based on tumor location.

This stage of disease has a 5-year survival rate of 60% to 70% after complete resection. The size of the primary tumor, a central location, and involvement of the visceral pleura are poor prognosticators. An ongoing American College of Surgeons Oncology Group randomized trial in early NSCLC is evaluating the effect on survival of complete mediastinal lymph node dissection versus selective sampling of various nodal stations in these early stages.

■ STAGE II (N1) DISEASE

Diagnosis and Staging

Clinical stage II (N1) disease is identified when enlarged (>1 cm) hilar lymph nodes (N1) are observed on preoperative imagining studies. Often enlarged lymph nodes may reflect other processes associated with adenopathy, however, such as postobstructive pneumonia or other inflammatory causes. In most instances, stage II (N1) disease is identified pathologically after surgical resection. PET, although sensitive and specific for the detection of mediastinal N2 lymph node metastasis, is yet of unknown value in accurately defining N1 disease.

Treatment and Results

The operation of choice is a complete anatomic dissection to obtain negative margins (e.g., lobectomy, sleeve lobectomy, bilobectomy, or pneumonectomy) with adequate sampling of the mediastinal node. At this stage of disease, pneumonectomy is required more frequently.

Stage II (N1) disease, surgically resected, has a 5-year survival of 40%, with two thirds of all relapses being systemic and presenting as disseminated disease. Evidence suggests a significant prognostic role of identifying occult disease within the locoregional lymph nodes or the bone marrow using molecular biology techniques (polymerase chain reaction, immunohistochemistry, flow cytometry). These may be responsible for locoregional and distant recurrence of disease and ultimately the relatively poor long-term results of early stage (stage I and stage II) NSCLC compared with other tumor systems.

To date, the effort to improve results using postoperative adjuvant chemotherapy or radiotherapy has been unsuccessful. A few trials adopting adjuvant low-dose and temporally prolonged regimens of nonalkylating agent–based chemotherapy (tegafur plus uracil) have shown a significant improvement in survival but require further confirmation. More recently, based on the apparent success of induction (preoperative) chemotherapy in advanced disease (stage III), similar trials are being conducted for earlier stage disease.

■ STAGE II (T3) DISEASE

Stage II NSCLC invades contiguous but resectable structures and can be subdivided into three variants: chest wall invasion, mediastinal invasion, and proximity to the carina or entire lung atelectasis.

Chest Wall Involvement

Complete resection is the goal when resecting any T3 tumor involving the chest wall. Multiple studies confirm the negligible 5-year survival after incomplete resection. As a general guideline, one rib above and one below the gross margin of the tumor should be taken to ensure negative margins. When the parietal pleura is minimally involved, an extrapleural approach may be sufficient, although multiple frozen sections are required to confirm the limited wall invasion. In superior sulcus tumors, preoperative radiotherapy has been adopted to improve operability and optimize local control. More recently, concurrent chemoradiotherapy has shown effectiveness with high rates of pathologic response and improved local control. Due to the lack of randomized trials, no significant long-term survival effect has been correlated to induction radiotherapy or chemoradiotherapy to date.

The role of adjuvant therapies has not been confirmed, although adjuvant radiotherapy is recommended if an incomplete R1 or R2 resection has been performed. Reconstruction of the defect depends on the stability of the chest after the resection. In general, defects up to three ribs in the paraspinous or scapular region usually do not need to be reconstructed. Large defects in the chest wall are repaired with synthetic meshes and appropriate reconstructive methods.

Marlex/methyl methacrylate sandwich technique readily restores stability and prevents paradoxical chest wall motion during breathing. A Gore-Tex patch, tightly stretched, also has acceptable results.

T3 tumors invading the diaphragm rarely are encountered at a stage when surgical resection is an option, but occasionally they can be resected completely for cure. With T3 chest wall invasion, the factors that affect survival include the extent of the chest wall involvement, the ability to resect the tumor completely, and the presence of lymph node involvement. The overall 5-year survival of T3N0M0 patients with chest wall involvement who undergo complete en bloc surgical resection is 35% to 60%. Specifically, invasion of the parietal pleura only has a 62% 5-year survival, whereas muscle and rib involvement has a 35% survival.

Mediastinal Invasion

T3 tumors with mediastinal involvement (mediastinal pleura, fat, nerves, and pericardium) notoriously have a poor outcome. They have lower rates of complete resection. If complete resection is possible, the 5-year survival rate is about 30%. An incomplete resection may be treated with intraoperative brachytherapy or external beam radiation, which provides a 10% salvage rate.

Carinal Proximities

T3N0M0 tumors, owing to their proximity to carina (within 2 cm but not involving it), are affected negatively by the peribronchial tissue invasion. The overall survival of these patients is about 35%, although patients without peribronchial tissue involvement have been reported to have a survival of 80% in early squamous cell tumors. Pneumonectomy or sleeve pneumonectomy may be required for complete excision, but, whenever possible, sleeve lobectomy should be employed. Lung-sparing surgical techniques should be adopted whenever possible: sleeve lobectomy or tracheobronchial sleeve lobectomy.

SUGGESTED READING

Allen MS, et al: Stage II (T3) lung cancer, *Chest Surg Clin N Am* 11:61, 2001.

Choy O, et al: Stage II (N1) lung cancer, *Chest Surg Clin N Am* 11:39, 2001.

Ginsberg RJ, Port JI: Surgical therapy of stage I and non-T3N0 stage II non-small cell lung cancer. In Pass H, et al, editors: *Lung cancer: principles and practice*, Philadelphia, 2000, Lippincott Williams & Wilkins, p 682.

Mountain CF: Revision in the International System for Staging Lung Cancer, *Chest* 111:1710, 1997.

Walsh GL, et al: Treatment of stage I lung cancer, *Chest Surg Clin N Am* 11:17, 2001.

NON–SMALL CELL LUNG CANCER—CHEST WALL INVASION

Joseph LoCicero III

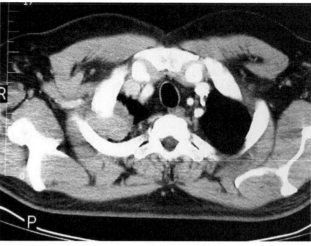

Figure 1
Computed tomography scan of a superior sulcus tumor in the anterior portion of the chest. This patient had right anterior chest pain extending down to the nipple.

Chest wall invasion by non–small cell lung cancer alone is not a sign of unresectability. It indicates that a more complex treatment is necessary to obtain an optimal survival rate. Often, but not always, neoadjuvant therapy is indicated. The operation may be lengthier, but the overall prognosis may be excellent.

■ PREOPERATIVE CONSIDERATIONS

Invasion of the chest wall connotes a T3 tumor. A superior sulcus tumor involves the upper chest wall at the apex of the lung. Because there are many structures in this area, these tumors often involve additional structures, such as the stellate ganglion, the brachial plexus, the subclavian artery or vein, the phrenic nerve, or the superior vena cava. Tumors also may involve the vertebral body, which would change the stage to T4.

Almost all tumors involving the chest wall invade the local intercostal nerve. They cause local pain syndromes with radiation forward and backward over the course of the nerve. Often tumors cause referred pain to other areas of the body leading to confusing symptoms. Frequently, these patients are treated for bursitis, shoulder pain, peripheral neuropathy, cervical radiculopathy, and angina before a chest radiograph shows the exact pathology.

Tumors in the superior sulcus of the chest with associated pain syndromes are called *painful apical tumors* (Figure 1). Tumors that involve the stellate ganglion causing Horner's syndrome are known as *classic Pancoast tumors* (Figure 2). These tumors also may involve the brachial plexus, the vertebral body, or the subclavian vessels.

Although pain is the most sensitive indicator of invasion, other methods are used. Computed tomography, magnetic resonance imaging, and ultrasound techniques have been touted as the best technique for confirming chest wall invasion. Thoracoscopy may be of benefit if there is continued question about whether there is true chest wall invasion. If the tumor is adherent to the chest wall, however, disturbing the planes at the time of thoracoscopy could cause tumor shedding into the pleura, which might affect adversely the patient's prognosis. Needle biopsy of the mass through the chest wall is the most direct and least invasive method of diagnosis. Bronchoscopy is of little benefit because the lesion is peripheral in the lung.

When evaluating the locoregional disease, the mediastinal nodes and the T stage must be evaluated. If the N2 nodes are involved, there are virtually no long-term survivors regardless of the location of the chest wall invasion. Pretherapy mediastinoscopy is essential in all patients to determine appropriate therapy. If the mediastinal nodes are involved, the prognosis is so poor that surgical therapy should be considered only in centers with aggressive investigational protocols.

■ PRESURGICAL THERAPY

Despite the propensity of many surgeons to administer multimodality therapy, there are no data that support giving neoadjuvant therapy to patients with isolated chest wall involvement except for patients with a Pancoast tumor. All trials to date for either preoperative or postoperative adjuvant therapy have been equivocal. Patients with a Pancoast tumor in whom preoperative radiation has been shown to be beneficial and to allow easier resection are an exception. In general, the radiation should be limited to less than 44 Gy, although success has been achieved with much higher doses. Operative complications are considerably less under these circumstances. When chemotherapy is added, the most common choice is a platin-based regimen. Paclitaxel-based therapy usually is not chosen because paclitaxel is a radiosensitizer. Concomitant chemoradiotherapy and sequential chemotherapy and radiotherapy have been applied.

■ OPERATION

The goal, as with all bronchogenic carcinomas of the lung, is complete resection (R0) of all gross and microscopic disease. The involved ribs and muscle must be resected with a reasonable margin. This margin varies among surgeons but should be enough so that there is no doubt either grossly or microscopically that the margins are clean. Practically, this

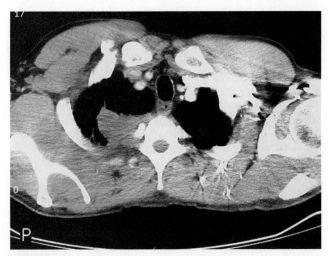

Figure 2
Computed tomography scan of a superior sulcus tumor in the posterior portion of the chest representing a classic Pancoast tumor. This patient had pain in the inner aspect of the upper arm and showed a classic Horner's sign.

is a minimum of 3 mm for the anterior and posterior margins. In general, the superior and inferior borders should include one segment of intercostal muscles that are free of tumor.

The pulmonary resection should be the standard resection for the tumor as though the chest wall were not involved. The minimum resection for cure is a lobectomy. The order of resection is not important but is determined by the ease of the conduct of the operation. Usually the chest wall is resected first followed by the lung. In the United States, most surgeons perform a complete node resection, either a full lymphadenectomy or a generous sampling of all stations.

When the tumor, chest wall, lung, and lymph nodes are removed, consideration of chest wall closure can be addressed. No decisions should be made until the appropriate curative resection is performed. The defect is assessed for size and location. Defects of the posterior and apical chest wall usually do not need reconstruction. When the posterior resection extends beyond the fifth rib, however, there is risk that the scapula may fall into the chest when the patient rotates the shoulder forward, and the defect should be reconstructed. Anterior defects of more than four ribs should be considered for reconstruction.

Most surgeons today choose thick (2 mm) polytetrafluoroethylene (PTFE) as the patch material of choice. PTFE can be stretched to fit tightly, is watertight, and does not stick to the surrounding tissue. It is secured with interrupted permanent sutures. PTFE sutures do not have to be used. When all of the rib is resected, the posterior portion of the patch usually is secured to the remaining paraspinous muscles. Perioperative antibiotics are given in the usual fashion. No additional antibiotics are necessary because of the patch.

Postoperative problems are no more common than with any standard pulmonary resection. Flail segments are not associated with increased risk of pulmonary failure as in blunt trauma because there is no associated pulmonary contusion.

■ RESULTS

Survival after therapy for chest wall tumors is comparable to other tumors of the same stage. In several series reported between 1999 and 2001, the 5-year survival for T3N0 lesions varied from 22% to 67%. The best results were achieved in patients with confirmed R0 resection. When the N1 nodes were involved, the 5-year survival ranged from 9% to 27%.

Controversy remains if the N2 nodes are involved. Many series report a dismal 5-year survival of 0% to 3%. Some isolated series report survival rates of 15% to 20%. In patients with true Pancoast's tumor, the 5-year survival is virtually nil. Resection of these lesions is inadvisable. Mediastinoscopy is suggested before attempts at surgical resection. For lesions in other parts of the chest wall, results are better, and resection is justified.

SUGGESTED READING

Curran WJ Jr, et al: Comparison of the Radiation Therapy Oncology Group and American Joint Committee on Cancer staging systems among patients with non-small cell lung cancer receiving hyperfractionated radiation therapy: a report of the Radiation Therapy Oncology Group protocol 83-11, *Cancer* 68:509, 1991.

Downey RJ, et al: Extent of chest wall invasion and survival in patients with lung cancer, *Ann Thorac Surg* 68:188, 1999.

Oda M, et al: Results of resection of T3N0-2M0 non-small cell lung cancer according to involved organ and nodal status, *Kyobu Geka* 51:902, 1998.

Okubo K, et al: Treatment of Pancoast tumors: combined irradiation and radical resection, *Thorac Cardiovasc Surg* 43:284, 1995.

Taniguchi Y, et al: A new method of reconstruction for chest wall resection, *Kyobu Geka* 53:396, 2000.

NON–SMALL CELL LUNG CANCER—STAGE III DISEASE

Robert J. Downey

Stage III lung cancer includes several anatomic subsets that vary considerably from one another in the likelihood that surgical resection will offer the patient a sustained benefit. Stage III represents primarily patients with intrathoracic extrapulmonary extension of a lung cancer. Stage IIIA includes subsets in which the disease is limited in extrapulmonary extent to the ipsilateral hemithorax: first, T3N1M0, which is a T3 primary (primary tumor directly invading locoregional nonvital structures, such as a rib) and lymphatic metastases limited to ipsilateral intrapulmonary nodes; and second, patients with a T1 or T2 primary tumor and metastases limited to the ipsilateral mediastinal (N2) nodes. Stage IIIB includes patients with a T4 classification (primary tumor directly invading locoregional vital structures such as the aorta, or a malignant pleural effusion) and/or N3 node metastases (involvement of the contralateral mediastinal, contralateral hilar, or any scalene or supraclavicular lymph node).

There is no role for surgical therapy in the management of a patient with stage IIIB NSCLC, including patients with N3 nodal metastases or with a malignant pleural effusion, and these are not discussed. Stage IIIA by virtue of T3N1M0 disease is considered in "Non–Small Cell Lung Cancer—Stage I and II Disease," which includes the majority of patients with T3 disease. This chapter focuses on the management of the patient with N2 nodal metastases or T4 primary disease.

■ N2 DISEASE

The concept of benefit from resecting N2 disease arises from published reports suggesting prolonged survival can be seen in 20% to 30% of patients with N2 disease if a complete resection can be performed. Careful analysis of these reports suggest benefit is most likely for patients with limited disease, specifically those who have a single node involved by microscopic metastases in a low paratracheal station or with a left upper lobe cancer with metastases to aortopulmonary window nodes. Several reports have documented that if the involvement in mediastinal lymph nodes can be identified by mediastinoscopy before thoracotomy, the likelihood of a complete resection being performed and a prolonged survival being achieved is only approximately 10% to 15%, which is not dissimilar to the rates for radiation therapy alone. By contrast, survival in patients who have had a negative mediastinoscopy but with resectable N2 disease identified at thoracotomy have a 5-year survival of 25% to 32%. Although it is true that there are convincing data that surgery is an important component of curative treatment in

any patient with lung cancer, it is also clear that every effort should be made to identify N2 disease preoperatively. This is because, first, an incomplete resection (even if leaving only microscopic residual disease) offers the patient no survival benefit; second, a lung resection may preclude the administration of adjuvant therapy for an extended period of time in the postoperative period, due to morbidity and possibly mortality; and, third, a combination of surgery with medical therapies such as chemotherapy and radiation therapy is likely to improve survival over surgery alone.

■ PREOPERATIVE STAGING

Currently, computed tomography (CT) of the chest is the imaging procedure of choice for the staging of the mediastinal lymph nodes. Plain chest radiographs or magnetic resonance images identify lymph node involvement poorly. It is highly likely that positron emission tomography with 18-fluorodeoxyglucose (FDG PET) will be soon be established as the most accurate noninvasive means of assessing the involvement of mediastinal lymph nodes, particularly if combined with CT images. Currently, neither CT nor PET may be taken as proof of mediastinal lymph node involvement for the majority of patients, with the gold standard remaining mediastinoscopy (used to assess the right and left paratracheal and the subcarinol lymph nodes), or mediastinotomy (also known as a "Chamberlain procedure," used to assess the aortopulmonary lymph nodes).

The procedure of mediastinoscopy is as follows: under general anesthesia, the patient is positioned with the neck extended, a 1-cm incision is made transversely in the suprasternal notch, and dissection is carried down through the subcutaneous tissue until the pretracheal plane below the thyroid is exposed. Digital palpation of the mediastinal structures allows the development of a tissue plane down into the mediastinum, into which the mediastinoscope is introduced and direct biopsies of paratracheal lymph nodes are performed. A complete sampling consists of biopsies of at least two right paratracheal lymph node stations, a subcarinal node, and one left paratracheal node. The procedure should have an associated mortality of much less than 1%. The major complications are primarily two—the first is injury to the right recurrent laryngeal nerve in the left tracheoesophageal groove, and the second is hemorrhage from injury to a mediastinal vessel. Repair of a mediastinal vessel injury may require sternotomy; therefore, the patient should be draped with the arms at the sides and a sternal saw readily available as needed.

If metastatic involvement of N2 nodes is proved, it is clear that the patient is likely to benefit from induction chemotherapy, after which local control is achieved with either surgery or radiation. It is likely that after chemotherapy has been completed patients could be stratified for treatment based on the amount of residual disease. Unfortunately, at this time, it is extremely difficult to assess whether the patient has had no response, significant response, or complete pathologic response based on CT scans, PET scans, or repeat mediastinoscopy. Currently, only thoracotomy with mediastinal lymph node dissections allows clear delineation of extent of residual disease after induction therapy. It is likely that if imaging modalities become available that would allow reassessment as to the amount of residual disease after chemotherapy, we will then be able to conduct trials to assess the efficacy of the alternate therapies of surgery or radiation. At this time, surgery and radiation therapy should probably be considered as equivalents. However, many patients do undergo a thoracotomy and an exploration in attempt to resect all residual disease after induction therapy. To completely resect all disease, a lobectomy, bilobectomy, or even pneumonectomy may be required. The risks of this surgical resection after chemotherapy probably approximate the risk of a resection in a patient who has never received chemotherapy, with the exception being possible increased mortality seen following a right pneumonectomy after induction therapy. A complete mediastinal lymph node dissection, as described later, should be performed, excising all of the fat lymph node–bearing tissue from the superior mediastinum, the subcarinal space, the paraesophageal region, and the inferior pulmonary ligament.

■ N2 DISEASE ENCOUNTERED AT THORACOTOMY

At the time of thoracotomy, in an attempt to perform a curative lung cancer resection, exploration of the entire chest cavity should be performed, including an assessment of the mediastinal lymph nodes. A visual assessment of the mediastinal lymph nodes for involvement by metastatic disease is inadequate, as approximately one half of enlarged lymph nodes are hyperplastic without metastatic involvement and approximately 5% to 10% of normal-sized lymph nodes contain microscopic metastatic disease. The generous use of a frozen section assessment for microscopic histology is reasonable. If metastases to mediastinal lymph nodes are detected and a complete resection can be performed, it is reasonable to continue with the expectation that approximately one third of patients will experience long-term benefit. It is also reasonable to terminate the operation at that point to administer chemotherapy, if the patient is otherwise able to receive it, with a planned reoperation for resection after the chemotherapy has been completed, although there are very little published data that support this approach. The difficulty patients have in tolerating chemotherapy after a lung resection limits the effectiveness of adjuvant therapy.

■ LYMPH NODE REMOVAL—SAMPLING VERSUS DISSECTION

Mediastinal lymph node removal has become a routine part of any potentially curative lung resection, both as a staging procedure and for possible survival benefit. However, the published descriptions of the techniques used for nodal removal vary widely; therefore, we briefly outline an overview of techniques, the accuracy in staging achieved, and the possible benefits and risks accruing to the patient with lung cancer.

The terms describing the techniques used have achieved a measure of consistent use within the literature. *Lymph node sampling* is taken to mean the removal of any lymph node that appears abnormal at the time of thoracotomy, leaving any apparently normal nodes or nodal-bearing tissue intact. *Systematic lymph node sampling* means the partial or complete removal of nodal tissue from multiple predetermined areas of the mediastinum, whether the lymph nodes in these regions are abnormal appearing or not. *Systematic lymph node dissection* is the complete removal of all node-bearing tissue from multiple predetermined sites within the lung and the mediastinum.

A systematic lymph node dissection would involve, on the right, the complete removal of all lymph node–bearing tissue from the hilum of the lung and the superior and inferior mediastinum. Complete removal from either the right or the left inferior mediastinum entails removal of all fatty tissue encompassing the subcarina and the perioesophageal and inferior pulmonary lymph nodes. Dissection of the superior mediastinum varies by the side involved. On the right, dissection of the superior mediastinum involves mobilization of the azygous vein with removal of all lymph node–bearing tissue from between the posterior aspect of the superior vena cava, the anterior aspect of the trachea, the superior aspect of the pericardial reflection onto the right main pulmonary artery, and the inferior aspect of the innominate artery. Some authors advocate incision of the pleura anterior to the superior vena cava, with exploration of the anterior mediastinum with removal of any fatty tissue or thymus that is encountered.

Dissection of the left superior mediastinum differs from that of the right because of the presence of the aortic arch and related structures. The majority of surgeons remove all node-bearing tissue lateral to the aortic arch, and superior to the pulmonary artery; this dissection may be continued superiorly along the course of the phrenic nerve, if tissue is apparent there. Other authors, primarily from Japan, advocate, in addition, mobilization of the aortic arch by division of one or multiple intercostal vessels, and division of the ligamentum arteriosum, to allow removal of the left peritracheal tissue in continuity with the aortopulmonary window lymph nodal tissue. Finally, after removal of all subcarinal tissue from either the right or the left, dissection can be performed along the contralateral bronchus to remove contralateral hilar lymph node tissue, if desired.

With this background material in mind, the important questions about mediastinal lymph node resection are as follows. First, does systematic mediastinal lymph node dissection stage patients better than mediastinal lymph node sampling? Second, does systematic mediastinal lymph node dissection improve survival of patients over sampling? Third, what are the probable morbidity and mortality associated with the performance of unilateral mediastinal lymph node dissection?

Mediastinal lymph node sampling is the removal of only those lymph nodes that appear abnormal by visual and tactile impression. There is evidence that such impressions are a very poor guide to the histologic composition of a node: enlarged nodal tissue will contain metastatic spread only 50% of the time, and grossly normal-appearing lymph nodes have a 4% chance of containing metastatic disease on microscopic examination.

Second, and similarly, there is very good evidence that even the smallest and most peripheral lesions can be associated with hilar and mediastinal nodal metastatic disease.

Of patients undergoing resection for clinical stage IA disease (tumors <3 cm in diameter), 25% will be found with either N1 or N2 nodal metastases. Finally, the complication rate of a mediastinal lymph node dissection is probably low, with the most significant problems being either injury to the recurrent laryngeal nerves (at the superior aspect of the removal of the right paratracheal fat pad around the innominate artery, and in the aortopulmonary window on the left) or bleeding (primarily from the subcarinal space whether approached from either the right or the left).

Overall, then, systematic unilateral mediastinal lymphadenectomy appears to be associated with low morbidity and mortality and offers more accurate staging for patients with lung cancer than mediastinal nodal sampling alone. Mediastinal lymphadenectomy may offer improved survival benefit to select patients with NSCLC, primarily those with microscopic foci of disease and single station disease and without extracapsular spread. The benefit to patients with multiple levels of nodal involvement is probably minimal to none.

■ T4 DISEASE

T4 is defined as a tumor of any size with invasion of the mediastinum (more than pleura) or involving the heart, great vessels, trachea, esophagus, vertebral body, or carina; with the presence of a malignant pleural or pericardial effusion; or with satellite tumor nodules within the same lobe of the lung (see "Extended Resection for Primary Lung Cancers"). A malignant pleural or pericardial effusion for which there is no known curative surgical therapy also falls within the T4 group, and these will not be discussed further. Resection of the great vessels is certainly technically feasible, although occasionally cardiopulmonary bypass is required.

The two resections that are common and reasonable to perform are resection of the aortic adventitia and the resection of the pulmonary vein in conjunction with the portion of the left atrium. Other resections, such as full-thickness resection of the aorta, the main pulmonary artery outflow tract, and resection of the innominate or subclavian vessels, are technical tours de force for aggressive tumors with a low probability of cure being achieved. Vertebrectomy for direct extension of malignant disease is performed in specialized centers; certainly resection of tumors with invasion into the ligaments overlying the vertebral bodies appears to be associated in some patients with extended benefit, but the extension of the tumor into the cancellous bone appears to be associated with a very poor outlook even if a complete resection and reconstruction are achieved. Tumors invading the carina certainly may be resectable, and if the patient survives the procedure, long-term survival may be anticipated.

SELECTED READING

Bunn PA, et al: Adjuvant and neoadjuvant chemotherapy for non-small cell lung cancer: a time for reassessment? *Chest* 117:119S, 2000.

Martin J, et al: Morbidity and mortality after neo-adjuvant therapy for lung cancer: the risks of a right pneumonectomy, *Ann Thorac Surg* 72:1149, 2001.

Martini N: The current state of the art in treating stage IIIA (N2) lung cancer, *Ann Oncol* 9:243, 1998.

Meko J, Rusch VW: Neoadjuvant therapy and surgical resection for locally advanced non-small cell lung cancer, *Semin Radiat Oncol* 10:324, 2000.

Roth JA, et al: Long-term follow-up of patients enrolled in a randomized trial comparing perioperative chemotherapy and surgery with surgery alone in resectable stage IIIA non-small-cell lung cancer, *Lung Cancer* 21:1, 1998.

Rusch VW, et al: Factors determining outcome after surgical resection of T3 and T4 lung cancers of the superior sulcus, *J Thorac Cardiovasc Surg* 119:1147, 2000.

NON–SMALL CELL LUNG CANCER—STAGE IV DISEASE

Virginia R. Litle
James D. Luketich

The majority of patients diagnosed with non–small cell lung cancer (NSCLC) present with advanced locoregional disease (IIIB) or distant metastases (stage IV) and are not candidates for curative surgical resection. In approximately

7% of patients with stage IV disease, only a solitary site of metastasis (M1 disease) is discovered at the time of staging. In highly selected patients with M1 disease, complete surgical resection of the primary tumor and definitive treatment of the solitary metastasis by surgery or radiotherapy may be curative. For most patients with metastatic disease, surgical resection is not an option due to multiple involved sites, and treatment is primarily directed at palliation of pain, shortness of breath, obstruction, or bleeding. Most randomized trials of chemotherapy versus best supportive care for patients with advanced NSCLC have not demonstrated dramatic survival advantages. However, some chemotherapy trials have demonstrated a marginal increase in survival accompanied by improved quality of life and less complications compared with supportive care only.

◼ EXTRATHORACIC METASTASES

Brain Metastases

Patients with solitary or limited brain metastases may be candidates for surgical resection with curative intent. Brain metastases are responsible for up to 25% of recurrences after resection of an apparent localized primary NSCLC. The Lung Cancer Study Group reported cerebral metastases as the sole site of first recurrence in 6.4% of patients after surgically resected NSCLC. Treatment options for brain metastases include chemotherapy, surgical resection, whole brain radiation (WBR), or stereotactic radiosurgery (SRS). Five-year survival rates after surgical resection of synchronous or metachronous solitary brain metastases range from 10% to 30%, with median survival rates for solitary cerebral metastases of 11 to 13 months (Table 1). Favorable prognostic factors for survival include solitary lesions, metachronous presentation, mild neurologic deficits, and no other sites of metastases. The operative mortality ranges from 1% to 6%. Local failure is reported in 30% of patients, and up to 60% die from systemic disease. Postcraniotomy WBR may provide additional survival and quality-of-life advantages. In the only prospective, randomized trial comparing surgery with adjuvant WBR versus WBR alone, the addition of surgery improved survival (median 40 versus 15 weeks) and quality of life after treatment of brain metastases from various primary tumors.

SRS, sometimes referred to as gamma knife therapy, is a relatively recent treatment option for solitary or limited brain metastases and has replaced surgical resection for many patients. SRS delivers approximately 1500 cGy of radiation to the tumor with relative sparing of surrounding brain parenchyma. In a retrospective report by Alexander et al in 1995 of 248 patients with brain metastases (105 with NSCLC), the median overall survival was 9.4 months with good local control in 65% of patients at a follow-up of 2 years. In this study, all of the patients also received WBR (3000 cGy). Benefits of SRS include minimal toxicity, ability to reach surgically inaccessible sites, and outpatient or short-stay treatment. Similar to surgically treated patients, negative prognostic factors after SRS include multiple cerebral metastases (more than three), systemic disease, male gender, and age greater than 60 years. Poor prognostic factors for local control with SRS include tumor volume greater than 3 cm or supratentorial lesions.

Patients with multiple brain metastases from NSCLC are generally treated with chemotherapy and WBR. Survival after WBR alone for multiple metastases approximates 6 months, with complications that include dementia and ataxia occurring in up to 8%. The addition of SRS after WBR for multiple metastases may improve local control in select cases, but no survival advantage has been demonstrated. When brain metastases and the primary NSCLC are detected concurrently, and both are deemed resectable, the brain metastases are treated first to avoid neurologic complications. In cases of a small intracranial lesion with minimal local effects and a primary lung tumor with pulmonary complaints such as hemoptysis or obstructive pneumonia, the lung resection should be carried out first.

Adrenal Metastases

Routine preoperative computed tomography scanning of the abdomen will identify a unilateral adrenal mass in up to 4% of patients with an otherwise operable NSCLC and up to 40% are considered metastatic. Positron emission tomography was shown to distinguish metastases from benign adenomas with a sensitivity approaching 100% and a specificity of 80%.

A number of case reports and a few small series have reported a possible survival advantage after surgical resection of isolated adrenal metastases. We previously reported in 14 patients a median survival of 31 months after adrenalectomy compared with only 8 months in patients treated with chemotherapy alone.

Extracranial, Extraadrenal Metastases

Isolated extracranial, extraadrenal metastases occur even more uncommonly. We reviewed 14 patients in whom successful treatment of solitary extracranial, extraadrenal metastases from NSCLC was demonstrated. The sites of metastases included extrathoracic lymph nodes (six cases), skeletal muscle (four), bone (three), and small bowel (one). Twelve of 14 patients underwent complete surgical resection of the isolated metastases, and 5 of 12 (42%) received postoperative radiation with or without cisplatin-based therapy. Two patients were treated with curative radiation therapy

Table 1 Outcome After Treatment of Brain Metastases With Surgical Resection, Whole Brain Radiation (WBR), and/or Stereotactic Radiosurgery (SRS)

AUTHORS, YEAR	TREATMENT	N (HISTOLOGY)	MEDIAN SURVIVAL (MO)	5-YEAR SURVIVAL (%)
Magilligan et al, 1986	Resection WBR (25 patients)	41 (4 SCLC, 37 NSCLC)	13	21
Wronski et al, 1995	Resection WBR	231 (NSCLC)	11	12.5
Alexander et al, 1995	SRS	248 (105 NSCLC)	9.4	NA
Kim et al, 1997	SRS + WBR (71 patients)	77 (NSCLC)	10	NA
Kondziolka et al, 1999	WBR WBR + SRS	14 (7 lung) 13 (5 lung)	7.5 11	NA

SCLC, small cell lung cancer; NSCLC, non–small cell lung cancer; NA, not available.

to the metastatic site. The overall 10-year actuarial survival was 86%. At a median follow-up of 101 months, 10 patients had no evidence of disease. This highly selected group of 14 patients was accumulated over a 10-year period at a specialized cancer center. Of note, the solitary metastases in this group occurred at a mean of 19 months after treatment of their primary lung cancer.

Intrathoracic Disease

Involvement of the tracheobronchial tree or pleural cavity by stage IV NSCLC can cause symptoms amenable to palliation. Common problems include airway obstruction, hemoptysis, pleural effusions, and chest wall invasion with pain. Several treatment options exist for palliation of intrathoracic progression of tumor, and the appropriate choice depends on the performance status and prognosis of the patient, the severity and acuity of the obstruction, previous treatments, and the location and nature of the obstructing tumor. In the end-stage patient with very poor performance status who has undergone previous treatment, supportive care only may be a reasonable choice. On the other hand, if the disease progression and symptoms are primarily related to intrathoracic disease, aggressive endoscopic or minimally invasive palliation may afford a significant improvement in symptoms and quality of life. These decisions require the input of an experienced thoracic surgeon or interventional pulmonologist, with the first step being flexible bronchoscopy with the capability of performing rigid bronchoscopy as needed.

Airway Obstruction with or without Mild Hemoptysis

External beam radiotherapy, endoluminal brachytherapy, endobronchial or tracheal stents, laser treatment with neodymium:yttrium–aluminum garnet laser (Nd:YAG), and nonthermal photodynamic therapy (PDT) all play important roles in relieving airway obstruction with or without mild hemoptysis, depending on the clinical scenario. When symptoms are relatively mild and are secondary to mediastinal involvement with airway compression or limited endoluminal disease, treatment with chemotherapy and external beam radiotherapy or radiation alone frequently leads to improvement. More rapid relief of obstruction or bleeding may be required for more severe symptoms and higher-grade airway obstruction. If obstruction is secondary to extrinsic compression of the airway and little endoluminal disease is present, an expandable metal stent offers excellent palliation for proximal airway obstruction at the tracheal, bronchial, or segmental level. A more consistent improvement in symptoms can be expected if one can document distal airway patency at the time of the diagnostic bronchoscopy.

The choice of stent depends on several considerations. Expandable metal stents have become increasingly popular due to their relative ease of insertion. They are available as covered or uncovered, with a variety of sizes that are available for trachea down to segmental bronchial levels. If minimal endoluminal disease is present and no fistula is anticipated, we primarily use uncovered expandable metal stents. One potential complication of uncovered metal stents is tumor in-growth causing recurrent obstruction. A covered stent avoids this problem, although it has the potential to dislodge in the airway. If a fistula is present to the esophagus,

a covered airway stent, possibly in combination with a covered esophageal stent, may give good results.

If the obstruction is primarily due to endoluminal disease, some form of laser ablation frequently yields good results. If there is a bulky component to a more central tracheal or main bronchial tumor with high-grade obstruction, rigid bronchoscopy with a "core out" of the endobronchial tumor may be the most effective first step. This can be followed by Nd:YAG or phototherapy laser ablation of residual disease. We prefer photodynamic therapy for this setting, because it is relatively easy to use, results in a deeper penetration than surface lasers, and has palliated mild to moderate hemoptysis in our experience. It is not advisable to use PDT as initial therapy for centrally located, near obstructing tumors because the initial edema may lead to a temporary worsening of the obstruction and acute airway blockage.

Mild hemoptysis due to central endobronchial metastases or local tumor extension can be treated with Nd:YAG, CO_2 laser, or PDT. Phototherapy causes thrombosis of the vasculature of endobronchial tumors and in our experience affords good palliation for mild hemoptysis. Massive hemoptysis is a surgical emergency and should be investigated with flexible and rigid bronchoscopy, followed by aggressive intervention, which may include Fogarty balloon occlusion of the site of bleeding or double-lumen intubation and selection ventilation and, in some cases following initial stabilization, bronchial artery embolization.

Malignant Pleural Effusion

Malignant pleural effusion results in varying degrees of dyspnea, cough, and chest pain depending on the volume. Pleural effusions can be treated with chest tube drainage followed by talc pleurodesis at the bedside or via videothoracic surgery (VATS) under general anesthesia. Regardless of the approach, near-complete expansion of the lung after drainage of the effusion leads to the best results because it allows good apposition of the parietal and visceral pleura. In a retrospective review, the recurrence rate after VATS talc pleurodesis from various malignancies was 6% in a series of 256 patients. Morbidity was acceptable and included prolonged drainage of greater than 14 days (4.7%), empyema (3.5%), reexpansion pulmonary edema (2.2%), and adult respiratory distress syndrome (ARDS) (1.3%). Bedside talc may be equally effective with good lung expansion, but VATS offers the advantage of less procedure-related pain and the ability to take down adhesions, which may allow more complete lung expansion in some cases. Currently, a randomized trial is under way that compares bedside talc pleurodesis with VATS.

If complete lung expansion cannot be obtained, several options may be considered. One is the insertion of an intraperitoneal catheter with the daily installation of air to result in a pneumoperitoneum designed to elevate the diaphragm, leading to better pleural apposition. In our experience, this has been effective, especially in the setting of a partially collapsed lower lobe with a limited intrathoracic space.

■ CONCLUSION

Selected patients with solitary metastases from NSCLC may be candidates for surgical and radiation therapy with intent to cure. Most patients with stage IV NSCLC should be managed palliatively. Interventions for symptoms such as pain, shortness of breath, or hemoptysis can lead to improved quality of life for many patients and should be considered in patients with good performance status.

SUGGESTED READING

Alexander E, et al: Stereotactic radiosurgery for the definitive, noninvasive treatment of brain metastases, *J Natl Cancer Inst* 87:34, 1995.

Burt M, et al: Prospective evaluation of unilateral adrenal masses in patients with operable non–small-cell lung cancer, *J Thorac Cardiovasc Surg* 107:584, 1994.

Kim YS, et al: Stereotactic radiosurgery for patients with non–small cell lung carcinoma metastatic to the brain, *Cancer* 80:2075, 1997.

Kondziolka D, et al: Stereotactic radiosurgery plus whole brain radiotherapy versus radiotherapy alone for patients with multiple brain metastases, *Int J Radiat Oncol Biol Phys* 45:427, 1999.

Luketich JD, et al: Successful treatment of solitary extracranial metastases from non-small cell lung cancer, *Ann Thorac Surg* 60:1609, 1995.

Luketich JD, Burt ME: Does resection of adrenal metastases from non-small cell lung cancer improve survival? *Ann Thorac Surg* 62:1614, 1996.

Magilligan DJ Jr, et al: Surgical approach to lung cancer with solitary cerebral metastasis: twenty-five years' experience, *Ann Thorac Surg* 42:360, 1986.

Reyes L, et al: Adrenalectomy for adrenal metastasis from lung carcinoma, *J Surg Oncol* 44:32, 1990.

Wronski M, et al: Survival after surgical treatment of brain metastases from lung cancer: a follow-up study of 231 patients treated between 1976 and 1991, *J Neurosurg* 83:605, 1995.

SUPERIOR SULCUS TUMORS

Philippe G. Dartevelle

Paolo Macchiarini

Superior sulcus lesions include a constellation of benign and malignant tumors (Table 1) invading the superior thoracic inlet and causing a steady, severe, and unrelenting shoulder and arm pain along the distribution of the eighth cervical nerve trunk and first and second thoracic nerve trunks; Horner's syndrome (ptosis, miosis, and anhidrosis); and weakness and atrophy of the intrinsic muscles of the hand, a clinical entity named *Pancoast-Tobias syndrome.* Non–small cell lung cancer is the most frequent cause of superior sulcus tumor and is the subject of this chapter.

■ CLINICAL PRESENTATION AND DIAGNOSTIC INVESTIGATIONS

Superior sulcus tumors arise from either upper lobe and in their natural course tend to invade the parietal pleura, endothoracic fascia, subclavian vessels, brachial plexus, vertebral bodies, and first upper ribs. Their clinical features are influenced by their local invasiveness. Tumors located anterior to the anterior scalenus muscle may invade the platysma and sternocleidomastoid muscles, external and anterior jugular veins, inferior belly of the omohyoid muscle, subclavian and internal jugular veins and their major branches, and scalene fat pad. They invade more frequently the first

intercostal nerve and first ribs rather than the phrenic nerve or superior vena cava, and patients usually complain of pain distributed to the upper anterior chest wall.

Tumors located between the anterior and middle scalenus muscles may invade the anterior scalenus muscle with the phrenic nerve lying on its anterior aspect, the subclavian artery with its primary branches except the posterior scapular artery, and the trunks of the brachial plexus and middle scalenus muscle. These tumors are likely to present with signs and symptoms related to the compression or infiltration of the middle and lower trunks of the brachial plexus (e.g., pain and paresthesia irradiated to the shoulder and upper limb). Tumors lying posteriorly to the middle scalenus muscles usually are located in the costovertebral groove and usually invade the nerve roots of T1, the posterior aspect of the subclavian and vertebral arteries, paravertebral sympathetic chain, inferior cervical (stellate) ganglion, and prevertebral muscles. Because of the peripheral location of the lung tumors, pulmonary symptoms, such as cough, hemoptysis, and dyspnea, are uncommon in the initial stages of the disease. Abnormal sensation and pain in the axilla and medial aspect of the upper arm in the territory of the intercostobrachial nerve are observed more frequently at these early stages. With further tumor growth, patients may present with full-blown Pancoast's syndrome.

Any patient presenting with signs and symptoms suggesting the involvement of the thoracic inlet should undergo a careful, detailed preoperative workup to establish the histologic diagnosis and to assess operability. These patients usually present with small apical tumors that are hidden behind the clavicle and the first rib on routine chest x-ray. The diagnosis is established by history and physical examination, biochemical profile, chest x-ray, bronchoscopy, sputum cytology, fine needle transthoracic or transcutaneous biopsy with aspiration, and computed tomography (CT) of the chest. Video-assisted thoracoscopy might be indicated to obtain

Table 1 Causes of Pancoast's Syndrome

NEOPLASMS	
Primary bronchogenic carcinomas	
Other primary thoracic neoplasms	Adenoid cystic carcinomas, hemangiopericytoma, mesothelioma
Metastatic neoplasms	Laryngeal carcinoma, cervical carcinoma, urinary bladder carcinoma, thyroid gland carcinoma
Hematologic neoplasms	Plasmacytoma, lymphoid granulomatosis, lymphoma
INFECTIOUS PROCESSES	
Bacterial	Staphylococcal and pseudomonal pneumonia, thoracic actinomycosis
Fungal	Aspergillosis, allescheriasis, cryptococcosis
Tuberculosis	
Parasitic	Hydatid cyst
MISCELLANEOUS CAUSES	
Cervical rib syndrome	
Pulmonary amyloidoma	

Adapted from Arcasoy SM, Jett JR: *N Engl J Med* 1370:337, 1997.

tissue proof when the other investigations are negative and to eliminate the presence of pleural metastatic diffusion. If there is evidence of mediastinal adenopathy on chest x-ray or CT, histologic proof is mandatory because patients with clinical N2 disease are not suitable for operation. Peripheral neurologic examination and electromyography delineate tumor extension to the brachial plexus, phrenic nerve, and epidural space. Vascular invasion is studied with Doppler ultrasound and magnetic resonance imaging (MRI). MRI also should be performed routinely when tumors approach the intervertebral foramina to rule out invasion of the extradural space.

■ SURGICAL INDICATIONS

Different surgical approaches have been described. The surgeon must be familiar with all of the approaches because the ultimate hope for cure depends on whether or not a complete resection is performed. Absolute surgical contraindications are the presence of extrathoracic sites of metastasis and clinically and histologically confirmed mediastinal lymph node involvement. Invasion of the brachial plexus above T1 as supported by sensitivity or motor deficits in the nerve distribution of the median and radial nerves indicates inoperability. Extensive involvement of the subclavian vessels is not a contraindication, provided that a complete surgical resection may be anticipated. Patients whose tumors abut the vertebral body should not be deemed inoperable unless invasion of the spinal canal through the intervertebral foramina is confirmed. The role of palliative incomplete resection is debatable and without any individual benefit.

■ OPERATIVE TECHNIQUES

Before operating on a patient with an apical tumor, the thoracic surgeon should be familiar with all approaches to these tumors. The ultimate hope for cure depends on whether or not a complete resection is performed, and to accomplish this, the most appropriate approach should be selected.

The goal of the operation is resection of the upper lobe along with the invaded ribs and transverse processes and all invaded structures, which may include the lower trunk of the brachial plexus, stellate ganglion, and upper dorsal sympathetic chain. Our philosophy is that any apical tumor without invasion of the thoracic inlet can be resected completely through the posterior Shaw-Paulson approach alone. Lesions with a high suspicion or proof of invading the thoracic inlet should be explored first by an anterior transclavicular approach, which may be followed by the Shaw-Paulson approach.

Posterolateral Approach (Shaw-Paulson)

The patient is placed in the lateral decubitus position, leaning slightly forward with the upper arm loosely supported by folded sheets and free to move as the scapula is elevated. The skin preparation is carried out from the base of the skull (included are the spinal processes above C7) and down to the iliac crest and past the midline posteriorly and anteriorly.

A long posterolateral thoracotomy is made. It starts superiorly at the midway between the spinous process of the seventh cervical vertebra and the posterior aspect of the scapula, describes a gentle arc between the thoracic spinous processes and the medial margin of the scapula, extends downward 2 cm below the inferior angle of the scapula, and ends 2 cm beyond it or just lateral to the breast in women. The incision is carried deeper with electrocautery. Anteriorly the latissimus dorsi and the fascia posterior to the serratus anterior muscle is incised along its posterior edge; the serratus anterior muscle is divided toward the lower margin of the incision. Posteriorly the trapezius muscle is divided along the full length of the incision. Below the trapezius muscle, the levator scapulae and rhomboideus minor and major muscles (from superior to inferior) are divided in the line of the incision. The rhomboid muscles insert into the medial border of the scapula, and care should be taken to avoid injury of the dorsal scapular nerve and satellite scapular artery, which run down the medial border of the scapula. The division of the rhomboid muscles elevates the medial border of the scapula from the chest wall. A right angle clamp is placed behind the upper digitations of the serratus anterior and serratus posterior superior muscles, then the muscles are divided by electrocautery. The scapula, fully mobilized from the chest wall, is retracted upward and forward.

The thorax is entered through the intercostal space below the lowest rib to be resected, as determined by preoperative chest x-ray, CT, or MRI (usually the third intercostal space). For local resection to be complete, one intact rib with its intercostal muscles below the lower margin of the lesion is removed. At this time, the interspace selected is opened only to an extent that permits inspection of the cavity and assessment of the resectability; the exact evaluation of tumor extension on the thoracic chest wall, thoracic inlet, lung, and mediastinum should be assessed. The chest wall resection should be started first, the rationale being that it can be released into the pleural cavity, permitting a safer pulmonary resection.

When resectability has been determined, the previously made intercostal incision is extended posteriorly toward the angle of the rib, taking care to keep the incision 2 to 3 cm away from the costovertebral angle. The erector spinae muscle is incised along its anterior border and retracted laterally and posteriorly from the first to the fifth thoracic vertebrae; this exposes the angle of the invaded ribs and transverse processes. Hemostasis usually is obtained by packing the space between the muscles and bony structures. A Tuffier rib spreader is placed, and the tumor is palpated from within the chest to determine the anterior (usually 4 cm away from the tumor) and inferior (usually includes one rib and intercostal muscle below) margins of the chest wall resection. All involved ribs should be resected en bloc; we do not recommend an extrapleural dissection without rib removal because this inevitably may lead to incomplete procedures. The division of the ribs is started anteriorly along the previously established margins of resection beginning with the healthy rib. Electrocautery is used to score the periosteum of all ribs to be resected except the first one. Using rib shears, the intercostal muscles and ribs are divided anteriorly in succession from below to above and labeled as the anterior margin of the resection. The intervening intercostal neurovascular pedicles are suture-ligated and divided. By performing gentle traction of the previously divided anterior margins of the invaded ribs, the anterior end of the first rib is exposed. The anterior and middle scalenus anterior muscles are divided with cautery, either at their insertion on the first rib or above the level of the tumor; the scalenus posterior muscle is divided where it crosses the outer border of the first rib. The superior margin of the first rib is freed in tumor-free margins after protection of the subclavian vein, artery, and brachial plexus by the operator's finger. Thereafter the relation of the apical tumor with the inlet structures is outlined, and the operation is continued posteriorly.

The previously placed pack between the erector spinae muscle and the bony structures is withdrawn, an erector spinae muscle retractor is placed, and the angle of the ribs is pushed toward the pleural cavity to improve exposure. After having dissected the angle of the invaded ribs, they are disarticulated or transected at the costotransverse or transverse level; this should be done while holding the operator's finger along the costovertebral groove to avoid injury of this region. If the parietal pleura is invaded but not the ribs or vertebrae, the invaded heads of the ribs are disarticulated from the transverse process without transecting them by using a periosteal elevator and after division of the costotransverse ligaments. Conversely, if the tumor erodes the ribs posteriorly, the transverse processes are transected along with the lateral cortex of the vertebrae using an osteotome. When completed, the entire intercostal bundles are sutured successively with polypropylene (Prolene) 3-0 and divided. Attempts to control bleeding at the costovertebral angle by electrocautery or packing the wound with oxidized but not pledgets of cellulose should be made gently to avoid migration of these elements into the spinal cord or occlusion of an anterior spinal artery. This posterior step of the resection is continued upward until the angle of the first rib is reached.

At this point, the roots of the eighth cervical nerve above and first thoracic nerve below the neck of the first rib, which join to form the lower trunk of the brachial plexus, and their relation with the tumor are seen. The head of the first rib is disarticulated from the costovertebral joint after transecting the respective transverse process. Most commonly the tumoral invasion is limited to the first thoracic nerve root; in this case, it should be divided as it emerges from the intervertebral foramen while keeping intact the eighth cervical nerve component. Little bleeding generally is encountered. If the lesion also involves the eighth cervical nerve, the lower trunk of the brachial plexus should be divided after its invasion. The nerve roots are secured with a ligature before transecting them at the intervertebral foramen to prevent cerebral fluid leakage. If that occurs, the foramen is packed gently or the erecta spinae muscle is transposed to the lateral aspect of the vertebral body to tamponade the leak.

Careful dissection of the subclavian artery usually can be done after a subadventitial plane. Local branches, such as the internal mammary artery and the thyrocervical trunk, are identified and ligated if necessary. If the subclavian vein and artery are encased or occluded by the tumor, efforts should be made to complete the operation by removing the segment of involved subclavian vein, which should be sutured and ligated but not revascularized. If the subclavian artery is invaded, it should be cross-clamped (after adequate systemic heparinization, e.g., 0.5 mg/kg) beyond the invaded segment and revascularized by an end-to-end anastomosis. The management of the subclavian vessels is hazardous through the posterior approach, however, because most tumoral invasion extends beyond the subclavian vessels into the planes of the anterior scalenus muscles and phrenic nerve. One option should be to continue the operation by an additional anterior approach.

The last step includes the eventual removal of part of the vertebral body of the upper thoracic vertebrae, depending on tumor attachment and frozen section of uncalcified periosteum; one quarter of the vertebral body may be resected without affecting stability. The sympathetic chain is divided above and below the tumor mass, and the stellate ganglia are removed. The segment of chest wall including the first, second, and third ribs and a portion of the vertebrae if necessary is dropped into the thorax, and hemostasis is secured. A standard upper lobectomy is the preferred extent of lung parenchyma resection even if the lesion is small and peripheral. This lobectomy usually is performable through the hole of the previously made chest wall resection. We suggest completing the lobar fissures with stapler instruments to avoid unnecessary air leaks. Complete nodal dissection of the upper mediastinum and subcarinal nodes is necessary.

Anterior Approaches
Transclavicular Approach (Dartevelle)

The patient is placed in the supine position with the neck hyperextended and head turned away from the involved side. A roll is placed behind the shoulder to elevate the operative field. The skin preparation extends from the mastoid downward to the xiphoid process and from the middle axillary line laterally to the contralateral midclavicular line medially.

An L-shaped cervicotomy is made and includes a vertical presternocleidomastoid incision extended horizontally below the clavicle up to the deltopectoral groove (Figure 1). The incision is deepened with cautery. Division of the sternal and clavicular attachments of the sternocleidomastoid muscle are made along with the upper digitations of the ipsilateral pectoralis major muscle; a myocutaneous flap can be folded back inferolaterally, giving full exposure of the neck, thoracic inlet, and upper part of the anterolateral chest wall. When the inferior belly of the omohyoid muscle is divided, the scalene fat pad is dissected and examined pathologically to exclude scalene lymph node micrometastasis. Inspection of the ipsilateral superior mediastinum is made by the operator's finger along the tracheoesophageal groove, after division of the sternothyroid and sternohyoid muscles. Tumor extension to the thoracic inlet is assessed carefully. We recommend resection of the internal half of the clavicle only if the tumor is deemed resectable.

Jugular veins are dissected first so that branches to the subclavian vein eventually can be divided. On the left side, ligation of the thoracic duct usually is required. Division of the distal part of the internal, external, and anterior jugular veins makes the visualization of the venous confluence at the origin of the innominate vein easier; one should not hesitate to suture-ligate the internal jugular vein to improve exposure of the subclavian vein. If the subclavian vein is involved, it can be resected easily after proximal and distal control has been achieved. Direct tumor extension to the innominate vein does not preclude resection.

Next the scalenus anterior muscle is divided either on its insertion on the scalene tubercle on the first rib or in tumor-free margins with cautery. If the tumor has invaded the upper part of this muscle, it needs to be divided at the insertion on the anterior tubercles of the transverse processes of C3 through C6. Before dealing with the anterior scalene muscle, the status of the phrenic nerve is assessed carefully because its unnecessary division has a deleterious influence on the postoperative course. It should be preserved whenever possible. Then the subclavian artery is dissected. To improve its mobilization, its branches are divided; the vertebral artery is resected only if invaded and provided that no significant extracranial occlusive disease was detected on preoperative Doppler ultrasound. If the tumor rests against the wall of the subclavian artery, the artery can be freed following a subadventitial plane. If there is invasion of the arterial wall, resection of the artery to obtain tumor-free margins is necessary. After obtaining proximal and distal control, the artery is divided on either side. Revascularization is performed at the end of the procedure with an end-to-end anastomosis after freeing the jugulocarotid and all branches of the subclavian arteries. The pleural space usually is opened by dividing Sibson's fascia.

The middle scalenus muscle is divided above its insertion on the first rib or higher as indicated by the extension of the tumor. It might require, especially for apical tumors invading the middle compartment of the thoracic inlet, division of its insertions on the posterior tubercles of the transverse processes of the second through seventh cervical vertebrae.

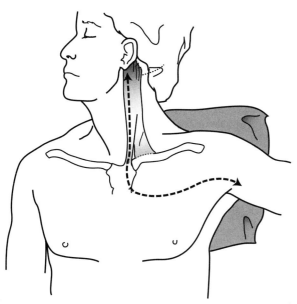

Figure 1
A left L-shaped cervicotomy is made and includes a vertical presternocleidomastoid incision extended horizontally below the clavicle up to the deltopectoral groove. To increase the exposure and make the entire resection through this incision only, however, the interception between the vertical and horizontal branches of the L-shaped incision is lowered at the level of the second or third intercostal space, as indicated by the level of tumoral invasion.

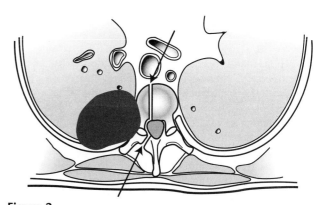

Figure 2
Right-sided apical tumor involving the costotransverse space and intervertebral foramen and part of the ipsilateral vertebral body; this tumor usually is approached first anteriorly as described in the text, then the operation is completed through a hemivertebrectomy performed through a posterior cervical midline approach.

The nerve roots of C8 and T1 are identified easily and dissected in an outside-to-inside fashion until the confluence forms the lower trunk of the brachial plexus. Thereafter the ipsilateral prevertebral muscles are resected along with the paravertebral sympathetic chain and stellate ganglion from the anterior surface of the vertebral bodies of C7 and T1. This permits an oncologic clearance of the major lymphatic vessel draining the thoracic inlet and the visualization of the intervertebral foramina. The T1 nerve root usually is divided beyond visible tumor, just lateral to the T1 intervertebral foramen. Although tumor spread to the brachial plexus may be high, neurolysis usually is achieved without division of the nerve roots above T1. Nerve damage of the lateral and long thoracic nerves should be avoided because this may result in winged scapula.

Before performing the upper lobectomy, the chest wall resection is completed. The anterolateral arch of the first rib is divided at the costochondral junction, whereas the second rib is divided at the level of its middle arch, and the third rib is scraped on the superior border toward the costovertebral angle. The specimen is progressively freed. The first ribs are disarticulated from the transverse processes of the first two or three thoracic vertebrae. It is through this cavity, although technically demanding, that the operation is completed by performing the upper lobectomy and complete nodal dissection (Figure 2). The cervical incision is closed in two layers after the sternal insertion of the sternocleidomastoid muscle is sutured and conventional postlobectomy drainage of the ipsilateral chest cavity is placed.

There is increasing concern regarding the functional and esthetic benefit that the preservation of the clavicle would have. We believe that the indications to preserve and reconstruct the clavicle are limited to the combined resection of the serratus anterior muscle and its nerve (long thoracic nerve) because if this occurs, the scapula rotates and draws forward. This entity, named *scapula alata,* combined with the resection of the internal half of the clavicle, pushes the shoulder anteriorly and medially and leads to severe cosmetic and functional discomfort. If this circumstance is anticipated, we recommend making an oblique section of the manubrium that fully preserves the sternoclavicular articulation, its intraarticular disk, and the costoclavicular ligaments rather than the simple sternoclavicular disarticulation. Clavicular osteosynthesis can be accomplished by placing metallic wires across the lateral clavicular edges and across the divided manubrium.

Hemi-Clamshell or Trapdoor Incision

The hemi-clamshell or trapdoor incision includes a partial sternotomy extended into an anterior thoracotomy. The patient is positioned supine, usually with the ipsilateral operative side elevated. An oblique incision is made along the lower third of the anterior border of the sternomastoid muscle to the midsternal notch. It is continued vertically in the midsternal plane to the third intercostal space, then laterally as a slightly curved incision in the axillary line, eventually below the breast line. The incision is carried deeper with cautery, and after a standard partial (up to the third interspace) median sternotomy, the internal mammary vessels are divided, and the lateral half of the sternum is transected transversely to meet the sternotomy incision. A rib-spreading retractor or sternal hook is placed, elevating the chest wall superolaterally; this allows exposure of the upper half of the superior mediastinum and apex of the thoracic cavity. The superior vena cava and ipsilateral innominate vein in the superior mediastinum are dissected until the subclavian vein is found. After having assessed the resectability, the clavicle can be removed for better exposure of the subclavian vessels and brachial plexus. The involved ribs are divided at the costochondral or costosternal junctions and the appropriate intercostal space below, and visible tumor is entered. The posterolateral aspects of the involved ribs are divided, and the specimen is released within the chest cavity, remaining attached to the apical fascia. The dissection and management of the subclavian vein and artery and brachial plexus are done as outlined previously by the transclavicular approach. The operation is completed by a standard closure of the incision after the chest tube has been inserted.

Masoaka Incision

The Masoaka incision includes a proximal median sternotomy extended to an incision in the anterior fourth intercostal space and above with a transverse cervical incision at the base of the neck (Figure 3). Management of this region thereafter is as in the previously described approaches.

■ RESULTS AND PROGNOSIS

The overall 5-year survival rates after combined radiosurgical (posterior approach) treatment for bronchogenic superior sulcus tumors range from 18% to 56%, with the best prognosis associated with lack of nodal involvement, T4 stage, or Horner's syndrome and having had a complete resection.

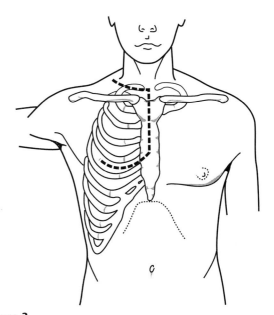

Figure 3
This approach includes a proximal median sternotomy (1) extending to the fourth anterior intercostal space below, (2) the base of the invaded neck above, and (3) transverse collar incision.

■ CONCLUSIONS

Superior sulcus tumors are uncommon neoplasms that have challenged many thoracic surgeons because of their anatomic location and the need for a technically demanding operation. It has become evident, however, that complete resection as part of combined modality treatment still gives the best ultimate hope for cure in selected cases. With the development of new treatment modalities and surgical techniques, the rate of incomplete resections has decreased dramatically. Thoracic surgeons should be fully knowledge-able about the different surgical options available to offer a complete resection to the individual patient.

SUGGESTED READING

Arcasoy SM, Jett JR: Superior pulmonary sulcus tumors and Pancoast's syndrome, *N Engl J Med* 1370:337, 1997.

Dartevelle P, et al: Anterior transcervical-thoracic approach for radical resection of lung tumors invading the thoracic inlet, *J Thorac Cardiovasc Surg* 105:1025, 1993.

Dartevelle P, Macchiarini P: Surgical management of superior sulcus tumors, *Oncologist* 4:398, 1999.

Rusch VW, et al: Induction chemoradiation and surgical resection for non-small cell lung carcinoma of the superior sulcus: initial results of Southwest Oncology Group Trial 9416 (Intergroup Trial 0160), *J Thorac Cardiovasc Surg* 121:472, 2001.

Shaw RR, et al: Treatment of the superior sulcus tumor by irradiation followed by resection, *Ann Surg* 154:29, 1961.

OCCULT LUNG CANCER

Brian T. Bethea
Stephen C. Yang

The vast majority of lung cancers are identified, localized, and diagnosed by findings on chest roentgenography or chest computed tomography. Occult lung carcinomas represent a very small subpopulation that is initially suspected due to malignant cells found on sputum cytology. Occult lung cancer is defined by the lack of any lesion by conventional radiographic means. Of note, between 10% and 30% of patients with abnormal sputum cytology and negative chest radiography will have a cancer of the upper airway.

Occult lung cancers have several interesting characteristics. First, almost all are squamous cell carcinomas, which are usually in situ or early invasive carcinoma while being node negative. Next, a significant number of patients will have a second primary lung carcinoma. Several studies have demonstrated that this patient population is at high risk for either synchronous or metachronous lesions. Finally, patients are generally asymptomatic and do not display any negative prognostic features (i.e., weight loss) that may predict poor outcome.

■ EVALUATION

The diagnostic evaluation of these patients should begin with a thorough head and neck examination to rule out any cancers of the upper airway. The patient should then undergo bronchoscopy, which may be challenging given the characteristically early stage of the disease and the associated minimal mucosal abnormalities. Each bronchopulmonary segment should be visualized and biopsy samples taken of any suspicious lesions. Further, any visible lesion should be described in detail regarding whether the entire lesion is endoscopically visible and its overall longitudinal length. These two factors provide important information in selecting the appropriate therapeutic option. If a suspicious lesion is not visualized, then a washing and/or brushing of each bronchopulmonary segment should be performed. This is a tedious procedure, because multiple protected brushed specimens must be labeled accurately. A carcinoma is considered localized when a single positive biopsy of a lesion is obtained at bronchoscopy or when bronchial brushings from the same segment are positive on two separate bronchoscopy examinations. Surgical resection (lobectomy) is then advocated, like for any other localized lesion. If the carcinoma cannot be localized, bronchoscopy should be repeated every 3 months.

Several relatively new methods for detecting and evaluating occult lung cancer are becoming available. The use of protein markers, such as MCM2, will aid in identifying malignant and premalignant cells on sputum cytology that have previously gone undetected. In addition, two new technologies that may also prove to be advantageous are transtracheobronchial ultrasonography (TUS) and the laser-imaging fluorescence endoscope (LIFE). TUS and LIFE are both believed to be superior to conventional endoscopy techniques in detecting and characterizing bronchopulmonary lesions. TUS also allows evaluation of the depth of tumor invasion, although the ability to detect relatively superficial invasions remains limited. However, both techniques are not readily available at all centers because of cost and lack of experience.

■ THERAPY

Several treatment options are available for the management of occult lung cancer, including surgery, photodynamic therapy (PDT), and brachytherapy. Other nonsurgical options are currently being investigated for the patient with limited pulmonary reserve or who is unable to tolerate surgery. As expected, the pulmonary preserving treatments are directly associated with a higher risk of recurrence. The two factors important in selecting the most appropriate therapeutic option are the abilities to visualize the entire lesion endoscopically and to know the overall longitudinal length. Lesions within endoscopic visibility have been described as having a much lower reported incidence of lymph node involvement compared with lesions that are beyond endoscopic visibility. Likewise, longitudinal extension has been shown to correlate with both depth of invasion and lymph node involvement. When the longitudinal extension is less than 10 mm, 90% of occult lung cancers will be limited to within the bronchial cartilage and be lymph node negative. However, when the greatest length is more than 30 mm, approximately 67% of occult cancers will involve the cartilaginous layer or have positive lymph nodes.

Surgery remains the gold standard for the treatment of occult lung carcinoma. Most occult lung cancers require large pulmonary resections due to their proximal locations despite their low pathological stage. In general, if a lesion is beyond endoscopic visibility, is greater than 10 mm, has nonsquamous histology, has extrabronchial extension, or has possible lymph node involvement, the patient should be considered for surgery if there are no medical contraindications. Surgical resection has been shown in several studies to have a 90% lung cancer–specific 5-year survival rate. Recently, the role of segmentectomy versus lobectomy was evaluated in a small series of patients. The candidates for segmentectomy have superficial lesions with no apparent extrabronchial extension or lymph node involvement but are not candidates for less invasive treatment modalities because of tumor size or location (i.e., >10 mm or beyond bronchoscopic visibility). All patients undergoing surgical resection should have regional and mediastinal lymph node sampling or dissection. Studies thus far have shown that patients undergoing segmentectomy have 5-year survival rates equivalent to those for lobectomy with no evidence of recurrence.

Nonsurgical therapies aimed at preserving pulmonary function should be considered when the lesion is of squamous cell histology, within endoscopic visibility, less than 10 mm, and with no evidence of extrabronchial extension or lymph node involvement. PDT is very effective at eliminating tumor cells located in the submucosa and should be considered when a lesion fits the appropriate criteria. Patients treated with PDT can expect to have a response rate of approximately 90% or greater but a recurrence rate of 0% to 20%. Endobronchial brachytherapy (EBBT) has been used mainly when patients are not surgical candidates because of medical reasons and when lesions are endoscopically visible and localized but may have extracartilaginous invasion. EBBT has been used less frequently than PDT mainly because of the complications associated with brachytherapy: mucosal ulcers, bronchial wall necrosis, and the development of secondary tumors. EBBT has reported response rates from 80% to 100% and recurrence rates from 0% to 25%. Larger studies involving these nonsurgical options are still needed to determine long-term survival rates and more accurate response and recurrence rates.

■ SUMMARY

Lung cancer continues to be the most deadly malignancy in the United States, with occult disease comprising a small subpopulation. In the future, however, the number of patients with radiographically occult lung cancer may increase as the ability to detect early lung cancer continues to improve. Surgery remains the gold standard of therapy, but several pulmonary preserving options have shown promising results. Patients with occult lung cancer have an overall favorable 5-year survival but require close surveillance due to the high incidence of a second primary lung cancer.

SUGGESTED READING

Cortese DA, et al: Roentgenographically occult lung cancer: a ten year experience, *J Thorac Cardiovasc Surg* 86:373, 1983.

Fujimura S, et al: A therapeutic approach to roentgenographically occult squamous cell carcinoma of the lung, *Cancer* 89:2445, 2000.

Saito Y, et al: Results of surgical treatment for roentgenographically occult bronchogenic squamous cell carcinoma, *J Thorac Cardiovasc Surg* 104:401, 1992.

Speiser BL: Strategies for treatment of occult carcinomas of the endobronchus, *Chest* 11:1159, 1997.

Weigel TL, Martini N: Occult lung cancer treatment, *Chest Surg Clin North Am* 10:751, 2000.

SLEEVE LOBECTOMY

Pierre R. Theodore
Stephen C. Yang

Parenchyma-sparing operations for carcinoma permit favorable long-term oncologic results, while maintaining functional lung tissue. Perioperative mortality appears equivalent in sleeve resections, and loss of respiratory function is less compared with pneumonectomy. The role of sleeve resection in thoracic surgery has progressed since its introduction in 1956 by Price Thomas. Complication rates are sufficiently low that sleeve techniques are considered within the spectrum of standard approach to centrally located tumors involving a main stem bronchus. Advances in lung transplantation, improved anesthetic techniques, and management of the complications of surgery of the main stem bronchi have paralleled the application of parenchyma-sparing resections for lung tumors.

Sleeve resections vary in complexity, potentially involving the pulmonary artery, carina, or superior vena cava resection. Cardiopulmonary artery bypass may be required for resections of tumors requiring reimplantation of both main stem bronchi. Sleeve lobectomy is technically more difficult than a routine lobectomy and is the focus of this chapter.

■ INDICATIONS

The overall indication for sleeve resection is straightforward: disease or tumor involving the origin of a lobar bronchus that is not amenable to simple lobectomy. Traditionally, sleeve resections have been performed on patients who, based on pulmonary function testing and preoperative evaluation, are thought incapable of undergoing pneumonectomy. Under the supposition that preservation of parenchyma is a worthwhile goal, however, many groups have liberalized the indications for sleeve resections to include patients who otherwise might tolerate pneumonectomy.

Sleeve resections are performed mainly for two pathologic groups: neoplasms and benign strictures. Bronchogenic carcinoma is the most frequent indication, followed by carcinoid tumors, endobronchial metastases, primary airway tumors, and bronchial adenomas. Bronchial stenosis that requires surgical resection is most often due to infection, usually from tuberculosis. Excision of the airway without removal of lung parenchyma usually can be accomplished in the left main stem bronchus. There also are four anatomic indications for neoplasms necessitating sleeve resection of the bronchial airway for clear margins: (1) tumor limited to the main stem bronchus (usually left) that would not require removal of lung parenchyma, (2) tumor growing outward from a lobar bronchus, (3) extrabronchial tumor infiltrating the bronchial tissue, and (4) peripheral tumor with hilar nodes invading the lobar bronchus.

Low complication rates of the bronchial anastomosis have been reported by several groups for bronchoplastic procedures in groups liberalizing the indications for sleeve resections. As centers gain experience in sleeve resections, the rate of parenchyma-sparing procedures increases, and the rate of pneumonectomy decreases. Sleeve resections in retrospective studies have been associated with shorter intensive care unit stays and periods of postoperative mechanical ventilation. More importantly, the incidence of locoregional recurrence is not higher compared with pneumonectomy in short-term and long-term follow-up. The sleeve resection technique often is required in the setting of preoperative chemoradiation therapy for N2 disease. These situations are fraught with higher rates of bronchial complications, however, and are technically more challenging due to the associated inflammation and destruction of clear tissue planes. For benign endobronchial lesions (i.e., carcinoid tumors or tuberculous bronchial stenosis), the excellent survival indicates sleeve resection as the procedure of choice in suitable candidates.

■ PREOPERATIVE EVALUATION

Pulmonary function tests are reviewed to determine not only if the lobectomy can be tolerated, but also pneumonectomy if required based on intraoperative findings. Patients who have total obstruction of the involved segment or lobe already have compensated clinically for the loss of that lung tissue and should tolerate surgical resection of the involved area.

Skilled preoperative bronchoscopy is key to the evaluation of the potential sleeve resection patient. Not only is tissue diagnosis essential, but also the pathology location is important with respect to lobar orifices and assessment of grossly clear margins. Computed tomography with intravenous contrast enhancement is routine in lung cancer patients, although magnetic resonance imaging and magnetic resonance angiography may be more helpful in defining vascular anatomy and involvement by tumor. The aim of sleeve resection includes adequate oncologic resection with tumor-free margins, while preserving functional lung parenchyma without compromising the airway to the remaining section of lung. Parenchymal preservation should not be performed at the expense of adequate resection, making the choice of proper candidates for sleeve resection crucial. The role of mediastinoscopy versus positron emission tomography scanning for evaluation of nodal status and extent of spread of primary lung cancers remains controversial, but proper nodal status to evaluate for N2 disease is important (ipsilateral paratracheal, paraesophageal, subcarinal, or posteroanterior window nodes) because patients who are responsive to chemoradiotherapy still may be candidates for sleeve resection with curative intent after neoadjuvant therapy. The use of preoperative steroids is controversial: Low-dose methylprednisolone (Solu-Medrol) has been associated with decreased edema at the bronchial anastomosis and improved healing.

■ OPERATIVE TECHNIQUE

All patients require lung isolation with either a double-lumen endotracheal tube or bronchial blocker. Classic teaching dictates that for double-lumen tubes the bronchial blocker should be directed to the opposite side of the pathology. Left-sided tubes can be used for almost all resections however, except for sleeve resections of the left main stem bronchus and carina. Alternatively, high-frequency jet ventilation can be used, particularly for resections close to the carina.

A posterolateral thoracotomy is the preferred approach. This approach gives wide access to airway and vascular structures in the hilum and mediastinum. Median sternotomy has been described for right-sided bronchoplastic procedures but is limited in its exposure to perform lymph node sampling or dissection for malignant processes.

A wide array of bronchoplasties can be performed. The simplest and "classic" sleeve lobectomy is that of the right upper lobe. Following in varying technical complexity are main stem bronchial resection without parenchymal involvement, left upper sleeve lobectomy, superior segmental resection of either lobe, right middle sleeve lobectomy, middle and lower bilobectomy, and Y-sleeve resections in which the upper lobe bronchus is reanastomosed to the proximal main stem bronchus after resection of the distal main stem bronchus with the lower lobe on the left or bilobectomy on the right.

For resections in which the neoplasm or stricture does not involve the pulmonary artery, lobectomy is performed in the standard fashion. The segmental pulmonary arterial and venous branches are tied off, and the fissures are completed. When arterioplastic procedures on the pulmonary artery are required, options include tangential resection with primary closure or reconstruction with pericardial tissue, complete segmental sleeve resection and primary reanastomosis, or reanastomosis of segmental arterial branches. These are described in more detail later.

Essential to the success of proper bronchial anastomotic healing is preservation of blood supply to the cut edges of bronchial tissue. In dissection of nodal tissue off the airway, care is taken not to skeletonize the bronchus. Before the airway is divided, traction sutures of 2-0 polyglactin 910 (Vicryl) are placed in the medial and lateral aspect of the cartilage just above and below the intended transection sites. The airway is cut sharply beginning with the cartilage, being cognizant of the bronchial blocker, and the segmental orifices for reimplantation. The amount resected is dictated by gross findings and intraoperative frozen sections. For strictures, the airway is cut a ring at a time, until a normal caliper of airway is seen. We leave an extra 2-mm edge of membrane on both sides to help reduce the tension on this fragile part of the airway during reanastomosis. Bleeding should be noted from both ends of the airway and should not be cauterized. The edges should be smooth—with ragged, severed, or frayed tissue removed. The line of resection should parallel closely the cartilaginous ring. Experience has shown that wedge resections of the airway result in kinking of the anastomosis.

Lymph node sampling or dissection is performed before reanastomosis of the bronchus to avoid unnecessary traction on the suture line. Care should be taken to preserve bronchial arterial supply. Often this is difficult, particularly in dissection of mediastinal and subcarinal lymph nodes.

Another premise essential to proper healing of the bronchus is a tension-free anastomosis. For upper lobe sleeve resections, the inferior pulmonary ligament should be released.

This is usually adequate for bronchial defects less than 2 cm. For more extensive defects, a circular pericardiotomy around the inferior pulmonary vein is performed and can be extended to mobilize the left atrium completely. On the right side, the distal pretracheal and carinal tissue can be mobilized, which requires division of the azygos vein, being careful not to disrupt the lateral segmental arterial supply to the trachea. On the left, the aortic arch can be mobilized by dividing the ligament of Botallo and Marshall's fold.

When these maneuvers fall short, a lobe transposition may be required. This technique transplants the lower lobe vein to the superior vein stump. Briefly, after systemic heparinization with 5000 U, pulmonary arterial inflow is clamped. With the pericardium circumferentially incised around both pulmonary veins, a vascular clamp is placed on the left atrium proximal to both pulmonary veins. The inferior vein is transected sharply, keeping as much vein as possible but leaving enough tissue behind on the left atrial side so that it can be closed without difficulty using a running 4-0 polypropylene suture (Prolene). The superior vein stump is opened and trimmed to accept an end-to-end anastomosis with the inferior pulmonary vein using a 5-0 or 6-0 polypropylene suture.

Airway Anastomosis

Bringing the two stay sutures on either side of the defect together helps to confirm a tension-free repair. We prefer to perform the anastomosis in an end-to-end fashion, telescoping the smaller distal airway into the larger proximal airway, which is almost always the situation. We use 4-0 or 5-0 polydioxanone suture (PDS) because of its smooth surface and small atraumatic needle. An interrupted row of sutures first is placed through the cartilaginous rings (about two rings from the edge), beginning on the lateral aspect at the cartilaginous-membranous junction first because of the difficult exposure. The cartilaginous ends must be aligned properly according to topography. The sutures are pulled up together at one time to approximate the two airway ends and tied from lateral to medial. The membranous airway is closed in a running fashion, passing the needle through the tissue carefully so as not to make a larger hole around the suture. When the reanastomosis is complete, the two stay sutures are tied to help reduce tension further.

Pneumostasis is checked by submerging the anastomosis under saline and inflating the lung to a pressure of 30 cm H_2O. Air leaks should be reinforced meticulously with the minimal amount of suture. Bronchoscopy is performed simultaneously to suction residual secretions and to confirm proper placement of the suture, correct orientation of the repair, and no compromise of the segmental bronchi. Potential vascular compromise to the anastomosis can exist, especially in patients who had extensive nodal dissection or received induction chemoradiation therapy. We routinely wrap the site with pleura, pericardial fat, or pericardium. Other tissue flaps can be used, such as diaphragm, intercostal muscle, omentum, or chest wall muscle. These can provide too much bulk to the site, however, and can cause distortion. Chest closure is performed in the standard fashion leaving one chest tube in place, and all patients are extubated in the operating room before transfer to a monitored care unit.

Pulmonary Arterioplasty

Most pulmonary artery sleeve resections are done with upper lobectomies, usually in combination with an airway sleeve procedure. Situations that require arterial resection and reconstruction include tumor or lymph node involvement, technical reasons (especially for left upper lobe airway sleeve resections), or trauma. This part of the procedure usually is performed just before removal of the specimen.

The most straightforward technique is tangential resection of the segmental branches with a portion of the sidewall of the artery. A vascular clamp to occlude partially the main pulmonary artery is applied to include the area of resection. If this cannot be applied safely, proximal and distal control is obtained after systemic heparinization. The pulmonary vein also is occluded. Mobilization of the proximal right or left main pulmonary artery is done in standard fashion, occasionally with division of the pericardial attachments. A gross margin of vessel around the tumor or nodes is cut sharply and sent en bloc with the lung specimen. The defect is primarily repaired if a large portion is not removed and does not compromise flow distally. Sleeve resection should be considered if more than 50% of the wall is removed. If possible, the arteriotomy is closed transversely with a running 5-0 or 6-0 polypropylene suture; alternatively the pericardium can be used for patch arterioplasty.

When sleeve resection of the artery is required, arterial and venous control is obtained similarly. An end-to-end anastomosis is done with the same suture in a running fashion, tying the opposite ends to prevent purse-string narrowing. In rare instances, segmental branches require transection (usually right middle lobe or lingula) and reanastomosis to the descending pulmonary artery. In this situation, interrupted sutures are used.

An airway and arterial sleeve resection are done simultaneously (double-sleeve resection), usually associated with the left upper lobe. The artery requires resection because of exposure issues, tumor involvement, or to prevent kinking when an extensive airway defect is closed. The bronchial reanastomosis usually is performed first, but exposure issues may preclude this. Either way, the airway and arterial suture lines must be separated with a viable tissue flap, similar to that described earlier to wrap the bronchial anastomosis.

Finally, a rare situation requires extracorporeal resection, in which a pneumonectomy is performed because the standard sleeve resection cannot be performed in situ due to technical reasons. The parenchymal resection is performed on the back table, and the noninvolved lobe is reimplanted usually with the lobe transposition technique.

■ COMPLICATIONS

Atelectasis is the most common complication postoperatively, occurring in around 15% of patients. All patients require aggressive pulmonary toilet similar to patients undergoing routine pulmonary resection. Blind nasotracheal suction should be avoided, however, and bronchoscopy performed early.

Bronchial complications, although the most feared concern, occur rarely after sleeve resection if a meticulous dissection and reimplantation was performed. These range from local ulceration to mucosal sloughing to full-thickness anastomotic necrosis. Repetitive bronchoscopy should be performed to monitor any progression of necrosis. Limited problems can be watched with a small risk of stenosis long-term that might require eventual dilation or stent insertion. Dehiscence requires completion pneumonectomy, especially if dark red hemoptysis occurs—a sign of pulmonary arterial fistulization.

Thrombosis at the arterial suture site is the only significant problem. Acute thrombosis may present identical to a pulmonary embolism—rapid clinical deterioration and hypoxia. The diagnosis should be made with spiral computed tomography or pulmonary angiography. Clot lysis or anastomotic revision rarely resolves the situation, requiring completion pneumonectomy. Chronic thrombosis may not present with any clinical symptoms, and management is conservative. When the pulmonary vein has been reimplanted, specific outflow problems (either due to suture narrowing or due to thrombosis) manifest as an acutely deteriorating patient, requiring complete pneumonectomy.

■ RESULTS

Reported operative mortality ranges from 0% to 12%. Higher mortality is associated with cancer operations and double-sleeve resections. Bronchopleural fistula and empyema occur at a rate of 8% and 3%.

In long-term evaluations of results after sleeve resections for carcinoma, survival rates compare favorably with pneumonectomy, suggesting that the oncologic result of parenchyma-sparing operations is equivalent. Perioperative mortality should be less than 5% in centers with experience with the techniques and with management of bronchial anastomosis complications. Overall, 5-year and 10-year survival rates are 50% and 25%, which mirrors mortality associated with pneumonectomy. Factors found to influence long-term survival are nodal status and bronchial stump tumor-free margins. Prognosis for carcinoid tumor patients is favorable.

SUGGESTED READING

Deslaurier J, et al: Long-term clinical and functional results of sleeve lobectomy for primary lung cancer, *J Thorac Cardiovasc Surg* 92:871, 1986.

Fadel E, et al: Sleeve lobectomy for bronchogenic cancers: factors affecting survival, *Ann Thorac Surg* 74:851, 2002.

Jensik RJ, et al: Sleeve lobectomy for bronchogenic carcinoma: the Rush-Presbyterian-St. Luke's Medical Center Experience, *Int Surg* 71:207, 1986.

Shrager JB, et al: Lobectomy with tangential pulmonary artery resection without regard to pulmonary function, *Ann Thorac Surg* 70:234, 2000.

CARINAL RESECTION

Simon K. Ashiku

Douglas J. Mathisen

Tumors of the carina resist conventional histologic classification schemes. One classification schema divides tumors into two main categories: bronchogenic carcinoma and other airway neoplasms. Bronchial carcinomas are by definition malignant; the other airway neoplasms may exhibit a wide range of behavior. As shown in Table 1, the most common histologies are squamous cell carcinoma and adenoid cystic carcinoma.

Surgical techniques have been developed that allow resection and primary reconstruction of the carina. Experience is limited, however. Grillo reported 36 resections in 1982, and in 1999, Mitchell expanded the series to 135 patients.

■ CLINICAL PRESENTATION

Patients commonly present with dyspnea and stridor due to tracheobronchial obstruction. Chest radiographs may show a mass in the tracheobronchial airway column. These findings are often subtle and usually are missed. As a result, patients commonly are given a diagnosis of adult-onset asthma, and diagnosis is delayed. Patients who present with symptoms of cough and hemoptysis usually are diagnosed more rapidly.

■ DIAGNOSTIC STUDIES

Chest radiographs can appear normal despite significant tracheobronchial obstruction, but careful evaluation often

Table 1 Diagnosis by Tumor Type in Primary Carinal Resection (n = 118)*

BRONCHOGENIC CARCINOMA (n = 58)	
Squamous cell carcinoma	42
Adenocarcinoma	10
Large cell carcinoma	4
Small cell carcinoma	1
Bronchioalveolar carcinoma	1
OTHER AIRWAY NEOPLASMS (n = 60)	
Adenoid cystic carcinoma	37
Carcinoid	11
Mucoepidermoid carcinoma	7
Malignant fibrosing histiocytoma	2
Fibrosarcoma	1
Mixed spindle cell carcinoma	1
Granular cell tumor	1

*Carinal neoplasms at the Massachusetts General Hospital from 1962-1996.

shows the outline of the mass within the airway column. Carinal tomograms reveal the location and extent of the lesion, permitting the assessment of the uninvolved proximal and distal airway. Metastatic workup should include chest computed tomography, head computed tomography, and bone scan to assess extraluminal extension; nodal basins; and liver, adrenal, brain, and bone metastases. Bronchoscopy allows tissue diagnosis and reveals the intraluminal extent of the tumor. Mediastinoscopy ideally is reserved for the day of resection to assess resectability and nodal status. This avoids the scarring and decreased mobility associated with a staged approach. Patients with bronchogenic carcinoma involving the carina and N2 disease should be considered to have unresectable disease, and surgery should be performed only in a protocol setting.

■ ANESTHESIA

An experienced anesthesiology team working in close cooperation with the surgical team is essential. Epidural anesthesia significantly decreases thoracotomy pain. When maintenance of the airway is a concern, induction with an inhalation agent is employed, and paralytics are given when the airway is secured. Anesthesia is maintained with total intravenous anesthesia using short-acting agents, such as remifentanil and propofol. This approach allows immediate extubation at the completion of the procedure. Endotracheal intubation is accomplished with an extra-long, armored endotracheal tube. Its flexibility allows bronchoscopic placement into one of the main stem bronchi. After transecting the airway, the orotracheal tube is pulled back into the trachea, and intermittent ventilation is performed with sterile cross-field equipment. Intraoperative deoxygenation can be alleviated by periodic partial inflation of the right lung. The orotracheal tube is advanced again when the anastomosis is completed. The anesthesiology team should be familiar with the techniques of high-frequency jet ventilation. Cardiopulmonary bypass is not helpful and only introduces unnecessary risks.

■ OPERATIVE PROCEDURE

When a high degree of obstruction exists, the airway can be reopened endoscopically. This allows a greater degree of preoperative assessment and preparation and the safe delivery of anesthesia. This reopening is accomplished using a ventilating rigid bronchoscope under general anesthesia, without respiratory paralysis. Using the tip of the bronchoscope as a coring device, the side with the least obstruction is cleared first. Significant bleeding is rarely a problem and can be handled with the usual techniques of rigid bronchoscopic tamponade and topical epinephrine solution.

Mediastinoscopy is performed on the day of proposed surgery not only to assess nodal status and resectability, but also to facilitate the resection and reconstruction by mobilizing the pretracheal plane, while visualizing the recurrent laryngeal nerve. Scarring of the pretracheal plane from prior mediastinoscopy limits airway mobility, complicates reconstruction, and increases the likelihood of injury to the left recurrent laryngeal nerve. Scar tissue also may be difficult to distinguish from tumor.

A standard right posterolateral thoracotomy in the fourth interspace creates excellent exposure of the carina and allows for most resections through a single incision. When tumor extension down the left main bronchus precludes carinal reconstruction after complete resection, median sternotomy, bilateral thoracotomies, or extended clamshell incision should be used because they permit sleeve pneumonectomy (Figure 1).

When the right lung is collapsed and retracted anteriorly, the pleura overlying the carina is incised, and the carina is exposed. Division of the azygos vein facilitates exposure. The carina should be freed circumferentially by dissecting on the airway and avoiding the left recurrent laryngeal nerve. Dissection should be kept to a minimum, and skeletonization of the airway should be limited to only the diseased segment to be resected. Likewise, a balance must be struck between achieving adequate lymphadenectomy and maintaining tracheobronchial blood supply. Tapes are placed around the trachea and both main stem bronchi. The inferior pulmonary ligament is released to allow greater mobility of the right lung, and equipment for cross-field sterile ventilation is prepared. The order of dividing the airway structures varies, but commonly the trachea is divided first. Preoperative bronchoscopic assessment by the surgeon directs the tracheal division to just proximal to the tumor. An adequate margin can be taken under direct visualization in the form of a complete ring sent separately for intraoperative frozen section. The endotracheal tube is removed to allow division of both main stem bronchi under direct

endobronchial visualization. Adequate margins are taken of both distal bronchi and sent separately for frozen section. Only the left main stem bronchus is reintubated, maintaining collapse of the right lung.

If mediastinoscopy was not performed, airway mobilization should be accomplished in the anterior plane up to the neck proximally and down the left main stem distally. Additional airway mobility can be obtained by hilar mobilization. This technique involves making a U-shaped incision in the pericardium below the inferior pulmonary vein. If required, the pericardium can be incised 360 degrees around the hilus for maximal mobility. In this event, the vascular and lymphatic pedicle to the main stem bronchus is left preserved behind the pericardium. Left-sided hilar release can be accomplished easily only through a median sternotomy by opening the pericardium anteriorly, bilateral thoracotomies, or an extended clamshell incision. As with most airway surgery, neck flexion is helpful. Laryngeal release has not been shown to produce meaningful mobility at the level of the carina.

Placement of 2-0 polyglactin 910 (Vicryl) lateral traction sutures in the trachea and both bronchi allows for easy handling of these structures during the reconstruction phase. The optimal mode of carinal reconstruction depends largely on the extent of resection. In the series from Massachusetts General Hospital (MGH) reported by Mitchell, 15 different modes of reconstruction were employed. The three most common methods (arranged in order of frequency) were (1) end-to-end anastomosis of trachea to the left main stem with reimplantation of the right main stem into trachea (Figure 2A), (2) end-to-end anastomosis of the trachea to the right main stem with reimplantation of the left main stem into the bronchus intermedius (Figure 2B), and (3) anastomosis of the trachea to reapproximated left and right main stem bronchi creating a "neocarina" (Figure 2C).

The neocarina method is the most simple but can be used in only limited resections because cephalad movement of the neocarina is limited by the aortic arch, requiring generous caudal displacement of the trachea. For this reason, end-to-end anastomosis of the trachea to the left main stem with reimplantation of the right main stem into the trachea is more commonly employed. A right hilar release maneuver facilitates this procedure. More extensive resections require end-to-end anastomosis of the trachea to the right main stem with reimplantation of the left main stem into the bronchus intermedius; this obviates the need for extensive left main stem mobility. When there is extensive endobronchial involvement, excessive lung destruction, or invasion of hilar vessels, carinal (sleeve) pneumonectomy is necessary. Experienced intraoperative judgment is required to determine the ideal approach.

The anastomosis is fashioned with interrupted simple 4-0 Vicryl sutures placed with knots tied outside the lumen. When reconstructed, the anastomoses are tested for air tightness to 40 torr. All suture lines are wrapped circumferentially with pedicled flaps of pericardial fat or a broad-based pleural flap. In high-risk patients, especially patients who have undergone prior radiotherapy, an intercostal flap stripped of all periosteum or an omentum pedicle is used. These flaps not only buttress the anastomoses, but also, more importantly, separate them from the hilar vessels, helping to prevent bronchovascular fistulas.

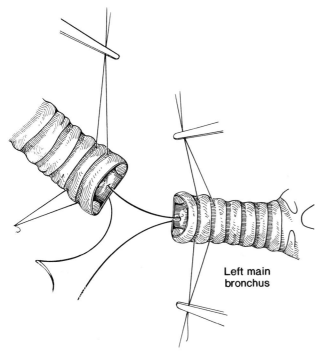

Left main bronchus

Figure 1
Technique of end-to-end anastomosis after right pneumonectomy sleeve resection.

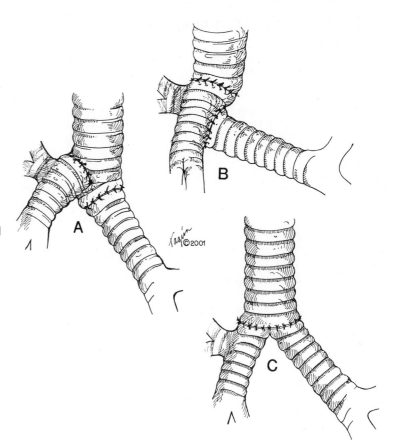

Figure 2
A-C, The three most common types of carinal reconstructions (see text for descriptions).

When the disease is too extensive for resection, tumor "core-out" with or without expandable covered stents is often helpful. External beam radiotherapy and brachytherapy remain the standard palliative treatment.

■ COMPLICATIONS

The current overall mortality for all types of carinal resections is 9%. Overall morbidity is 39%. Major postoperative complications are higher after carinal pneumonectomy than after carinal resection. In the MGH series, the two major types of complications were anastomosis-related problems and acute respiratory distress syndrome (ARDS). Anastomotic complications occurred in 17% of patients. Early complications were necrosis, separation, and mucosal sloughing. Late complications were stenosis, excessive granulation tissue, and recurrent postobstructive pneumonia. Most of these required intervention. Anastomosis-related complications were associated with a 44% mortality rate. ARDS occurred in 10% of patients, usually after carinal pneumonectomies, and was associated with a 90% mortality rate. The cause of ARDS is unclear, but it may result from intraoperative overhydration and lung overinflation. This situation may induce lung injury and interstitial edema in a lung that already has a disrupted lymphatic drainage system. When ARDS develops, inhaled nitric oxide may be beneficial.

■ PROGNOSIS

Carinal neoplasms are a rare and heterogeneous group, which limits the ability to determine prognostic factors. In our series of bronchogenic carcinomas involving the carina, 57% presented with N0 disease, 25% had N1 disease, and 18% had N2/N3 disease. The overall 5-year survival was 42%. Lymph node status strongly influenced survival. The 5-year survival of N0, N1, and N2/N3 patients was 51%, 32%, and 12%. Microscopically positive margins did not affect survival. Isolated carinal resection resulted in a more favorable prognosis than more extensive resections, with a 5-year survival of 51%.

The long-term survival data for resected adenoid cystic carcinoma of the carina has not been as well defined, partly because of its proclivity for late recurrence. The published experience of all tracheal adenoid cystic carcinomas, which includes carinal involvement, suggests a much more favorable prognosis than bronchogenic carcinomas. Lymph node and margin status do not seem to affect survival significantly.

Postoperative radiation therapy is recommended in all cases of bronchogenic or adenoid cystic carcinoma, unless contraindicated by performance status or anastomotic complications. The role of chemotherapy has not been established.

SUGGESTED READING

Grillo HC, Mathisen DJ: Primary tracheal tumors: treatment and results, *Ann Thorac Surg* 49:69, 1990.

Mathisen DJ, Grillo HC: Endoscopic relief of malignant airway obstruction, *Ann Thorac Surg* 48:469, 1989.

Mitchell JD, et al: Clinical experience with carinal resection, *J Thorac Cardiovasc Surg* 117:39, 1999.

Mitchell JD, et al: Resection of bronchogenic carcinoma involving the carina: long-term results and the effect of nodal status on outcome, *J Thorac Cardiovasc Surg* 121:465, 2001.

Regnard JF, et al: Results and prognostic factors in resections of primary tracheal tumors: a multicenter retrospective study, *J Thorac Cardiovasc Surg* 111:808, 1996.

SUPERIOR VENA CAVA SYNDROME

Juan P. Arnoletti

Melvyn Goldberg

The superior vena cava (SVC) is a low-pressure, thin-walled vessel, surrounded by relatively rigid structures and easily compressible in the middle mediastinum. The signs and symptoms of SVC obstruction are called *superior vena cava syndrome* (SVCS). Symptoms caused by SVC obstruction include face, neck, and upper extremity edema; dyspnea; orthopnea; and cough. Patients with SVCS may have a plethoric or cyanotic face and can present with hoarseness, stridor, dysphagia, nasal congestion, and headache. SVCS symptoms have positional worsening and result in fatigue and sleep deprivation. Findings on the physical examination of these patients include facial and upper extremity edema, upper body superficial venous distention, and cyanosis. The onset of SVCS is usually insidious with symptoms present for several weeks before a diagnosis is reached. Depending on the underlying disease process, however, SVCS may develop rapidly with cephalic venous congestion, laryngeal edema, and possible airway compromise.

Pathologic processes arising in any of the surrounding structures may result in SVC obstruction by extrinsic compression, direct invasion, or thrombosis of this vessel. Multiple series since the 1950s have shown that SVCS is caused most often by malignancy (90% to 95% of SVCS cases). The tumor types most frequently associated with this syndrome are bronchogenic carcinoma (>80% of cases, two thirds of which are non–small cell lung cancer), non-Hodgkin's lymphoma, and mediastinal metastatic disease from various primary cancers (breast, testicular, gastrointestinal). Although much less frequent, multiple nonmalignant causes for SVCS have been described, including idiopathic fibrosing mediastinitis, tuberculosis, sarcoidosis, aortic aneurysms, benign tumors of the mediastinum, and pericarditis. Indwelling central venous catheters and pacemaker wires can cause SVC thrombosis, and the incidence of this condition has increased with the widespread use of such devices.

◾ DIAGNOSIS

The diagnosis of SVCS essentially is based on the described clinical findings. A chest x-ray can provide useful information in most patients. Computed tomography or magnetic resonance imaging of the chest with intravenous contrast material can characterize further the SVC obstruction and its cause. A two-projection venogram provides valuable information for therapeutic planning. Based on venographic findings, four patterns of collateral circulation in SVCS patients have been described:

Type I: 90% SVC stenosis with patent azygos vein

Type II: near-complete to complete SVC obstruction with antegrade flow in the azygos vein

Type III: near-complete to complete SVC obstruction with reversal of azygos vein flow

Type IV: complete obstruction of the SVC and its major tributaries

Most patients with severe symptoms have type III or IV SVC obstruction.

The diagnosis of the specific underlying cause of SVCS should be obtained before the institution of therapy. Tissue diagnosis should not delay therapy in patients with severe symptoms.

◾ TREATMENT

There are multiple treatment modalities for patients with SVCS, and therapy must be tailored to the individual patient. Because most patients have an advanced underlying malignancy, the most adequate form of palliation must be sought. Most cancer patients with SVCS carry a poor prognosis with a median survival of less than 1 year. The treatment modalities currently available for SVCS include (1) conservative medical therapy, (2) radiation therapy, (3) chemotherapy, (4) surgery, and (5) endovascular therapy.

Symptoms caused by SVC obstruction can be relieved initially by simple conservative measures, such as elevation of the head of the bed and supplemental oxygen. The use of steroids and diuretics has been described, but evidence is lacking regarding their efficacy. SVCS almost always is associated with some degree of SVC thrombosis, and anticoagulation can help prevent propagation of the clot. Anticoagulation has not been shown to be effective in symptom relief but frequently is used as an adjunctive measure.

Radiation therapy is standard treatment for SVCS caused by bronchogenic carcinoma or lymphoma, and it can prolong survival significantly in that subgroup of patients. Histologic diagnosis is required before treatment, and most patients receive a total of 20 to 30 Gy, reporting symptomatic relief within a few days. Initial response rates reach 80% to 90%, but recurrence rates of 50% have been reported. Besides the general side effects of radiation, SVCS patients may develop pulmonary and mediastinal fibrosis, tumor necrosis with fever, bleeding, and perforation of the SVC.

Chemotherapy, either alone or in combination with radiation therapy, can be effective in the treatment of SVCS, particularly in patients with small cell lung cancer and lymphoma. Proposed regimens include cyclophosphamide, doxorubicin, vincristine, etoposide, paclitaxel, and platin-based agents. Morbidity is usually significant with partial response rates that provide only temporary relief.

Surgical bypass is a safe, long-term solution for selected patients with SVCS due to benign causes. Various types of bypass procedures to the right atrial appendage can be performed from the jugular, innominate, or azygos vein, with the purpose of relieving the SVC obstruction. The conduits most frequently used are autogenous saphenous vein (spiral graft) and prosthetic grafts (polytetrafluoroethylene). Surgical bypass for SVCS is associated with low morbidity and high patency rates, but this type of procedure hardly can be justified as palliation for the terminally ill patient.

Endovascular techniques have become the mainstay of therapy for patients with SVCS, particularly for patients with underlying malignancy who are poor surgical candidates. Endovascular treatment modalities, especially when used in combination, provide rapid symptom relief, and they include thrombolytic therapy, angioplasty, and stent placement.

Thrombolytic therapy may be used for patients who show evidence of SVC thrombosis, usually associated with indwelling central venous catheters. Catheter removal followed by urokinase or tissue-type plasminogen activator infusion has been shown to be effective in clot lysis. Clot lysis also is beneficial in many SVCS patients as adjunctive therapy to help relieve the obstruction, further delineate the morphology of the lesion, and allow angioplasty and stent placement. The potential hemorrhagic complications of this kind of therapy and its formal contraindications must be kept in mind.

Angioplasty of the SVC is useful in SVCS caused by benign conditions. Balloon dilation alone often has a high failure rate, however, and requires combination with stent placement. Several stent models are currently available, and they can be either self-expandable or balloon-expandable. The most common approach for stent placement is through the right femoral vein, and the procedure has a high technical success rate (>90%). Incidence of complications is low, but stent migration, pulmonary embolus, and congestive heart failure have been reported. The long-term patency rate of SVC stents is not known because most SVCS patients have relatively short life expectancy. Most stents have been shown to remain patent for the lifetime of the patient. The indication for anticoagulation after stent placement is a subject of debate; anticoagulation has not been shown to improve stent patency. Nevertheless, long-term anticoagulation and antiplatelet agents are used often in this setting. Patients with SVCS caused by benign conditions should be evaluated carefully on an individual basis for either surgical bypass or a combination of endovascular techniques.

■ SUMMARY

Most patients with SVCS have underlying malignancy, and their prognosis is poor. Adequate palliation can be provided with a multidisciplinary approach mainly based on endovascular techniques and radiation therapy. Anticoagulation, chemotherapy, and surgical bypass should be used selectively.

SUGGESTED READING

Abner A: Approach to the patient who presents with superior vena cava obstruction, *Chest* 103:394S, 1993.

Chen JC, et al: A contemporary perspective on superior vena cava syndrome, *Am J Surg* 160:207, 1990.

Nieto AF, Doty DB: Superior vena cava obstruction: clinical syndrome, etiology, and treatment, *Curr Probl Cancer* 10:441, 1986.

Schindler N, Vogelzang RL: Superior vena cava syndrome, *Surg Clin North Am* 79:683, 1999.

Yin CD, et al: Superior vena cava stenting, *Radiol Clin North Am* 38:409, 2000.

SPIRAL SAPHENOUS VEIN BYPASS GRAFT FOR SUPERIOR VENA CAVA OBSTRUCTION

John R. Doty
Donald B. Doty

Obstruction of the superior vena cava (SVC) can present either as a chronic, progressive syndrome or as an acute, life-threatening process. Most cases are caused by malignancy, with lung carcinoma and lymphoma the most common tumors. Lung cancer in particular has a propensity to cause obstruction of the SVC, with reports of 5% to 15% of patients with bronchogenic carcinoma developing superior vena cava syndrome (SVCS). Benign causes are less common, with fibrosing mediastinitis and fungal diseases as the leading etiologies. More recently, an increasing number of infectious causes of SVCS have been reported, however, in the setting of immunosuppression. Thrombosis of the SVC results in the most dramatic presentation and is becoming more prevalent with the increasing use of central venous access catheters and invasive monitoring devices.

The symptoms of SVC obstruction are typically insidious in onset and are characterized by gradual dilation and tortuosity of the veins in the neck and upper thorax. Progressive obstruction results in facial edema, cyanosis, proptosis, and laryngeal edema; the most severe degree of obstruction produces symptoms of cerebral edema, such as headache, convulsions, altered mental state, and coma. Ultrasonography, computed tomography, and contrast venography should be used to guide medical and surgical therapy, with venography having particular importance for stratifying patients for surgical intervention. Patients with type III (near-complete to complete obstruction of the SVC with reversal of azygos blood flow) pattern of obstruction on venography are the best candidates for caval bypass operations.

Most cases of SVCS are treated effectively with medical therapy, especially if the cause is infectious or malignant. Radiation therapy has a central role in the treatment of acute SVC obstruction from malignancy, but a tissue diagnosis should be sought before initiation of radiation. Pleural fluid cytology, lymph node biopsy, bronchoscopy, mediastinoscopy, and thoracotomy may be required to obtain a tissue diagnosis to guide therapy accurately. Thrombolytic therapy has been shown to be useful in resolving SVC obstruction secondary to clot formation and is most effective in lysis of thrombus associated with a central venous catheter. Percutaneous placement of intravascular stents has a role in SVC obstruction secondary to malignancy, although these stents are prone to thrombosis. Simple balloon angioplasty has inferior results to operative reconstruction and requires multiple attempts to approach the long-term success of surgery.

■ INDICATIONS FOR SURGERY

The operative indications for surgical treatment of SVC obstruction are not completely defined and depend to some degree on the underlying cause and the rapidity of the obstructive process. Most commonly, surgical reconstruction is required in the chronic form of SVC obstruction. Some of the so-called benign causes of SVC obstruction are severe and relentless fibrotic processes that result in recurrent obstruction. Malignant diseases that result in acute, sudden obstruction and thrombosis of the SVC may not resolve with thrombolytic and radiation therapy. Acute obstruction of the SVC associated with signs of cerebral or laryngeal edema is indicative of death within 6 weeks and demands urgent surgical intervention. Invasion of the SVC by malignant or benign tumor may be resistant to chemotherapy and produce a persistent obstruction to flow. Any patient being considered for surgical reconstruction should have contrast venography documentation of complete obstruction of the SVC with inadequate collateral circulation. Current indications for surgical reconstruction in SVC obstruction include the following:

1. Persistent chronic SVC obstruction with SVCS due to benign process
2. Acute SVC obstruction due to benign or malignant process with signs of cerebral or laryngeal edema
3. Palliation of SVCS due to a malignant process
4. Failure of medical therapy to resolve SVC obstruction

Contraindications to surgical reconstruction include patients in whom collateral circulation has formed adequately to provide upper compartment venous decompression. Patients with large, bulky tumors of the mediastinum are unsuitable candidates for operative intervention, as are patients with limited life expectancy from associated medical disorders.

■ OPERATIVE TECHNIQUE

Operative reconstruction for SVC obstruction ideally should be performed with autogenous tissue to provide the optimal long-term outcome. Options for autogenous venous conduits include spiral saphenous vein, femoral vein, straight saphenous vein, and composite vein grafts. In unusual settings and according to individual patient anatomy, alternative venous conduits, such as azygos vein–inferior vena cava or jugular vein–femoral vein grafts, can be constructed. In the absence of autogenous venous tissue, aortic homograft, venous homograft, and pericardial tube construction can serve as conduits. Prosthetic graft materials are generally inferior to autogenous tissue grafts.

The ideal graft to replace the SVC should match closely the diameter of the native SVC to prevent residual obstructive flow gradients. As a practical matter, however, the size of the SVC usually is destroyed by the disease process so that replacement is seldom possible, and bypass of the obstructed SVC is usually the best option. Success with bypass grafting of the SVC depends primarily on two main factors: adequate size of the conduit and proper orientation. The graft should be measured carefully for length so that the diameter precisely matches that of the inflow vein and so that the completed conduit does not have redundancy, which can result in graft kinking and obstruction. The inflow and outflow of the graft should be free of intraluminal obstructions, such as atrial trabeculations and venous thrombosis.

The most extensive experience with venous bypass grafts for relief of SVC obstruction has been with the spiral saphenous vein graft, a concept developed by Chiu et al in 1974. We reported the first use of the spiral vein graft in humans in 1976 in a patient with SVC obstruction secondary to granulomatous mediastinitis. Twenty-three years later, the graft was patent and the patient remained asymptomatic.

The spiral vein graft is constructed from the patient's own saphenous vein and is used as a bypass graft from the innominate or jugular vein to the right atrium. After performing a sternotomy, the distance from the confluence of the left internal jugular vein and the left subclavian vein to the right atrial appendage is measured. The diameter of the innominate vein is measured as the eventual diameter of the spiral vein graft. The saphenous vein is exposed, and its diameter is measured. The length of the saphenous vein to be removed is calculated using the following simple formula:

$$\frac{\text{Innominate vein diameter (mm)}}{\text{Saphenous vein diameter (mm)}} \times \text{Length to right atrial appendage (cm)}$$

For example, if the innominate vein is 15 mm in diameter, the saphenous vein is 3 mm in diameter, and the length to the right atrial appendage is 8 cm, the proper length of saphenous vein to be harvested is 40 cm ($15/3 \times 8$).

The saphenous vein is removed and incised in a longitudinal fashion throughout its entire length. A thoracostomy tube is chosen that is the same diameter as the innominate vein as a stent to form the bypass graft. The saphenous vein is flattened and wrapped in a spiral fashion around the stent, and the edges are joined using a continuous suture of 7-0 polypropylene (Figure 1). This forms a large conduit

with a diameter that closely matches the innominate vein and a length that approximates the distance from the jugular-subclavian confluence to the right atrial appendage.

Heparin (200 to 300 U/kg) is administered intravenously. A soft jaw vascular clamp is applied at the jugular-subclavian confluence, and the innominate vein is divided. Abnormal intimal tissue and thrombus are removed from the innominate vein. The innominate vein is ligated or oversewn on the SVC end (Figure 2). The spiral vein graft is pushed slightly off the stent, and an end-to-end anastomosis is performed to the innominate vein using continuous 7-0 polypropylene suture. The stent is removed from the graft, and a curved vascular clamp is placed on the right atrial appendage. The tip of the right atrial appendage is excised, and obstructing trabeculae are removed to ensure unrestricted blood flow out of the graft. The graft is anastomosed to the right atrial appendage using continuous 5-0 polypropylene suture.

Long-term follow-up of patients receiving spiral saphenous vein grafts for SVC obstruction has shown excellent results. Our series reported in 1999 of patients treated with spiral vein bypass grafting for benign disease showed patency in 14 of 16 patients (88%) at a mean follow-up of 11 years. Three separate individuals in the series showed patency of the spiral vein graft at 20, 21, and 23 years. Alimi et al also reported a favorable patency rate of 70% at 8 years in 12 patients.

Spiral vein bypass grafting also is useful in the setting of SVC obstruction from malignancy. We reported six patients with spiral vein grafting, all with bronchogenic carcinoma; symptoms of SVC obstruction were relieved in all six patients. Long-term survival in these patients understandably is reduced due to the underlying malignant process, but acute mortality from SVCS was abolished in this series. All but one patient died from metastatic carcinoma, and all patients had patent grafts at the time of death. Smith and Brantigan also reported successful use of a spiral vein bypass graft in the setting of SVC obstruction from bronchogenic carcinoma. Spiral vein graft has been used in two separate

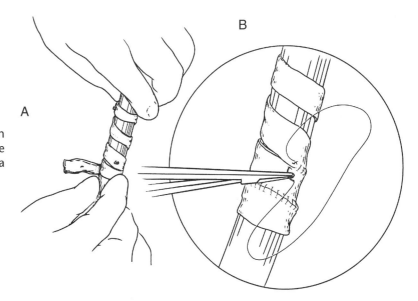

Figure 1
The saphenous vein is flattened and wrapped in a spiral fashion around the thoracostomy tube stent **(A)**, and the edges are joined using a continuous suture of 7-0 polypropylene **(B)**.

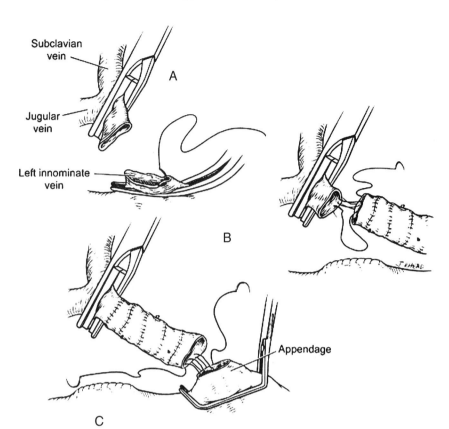

Figure 2
Anastomotic technique for creation of spiral vein bypass graft. **A,** A soft jaw vascular clamp is applied at the jugular-subclavian confluence, and the innominate vein is divided. Abnormal intimal tissue and thrombus are removed from the innominate vein, and the proximal end is oversewn. **B,** The spiral vein graft is anastomosed in an end-to-end fashion to the innominate vein using continuous 7-0 polypropylene suture. **C,** The tip of the right atrial appendage is excised, and obstructing trabeculae are removed to ensure unrestricted blood flow out of the graft. The graft is anastomosed to the right atrial appendage using continuous 5-0 polypropylene suture.

case reports as an interposition graft to reconstruct the SVC after resection of a leiomyosarcoma.

The spiral vein graft has been shown by Brandt et al to be useful in children and adults, as evidenced by their case report of successful treatment of SVC obstruction secondary to intraatrial baffle for transposition of the great arteries. The saphenous vein was of adequate caliber in this child to form a spiral vein bypass graft from the innominate vein to the left atrial appendage. Although most cases of SVCS secondary to sarcoidosis are treated medically, Narayan et al reported use of a spiral vein conduit for reconstruction in a patient with severe symptoms refractory to medical therapy.

Most patients undergoing spiral vein bypass grafting for SVC obstruction can be followed clinically for graft patency. Prompt resolution of symptoms indicates successful decompression, and stenosis or occlusion of the graft typically is heralded by return of the obstructive syndrome. Ultrasonography, computed tomography, venography, and magnetic resonance imaging are useful adjuncts for evaluating spiral vein bypass grafts when the clinical presentation is less clear.

■ CONCLUSION

Surgical treatment of SVC obstruction requires a careful evaluation of the etiology and progressive course of the patient's symptoms. Although most patients with SVC obstruction are not candidates for surgery, operative

decompression of patients with acute and severe obstruction from either benign or malignant causes allows for a more orderly subsequent treatment of the underlying disease. Thorough investigation of the degree of SVC obstruction, the development of venous collaterals, and the patterns of thoracic venous blood flow should be performed before operative intervention.

Large-caliber spiral saphenous vein bypass grafts offer the best current solution for long-term conduit patency and resolution of obstructive symptoms. Alternatively, femoral vein grafts or multiple saphenous vein grafts can be used to bypass or reconstruct the SVC and its major branches. Recurrent obstruction is uncommon for either benign or malignant SVC obstruction and is diagnosed easily on clinical examination.

SUGGESTED READING

Chiu CJ, et al: Replacement of superior vena cava with the spiral composite vein graft, *Ann Thorac Surg* 17:555, 1974.

Doty JR, et al: Superior vena cava obstruction: bypass using spiral vein graft, *Ann Thorac Surg* 67:1111, 1999.

Narayan D, et al: Surgical management of superior vena caval syndrome in sarcoidosis, *Ann Thorac Surg* 66:946, 1998.

Stanford W, Doty DB: The role of venography and surgery in the management of patients with superior vena cava obstruction, *Ann Thorac Surg* 41:158, 1986.

Wisselink W, et al: Comparison of operative reconstruction and percutaneous balloon dilatation for central venous obstruction, *Am J Surg* 166:200, 1993.

LIMITED RESECTION PROCEDURES FOR LUNG CANCER

L. Penfield Faber

A limited pulmonary resection is one in which less than a complete lobe is removed. The two procedures fitting this definition are segmentectomy and wedge resection. Segmentectomy is an anatomic pulmonary resection of the pulmonary artery, vein, bronchus, and parenchyma of a particular segment of the lung. Wedge resection is a nonanatomic removal of a portion of lung parenchyma that may or may not traverse segmental planes. Limited pulmonary resections for lung cancer can be considered for primary, synchronous, and second primary tumors.

■ INDICATIONS

The goal of any surgical procedure for lung cancer is to achieve a complete resection with the removal of regional lymph nodes. The procedure must be planned to achieve satisfactory long-term results with minimal morbidity and mortality. Lung cancers that can be considered for limited resection are tumors that are less than 3 cm in size and located in the peripheral aspect of the lung with regional lymph nodes free of metastatic cancer. Controversy exists regarding limited resection as an operation of choice for the patient who would tolerate lobectomy. Long-term survival and local-regional recurrence must be considered. The clinician must be completely aware of the advantages and disadvantages of limited resection when considering these procedures.

The chest x-ray and computed tomography scan provide the first indication that a limited resection might be possible. A favorable lesion is located in the periphery of the lung and is less than 3 cm in diameter. Lesions located in the central portion of the lobe usually are not amenable to limited resection, and lobectomy becomes a required procedure. Cervical mediastinoscopy is carried out if mediastinal lymph nodes are greater than 1 cm in diameter, and a positive mediastinoscopy contraindicates a limited resection as a curative procedure. Positron emission tomography can be helpful in assessing the status of hilar and mediastinal lymph nodes. Bronchoscopy is done preoperatively or at the time of the planned resection to be certain that the tumor does not involve the segmental or lobar bronchus. In this instance, lobectomy is required to obtain a cancer-free proximal margin of resection.

Histology of the tumor does not indicate or contraindicate segmental resection. Bronchioloalveolar carcinoma in its limited and nodular form is a tumor that should receive consideration for limited resection. These lesions are frequently multicentric, and second and third primary tumors of this histologic type are commonplace. Peripheral squamous cell carcinomas and adenocarcinomas are amenable to limited resection.

Decreased cardiopulmonary reserve is a major consideration for carrying out a limited pulmonary resection. A patient's history of cardiac problems, such as angina pectoris, prior myocardial infarction, or congestive heart failure, indicates consideration for echocardiogram, thallium scan, stress test, and possible coronary angiography. Decreased left ventricular function in association with decreased pulmonary function may preclude resection.

Spirometry values that indicate a high risk for increased postoperative morbidity and mortality include a vital capacity less than 50% predicted, forced expiratory volume in 1 second (FEV_1) less than 50% predicted, maximal voluntary ventilation less than 40% predicted, and carbon monoxide diffusion in the lung less than 50%. Blood gas analysis is always obtained in high-risk patients. A $Paco_2$ greater than 45 torr indicates advanced lung disease with an increased risk of postoperative complications, and a Pao_2 less than 75 torr suggests chronic lung disease. Patients with a Pao_2 of 60 torr can tolerate limited resection if the $Paco_2$ is not significantly elevated.

Miller and Hatcher reported 32 limited resections in patients who had an FEV_1 equal to or less than 1 liter, forced expiratory flow at 25% to 75% of forced vital capacity equal to or less than 0.6 liters, and a maximum breathing capacity less than 40% of predicted. Ten segmentectomies and 22 wide wedge resections were performed in these patients, with no deaths.

Other factors to consider when assessing a patient for type of pulmonary resection are age, prior pulmonary resection, obesity, renal function, and patient motivation. A patient with limited function requires a limited resection, and if the anatomic extent of the lesion is not favorable, thoracotomy is not carried out. A decision for resection in a compromised patient requires clinical judgment with a synthesis of all factors that come into play—history, physical examination, laboratory testing, and clinical staging. No one factor renders a patient inoperable.

■ RESECTION TECHNIQUE

A muscle-sparing incision through the fourth or fifth intercostal space is used for a planned limited resection. The fourth intercostal space provides access to all portions of the right or left lung, and the fifth intercostal space is used only for lesions in the lower portion of either lower lobe.

Segments commonly resected on the right are the anterior, apical, or posterior segment of the right upper lobe or the apical segment in continuity with either the posterior or anterior segment; the posterior segment of the right upper lobe and superior segment of the right lower lobe in continuity; and the four basal segments of the right lower lobe in one unit. The medial basal segment of the right lower lobe is easily resected, but the three remaining basal segments require careful dissection so that the vascular or bronchial supply to the remaining basal segments is not compromised. Individual basal segments of either lower lobe usually are resected singularly only when maximum lung tissue is required.

Segmental resections of the left lung include the apical posterior, anterior, or lingular segments of the left upper lobe; superior anteromedial basal segment of the left lower lobe; and basal segments of the left lower lobe in continuity. The apical-posterior segment of the left upper lobe and superior segment of the left lower lobe also can be resected in continuity. The left upper lobe bronchus commonly bifurcates, creating a superior and inferior division of the left upper lobe. The superior division, consisting of the apical-posterior and anterior segments of the left upper lobe, is resected easily as a segment. The lingula or inferior division is also a common segmental resection (Figure 1).

After the chest is opened, the precise anatomic location of the tumor is identified. This assessment is done with the lung inflated so that margins of resection and precise segmental anatomy are determined. If a diagnosis of cancer has not been established, wedge resection by cautery or stapling technique can remove a peripheral tumor for frozen section study. Needle aspiration cytology is appropriate for deeper seated lesions in which a wedge resection would destroy the planes of the planned segmentectomy or compromise the central anatomy of the hilum.

The hilar dissection is begun, and exposure is facilitated by having the lung deflated. The pulmonary artery to the segment or segments to be resected is dissected free, ligated, and transected. The segmental bronchus is freed of adventitial tissue by sharp scissor dissection. A right-angled clamp is passed around the bronchus to identify better which segment it is supplying and to be certain that it is the correct bronchus to be transected. Segmental lymph nodes always are encountered in this phase of dissection, and they may be sent to pathology for frozen section analysis. If microscopic tumor is identified in these lymph nodes, lobectomy must be considered. The patient's physiologic impairment may necessitate segmentectomy, however, and in this instance, appropriate lymphadenectomy and postoperative adjunctive therapy are considered. The segmental bronchus is not clamped to visualize distal atelectasis of that segment because when the lung is inflated, collateral ventilation from the adjacent segments inflates the segment of the clamped bronchus. When the proper segmental bronchus has been identified, it can be transected and closed with staples or interrupted fine absorbable sutures. After the bronchus and pulmonary artery have been divided, the pulmonary vein draining that segment is dissected free, ligated, and transected. If the surgeon is unsure of the venous drainage of the segment to be removed, the encountered venous branches can be ligated or stapled as the segment is removed.

The classic method of completing a segmental resection was described by Fell and Kirby. This method of completion of the segmental plane has been rendered almost obsolete, however, by the advent of the stapling technique. The almost standard method of completing the intersegmental plane is now with one or two applications of a 90-mm stapling instrument. Staple transection

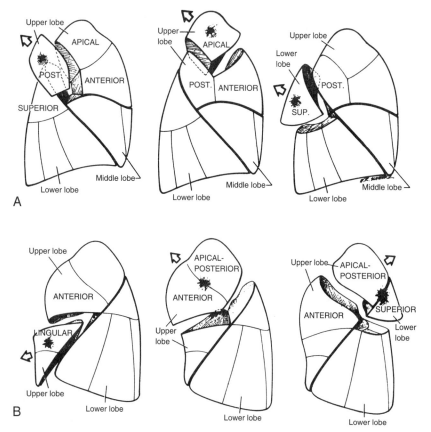

Figure 1
Types of segmental resections. **A,** Right lung. **B,** Left lung. (*From Faber LP, Jensik RJ: Limited pulmonary resection. In Baue AE, editor: Glenn's thoracic and cardiovascular surgery, vol 1, ed 5, Norwalk, CT, Appleton & Lange, 1991, p 391; with permission.*)

and closure of the intersegmental plane should be carried out only after the pulmonary artery and bronchus have been transected. This aspect of the dissection allows proper lymph node assessment and ensures that anatomic segmentectomy is completed. Nonanatomic segmentectomy can only enhance local recurrence.

Stapling of the intersegmental plane is accomplished with the lung deflated or partially inflated because the lung is passed more easily into the jaws of the stapling device. Stapling is particularly effective for the apicoposterior segment of the left upper lobe, the superior or inferior division of the left upper lobe, the anterior segment of the right upper lobe, the posterior segment of the right upper lobe, and the superior segment of either lower lobe. The lung is inflated gently after completion of the segmentectomy to avoid disruption of the staple line, and any defects of the staple line are closed with interrupted absorbable sutures. Staple line closure of the segmental surface minimizes postoperative air leaks and permits early chest tube removal. Compression of adjacent lung tissue does not seem to be a significant problem, and proper use of the stapling instrument minimizes distortion of the residual lobar tissue. After completion of the segmentectomy, regional lymph nodes are sampled or removed. This procedure ensures proper staging. Chest tubes are placed to maximize postoperative expansion and minimize space complications. Suction or water seal alone is used at the surgeon's discretion.

WEDGE RESECTION

A wedge resection is the nonanatomic resection of a small portion of lung tissue with the tumor preferably located in the central portion of the wedge with a 1.5- to 2.0-cm margin. A wedge resection can be accomplished by open surgery or video-assisted thoracic surgery (VATS). A muscle-sparing thoracotomy provides adequate exposure for open wedge resections. Stapling techniques are ideally suited for lesions on the more peripheral part of a lobe. The lung is deflated partially to palpate the precise anatomic extent of the tumor, and two to three applications of the stapling device accomplish the wedge resection. Absorbable sutures are used to close any air leaks from the staple line. If a lesion lies on the flat surface of the lobe, the stapling technique cannot be accomplished safely. In this instance, the cautery technique of wedge resection can be effective. Needle-tip cautery is recommended because it is effective in cauterizing smaller vessels. Larger vessels and bronchi are ligated individually as they are encountered. After completion of the wedge resection, the lung tissue is reapproximated with interrupted absorbable sutures. For deeper cautery excisions, fibrin glue is used to coat the raw surface to minimize hematoma formation and to enhance approximation of the deeper tissue. Neodymium:yttrium-aluminum-garnet laser excision and the Cavitron ultrasonic aspirator have not received wide acceptance and are not recommended. Regional lymph nodes should be sampled for any evidence of metastatic carcinoma and pathologic staging. It is recommended to carry out cautery wedge resection with the lung inflated to minimize the amount of lung tissue removed.

The VATS approach is readily applicable to wedge resection of lesions on the periphery of the lung (<1 cm deep to the visceral pleura) and smaller than 3 cm in diameter. Lesions on the flat surface or beneath the surface of the lung in a central position are technically difficult or hazardous to remove by the VATS technique. Single-lung anesthesia is required, and when dealing with a primary lung cancer, technical concerns are margin adequacy, regional lymph node sampling, and localizing a deep-seeded lesion. The thoracic surgeon should be familiar with the many techniques that have been described to localize lesions that are not readily visible through the thoracoscope.

RESULTS

In 1973, Jensik and Faber reported 69 patients who underwent a curative segmentectomy for primary bronchogenic carcinoma with an actuarial survival rate of 56% at 5 years and 27% at 15 years. Resections were not limited to stage I disease. Subsequent analysis of 348 limited resections for stage I and II primary bronchogenic carcinoma at the Rush–Presbyterian–St. Luke's Medical Center revealed an actuarial survival of 54% at 5 years, 30% at 10 years, and 12% at 15 years. There were 84 lesions larger than 3 cm in diameter, and positive lymph nodes were identified in 26 patients. Surgical mortality was 1.1% (4 of 348). Read et al in 1990 analyzed 255 patients who underwent lobectomy (n = 131) or segmentectomy/wedge resection (n = 113) for T1N0 non–small cell lung cancer (NSCLC). In the limited resection group, 107 patients had segmental resection. The results of conservative resection showed no statistically significant differences from that of lobectomy. Survival data were calculated using only deaths as a result of the primary cancer, and Kaplan-Meier survival for the limited resection group was 92% at 5 years compared with 73% for the lobectomy patients. Mortality for limited resection was 3.5% (4 of 113). Kodama et al in 1997 reviewed 46 patients with good pulmonary function who underwent intentional segmentectomy. Lymph node dissection was completed before pulmonary resection, and conversion to lobectomy was done if mediastinal nodes were positive. Results were compared with 77 patients who underwent lobectomy and mediastinal lymph node dissection. Actuarial 5-year survival was 93% in the segmentectomy group and 88% in the standard lobectomy group. Tumor size and age were independent predictors of survival. Local-regional recurrence in the segmentectomy patients was 8.7% (4 of 46); in 3 patients, recurrence was in the mediastinum.

These studies were retrospective analyses. The Lung Cancer Study Group reported the first randomized trial of lobectomy versus limited resection for T1N0 NSCLC. There were 122 patients randomized to a limited resection (82, segmental; 40, wedge) and 125 lobectomies. Survival was improved in the lobectomy group but was of borderline statistical significance. Local-regional recurrence rate showed a 3-fold increase with wedge resection, however, and a 2.4-fold increase with segmental resection compared with lobectomy. The increase in local-regional recurrence rate was postulated to be related to occult intrapulmonary and lymphatic mediastinal nodal disease. There was no statistical difference in survival related to tumor size. The requirement for lymph node dissection was illustrated by the finding that 25% (122 of 427) of patients clinically staged as T1N0 were found to have positive mediastinal lymph nodes. The conclusion of Ginsberg and Rubenstein was that "lobectomy with systematic hilar and mediastinal lymph node sampling or dissection should remain the standard surgical treatment for clinical T1N0 tumors."

Warren and Faber compared the results of 66 patients with stage I (T1N0, T2N0) NSCLC versus 105 patients with the same stage undergoing lobectomy. There was no difference in survival when comparing segmentectomy with lobectomy for tumors 3.0 cm or smaller in diameter. A survival advantage was noted for lobectomy patients when the tumor was larger than 3.0 cm. Of critical importance, it was found that local-regional recurrence was 22.7% (15 of 66) after segmental resection versus 4.9% (5 of 103) after lobectomy. Histologic tumor type, original tumor diameter, and segment resected revealed no risk factors that were predictive of recurrence.

Complete mediastinal and hilar lymph node dissection provides accurate pathologic staging, may decrease local recurrence, and may improve long-term survival. The question arises as to how complete a lymphadenectomy should be done with segmental resection. In 1997, Takizawa et al reviewed 157 patients undergoing lobectomy and complete hilar/mediastinal lymphadenectomy for NSCLC tumors 1.1 to 2.2 cm in diameter. Pathologic staging revealed lymph node metastases in 27 (17%) patients, and positive nodes were not identified during the operation by gross inspection or frozen section in 19 of 27 patients. Lymph node metastases occur with small peripheral tumors, as described by Konaka et al in 1998. In 171 consecutive patients with T1N0 NSCLC 2 cm or less in diameter, 5.8% (10 of 171) had positive N1 nodes, and 11.7% (20 of 171) had positive N2 nodes. These data indicate that mediastinal and hilar lymph node dissection is indicated for patients with a tumor diameter less than 2 cm. It also was noted in this latter study that tumors less than 1.0 cm in diameter had no positive nodes (n = 19).

Martini et al reviewed 598 patients who underwent resection for stage I NSCLC. There were 511 lobectomies and 62 wedge resections or segmentectomies. Five-year survival for the limited resection group was 59% and for the lobectomy group was 77%. The wedge/segmentectomy group had higher recurrence rates and reduced survival.

Errett et al evaluated 197 patients who had stage I NSCLC. There were 100 wedge resections and 97 lobectomies. For the wedge resection group, 30-day operative mortality was 3% (3 of 100), and for the lobectomy group, mortality was 2.1% (2 of 97). Actuarial survival was 72% in the wedge group and 74% in the lobectomy group at 2 years. There was no reported difference in local recurrence.

Harpole et al evaluated 289 consecutive patients with stage I and II disease. There were 75 wedge resections, and when compared with 193 lobectomies, the limited resection group showed a trend toward an increased rate of local-regional recurrence with no difference in survival. Landreneau et al analyzed 219 consecutive patients with stage I NSCLC who underwent open wedge resection (n = 42), VATS wedge resection (n = 60), and lobectomy (n = 117).

Projected 5-year survival was 58% for open wedge resection, 65% for VATS wedge resection, and 70% for lobectomy. There were significantly more non–cancer-related deaths among the wedge resection patients, however, due to their older age and reduced pulmonary function.

■ SECOND PRIMARY

Segmentectomy plays a significant role in the management of patients with a second primary lung cancer. Adequate pulmonary function must be preserved, and this can be achieved by anatomic segmental resection.

Faber reported 66 segmentectomies for resection of second or third primary lung cancers with a mortality of 6.6% (4 of 66) and an actuarial survival of 35% at 5 years and 22% at 10 years. Segmentectomy also should be considered when contemplating staged bilateral thoracotomy for synchronous primary lung cancers. Ferguson reported a 2-year survival of 60% and a median survival time of 27 months in synchronous stage 1 lung cancers. Segmental resection played a significant role in accomplishing these procedures without mortality. We have performed 12 segmentectomies and 15 wedge resections in patients who had prior pneumonectomy for NSCLC. Operative mortality was 4% (1 of 27), and 6 patients have survived 5 years after the second resection. Limited resection can be appropriate therapy for patients with second and third primary NSCLC.

■ WHAT TO DO

The planned surgical resection for every patient with lung cancer must be individualized. The magnitude of the resection is guided by the patient's general and cardiophysiologic status, clinical stage of the cancer, and associated disease entities. Only patients with clinical stage I cancer (T1N0, T2N0) are possible candidates for a curative limited resection. The trend of data indicates, however, that it may not be an operation of choice in the low-risk patient. There is no question that segmentectomy is the operation of choice in patients with marginal function because mortality is lower, and almost comparable long-term survival is achieved.

An anatomic resection (segmentectomy) is favored for a limited resection for several reasons. Lymphatics drain centrally toward the hilum in a segmental anatomic plane, and they are removed accordingly. Regional lymph nodes can be resected when the segmental artery and bronchus are dissected free and transected, and mediastinal lymphadenectomy can be carried out during open thoracotomy. Parenchymal margins of resection are identified more cleanly when an anatomic resection is accomplished and a longer length of bronchus is removed, negating the opportunity for local bronchial recurrence.

The wedge resection crosses lymphatic channels, does not remove the originating bronchus, and does not permit adequate regional lymph node resection, and parenchymal margins are in close proximity to the tumor. All these factors negate wedge resection as a planned curative procedure for primary lung cancer. It remains to be proved whether localized parenchymal radiation after wedge resection will be of benefit. The incidence of radiation fibrosis associated with this form of adjunctive therapy remains unreported.

Lesions less than 2 cm in diameter and tumors of squamous histology offer better long-term prognosis for a limited resection. If for whatever reason a wedge resection were to be done, this would be the favorable lesion. Segmentectomy remains the operation of choice for compromised patients and lobectomy is currently the operation of choice in noncompromised patients.

SUGGESTED READING

Fell S, Kirby TJ: Segmental resection. In Pearson FG, et al, editors: *Thoracic surgery*, ed 2, Philadelphia, 2002, Churchill-Livingstone, p 991.

Ginsberg RJ, Rubenstein LV (Lung Cancer Study Group): Randomized trial of lobectomy versus limited resection for T1N0 non-small cell lung cancer, *Ann Thorac Surg* 60:615, 1995.

Jensik RJ, et al: Segmental resection for lung cancer, *J Thorac Cardiovasc Surg* 66:563, 1973.

Warren WH, Faber LP: Segmentectomy versus lobectomy in patients with stage 1 pulmonary carcinoma, *J Thorac Cardiovasc Surg* 107:1087, 1994.

EXTENDED RESECTION OF PRIMARY LUNG CANCERS INVOLVING GREAT VESSELS OR HEART

David S. Schrump
Dao M. Nguyen

Primary lung cancers that invade the great vessels or heart pose considerable therapeutic challenges. An aggressive surgical approach to these tumors is indicated, particularly for tumors involving the left atrium to prevent sudden death or debilitating complications related to stroke. Under appropriate conditions, extended resections can be performed with acceptable morbidity and mortality, enabling significant palliation and, occasionally, long-term survival. The indications for and expected outcomes of these procedures must be defined clearly relative to the histology and stage of the malignancy, the presence of comorbid conditions, and the availability of additional treatment modalities.

Although resection of tumors involving the great veins is relatively straightforward, malignancies involving the aorta, central pulmonary artery, or heart are technically more challenging; in most instances, extirpation of these tumors requires extracorporeal circulatory support. Although cardiopulmonary bypass has been used to facilitate resection of thoracic malignancies for nearly 40 years, experience with extended resections for primary lung cancer remains limited. In 1965, Neville et al used extracorporeal support to perform extended resections in seven lung cancer patients, six of whom died in the immediate postoperative period from bleeding, heart failure, or pulmonary edema. Shortly thereafter, Bailey et al performed left pneumonectomy in conjunction with resection of the left atrium, descending aorta, or main pulmonary artery in two individuals, one of whom survived 14 months before dying of metastatic disease.

Stage IIIB (T4) lung cancers comprise a heterogeneous group of locally advanced neoplasms associated with malignant pleural effusions or directly involving carina, great vessels, heart, esophagus, or spine. As such, survival rates for patients with these malignancies can vary significantly. Although patients with cancers associated with malignant pleural effusions or esophageal invasion typically cannot be salvaged, nearly 30% of patients undergoing carinal pneumonectomies achieve long-term survival. At present, the efficacy of resections involving great vessels or the heart remains less clearly defined, primarily due to the extent of mediastinal invasion and the frequency of lymph node metastases associated with these lesions. Aortic involvement occurs in approximately 10% to 20% of lung cancers with mediastinal invasion, and approximately one third of these tumors exhibit simultaneous involvement of the main pulmonary artery. Although most individuals with these cancers have mediastinal lymph node metastases, a small subset of patients may have more favorable tumors. Martini et al described more than 100 patients with T3 or T4 tumors without mediastinal lymph node metastases, 16 of whom had aortic involvement as the sole T4 site. Although none of these individuals underwent surgery, available data suggest that patients with primary lung cancers that invade the great vessels or atrium without mediastinal lymph node involvement may benefit from extended resections in the context of aggressive multimodality treatment regimens. Extended resections also may be appropriate in patients with neoplasms of nonthoracic origin that are metastatic to the hilum or mediastinum as a means to control local disease, palliate symptoms, and prevent sudden death or stroke.

▪ PATIENT SELECTION AND SURGICAL TECHNIQUE

The principles of en bloc excision of primary lung cancers invading the great vessels or heart should follow a clearly defined algorithm during which the patient is staged thoroughly preoperatively and intraoperatively before definitive resection. In general, any evidence of mediastinal node or distant metastases should preclude resection. The preoperative evaluation should include standard imaging studies (chest x-rays and computed tomography scans of the chest, abdomen, and pelvis and brain magnetic resonance imaging). In addition, a fluorodeoxyglucose positron emission tomography scan should be obtained to rule out occult metastatic disease. If these preliminary studies indicate a potentially favorable tumor, and provided that the patient has adequate cardiopulmonary reserve to tolerate resection, magnetic resonance imaging of the chest should be obtained to delineate further the extent of mediastinal invasion. Patients with tumors invading the atria or aorta should undergo transesophageal echocardiography to determine the extent of cardiac involvement, including the proximity of tumor to the conduction system, valves, and coronary circulation; transesophageal echocardiography also is useful for assessing the extent of atherosclerotic disease in the aorta, which could complicate cannulation or graft reconstruction during cardiopulmonary bypass. Bronchoscopy should be performed to document histologically normal mucosa at the line of the intended bronchial resection, and cervical mediastinoscopy should be performed to rule out metastatic disease involving the subcarinal and paratracheal nodal stations. If nodal metastases are not detected by mediastinoscopy, additional intraoperative staging should be performed during mobilization of the lung and great vessels.

The surgical approach and methods of extracorporeal support, if indicated, vary relative to the location of the primary tumor and the extent of mediastinal invasion. Right-sided neoplasms with superior vena cava (SVC) or atrial invasion can be approached via posterolateral thoracotomy or median sternotomy; left-sided neoplasms with atrial or aortic invasion are approached best via posterolateral thoracotomy. Tumors extending to the main pulmonary artery are approached best via median sternotomy or clamshell incision. In general, tumors invading the great veins can be resected without cardiopulmonary bypass; occasionally, extracorporeal support is required for resection of extremely large central neoplasms or massive chest wall sarcomas compressing mediastinal structures. Left-sided neoplasms involving the distal arch or descending aorta can be resected either with partial left heart bypass using a BioMedicus circuit (Medtronic-BioMedicus Inc., Eden Prairie, MN) from the left atrium to the descending aorta or with a shunt from the distal arch or subclavian artery to the descending aorta. In most instances, resection of tumors invading the central pulmonary artery or left atrium requires full cardiopulmonary bypass, which is accomplished readily by femoral-femoral cannulation or by ascending aorta-bicaval cannulation techniques. In cases requiring cardiopulmonary bypass, as much dissection as possible should be accomplished off-pump to minimize bleeding and the propensity for postthoracotomy pulmonary edema, the significance of which should not be underestimated in patients with long-standing tobacco exposure or prior chemotherapy and radiation treatment. Fluids and blood products must be minimized and patients diuresed aggressively after the pump run.

In the absence of intrapleural dissemination or mediastinal nodal involvement, and under circumstances in which there is direct tumor invasion of the great vessels or heart, extended lung cancer resections can be performed safely. The location of the tumor typically dictates the extent of pulmonary resection. Most tumors in the aortopulmonary window require pneumonectomy. Fixation of the tumor to the distal arch and the proximal descending aorta significantly limits manipulation of the hilum. The dissection proceeds in an intrapericardial manner with mobilization of the left pulmonary artery and pulmonary veins. The arch of the aorta is mobilized, and the distal arch and left subclavian artery are controlled. The descending aorta is similarly mobilized and encircled at the level of the inferior pulmonary vein. The left pulmonary veins and left pulmonary artery are ligated and divided intrapericardially. The posterior pericardium is incised and left main stem bronchus transected flush with the carina after staple closure. The left atrium and descending aorta (or femoral artery) are cannulated, and left heart bypass is initiated using a BioMedicus pump or shunt established from the aortic arch or left subclavian artery to the distal descending aorta. The aorta is transected approximately 1 cm proximal and distal to the tumor, allowing en bloc removal of the left lung; posterior pericardium; periesophageal, low paratracheal, and hilar nodal tissues; and descending aorta. Frozen sections are obtained to verify negative margins at the line of resection on the aorta and the left main stem bronchus, and additional lymphadenectomy is performed. The aorta is repaired with a woven Dacron interposition graft, and the pericardium is repaired with Gore-Tex or polypropylene (Prolene) mesh.

The vascular aspects of resections involving the innominate veins and SVC are more straightforward. Typically, lung cancers invading the SVC that are amenable to resection with curative intent arise in the right upper lobe and directly extend to the SVC; less commonly, isolated metastases in right paratracheal nodes that invade the SVC may be resectable. The algorithm for resecting these tumors is analogous to that described for tumors involving the aorta. Specifically, after comprehensive intraoperative staging, intrapericardial dissection enables control of the right pulmonary artery and pulmonary veins. The pulmonary dissection (right upper lobectomy or pneumonectomy) is completed. When the azygos vein has been divided, vascular control is achieved at the level of the innominate veins or proximal SVC and the cavoatrial junction, enabling en bloc resection of pulmonary parenchyma, ipsilateral nodal tissue, and SVC; additional pretracheal and left paratracheal node dissection can be completed after removal of the primary tumor mass. Typically, vascular shunts are not required for these procedures, and completion of the pulmonary dissection before transection of the SVC minimizes hemodynamic instability, upper body edema, and cross-clamp times required for vascular reconstruction. Using this approach, clamp times typically approximate 20 minutes. Depending on the extent of the vascular resection, the SVC is repaired with a Gore-Tex patch or a ringed polytetrafluoroethylene (PTFE) interposition graft (usually size 12 Fr or 14 Fr) from the proximal SVC to the cavoatrial junction. For restoration of venous flow directly from the innominate veins to the right atrium, dual ringed interposition grafts are preferable to Y-shaped grafts; individual grafts are less prone to kinking after closure of the chest, and occlusion in one arm of a Y-graft may propagate into the other arm, resulting in SVC syndrome. All patients receiving prosthetic graft reconstruction of the SVC system should remain anticoagulated indefinitely.

Resection of primary lung cancers invading the main pulmonary artery typically requires full cardiopulmonary bypass. The approach and extent of pulmonary resection are determined by the site of the primary tumor and the involvement of adjacent vascular structures. The algorithm for resection of these malignancies is analogous to that described previously. Frequently, complete resection is not achievable in patients with these tumors due to the extent of direct mediastinal invasion and nodal metastases.

In many instances, primary lung cancers and metastatic neoplasms that involve the heart extend as polypoid masses via the pulmonary veins into the left atrium. These masses can become large before becoming symptomatic. Lung cancers with direct invasion of the epicardial surface of the left atrium and small polypoid masses in the left atrium can be removed without extracorporeal support. Given the friability of most endoluminal tumor masses and the potentially disastrous complications resulting from embolization, large left atrial tumors are resected most safely using extracorporeal support and mechanical arrest achieved via cold fibrillation or cardioplegia techniques. When mechanical arrest has been achieved, an elliptical atriotomy is performed, enabling removal of the atrial tumor mass en bloc with the pulmonary parenchyma from which the neoplasm originated, followed by atrial repair with pericardium or Gore-Tex patch.

■ OUTCOME OF EXTENDED RESECTIONS

Most more recent data pertaining to resection of lung cancers invading the great vessels or heart are derived from the Japanese and European literature. Tsuchiya et al summarized their results of extended resection in 101 patients with T4 lung cancers. Of patients, 72 required pneumonectomy; resections included left atrium (44 patients), SVC (32 patients), adventitia of aorta (21 patients), aorta (7 patients), and central pulmonary artery (7 patients). None of the patients undergoing left atrial resection required cardiopulmonary bypass, indicating limited atrial invasion. Of 32 patients with SVC invasion, 21 had partial caval resections with patch repair. Five of seven patients undergoing aortic resections required interposition grafts, whereas two patients had patch aortoplasties. Overall operative mortality was 8%, with an in-hospital death rate of 13%. The overall 5-year survival was 13%, with a median survival time (MST) of 9.2 months. Patients undergoing complete resections had a 5-year survival rate of 19% and an MST of 13.8 months. Patients undergoing left atrial resections had a 22% 5-year survival rate. Although 67 patients had no gross

residual disease, only 31 had pathologically complete (R0) resections. Thirteen patients undergoing potentially curative procedures (including 7 undergoing left atrial resections, 2 having SVC resections, and 4 undergoing resections of aorta or adventitia of aorta) survived 3 or more years; 10 patients survived at least 5 years. Multivariate analysis revealed that postoperative pneumonia, bleeding, complete resection, and pathologic N status correlated with survival.

In an additional series, Kodama et al examined their results of extended resections performed in 127 lung cancer patients. Of patients, 35 received induction chemotherapy, whereas 92 received surgery alone. Twenty-nine patients had tumors involving heart or great vessels. Three patients, including one undergoing left atrial resection and two receiving aortic resections, were long-term survivors.

Spaggiari et al reported results of 25 lung cancer patients undergoing resection of the innominate veins or SVC. Of patients, 12 underwent pneumonectomy, 10 had lobectomy, and 3 underwent segmental lung resection. Seven patients had complete resection of the SVC with PTFE interposition graft repair, 12 patients had tangential resection, 1 patient had pericardial patch repair, and 5 patients had resection of the right subclavian vein. No postoperative graft occlusions were observed. Final pathologic nodal status was N0 in 8 patients, N1 in 3 patients, and N2 in 14 patients. Resection was incomplete in five patients. Overall, MST was 11.5 months, with a 5-year actuarial survival rate of 29%; four patients were alive 5 years after resection. The MST was 14 months for patients with N0 tumors compared with 5 months for patients with N2 disease. Patients undergoing pneumonectomy tended to have diminished survival relative to patients undergoing lobectomy or segmental lung resection. No significant survival differences were noted in patients undergoing partial versus complete SVC resection; patients whose pulmonary procedure required resection of carina or left atrium in addition to the SVC had survivals comparable to patients undergoing more limited pulmonary and SVC resections.

In an additional study, Fukuse et al analyzed results of 42 patients undergoing resection of lung cancers invading the great veins or left atrium. Thirteen individuals had tumors invading SVC or innominate vein, 15 had tumors involving aorta or left subclavian vein, and 14 had tumors extending to the left atrium. Thirteen patients underwent induction therapy, and 22 received adjuvant therapy. Sixteen patients underwent pneumonectomy, whereas 26 patients had lobectomies. Three patients had total replacement of the aorta; 9 patients had a focus of tumor left on the aorta. One patient with involvement of the left subclavian artery had complete resection and reconstruction of the artery, 8 patients had replacement or partial resection of the SVC, and 13 patients with tumor involving the left atrium had resection without cardiopulmonary bypass. The operative mortality was 2.4%. Resection was complete in 15 patients. Of the 15 patients undergoing complete resections, 6 had aortic invasion, 4 had SVC invasion, and 5 had left atrial invasion. Patients with complete resections had an MST of 36 months (3-year survival 40%). Induction or adjuvant therapy did not seem to influence survival. Six patients survived 3 or more years. Overall survival was 17% at 3 years (MST 14 months). Patients with cancers invading the great veins or aorta had median survival times of approximately 20 months compared with 10 months for patients with tumors invading the left atrium. Patients with T4N0/1 tumors experienced an MST of 22 months compared with 9 months for patients with T4N2 cancers. Cox regression analysis revealed that pathologic nodal status, completeness of resection, and preoperative and postoperative radiation therapy correlated with survival.

Doddoli et al reported their experience with 29 patients undergoing extended resections for lung cancer. Of patients, 25 underwent pneumonectomy, whereas 4 had lobectomy. The resections were extended to involve SVC (17 patients), aorta (1 patient), left atrium (5 patients), or carina (6 patients). Seventeen patients received postoperative radiation therapy, with or without chemotherapy. Complete (R0) resections were achieved in 25 patients, with an operative mortality of 7%. MST of the 18 patients with N0/1 disease was 16 months, whereas the MST in the 11 patients with N2 disease was only 9 months. Collectively, these data indicate that extended resections may be justified in lung cancer patients with N0/1 tumors. In the absence of a means to control microscopic metastatic disease, extended resection should not be performed routinely in patients with documented N2 disease.

■ SUMMARY

Rigorous adherence to treatment algorithms excludes most lung cancer patients from extended resections due to mediastinal lymph node metastases. Given the lack of large single-institution series and incomplete information regarding final pathologic status relative to surgical procedures in the literature, it is difficult to ascribe accurately morbidity and survival rates for extended resections. Patients undergoing extended resections are highly selected; despite this fact, complete resections have been accomplished in less than 50% of patients undergoing these procedures. In experienced hands, morbidity of extended procedures seems to be in the range of 30%; in patients undergoing extended resections without the use of cardiopulmonary bypass, morbidity does not seem to be significantly increased compared with that observed in patients undergoing comparable pulmonary resections alone. Available data indicate that survival is contingent on completeness of resection and final pathologic

stage; histology has not proved to be a significant prognostic factor. MST for patients with completely resected T4N0/1 tumors seems to be in the range of 16 to 20 months compared with 9 months for patients with T4N2 cancers. These survival rates approximate those reported for patients receiving chemotherapy and surgery for stage IIIA non–small cell lung cancers. Radiation therapy has not proved to be beneficial in terms of improving patient survival after resection; however one cannot exclude the possibility that an occasional patient with microscopic residual disease may be salvaged by postoperative mediastinal irradiation. None of the series has sufficient numbers of patients to enable appropriate subset analysis.

Continued evolution of cardiac surgery techniques and improved imaging modalities for lung cancer now enable better selection of patients for extended resections with curative intent. The indications for extended resections should be weighed in terms of potential perioperative complications and the expertise of the surgical team. These procedures should be undertaken only in the context of multimodality treatment regimens that may improve long-term survival. Ideally, extended resections for primary lung cancers involving the great vessels or heart should be performed in the context of a prospective multiinstitutional trial using standardized preoperative staging studies and consistent multidisciplinary therapy. In the absence of a protocol, it seems reasonable to use induction therapy regimens currently administered for stage IIIA non–small cell lung cancers. Under appropriate conditions, significant local control and possibly long-term survival may be achieved after aggressive resections in patients with lung cancers invading the great vessels and heart.

SUGGESTED READING

Doddoli C, et al: Is lung cancer surgery justified in patients with direct mediastinal invasion? *Eur J Cardiothorac Surg* 20:339, 2001.

Fukuse T, et al: Extended operation for non-small cell lung cancer invading great vessels and left atrium, *Eur J Cardiothorac Surg* 11:664, 1997.

Kodama K, et al: Survival and postoperative complications after extended surgery for non-small-cell lung cancer, *Jpn J Thorac Cardiovasc Surg* 47:546, 1999.

Spaggiari L, et al: Extended resections for bronchogenic carcinoma invading the superior vena cava system, *Ann Thorac Surg* 69:233, 2000.

Tsuchiya R, et al: Extended resection of the left atrium, great vessels, or both for lung cancer, *Ann Thorac Surg* 57:960, 1994.

MEDIASTINAL LYMPH NODE DISSECTION FOR LUNG CANCER

Keith D. Mortman
Steven M. Keller

There are three approaches to the intraoperative assessment of mediastinal lymph nodes: systematic sampling (SS), complete lymph node dissection, and extended lymph node dissection. SS involves biopsy of selected lymph nodes at each of the mediastinal lymph node stations. Complete mediastinal lymph node dissection (MLND) entails removal of all the mediastinal lymph nodes within the ipsilateral hemithorax. Extended lymph node dissection refers to dissection of lymph nodes beyond the ipsilateral hemithorax or removal of mediastinal lymph nodes via a separate incision. SS and MLND are equally efficacious for accurate staging. However, MLND can be used to identify more levels of N2 disease in those patients who have metastases to the mediastinal lymph nodes.

We commonly perform MLND after pulmonary resection while waiting for frozen section results of the bronchial margin. Alternatively, MLND may be performed before resection of the lung if the presence of metastases would change the extent of the operation. If MLND is performed before resection, intraoperative frozen section analysis of the lymph nodes is critical. Otherwise, routine submission of appropriately labeled lymph nodes is sufficient. Regardless of the technique that is used, a minimum of levels 4, 7, and 10 should be sampled or removed during a right thoracotomy and levels 5, 6, and 7 during a left lung resection.

A vertical muscle-sparing lateral thoracotomy permits excellent exposure of all mediastinal lymph node stations and is our preferred incision. Epidural anesthesia minimizes postoperative pain and pulmonary dysfunction. A double-lumen endotracheal tube is routinely used to facilitate exposure and dissection. Clips are used for hemostasis adjacent to nodal tissue to avoid distortion of histologic architecture caused by electrocautery. The current lymph node level definitions accepted by the American Joint Committee on Cancer (AJCC) and Union Internationale Contre le Cancer (UICC) are used to ensure standardization and reproducibility.

■ RIGHT HEMITHORAX

With the patient in the left lateral decubitus position, the chest is entered in the fourth or fifth intercostal space. Ventilation of the right lung is terminated before entering the chest. After exploration of the hemithorax, the lung is retracted superiorly and the inferior pulmonary ligament is divided between hemoclips to the level of the inferior pulmonary vein. Level 9 lymph nodes are removed and labeled appropriately. The pleura is opened anterior and posterior to the hilum with electrocautery in preparation for pulmonary resection.

After pulmonary resection, the remaining lung is retracted inferiorly to allow access to the superior mediastinum. The pleura above the azygos vein is incised midway between the trachea and superior vena cava from the cephalad border of the azygos vein to the level of the innominate artery. The anterior and posterior pleural flaps are sequentially retracted to provide countertraction as the underlying fat pad is bluntly dissected from the trachea and superior vena cava with a peanut sponge. Small vessels entering the lymph nodes should be sought and clipped. The lymph node–bearing fat pad is then clipped cephalad to the azygos vein and removed. The lymph nodes between the cephalad border of the azygos vein and the arch of the aorta (approximated by the entry of the internal mammary vein into the superior vena cava) are labeled right level 4 superior. Those lymph nodes above the aortic arch and below the innominate vein are considered right level 2. Care should be taken to identify and preserve the vagus nerve.

A vein retractor is used to elevate the azygos vein superiorly. Lymph nodes between the caudal aspect of the azygos vein and the origin of the right upper lobe bronchus are grasped with an empty sponge stick and bluntly dissected from the surrounding tissues with a peanut sponge. Hemoclips are applied to feeding vessels and the specimen is removed. These lymph nodes are labeled as right level 4 inferior. A 4 × 4 sponge packed in the region of dissection aids hemostasis.

The right level 10 lymph nodes are located anterior to the bronchus intermedius distal to the right upper lobe bronchus and exposed by retracting the pulmonary artery. Right level 11 lymph nodes are found between the lobar bronchi and should be labeled after removal. Level 12 peribronchial lymph nodes are removed with the lobectomy specimen.

Attention is next directed to the subcarinal space (level 7). The pleura midway between the anterior border of the esophagus and the medial border of the bronchus intermedius is incised (Figure 1). After development of a space anterior to the esophagus, a narrow malleable retractor is inserted and the esophagus retracted posteriorly. The carina, subcarinal lymph nodes, and right main stem and proximal left main stem bronchi are visualized. Branches of the vagus nerve and accompanying blood vessels enter the subcarinal space and should be clipped. A 4 × 4 sponge is temporarily packed in the region of the subcarinal dissection.

The pleura overlying the esophagus is opened midway between the azygos vein and the diaphragm. Ring forceps are used to grasp and remove the right level 8 paraesophageal lymph nodes. All gauze sponges are removed, and the right hemithorax is thoroughly irrigated with warm saline. The lymph node beds are inspected for hemostasis, and additional clips are applied where appropriate.

■ LEFT HEMITHORAX

After placement of a double-lumen endotracheal tube, the patient is placed in the right lateral decubitus position. The left chest is entered in the fourth or fifth intercostal

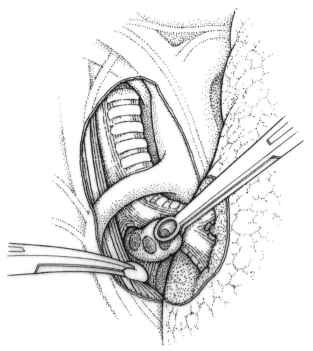

Figure 1
Dissection of level 7 lymph nodes from the right. The pleura overlying the esophagus is grasped with a right-angled clamp and retracted posteriorly as blunt dissection is begun with a peanut sponge. The level 7 lymph nodes are grasped with a ring forceps or ring clamp and separated from the surrounding tissue.

space via either a vertical thoracotomy or a posterolateral thoracotomy. The inferior pulmonary ligament is divided with electrocautery between hemoclips. The level 9 lymph nodes are grasped with ring forceps and removed. The pleura surrounding the hilum is opened, and pulmonary resection is performed in the usual fashion.

The remaining left lung is retracted inferiorly, and the mediastinal pleura between the phrenic and vagus nerves at the level of the aortic arch is opened, exposing the aortopulmonary window. The location of the phrenic and vagus nerves must be repeatedly checked to avoid iatrogenic injury. The lymph nodes are grasped with a ring forceps and bluntly dissected from the surrounding tissues. Level 5 lymph nodes are located lateral to the ligamentum arteriosum; level 6 lymph nodes are situated anterior to the ligamentum arteriosum. Small blood vessels entering the lymph nodes are clipped. The phrenic and vagus nerves should be identified before application of the hemoclips. The recurrent laryngeal nerve is usually not visualized because dissection in the region of the ligamentum arteriosum is not commonly necessary. Use of the electrocautery should be avoided in this region to minimize the risk of nerve injury.

The mediastinal pleura overlying the aorta is grasped with a right-angled clamp and retracted posteriorly as the lung is retracted anteriorly. A narrow malleable retractor

is particularly useful in retracting the aorta and esophagus posteriorly as the subcarinal space is deeper when approached from the left hemithorax. The lymph nodes are bluntly dissected from the underlying pericardium and grasped with a ring clamp. Further blunt dissection is required to elevate the lymph nodes from the left and right main stem bronchi. Small vessels entering the lymph nodes are clipped before transection. An arterial vessel usually enters the lymph nodes at the level of the carina and should be sought to avoid postoperative hemorrhage. A 4 × 4 sponge temporarily packed in the subcarinal space aids hemostasis.

Level 8 paraesophageal lymph nodes are located between the aortic arch and diaphragm. These lymph nodes are teased from the esophagus with a peanut sponge and clipped at their base. All sponges are removed, the chest is irrigated, and hemostasis is ascertained.

Clear communication with the operating room personnel responsible for completing the pathology submission forms is essential to ensure proper labeling of the lymph node specimens. In addition, the pathologist must identify and appropriately label lymph nodes contained within the resected pulmonary tissue (usually levels 12 to 14). This is particularly important after a pneumonectomy, when levels 4, 7, and 10 may be included in continuity with the lung parenchyma and not submitted from the operating room as separate specimens.

■ EXTENDED LYMPH NODE DISSECTION

Extended lymphadenectomy generally entails removal of all the locoregional lymph node groups in addition to those located within the ipsilateral mediastinum. The indications and techniques vary and are typically determined by tumor location, histology, and stage. For instance, Hata et al dissects the ipsilateral scalene lymph nodes during resection of a right lung cancer if the most cephalad right paratracheal lymph nodes (levels 1, 2, and 4) contain metastases. The supraclavicular dissection is broadened to include the left scalene lymph nodes if anterior mediastinal lymph node (level 3a) involvement is documented. Patients with clinical stage I squamous cell cancers of the left lung undergo a posterolateral thoracotomy. The ligamentum arteriosum is divided, and the aortic arch is mobilized to gain access to left lymph node levels 2 and 4. Patients with more advanced stages and other histologies undergo median sternotomy followed by bilateral paratracheal lymphadenectomy (levels 1 to 4). Exposure is obtained by retracting the ascending aorta to the left and the superior vena cava to the right. Caudal retraction of the right main pulmonary artery exposes the subcarinal lymph nodes (level 7). The left lobe of the thymus is resected to uncover the aortopulmonary window lymph nodes, which are removed to the ligamentum arteriosum. Left upper lobectomy and pneumonectomy are performed via sternotomy, whereas a left lower lobectomy is accomplished through an additional anteroaxillary thoracotomy. A cervical dissection is performed if metastatic disease is found in the highest mediastinal, supraclavicular, or scalene lymph nodes.

■ RESULTS OF MEDIASTINAL LYMPH NODE DISSECTION

SS or MLND is necessary to achieve precise pathologic staging, because mere inspection or palpation of lymph nodes is inaccurate. Furthermore, the lack of metastases in the lymph nodes contained within the resected specimen does not guarantee the absence of metastases in the mediastinal lymph nodes. Noncontiguous or "skip metastases" have been identified in 35% to 41% of patients with N2 disease. Although SS and MLND each reflect the correct pathologic stage of the patient, MLND detects more levels of N2 disease.

Complete MLND may be associated with improved survival in patients with N1 and N2 disease compared with SS. Analysis of the randomized, prospective, adjuvant therapy trial in patients with completely resected stages II and IIIa non–small cell lung cancer conducted under the direction of the Eastern Cooperative Oncology Group by the type of lymph node dissection demonstrated significantly improved survival for those patients who had undergone MLND. Median survival was 58 months for those patients who had undergone MLND and 29 months for those who had SS. However, the benefit was limited to right lung tumors. A randomized prospective trial of MLND versus SS in 169 patients with stages I-IIIa NSCLC conducted by Izbicki et al also demonstrated a survival advantage for the subgroup of patients with N1 and N2 disease.

■ MORBIDITY

Some surgeons are hesitant to perform an MLND for fear of complications that might result from interrupting the blood supply to the bronchial stump or removing a large portion of the intrathoracic lymphatics. The sequelae of SS and MLND were compared in a randomized prospective study (n = 182) conducted by Izbicki et al. Although MLND extended the operative procedure by approximately 20 minutes compared with SS, there was no increase in blood loss, mortality, or need for reoperation. One chylothorax occurred in each group. Six patients who underwent SS and five patients who underwent MLND had recurrent laryngeal nerve injury. Chest tube drainage and length of hospitalization were similar in both groups. Hata et al reported two left recurrent laryngeal nerve injuries and one phrenic nerve paralysis in 50 patients who underwent extensive mediastinal lymph node dissection.

■ FUTURE DIRECTIONS

The American College of Surgeons–Oncology Group is conducting a randomized prospective trial designed to evaluate the role of lymph node dissection (ACOS-OG Z0030). After intraoperative histologic documentation of the absence of N2 disease, patients with T1-2, N0-1 NSCLC are randomization to either MLND or SS. The end points of the trial include local recurrence and overall survival.

SUGGESTED READING

Bonner JA, et al: Frequency of noncontiguous lymph node involvement in patients with resectable nonsmall cell lung carcinoma, *Cancer* 86:1159, 1999.

Hata E, et al: Rationale for extended lymphadenectomy for lung cancer, *Theor Surg* 5:19, 1990.

Izbicki JR, et al: Radical systematic mediastinal lymphadenectomy in non-small cell lung cancer: a randomized controlled trial, *Br J Surg* 81:229, 1994.

Izbicki JR, et al: Effectiveness of radical systematic mediastinal lymphadenectomy in patients with resectable non-small cell lung cancer, *Ann Surg* 227:138, 1998.

Keller SM, et al: Mediastinal lymph node dissection improves survival in patients with stages II and IIIa non-small cell lung cancer, *Ann Thorac Surg* 70:58, 2000.

CHEMOTHERAPY FOR LUNG CANCER

W. Thomas Purcell

Julie R. Brahmer

David S. Ettinger

Lung cancer treatment uses three modalities: surgery, ionizing radiation, and chemotherapy. Chemotherapy treatment decisions are based on the pathologic type and stage of disease. The two main pathologic categories of lung cancer are non–small cell lung cancer (NSCLC) (approximately 80% of total number of lung cancers) and small cell lung cancer (SCLC) (approximately 20% of total number of lung cancers). NSCLC can be divided further into three main pathologic types: squamous cell, adenocarcinoma, and large cell. Chemotherapy for the three main types of NSCLC is essentially the same. Because of the pathologic differences between NSCLC and SCLC, however, chemotherapy treatment for NSCLC is different from that for SCLC. This chapter outlines the recommended chemotherapy for each tumor and staging category.

■ CHEMOTHERAPY FOR NON–SMALL CELL LUNG CANCER

Approximately 80% of lung cancer cases are NSCLC with most patients presenting with late stage disease. Of patients with NSCLC, 25% present with stage I or II disease, whereas 30% present with stage III disease and 40% with stage IV disease. The standard TNM staging is used to determine the staging for NSCLC. Patients with stage I NSCLC have approximately a 60% 5-year survival. Stage II NSCLC patients have approximately 20% to 40% 5-year survival. Stage IIIA NSCLC patients have approximately 15% 5-year survival. Stage IIIB NSCLC patients have approximately 7% 5-year survival. Patients with stage IV NSCLC have 20% to 41% 1-year survival and less than 2% 5-year survival. Chemotherapeutic treatment strategies are based on the stage of disease and are described subsequently.

Stage I (T1/2N0M0) and Stage II (T1/2N1M0 or T3N0M0) NSCLC

Surgical resection remains the mainstay curative treatment for stage I and II patients. Of stage I patients, 30% to 40%, despite having detected no initial local lymph node involvement, relapse with distant, metastatic disease. Of stage II patients, 70% relapse. These recurrences are due to occult micrometastatic disease not seen before surgical resection. To attempt to eradicate micrometastatic disease, a rational approach to minimize this risk of relapse seems to be adjuvant or neoadjuvant systemic chemotherapy.

Many adjuvant studies and meta-analyses performed to date have not shown a survival benefit with this approach, however.

Newer chemotherapy agents have shown increased in vitro and in vivo biologic activity against NSCLC leading the way for future adjuvant and neoadjuvant studies. A prospective randomized study with 323 stage I and II patients performed in Japan showed overall 5-year survival rates of 60% (cisplatin plus vindesine followed by ftorafur plus uracil for 1 year) and 64% (ftorafur plus uracil alone for 1 year) for patients who received adjuvant chemotherapy versus 49% for the control group. A randomized phase III trial of preoperative and postoperative chemotherapy in NSCLC was published by Depierre et al. The study included 335 patients (stage I [except T1N0], II, and IIIA patients) who received two cycles of neoadjuvant chemotherapy (mitomycin, cisplatin, and ifosfamide), surgery, then two cycles of postoperative chemotherapy (preoperative responders only [65% of patients]) versus surgery alone. In both treatment arms, adjuvant radiation therapy was administered to patients who were T3 or N1/2. Median survival in chemotherapy patients versus surgery alone was 37 months versus 26 months ($p = .15$). Subset analysis of the stage I/II patients showed a statistically significant improved survival. Postoperative mortality was 6.7% in patients who received chemotherapy and 4.5% in patients who received surgery ($p = .38$). Because these results are from a subset analysis, confirmation with other studies is ongoing.

With newer highly active cytotoxic agents, such as paclitaxel, docetaxel, carboplatin, gemcitabine, and irinotecan, and other novel targeted chemotherapy compounds, such as Iressa (an investigational tyrosine kinase inhibitor) becoming available, stage I and II patients should be considered for further neoadjuvant and adjuvant clinical trials. Neoadjuvant trials are particularly of interest given that biologic activity can be assessed at the time of surgical resection. Currently a large prospective randomized intergroup (S9900) neoadjuvant chemotherapy trial in the United States is under way. The trial compares surgery alone with three cycles of neoadjuvant carboplatin and paclitaxel followed by surgery.

Other studies have looked into chemoprevention strategies to prevent relapse. An Intergroup study comparing 13-cis-retinoic acid with placebo in surgically resected, stage I NSCLC patients has completed accrual, and results of that trial are pending. A successor Intergroup trial is under way comparing high selenium yeast with placebo yeast in stage I NSCLC resected patients with treatment planned for 4 years. Until the results from these studies emerge, the standard of care of stage I and II patients remains surgery alone. Future treatment likely will include some form of systemic neoadjuvant or adjuvant chemotherapy, however.

Stage IIIA (T1/3N2M0 or T3N1M0) NSCLC

Patients who present with stage IIIA NSCLC have locally advanced disease, but many patients are still candidates for surgical resection. Several studies have shown improvement in survival in stage IIIA patients with preoperative (neoadjuvant) chemotherapy. Patients who are considered resectable or unresectable with stage IIIA NSCLC and have a good performance status should receive neoadjuvant chemotherapy. There currently is no standard regimen for neoadjuvant chemotherapy, but three cycles of paclitaxel (225 mg/m^2) and carboplatin (6 area under the curve [AUC]) every 21 days is one of the most widely used regimens. Other combination regimens can be used as well with gemcitabine, vinorelbine, irinotecan, cisplatin, or docetaxel. After neoadjuvant chemotherapy, patients should undergo surgical resection, if technically feasible, and complete mediastinal lymphadenectomy. If there is residual tumor present within the mediastinal lymph nodes, postoperative radiation therapy is recommended to prevent overt local recurrence. Radiation therapy has not been shown to improve survival but has been shown to improve local control of disease. Patients with N2-positive NSCLC whose nodal disease is eradicated after neoadjuvant therapy and surgery have significantly improved cancer-free survival. These data support surgical resection for patients downstaged by induction therapy. The number of N2-positive mediastinal lymph nodes has been shown to have prognostic significance. Patients with N2-negative nodes have a lower risk of recurrence than patients with two or more N2-positive nodes. Additional chemotherapy given concurrently with radiation or sequentially is controversial.

Some patients initially thought to have stage I or II disease before surgery are found to have pathologic stage IIIA disease (usually N2-positive nodes found during mediastinal lymphadenectomy) and should be considered for adjuvant chemotherapy or combined chemoradiation therapy. Several phase II studies have shown significant response rates with weekly paclitaxel (50 mg/m^2) and carboplatin (2 AUC) in combination with radiation therapy for 6 weeks. Other chemotherapeutic agents, such as gemcitabine, docetaxel, vinorelbine, irinotecan, cisplatin, and etoposide, also have been used in combination with radiation for stage IIIA patients.

Stage IIIB (T1/4N3M0 or T4N0/3M0)

Patients who present with stage IIIB NSCLC have locally advanced, unresectable disease. The mainstay of initial treatment of these patients is chemotherapy and radiation therapy. In the past, treatment was either sequential chemotherapy followed by radiation therapy or vice versa. More recently, studies show the advantage of using concurrent chemotherapy and radiation therapy over sequential therapy in the treatment of unresectable stage IIIB disease. Stage IIIB patients can receive combination chemoradiation for 6 weeks as described previously with stage IIIA patients. Typically, these patients are given two cycles of induction combination chemotherapy (e.g., carboplatin plus paclitaxel) before combined chemoradiation or chemoradiation followed by two cycles of combination chemotherapy. Some stage IIIB patients who are given neoadjuvant chemotherapy or chemoradiation therapy and have a clinical response may undergo clinical down-staging significant enough to attempt surgery for possible resection.

Stage IV (T1/4N0/3M1)

Approximately 40% of patients with NSCLC present with incurable, stage IV, metastatic disease. Except for patients who initially present with isolated single brain or adrenal metastasis, treatment for stage IV patients is palliative, and

surgery is considered contraindicated. Combination chemotherapy has been shown, however, to improve median survival (30 weeks versus 17 weeks for best supportive care) and 1-year survival (20% versus 10% for best supportive care). Many combinations have been studied. The most commonly used regimens include paclitaxel plus carboplatin, gemcitabine plus cisplatin, docetaxel plus carboplatin, vinorelbine plus cisplatin, and several three-drug combinations. In general, compared with single-agent regimens, combination chemotherapy has a higher response rate, but also more significant toxicities. For such regimens, the median survival ranges from 8 to 10 months. Survivals of 1 year and 2 years are approximately 30% and 8% to 12%. Patients treated with nonplatinum chemotherapy regimens have a trend toward poorer survival than patients who receive platinum combination chemotherapy.

A phase III randomized study by the Eastern Cooperative Oncology Group (ECOG) showed no significant survival difference between four commonly used regimens. The paclitaxel plus carboplatin regimen was found to be least toxic among the four, however. The initial treatment for stage IV NSCLC for patients with acceptable performance status is a platinum-containing combination, taking into account side effects of the individual regimens to determine which is most applicable. In the United States, the most popular first choice seems to be paclitaxel plus carboplatin. Patients usually are treated for four to six cycles or until disease progression.

For patients who have tumor progression after first-line chemotherapy or who cannot tolerate combination chemotherapy, single-agent chemotherapy is widely used. Perhaps the most used agent is docetaxel given on a weekly or every-3-week basis. In a prospective randomized trial that compared docetaxel (100 mg/m^2 and 75 mg/m^2) with best supportive care in 103 patients who had progressed after platinum-based first-line chemotherapy, Shepherd et al showed that single-agent docetaxel (75 mg/m^2 every 3 weeks) improved survival compared with best supportive care (7.5 months versus 4.6 months). There was one death from neutropenic fever in the docetaxel 75 mg/m^2 group compared with three deaths in the docetaxel 100 mg/m^2 group. Other risks to chemotherapy were minimal. In a community-based phase II trial conducted in 39 elderly or poor performance status patients with stage IV NSCLC, weekly docetaxel, 36 mg/m^2, produced a response rate of 20%. The response rate was 26% in patients with an ECOG performance status of 0 or 1. Actuarial 1-year survival was 28%, and actuarial 2-year survival was 15%. These results are similar to results achieved with other active single agents, such as gemcitabine, paclitaxel, etoposide, irinotecan and vinorelbine.

■ SUPERIOR SULCUS PANCOAST'S TUMORS

Most superior sulcus tumors are NSCLC that are located in the apical, pleuropulmonary groove adjacent to the subclavian vessels. They present a particular challenge in that complete resection is difficult and can cause significant morbidity given the important biologic structures that are close by. In the past, for patients without locally advanced disease (N2-negative), preoperative radiation therapy followed by surgery was the standard of care. A phase II Intergroup study showed, however, that induction with combined chemoradiation followed by surgery showed promising results. Specifically, patients received two cycles of cisplatin plus etoposide and concurrent 45 cGy of thoracic radiation. Of the 95 patients eligible for surgery, 83 underwent thoracotomy, 2 (2.4%) died postoperatively, and 76 (92%) had a complete resection. Of thoracotomy specimens, 54 (65%) showed either a pathologic complete response or minimal microscopic disease. The 2-year survival was 55% for all eligible patients and 70% for patients who had a complete resection. Patients with locally advanced (N2-positive) nodes are similar to patients with stage IIIB NSCLC.

■ CHEMOTHERAPY FOR SMALL CELL LUNG CANCER

Accurate initial staging determines the chemotherapeutic treatment approach for SCLC. Surgical TNM staging for SCLC is similar to that of NSCLC. Two broader staging categories are used to classify SCLC patients for treatment purposes, however. The two disease categories are (1) limited stage SCLC and (2) extensive stage SCLC. Approximately 30% to 40% of patients with SCLC have limited stage disease at the time of initial diagnosis. Limited stage patients are defined as patients with disease confined to the ipsilateral hemithorax and within a single radiotherapy port. These patients are potentially curable and undergo aggressive combined chemoradiation, as discussed subsequently. The median survival for limited stage SCLC patients is 14 to 20 months, and the 5-year survival is approximately 20%. At the time of initial diagnosis, 60% to 70% of patients with SCLC have extensive stage disease. This includes disease detected outside the ipsilateral hemithorax, including the contralateral hemithorax, and other common areas of metastasis, such as brain, adrenal glands, liver, pleural cavity (malignant pleural effusion), and bone marrow. The median survival for extensive stage patients is 8 to 13 months with the 5-year survival less than 5%.

SCLC usually widely disseminates early in the disease course, and patients with limited stage disease usually die of distant relapse. Regardless of the initial disease stage, all patients with SCLC require systemic chemotherapy. SCLC usually is remarkably chemosensitive when initially treated with chemotherapy. There is a high relapse rate (median duration of response approximately 6 months) with development of chemotherapy resistance. In an attempt to reduce resistance, combination chemotherapy with at least two agents is used for initial treatment. Radiation therapy often is given for local control and possible synergy, especially in limited stage disease. Surgical resection also is used in limited stage patients, but the precise indications for surgery of these patients remains controversial. SCLC also is associated with several paraneoplastic syndromes, such as syndrome of inappropriate secretion of antidiuretic hormone, Cushing's syndrome, Lambert-Eaton myasthenic syndrome, cerebellar degeneration, encephalomyelitis, and sensory neuropathies. SCLC, in contrast to NSCLC, rarely causes hypercalcemia.

Limited Stage SCLC

Patients with limited stage disease (N1/3M0) and good performance status should undergo concurrent chemotherapy and radiation therapy as initial treatment. Treatment usually includes cisplatin (60 mg/m^2 on day 1) and etoposide (120 mg/m^2 on days 1 to 3) given every 21 days for four cycles. Radiation therapy directed to the involved field usually is given concurrently during the first two cycles (42 days). After completion of four cycles of chemotherapy and concurrent radiation, resection of an unresponsive, residual tumor is controversial. These lesions could represent a "mixed" tumor with an NSCLC component and would warrant resection. A prospective, randomized trial by Lad et al showed, however, that resection of residual tumor in patients with partial response provided no survival benefit. The result has been confirmed by other studies as well.

Rarely (<5% of SCLC), "very limited" SCLC disease presents as a peripheral, solitary pulmonary nodule (T1N0M0) with no hilar adenopathy. Usually these patients are diagnosed after biopsy or surgical removal of the nodule for diagnosis purposes and should have mediastinoscopy before resection to confirm N0 nodal status (see chapter on "Surgical Approach for Small Cell Lung Cancer"). These patients should be treated as limited stage patients with chemotherapy even in the postoperative setting. If the patient does not have hilar or mediastinal lymphadenopathy, radiation therapy may not be necessary.

Extensive Stage SCLC

Extensive stage SCLC (M1) is defined by SCLC outside the ipsilateral hemithorax, including the contralateral hemithorax. Patients with good performance status should be treated systemically with combination chemotherapy. Platinum-containing agents (either cisplatin or carboplatin) and etoposide are considered the first-line chemotherapy. Carboplatin can be substituted for cisplatin in the extensive disease regimen because it seems to have equivalent activity, fewer mucosal and neuropathic toxic effects, but increased myelosuppression compared with cisplatin. Carboplatin has not been studied extensively in limited stage patients. A randomized phase III trial of 154 Japanese patients with extensive stage SCLC was reported in *The New England Journal of Medicine*. Patients were treated with either cisplatin plus etoposide or cisplatin plus irinotecan. The median survival was 12.8 months in the cisplatin plus irinotecan group and 9.4 months in the cisplatin plus etoposide group ($p = .002$). Two-year survival was 19.5% in the cisplatin plus irinotecan group and 5.2% in the cisplatin plus etoposide group. The study had several limitations and will need to be confirmed with other studies. It does show, however, that cisplatin plus irinotecan is an active regimen in extensive stage SCLC. For either regimen, treatment is given for two cycles, then imaging is performed to determine radiographic response. Patients usually receive a total of four cycles if their disease is initially responsive.

Prophylactic Cranial Irradiation for SCLC Patients

Approximately 35% to 60% of patients with successfully treated SCLC develop central nervous system metastasis within 2 years of initial treatment. Auperin et al performed a meta-analysis of the efficacy of prophylactic cranial irradiation (PCI) in 847 patients with limited disease and 140 patients with extensive disease. The meta-analysis confirmed a small, absolute survival advantage for limited stage and extensive stage patients who receive PCI. PCI is considered standard of care, especially for limited stage patients, given the improved survival for those patients. PCI may cause some neurocognitive deficits in some patients, however. This side effect is minimized by administering the radiation therapy in smaller fractions and by giving PCI after the completion of the initial combined therapy.

Salvage Chemotherapy After SCLC Relapse

For limited and extensive disease, many SCLC patients relapse. When relapse occurs, the median survival is approximately 4 months. Patients who initially respond, then relapse more than 3 months after the initial chemotherapy treatment have a greater than 30% response to chemotherapy. Patients who relapse less than 3 months after therapy have a 10% response to additional chemotherapy. Depending on performance status, patients may be treated with topotecan, or other single cytotoxic agents can be considered.

■ CONCLUSION

Most lung cancer patients die from metastatic disease, including approximately 30% to 40% of patients with stage I NSCLC. It is hoped that newer chemotherapeutic agents and better treatment techniques (e.g., neoadjuvant treatment) will improve survival. Only innovation by investigators and aggressive participation in clinical trials will ensure that improvement occurs.

SUGGESTED READING

Bunn PA Jr, et al: Adjuvant and neoadjuvant chemotherapy for non-small cell lung cancer: a time for reassessment? *Chest* 117(4 Suppl 1):119S, 2000.

Depierre A, et al: Preoperative chemotherapy followed by surgery compared with primary surgery in resectable stage I (except T1N0), II, and IIIa non-small-cell lung cancer, *J Clin Oncol* 20:247, 2002.

Schiller JH, et al: Comparison of four chemotherapy regimens for advanced non-small-cell lung cancer, *N Engl J Med* 346:92, 2002.

Turrisi AT III, et al: Twice-daily compared with once-daily thoracic radiotherapy in limited small-cell lung cancer treated concurrently with cisplatin and etoposide, *N Engl J Med* 340:265, 1999.

Wagner H Jr: Postoperative adjuvant therapy for patients with resected non-small cell lung cancer: still controversial after all these years, *Chest* 117:110S, 2000.

RADIOTHERAPY FOR LUNG CANCER

Lawrence Kleinberg

Radiotherapy (RT) uses ionizing radiation, generally x-rays, in the therapy of malignant disease. The energy of these x-rays generally exceeds the energies used in diagnostic radiology, and this enables the radiation beams to penetrate effectively into the body. Success of RT of malignant disease is a consequence of several important properties. Radiation beams have predictable characteristics that allow them to be aimed at the targeted tissue such that only nearby or overlying tissues will receive a substantial dose while protecting distant normal tissues. Additionally, ionizing radiation has a greater chance of killing malignant or rapidly dividing cells than normal body tissues. These factors form the basis of a favorable therapeutic ratio.

Typically, normal tissues are protected by aiming the beams from several different directions. Where all the beams cross, a high dose of RT will be deposited. In addition, the actual beam is shaped with lead alloy, deflecting rays to that area needing treatment and further protecting normal tissues. The increasing availability of high-powered desktop computers has substantially improved radiation planning over the past decade, such that the treatment is much more precise. RT is given in fractionated doses over 6 weeks because at low daily doses, the differential effect of the radiation on normal tissues and tumor tissues is at its greatest. If treatment were shortened and high daily doses given, the risk of injury to normal tissues would be greater. In palliative treatment, higher daily doses are used with a substantially lower total dose as maximal killing of tumor may not be critical in the palliative setting and more prolonged treatment is not respectful of the patient's limited time.

For the patient, the radiation procedure starts with a simulation procedure. During the simulation, radiographs or computed tomography scans are obtained in the position in which the patient will be treated on a daily basis. This position is selected for reproducibility. Available diagnostic data are used in combination with imaging taken at simulation to identify the area to be treated. Reference marks are placed on the patient to guide the day-to-day delivery of treatment. Computerized treatment planning is used to define how much of the radiation dose will be deposited in tumor and normal tissues each day. During formal therapy, the patient is placed in the treatment position using the reference mark. Treatment itself generally takes only several minutes. There is no abnormal sensation generally associated with actual treatment delivery, but toxicity develops from the cumulative effect of radiation through the weeks of treatment. The short-term toxicities of RT, outlined in the sections later, may take weeks to months to fully resolve. Long-term toxicity generally develops as late effects over months to years after RT is complete.

The objective of an RT plan is to deliver a sufficient dose to control tumor while limiting injury to normal tissue. In general, a higher dose will increase the chance of controlling the tumor, although resistant disease and the possibility of mortality from treatment injury limit the optimal dose. When radiation is used in definitive therapy of gross tumor, generally a dose of 60 to 70 Gy is used. The use of higher doses, especially in lung cancer, is under evaluation. Although higher doses should improve the higher chance of controlling tumor, the effects of increasing toxicity and/or the presence of resistant cells may limit the success of that approach. For example, dose escalation used in concurrent chemoradiation for esophageal cancer has not improved outcome beyond 50 Gy. Another objective is to clear areas at risk for subclinical extension of tumor. In general, 45 to 50 Gy over approximately 5 weeks is sufficient to treat subclinical microscopic disease with success. For example, lymph nodes irradiated electively in lung cancer are generally given this dose, although involved nodes would be treated like gross disease.

When radiation is used as an adjuvant to surgery, a dose of 45 to 50 Gy is the goal to control subclinical extension of tumor, but not achieve a complete response of gross disease. In addition, higher preoperative doses increase the complications after surgery, including increased wound complications, bronchial stump leaks, and adult respiratory distress syndrome (ARDS), particularly if a large volume of lung is irradiated. The theoretical advantages of preoperative RT depend on the circumstances in which it is used but include increasing the chances of resection with clear tumor margins, reducing the need for extensive surgery, and immediate administration of therapy to areas at risk for subclinical involvement. Postoperative RT has the potential advantage that the decision to administer treatment is based on pathologic findings rather than radiographic evidence of extent of disease. However, disadvantages include delay in treatment to areas that may have been subclinically involved with consequent risk of progression, the concern that tumor cells with a less-vascularized postoperative bed may be resistant to RT, and the potential loss of opportunity to achieve a total resection in some patients. When possible, areas of known positive margins are generally treated to higher doses used for gross disease.

Definitive RT given in combination with concurrent chemotherapy has resulted in improved long-term survival compared with radiation alone. A landmark multiinstitutional trial by the Radiation Therapy Oncology Group compared patients treated with 64 Gy of RT alone with patients treated with 50 Gy of RT given concurrently with two cycles and followed by an additional two cycles of cisplatin

75 mg/m^2 and 5-fluorouracil 1000 mg/m^2 per day for 4 days. With the addition of chemotherapy, 3- and 5-year disease-specific survival was improved.

■ RADIOTHERAPY FOR LUNG CANCER

RT for lung cancer has limited but definite efficacy. For non–small cell lung cancer (NSCLC), RT is appropriately used as an adjunct to surgery for patients with advanced disease or positive margins, as an alternative to surgery for patients with medically inoperable early stage disease, as definitive therapy for advanced disease, as preoperative therapy for Pancoast's tumor, and as palliative therapy. The barriers to success include the size and extent of the tumors; the high risk of distant metastases not encompassed by radiation; the limitations on radiation dose due to surrounding normal tissue (lung, heart, esophagus, and spinal cord); and the geometric complexity of the tumors. In limited stage small cell lung cancer, radiation is an important part of definitive therapy.

Definitive Radiotherapy: Early Stage Medically Inoperable Lung Cancer (Non–Small Cell Lung Cancer)

Radiation therapy may be used as an alternative to surgery for patients who have early stage NSCLC but are medically inoperable. The decision to use RT in this situation should be based on assessing the risks of morbidity and mortality if the patient does not undergo surgery, against that from concurrent medical illnesses. When RT is used, 5-year survival has generally been in the range of 20% to 30% (higher in some series with carefully selected patients) with substantial risk of death due to progression of disease. RT is likely to also result in at least some decrement in pulmonary function. Consideration of the patient's current pulmonary function and possible deterioration should be taken into account. When the decision to proceed is questionable, patients can be watched without therapy, with treatment instituted for palliation only if the tumor is growing rapidly or symptoms develop.

When treatment is instituted, the smallest localized field is used and a dose of 60 to 70 Gy is administered. If pulmonary function is especially poor, care should be taken to limit the treatment volume to the primary tumor with a small margin. To limit toxicity, the clinically and radiographically uninvolved nodes are not treated. Although elective nodal irradiation may be considered for patients with good performance status, adequate pulmonary function, and high-risk disease (large, central lesions), the existing retrospective studies do not suggest any potential benefit in survival.

Definitive Radiation Therapy: Advanced Lung Cancer (Non–Small Cell Lung Cancer)

RT is the mainstay of treatment for clinical stage III lung cancer patients who are not candidates for surgery because the mediastinal nodes are involved or the primary tumor is unresectable. Generally, a dose of 60 Gy or higher is used. A landmark randomized trial done by the Cancer and Leukemia Group B and reported by Dillman in 1990 revealed that median survival with RT alone was 9.7 months but increased to 13.6 months when cisplatin and vinblastine chemotherapy was given before the radiation. More importantly, 5- and 7-year survival were improved from 7% and 6% to 19% and 13%, respectively. Since then, other trials have confirmed that there is a benefit to adding chemotherapy in this setting, which has now become standard therapy for this stage of tumors. Most trials that have demonstrated a benefit of combined chemoradiation are generally administered to patients with limited weight loss (no more than 5% to 10% of body weight) and a performance status of 70 or greater. Caution should be used in recommending chemotherapy with definitive RT to patients with a poor prognosis, with significant weight loss, or requiring substantial care. Randomized studies have been performed comparing chemotherapy before radiation with more toxic regimens of radiation given concurrently with chemotherapy. Final results of these definitive trials are not available, but the potential benefit should be balanced against the significant increase in toxicity with concurrent therapy. The incidence of esophagitis resulting in weight loss and myelosuppression may be increased with concurrent RT.

Postoperative Radiation

Postoperative RT should not be used in early stage node-negative NSCLC. In fact, meta-analysis of randomized trials including such patients has suggested a decrement in survival with postoperative RT. This meta-analysis carved out by the Postoperative Radiotherapy (PORT) Meta-analysis Trialists Group demonstrated an absolute decrement in survival of 7% at 2 years with postoperative RT, an effect confined to stage I and II tumors only. Therefore, postoperative RT should not be used in early stage lung cancer. The results of the PORT meta-analysis have been questioned because similar trials used older suboptimal radiation techniques that may have increased the risks of toxicity while decreasing the possible benefits; however, individual trials do not suggest any potential improvement in outcome. Postoperative RT is warranted for early stage disease when there is a positive margin.

Postoperative RT for patients with pathologically confirmed N1 disease is highly controversial. Recent randomized data do not suggest a survival benefit with adjuvant radiation, although some trials have demonstrated improved local control. The value of local control as an end point given the high rate of early distant failure is questionable. The Lung Cancer Study Group conducted a randomized trial addressing this issue for patients with only squamous cell carcinoma. Most patients had N1 disease. Local failure at the initial site was reduced from 19% to 1% with the addition of postoperative RT, although other trials have failed to confirm this benefit. Nevertheless, based on these data, RT is a standard option for N1 disease lung cancer. These randomized data have been criticized for combining patients with N1 and N2 disease, varying eligibility criteria, and having differing criteria for nodal sampling/dissection and possibly flawed RT technique.

Similarly, the value of postoperative RT is uncertain for patients with N2 disease. The randomized trials have the same weakness as described above for N1 disease and have not confirmed or ruled out a benefit to postoperative RT. Because there are significant retrospective data demonstrating a survival benefit despite flawed randomized trials, postoperative RT for N2 disease is frequently used. Sawyer reported a retrospective analysis on outcome for 224 patients treated at the Mayo Clinic for N2 lung cancer. An actuarial 4-year local recurrence rate was 60% with surgery alone, but only 17% if adjuvant RT was administered. Actuarial 4-year survival was improved from 22% to 43% ($p = .005$).

The potential benefit of RT in these settings is limited by the high incidence of distant failure from micrometastases that are present but undetectable at the time of surgery. These systemic micrometastases cannot be addressed by local RT. As better systemic therapies are developed that may effectively treat micrometastases and improvement in radiologic techniques such as positron emission tomography scanning to detect smaller metastases, the value of postoperative RT will be reassessed.

Preoperative Radiation

Preoperative RT is not generally used (except for Pancoast's tumor), because early randomized trials did not suggest a benefit. Preoperative combined RT/chemotherapy is a current subject of study. Numerous uncontrolled trials have raised the questions of survival benefit with preoperative chemoradiotherapy, but definitive randomized trials are clearly needed.

Attention to patient selection and radiation technique is required when preoperative chemoradiation is used. Care should be taken to select patients with adequate pulmonary function relative to the treatment volume. Doses up to 45 Gy at 1.8 to 2.0 Gy/day do not seem to increase surgical complications significantly, but the incidence of ARDS and bronchial stump leaks may increase with higher doses.

Preoperative RT is a standard management option for T3N0 superior sulcus (Pancoast's) tumor. In this situation, preoperative RT has been used for several decades as it adds to the chance of obtaining a complete resection in these tumors that abut or encase the neurovascular structures in the superior sulcus and has lowered the incidence of local failure observed with surgery alone. With this regimen, the survival is reported as high as 40% to 50% in well-selected patients. There have been no prospective studies comparing preoperative RT with RT or surgery alone for superior sulcus tumors. Definitive RT should used in settings when surgery is unlikely to lead to a complete resection (T4 tumors) with negative margins or when there is evidence of mediastinal lymph node (N2 or N3) involvement. As chemotherapy appears beneficial in other clinical situations for advanced lung cancer, there is sound rationale for combination chemoradiotherapy for superior sulcus tumor. Postoperative radiation treatment also may be used in similar scenarios described previously.

Palliative Radiotherapy in Lung Cancer (Non–Small Cell Lung Cancer)

Radiation is of palliative benefit in lung cancer. Symptoms resulting from the primary tumor such as hemoptysis, pain, and dyspnea due to airway obstruction can be successfully palliated with minimal morbidity. Symptoms of metastatic disease, such as pain from bone metastasis or neurologic symptoms from brain metastasis, can also be irradiated with a high degree of success. Constitutional symptoms such as weight loss and malaise are not well alleviated. Regimens of limited duration, such as 30 Gy in 10 treatments or 35 Gy in

14 treatments, are used, because symptoms are only palliative and shorter courses are more respectful of the limited time available to patients with a poor prognosis.

■ SMALL CELL LUNG CANCER

For several years, chemotherapy was the standard treatment for limited stage small cell lung cancer (SCLC). A meta-analysis of randomized trials by Pignon and colleagues in 1993 including 2103 patients assessed the value of adding thoracic RT to chemotherapy. An absolute improvement of 5.4% in 3-year survival was demonstrated. Therefore, thoracic RT is now considered a standard component to chemotherapy for patients with limited disease. Because SCLC is exquisitely sensitive to RT, a standard dose of approximately 45 Gy at 1.8 Gy to 2.0 Gy/day is used. Although randomized trials in the past have yielded conflicting results on whether RT should be given concurrently at the start of chemotherapy or later in the course of therapy, the best results in recent trials have been achieved with early concomitant chemoradiotherapy. Therefore, RT should generally be integrated early into the treatment course, although an initial one to two cycles of chemotherapy may shrink the tumor, allowing a smaller volume to be treated. Radiation after chemotherapy should be reserved for patients judged unable to tolerate concurrent therapy.

Benchmark outcome results are provided by a recently reported randomized trial of the RTOG and the Eastern Cooperative Oncology Group. RT began at the initiation of four cycles of cisplatin and VP16 chemotherapy. The patients were randomized to receive 45 Gy at 1.8 Gy/day or 1.5 Gy twice a day, with the latter being a more intensive regimen. Local failure was reduced from 61% to 48% with twice-a-day RT, but 2-year survival was unimproved at 41% and 44%, respectively. Clearly, treatments better able to prevent both local and distant failure are required.

For patients achieving a complete response, prophylactic cranial RT is added to prevent brain metastasis. Randomized trials have demonstrated a substantial reduction in the incidence of brain metastasis. A meta-analysis using individual patient data on 987 patients in randomized trials demonstrated that the cumulative incidence of cranial recurrence at 3 years was reduced from 58.6% to 33.3% with the addition of RT. Although individual trials have not demonstrated a survival benefit, this meta-analysis showed an absolute improvement in survival of 5.4% at 3 years after randomization. Therefore, prophylactic cranial irradiation is a standard component of therapy for the SCLC patient who achieves a complete response of chest disease. Although neurocognitive effects of RT have been a concern, modern RT approaches and the administration of RT treatments after the completion of all chemotherapy has minimized this problem.

■ COMPLICATIONS OF RADIATION THERAPY

Common short-term side effects may include local skin reactions (erythema, irritation and darkening), esophagitis, fatigue, decreased blood counts, and temporary alopecia to the area. Uncommon side effects may include pneumonitis, resulting in fever, cough, and shortness of breath, which could be severe. Pneumonitis generally occurs 4 to 12 weeks after RT and results in an infiltrate shaped like the radiation fields. Treatment consists of corticosteroids. For severe cases (in up to 5% of patients), doses of 1 mg/kg prednisone may be used, but the taper should be cautious as symptoms may recur.

The most common long-term side effect is shortness of breath, especially with exertion, usually resulting from fibrosis of the treated area of functional lung. The risk of both short-term pneumonitis and long-term fibrosis causing significant disability is greatly increased when large volumes of normal lung are irradiated, particularly in patients with marginal to poor pulmonary function. In these situations, limited field volumes should be used whenever feasible and patients should certainly be informed of the risks of injury as well as a realistic view of the benefits of RT to help guide the decision to proceed. Rare side effects include cardiac injury, permanent esophageal injury, rib fracture, radiation-induced cancer, nerve or spinal cord damage, or eventual death from pulmonary fibrosis or pneumonitis.

■ FUTURE DIRECTIONS IN RADIOTHERAPY

Efforts are continually ongoing to improve the therapeutic benefits of RT. Efficacy can potentially be improved by optimizing the targeting of RT, developing improved schedules for RT administration, escalating the radiation dose, and adding agents that may sensitize tumor cells to the effects of RT. In addition, the therapeutic ratio can be improved by better protecting normal tissues. If a lower proportion of the radiation dose can be directed away from normal tissues, toxicity can be reduced, while escalating radiation doses to the tumor bed and thereby maintaining the current level of toxicity. In addition, other agents are being evaluated that may selectively protect normal tissues from the effects of RT. Some of these areas of investigation are briefly described as follows.

First, the increased power and decreased costs of desktop computing have allowed profound improvements to occur in the planning of RT. Conventional treatment planning involves computations that depict the distribution of radiation dose in, at most, several planes through the involved region. The physician must make assumptions about the radiation dose in the intervening areas. Three-dimensional treatment planning provides information on how radiation is deposited in every pixel of the area of interest, including tumor and surrounding normal tissues, so that the treatment plan can be optimized. In addition, this planning allows a greater complexity of beam arrangements and directions to be used. Several studies have demonstrated that, with the complex geometry of treating advanced lung cancer while protecting normal tissues, portions of the tumor are likely to be significantly underdosed using conventional treatment planning as opposed to three-dimensional treatment planning. This may play a role in treatment failure. In addition, studies are under way to use the improved accuracy of three-dimensional treatment planning to significantly escalate the dose given to the tumor while maintaining safe doses to surrounding critical structures.

Second, investigation also continues into improving the dosing regimens for RT. The intensity of RT has been guided by a regimen called CHART (continuous hyperfractionated accelerated radiotherapy). In this regimen, 1.5 Gy is given three times a day for 12 consecutive days to a total dose of 54 Gy. Each treatment is given at least 6 hours apart, which allows sufficient time for some repair of normal tissue. Saunders reported a large randomized trial of 563 patients with advanced NSCLC comparing the CHART regimen with standard RT. He demonstrated improved 2-year survival of 29% versus 20% and improved local control of 23% versus 15%, respectively. This trial, performed in the United Kingdom, included 45% of patients who were stage I and II and when chemotherapy was not used. A trial to confirm this benefit with a similar regimen confined to advanced lung cancer is ongoing in the United States.

Third, developing agents that may sensitize tumor cells to the effects of radiation is a particularly important area of investigation. Many of the newer chemotherapy agents, such as paclitaxel, gemcitabine, and irinotecan, are under evaluation for this purpose. There are also true radiosensitizers (drugs that may sensitize cells to radiation but do not themselves kill tumor cells). An example is RSR13, an agent that binds to hemoglobin, shifts the hemoglobin oxygen dissociation curve to the right, and causes oxygen release into tissues. It has long been known that hypoxic cells within tumors are resistant to RT. Previous methods that have been tested to reverse this hypoxia have been of limited potential efficacy as a result of limited physiologic effects at tolerable doses. However, by using hemoglobin, RSR13 has the potential to substantially increase oxygen delivery and is under evaluation in lung cancer as well as other tumor types. Of note, only a minimal concentration of oxygen is needed to fully sensitize cells, such that already well-oxygenated normal tissues would not be sensitized by this agent.

Finally, the protection of normal tissues remains another area of active research. Improvements in radiation treatment planning or targeting were discussed earlier. Amifostine is a potential radioprotector that was initially identified by the Defense Department during a search for agents that might be useful in the battlefield. Although this intravenous agent might not be useful in any practical sense during a wartime situation, it may potentially protect against the injury of therapeutic radiation by scavenging radiation-induced free radicals before they can injure the DNA. This agent differentially accumulates in normal tissue as opposed to tumor and therefore may not protect neoplastic cells. Randomized trials have indeed confirmed that this agent can reduce toxicities of head and neck RT without compromising control of tumor. Preliminary data suggest that amifostine may protect against the toxicities of RT seen for lung and possibly esophageal cancer. Reducing radiation toxicities could improve patient survival by allowing fewer treatment interruptions and thus higher dose escalations. Randomized trials using amifostine in lung cancer are under way.

SUGGESTED READING

Dillman RO, et al: A randomized trial of induction chemotherapy plus high-dose radiation versus radiation alone in stage III non-small-cell lung cancer, *N Engl J Med* 323:940, 1990.

Pignon JP, et al: A meta-analysis of thoracic radiotherapy for small-cell lung cancer, *N Engl J Med* 328:1425, 1993.

PORT Meta-analysis Trialists Group: Postoperative radiotherapy in non-small-cell lung cancer: systematic review and meta-analysis of individual patient data from nine randomised controlled trials, *Lancet* 352:257, 1998.

Rusch VW, et al: Induction chemoradiation and surgical resection for non-small-cell lung carcinomas of the superior sulcus: initial results of Southwest Oncology Group Trial 9416 (Intergroup Trial 0160), *J Thorac Cardiovasc Surg* 121:472, 2001.

Sawyer TE, et al: The impact of surgical adjuvant thoracic radiation therapy for patients with nonsmall cell lung carcinoma with ipsilateral mediastinal lymph node involvement, *Cancer* 80:1399, 1997.

PULMONARY METASTASES

Joe B. Putnam, Jr.

Systemic metastases frequently represent failure of local and systemic control of a primary neoplasm and herald a rapid demise for the patient. In some patients, metastatic disease confined to one or two particular organs may not carry such an ominous prognosis. Patients with metastases to a single organ, such as the lung, liver, brain, or rarely other organs, may undergo resection with an associated prolonged survival.

The biologic factors and clinical factors that contribute to this unique situation are not clear. Clinical and biologic factors have been identified previously, which assists the clinician in identifying selected patients with improved survival. Still the heterogeneity of pulmonary metastases does not provide consistent or predictable outcomes with standard surgical therapy. Metastases that are located entirely within the lungs and are potentially resectable may be resected with associated improved survival compared with unresectable metastases. In general, patients undergoing complete resection of all pulmonary metastases have an improved survival, regardless of the histology of the primary, compared with patients with unresectable metastases.

A prospective trial evaluating overall survival with medical management versus complete resection in patients with resectable pulmonary metastases (from the time of diagnosis of metastases) has never been performed. The morbidity of resection is low, and mortality is almost zero. Withholding potentially curative resection in patients with isolated and resectable pulmonary metastases makes such a trial unlikely. Survival after complete resection of pulmonary metastases may be long-term in 40% of patients.

■ DEVELOPMENT OF RESECTION FOR PULMONARY METASTASES

The history of surgical resection for pulmonary metastasis has been reviewed. Although sporadic isolated reports of resection of solitary metastases were first made in the late 1800s and early 1900s, it was not until Alexander and Haight reported the first selected series of patients with resection of pulmonary metastasis that the concept of "resection for cure" emerged. Resection of multiple pulmonary metastases and multiple resections for recurrent metastases also were developed. Repeat resection of metastases can be performed with minimal morbidity. More recently, techniques to preserve the lung parenchyma while still treating micrometastatic disease have been proposed. These strategies have incorporated resection after preoperative chemotherapy. Preoperative chemotherapy for sarcomatous metastases may be a valid consideration given the high potential for recurrence in these patients, particularly patients with multiple metastases. Complete resection of pulmonary metastases remains the standard of care for treatment of patients with resectable pulmonary metastases.

■ IDENTIFICATION OF METASTASIS AND RADIOLOGIC EVALUATION

All patients with a primary nonthoracic neoplasm (with the exception of nonmelanoma skin cancer) should have a screening chest radiograph to identify occult metastases or a new lung cancer. A chest radiograph is more specific but less sensitive than computed tomography (CT). Plain chest radiographs cannot identify occult or small lesions, multiple lesions, or early metastasis. CT is performed most frequently to evaluate abnormalities that are identified on the screening chest x-ray. In patients with osteogenic or soft tissue sarcomas, a baseline CT scan of the chest is performed to evaluate for occult pulmonary metastases. CT also may be used to evaluate the response to perioperative chemotherapy. After therapy, a periodic screening chest x-ray should be obtained. CT is necessary for patients with primary sarcomas (soft tissue sarcomas or osteogenic sarcomas) or to confirm chest radiograph changes. Chest CT should be performed whenever a patient is restaged for recurrent disease.

Magnetic resonance imaging (MRI) is rarely helpful in identifying occult metastases within the lung parenchyma. MRI is helpful, however, to evaluate the extent of mediastinal

or thoracic structure abutment, compression, or invasion from large bulky metastasis. MRI can assist the clinician in estimating tissue-tumor interaction and in planning the approach and extent of resection for these complex thoracic problems.

Positron emission tomography (PET) may be helpful in identifying patients with occult metastases elsewhere in the body. PET may aid in determining if there is residual metabolic activity remaining in the lung nodules identified on preoperative radiographs. PET is less sensitive than CT but can identify other sites of metastases and may be of value in identifying the extent of disease in patients with metastases from other solid tumor histologies, such as adenocarcinoma and squamous cell carcinoma.

■ SELECTION OF PATIENTS FOR SURGERY

The selection criteria of patients for resection of pulmonary metastases are well established and are listed in Table 1. Prognostic indicators are objective clinical descriptors, which can assist the clinician in identifying patients who optimally would benefit from resection of pulmonary metastasis. Current prognostic indicators are crude clinical characteristics, which may be used to define better the specific biologic characteristics of metastases. Patients with a combination of favorable prognostic indicators (e.g., slower tumor doubling time, fewer numbers of nodules, long disease-free interval) tend to have a better long-term survival than patients with unfavorable prognostic indicators (e.g., rapid tumor doubling time, multiple numbers of nodules, short disease-free interval, aggressive histology). Patients should not be excluded from resection on the basis of any single prognostic indicator. Rather, patients should be counseled as to the potential benefit of surgical resection in their unique situation.

Multiple pulmonary metastases suggest undetectable micrometastases. Although a surgeon removes all the metastases visualized or palpated, the surgeon cannot identify micrometastases at the time of surgery. Systemic chemotherapy may be considered in patients with multiple

---

Table 1 Selection Criteria for Resection of Pulmonary Metastasis

1. Pulmonary nodules consistent with metastasis
2. No uncontrolled metastases outside the chest
3. Primary tumor control
4. Potential for complete resection of all clinical disease
5. Adequate functional pulmonary parenchymal reserve after resection
6. Evaluate effects of chemotherapy on remaining disease
7. Establish a diagnosis
8. Obtain tissue for study of molecular markers, experimental vaccine therapy, or other histologic/immunohistochemical analysis
9. Palliate clinical symptoms (e.g., pain, dyspnea, obstruction)
10. Decrease tumor burden

metastases before surgery. In patients with multiple pulmonary metastases, chemotherapy may be considered before resection to establish a biologic response profile. In sarcomas, doxorubicin and ifosfamide are two active agents that have a positive dose-response profile. In patients with a significant biologic response (e.g., reduction in size or number of the metastases), chemotherapy may be maintained until the tumor nodules (or residual scar) have stabilized. Then resection can be done. In patients with bulky metastases from soft tissue sarcomas, this treatment may reduce the size of the tumor and allow a complete resection to be performed. In patients with a significant response before resection, chemotherapy may be applied postoperatively for 2 to 6 months for treatment of residual micrometastatic disease. Other studies have not shown value from systemic chemotherapy for pulmonary metastases from osteogenic sarcoma.

■ PROGNOSTIC INDICATORS

Use of prognostic indicators suggests that some patients could benefit more from resection than others. In patients with adverse prognostic factors, a multimodality approach to the disease process is recommended. In my institution, patients with pulmonary metastasis from sarcoma, gastrointestinal origin, melanomas, or breast carcinoma are discussed in a multidisciplinary fashion. Protocol participation or entry into a clinical study is presented to all patients who meet inclusion criteria. The medical oncologist, the radiation oncologist, and the thoracic surgeon discuss the range of options for the patient. A "best" strategy or plan is decided on along with appropriate alternatives to be discussed with the patient. The primary attending physician discusses the options with the patient, and together the patient and physician decide on the "best" treatment for the patient and family.

The results of resection of various pulmonary metastases have been reported. The characteristics of the primary tumor (histology, grade, location, or stage), patient characteristics (age, sex, disease-free survival), and characteristics of the metastases (number of nodules on preoperative radiologic studies, single or multiple metastases, unilateral or bilateral metastases, tumor doubling time, synchronous or metachronous metastases, and overall survival since diagnosis of the primary) all have been evaluated and examined. Regardless of the characteristics identified preoperatively, complete resection is associated most consistently with prolonged survival. Use of other modalities to achieve complete resection may provide a significant survival and local control value to the patient.

Stage or location of the primary tumor, age, and gender usually are not considered prognostic factors. Patients with soft tissue sarcoma or osteogenic sarcoma frequently metastasize to the lungs. Histology of the primary tumor is important because patients with differing histologies of soft tissue sarcomas have a different survival. The disease-free interval (the interval calculated from the time of the controlled primary neoplasm until the diagnosis of metastatic disease in the lungs) is an indirect measure of the biologic virulence of the tumor. Patients with a long disease-free interval may have a less aggressive tumor compared with patients with a short disease-free survival. Similarly, larger numbers of nodules on CT, the number of metastases resected, and the tumor doubling time all are indirect measures of the complex interactions of the host with the tumor. This tumor biology may suggest that resection alone may be optimal or that additional strategies may provide more value (chemotherapy before surgery for patients with multiple metastases from soft tissue sarcoma).

Although the individual characteristics may assist the clinician in selecting patients for resection, the ability to predict survival may be determined better with multivariate analysis of prognostic factors. Longer disease-free interval, longer tumor doubling time, and small numbers of nodules on preoperative studies were better predictors of postthoracotomy survival than any single factor.

The use of prognostic indicators was reviewed extensively in an international series of patients with pulmonary metastasis. In this series of more than 5000 patients, Pastorino et al reviewed the results of resection in patients with solitary or multiple metastases from various histologies. In this international series, overall actuarial 5-year survival was 36%, 10-year survival was 26%, and 15-year survival was 22%. Patients with a solitary pulmonary nodule, a disease-free interval of 3 years or greater, and complete resection had a significantly improved survival compared with patients who did not meet these criteria. Patients with germ cell neoplasms and complete resection had the most favorable histology of all. This international registry confirmed that patients with complete resection of pulmonary metastases have an associated long-term survival. Almost half of the patients in this registry had only a solitary metastasis resected.

■ METHODS OF RESECTION

Various incisions may be used for complete and successful resection of pulmonary metastasis. Median sternotomy commonly is performed for patients with bilateral peripheral lesions. Bilateral thoracic extirpations can be performed with one incision. There is typically less patient discomfort than with separate bilateral thoracotomies. Metastases near the hilum are difficult to resect through a median sternotomy, particularly within the left lower lobe, or in patients with comorbid conditions, such as obesity, cardiomegaly, or an elevated left hemidiaphragm.

The posterolateral thoracotomy with a latissimus dorsi muscle-sparing or muscle-cutting approach commonly is performed to expose all areas of the hemithorax. This incision provides excellent exposure to all components and areas of the chest, but has potentially more patient discomfort than median sternotomy. Typically, only one operation is performed at a time. A second and subsequent operation is needed for resection of contralateral metastasis.

The transverse sternotomy (clamshell) incision allows excellent exposure of both hemithoraces and both hila. The incision is larger than thoracotomy or median sternotomy. This technique commonly is used when the metastasis compresses the heart or involves both lungs or both hila. Access to the great vessels and the heart for cardiopulmonary bypass (e.g., to aid in support of decompression of the heart for mobilization and exposure) is facilitated by this approach and may be preferable to median sternotomy, particularly if significant hilar dissection or mobilization or both are required. A "hemi-clamshell" approach may be helpful for large, bulky metastases involving the hilum and the antero-lateral aspects of the middle mediastinum.

Thoracoscopy or video-assisted thoracic surgery (VATS) provides excellent visualization and potentially less morbidity and discomfort than open thoracotomy. Visceral and parietal pleural metastasis can be identified easily. VATS is ideally suited for diagnosis or staging in patients with metastatic disease. In contrast to open thoracotomy, in which the surgeon can evaluate carefully the lung by palpation to confirm or exclude occult metastases, patients undergoing thoracoscopy are constrained by the surgeon's inability to palpate completely all the lung parenchyma. If parenchymal metastases are subpleural and not easily identified, incomplete resection is likely. Subsequent resection may be required. Alternative techniques to assist with palpation of the parenchyma have been developed, such as the subxiphoid incision for substernal/retrosternal entry into the right or left hemithorax to allow palpation of the lung with thoracoscopic guidance. Although some authors have suggested that incomplete excision may yield similar outcomes to complete excision, this has not been confirmed in prospective studies. A selected approach may be optimal. In my opinion, patients with solitary, peripheral, nonsarcomatous metastasis identified on high-resolution CT may benefit from initial thoracoscopy for diagnosis, staging, and treatment.

The surgeon also must consider whether a solitary adenocarcinoma or squamous cell carcinoma "metastasis" may represent a primary lung cancer. In this situation, a lobectomy and mediastinal lymph node dissection are recommended.

■ INTRAOPERATIVE AND POSTOPERATIVE THERAPY

In preparation for surgery, adequate general endotracheal anesthesia is obtained, and selective ventilation is accomplished with the use of a double-lumen endotracheal tube. The position of the double-lumen endotracheal tube is confirmed with flexible fiberoptic bronchoscopy. After the thoracic incision is made, the lung is deflated sequentially for palpation and resection. In a patient undergoing thoracotomy, only the exposed lung is deflated. The contralateral lung continues ventilating. The surgeon palpates all areas of the lung and identifies the pulmonary metastases in question or identifies metastases on the preoperative CT scan. More recently, high-speed thin-section (3.8 mm) tomography allows accurate identification of small metastases. The surgeon must palpate the lung to identify physically all nodules visualized on preoperative CT and to identify occult metastases or other metastasis-like abnormalities, all of which also must be resected. Many of these are metastases. Many objective but small lesions may be identified and resected that may reveal a benign process after pathologic examination. Nodules are resected with a small rim of normal tissue. Nodules are completely resected. The nodules

are not "shelled out." The surgeon must determine the adequacy and completeness of the margin. Distortion of the lung parenchyma by the pathologist may give a false-positive margin.

Although mediastinal lymph nodes are not routinely resected, the hilum should be inspected, and if enlarged or hard lymph nodes are identified, a mediastinal lymph node dissection or sampling should be performed. Mediastinal lymph node metastases from pulmonary metastases are rare. Presence of hilar or mediastinal nodal metastases from intraparenchymal metastases suggests extensive systemic disease and an ominous prognosis.

Techniques of resection may vary depending on the needs of the patient and the requirement to obtain complete resection. Usually, use of a surgical stapling device is all that is required. Occasionally, use of the laser may be required to minimize distortion of the lung tissue. Electrocautery could be considered for small parietal pleural lesions. Topical sealants may minimize the resultant air leak. The laser may prevent the distortion of the lung parenchyma commonly found in patients having multiple wedge resections using surgical staplers.

During the postoperative convalescence, pulmonary hygiene and adequate pain relief are paramount. Ambulation, respiratory therapy, and adequate pain control with a thoracic epidural infusion system or a patient-controlled analgesia system all are crucial components for adequate pain relief and minimizing in-hospital convalescence.

■ RESECTION OF RECURRENT PULMONARY METASTASES

Resection of recurrent pulmonary metastases may be accomplished with similar morbidity and equally good survival results (postthoracotomy survival) in patients undergoing an initial resection, especially for patients with soft tissue sarcomas. Patients are selected for surgery based on the same criteria listed in Table 1 used for an initial resection. Complete resection remains the predominant prognostic indicator associated with prolonged survival even in patients with recurrent metastases.

■ EXTENDED RESECTION OF PULMONARY METASTASES

To achieve complete resection of isolated pulmonary metastases, larger operations and wedge resection may be required. Although unusual, pneumonectomy or resection of a metastasis contiguous with mediastinal components may be required. Resection of metastasis with chest wall, superior vena cava, pericardium, or diaphragm can be accomplished with 5-year survival of greater than 25% and a median survival (after resection) of 27 months. Pneumonectomy also may be performed with associated long-term survival.

Resection of selected metastases may be indicated if local control cannot be achieved with chemotherapy or other techniques. Resection of large tumors obstructing the bronchus or tumors compressing the mediastinum can be performed with improvement in symptoms, although overall survival (from the metastases) may not be improved.

Combination procedures, such as pulmonary resection and hepatic resection of metastases from colorectal carcinoma, may be performed with improved survival compared with patients with incomplete resection. The surgeon must balance the physiologic fitness of the patient with the potential morbidity or mortality of the operation and the potential to achieve meaningful improvements in survival or local control. This aggressive resection must be tailored to the individual patient.

Partial cardiopulmonary bypass may be required for bulky tumors compressing the heart and mediastinum. Decompression of the heart may be necessary for mobilization, dissection, and separation of the tumor from the mediastinum. Complete cardiopulmonary bypass may be needed for resection and repair (or reconstruction) of the heart.

Radiofrequency ablation techniques, commonly used for liver tumors, have been applied to pulmonary metastases. Radiofrequency ablation techniques create safe, reproducible lesions in normal porcine lung parenchyma. The application of controlled thermal injury to normal or neoplastic lung lesions for therapy requires rigorous preclinical and clinical studies. This experimental technique has the potential to injure adjacent pulmonary structures, including the bronchus, pulmonary vasculature, and mediastinal structures. The ability to achieve consistently ablation of all viable tumor within the pulmonary metastasis is not known. In contrast to liver metastases, which have a high water content, pulmonary metastases have variable amounts of water and fibrosis. Consistent spacing of the needle array from the radiofrequency catheter cannot be achieved in patients with osteogenic or soft tissue sarcomas or other fibrous-like pulmonary metastases.

■ EXPERIMENTAL TREATMENT STRATEGIES

Mechanical techniques for resection of pulmonary metastases do not provide consistent benefit to patients. The use of mechanical solutions for such a complex biologic problem assists some patients and does not assist others. Although prognostic indicators can assist in the clinical selection of patients, identification of specific markers of metastasis, apoptosis, or invasion may identify patients who optimally would benefit from chemotherapy, targeted biologic therapies, or systemic control in addition to surgery for enhanced local control. Mutations of the *p53* gene (a tumor-suppressor gene) have been identified in soft tissue sarcomas. Transduction of the normal or wild-type *p53* in soft tissue sarcoma cells resulted in decreased cell proliferation, decreased colony formation in soft agar, and decreased tumor formation in a nude mouse model. Restoration of normal *p53* function in soft tissue sarcomas may be considered a future therapy. *p53* mutations may differ between the primary tumor and the metastases. Specific molecular markers of the primary tumor and the metastasis may aid in better selection of therapy for patients who would or would not benefit from surgery, chemotherapy, targeted biologic therapies, or other treatment modalities.

Other strategies may include other types of gene therapy (thymidine kinase/ganciclovir/acyclovir), liposome-encapsulated muramyl tripeptide (LMTP-E), nebulized liposomes, and isolated lung perfusion. Although such therapies are exciting, all suffer from the inability to deliver sufficient drug or active pharmaceutical to the target metastases. Hurdles that must be overcome include (1) selective targeting of the metastasis, rather than host tissue; (2) protection of normal tissue; (3) minimal morbidity; (4) no systemic toxicity; (5) independent physical function after treatment; (6) prolonged treatment effect; (7) the ability to repeat the treatment if necessary; and (8) the ability to deliver high concentrations of therapeutic agent to the metastasis. Strategies to examine the biologic characteristics, molecular markers, inhibition of pathways crucial to progression of metastasis, or other perhaps yet undescribed techniques will be needed to treat these metastases accurately and repeatedly. Although models of micrometastases from intravenous injection have shown promising results with various types of inhalational or perfusional therapies, the value of these treatments for macroscopic disease that may have a component of pulmonary arterial and systemic arterial blood supply will pose a challenge to investigators.

Targeted therapy with Gleevec (a signal transduction inhibitor imatinib mesylate [previously STI571]; Novartis Pharmaceuticals Corp, East Hanover, NJ) has cured patients with gastrointestinal stromal tumors. These tumors have overexpression of a transmembrane receptor, a product of the *c-kit* protooncogene. Inhibition of the *c-kit* gene is the proposed (and successful) mode of action for tumors having overexpression of *c-kit*. Other targeted therapies may be equally effective in patients with pulmonary metastases of specific molecular characteristics.

■ CONCLUSION

Patients with isolated and resectable metastases to the lung represent a unique but salvageable group of patients with cancer. The unique characteristics of this patient population demand the careful attention of surgical and medical oncologists. Combinations of local and systemic control or targeted drug treatment (e.g., gene therapy, inhalational agents, regional drug perfusion) eventually may prove superior to surgery alone. Patients with complete resection of metastasis isolated to the lung have associated long-term survival greater than patients who have unresectable metastases, regardless of primary histology. These patients should undergo resection to render them disease-free. Surgery alone for treatment of pulmonary metastasis fails in a significant number of patients. Even with extended resection, resection of recurrent metastases, or other aggressive approaches, surgery fails to change the fundamental biology of the neoplastic or metastatic process. Chemotherapy as an adjuvant or neoadjuvant modality commonly is used for soft tissue sarcomas at my institution. Other strategies incorporating a systemic and local control modality for pulmonary metastasis appear sound and potentially of greater benefit to surgery alone. Novel therapies are needed to improve the systemic and local control of patients with pulmonary metastases.

SUGGESTED READING

Billingsley KG, et al: Multifactorial analysis of the survival of patients with distant metastasis arising from primary extremity sarcoma, *Cancer* 85:389, 1999.

Casson AG, et al: Efficacy of pulmonary metastasectomy for recurrent soft tissue sarcoma, *J Surg Oncol* 47:1, 1991.

McCormack PM, et al: Role of video-assisted thoracic surgery in the treatment of pulmonary metastases: results of a prospective trial, *Ann Thorac Surg* 62:213, 1996.

Pastorino U, et al: Long-term results of lung metastasectomy: prognostic analyses based on 5206 cases. The International Registry of Lung Metastases, *J Thorac Cardiovasc Surg* 113:37, 1997.

Putnam JB Jr, et al: Analysis of prognostic factors in patients undergoing resection of pulmonary metastases from soft tissue sarcomas, *J Thorac Cardiovasc Surg* 87:260, 1984.

Putnam JB Jr, et al: Extended resection of pulmonary metastases: is the risk justified? *Ann Thorac Surg* 55:1440, 1993.

UNUSUAL PRIMARY MALIGNANT NEOPLASMS OF THE LUNG

Ara A. Vaporciyan

Most primary malignancies arising in the lung are either the small cell or the non–small cell subtype. Rarely the clinician encounters other malignant neoplasms arising in the lung. These tumors account for less than 2% of all primary pulmonary malignancies and vary by their histologic features. Many malignancies occur more frequently as extrapulmonary tumors and only in rare cases arise solely in the lung.

To promote the adoption of a uniform terminology, the World Health Organization (WHO) developed the International Histological Classification of Tumors. Under this system of classification, all small cell lung cancers (SCLCs) and non–small cell lung cancers (NSCLCs) are designated *malignant epithelial tumors*. There are numerous variants of the classically described SCLCs and NSCLCs (squamous cell carcinoma, adenocarcinoma, and large cell carcinoma). Many of these variants are rare, with a limited number of reports in the literature. This chapter discusses the epithelial tumor variants not considered to be part of classic SCLC or NSCLC and other primary malignancies of the lung that are classified as soft tissue tumors, lymphoproliferative diseases, and miscellaneous tumors. The goal of this chapter is to familiarize the reader with the variety of rare malignancies that can occur in the lung and the general principles involved in managing these lesions.

■ COMMON FEATURES

Unusual primary pulmonary malignancies can occur as an isolated pulmonary nodule, rendering them difficult to distinguish from NSCLC. The symptoms and radiographic appearances also often are indistinguishable from NSCLC. The most common symptoms, which are present in 50% to 85% of cases, are cough, dyspnea, chest pain, and hemoptysis. Systemic symptoms, such as fever, fatigue, and weight loss, occur less commonly. A specific diagnosis usually is made at surgery because bronchoscopic or transthoracic fine needle aspiration (FNA) renders, at best, a diagnosis of malignancy without further detail. In cases in which these tumors are multifocal, such as lymphoproliferative disorders and pulmonary epithelioid hemangioendothelioma, the evaluation is considerably different. After excluding infectious and benign etiologies, a surgical or video-assisted thoracoscopic lung biopsy usually is required, although occasionally less invasive means may be possible to diagnose the lesion.

■ EPITHELIAL TUMORS

Carcinoma with Pleomorphic, Sarcomatoid, or Sarcomatous Elements

Carcinomas with pleomorphic, sarcomatoid, or sarcomatous elements are thought to be epithelial in origin and are malignant epithelial tumors under the new system outlined by the WHO. These carcinomas have been subcategorized into three major groups: carcinoma with spindle or giant cell, carcinosarcoma, and pulmonary blastoma.

Carcinoma with Spindle or Giant Cell and Carcinosarcoma

The clinical features at presentation and the prognosis of carcinoma with spindle or giant cell elements are similar to those of carcinosarcoma. Carcinoma with spindle or giant cell elements and carcinosarcoma have initial clinical features similar to those of NSCLC. The evaluation and treatment should proceed as they would for common forms of NSCLC. These tumors tend to be difficult to diagnose on preoperative workup unless they are endobronchial and biopsy specimens are obtained at the time of bronchoscopy. Most commonly, a nonspecific diagnosis of NSCLC results from the biopsy. As in cases of more common variants of

NSCLC, the next step should include an assessment of stage. Patients with stage I or II tumors are offered resection if they have adequate pulmonary reserve. Stage IIIA tumors are treated on protocol, if available, or with combination chemotherapy and radiotherapy if the patient has a good performance status. Advanced disease is treated with chemotherapy, radiotherapy, or both.

The natural history of these tumors has been debated. We examined all cases at our institution of precipitous recurrence (<9 months) after resection of stage I and II NSCLC and compared the cases with a group of cases in which stage-matched control subjects remained disease-free 3 years after resection. Only weight loss and unusual histology including carcinosarcoma were found to predict early relapse. If the diagnosis of carcinosarcoma is made preoperatively, neo-adjuvant or adjuvant systemic therapy should be considered even if the tumor is completely resected.

Pulmonary Blastoma

A pulmonary blastoma consists of immature mesenchyme or epithelium that morphologically mimics the embryonal structure of the lung. Initially described as an "embryoma of the lung," the lesion later was named *pulmonary blastoma* because of its similarity to nephroblastoma. Pulmonary blastomas have been categorized into the following three variants based on their histologic appearance: biphasic blastoma, well-differentiated fetal adenocarcinoma (WDFA), and pleuropulmonary blastoma. Biphasic blastoma is a mixture of malignant mesenchyme and malignant epithelium, with one or both resembling embryonal lung between 10 and 16 weeks' gestation. WDFA is the epithelial variant, which consists of neoplastic but well-ordered glandular epithelium with an embryonal appearance. Pleuropulmonary blastoma is the mesothelial variant, which consists of malignant mesothelial components only. Biphasic blastoma and WDFA occur in adults in their 20s and 30s, whereas pleuropulmonary blastoma is a pediatric tumor that occurs in the first decade only. Molecular distinctions also exist between the three variants, with varying frequencies and types of genetic mutations identified by immunohistochemistry and molecular studies. No mutations have been found in WDFA, which is why the WHO categorizes WDFA as a variant of adenocarcinoma.

Despite the debate regarding the classification of pulmonary blastomas, all variants tend to present classically in a similar fashion. In nearly all patients with pulmonary blastoma, the mass is unilateral, and only 50% to 60% are symptomatic. The primary symptoms are cough, chest pain, and hemoptysis. Biphasic and pleuropulmonary blastomas tend to be larger and have a worse prognosis than WDFA, although nodal metastases are uncommon for all these tumors, with an incidence of less than 10% in the largest reported series. The treatment for pulmonary blastoma consists of complete surgical resection. Some response to chemotherapy has been reported with multidrug regimens, although data regarding response to radiotherapy are scarce. The overall 5-year survival rate after surgical resection for pulmonary blastoma has been reported to be 45% to 50%; the WDFA variant seems to confer a better prognosis, however. Adverse prognostic signs in patients with pulmonary blastoma include the presence of lymph node or systemic metastasis, pathologic stage II after surgical resection, and tumor recurrence.

■ SOFT TISSUE TUMORS

Isolated pulmonary soft tissue tumors are exceedingly rare. With the exception of pulmonary epithelioid hemangioendothelioma, soft tissue tumors include various rare histologic subtypes of sarcoma. These sarcomas arise much more commonly in extrapulmonary sites.

Pulmonary Epithelioid Hemangioendothelioma

Pulmonary epithelioid hemangioendothelioma previously was referred to as an *intravascular sclerosing bronchoalveolar tumor* or an *intravascular bronchoalveolar tumor* because the initial report of this subtype included many patients with bilateral tumors and one patient with concurrent bronchoalveolar cancer. The later identification of Weibel-Palade bodies in the cytoplasm of tumor cells revealed their endothelial origin, however. The pulmonary epithelioid hemangioendothelioma is described best as a low-grade sarcoma and is grouped with the soft tissue tumors. Most patients are young women, with 85% of these lesions occurring in women, 40% being younger than 30 years of age (median age 35 years). Most patients present with multiple nodules less than 2 cm in size. Distant metastases have developed in 24% of the reported cases, with the liver being the dominant site of failure. The disease in half of the reported cases was asymptomatic; in two thirds of the remaining cases, the symptoms were mild and relatively minor.

The role of surgery for pulmonary epithelioid hemangioendothelioma is limited to tissue diagnosis. Although a patient in the literature with an isolated case of the disease did undergo successful resection, most patients present with multifocal disease, and the surgeon's role generally is limited to performing a lung biopsy. Despite its multifocal presentation, the disease has an indolent course. Multiple chemotherapy combinations have been tried without significant success. Lung transplantation has been considered because of the tumor's propensity for slow growth and usually localized disease. The natural history of the disease may span 5 to 10 years, and reports of spontaneous regression do exist.

Sarcoma

Although primary pulmonary sarcoma is rare, the complete list of histologic subtypes that have been described arising within the lung is considerable (Table 1). Metastasis from an extrapulmonary primary site is more common, however, than primary pulmonary sarcoma. Any diagnosis of sarcoma within the lung should prompt an aggressive search for an occult extrathoracic primary tumor, especially if the pulmonary lesions are multiple.

The age range at the time of presentation with primary pulmonary sarcoma is 5 to 78 years (median 50 years). Patients generally have symptoms, with most series reporting only 11% to 32% of patients being asymptomatic. Most symptoms are related to the mass effect, with cough,

Table 1 Unusual Primary Malignant Neoplasms of the Lung

EPITHELIAL TUMORS
Carcinoma with pleomorphic, sarcomatoid, or sarcomatous elements
    Carcinoma with spindle and/or giant cell
    Carcinosarcoma
    Pulmonary blastoma
        Biphasic blastoma
        Well-differentiated fetal adenocarcinoma (previously termed *fetal lung type adenocarcinoma*)
        Pleuropulmonary blastoma
SOFT TISSUE TUMORS
Pulmonary epithelioid hemangioendothelioma (previously termed *intravascular bronchioalveolar tumor*)
Sarcoma
    Fibrosarcoma, neurogenic sarcoma, angiosarcoma, lymphangiosarcoma, leiomyosarcoma, malignant fibrous histiocytoma,
        hemangiopericytoma, Kaposi's sarcoma, chondrosarcoma, osteosarcoma, liposarcoma, rhabdomyosarcoma, alveolar soft part
        sarcoma, synovial sarcoma, primitive neuroectodermal tumor, and desmoplastic round cell tumor
LYMPHOPROLIFERATIVE DISEASES
BALT lymphoma
    Low-grade, small B-cell lymphoma (previously termed *pseudolymphomas*)
    High-grade, large B-cell lymphoma
Angiocentric lymphoma (previously termed *lymphomatoid granulomatosis*)
Primary pulmonary Hodgkin's disease
Extramedullary plasmacytoma
Primary pulmonary Langerhans cell histiocytosis (previously termed *eosinophilic granuloma*)
MISCELLANEOUS TUMORS
Germ cell tumors
    Malignant teratoma
    Choriocarcinoma
Thymoma
Malignant melanoma

chest pain, and dyspnea predominating. The radiographic evaluation does not differentiate these tumors from other forms of lung cancer, although these tumors tend to have smooth borders and are large (median 5 cm). Specific histologic identification rarely is made preoperatively but should be attempted with transthoracic FNA or bronchoscopy. Reported overall resection rates are 69% to 89%. Cytoreduction with neoadjuvant chemotherapy sometimes can increase resectability, but radiotherapy is reserved for cases in which surgery has failed. The 5-year survival rates in most series (which included unresectable tumors) ranged from 30% to 40%, although survival rates of 80% have been reported in series including totally resected tumors. Obtaining an R0 surgical resection and the disease stage (i.e., presence or absence of metastases) seem to corollate with survival. In general, in the absence of metastases, every attempt should be made to obtain a complete resection. The most common histologic subtype of pulmonary sarcoma is malignant fibrous histiocytoma. Other commonly seen varieties include leiomyosarcoma, synovial sarcoma, and angiosarcoma arising from the pulmonary arteries.

■ LYMPHOPROLIFERATIVE DISEASES

Previous reports have differentiated between pseudolymphoma, Hodgkin's lymphoma, and non-Hodgkin's lymphoma of the lung. Further investigation has revealed, however, that many lesions diagnosed as pseudolymphomas were low-grade lymphomas of bronchus-associated lymphoid tissue (BALT). These lesions are similar to intestinal lymphomas derived from mucosa-associated lymphoid tissue (MALT). More recent classifications have differentiated between BALT lymphoma and other forms of non-Hodgkin's lymphoma.

BALT Lymphoma

Most (75% to 90%) non-Hodgkin's lymphomas are diagnosed as low-grade, small B-cell lymphoma. These lesions previously were called *pseudolymphomas*. Patients with low-grade small B-cell lymphoma may have nodules (single, bilateral, or multiple) or, in rare cases, a diffuse infiltrate. Symptoms are absent in half of patients and when present are nonspecific (e.g., cough, dyspnea, and hemoptysis). The prognosis depends on the stage of disease at presentation. Indolent, slow-growing, usually solitary tumors generally are cured with surgery alone. Chemotherapy and radiation therapy are indicated when complete resection is not possible. Recurrence in local or other extrapulmonary MALT sites can occur, as can transformation to the more aggressive form of BALT lymphoma, high-grade large B-cell lymphoma. This latter type accounts for 6% to 20% of pulmonary lymphomas. Most occur as solitary masses greater than 3 cm in diameter, but these lesions occasionally are multinodular or diffuse. The resection of solitary lesions with complete nodal dissection should be attempted. The reported 5-year survival rate is 45% compared with 87% for patients with low-grade small B-cell lymphoma. For this reason, adjuvant chemotherapy often is administered to patients with high-grade large B-cell lymphoma.

Angiocentric Lymphoma

Angiocentric lymphoma can be difficult to distinguish from other lymphomas, although strict histologic criteria indicate that this subtype tends to affect predominantly men in their 40s. Nonspecific symptoms of cough, dyspnea, and chest pain are common. The typical radiographic appearance is of bilateral nodules that may contain cavities with thick walls. Surgery, usually lung biopsy, is diagnostic, with chemotherapy being the primary mode of treatment.

Primary Pulmonary Hodgkin's Disease

The incidence of primary pulmonary Hodgkin's disease by strict diagnostic criteria is rare, representing less than 0.6% of all cases of Hodgkin's disease. The strict diagnostic criteria include (1) histologic features of Hodgkin's disease; (2) restriction of the disease to the lung, with minimal or no thoracic nodal involvement; and (3) absence of disease at extrathoracic sites. Two thirds of patients with primary pulmonary Hodgkin's disease present with a solitary nodule; the rest have multiple unilateral or bilateral nodules. The standard treatment for Hodgkin's disease of the lung includes combination chemotherapy and radiotherapy. A resection with complete node dissection can be performed, however, for isolated disease that meets the strict diagnostic criteria. For patients with multiple sites of pulmonary disease, the surgeon's role typically involves tissue biopsy only.

Extramedullary Plasmacytoma

Solitary plasmacytoma of the lung is rare. This lesion usually is not associated with elevated serum or urine paraproteins. Curative resection can be achieved, but delayed progression to disseminated multiple myeloma has been reported.

Primary Pulmonary Langerhans Cell Histiocytosis

Primary pulmonary Langerhans cell histiocytosis is more commonly part of a systemic disease process but can be limited to the lung. The presentation of patients with this lesion varies, with the entire spectrum of solitary to interstitial infiltrates seen. Most solitary lesions can be cured with resection. Multiple lung lesions are not resectable and usually progress to advanced disease, although reports of stabilization or spontaneous regression do occur. Progressive disease may respond to radiation therapy, chemotherapy, or a combination of both.

■ MISCELLANEOUS TUMORS

Germ Cell Tumors

Germ cell tumors are broadly grouped into malignant teratomas and choriocarcinoma.

Malignant Teratomas

Malignant teratomas are exceedingly rare; fewer than 20 cases have been documented. Patients with malignant teratoma present with a solitary nodule. Therapy for this lesion should parallel that for NSCLC. If a malignant teratoma is large and a diagnosis can be obtained preoperatively, the patient would benefit from preoperative chemotherapy. Extension of a mediastinal teratoma into the lung is more common than a primary malignant teratoma of the lung.

Choriocarcinoma

Primary choriocarcinoma is also rare. Most reported cases are pleomorphic ectopic carcinomas (a variant of spindle or giant cell carcinoma) that produce β-human chorionic gonadotropin. Of primary lung cancers, 6% can produce β-human chorionic gonadotropin. The evaluation and treatment of primary choriocarcinoma of the lung are similar to those of other NSCLCs.

Thymoma

When a suspected thymoma of the lung occurs, an aggressive search for a mediastinal primary tumor should be performed because primary pulmonary thymoma is extremely rare. Treatment consists of surgical resection. Myasthenia gravis can occur in association with pulmonary thymoma.

Malignant Melanoma

Although a solitary pulmonary metastasis from malignant melanoma is unusual, it is still more common than primary pulmonary melanoma. When a pulmonary melanoma is found, workup for an extrathoracic primary tumor site is required (e.g., skin, ocular, oral, anal). Primary pulmonary melanoma tends to be central endobronchial and frequently metastasizes to the mediastinal nodes. Anatomic resection with complete nodal dissection has been recommended. Long-term survivors have been reported.

SUGGESTED READING

Burt M, Zakowski M: Rare primary malignant neoplasms. In Pearson FG, et al, editors: *Thoracic surgery,* New York, 1995, Churchill-Livingstone, p 807.

Pietra GG, Salhany KE: Lymphoproliferative and hematologic diseases involving the lung. In Fishman AP, et al, editors: *Fishman's pulmonary diseases and disorders,* New York, 1998, McGraw-Hill, p 1861.

COMPLICATIONS OF PULMONARY RESECTION

Robert J. Cerfolio

The key to treating most postsurgical complications is prevention. Complications from pulmonary resection are no different—most can be prevented in the operating room. Even with meticulous preoperative selection, intraoperative techniques, and diligent postoperative care, however, some complications after elective pulmonary resections are unavoidable. This chapter reviews the most common preventable complications by describing the problem, discussing intraoperative techniques to help avoid it, and discussing the optimal postoperative management. Other common complications that cannot be avoided in the operating room, such as pneumonia, aspiration, and other pulmonary sequela, are not discussed. Postoperative empyema and fistula are described elsewhere.

■ AIR LEAKS

Air leaks are the most common complication after elective pulmonary resection, with prolonged leaks (>7 days) occurring in 15% of patients. Despite this fact, there has been little to no literature concerning the prediction, prevention, and treatment of air leaks. A classification system was not even present. We have conducted clinical trials that have led to a better management and classification system for air leaks. A synopsis of this work and of intraoperative techniques that help avoid air leaks is presented.

Intraoperative Techniques to Prevent Air Leaks

To prevent air leaks, one first must know who is most at risk of developing them. We have found that patients with emphysema (specifically a low forced expiratory volume in 1 second and diffusing capacity of lung for carbon monoxide), patients with insulin-dependent diabetes, patients on steroids preoperatively, and patients who undergo lobectomy or lung volume reduction surgery are at increased risk. In these patients, prophylactic measures should be used in the operating room to help prevent leaks. One of the most important ways to accomplish this goal is a fissureless technique of pulmonary surgery. This surgical approach avoids dissection through the lung. There should be no dissection in an incomplete fissure to find the pulmonary arterial branches. Instead the dissection starts in the hilum. The vein is taken first, the arterial branches are taken second, and the bronchus is divided last. The fissures are completed last with staplers, and this completes the lobectomy. This fissureless technique can be employed for almost any type of pulmonary resection.

A second method that helps prevent air leaks is buttressing the staple line. We often use bovine pericardial strips (Peri-Strips; Biovascular, Minneapolis, MN) if the lung is emphysematous or if the patient has other risk factors for developing an air leak. Before closing the chest, the lung is reinflated, and warm water is squirted over it to identify and pinpoint small air leaks. These air leaks should be oversewn. If the leaks persist, we use FocalSeal, a sealant approved by the Food and Drug Administration. This sealant has been highly successful in allowing us to leave the operating room without an air leak. In the patient with significant risk factors to develop a leak after surgery, we often have applied FocalSeal as a prophylactic measure as well.

Postoperative Techniques to Help Seal Air Leaks

A major area of our clinical research has been in chest tube management. We have found that water seal is safe for patients with air leaks. We have found that water seal is superior to suction for helping air leaks to resolve after surgery. In patients with large leaks greater than 4/7 (as measured on the only commercially available air leak meter, Deknatel [Sahara, Boston, MA]), a pneumothorax can occur, however. If this happens or if an enlarging pneumothorax or subcutaneous air develops while on water seal, some suction is needed. In this situation, we apply the least amount of suction needed to eliminate the symptomatic pneumothorax or to eradicate the subcutaneous emphysema. This approach minimizes the size of the air leak and helps achieve contact between the visceral and parietal pleura, which we believe is an important element for the sealing of air leaks.

Treatment of Persistent Air Leaks

We also have studied the best treatment of air leaks that still are present on postoperative day 3 or 4. In our fast-tracking protocol after pulmonary resection, patients are usually ready for discharge by postoperative day 3 or 4. We remove all but one chest tube via a technique we call *serial chest tube clamping*. This technique enables the surgeon at the bedside to determine which tubes are best controlling the air leak and the pleural space. The one remaining tube that is left in is placed to a Heimlich valve. Patients are discharged home the next day. This practice has been extremely successful in allowing patients to leave the hospital on time. Most patients are able to tolerate conversion from water seal to a Heimlich valve. Some patients develop a new or enlarging pneumothorax or subcutaneous emphysema on the Heimlich valve, however. Air leaks that are expiratory and greater than 5/7 on the leak meter or air leaks that are continuous probably will fail a Heimlich valve. These patients need to be returned to water seal or to some suction, usually −10 cm H_2O.

Finally, we have found that patients who still have a persistent air leak after 2 weeks on a Heimlich valve can have their chest tubes removed. Although there still may be a small leak, the patients do not develop a pneumothorax with chest tube removal. This is probably due to pleural adhesions that compartmentalize the pleural space and that prevent a tension pneumothorax or an enlarging, symptomatic pneumothorax to occur.

POSTOPERATIVE BLEEDING

Postoperative bleeding is prevented by meticulous intra-operative technique. In general, if the pulmonary artery is handled carefully (we prefer double ligation) and the vein is either stapled or doubly ligated, few if any patients ever return to the operating room for life-threatening bleeding. We have performed more than 3000 operations over 5 years, and no patients have returned for bleeding from the artery or vein. Chest wall bleeding after a redo thoracotomy, bleeding from the base of lymph nodes, coagulopathy, or bleeding from the bronchial arteries can occur. Just before closure of the chest, the main vascular structures and bronchus should be rechecked for hemostasis. Then each lymph node station should be checked. For both chest cavities, special attention should be given to the inferior pulmonary ligament lymph nodes (no. 9 station) and the subcarinal lymph nodes (no. 7 station). The aortopulmonary window lymph nodes (no. 5 and no. 6) on the left and the paratracheal nodes (no. 2 and no. 4) on the right also should be rein-spected carefully. Other areas that require special attention are the posterolateral aspect of the right main stem bronchus (where the branches of the vagus nerve and the bronchial arteries enter the lung), the chest tube insertion site, parietal pleural surface (from adhesions or pleural flap), and the periosteal sutures for rib approximation. Vessels in the area of the bronchial arteries should be clipped or tied and not coagulated.

If bleeding does occur, early recognition and intervention is mandatory. In the postoperative period, if the chest tube output is high (>800 ml/24 hr or >250 ml/hr for 3 consecutive hours), a hemoglobin level should be checked from the serum and chest tube drainage. An international normalized ratio (INR), partial thromboplastin time, and platelet count also should be drawn. If the hemoglobin is stable, one can send the fluid for a triglyceride level to help rule out chylothorax. A final consideration of a high unexplained chest tube output is a subarachnoid pleural fistula, which is exceedingly rare. A chest radiograph also should be performed to ensure that the chest tubes have not clotted, resulting in a pleura full of blood. If the effluent from the chest tubes is frank or bright red blood, immediate return to the operating room is mandatory, if the INR, partial thromboplastin time, and platelet count are normal.

TORSION OF THE MIDDLE LOBE

Torsion or gangrene of the right middle lobe (RML) after right upper lobe (RUL) or right lower lobe (RLL) lobectomy with resultant gangrene is a rare but often fatal complication after pulmonary resection. Torsion has been reported to occur in the other lobes, but to a lesser degree. It is almost always preventable in the operating room. It is more common after RUL lobectomy because the fissure between the RML and RLL is usually relatively complete. In contrast, the fissure between the RUL and RML is almost never complete. This complete fissure helps anchor the RML to the RUL and makes RML torsion after RLL lobectomy extremely unusual.

After RUL lobectomy, the RML can twist 360 degrees. This twisting leads to arterial and/or venous embarrassment. If undetected within several hours (a clue is often seen on chest x-ray that shows a new infiltrate with volume loss or a relapsing then recurring infiltrate), the patient can become acidotic and critically ill. Immediate return to the operating room with RML lobectomy is the treatment of choice.

Prevention of this devastating complication is performed best and easily at the time of chest closure. Before rib approximation after an RUL lobectomy, the remaining lung should be reinflated and inspected to ensure that there are no twists to the RML. For proper alignment, the edge of the RML along the oblique fissure only should be seen; if staplers were used to complete the fissure, they should be out of the visual field from the thoracotomy incision. If the patient has undergone an RUL lobectomy, a tacking stitch between the RML and the RLL should be placed if it appears that the RML twists easily around its hilum after reinflation. The two lobes can be stapled together, but we believe this prevents the RML from fully rising into the apex of the right chest. We prefer one or two tacking stitches using 4-0 polypropylene (Prolene) between the lateral aspect of the RML and the posterior segment of the RLL. These same observations and principles can be applied after an RLL lobectomy if the fissure is relatively incomplete between the RUL and RML.

ARRHYTHMIAS

Arrhythmias after pulmonary resection continue to be a common and often frustrating complication. The incidence has been reported to be 5% to 40%, depending on how carefully the patients are monitored. Atrial fibrillation is the most common arrhythmia (75%), followed by supraventricular tachycardia and atrial flutter. Of arrhythmias, 80% occur within the first 3 days after surgery. Pneumonectomy is associated with a fivefold increase in atrial arrhythmias. Half may be recurrent or refractory to medical management.

Data suggest that the prophylactic use of calcium channel blockers can decrease the incidence of atrial fibrillation or flutter in patients who undergo pneumonectomy or radical or intrapericardial pneumonectomy. These data have never been extrapolated to patients who undergo lobectomy, however. If patients have a history of atrial fibrillation or atrial flutter preoperatively, they are at even higher risk of developing this problem postoperatively.

Factors that have been associated with arrhythmias include hypoxia, intrapericardial dissection, pericardial manipulation, vagal irritation, pulmonary hypertension, and preexisting cardiac disease. Chest tubes should be placed carefully so that they are not lying on or irritating the pericardial surface.

When a patient has any sign of an atrial arrhythmia, medications such as digoxin, a calcium channel blocker, or amiodarone should be given. Immediate cardioversion is required for hemodynamically unstable patients. Underlying causes, such as hypoxia, electrolyte abnormalities, or even silent myocardial ischemia, should be ruled out. If the arrhythmia continues for 48 hours, the risks and benefits of anticoagulation and cardioversion should be considered.

■ CHYLOTHORAX

Chylothorax after pulmonary resection is a relatively uncommon complication and another example of a post-operative complication that can be prevented in the operating room. Lymph node biopsy or even complete thoracic lymphadenectomy (our preference) from all lymph node stations (mandatory with all resections for bronchogenic malignancies) can be performed with a low incidence of chylothorax. Patients with N2 disease (especially gross extracapsular N2 disease) are at increased risk of developing a chylothorax. This is likely due to lymphatic obstruction from metastatic cancer.

Before closing the chest, each thoracic lymph node station should be examined carefully to ensure that there is no evidence of a clear or milky effluent. If this is present, the base of the offending node should be clipped. If a complete thoracic lymphadenectomy is performed, the feeding collateral lymphatic channel should be identified and clipped. If significant drainage is present and the effluent cannot be well visualized, a nasogastric tube should be placed by the anesthesiologist into the stomach. Cream or a liquid that is high in fat should be delivered down the naso-gastric tube. Within several minutes, the leaking collateral channel usually is seen easily and should be clipped. If sutures are used, we prefer 5-0 polypropylene, buttressed by felt pledgets. When the duct is closed, a surgical sealant, such as fibrin glue, also could be placed prophylactically over the offending area. Chemical pleurodesis or mechanical pleurodesis can be added to help sclerose the pleural space and discourage any space for a chylothorax to accumulate.

If a patient develops a chylothorax after pulmonary surgery, we have found the natural history to be relatively benign. After pulmonary resection, in contrast to esophageal resection, injury to the main duct is uncommon. This type of chylothorax, which is usually from collateral branches, stops with a medium-chain triglyceride diet. Total parenteral nutrition rarely is needed.

■ CARDIAC HERNIATION

Although a rare complication, cardiac herniation can be fatal. It is seen most commonly after a right pneu-monectomy that repaired intrapericardial dissection or partial pericardiectomy. The diagnosis often is made in the recovery room. The patient develops hemody-namic instability because the inferior or superior vena cava becomes kinked by the herniation. If the patient is stable, the diagnosis often can be confirmed by a portable chest x-ray. If unstable, the patient should be returned immediately to the operating room and the defect closed.

Prevention is mandatory. At initial operation, if any pericardium has been resected, the defect should be closed. A patch of bovine pericardium or a Gore-Tex patch can be used and sewn around the defect. Even if just a small part of the pericardium has been resected (especially on the right), we prefer to close it.

■ POSTPNEUMONECTOMY SYNDROME

Postpneumonectomy syndrome is another unusual compli-cation that involves herniation of the mediastinum, heart, and contralateral lung into the postpneumonectomy space. It usually is associated with a right pneumonectomy. For either side, the main stem bronchus is stretched and com-pressed by the vertebral body and descending aorta. Patients usually present months to years after pneumonectomy, with audible stridor, dyspnea, and recurring pulmonary infec-tions. Plain chest radiographs and computed tomography scans reveal marked deviation of the mediastinal contents rotating posteriorly. Bronchoscopy shows the tracheal devi-ation, with severe bronchial obstruction and malacia.

It is impossible to predict who will develop this complica-tion. If chest tubes are used after resection, most surgeons do not use suction and keep the tubes clamped to prevent acute mediastinal shifting. Correction of this problem is aimed at repositioning the mediastinum. This can be accomplished by suturing the pericardium (anterior to the phrenic nerve) to the posterior shelf of the sternum and placing expandable saline breast implants in the postpneumonectomy pleural space, which usually is spared of any adhesions. If after repositioning the mediastinum the bronchial segment remains malacic, endobronchial stents are inserted. Long-term results are good.

■ LUNG HERNIATION

Herniation of the lung through a rib interspace is an uncommon complication that begins early after thoracot-omy, but it usually does not manifest clinically for several years. The herniation is due to dehiscence or incomplete clo-sure of the intercostal space. Factors that might be associated with this complication are those associated with poor wound healing (steroids, diabetes, immunosuppressed state, preoperative chemotherapy or radiotherapy) and structural problems, such as osteoporosis and hyperinflation of the chest cavity. Proper closure is paramount, regardless of the type of suture used. If poor wound healing is suspect at the time of initial closure, some surgeons recommend the use of wire for additional support of the intercostal space.

Most patients present with pain or tenderness, and if the defect is large, they are able to cause protrusion of the lung with a Valsalva maneuver. A chest x-ray or computed tomography scan may reveal extrathoracic herniation of pulmonary tissue. Asymptomatic patients may be watched expectantly. Patients with large or symptomatic hernias require surgical closure, usu-ally with a prosthetic patch of Gore-Tex or bovine pericardium.

SUGGESTED READING

Cerfolio RJ, et al: Predictors and treatment of persistent air leaks, *Ann Thorac Surg* 73:1727, 2002.

De Decker K, et al: Cardiac complications after noncardiac thoracic surgery: an evidence-based current review, *Ann Thorac Surg* 75:1340, 2003.

Grillo HC, et al: Postpneumonectomy syndrome: diagnosis, management and results, *Ann Thorac Surg* 54:638, 1992.

Wagner RB, Nesbitt JC: Pulmonary torsion and gangrene, *Chest Surg Clin N Am* 2:839, 1992.

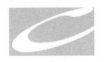

ACTINOMYCOSIS AND NOCARDIAL INFECTIONS OF THE LUNG

Cleveland W. Lewis
Walter G. Wolfe

The phylogenic order of Actinomycetaceae includes the Actinomycetaceae and Nocardiaceae, and this family of organisms is known to be bacterial in origin. However, they were once considered to be fungi and were acknowledged as the most common etiology of fungal infection in humans. Similar to fungi, these organisms are slow-growing, form-branched filaments ex vivo and produce chronic illness in humans. This error in classification lasted until the 1970s. Histologic and biochemical investigations revealed that these organisms are true bacteria. The presence of lysine and muramic and diaminopimelic acids, and the lack of fungal cell wall chitin is evidence of their bacterial origin. Reproduction occurs via fission, not via spores or buds as in fungi. Both organisms lack a nuclear membrane and mitochondria, which are prokaryotic traits, and they are susceptible to antibacterial agents (e.g., penicillin), not antifungal agents. Both organisms are capable of producing chronic pulmonary infections that are clinically indistinguishable but are treated with different antimicrobial agents.

■ ACTINOMYCOSIS

Actinomycosis is a chronic suppurative and granulomatous infection that forms multiple sinus tracts that produce "sulfur granules." This infection does not adhere to normal anatomic barriers and is able to invade and destroy bone. This destruction of bone can lead to significant skeletal and cosmetic disfigurement. Slow, but progressive, hematogenous spread may occur if local infection has been established. These organisms do not exist alone in nature but colonize the human oral cavity and can also be found in tonsillar crypts and the female genital tract. This disease favors the cervicofacial region over 60% of the time. Abdominal and thoracic infections are less frequent sites of involvement—25% and 15% of cases, respectively. Mediastinal and cardiac actinomycosis usually occur secondary to direct extension of pulmonary disease. Pericarditis is the most common clinical finding of cardiac involvement. Endocarditis has been described, but myocardial involvement is rare.

Epidemiology
The first reported actinomycotic infection was described in 1826 as an "osteosarcoma of the jaws of cattle." Initially, this disease was thought to be an exogenous infection, the responsible organism arising from the ground and soil. The first described case of thoracic actinomycosis was in 1882; the first successful surgical treatment of this disease occurred in 1923; and the first successful pulmonary resection for this disease was done in 1932 by Wangensteen.

Microbiologists have been able to clearly show that *Actinomyces* are part of the natural flora of mammalian mucous membranes. *Actinomyces israelii* can always be isolated from the human oral cavity if cultured in anaerobic conditions. Infections are more common in males than in females by an approximately 3:1 ratio. The peak incidence of this disease is seen in middle-aged persons, although infection can occur at all ages. No person-to-person transmission has ever been reported in the literature. Since the emergence of successful antibiotic therapy, the incidence of actinomycotic infections has significantly decreased. Also, better dental hygiene probably has contributed to the fall in the number of cases of actinomycotic infections. There has been an increased incidence of infections seen in immunocompromised hosts. Cases in the literature include reports of actinomycotic infections complicating acute lymphocytic leukemia during chemotherapy, lung transplantation, steroid use, and human immunodeficiency virus (HIV) infection.

Morphology and Pathology
Actinomyces are filamentous bacteria that are 0.5 to 1.0 μm in diameter and 2 to 30 μm in length; in culture, they display lateral and dichotomous branching. These organisms are gram-positive, anaerobic or microaerophilic bacteria that fragment to form both bacillary and coccoid elements. Classic actinomycotic infection is characterized by the development of a fibrotic nodule that has a dense cellular infiltrate. However, this intense fibrotic reaction may be minimal in pulmonary or central nervous system (CNS) infections. This lesion will progress into a noncaseating granuloma that suppurates centrally and creates interconnecting channels that often form sinus tracts to the skin or adjacent structures. Disseminated hematogenous spread can occur from these sites of local infection but is now rare since the arrival of effective antibiotic therapy. Disseminated disease is most commonly seen in patients with thoracic actinomycosis; the incidence has been reported to be as high as 50%.

Histologically, the region of intense fibrotic reaction consists of an outer zone of collagen fibers and fibroblasts.

Within an area of central suppuration, sulfur granules, up to 2.5 mm in diameter, can be found. These organisms coalesce to form granules. Finding these sulfur granules within a lesion is diagnostic, but they are rarely found in sputum samples.

Pathogenesis

Present among the normal human flora, *Actinomyces* are not virulent organisms. Located in dental caries, plaque, periodontitis, and tonsillar crypts, infection occurs when there is a break in the oral mucosa. Pulmonary infection occurs when organisms are aspirated, and only in rare occasions does thoracic disease arise from direct extension of cervicofacial disease, esophageal disease, or an intraabdominal, transdiaphragmatic process.

Approximately 25% of patients with thoracic disease experience the complication of bony destruction as a result of direct extension. The bones typically involved include the ribs, sternum, shoulder, scapula, and vertebral column. Grossly, bony involvement ranges in appearance from intense periosteal reaction to actual lytic lesions. *Actinomyces* infections are more likely to exhibit bony involvement compared with *Nocardia asteroides*. Less common complications include pleuropulmonary disease, empyema, and pericardial and myocardial disease. Complications such as superior vena cava syndrome and tracheoesophageal fistula are rarely seen.

Clinical Features

Thoracic actinomycosis accounts for approximately 15% of all actinomycotic infections. The usual source of infection is the aspiration of organisms from the oropharynx. Direct spread of organisms from an extrathoracic site of infection is rare in the days of effective antibiotic therapy. The classic clinical picture is a patient with poor oral hygiene who experiences an indolent, but progressive course of fever, night sweats, weight loss, dyspnea, and productive cough. Mild hemoptysis or blood-streaked sputum occurs when there is parenchymal destruction. Sinus tract formation, once common, is now rarely seen in thoracic disease. The occasional patient may even be asymptomatic. Given the infrequency and chronicity of this disease, diagnosis can be delayed 1 to 5 months after the onset of symptoms. Patients who are diagnosed with thoracic actinomycosis tend to have a history of one or more of the following processes: tuberculosis, coccidioidomycosis, chronic bronchitis, emphysema, chronic pneumonitis, and bronchiectasis. The clinical findings are nearly indistinguishable from those of bacterial pneumonia.

No specific radiographic signs are associated with this disease, and any lobe may be involved. The common appearance is an enlarging mass lesion, pneumonitis, or massive consolidation with variable pleural involvement. This disease has a tendency to appear in the lung bases and near the hila and can be bilateral. Bronchopleurocutaneous fistula, once a common presentation in the preantibiotic era, is rarely seen now in developed countries. A patchy, pneumonia-like infiltrate may also be seen. Specimens for histologic examination may be obtained from sinus tract drainage, transbronchial biopsies, transthoracic needle aspirations, and surgical resection tissue. A sputum culture positive for *Actinomyces* has to be correlated to clinical findings, knowing that the organism is part of the endogenous oral flora. In treating an actinomycotic infection, both aerobic and anaerobic cultures should be obtained because concurrent infection with aerobic organisms is often present. Routine cultures often do not grow *Actinomyces*, and the delay in diagnosis may account for the increased incidence of dissemination seen in thoracic disease. The presence of sulfur granules in the examined tissue or purulent exudate allows a tentative diagnosis, but microbiologic identification of *Actinomyces* usually requires 4 to 7 days of growth.

Therapy

Before the use of penicillin therapy for this disease in 1941, actinomycosis was associated with a mortality rate of 75% to 100%. Most survivors in the preantibiotic era had persistent, chronic infection. Current therapy has changed very little since the 1960s. Most antibiotic therapeutic regimens include high doses of penicillin and a long period of treatment. Large doses (10 to 20 million units) of penicillin are administered intravenously for 2 to 6 weeks, followed by oral penicillin V at 500 mg four times a day for 6 to 12 months. The length of therapy is important to prevent the relapse of disease. This regimen is also adequate initial regimen for immunocompromised patients, but refractory disease may occur and has been described in HIV-infected patients. For penicillin-allergic individuals, erythromycin, tetracycline, and doxycycline have been used with success. Imipenem has also been shown to be efficacious. The initial treatment for pulmonary actinomycosis is penicillin. Disease complicated by sinus tracts, abscesses, or empyema necessitate surgical intervention in addition to antibiotic therapy. An aggressive surgical approach is warranted, with some patients requiring lobectomy or even pneumonectomy. Failure to adequately débride all affected tissue can result in a postoperative bronchopleural fistula, systemic dissemination, or empyema. The combination of surgery and antibiotic therapy has resulted in a survival rate from thoracic actinomycosis that exceeds 90%.

■ NOCARDIOSIS

Nocardiosis can be a transient, subclinical, acute or chronic suppurative disorder. The isolated clinical pathogens most commonly responsible for nocardiosis are *Nocardia asteroides*, *Nocardia brasiliensis*, *Nocardia otitidis-caviarum*, and possibly *Nocardia transvalensis*. These organisms belong to the genus of aerobic, soil-borne actinomycetes. Documented cases of nocardiosis have risen substantially in the past two decades secondary to an increasing number of immunocompromised hosts and microbiologic identification. The three primary forms of the disease are cutaneous, subcutaneous, and pulmonary, with the latter accounting for almost 75% of the primary cases. Dissemination is also most prevalent with pulmonary disease, with central nervous system involvement present in approximately 30% of patients with disseminated nocardiosis. Pulmonary nocardiosis usually arises as an opportunistic infection in immunocompromised hosts in more than 85% of documented cases. *N. asteroides* and *N. otitidis-caviarum* are opportunistic organisms, whereas *N. brasiliensis* is more virulent, possessing opportunistic and pathogenic capabilities. *N. asteroides* is responsible for approximately 95% of cases of pulmonary nocardiosis, whereas *N. otitidis-caviarum* and *N. brasiliensis* are usually causative agents in cutaneous and subcutaneous infections.

Epidemiology

In 1888, Nocard first described an aerobic actinomyces infection in Guadeloupean cattle with pulmonary lesions, draining sinuses, cutaneous abscesses, and cachexia. The first human infection was noted in 1891 and was found to be highly susceptible to sulfonamides in 1944. *Nocardia* are ubiquitous, aerobic organisms found in soil, organic matter, and water. Direct tissue inoculation or inhalation is the usual method of infection. *N. brasiliensis* is most commonly responsible for nocardiosis in tropical regions, whereas *N. asteroides* is the usual causative agent in other regions of the world. Although nocardiosis is a well-known agent of infection in animals (e.g., bovine mastitis), no animal-to-human or human-to-human transmission has been reported. Outbreaks of nocardiosis in hospital oncology and transplant wards and during hospital construction work have been described.

Morphology and Pathology

Nocardia appear as gram-positive, beaded, multibranched filaments on gram-stain evaluation. Using special methods, *Nocardia* will stain acid-fast using a modified Ziehl-Neelsen stain, whereas other species of Actinomycetes will not. Purulent material draining from a sinus tract or an abscess is usually sufficient to yield a histopathologic diagnosis. This organism can be readily cultured on Sabouraud's glucose or blood agar, especially in the presence of 10% carbon dioxide. *Nocardia* is a slow-growing bacteria and usually requires 4 to 21 days of growth for accurate identification.

The most common gross appearance is multiple abscesses that can coalesce to form draining sinuses. The intense fibrotic reaction is associated with actinomycosis. Pulmonary disease may be characterized by consolidation, diffuse and nodular lesions, effusion, "fungus ball," and empyema; these findings may be the initial presentation of disease. Peribronchial lymphadenopathy is also usually present to some degree. Suppuration and cavitation may occur, but granulation, caseation, and giant cell formation are rarely seen. Sulfur granules are seen less often in nocardiosis than with actinomycosis, with *N. brasiliensis* and *N. otitidis-caviarum* infections more often displaying sulfur granules than *N. asteroides*.

Pathogenesis

Nocardia organisms are soil-inhabiting bacteria whose entry is gained into the host through inhalation or traumatic introduction. *N. brasiliensis* is the most virulent of all species of *Nocardia*, whereas *N. otitidis-caviarum* and *N. asteroides* are usually considered opportunistic organisms. Established cutaneous infection can occur with relatively small injuries: insect and animal bites, puncture wounds and abrasions. The *Nocardia* species elicit a primary T cell–mediated immune response with little or no humoral response. Therefore, nocardiosis is more prevalent in immunocompromised patients with impaired cell-mediated immunity. Serious disseminated infection can occur in these patients and is most commonly reported in transplant patients and those with lymphoreticular neoplasia. A recent report that examined 1000 random cases of nocardiosis determined that more than 60% of the cases occurred in patients who exhibited some evidence of immunosuppression. Approximately 12% of patients who contract pulmonary nocardiosis have underlying pulmonary disease. Patients at risk include those with chronic pulmonary disease, including pulmonary alveolar proteinosis, chronic obstructive pulmonary disease, and tuberculosis. Patients undergoing long-term corticosteroid use also are at risk for nocardiosis infections. A slight increase in prevalence has also been reported in patients with AIDS, but the overall incidence is low, not explained by the use of sulfonamide prophylaxis for *Pneumocystis carinii* pneumonia.

Clinical Features

The predominant clinical manifestation is pulmonary disease (>40% of cases), and *N. asteroides* accounts for approximately 89% of cases of pulmonary nocardiosis. Symptoms, although present in more than 75% of affected patients, are usually nonspecific. Anorexia, productive cough, night sweats, malaise, fever, dyspnea, and hemoptysis can occur with nocardiosis.

Pulmonary nocardiosis also has no specific radiographic findings. Radiologic findings include solitary or multiple irregular nodules, bronchopneumonia (reticulonodular or diffuse patterns), cavitation, and pleural effusion. Prolonged disease may be complicated by empyema, pulmonary mycetoma (lung abscess), and severe cavitation with extension to the chest wall. Mediastinal adenopathy is commonly seen and can be great enough to cause superior vena cava syndrome. If pulmonary nocardiosis is inadequately treated, progressive pulmonary fibrosis may occur. Bony involvement is seen less commonly than with actinomycotic infection but is seen occasionally with *N. brasiliensis* infections. Approximately one third of patients with pulmonary nocardiosis may have CNS involvement and may be the only source of symptoms in these patients. CNS involvement is most frequently manifested by brain abscesses, either uniloculated or multiloculated. Pulmonary nocardiosis may be the terminal event in advanced HIV infection, appearing as pulmonary infiltrates. In the immunocompromised patient, the process may demonstrate relentless clinical progression, or it may be a chronic, indolent disease. Subsequent involvement of contiguous structures or the CNS should alert the clinician to the possibility of a *Nocardia* etiology.

Diagnosis

One must always consider *Nocardia* as a pathogen in any immunocompromised patient with a pulmonary infiltrate. Most diagnoses are made on Gram and modified Ziehl-Neelsen stains of purulent material or sputum. Sputum analysis is usually diagnostic. Direct microscopic smears of purulent sputum material usually reveal gram-positive, beaded, branching filaments that can be acid-fast. *Nocardia* will grow on most nonselective media and appear as pigmented waxy rounded colonies. With special techniques, many of these colonies will stain acid fast, distinguishing them from actinomycotic organisms. Growth of *Nocardia* species may take up to several weeks, but usually colonies appear within 3 to 5 days.

Therapy and Prognosis

During the preantibiotic era, nocardiosis was associated with a high rate of mortality. Lyons was the first to report the successful treatment of a patient with nocardiosis using sulfonamides. The use of sulfa drugs has significantly diminished the mortality rate previously associated with this disease. The sulfonamides continue to be the mainstay of therapy. Trimethoprim-sulfamethoxazole is the most preferred drug combination and is the treatment of choice for infections caused by *N. brasiliensis*, *N. asteroides*, and *N. transvalensis*. The recommended dose is 5 to 10 mg/kg of trimethoprim and 25 to 50 mg/kg of sulfamethoxazole in two divided doses for 3 to 12 months given the extent of the disease. Higher doses may be needed in patients with cerebral abscesses, systemic spread, or advanced HIV infection. Other alternative drugs that have shown efficacy in the treatment of nocardiosis are imipenem and amikacin. The addition of surgical drainage for persistent infections or abscesses may be necessary for complete resolution of disease. In patients with normal immune systems, pulmonary nocardiosis should be treated for at least 6 months. If CNS involvement is present, then a 12-month regimen of therapy is warranted. Immunosuppressed patients without HIV infection should be treated for no less than 12 months, depending on the severity and length of immunosuppression. Patients with HIV infection or those who require long-term immunosuppression should be considered for life-long low-dose maintenance therapy once primary therapy is completed, given the significant rate of relapse associated with nocardiosis in these patients.

Almost 90% of patients with pulmonary disease can be cured with a combination of appropriate drug therapy and surgery if necessary. However, mortality rises significantly in immunosuppressed patients and approaches 50% to 55%, even in treated cases. Transplant patients who require continuing immunosuppression can be adequately treated without cessation of immunosuppressive drugs. Early diagnosis and adequate length of antibiotic therapy and surgical therapy if needed are paramount to successful eradication of this disease.

SUGGESTED READING

Balikian JP, et al: Pulmonary nocardiosis, *Radiology* 126:145, 1978.

Bassiri AG, et al: *Actinomycosis odontolyticus* thoracopulmonary infections, *Chest* 109:1109, 1996.

Bates M, Cruickshank G: Thoracic actinomycosis, *Thorax* 12:99, 1957.

Beaman BL, et al: Nocardial infections in the United States, 1972-1974, *J Infect Dis* 134:286, 1976.

Beaman BL, et al: Nocardia, Rhodococcus, Streptomyces, Oerskovia, and other aerobic actinomycetes of medical importance. In Murray PR, et al, editors: *Manual of clinical microbiology*, ed 6, Washington, DC, 1995, ASM, p 379.

Beaman L, Beaman BL: Nocardia species: host-parasite relationships, *Clin Microbiol Rev* 7:213, 1994.

Benbow EP, et al: Sulfonamide therapy in actinomycosis, *Am Rev Tuberc* 49:395, 1944.

Bigland AD, Sergeant FCH: A case of actinomycosis with recovery, *Br Med J* 2:61, 1923.

Brown JR: Human actinomycosis: a study of 181 subjects, *Hum Pathol* 4:319, 1973.

Cendan I, et al: Pulmonary actinomycosis. A cause of endobronchial disease in a patient with AIDS, *Chest* 103:1886, 1993.

Cherian G, et al: Myocarditis. In *Cardiology*, Philadelphia, 1987, JB Lippincott.

Cope VZ: *Actinomycosis*, London, 1939, Oxford University Press.

Cutler EC, Gross RE: Actinomycosis of the lung and pleura, *Am Rev Tuberc* 41:358, 1940.

Eppinger H: Ueber eine neue, pathogene Cladothrix und eine durch Sie hervorgerufene Pseudotuberculosis (cladothrichica), *Beitr Pathol Anat Allgemein Pathol* 9:287, 1890.

Feigin DS: Nocardiosis of the lung: chest radiographic findings in 21 cases, *Radiology* 159:9, 1986.

Gaffney RJ, Walsh MA: Cervicofacial actinomycosis: an unusual cause of submandibular swelling, *J Laryngol Otol* 107:1169, 1993.

Gallant JE, Ko AH: Cavitary pulmonary lesions in patients infected with human immunodeficiency virus, *Clin Infect Dis* 22:671, 1996.

Garrod LP: Actinomycosis of the lung. Aetiology, diagnosis and chemotherapy, *Tubercule* 33:258, 1952.

Harz CO: *Actinomyces bovis*: ein neue Schimmel in dem Gewebe des Rindes, *Jahresber Konigl Cental Thierarneischule Munchen* 5:125, 1877.

Hennrikus EF, Pederson L: Disseminated actinomycosis, *West J Med* 147:201, 1987.

Hsieh M-J, et al: Thoracic actinomycosis, *Chest* 104:366, 1993.

Israel J: Neue Beobachtungen auf dem Gebiet der Mykosen des Menschen, *Virchows Arch [B]* 74:15, 1878.

Jordon HV, et al: Enhancement of experimental actinomycosis in mice by *Eikenella corrodens*, *Infect Immun* 46:367, 1984.

Kay EB: Pulmonary actinomycosis: its treatment by pulmonary resection in conjunction with chemotherapy, *Ann Surg* 124:535, 1946.

Kinnear WJM, MacFarlane JT: A survey of thoracic actinomycosis, *Respir Med* 84:57, 1990.

Kramer MR, Uttamchandani RB: The radiographic appearance of pulmonary nocardiosis associated with AIDS, *Chest* 98:382, 1990.

Lam S, et al: Primary actinomycotic endocarditis: case report and review, *Clin Infect Dis* 16:481,1993.

Lerner PI: Actinomycosis and Arachnia species. In Mandell GL, et al, editors: *Principles and practice of infectious diseases*, ed 3, New York, 1986, Churchill Livingstone.

Lerner PI: Nocardia species. In Mandell GL, et al, editors: *Principles and practice of infectious diseases*, ed 3, New York, 1986, Churchill Livingstone.

Lerner PI: Nocardiosis, *Clin Infect Dis* 22:891, 1996.

Lord FT: Presence of actinomycosis in contents of carious teeth and tonsillar crypts of patients without actinomycosis, *JAMA* 55:1261, 1910.

Lucas SB, et al: Nocardiosis in HIV-positive patients: an autopsy study in West Africa. *Tuber Lung Dis* 75:301, 1994.

Lyons C, et al: Sulfonamide therapy in actinomycotic infections, *Surgery* 14:99, 1943.

Manfredi R, et al: Progressive intractable actinomycosis in patients with AIDS, *Scand J Infect Dis* 27:405, 1995.

McNeil MM, Brown JM: The medically important aerobic actinomycetes: epidemiology and microbiology, *Clin Microbiol Rev* 7:357, 1994.

Murray JF, et al: The changing spectrum of nocardiosis, *Am Rev Respir Dis* 83:315, 1961.

Neu HC, et al: Necrotizing nocardial pneumonitis, *Ann Intern Med* 66:274, 1967.

Nichols DR, Herrell WE: Penicillin in the treatment of actinomycosis, *J Lab Clin Med* 33:521, 1948.

Niedt GW, Schinella RA: Acquired immunodeficiency syndrome, *Arch Pathol Lab Med* 109:727, 1985.

Nocard E: Note sur la maladie des boeufs de la Guadeloupe, conne sous lenom defarcin, *Ann Instit Pasteur* 2:293, 1888.

O'Sullivan RA, et al: Pulmonary actinomycosis complicated by effusive constrictive pericarditis, *Aust N Z J Med* 21:879, 1991.

Palmer DL, et al: Diagnostic and therapeutic considerations *in Nocardia asteroides* infection, *Medicine* 53:391, 1974.

Peabody JW, Seabury JH: Actinomycosis and nocardiosis, *J Chronic Dis* 5:374, 1957.

Persson E: Genital actinomycosis and *Actinomyces israelii* in the female genital tract, *Adv Contracept* 3:115, 1987.

Peterson PK, et al: Infectious diseases in hospitalized renal transplant recipients: a prospective study of a complex and evolving problem, *Medicine* 61:360, 1982.

Ponflick E: *Die Actinomykose des Menschen*, Berlin, 1882, Hirschwald.

Pritzker HG, MacKay JS: Pulmonary actinomycosis simulating bronchogenic carcinoma, *Can Med Assoc J* 88:785, 1963.

Rippon JW, Kathuria SK: *Actinomycoses meyeri* presenting as an asymptomatic lung mass, *Mycopathologia* 84:187, 1984.

Rippon JW: Introduction to the pathogenic actinomycetes. In *Medical mycology*, ed 3, Philadelphia, 1988, WB Saunders, p 15.

Rippon JW: Nocardiosis. In *Medical mycology*, ed 3, Philadelphia, 1988, WB Saunders.

Robby SJ, Vickery AL: Tinctorial and morphologic properties distinguishing actinomycosis and nocardiosis, *N Engl J Med* 282:593, 1970.

Sahathevan M, et al: Epidemiology, bacteriology and control of an outbreak of *Nocardia asteroides* infection on a liver unit, *J Hosp Infect* 18(Suppl A):473, 1991.

Simpson GL, et al: Nocardial infections in the immunocompromised host: a detailed study in a defined population, *Rev Infect Dis* 3:492, 1981.

Singh M, et al: Comparison of paraffin baiting and conventional culture techniques for isolation of Nocardia asteroides from sputum, *J Clin Microbiol* 25:176, 1987.

Smego RA Jr, et al: Trimethoprim-sulfamethoxazole therapy for Nocardia infections, *Arch Intern Med* 143:711, 1983.

Sorrell TC, et al: *Nocardia* Species. In Mandell GL, et al, editors: *Principles and practice of infectious diseases*, ed 5, New York, 2000, Churchill Livingstone.

Takeda H, et al: Cutaneous disseminated actinomycosis in a patient with acute lymphocytic leukemia, *J Dermatol* 25:37, 1998.

Waksman SA, Henrici AT: The nomenclature and classification of the actinomycetes, *J Bacteriol* 46:677, 1943.

Wallace RJ Jr, et al: Use of trimethoprim-sulfamethoxazole for treatment of infections due to Nocardia, *Rev Infect Dis* 4:315, 1982.

Wangensteen OH: The role of surgery in the treatment of actinomycosis, *Ann Surg* 104:752, 1936.

Warren NG: Actinomycosis, nocardiosis, and actinomycetoma, *Dermatol Clin* 14:1, 1996.

Weese WC, Smith IM: A study of 57 cases of actinomycosis over a 36-year period, *Arch Intern Med* 135:1562, 1975.

PULMONARY FUNGAL INFECTIONS

Edmund Kassis
Stephen C. Yang

Pulmonary fungal infections are an increasingly important problem facing the thoracic surgeon. The prevalence of human immunodeficiency virus/acquired immunodeficiency syndrome (HIV/AIDS) and the use of immunosuppressive agents have led to an increase in opportunistic fungal infections. Although most clinically significant infections are treated medically, the thoracic surgeon frequently is called on to aid in the diagnosis and definitive treatment of these infections.

Fungal organisms can be classified as either pathogenic or opportunistic (Table 1). Pathogenic fungi are usually endemic to a particular geographic area in the United States. They afflict immunocompetent and immunocompromised patients who inhale a sufficient number of organisms. In the immunocompetent host, pulmonary involvement may be subclinical and self-limited. Likewise, opportunistic organisms can infect immunocompetent and immunocompromised patients, with more pronounced clinical symptoms in the latter. Lung tissue damaged by previous disease can be affected. If a diagnosis cannot be made by less invasive means

(e.g., sputum, bronchoscopy), surgery usually is required to eliminate carcinoma when a pulmonary nodule appears. As the fungal disease progresses, surgical intervention may be required to treat complicated sequelae, such as cavitation, pneumothorax, bronchopulmonary fistula, hemoptysis, empyema, effusions, bronchiectasis, broncholithiasis, and fibrosing mediastinitis (usually due to histoplasmosis).

■ PATHOGENIC FUNGAL ORGANISMS

Histoplasmosis

Histoplasmosis is the most common cause of pulmonary fungal diseases. Most infections are self-limited in the immunocompetent host and when present usually affect the lungs, pericardium, or joint space. In the immunocompetent host, histoplasmosis is usually indolent and asymptomatic; conversely, histoplasmosis can progress to disseminated infection in immunocompromised patients and is a common sequela of AIDS. If symptoms do occur, they include fever, chills, sweats, anorexia, cough, chest pain, and dyspnea. Disease progression usually leads to respiratory failure and death. Typically the severity of symptoms depends on the

Table 1 Classification of Pulmonary Fungal Diseases

PATHOGENIC	OPPORTUNISTIC
Histoplasmosis	Aspergillosis
Coccidioidomycosis	Candidiasis
Blastomycosis	Mucormycosis
	Cryptococcosis

degree of exposure. In advanced disease, chest radiographs show hilar and mediastinal adenopathy with diffuse reticulonodular infiltrates. Patients with lesser degrees of exposure may be asymptomatic or present with a milder form of the aforementioned symptoms. Of patients, 20% develop a chronic form of pulmonary histoplasmosis. Characteristically, this is a solitary pulmonary nodule that grows slowly and calcifies. Other forms include chronic cavitary disease, mediastinal granuloma, and fibrosing mediastinitis. Patients with chronic manifestations are typically asymptomatic and come to the attention of the thoracic surgeon when these lesions are found incidentally during the workup of an unrelated issue.

Mediastinal Granuloma

Reactive mediastinal lymph nodes are common in patients with pulmonary histoplasmosis. These lymph nodes may impinge on adjacent pulmonary structures, leading to chest pain, cough, dysphagia, and dyspnea. These mediastinal lymph nodes may calcify and erode into adjacent mediastinal structures, leading to severe hemoptysis and obstructive pneumonia. When there is communication with the airway, broncholithiasis ("coughing up rocks") occurs.

Diagnosis

Histoplasma antigen is detected in most patients with diffuse pulmonary involvement. The antigen can be found in the blood, urine, or bronchoalveolar lavage fluid. Fungal cultures are useful in patients with diffuse pulmonary involvement or disseminated disease. Cultures are unreliable in patients with milder forms of the disease, however. Patients with acute histoplasmosis eventually develop antibodies 4 to 8 weeks after initial exposure, making antibody detection a less practical method in this situation.

Treatment

Patients who are mildly symptomatic and have localized disease do not require treatment because symptoms usually resolve in 4 to 6 weeks. If symptoms do not resolve after this time, itraconazole therapy should be started. Patients with diffuse pulmonary involvement and severe symptoms should receive amphotericin B and later be converted to itraconazole after an initial response. In this setting, corticosteroids may be beneficial in reducing the acute inflammatory process. Patients with milder symptoms and diffuse pulmonary involvement may be treated with itraconazole alone.

Treatment of mediastinal granuloma is controversial because many patients spontaneously improve. Patients usually are treated medically if the patient is experiencing mild symptoms of mediastinal impingement. If the symptoms are severe or progressive despite aggressive medical therapy, surgery is indicated. Common indications requiring surgical intervention include resection for middle lobe syndrome, esophagotracheal fistula, bronchostenosis, and hemoptysis.

There is no consensus about how best to treat cavitary histoplasmosis. If the diagnosis is made before resection, some advocate therapy with amphotericin B alone. The argument for this approach is that surgery in this setting has not been shown to improve survival or lessen the risk of recurrence. Some centers advocate resection of known cavitary histoplasmosis. Finally, in patients in whom the diagnosis of active histoplasmosis is made after resection of a cavitary lesion, it is recommended that they be treated with 1 month of amphotericin B. There are no prospective data, however, to support any of these recommendations.

Patients with undiagnosed pulmonary granuloma that presents as a solitary pulmonary nodule often require surgery for diagnostic reasons and to exclude neoplastic disease. Surgery also is indicated to address fibrosing mediastinitis. Options include (1) spiral vein graft interposition for superior vena cava syndrome; (2) pulmonary resection for pulmonary venous obstruction; and (3) dilation, stenting, or bronchoplastic procedures for bronchostenosis.

Coccidioidomycosis

The incidence of coccidioidomycotic infections has risen steadily since the 1970s. *Coccidioides immitis* has the potential to cause serious pulmonary infections, especially in the immunocompromised host. Although pulmonary illness is most common, immunosuppressed patients may develop disseminated disease, which is often progressive and fatal. In AIDS patients, the disease is quite fulminant, with a 6-month survival of only 40%. Although 60% of patients are asymptomatic, the rest with pulmonary involvement complain of fever, cough, and chest pain. If the pulmonary infection is diffuse, dyspnea and respiratory failure may result.

Coccidioidomycosis predominantly affects the upper lobes. Greater than 90% of symptomatic patients have some degree of parenchymal involvement manifested as patchy infiltrates on computed tomography scan. In other patients, imaging studies may show a solitary nodule without calcification, multiple nodules, or cavitary lesions. In areas such as the southwestern United States, where the fungus is endemic, 50% of pulmonary nodules are coccidioidomas. The cavitary lesions frequently enlarge and are at risk for rupture.

Diagnosis

The diagnosis of coccidioidomycosis can be made by isolation of the organism by fungal culture. Serologic tests are helpful in making the diagnosis of infection with *C. immitis*. Skin tests are frequently positive several weeks before the development of serum antibodies and are helpful in making the diagnosis of the acute infection.

Treatment

Surgery is indicated most often when patients present with a solitary pulmonary nodule, and resection is required to exclude a neoplastic process. Resection is required for cavitary disease, especially if it is enlarging or a secondary infection such as aspergillosis is identified. Ruptured cavities resulting in hemoptysis and pyopneumothorax also are indications for surgery.

Patients with identified pulmonary infections and patients with severe infection should be treated with amphotericin B. If initial therapy with amphotericin B is successful, patients may be converted to either fluconazole or itraconazole.

Blastomycosis

Blastomycosis is an uncommon fungal infection but one that can affect the immunocompromised host. Common forms of the illness include acute and chronic pulmonary infections, cutaneous involvement, and disseminated disease.

Patients with pulmonary infections present with fever, cough, dyspnea, chest pain, or weight loss. The course is variable; immunocompetent patients experience a self-limiting course, whereas others have a progressive, chronic form of the disease. The fungus may affect the tracheobronchial tree, lung parenchyma, or the pleural space. Similar to coccidioidomycosis, radiographic findings show upper lobe predominance. Asymptomatic patients present with single or multiple nodules that require resection to exclude bronchogenic carcinoma. Patients with symptoms may have focal or diffuse infiltrates. If fulminant pneumonitis occurs, mortality is 50%.

Diagnosis

There are no reliable serologic tests to make the diagnosis of blastomycosis. The diagnosis usually is made by culture or fungal stain of samples obtained by bronchoalveolar lavage, biopsy, or surgical resection.

Treatment

Therapy is indicated in immunosuppressed patients with blastomycosis to prevent overwhelming pneumonia. Mild to moderate cases can be treated with oral itraconazole. Patients with life-threatening illness require treatment with amphotericin B and have a 97% cure rate. Surgical management is not indicated in the routine treatment of pulmonary blastomycosis but as with solitary nodules may be required to exclude a neoplastic process.

■ OPPORTUNISTIC FUNGAL ORGANISMS

Aspergillosis

Aspergillosis is the third most common fungal infection requiring medical attention. There are three classifications for the disease: aspergilloma, invasive infection, and noninvasive bronchial allergic. Immunosuppressed patients are at highest risk for invasive and pulmonary infections. The prognosis of patients with invasive aspergillosis is poor.

Aspergilloma

An aspergilloma represents colonization of the lung with *Aspergillus*. This is the most common form of aspergillus infections, accounting for 70% of all cases. There are two types of aspergillomas. The simple form has normal-appearing lung parenchyma surrounding it. The complex type has associated chronic lung disease around it, such as tuberculosis, sarcoidosis, lung abscess, or bronchiectasis. Most of these are found in the upper lobes or superior segments and can be multiple 20% of the time.

Patients may be asymptomatic or may develop hemoptysis, which is the presenting symptom in approximately 70% of cases. Other symptoms include cough, wheezing, and shortness of breath. Patients at highest risk for developing the disease are those with prior lung injury. Imaging studies show a central mass located within a pulmonary cavity. This represents the classic "fungus ball" associated with pulmonary aspergilloma.

If a pulmonary aspergillosis is suspected, early diagnosis and treatment are essential. There are currently no validated or reliable serologic tests to diagnose pulmonary aspergillosis.

The diagnosis of either aspergilloma or invasive aspergillosis relies primarily on patient presentation and proper imaging studies. Occasionally, bronchoalveolar lavage may aid in isolation of *Aspergillus*.

Although there are no controlled studies comparing medical versus surgical management of aspergilloma, it generally is believed that medical treatment is ineffective. Although surgery is the treatment of choice, most centers do not advocate routine resection of these lesions. The major indication for surgical resection is severe or recurring hemoptysis. Patients with even minor recurring hemoptysis should undergo surgical resection because 30% progress to massive life-threatening hemoptysis, with an associated mortality rate of 25%. In addition, surgery is recommended when there is chronic symptomatic disease, progressive infiltrate around a mycetoma, or a solitary pulmonary nodule when a neoplasm cannot be excluded. Because patients at highest risk for aspergilloma are those with prior lung injury, the underlying pulmonary function is crucial in deciding if surgical management can be performed safely. Lobectomy is performed most commonly. As with other pulmonary resection procedures, all disease must be removed sparing as much normal lung tissue as possible, there should be no residual space, and the bronchial stump should be covered with a vascularized pedicle of tissue.

Invasive Pulmonary Aspergillosis

Patients with the invasive form of disease in the lungs typically present with chest pain, cough, and hemoptysis. These symptoms in an immunocompromised patient with cultures positive for aspergillosis are almost pathognomonic of invasive disease. Chest radiographs classically show either focal or diffuse infiltrates, nodular lesions, or wedge-shaped infarcts. Computed tomography scan of the chest is more sensitive than chest radiographs in identifying these lesions.

Amphotericin B is the treatment of choice for invasive pulmonary aspergillosis. Studies have shown that the addition of 5-fluorocytosine provides no additional benefit. Surgery usually is not indicated in patients with invasive aspergillosis, unless tissue diagnosis is required.

Noninvasive Bronchial Allergic Disease

Noninvasive bronchial allergic disease is the least common form and usually is diagnosed by bronchoscopy. Patients require surgery only if they develop clinically significant bronchiectasis, which occurs rarely in this form.

Candidiasis

Candida is the second most common opportunistic fungus affecting the lungs. These infections usually affect immunosuppressed patients, patients who have long-term indwelling catheters (Foley, central lines, drains), and patients on long-term antibiotics. *Candida* is obtained in 50% of bronchial aspirates of uninfected patients. It is also difficult to differentiate between colonization and tissue invasion. *Candida* sepsis therapy is aimed at removal of any potential catheter source and is with amphotericin B. Pulmonary involvement by *Candida* requires surgery only when tissue diagnosis is needed before amphotericin B therapy. Patients with mild forms of *Candida* esophagitis are treated initially with oral nystatin, ketoconazole, or itraconazole. Fluconazole should be used for more advanced disease; if there is a response failure, amphotericin B is used in synergy with 5-fluorocytosine.

Mucormycosis

Mucormycosis is an uncommon fungus, causing pulmonary problems particularly in immunosuppressed patients with hematologic malignancies, organ transplantation, and HIV/AIDS. It is of the fungal class Zygomycetes and is associated with *Rhizopus*. This inhaled spore penetrates the bronchial walls and invades the pulmonary vessels. As thrombosis occurs, the most significant sequela is hemoptysis, which is fatal in one third of all patients. Other symptoms include fever, chills, cough, and dyspnea. Neutropenic patients are most susceptible to pulmonary involvement, which manifests as diffuse, alveolar infiltrates limited to one lobe or affecting the airway and causing endobronchial obstruction. It can act as a secondary infection of a preexisting cavity or pneumonic process.

Diagnosis is based primarily on identification of the organism during pathologic evaluation of biopsy specimens. The fungus is isolated only 40% of the time antemortem. There are no available serologic tests for diagnosis. All patients are started on amphotericin B. Surgical resection is indicated when there is no response after 72 hours of therapy because of its aggressive behavior. With limited involvement, lobectomy is recommended. In the rare instance when there is endobronchial involvement, yttrium aluminum garnet (YAG) laser débridement is performed. With aggressive management of antimicrobial therapy and surgery, survival is only 50% and drops to 10% when inoperable.

Cryptococcosis

Infection with *Cryptococcus neoformans* in the immunocompetent host is uncommon and usually a self-limiting process when it occurs. Pulmonary involvement is less frequent and asymptomatic and usually the only site of infection in the normal host. The lower lobe is affected most often; characteristically, chronic granuloma presents as a peripheral nodule, but it also may present as a well-defined infiltrate.

In contrast, cryptococcosis occurs predominantly in immunosuppressed patients, manifesting most commonly as meningitis. Cryptococcal infection occurs in approximately 10% of AIDS patients and is the presenting problem in 40%. Symptoms are usually present, consisting of cough, dyspnea, and fever; this may progress to hypoxia and respiratory failure. Also in contrast to the normal host, these patients develop more diffuse interstitial or alveolar disease in the lower lobes. Cavitation is rare.

Diagnosis

Cryptococcal pneumonia is diagnosed by culturing the organism from sputum or biopsy specimens or by special staining on histopathology. Diagnosis of cryptococcal granuloma typically is made histologically after bronchoscopic or surgical lung biopsy.

Treatment

Asymptomatic, immunocompetent patients with isolated pulmonary disease may be observed without therapy. If the patient becomes symptomatic, amphotericin B is begun. Immunosuppressed patients, regardless of symptoms, also should be treated aggressively. After initial therapy, patients may be converted to fluconazole. Patients with lesser degrees of immunosuppression and mild infections (without central nervous system involvement) may be treated initially with fluconazole and close follow-up. Surgery often is required to diagnose the solitary pulmonary nodule (e.g., chronic granuloma), or lung biopsy is required to help guide therapy for pulmonary infiltrates unresponsive to therapy.

SUGGESTED READING

American Thoracic Society statement: chemotherapy of the pulmonary mycoses, *Am Rev Respir Dis* 138:1078, 1988.

Ampel NM, et al: Coccidioidomycosis: clinical update, *Rev Infect Dis* 11:897, 1989.

Daly RC, et al: Pulmonary aspergilloma: results of surgical treatment, *J Thorac Cardiovasc Surg* 92:981, 1986.

Reed CE, et al: Surgical resection for complication of pulmonary tuberculosis, *Ann Thorac Surg* 48:165, 1989.

Tedder M, et al: Pulmonary mucormycosis: results of medical and surgical therapy, *Ann Thorac Surg* 57:1044, 1994.

LUNG ABSCESS

Wickii T. Vigneswaran

The incidence and need for surgical intervention for abscess cavities of the lung parenchyma have decreased dramatically with the use of antibiotics. However, these problems are still quite prevalent, particularly with the overuse of antibiotics, immunosuppressive states, changing technologies, and persistent public health issues.

A lung abscess can be defined as subacute focal pneumonia with some degree of tissue necrosis and destruction. There may be continuity with the airway, leading to partial drainage and an air-fluid level on plain radiographs. If erosion into the pleural cavity occurs, an empyema results with an associated bronchopleural fistula. There are many potential infections that cause lung abscesses, but anaerobic infections remain the most frequent and account for approximately 5 patients per 10,000 hospital admissions.

Lung abscesses are generally classified as primary or secondary. A primary lung abscess is defined as one in a previously healthy individual with no underlying lung pathology, whereas a secondary abscess occurs in an individual with an underlying disease, a predisposing condition, or immunocompromised state. Parenchymal involvement typically occurs in a segmental distribution—usually those portions that are dependent when the patient is in a recumbent position. These include the posterior segments of the upper lobes and superior segments of the lower lobes and, most frequently, right-sided segments due to the bronchial anatomy. In the prone position, the lingula and right middle lobe are at risk.

The clinical presentation typically includes intermittent fevers, hemoptysis, cough, weight loss, malaise, and night sweats. When cavitation of the abscess occurs and there is communication with the bronchus, putrid expectoration (vomica) is not uncommon and is especially pronounced in patients with anaerobic infections. Hemoptysis may be brisk. On physical examination, signs of advanced disease or toxemia might be present, including tachypnea, tachycardia, and cyanosis. Consolidation of the lung yields decreased or cavernous breath sounds, dullness to percussion, and localized chest wall tenderness, an ominous sign of pleural involvement.

Sputum cultures should be obtained; they are often helpful in identifying the causative organism. Anaerobic organisms tend to be the most frequent isolates in immunocompetent patients, whereas aerobic organisms are found more in the immunocompromised. Postpneumonic lung abscesses are usually associated with the debilitated elderly patient, children, and immunosuppressed host. They can occur anywhere in the bronchial tree, and are often multiple. The dominant organisms include *Staphylococcus aureus,* β-hemolytic streptococci, *Pseudomonas,* and *Klebsiella pneumoniae*. Obstructing lesions such as neoplasms, foreign bodies, or broncholiths may be the cause of distal suppuration. Other less common causes include posttraumatic pulmonary contusions, hematomas, and infected bullae and cysts. If multiple lesions occur, septic pulmonary emboli should be considered from multiple causes, such as right-sided endocarditis, infected venous thrombosis, and embolic debris from drug abuse.

Early in its course, lung abscesses are difficult to distinguish radiographically from pneumonitis on plain chest radiographs. However, when communication with the bronchus occurs, it assumes the characteristic cavitary lesion within the lung parenchyma and an air-fluid level. Loculated empyemas with airway fistulization may be mistaken for lung abscesses. Computed tomography is always performed and may help distinguish between the two. It is necessary to consider other potential causes of cavitary lesions in the lung in the differential diagnosis, including other infectious processes such as fungus or tuberculosis, and especially neoplastic processes (particularly if the cavity is thick walled and eccentric).

In most cases, fiberoptic bronchoscopy is useful in the diagnostic evaluation and should be performed early if considered. Protected specimen collection during bronchoscopy for culture has a better yield in identifying the causative organism than sputum culture and helps to direct the antimicrobial treatment. Although therapeutic bronchoscopy for drainage of the abscess is controversial and perhaps harmful by contaminating the remaining lung, it becomes crucial in cases when the presentation is atypical, to exclude endobronchial obstruction by foreign bodies or benign or malignant lesions.

■ MEDICAL MANAGEMENT

The initial management of a lung abscess is antibiotic therapy. With the discovery of previously unknown organisms and the introduction of newer antibiotics, the choice of therapy will evolve and change over time. Antibiotic therapy should be directed by the culture and sensitivity of the causative organism. When empirical therapy is required, the historical data suggest high-dose penicillin and clindamycin to be the superior agents. The initial therapy should be intravenous, unless the patient is minimally symptomatic, when oral antibiotics with equally high absorption could be used. After the initiation of therapy, the clinical, radiologic, and laboratory response, including the white blood cell count and sedimentation rate, should be monitored. Although improvement may be gradual, the trend in response is more important. If there is no response after a week of therapy, more aggressive therapy is warranted. If, however, the patient continues to improve, antibiotic therapy is continued for 6 to 8 weeks. More than 90% of primary lung abscesses will respond to antibiotic therapy alone. Because most abscesses communicate with the tracheobronchial tree and drain spontaneously, pulmonary clearance techniques, including humidification, expectorants, chest physiotherapy, and postural drainage, are useful adjuncts. However, bronchoscopy may be needed to exclude an airway obstruction from tumor or foreign body or be used therapeutically (even repetitively) to help clear the infectious process.

■ SURGICAL MANAGEMENT

Surgical intervention including external drainage or abscess/lung resection is indicated if symptoms persist despite aggressive antibiotic therapy, the cavity fails to collapse, or if obstructing endobronchial lesions exist. External drainage is usually required in an immunocompromised host, in an abscess cavity greater than 6 cm, or in the presence of necrotizing pneumonia. Chest tube thoracostomy should be avoided to prevent pleural contamination, especially if pleural symphysis has not occurred. Percutaneous external drainage with radiographically guided catheters is safe and effective. This is used as an alternative for resection or to stabilize a critically ill patient before thoracotomy. It is seldom complicated by empyema, pneumothorax, or hemorrhage. However, the most common complication is bronchopleural fistula. Fortunately, this is an infrequent complication, although it occurs more often in ventilated patients and usually is self-limiting, rarely requiring surgical repair.

An intermediate alternative to major thoracotomy is the pneumonotomy or cavernostomy. This was once the mainstay of surgical therapy before percutaneous drainage catheters and now is rarely used. It should be considered for those patients for whom radiologically placed drains fail or for an elderly or a debilitated patient who is too sick for thoracotomy and pulmonary resection. This approach requires precise localization of the abscess on the chest wall. A limited thoracotomy incision is made, a subperiosteal rib resection done, and pleural symphysis confirmed. Needle aspiration is performed to enter the abscess cavity, the overlying pleura and compressed lung are excised, and a large-bore chest tube is placed and connected to the water seal chamber. The wound is then closed loosely around the tube. If pleural symphysis is not present, the wound is packed and changed with iodoform gauze or iodine-impregnated gauze for 7 to 10 days before cavernostomy is attempted.

Definitive indications for thoracotomy and resection of the abscess are failure to respond to 6 to 10 weeks of medical therapy, inadequate external drainage, massive hemoptysis, rupture into the pleural space causing pyopneumothorax, the inability to exclude bronchogenic carcinoma, or the presence of an obstructing endobronchial lesion. Roughly one third of patients undergoing percutaneous drainage will require thoracotomy. All patients should undergo flexible bronchoscopy at the time of surgery. During surgery, it is important to isolate the lung early with a double-lumen endotracheal tube or bronchial blocker to avoid contaminating the contralateral lung with purulent material. Steps should be taken to avoid gross contamination of the pleural cavity, and the pleural space should be irrigated at the end of the procedure to reduce contamination.

Usually the inflammatory process is so extensive that it precludes a lesser resection such as wedge or segmentectomy. Lobectomy is typically required because of the size and location of the abscess. Extensive pleural adhesions may be present, and in light of minimizing bronchopleural fistula formation and to circumvent all the disease, an extrapleural pneumonectomy may be required in rare cases. If an anatomic lung resection is required, the bronchial stump should be covered with vascularized tissue (pleural flap, pericardial fat, thymic tissue, intercostals, or chest wall muscle) to prevent the development of a bronchopleural fistula. If a previous drainage or cavernostomy procedure was performed, an extensive resection as described earlier is required with revision of the chest wall sinus. Failure rate and complications are much higher in this group of patients, including empyema and bronchopleural fistula. If these occur, other adjunct procedures may be required, including redo drainage, thoracoplasty, or muscle flap coverage.

■ RESULTS

Although the majority of patients with lung abscesses respond to medical therapy alone, approximately 10% require external drainage, and a smaller percentage (1%) undergo a major pulmonary resection. With better antibiotics and interventional methods, morbidity and mortality rates in the limited literature are less than 15% and 5%, respectively. Factors that are associated with a higher mortality rate include abscess size, location (right lower lobe), immune deficiency, and organism type (*Pseudomonas aeruginosa, Staphylococcus aureus,* and *Klebsiella pneumoniae*—in decreasing order of mortality). Operative complications such as bronchopleural fistulas are not significantly increased.

■ SUMMARY

The treatment of abscess cavities involving the lung parenchyma is primarily medical. Surgical resection is indicated when medical therapy fails, in the presence of a large abscess, and with complications such as massive hemoptysis or empyema, the need to exclude malignancy, or a residual cavity. The prognosis for primary lung abscess is excellent with medical or surgical therapy.

SUGGESTED READING

Davis B, Systrom DM: Lung abscess: pathogenesis, diagnosis and treatment, *Curr Clin Top Infect Dis* 1998;18:252-73.

Hirshberg B, et al: Factors predicting mortality of patients with lung abscess, *Chest* 1999;115:746-50.

Le Roux BT, et al: Suppurative diseases of the lung and pleural space, Part 1: empyema thoracis and lung abscess, *Curr Probl Surg* 1986; 23:1-89.

Tan TQ, et al: Pediatric lung abscess: clinical management and outcome, *Pediatr Infect Dis J* 1995;14:51-5.

Wiedemann HP, Rice TW: Lung abscess and empyema, *Semin Thorac Cardiovasc Surg* 1995;7:119-28.

BRONCHIECTASIS

Daniel L. Miller

Bronchiectasis is defined as abnormal, irreversible dilation of the bronchi. It is not a disease per se, but it represents the end stage of a variety of pathologic processes. Laennec first described the clinical entity of bronchiectasis in 1819. Bronchiectasis develops as a result of an inflammatory response of the bronchi to an infectious insult; this inflammatory reaction damages the bronchial wall permanently. The injured bronchial wall experiences abnormal traction secondary to surrounding atelectatic lung, augmented by trapped secretions, which leads to persistent dilation and chronic relapsing infection.

The clinical pattern of bronchiectasis changed in the last half of the 20th century due to earlier treatment of necrotizing pneumonia; better control of tuberculosis; and prevention of predisposing pulmonary infections by routine immunization against measles, pertussis, and diphtheria. Advances in medical treatment also have led to an increased survival to adulthood of patients with cystic fibrosis, hypogammaglobulinemia, and immotile cilia syndrome, all of which predispose to bronchiectasis. An underlying cause of bronchiectasis is not found, however, in one third of patients.

Bronchiectasis has been described as an orphan disease, with a low prevalence that is estimated to be decreasing. The true prevalence of bronchiectasis likely is underestimated, however, because less severe asymptomatic forms of bronchiectasis are found incidentally with the increased use of high-resolution computed tomography (CT). High-resolution CT features alone do not allow a confident distinction between idiopathic bronchiectasis and known causes of bronchiectasis.

Clinical findings in patients with bronchiectasis are not specific but may be characteristic. Most patients experience chronic cough with daily mucopurulent sputum production and recurrent infectious exacerbations. Dyspnea, wheezing, and pleuritic chest pain may be present but usually late in the disease process. Hemoptysis is the most common characteristic feature for which patients seek medical care.

Complications of bronchiectasis changed with the introduction of antibiotic therapy. Before antibiotics, most patients died as a direct result of the pulmonary disease. The complications experienced by these patients included brain abscess and amyloidosis. After the introduction of antibiotics, these complications disappeared; most patients with bronchiectasis do not die of pulmonary disease except for patients with cystic fibrosis. Complications now include recurrent pulmonary infections, hemoptysis, lung abscess, empyema, respiratory failure, and cor pulmonale.

The most commonly cited classification of bronchiectasis was based on bronchographic and autopsy findings and included three patterns: cylindrical, varicose, and saccular or cystic. The clinical usefulness of designating bronchiectasis into one of these patterns is questionable, and no study to date has shown a clinical, epidemiologic, or pathophysiologic difference between these patterns. Associated with these bronchial changes are varying degrees of scarring and fibrosis of the lung parenchyma.

Chest radiographic findings that are suggestive but nondiagnostic of bronchiectasis include stranding, cystic lesions, volume loss with crowding of pulmonary vasculature, and areas of infiltrates and atelectasis. Bronchography, for many years the imaging method of choice for bronchiectasis, is now obsolete in part because of lack of suitable contrast medium and associated complications, such as allergic reaction and temporary ventilation impairment. High-resolution CT (Figure 1) largely has replaced bronchography as the diagnostic tool of choice. Bilateral lung involvement is found in 10% to 20% of patients.

The treatment of bronchiectasis is centered on airway management (secretions) and control of recurrent infection (bacterial). The initial treatment of patients with symptomatic bronchiectasis is primarily medical, with the goal being to reduce airway obstruction and to eliminate bacteria from the lower respiratory tract. Postural drainage, chest percussion, and assisted cough techniques facilitate clearance of secretions. Bronchodilators are used for associated obstructive airway symptoms. Corticosteroids are reserved for acute exacerbations only when worsening obstructive symptoms are present; long-term corticosteroid therapy is usually not warranted. Antibiotic therapy should consist of rotating antimicrobial agents. Broad-spectrum antibiotics should be instituted for acute respiratory infection and exacerbations of chronic infection.

■ SURGICAL THERAPY

The role of pulmonary resection has evolved from early curative resection for all patients to a more palliative approach

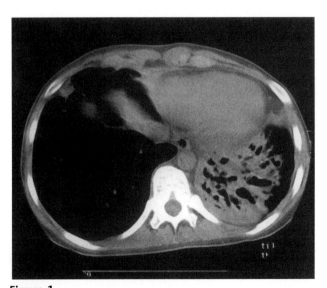

Figure 1
High-resolution computed tomography scan shows saccular bronchiectasis of the left lower lobe.

limited to either patients who have medically resistant disease or patients who develop complications. In a series from our institution, only 3.4% of patients with bronchiectasis underwent surgical intervention over a 17-year period.

The goal of surgical therapy for bronchiectasis is to improve the quality of life for patients who have failed medical treatment; resolve complications, such as severe or recurrent hemoptysis, lung abscess, and empyema; or remove a potential malignancy. The indications for pulmonary resection in our series were failure of medical therapy in 63.4%, recurrent or massive hemoptysis in 19.4%, lung abscess in 9.0%, and indeterminate mass in 8.2%.

Appropriate selection of patients is crucial for optimal results. Acute suppurative bronchitis should be treated aggressively preoperatively. Preoperative bronchoscopy should be performed to rule out an endobronchial lesion, foreign body, or stricture. Early pulmonary resection while the disease is localized is preferred. Complete and anatomic resection should be done with preservation of as much lung function as possible to avoid cardiopulmonary limitations. Pulmonary function studies rarely are indicated in patients with localized disease, but they should be obtained when more extensive or repeat resection is considered. Complete resection of all bronchiectasis was performed in 81.0% of our patients; 99.1% of these patients had complete resection for unilateral disease, whereas only 3.8% had complete resection of all bronchiectasis with bilateral involvement.

The operation should be performed with a double-lumen endotracheal tube in place to decrease the risk of contaminating the contralateral lung. When indicated, intrapericardial isolation of the pulmonary hilum should be performed, and bronchial reinforcement is recommended. A completion pneumonectomy may have an associated higher mortality compared with the same procedure for primary lung cancer or metastatic disease. Operative mortality should be low (2.2% in our series), but morbidity may be significantly increased because of the chronic debilitating condition of the patient and urgency of the surgical procedure. In our series, more than 80% of patients had total relief or substantial improvement of preoperative symptoms.

■ CONCLUSION

Surgical resection for bronchiectasis should be limited to patients with localized disease, unless life-threatening complications or medically refractory disease is present. Complete resection should be performed whenever possible to achieve maximum benefit. In properly selected patients, pulmonary resection can be performed with acceptable morbidity and low mortality.

SUGGESTED READING

Agasthian T, et al: Surgical management of bronchiectasis, *Ann Thorac Surg* 62:976, 1996.

Miller DL, et al: Completion pneumonectomy: factors affecting mortality and cardiopulmonary morbidity, *Ann Thorac Surg* 74:876, 2002.

Nicotra MB: Bronchiectasis, *Semin Respir Infect* 9:31, 1995.

Tasker AD, Flower CDR: Imaging the airways: hemoptysis, bronchiectasis, and small airway disease, *Clin Chest Med* 20:761, 1999.

TUBERCULOUS DISEASES OF THE CHEST

Marvin Pomerantz

When discussing tuberculous diseases, one has to include tuberculosis as well as other mycobacterial diseases that affect the lung. These other mycobacterial diseases have been called *atypical tuberculosis, nontuberculosis mycobacterial disease, mycobacterium other than tuberculosis (MOTT)*, and, more recently, *environmental mycobacterial infections*.

Tuberculosis primarily attacks the lung; however, it can invade every organ system in the body. Tuberculosis can be transmitted from human to human by airborne droplets without any intermediate vector. The *Mycobacterium tuberculosis* organism is virile and can invade and destroy normal lung tissue. The other mycobacterial infections, which for the remainder of this chapter are called *MOTT*, are not transmitted from human to human and most often colonize previously damaged lung. Although not as virulent as *M. tuberculosis*, infections with MOTT are usually indolent and often difficult to eradicate.

It has been estimated that the tuberculosis organism is about 15,000 years old and probably mutated from *Mycobacterium bovis*. It was not until the late 19th century, however, that Koch isolated the tuberculosis bacillus.

Typically, tuberculosis is a disease of poverty, overcrowding, and malnutrition. Approximately 10% of patients infected with *M. tuberculosis* develop the overt disease. Between one third and two fifths of the world's population have been infected with tuberculosis and remain a latent source for later disease. Currently, 3 million people in the world die yearly of tuberculosis. It is estimated that in India 1000 people die of tuberculosis daily. Most of these deaths are from drug-sensitive tuberculosis and could be treated if adequate antibiotic therapy became available.

The primary treatment of tuberculosis is medical. There are five primary drugs: isoniazid, rifampin, streptomycin, ethambutol, and pyrazinamide. A 4- to 6-month course with rifampin and isoniazid with 2 months of pyrazinamide is a standard treatment regimen. The use of directly observed therapy for compliance is important because side effects to these drugs are common, and left on their own patients often do not take a drug that has serious side effects. The end result of this is the development of resistant strains. Strains that become resistant to isoniazid and rifampin are classified as multidrug-resistant tuberculosis. The treatment of tuberculosis before the antibiotic era was rest and fresh air. To achieve this, sanatoria systems were built throughout the United States and elsewhere.

Before the introduction of chemotherapy, the surgical treatment of tuberculosis was that of collapse therapy. This therapy was effective because *M. tuberculosis* is an obligate aerobe. With cavitary disease, billions of organisms reside within the cavities, and by collapsing the cavity and depriving the mycobacteria of oxygen, the organisms die, in effect controlling the tuberculosis infection. There were various forms of collapse therapy. Thoracoplasty was used most commonly; however, plombage with Lucite balls, wax plombage, induced pneumothorax, or pneumoperitoneum also was employed.

Rifampin was introduced into clinical use in 1966. This drug markedly improved the treatment of tuberculosis and eliminated the need for surgical intervention in most cases. Around the same time, resection replaced collapse therapy as the treatment for patients with tuberculosis requiring surgery.

Surgical indications for drug-sensitive tuberculosis in the post-rifampin era included massive hemoptysis, bronchopleural fistula, bronchostenosis to rule out cancer, and in some cases to decorticate a trapped lung. The last-mentioned indication usually results when there is a tuberculous effusion that gets contaminated by frequent taps or by tube placement.

There are an increasing number of patients with multidrug-resistant tuberculosis. These infections are difficult to treat, and if there is cavitary disease, if there is destroyed lung, or if the sputum remains positive after chemotherapy, resection of localized disease is advocated. In these cases, chemotherapy after surgery should be continued for 12 to 24 months.

The epidemiology of MOTT infections is more complex than that of tuberculosis. As mentioned earlier, previously damaged lungs are predisposed to infections with MOTT organisms.

Surgical indications for patients with MOTT are similar to those for patients with tuberculosis. The most common MOTT organism belongs to the *Mycobacterium avium* complex. There appears to be an increasing number of patients infected with "rapid growers," however, such as *Mycobacterium chelonae* and *Mycobacterium abscessus*. There are many other MOTT organisms, but their clinical implications are less. With *M. avium* complex and other MOTT infections, careful culture and sensitivity data are important because these organisms, similar to multidrug-resistant tuberculosis, can develop resistance and are difficult to treat.

Infections with *M. chelonae* and *M. abscessus* are less likely to respond to antibiotic therapy due to the fact that there are few good antibiotics to treat these infections. Surgery for localized disease can be helpful in the treatment of these infections. These rapid growers have a tendency to infect soft tissues, and wound infections are common.

MOTT infections of the middle lobe or lingula occur primarily in women. Although it is possible to have these infections in men, in our series of about 40 patients, this has not been found. These women often have skeletal abnormalities, such as pectus excavatum or scoliosis, and have signs of mitral prolapse. These infections are difficult to treat by antibiotic therapy alone, and when the antibiotics are stopped, clinical infection recurs. When these areas are resected, they invariably are nonaerated and act as a culture medium for continued infection.

The surgical principles include treatment with the best available antibiotics for 2 to 3 months before surgery. All gross disease should be removed; this includes cavitary disease and destroyed lung. The surgery is difficult, often due to dense scarring and absence of good tissue planes. Adequate pulmonary function should remain after a resection, and antibiotic therapy should be continued postoperatively for 18 to 24 months.

Surgery for mycobacterial infections can be performed with a mortality rate of less than 5%. Complications are high, however. Bronchopleural fistula after right pneumonectomy is the most dreaded complication. Although decreased by stump coverage with muscle, it still occurs in many patients. Poor nutrition is a major cause of surgical complications. Massive pleural contamination, previous radiation therapy, diabetes, and prior surgery also add to morbidity. Other complications are wound infections with rapid growers, damage to the recurrent laryngeal nerve with extrapleural resections, and respiratory failure. To prevent some of these complications, Eloesser flaps are used when there is massive contamination, and half-strength Dakin's solution is used in the packing, which is changed daily over a 4- to 6-week period. The Eloesser flap is closed, and Claggett's solution instilled into the pleural space. Omental flaps also can be used to cover the bronchus when there is massive contamination.

Postoperatively, nutrition is the most important intervention. If patients are not eating well, enteral feeding should supplement oral intake. Invariably, these patients are below ideal body weight and do not do well if catabolic postoperatively.

■ SUMMARY

Mycobacterial infections still are a significant health hazard in the United States and worldwide. Surgical intervention is appropriate in many cases. Careful preoperative preparation and postoperative care are required.

SUGGESTED READING

Bradham RR, et al: Chronic middle lobe infection: factors responsible for its development, *Ann Thorac Surg* 2:612, 1966.

Crofton J, et al: *Guidelines for the management of drug-resistant tuberculosis,* Geneva, 1997, World Health Organization.

Iseman MD: *A clinician's guide to tuberculosis,* Baltimore, 2000, Lippincott Williams & Wilkins.

Iseman MD, DeGroote M: Environmental mycobacterial (EM) infections. In Gorbach SL, et al, editors: *Infectious diseases,* ed 3. Baltimore, Lippincott Williams & Wilkins (in press).

Pomerantz BJ, et al: Pulmonary resection for multi-drug resistant tuberculosis, *J Thorac Cardiovasc Surg* 121:448, 2001.

Pomerantz M, et al: Resection of the right middle lobe and lingula for mycobacterial infection, *Ann Thorac Surg* 62:990, 1996.

LUNG AMEBIASIS

Hasan F. Batirel
Scott J. Swanson

Amebiasis, the parasitic disease caused by the protozoan, *Entamoeba histolytica,* is endemic in tropical countries such as Vietnam, Mexico, and India. Approximately 500 million people are infected worldwide with *E. histolytica.* The trophozoites form colonies in the human large bowel and cause the infection. Sporadic cases have been reported in the United States. Ten percent of patients develop amebic colitis and are at risk of developing amebic hepatic abscess. In 20% to 35% of patients with amebic hepatic abscess, pleuropulmonary complications occur. Solitary lung involvement is rare.

Four theoretical mechanisms have been suggested for intrathoracic spread of amebiasis: (1) rupture of an amebic hepatic abscess directly through the diaphragm, (2) transdiaphragmatic spread of amebic abscess or hepatitis through lymphatic channels, (3) hematogenous embolic dissemination of *E. histolytica* to lung and/or pleura from liver or colon, and (4) inhalation of cysts of *E. histolytica.*

Symptoms are cough and pleuritic pain on the affected side. Associated symptoms include high fever and diarrhea.

Amebic colonization can be confirmed by direct visualization of trophozoites in a fresh stool sample or pleural fluid. In geographic areas where the disease is endemic, the sensitivity of direct examination in experienced laboratories is as high as 85%. Measurement of serum indirect hemagglutination antibody is the gold standard and leads to diagnosis in almost all cases.

■ CURRENT MANAGEMENT

Management of hepatic and pleuropulmonary amebiasis is mainly medical. Surgical interventions are reserved for the advanced stage of the disease such as in the case of superinfection or an uncontrolled course resulting from a delay in diagnosis. In a series of 140 patients with pleuropulmonary amebiasis by Cameron in 1978, only 50 (36%) patients needed surgical intervention. Thirty-one of these interventions were simple chest tube drainage, four open drainage, eight decortications, and seven lung resections. Ninety (64%) patients healed without any surgical intervention from pleural effusion (n = 12), amebic empyema (n = 4), superinfected amebic empyema (n = 8), and pulmonary lesions (n = 66).

Metronidazole is the standard medical treatment (750 mg intravenously three times a day for 5 to 10 days). It is effective in 90% of patients, with pain and fever alleviated within 3 days. It has good penetration into the liver and pleural space and can be used safely in pregnant women. Chloroquine and dehydroemetine were used in the past. Chloroquine (300 to 600 mg once a day) can only be administered orally and sometimes retinopathy occurs with higher doses. Dehydroemetine (1 to 1.5 mg/kg, maximum 90 mg/day) can be given intramuscularly or intravenously. It is cardiotoxic above 90 mg, with prolongation of QT intervals and inversion of T waves seen on electrocardiogram. It also causes hypotension and tachycardia.

Surgical treatment is indicated in the following cases: (1) the lung cannot be reexpanded, (2) the presence of a persistent bronchobiliary fistula, (3) uncontrollable superinfection, and (4) damaged pulmonary tissue (persistent lung abscess, bronchiectasis, or fistula) that produces a continuous morbid state.

■ PLEURAL EFFUSION

Pleural effusion due to amebiasis is typically right sided and serous in character. It results from the inflammatory process in the liver. Patients respond to antiamebic treatment with metronidazole, and the fluid regresses within a few days. If the fluid is massive, thoracentesis can relieve the symptoms. However, a treatment strategy should also be planned for the amebic abscess in the liver. It may need percutaneous drainage if the medical treatment is not effective.

■ AMEBIC EMPYEMA

Amebic empyema results from the rupture of an amebic abscess in the liver into the pleural space. This is an acute

Table 1 Published Major Series of Thoracic Amebiasis

AUTHORS	YEAR	NO.	AMEBIC EMPYEMA (n)	BRONCHOHEPATIC FISTULA (n)	LUNG ABSCESS (n)	MORTALITY (n)
Stephen and Uragoda	1970	40	22	7	10	NS
Cameron	1978	140	35	NS	7	5 (4%)
Verghese et al	1979	34	19	1	5	10 (36%)
Ibarra-Perez	1981	501	106	175	NS	41 (8.3%)
Vickers et al	1982	40	24	3	6	4 (10%)

NS, not stated.

event with the sudden onset of sharp pain in the right upper quadrant. Thoracentesis typically shows a maroon-colored pleural fluid. Medical treatment with metronidazole should begin immediately. The course of the amebic empyema can be unpredictable. Because impending superinfection complicates the treatment, early drainage and medical treatment are important. Delay in diagnosis leads to advanced disease and major surgical interventions such as decortication, which carries significant mortality.

Ibarra-Perez published a series of 85 patients with amebic empyema . Thirty-eight (45%) were definitively treated with chest tube drainage (n = 36) or thoracentesis (n = 2). Simple thoracentesis is generally ineffective because the pleural fluid is thick. Another nine (11%) patients who underwent thoracentesis subsequently required chest tube drainage. In eight cases (9%), aspiration of liver abscess was necessary together with other thoracic procedures. Open thoracostomy with chest tube and/or thoracentesis was performed in four patients (5%). In 31 patients (36%) treated before 1970, decortication was done during which the diaphragmatic perforation site was left open to allow further drainage of liver abscess into the pleural space. Current practice is to enlarge the diaphragmatic perforation site and remove the abscess contents from the liver. The patients who underwent decortication and open thoracostomy in this series were from the authors' early experience.

Metronidazole together with chest tube drainage, and in select cases simple thoracentesis, is the typical treatment and achieves success in more than 90% of the patients in the present era. If chest tube placement is indicated, a large-bore chest tube (32 Fr) should be used and connected to −20 cm H_2O suction. In the case of superinfection, appropriate antibiotic therapy should be added to the regimen. Although rare, left-sided empyemas may occur as a result of the rupture of a hepatic abscess in the left lobe of the liver.

The overall mortality of amebic empyema ranges from 4% to 40% in different series (Table 1). Mortality is mainly due to sepsis and respiratory failure. Most of these patients had disseminated disease (associated with superinfection) with impending sepsis and were cachectic with multiple comorbidities.

■ BRONCHOHEPATIC FISTULA

Bronchohepatic fistula is the result of rupture of an amebic liver abscess into a bronchus. The patient typically expectorates anchovy paste–like material and/or maroon-colored sputum. This complication is rare and seen in 1% to 2% of all cases with amebic liver abscess. Treatment consists of chest tube drainage and metronidazole. Low-pressure suction should be applied (−10 cm H_2O). The fistula can persist for up to 6 weeks. Decortication, thoracoplasty, or lung resection may be necessary if the fistula and pneumothorax persist for more than 6 weeks.

■ SOLITARY LUNG NODULE, LUNG ABSCESS, AND PNEUMONIA

Pulmonary involvement is evident in nearly 30% of pleuropulmonary amebiasis cases. Treatment of pulmonary conditions is again medical. The mortality of patients with amebic lung abscess and pneumonia was 30% in a series by Verghese et al. Most of these patients died as a result of septicemia and respiratory failure. Surgery was recommended by Ragheb in cases of lung abscess due to amebiasis but was not advocated by other authors. Most authors agree that lung abscesses are secondary to rupture of liver abscess to the lung. Drainage of liver abscess and medical treatment is successful in 80% to 90% of the patients.

■ PERICARDIAL EFFUSION AND TAMPONADE

Amebic abscess of the liver can rupture into the pericardium in 1% of the cases. This rupture is associated with significant mortality (40% to 60%). Immediate pericardiocentesis or pericardiotomy through a subxiphoid incision or thoracoscopy should be performed. Again, metronidazole and surgical drainage are the standard treatment.

Acknowledgment
The authors thank Mary S. Visciano for editorial assistance.

SUGGESTED READING

Cameron EWJ: The treatment of pleuropulmonary amebiasis with metronidazole, *Chest* 73:647, 1978.

Ibarra-Perez C: Thoracic complications of amebic abscess of the liver. Report of 501 cases, *Chest* 79:672, 1981.

Ibarra-Perez C, Selman-Lama M: Diagnosis and treatment of amebic empyema, *Am J Surg* 134:283, 1977.

Lyche KD, Jensen WA: Pleuropulmonary amebiasis, *Semin Respir Inf* 12:106, 1997.

Ragheb MI, et al: Intrathoracic presentation of amebic liver abscess, *Ann Thorac Surg* 22:483, 1976.

Stephen SJ, Uragoda CG: Pleuropulmonary amoebiasis: a review of 40 cases, *Br J Dis Chest* 64:96, 1970.

Verghese M, et al: Management of thoracic amebiasis, *J Thorac Cardiovasc Surg* 78:757-60, 1979.

Vickers PJ, et al: Hepatopulmonary amebiasis—a review of 40 cases, *Int Surg* 67:427, 1982.

BRONCHOLITHIASIS

Alene Wright
Walter J. Scott

Broncholiths are calcified peribronchial lymph nodes that produce clinical symptoms by either distorting or eroding into the tracheobronchial tree. Most broncholiths develop as a result of fungal (e.g., *Histoplasmosis* spp.) or mycobacterial infections, with silicosis being a rare, noninfectious cause. Distortion of the bronchial tree occurs as a result of the inflammatory reaction surrounding peribronchial lymph nodes. The repeated motions of breathing, swallowing, and cardiac activity promote the erosion of these calcified lymph nodes into the bronchial tree. Bronchial impingement and erosion by broncholiths can cause symptoms such as cough, hemoptysis, dyspnea, expectoration of broncholiths (lithoptysis), and recurrent pneumonia. Complications such as massive hemoptysis, lung abscess, and fistula formation between a bronchus and the esophagus can also occur.

■ DIAGNOSIS

Although symptomatic broncholithiasis is uncommon, the diagnosis should be considered whenever calcified hilar or mediastinal granulomas are seen on imaging studies in association with respiratory symptoms or other radiologic abnormalities such as atelectasis or infiltrates. Bronchoscopy is often the only test to document the diagnosis of broncholithiasis in patients who do not report lithoptysis. Typical bronchoscopic findings of eroding peribronchial lymph nodes include the presence of granulation tissue and bronchial stenosis, an appearance similar to that of carcinoma. The surgeon should remember to include broncholithiasis in the differential diagnosis along with carcinoma in this situation if brushings and washings come back as negative. Sometimes the calcified lymph node is more obviously visualized, protruding into the bronchial

lumen. This can be confirmed by observing the gritty feel of the underlying stone at the time of bronchoscopic biopsy of granulation tissue.

The report by a patient of dysphagia and/or cough when swallowing liquids should alert the physician to the presence of a bronchoesophageal fistula. It can be difficult to identify the presence of a bronchoesophageal fistula during a bronchoscopic examination. Granulation tissue and secretions tend to obscure the bronchial side of the opening. Contrast examination of the esophagus or esophagoscopy may be necessary to rule out a bronchoesophageal fistula. Even in patients without clear symptoms such as dysphagia or coughing when swallowing liquids, routine contrast examination in the presence of extensive subcarinal broncholithiasis may be advisable to diagnose small traction diverticula of the esophagus or a small fistulous tract.

■ THERAPEUTIC ALTERNATIVES

The natural history of broncholithiasis is poorly documented. In addition, current recommendations for treatment are based largely on retrospective studies. These options must be altered as necessary to take into account the condition of the patient and the capabilities and experience of the treating physicians. Treatment options in the literature include observation, bronchoscopic stone removal and other interventional bronchoscopic techniques, and surgical resection.

■ OBSERVATION

Some authors have recommended observation alone for patients with symptomatic broncholithiasis, but only under very specific clinical circumstances. Lithoptysis, unaccompanied by other symptoms, may often be self-limiting (i.e., coughing up a broncholith can be curative). Such patients may be observed but should undergo a chest radiograph and chest computed tomography (CT) scan to determine the relationship of any remaining broncholiths to adjacent blood vessels. This information may be helpful in deciding whether to intervene should symptoms recur. Another group for which observation has been recommended consists of patients with broncholith-related bronchial compression and obstructive pneumonia. In this group, directing the initial treatment toward the pneumonia is reasonable if there are no other associated symptoms. If obstructive pneumonia persists or recurs, relief of the broncholith-related compression becomes important to prevent chronic infection (i.e., bronchiectasis) and loss of significant amounts of functional lung tissue.

Recommendations for observation in other clinical settings are based on questionable assumptions regarding the benign natural history of symptomatic broncholithiasis. Some authors believe that the rare number of reports in the literature describing fatalities from broncholith-related hemoptysis supports an initial strategy of observation in patients with broncholiths and hemoptysis. They also note that in many cases, hemoptysis may be produced as a result of bleeding from friable granulation tissue surrounding a broncholith that has eroded into a bronchus. However, broncholith-related hemoptysis of any degree has traditionally resulted in referral of the patient for some type of intervention. Therefore, the paucity of reports of fatal hemoptysis following observation of patients with suspected broncholithiasis is not reliable evidence of the safety of this approach. Most authors would not recommend observation for symptomatic broncholithiasis other than for patients with isolated lithoptysis, during the initial episode of pneumonia from broncholith-caused external compression of the bronchial tree, or in those patients with significant comorbid conditions in whom intervention would be accompanied by a high morbidity and mortality rate.

■ BRONCHOSCOPIC INTERVENTIONS

The success of bronchoscopic techniques used for the treatment of broncholithiasis (and therefore the indications for performing those techniques) depends on several factors. The location and other characteristics of the broncholith determine how easily and safely it can be removed. A large retrospective series reported a 100% success rate (defined as complete removal of all calcified material from within the bronchial lumen) for bronchoscopic removal of symptomatic broncholiths that were sitting freely in the bronchial tree. In contrast, the success rate for removing partially eroding broncholiths (those that were protruding into the bronchial lumen but still embedded in the bronchial wall) was approximately 49%. Reasons for abandoning the attempt at bronchoscopic removal included a firmly embedded broncholith, difficulty grasping a broncholith, and concerns over bleeding related to manipulation of a broncholith. (Before attempting bronchoscopic stone removal, the authors recommended determining the location of the broncholith with respect to adjacent vascular and mediastinal structures by reviewing a recent chest CT scan.)

Operator experience and familiarity with the full range of bronchoscopic techniques were important as well. For example, there was a higher success rate for completely removing partially eroding broncholiths when rigid bronchoscopy was used (67%) compared with flexible bronchoscopy (33%). Finally, the setting and the availability of thoracic surgical backup were important because in one instance (2% of those in this series undergoing bronchoscopic stone removal), a patient developed severe bleeding during a third attempt at bronchoscopic broncholithectomy and was referred for urgent surgical intervention.

Other advanced bronchoscopic techniques have been helpful in certain situations. The literature contains case reports and anecdotal references to the use of the neodymium:YAG (Nd:YAG) laser to fracture obstructing broncholiths that cannot be removed by more standard bronchoscopic techniques. The theoretical advantages of laser therapy include both the adequate removal of the intraluminal portion of a broncholith without resorting to surgery and the ability to coagulate any bleeding granulation tissue. The broncholith is shattered by the laser energy, and the pieces must then be removed with conventional techniques. The shattering effect is achieved by applying high laser power (80 to 100 W to the smallest surface area) and very short pulses (0.2 to 0.3 second) interspersed by rest periods (2 to 5 seconds) to avoid excessive heating of the broncholith and damage to the bronchus and surrounding tissues.

Bronchoscopic removal of loose broncholiths, those lying freely in the bronchial lumen, appears to be safe and effective therapy. However, even those physicians with experience in both flexible and rigid bronchoscopy should use caution when approaching broncholiths that are partially embedded in the bronchial wall. The relation of the broncholith to adjacent vascular and mediastinal structures such as the esophagus should be defined by computed tomography before attempting bronchoscopic removal in order to minimize the likelihood of hemorrhage or fistula formation during endoscopic removal. We recommend that thoracic surgical backup should be immediately available whenever endoscopic removal of partially embedded broncholiths is attempted. Because broncholiths are frequently multiple, the removal of only one stone or of intraluminal stones does not mean that symptoms will not recur from any residual, extraluminal stones.

■ SURGERY

Indications for Surgery

Indications for thoracotomy include severe or recurrent hemoptysis, chronic infection, bronchoesophageal fistula formation, the inability to rule out the presence of bronchogenic cancer, and the treatment of complications from attempted bronchoscopic broncholithectomy. While granulation tissue surrounding an eroding broncholith may be the source of hemoptysis, a developing fistula between the airway and a major blood vessel that can eventually lead to massive bleeding cannot be ruled out. Infected broncholiths represent a type of "infected foreign body" and will continue to cause recurrent symptoms unless they are completely removed. Similarly, a bronchoesophageal fistula is unlikely to heal unless the infected broncholiths are removed. The decision to pursue surgical therapy is based on the severity of symptoms (or the presence of recurrent symptoms) and on the age and general condition of the patient.

General Considerations

The goal of surgical therapy for the treatment of broncholithiasis is the complete removal of broncholiths to decrease the likelihood that symptoms will recur. Surgical removal can be difficult because the process that caused the broncholiths often produces inflammatory adhesions that can obscure tissue planes. Patients and their families should be informed about potential complications or a possible lengthy or difficult procedure. Bronchoscopy performed before thoracotomy is useful for planning the specific operative approach and the extent of any possible resection. (Intraoperative bronchoscopy can also be useful for removing secretions and for checking the status of the airway after a sleeve resection or other bronchoplastic procedure.) Preoperatively, the surgeon should also review the chest CT scan to identify the structures in the immediate vicinity of the broncholith(s). A generous thoracotomy is recommended to provide adequate exposure to both the anterior and posterior hilar regions. Isolating one lung by using a double-lumen endotracheal tube or its equivalent will also improve exposure. The surgeon should discuss the need for more sophisticated airway management strategies with the anesthesiologist beforehand. Because this is not a malignant process, removing only the grossly involved tissue will preserve as much pulmonary function as possible. Therefore, lesser resections than lobectomy have an important role in the treatment of these patients as do sleeve resections and other bronchoplastic procedures. When confronted with a difficult dissection because of the obliteration of tissue planes, the surgeon should not hesitate to take the time to get proximal control of the pulmonary artery before proceeding.

Specific Surgical Techniques

The surgeon should be capable of performing node removal, bronchial repair, segmentectomy, lobectomy, sleeve resections, pneumonectomy, and esophageal repair. It may be possible to remove a calcified lymph node that is distorting a bronchus but not eroding into it. For anatomic reasons, broncholithectomy without pulmonary resection is most applicable for broncholiths eroding into either main stem bronchus, the bronchus intermedius, or the right upper lobe and right lower lobe bronchi. In many cases, the area of erosion is limited and a minimum of bronchus needs to be removed. In these situations, a reanastomosis or other bronchoplastic procedure can be successfully accomplished provided healthy tissue can be approximated without tension.

Most of the patients in large surgical series underwent broncholithectomy with pulmonary resection. Segmentectomy is the procedure of choice whenever a broncholith obstructs a segmental bronchus. Resection of the segmental bronchus until healthy tissue is reached is mandatory. If there is any doubt about this, a lobectomy should be performed. Similarly, an adequate length of viable bronchus must be present for the use of a stapling device. The surgeon should be comfortable with techniques for suture closure of the bronchus in those instances when the use of a stapler is not possible.

Lobectomy and sleeve resection can be performed to avoid pneumonectomy (in the case of upper lobe involvement with broncholithiasis) or even to avoid bilobectomy (in the case of resection of an involved middle lobe). Sleeve resection of the bronchus intermedius has been reported, allowing all three lobes on the right to be spared. As mentioned, broncholiths invading the main stem bronchi can usually be excised and the bronchus repaired with a resection

and reanastomosis, thereby avoiding pneumonectomy. Careful attention to preserving the blood supply of the bronchus, to adjusting for any size differences in the caliber of the bronchial segments by careful suture placement, and to avoiding tension during construction of the anastomosis helps to prevent stenosis caused by ischemic stricture or the formation of granulation tissue. Many satisfactory suture techniques have been described. The bronchial repair or bronchial anastomosis can be reinforced with healthy, vascularized tissue flaps from the parietal pleura, pericardial fat, intercostal muscle, or omentum. On completion of the anastomosis, intraoperative bronchoscopy is always performed to evaluate the patency of the bronchial lumen and also to remove any retained secretions. Patients may need periodic bronchoscopy for removal of retained secretions in the postoperative period. Many centers routinely perform bronchoscopy on the first postoperative day after a sleeve resection to clear any secretions and to examine the anastomosis.

The inflammatory reaction around subcarinal lymph nodes can produce traction diverticula of the esophagus. When removing broncholiths in this region, it is possible to transect a small diverticulum. Therefore, it is important to be alert for this possibility and to test for any esophageal leak after removing broncholiths in this area. Placement of a nasogastric tube or esophageal dilator helps to identify the esophagus in these situations or whenever a bronchoesophageal fistula is known to be present. Once the fistula is identified, usually by transecting the inflammatory lymph node mass, it is dissected down to the wall of the esophagus. The opening in the esophageal wall is trimmed back to healthy tissue and closed in two layers. The required bronchial repair or resection is then carried out. Once again, all of the infected inflammatory and calcified lymph nodes must be resected to minimize the chance of the development of a recurrent fistula. The placement of a vascularized tissue flap between the esophageal and bronchial repair sites is mandatory to prevent recurrence of the bronchoesophageal fistula.

Results of Surgical Therapy

Resections performed to treat broncholithiasis, although most often successful, can be associated with serious complications. Numerous series have documented complications such as major hemorrhage from pulmonary artery tears in addition to both esophageal and bronchial injuries during surgical attempts to remove broncholiths. Serious operative complications such as these occurred in almost 12.7% of patients in one recent series. Despite these difficulties, the authors reported no operative (30-day) mortality for that particular group of patients. In surgical series reported from 1971 to the present, operative mortality rates are uniformly low, varying from 0% to 2.9%. The rate of postoperative complications reported in the recent surgical literature varies from 6% to 34%.

Follow-up

Recurrent symptoms caused by residual broncholiths or the formation of new broncholiths occur after both bronchoscopic and thoracic surgical removal of broncholiths. In one recent report, 48 patients underwent an attempt at endoscopic broncholith removal during 61 bronchoscopy sessions, with 1 patient requiring 4 sessions over a 14-month period to remove recurrent calcified material from the bronchial tree. Good long-term data are not available in the literature for those patients who undergo bronchoscopic broncholithectomy as initial treatment; more data exist regarding the long-term results of surgical treatment of broncholithiasis.

In one surgical series, 59 patients were followed an average of 10 years postoperatively. Fifty (85%) remained asymptomatic, while seven developed symptoms, consisting of recurrent broncholithiasis in one patient, recurrent bronchoesophageal fistula in two patients, and empyema secondary to bronchopleural fistula in two patients. The remaining two patients were thought to be symptomatic from the development and progression of chronic obstructive pulmonary disease. A more recent series reported recurrent respiratory symptoms after surgical treatment in 12 of 46 (26%) patients, with recurrent broncholithiasis documented in 6 of 46 (14.6%). Three patients with recurrent

broncholithiasis were observed; two were eventually treated with bronchoscopic procedures and one with bilobectomy.

Concerns about the long-term development of bronchogenic cancer in these patients exist, but clear evidence that broncholithiasis is an independent risk factor for the development of lung cancer is lacking. However, most authors recommend regular follow-up of these patients.

SUGGESTED READING

Arrigoni MG, et al: Broncholithiasis, *J Thorac Cardiovasc Surg* 62:231, 1971.

Faber LP, et al: The surgical implications of broncholithiasis, *J Thorac Cardiovasc Surg* 70:779, 1975.

Olsen EJ, et al: Therapeutic bronchoscopy in broncholithiasis, *Am J Respir Crit Care Med* 160:766, 1999.

Potaris K, et al: Role of surgical resection in broncholithiasis, *Ann Thorac Surg* 70:248, 2000.

DIFFUSE LUNG DISEASES

Albert J. Polito

Many acute and chronic disorders with variable degrees of pulmonary inflammation and fibrosis have been identified, and they often are grouped under the heading of *interstitial lung disease*. The *interstitium* refers to the microscopic anatomic space bounded by the basement membranes of epithelial and endothelial cells. These diseases are not restricted to the interstitium, however, and all of the cellular and extracellular matrix components of the pulmonary parenchyma are involved in the pathogenesis of alveolitis and fibrosis. The term *interstitial* is misleading, and the growing trend is to call this heterogeneous group of disorders *diffuse parenchymal lung diseases*. More than 150 agents and clinical situations compose the broad spectrum of these diseases (Table 1), but remarkably, many patients share a similar constellation of clinical features on presentation. Classic characteristics of diffuse lung diseases include exertional dyspnea, diffuse bilateral infiltrates on chest radiographs, and abnormal pulmonary function tests showing restrictive physiology and a gas transfer defect.

■ NONINVASIVE CLINICAL APPROACH

History

Although surgical lung biopsy has become an increasingly used tool in the diagnosis of diffuse lung disease, the value of noninvasive approaches must be emphasized. A thorough history is essential and can rule in or out immediately many of the diseases in the differential diagnosis. The onset and duration of dyspnea and cough and the presence of constitutional or extrapulmonary symptoms provide important clues. Idiopathic pulmonary fibrosis (IPF) is the most common of the diffuse lung diseases, comprising approximately 30% of incident cases. Patients typically have symptoms for at least 6 months and sometimes years before presentation, and there is a distinct lack of extrathoracic findings. In contrast, bronchiolitis obliterans organizing pneumonia (BOOP) and hypersensitivity pneumonitis may follow a more acute presentation over 4 to 6 weeks, with associated fever.

Occupational exposures must be elicited in the history and may obviate the need for invasive testing. The pneumoconioses, including silicosis and asbestosis, are a broad group of diseases in which the accumulation of dust in the lungs leads to a tissue reaction. Many individuals are at risk for these disorders through their work. Silicosis is the most prevalent occupational diffuse lung disease in the world, and settings for exposure to crystalline silica include mines, foundries, brickyards, and sandblasting sites. Asbestosis specifically is defined as pulmonary fibrosis resulting from exposure to asbestos and does not include simple asbestos-induced pleural plaque formation, which is typically asymptomatic.

Table 1 Diffuse Parenchymal Lung Diseases*

ENVIRONMENTAL/OCCUPATIONAL DISORDERS
Asbestosis
Silicosis
Hypersensitivity pneumonitis (farmer's lung, pigeon
 breeder's lung)
Berylliosis
Hard metal pneumoconiosis
COLLAGEN VASCULAR DISEASES/VASCULITIS
Rheumatoid arthritis
Systemic lupus erythematosus
Scleroderma
Sjögren's syndrome
Polymyositis/dermatomyositis
Wegener's granulomatosis
Goodpasture's syndrome
**SYSTEMIC DISEASES (OTHER THAN COLLAGEN
VASCULAR DISEASES)**
Langerhans cell granulomatosis
Lymphangioleiomyomatosis
Tuberous sclerosis
Gaucher's disease
DRUGS/THERAPIES
Bleomycin
Methotrexate
Amiodarone
Gold
Penicillamine
Nitrofurantoin
Diphenylhydantoin
External beam radiation therapy
IDIOPATHIC PULMONARY DISORDERSòò
Sarcoidosis
Bronchiolitis obliterans organizing pneumonia
Chronic eosinophilic pneumonia
Idiopathic pulmonary fibrosis

*Representative sample.

Brief, low-level exposure does not predispose to the development of asbestosis, whereas patients with regular occupational exposure over at least 10 years are definitely at risk (e.g., pipefitters, boilermakers, shipbuilders, insulation workers). Environmental exposures are equally important but may be more difficult to identify than occupational exposures. These include farmer's lung and pigeon breeder's lung, the prototypes of hypersensitivity pneumonitis.

A full review of the patient's medications may uncover an iatrogenic cause for the diffuse parenchymal lung disease. Chemotherapeutic agents, including bleomycin and methotrexate, are well known to produce forms of interstitial lung disease. Among the many other drugs that can cause such changes, some of the most important are amiodarone, nitrofurantoin, diphenylhydantoin, gold, and penicillamine. Intravenous drug abuse can result in foreign body granulomatosis (talcosis) from an inflammatory reaction to the particulate matter mixed in with illicit drugs. Medications are not the only form of therapy to cause interstitial lung disease; external beam radiation therapy also can induce pneumonitis and fibrosis.

Finally, a thorough family history may provide useful information. A few patients with IPF are believed to have a familial predilection, with autosomal dominant transmission and variable penetrance. Collagen vascular diseases and sarcoidosis also can cluster in families.

Radiographic Studies

Rarely, chest radiographs in these patients are normal, but more typically they show bilateral infiltrates. The distribution of abnormalities can help narrow the differential diagnosis. Peripheral infiltrates that spare the central lung zones (the "photographic negative of pulmonary edema") are most suggestive of chronic eosinophilic pneumonia but also may be seen in BOOP. Interstitial changes that primarily affect the upper lobes suggest sarcoidosis, silicosis, Langerhans cell granulomatosis, and chronic hypersensitivity pneumonitis. In contrast, lower lobe interstitial infiltrates classically are seen in IPF, asbestosis, and the pulmonary syndromes of the collagen vascular diseases. A review of previous chest radiographs in a patient with IPF often reveals that the lower lobe abnormalities were visible, albeit to a lesser degree, for several years before the development of symptoms.

Although standard chest radiographs are useful, high-resolution computed tomography (HRCT) of the chest is currently the imaging modality of choice. HRCT allows for a detailed evaluation of the lung tissue using 1- to 2-mm–thick slices and can identify the ground-glass infiltrates and honeycomb changes that are thought to represent the two ends of the spectrum of lung inflammation—active, possibly reversible inflammation and end-stage, irreversible fibrosis. Controversy exists as to how closely ground-glass attenuation correlates with active alveolitis.

The HRCT appearance of IPF is characterized by patchy, predominantly lower lobe, reticular changes, concentrated in the subpleural regions. Ground-glass infiltrates may be present but are not typically extensive, whereas honeycombing is a major component. Asbestosis and the collagen vascular diseases (particularly rheumatoid arthritis and scleroderma) show similar features except that asbestosis also may be accompanied by calcified pleural plaques. Extensive ground-glass opacities are seen in desquamative interstitial pneumonia, nonspecific interstitial pneumonia, and respiratory bronchiolitis–associated interstitial lung disease.

Pulmonary Function Testing

Most of the diffuse parenchymal lung diseases are characterized by a restrictive ventilatory defect and a gas transfer defect. Pulmonary function tests do not generally aid in narrowing the differential diagnosis. The diffusing lung capacity (DLCO) is a relatively sensitive (but nonspecific) reflection of the severity of lung disease, and it frequently is decreased out of proportion to the degree of restriction. In a patient with symptomatic or radiographic evidence of interstitial lung disease, but with normal lung volumes and a normal DLCO, the earliest and most sensitive physiologic abnormality is oxygen desaturation in response to exercise.

■ BIOPSY TECHNIQUES

Not all individuals with a diffuse lung disease require a lung biopsy. In a patient who has worked for many years as a pipefitter, the development of exertional dyspnea, restrictive physiology, and lower lobe interstitial infiltrates (especially if calcified pleural plaques are also present) is strongly supportive of a diagnosis of asbestosis. A biopsy in this situation likely would not be indicated. In many clinical scenarios, however, a biopsy provides an invaluable means of making a definitive diagnosis of one of the diffuse lung diseases. The choice of biopsy technique is just as important as the choice of whether or not to do the biopsy.

Transbronchial Biopsy

A transbronchial biopsy specimen obtained via fiberoptic bronchoscopy is most useful when the disease has a characteristic distribution along the bronchovascular bundles. Sarcoidosis classically follows this pattern, and it is diagnosed most commonly by transbronchial biopsy. The standard approach is to obtain four to seven biopsy specimens in affected areas of the lungs. Lymphangitic carcinomatosis and lymphangioleiomyomatosis also tend to follow the bronchovascular bundles and may be diagnosed in this way. In some circumstances, a pulmonary infection may be identified by bronchoscopic biopsy after being erroneously suspected as one of the diffuse lung diseases.

The major limitation in the usefulness of transbronchial biopsies is the actual size of the specimens obtained (2 to 5 mm). Although the samples allow ready identification of granulomas and malignant cells, they are too small to permit accurate pathologic descriptions of the major interstitial pathologies (see later). A "nondiagnostic" transbronchial biopsy simply may reflect sampling error.

Surgical Lung Biopsy

There has been an increasing trend to perform surgical lung biopsy to diagnose diffuse parenchymal lung disease definitively. This trend has paralleled the development of a consistent classification system of interstitial lung disease pathology and the recognition that the various pathologies have clinical implications for response to therapy and prognosis. Usual interstitial pneumonia (UIP) has been identified as the pathologic hallmark of the clinical diagnosis of IPF, and it is only with the larger piece of tissue provided by a surgical lung biopsy that this pathology can be confirmed. The biopsy permits UIP and its attendant poor prognosis to be differentiated from one of the other idiopathic interstitial pneumonias (Table 2) and from lymphocytic interstitial pneumonia and BOOP.

Either an open lung biopsy or a video-assisted thoracic surgical (VATS) lung biopsy may be performed. The VATS procedure is preferred because it is associated with decreased morbidity, shorter duration of chest tube drainage, and reduced length of hospital stay. The biopsy specimen should be taken not only from a site where there is gross involvement, but also from a less affected area of lung tissue. This approach allows a more accurate interpretation of the findings by the pathologist and avoids the pitfall of identifying just nonspecific end-stage fibrotic changes when a grossly affected area is the only site biopsied.

Not all patients are suitable candidates for surgical lung biopsy, and not all patients need it. A major question that needs to be answered in the field of diffuse lung diseases is how to identify patients who would benefit the most from the procedure. An individualized approach to this question is important to balance the potential risks (and cost) of surgical lung biopsy and delay of medical therapy against the certainty of having a pathologic diagnosis and the likelihood that the subsequent course of treatment would be influenced by that diagnosis. Comorbid conditions, including age greater than 65 years, obesity, cardiac disease, and poorly controlled diabetes mellitus, may increase the risk of surgical complications and outweigh the benefits of a definitive pathologic diagnosis. There also are situations in which the preponderance of noninvasive data points to a specific disease entity, and biopsy would be expected to add little additional information (e.g., UIP would be strongly suspected in a dyspneic elderly individual with slow progression of lower lobe interstitial infiltrates over several years, restrictive lung physiology, a low D_{LCO}, and patchy, subpleural honeycomb changes on HRCT).

In younger patients (<65 years old), a surgical biopsy is often indicated, especially if the full noninvasive workup has failed to narrow the differential diagnosis to only one pulmonary process. Certain clinical features raise the potential benefit of pursuing a surgical biopsy, including the presence of constitutional symptoms, significant extrapulmonary manifestations, hemoptysis, a family history of interstitial lung disease, and rapidly progressive disease.

The need for biopsy has been debated most extensively in the diagnosis of IPF. The diagnosis of IPF (UIP on a lung biopsy specimen) can be determined accurately in some patients without a lung biopsy. The degree of accuracy remains an unanswered question, however, with published studies suggesting a range between 58% and 90%.

■ TREATMENT

Therapy for the various diffuse parenchymal lung diseases is highly variable, and specific protocols are beyond the scope of this chapter. When a causative agent for the disease has been identified, initial treatment should focus on avoidance of further exposure (e.g., discontinuation of an offending drug; removal of the patient from an environment causing hypersensitivity pneumonitis). Beyond this, many of the therapeutic interventions are aimed at reducing inflammation through the use of corticosteroids and other immunosuppressive agents. Some of the diffuse lung diseases, including sarcoidosis, BOOP, and desquamative interstitial pneumonia, generally respond more favorably to such therapy. In contrast, UIP has a poor response rate. Lung transplantation

Table 2 Idiopathic Interstitial Pneumonias	
NAME	**ACRONYM**
Usual interstitial pneumonia	UIP
Desquamative interstitial pneumonia	DIP
Respiratory bronchiolitis–associated interstitial pneumonia	RBILD
Acute interstitial pneumonia	AIP
Nonspecific interstitial pneumonia	NSIP

Adapted from Katzenstein A-LA, Myers JL: *Am J Respir Crit Care Med* 157:1302, 1998.

must be considered in selected patients with these disorders who progress despite medical therapy.

SUGGESTED READING

American Thoracic Society, European Respiratory Society: Idiopathic pulmonary fibrosis: diagnosis and treatment: international consensus statement, *Am J Respir Crit Care Med* 161:646, 2000.

Grenier P, et al: Chronic diffuse interstitial lung disease: diagnostic value of chest radiography and high-resolution CT, *Radiology* 179:123, 1991.

Hunninghake GW, et al: Utility of a lung biopsy for the diagnosis of idiopathic pulmonary fibrosis, *Am J Respir Crit Care Med* 164:193, 2001.

Katzenstein A-LA, Myers JL: Idiopathic pulmonary fibrosis: clinical relevance of pathologic classification, *Am J Respir Crit Care Med* 157:1301, 1998.

Reynolds HY: Diagnostic and management strategies for diffuse interstitial lung disease, *Chest* 113:192, 1998.

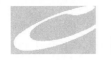

PULMONARY EMPHYSEMA

SURGERY FOR GIANT BULLOUS DISEASE

Stephen R. Hazelrigg
Ibrahim B. Cetindag

The term *giant bullous emphysema* is defined as a situation in which there is a dominant bulla that encompasses at least one third of a hemithorax. Typically, this degree of bullous disease results in symptoms, the most prominent of which is dyspnea. Occasionally, these bullae present because of rupture and pneumothorax, infection, hemoptysis, or pain. Bullae are distinguished from blebs by size, with bullae being larger than 1 cm, and they are produced by the progressive destruction of alveolar walls that eventually results in a large "air sac" that no longer functions in air exchange.

Typically, giant bullae occur in patients with long smoking histories who have emphysematous changes in other parts of the lung, although an occasional patient presents with an isolated bulla. Most bullae are located apically except in α_1-antitrypsin-deficient patients, in whom basilar bullae predominate. Because heavy smoking and lung damage typically coexist, the risk of an incidental lung cancer is estimated at 4% to 8%, and any noncalcified lung nodules should be investigated carefully.

■ PATHOPHYSIOLOGY

Simplistically, giant bullae are air-filled sacs that do not participate in gaseous exchange and do not participate in respiration. They cause compression of the surrounding lung, impairing its function. The larger the bulla and the greater the degree of hyperinflation, the more symptomatic the patient becomes and the greater the likelihood of a good surgical outcome. Hyperinflation also causes downward pressure on the hemidiaphragm (producing flattening on x-ray) and impairs its function.

Air enters the bulla on inspiration, but because the airways collapse, a ball-valve phenomenon exists whereby the air gets trapped, leading to increased pressure in the bulla. The bulla becomes an area of air trapping on ventilation studies and is typically poorly perfused, resulting in shunting and hypoxia.

■ OPERATIVE INDICATIONS

Giant bullae represent an operative indication just by their presence. Contraindications to surgery are the usual comorbid diseases in other systems that make surgery a prohibitive risk. Most patients are symptomatic, but an occasional patient has a giant bulla on x-ray but does not have dyspnea. In this instance, common sense should prevail, and observation may be prudent.

Rupture of the bulla results in a pneumothorax. This is referred to as a *secondary spontaneous pneumothorax* and often results in severe dyspnea until a chest tube is placed. It is estimated that one third of patients with giant bullae develop a pneumothorax with a mortality up to 16%. Options for treatment include chest tube, pleurodesis, and surgical treatment. The treatment decision depends on the patient's overall suitability for surgical intervention. If chest tube placement results in a prolonged leak (>5 days), we generally favor thoracoscopic treatment except in extremely poor-risk patients. Typically a pleurodesis (mechanical or chemical) is added to bullectomy to decrease further the risk of recurrence.

Air-fluid levels in a bulla may be from inflammation or true infection. An infected bulla is less common than inflammation but when present is treated as a lung abscess. Failure to respond to antibiotics may require surgical excision, but lung resection in the face of active infection is fraught with potential problems.

Hemoptysis is unusual but may occur from erosion into a bronchial artery due to infection or carcinoma. Massive bleeding requires embolization or resection. Bleeding in the region of a giant bulla probably is treated best with resection.

■ PREOPERATIVE EVALUATION

In addition to the usual evaluation of the patient's suitability for a general anesthetic, we routinely obtain computed tomography (CT) scans, pulmonary function tests, and room air arterial blood gas determinations. The CT scan provides anatomic information about size and location of the bulla and any masses in the lung as well as some idea of the degree of surrounding compression. Pulmonary function tests quantitate hyperinflation, whereas diffusing lung capacity (DLCO) gives valuable information on how well the remaining lung tissue works. A DLCO of less than 25% predicted is considered a relative contraindication. A 6-minute walk test may be used (as it is in the candidate for lung volume reduction surgery) for a general physiologic test and may be helpful in evaluating progress postoperatively. If the

6-minute walk distance is less than 600 feet, we have found operative risk to be elevated, and a preoperative pulmonary rehabilitation program is recommended.

In the past, pulmonary angiography was used to evaluate crowding of vessels and compression, but we rarely use it today. CT scans can give this information. Giant bullae essentially always cause compression. Ventilation-perfusion scans may provide useful information but are more applicable in lung volume reduction candidates than in giant bullectomy candidates. Tobacco use in the last 6 months, severe obesity or cachexia, unstable cardiac disease, active infection, severe carbon dioxide retention, and extreme age are considered contraindications for surgery.

■ SURGICAL TREATMENT

The surgical options presently include (1) some form of intracavitary drainage, (2) thoracoscopic excision or shrinkage, and (3) open surgical excision. Intracavity drainage of bullae often is called the *Monaldi procedure*. This originally was used to relieve tension in tuberculosis cavities but has been adapted to emphysema. Under local anesthesia (or general), a segment of rib is resected overlying the large bullae. This cavity may be packed for several days (≤2 weeks) to cause the underlying bulla to adhere to the pleura. After adherence, an incision is made into the bulla, and a tube is placed to suction. This suctioning decompresses the bulla and allows the compressed lung to reexpand. A modification of this procedure to one-stage in which a purse-string suture is placed incorporating the bulla and pleura has been reported. Often a Foley catheter is positioned inside the bullae and placed to 5 to 20 mm Hg of suction for 2 days, then water seal for 2 to 3 weeks.

The Monaldi procedure has been successful but may result in prolonged bronchopleural fistulas and extended hospital stays. Presently, we consider this procedure only in poor-risk patients with demonstrated compressed normal lung.

The surgical principles of excision of giant bullae are largely the same for video-assisted thoracic surgery (VATS) and open procedures. Thoracotomy adds to the magnitude of the operative procedure and early postoperative pain, however. Sternotomy is tolerated better than thoracotomy with less respiratory compromise. We favor thoracoscopy for most unilateral cases. Bilateral procedures may be performed by VATS or sternotomy without a clear advantage to either approach from a morbidity point of view.

■ BULLECTOMY

The patient is intubated with a double-lumen endotracheal tube and positioned in the full lateral position. Thoracoscopy typically is performed with three 10-mm ports, all placed anterior to the posterior axillary line and typically below the fourth intercostal space. A 10-mm, 0-degree thoracoscope is used, although a 30-degree scope is acceptable. Smaller sized scopes work fine; however, they have less light and less visualization.

With single-lung ventilation, the bullous areas tend to remain inflated compared with well-perfused lung, in which resorptive atelectasis occurs. The bullae are identified and resected using an endoscopic stapler at the base of the bulla. We generally recommend using a buttress on the staple line to decrease the risk of air leak. Pericardial and Gore-Tex sleeves have worked well and on average shorten hospital stay by about 2 days. The goal is to resect diseased lung, preserving all nonbullous lung tissue. The more narrow the base of the bulla, the simpler the resection and the more likely that minimal functional lung is resected. Ligation of narrow bullae is possible, but we prefer stapling as the most secure method.

Other techniques of management of bullae have been described. With open incisions, one can open the bulla and peel back the edges so that it can be used as a buttress for a staple line or suture closure. Similarly, some have recommended various rolling methods that bunch up the bulla or twist it into a narrow neck. Although these methods work, there does not seem to be any clear advantage to this type of resection.

Bilateral bullous disease can be managed simultaneously either via a median sternotomy or bilateral VATS approach. Although a supine position is possible for a bilateral VATS approach, we prefer to reposition in the full lateral position, being careful that the chest tube is not kinked on the side just completed. Based on studies pertaining to lung volume reduction, there is no advantage to staging unilateral procedures versus doing both sides at one setting. Likewise, there does not seem to be any great advantages of either bilateral VATS or sternotomy for a bilateral procedure.

■ POSTOPERATIVE MANAGEMENT

Postoperative management includes early mobilization and attention to pulmonary toilet. Essentially all patients are extubated in the operating room or shortly thereafter. Often carbon dioxide retention is seen in the early recovery period, but it is not treated as long as the patient is alert and oxygenating well. Oxygen is given only to maintain arterial saturation in the low 90s, being alert for the occasional patient with a hypoxic drive for ventilation. Chest tubes are left to water seal even if small-to-moderate apical spaces exist on x-ray. Avoidance of suction seems to decrease the length of postoperative air leaks, which are the main postoperative complication and reason for prolonged hospitalization. Heimlich valves are used early to aid in mobilization and even for early discharge in selected patients. Postoperative narcotics are limited due to increased gastrointestinal complications.

■ RESULTS

With proper selection and patient preparation, the results of surgery in giant bullous emphysema are gratifying. Most patients (>80%) show impressive improvement in pulmonary function tests, 6-minute walk distances, and general health. Similar results can be attained with lung volume reduction for patients with heterogeneous emphysema, severe hyperinflation (residual volume >200% predicted), and acceptable preoperative exercise capability (6-minute walk ≥ 600 feet). Over time, there is a gradual erosion of the improvement with progression of the emphysema, but recurrent bulla formation is unusual.

SUGGESTED READING

Deslauriers J, LeBlanc P: Management of bullous disease, *Chest Surg Clin N Am* 4:539, 1994.

Hazelrigg SR: Thoracoscopic management of pulmonary blebs and bullae, *Semin Thorac Cardiovasc Surg* 5:327, 1993.

Hazelrigg SR, et al: Comparison of staged thoracoscopy and median sternotomy for lung volume reduction, *Ann Thorac Surg* 66:1134, 1998.

Pearson MG, Olgilvie C: Surgical treatment of emphysematous bullae: late outcome, *Thorax* 38:134, 1983.

LUNG VOLUME REDUCTION SURGERY—VIDEO-ASSISTED THORACOSCOPIC APPROACH

Joseph B. Shrager

Larry R. Kaiser

Lung volume reduction surgery (LVRS) was pioneered as a surgical treatment for emphysema in the 1950s by Otto Brantigan. The inability at that time to objectively document improvements in pulmonary function and the operative mortality rate of 16%, however, soon led to abandonment of the procedure. Joel Cooper modified and reintroduced the operation in the early 1990s. With the benefit of surgical staplers and advances in perioperative care, Cooper and many others have now demonstrated in uncontrolled series that highly selected emphysema patients can benefit from dramatic improvements in dyspnea, pulmonary function, and quality of life following LVRS, with acceptable morbidity and mortality rates. Although there is still significant controversy surrounding the procedure and although several multicenter, randomized clinical trials are still under way, at the time of this writing there are four small, randomized, published studies available that document the effectiveness of LVRS.

The basic physiologic rationale for LVRS is as follows: parenchymal destruction in emphysema results in loss of the normal elastic recoil of the lung and progressive lung distention. The loss of recoil decreases both expiratory driving force and the mechanical support that holds airways open, resulting in decreased expiratory flows. The lung distention places the diaphragm and other inspiratory muscles at a mechanical disadvantage, resulting in decreased inspiratory force and respiratory muscle inefficiency.

Together these result in increased work of breathing and the sensation of dyspnea. By removing the most diseased portions of lung—those that contribute little to gas exchange—LVRS improves the elastic recoil of the remaining tissue and returns the muscles to more physiologic positions. The work of breathing is thus diminished and the dyspnea ameliorated. Other benefits may include decreased ventilation/perfusion mismatch resulting in improved gas exchange and improved cardiac hemodynamics as a result of decreased intrathoracic pressures and/or reduced pulmonary artery pressures.

LVRS can be performed unilaterally or bilaterally, and it can be done via median sternotomy or video-assisted thoracic surgery (VATS). Most surgeons, the authors included, now favor the bilateral procedure in the vast majority of patients. The question of the best incision(s), however, remains unsettled. For reasons discussed further later, we perform the procedure by both techniques, depending on the particular patient's characteristics. This chapter describes our technique of LVRS by VATS.

■ PATIENT SELECTION

The selection of patients is at least as important to a favorable outcome after LVRS as the technical performance of the procedure itself. We offer the procedure to selected patients with emphysema severe enough to markedly diminish their quality of life. The patients must be dramatically hyperinflated (residual volume at least >220% of the predicted value) and have sufficient reduction in forced expiratory volume in 1 second (FEV_1) (<45% predicted) to provide objective confirmation of their symptomatic state.

Although other selection criteria continue to undergo refinement, several principles have become increasingly clear. First, patients with predominately chronic bronchitis—the classic "blue bloater," with reactive airways and copious sputum production—certainly do less well with LVRS than patients whose disease more closely approximates the "pure emphysematous" type of chronic obstructive pulmonary disease. These better candidates—"the pink puffers"—have disease that is primarily due to the structural, mechanical changes of emphysema and have minimal airway inflammation. They tend to be thin and have visibly hyperexpanded chest walls, and they have little sputum production. They generally have none or little postbronchodilator improvement in their FEV_1.

Second, the best candidates have "target" areas—regions of lung that demonstrate more marked emphysematous changes by some combination of chest radiography, computed tomography scanning, and quantitative perfusion scanning. These patients have other areas in their lungs that are more or less well preserved, allowing resection to be targeted to the areas that participate minimally in gas exchange. Ideally, the targeted third of each lung will have perfusion of less than 10% of the total bilateral lung perfusion. There is some evidence that patients with targets in the apices do better than those with targets elsewhere, but this may merely be a function of the fact that the apices are more easily approached surgically by both sternotomy and VATS.

Other selection criteria are also available that seem to be important. Patients with markedly elevated P_{CO_2} or markedly diminished D_{LCO} are at higher risk after the operation. We prefer patients with P_{CO_2} <45 mm Hg and have operated on very few patients with P_{CO_2} >50 mm Hg. A D_{LCO} <20% of predicted is a virtual contraindication. Similarly, those with markedly elevated pulmonary artery pressures and those who are severely malnourished are poor candidates. We use no fixed age limit, but patients over 70 years old should be approached with caution and certainly be done by VATS as opposed to sternotomy, and we have operated on very few patients over age 75. Patients who have had previous thoracotomy cannot safely undergo LVRS on that side. Patients who have had previous sternotomy are at higher risk, but we have successfully operated on a number of such patients by a VATS approach.

CHOICE OF VIDEO-ASSISTED THORACIC SURGERY VERSUS STERNOTOMY

As mentioned earlier, it is not yet clear whether there is one approach—median sternotomy or VATS—that is optimal for LVRS. Our review of all published, nonrandomized series of bilateral LVRS performed exclusively by one approach or the other reveals a mean operative mortality of 4.4% for sternotomy versus 1.0% for VATS, a length of stay of 15 days for sternotomy versus 12 days for VATS, and a percentage increase in FEV_1 of 58% for sternotomy versus 49% for VATS. Certainly, however, most of the studies using sternotomy were carried out earlier than those using VATS, when surgeons were still on the steep portion of the learning curve for the procedure.

Recent studies from our institution (Roberts JR, et al) confirm that very similar improvements in pulmonary function can be achieved by VATS or sternotomy. Although there were significantly greater rates of morbidity and mortality in the sternotomy group as a whole, virtually all of the sternotomy deaths occurred in patients over age 65. Furthermore, when comparing contemporaneous cohorts of VATS and sternotomy cases performed later in the LVRS experience after the learning curve had presumably been completed, only number of ICU days, percent of patients with respiratory complications, and percent with "life-threatening" complications reached statistical significance between the groups. Mortality differences, although favoring VATS, did not reach statistical significance. It should be noted, furthermore, that three of the four randomized studies supporting LVRS used predominantly a median sternotomy approach.

In sum, it appears that functional improvements after LVRS by VATS or sternotomy are very similar. The VATS approach is likely somewhat better tolerated overall; it is certainly better tolerated in patients over 65 years of age. Given these findings, our practice is that older patients and those who are more severely compromised (by a variety of the criteria discussed earlier under "patient selection") should undergo the operation by VATS if the surgeon is comfortable with this approach. Younger and less severely compromised patients may undergo the procedure safely by either approach.

■ PREOPERATIVE PREPARATION

All patients complete at least 6 weeks of vigorous pulmonary rehabilitation before surgery to optimize their physical conditioning. Nutritional supplementation is provided as necessary to reach 80% of ideal body weight. An attempt is made to wean oral corticosteroids completely, but patients who are only able to get as low as 5 mg daily are accepted for surgery. Smoking must have ceased at least 3 months before surgery.

■ OPERATIVE PROCEDURE

Anesthesia
Preoperative placement of a thoracic epidural catheter is critical for postoperative pain management. Inspiratory pressures must be carefully limited throughout the procedure and kept to less than 25 cm H_2O, particularly when ventilating the lung that has been operated on first and has fresh staple lines. The inspiratory time/expiratory time ratio must be decreased in these patients to prevent the development of auto-PEEP. Flexible bronchoscopy is performed before the incision to rule out unexpected malignancy or active infection that would preclude proceeding with operation. A sputum sample taken at this time is often useful in guiding antibiotic therapy if the patient develops an infiltrate postoperatively.

We perform the procedure with the patient in the lateral decubitus position despite the fact that this requires that the patient be repositioned before working on the second side. Although the operation *can* be performed with the patient supine without the need for repositioning, we see no advantage to this since virtually all patients benefit from a period of two-lung ventilation to reduce P_{CO_2} before beginning on the second side (see later).

The side with the more severe disease is operated on first so that single lung ventilation is maintained for the shortest possible time on this lung.

Incisions
For the usual patient with upper lobe predominant disease, the initial incision is made just posterior to the anterior superior iliac spine in approximately the seventh intercostal space. An introducer for the 0-degree, 10-mm videothoracoscope is placed here and the chest is visually explored. Two additional incisions are placed under direct vision from within for placement of a ring clamp for grasping the lung and the linear stapler, respectively (Figure 1). The incision for grasping is made one to two ribs craniad and slightly posterior to the first incision (usually just below the tip of

the scapula); the incision for stapling is made at the same level as the first incision but approximately 8 cm anterior to it. This arrangement of ports facilitates visibility and provides a reliable angle that allows removal of large wedges of parenchyma from the upper lobe and the superior segment of the lower lobe. The placement of the camera and stapling ports near one another allows the surgeon the ideal view to be sure that each staple line is placed immediately at the crotch created by the previous staple line. We believe this minimizes postoperative air leaks. The location of the ports must be altered in the occasional patients whose target areas are not apical.

Exploration and Lysis of Adhesions

Many patients have scattered areas of filmy adhesions, which may be vascular, as a result of past infectious or inflammatory processes. The surgeon must take great care with these, as overly aggressive retraction may cause the lung to tear, rather than the adhesion, and this is another cause of a prolonged postoperative air leak. The lung must be retracted gently and the adhesions divided with electrocautery, staying well away from the visceral pleural surface. All adhesions should be taken down before beginning the parenchymal excision. On rare occasion, one may encounter unanticipated, extremely dense adhesions that may require conversion to thoracotomy or even abortion of the procedure on that side.

Parenchymal Excision

The goal of the operation is to remove one to three large strips of lung parenchyma, totaling approximately 20% to 30% of the lung volume on each side. The ideal amount of lung to resect cannot be easily quantified—more should be removed, certainly, in hemithoraces containing more areas of severely diseased lung; less is removed in those containing less severely diseased lung. If too much functioning lung is resected, postoperative gas exchange may be compromised; too little and one fails to accomplish the intent of the procedure. One index that can be used is that the resection should result in a small residual apical space when the lung is reinflated. If no such space is visible after initial reinflation, one should consider removing more tissue. Early in one's experience, the tendency is certainly to resect too little parenchyma rather than too much. This tendency is compounded by the magnification provided by the video camera.

The resection is targeted to the areas of most severe emphysema as determined by ventilation/perfusion scan, CT scan, and visual inspection at operation. These areas generally remain inflated longer than the areas of more normal lung tissue due to air trapping within them, and this fact aids in their identification.

Although via the median sternotomy approach to LVRS usually a single, large strip of tissue is resected from the upper lobe, at VATS it is more difficult to remove enough tissue with a single wedge due to the limited jaw opening of currently available endoscopic staplers. Thus, two or three wedges are more often removed by the VATS approach. Further, because the VATS approach is lateral rather than anterior, we have found it easiest to remove the initial strip from the *posterior* aspect of the upper lobe, beginning near the confluence of the fissures (or midway along the major fissure on the left) and proceeding around the apex. Common sites for additional excisions in the patient with apical predominant disease are as shown in Figure 2

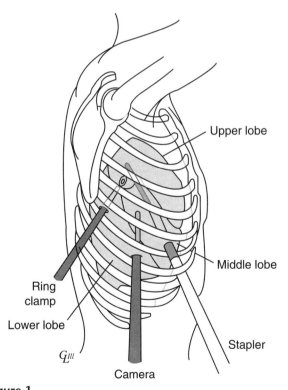

Figure 1
Placement of port sites on the right in the typical patient with apical predominant disease (*Adapted from Rob and Smith's* Operative thoracic surgery, *in press.*)

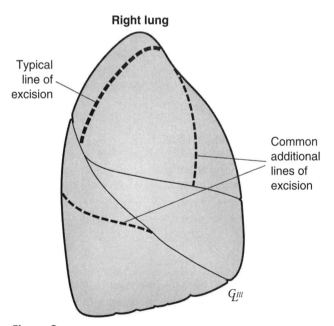

Figure 2
Typical first line of excision and common additional lines of excision for the right lung. (*Adapted from Rob and Smith's* Operative thoracic surgery, *in press.*)

from the anterior aspect of the upper lobe and the superior segment of the lower lobe on the right. On the left lung, the usual additional area for excision, as shown in Figure 3, is the superior segment. It is often useful to compress the poorly collapsing lung tissue with a long Kelly clamp to "thin" it before placement of the stapling device. We have not routinely buttressed the staple lines during VATS LVRS because of the current lack of availability of strips to conveniently fit and easily remove from the endoscopic staplers.

It is difficult and may be counterproductive to evaluate for air leaks by submerging the lung in saline during VATS. We do not attempt this, but rather we try to prevent air leaks in the first place by gentle handling of the emphysematous lung tissue throughout and adherence to the principles of adhesiolysis and parenchymal resection described above.

Closure

A 28 Fr straight chest tube is placed to the apex of the chest, posteriorly and kept to water seal. This tube is tunneled submuscularly, then into the chest at the intercostal incision made for the camera (because placing the tube directly through the port incision without tunneling can lead to air entry when the tube is removed in these often very thin patients). The lung is reinflated under direct vision. We are extremely careful to keep peak inspiratory pressures less than 25 cm H_2O at the time of reinflation and from this point forward during the procedure to prevent staple line

disruption. The port sites are closed in layers with polyglycolic acid suture.

Repositioning

After completing the first side, the patient is placed supine before repositioning to the opposite lateral decubitus position. An arterial blood gas is checked at this time while the patient is ventilated on both lungs. If severe hypercarbia (PCO_2 >70 mm Hg) is present, we ventilate both lungs for up to 15 minutes to reduce this value toward normal before reinstituting single-lung ventilation and operating on the second lung. The opposite lung is then collapsed, and the procedure described earlier is repeated in similar fashion on this second side. To reiterate, pressures on the previously operated lung that is now being ventilated are kept at a minimum.

■ POSTOPERATIVE MANAGEMENT

We have never been unable to extubate a VATS LVRS patient in the operating room. It is of great importance to achieve early extubation to minimize prolonged positive pressure on the staple lines that may result in tears and prolonged air leaks. One must occasionally wait up to 30 minutes in the operating room for a major respiratory acidosis with CO_2 narcosis to improve before extubation. It is remarkable, however, how well these patients do when extubated with PCO_2 levels even in the 80s and pH values as low as 7.20, as long as they have a reasonable mental status at the time of extubation.

All patients are mobilized early and instructed and helped in vigorous pulmonary toilet from the time they arrive in the recovery room. Ambulation is begun thrice daily on postoperative day 1. Patient-controlled thoracic epidural analgesia is used for 5 days at a minimum. Patients are encouraged to cough and to use the incentive spirometer, and chest physiotherapy is used when there is any difficulty clearing secretions. We have occasionally used bronchoscopy on a patient who is unable to clear secretions, and if this is required more than once, we place a minitracheostomy to allow frequent suctioning. Nebulized bronchodilators are used for at least 48 hours before converting to the patient's preoperative inhaled bronchodilators. Antibiotics are used routinely for only 24 hours perioperatively, but we have a low threshold to restart them on any indication of tracheobronchitis. Cultures sent at the time of the preoperative bronchoscopy are often useful to direct this therapy.

The chest tubes must be placed to water seal rather than suction. This appears to allow air leaks to heal more rapidly and avoids any major tears that may result from applying suction to this fragile lung tissue. We often tolerate an initial postoperative apical space of up to 20% without adding suction. These small pneumothoraces generally resolve over the first 2 to 4 postoperative days if there is not a large associated air leak. If a space greater than 20% develops, we place the tube on that side to −10 cm H_2O and increase the suction gradually and only as necessary to reexpand the lung. Once leaks have resolved, we remove chest tubes despite the frequent presence of a small residual space. If there is any question of a small air leak, we clamp the tube for a few hours

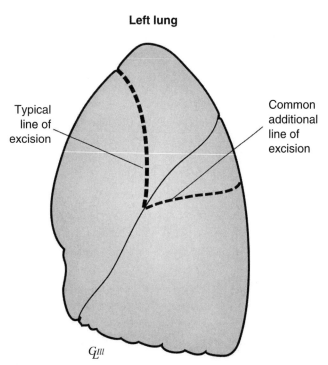

Left lung

Typical line of excision

Common additional line of excision

G_{III}

Figure 3
Typical first line of excision and common additional line of excision for the left lung (*Adapted from Rob and Smith's Operative thoracic surgery, in press.*)

and check for stability on chest radiogram before tube removal.

Unilateral air leaks persisting beyond 1 week after operation occur in approximately 10% of patients. We usually make one attempt at sealing such a leak through pleurodesis with doxycyline. This is effective in approximately half of attempts. In the remaining patients, if they are otherwise well, we cut the chest tube and attach a Heimlich valve. The patients are then discharged with the valve in place, on oral antibiotic prophylaxis, to follow-up in the office twice weekly until the leak resolves and the tube can be removed.

LUNG VOLUME REDUCTION SURGERY—MEDIAN STERNOTOMY APPROACH

Sunil Singhal
Stephen C. Yang

Chronic obstructive pulmonary disease afflicts 15 million Americans to varying degrees and is the fourth leading cause of death. Medical management includes bronchodilators, antiinflammatory drugs, and antibiotics. The only medical therapy proved to prolong life is oxygen therapy.

During the past 50 years, many operations have been described to manage emphysema surgically. Earliest techniques included procedures such as costochondrectomy, thoracoplasty, phrenic nerve paralysis, and the creation of a pneumoperitoneum to allow manipulation of thoracic cage dynamics. Surgeons have reinforced the membranous portion of the trachea and main bronchi by suturing bone graft and various prostheses to airway walls to prevent expiratory collapse. Needle aspiration and injection have been used to eliminate emphysematous bullae. There have been unsuccessful attempts at preventing the bronchospastic component of emphysema by resecting autonomic nerves such as the vagus. Other interesting approaches to treat emphysema include increasing the blood supply to the lung by stimulating collateral circulation from the chest wall through parietal pleurectomy or talc pleurodesis.

In the late 1950s, Brantigan and Mueller in Baltimore were the first to introduce the idea of lung reduction for emphysema. Although 75% of patients reported clinical improvement, the lack of rigid benefit criteria and an operative mortality rate of 18% prevented widespread acceptance. A recent resurgence in 1993 using their operative techniques by Cooper and colleagues has caused new interest in the field. Lung volume reduction is postulated to improve respiratory mechanics. The loss of elasticity of lung tissue in emphysema prevents bronchioles from being pulled open during lung expansion, causing a collapse of the airway. By reducing lung volume, the circumferential pull on the bronchioles can be restored. The deleterious effects of bullae, such as compression of the adjacent parenchyma and right-sided heart compression, can be prevented. By reducing the lung volume, one can raise the diaphragm and make more efficient use of the intercostal muscles. The diaphragmatic length-tension curve also shifts back to normal physiologic proportions and improves respiratory muscle efficiency.

■ INDICATIONS FOR MEDIAN STERNOTOMY APPROACH

Lung volume reduction surgery (LVRS) is a palliative procedure for medically optimized patients with disabling emphysema. Current indications include crippling dyspnea associated with hyperinflation, diaphragmatic dysfunction, and heterogeneous disease distribution. Approximately 20% of the patients with COPD qualify for LVRS. The most common reasons for exclusion are poor pulmonary function, homogeneous pulmonary disease, and insufficient target areas. Patients under consideration for LVRS are assessed by pulmonary function tests, chest computed axial tomography (CT) scans, isotope perfusion scans, and noninvasive and invasive cardiac evaluation.

Patients being considered for LVRS should have pulmonary function tests that suggest severe airflow obstruction. Some of the commonly accepted parameters include a forced expiratory volume in 1 second (FEV_1) of less than 30% predicted with bronchodilator response, total lung capacity greater

SUGGESTED READING

Brantigan OC, et al: The surgical approach to pulmonary emphysema, *Dis Chest* 39:485, 1961.

Cooper JD, et al: Bilateral pneumectomy (volume reduction) for chronic obstructive pulmonary disease, *J Thorac Cardiovasc Surg* 109:106, 1995.

Roberts JR, et al: Comparison of open and thoracoscopic bilateral volume reduction surgery: complications analysis, *Ann Thorac Surg* 66:1759, 1998.

Shrager JB , Kaiser LR: Lung volume reduction surgery, *Curr Probl Surg* 37:253, 2000.

than 120% predicted, and residual volume greater than 250% predicted. Diffusion abnormalities in this population are common but often are not reliable or reproducible because of the technique used in these dyspneic patients. If performed accurately, values are usually less than 50% of predicted.

The CT scan provides a detailed examination of the anatomy of the lung parenchyma and is routinely ordered on all patients. Candidates for LVRS are at an increased risk for malignancy and must be ruled out for suspicious lesions. Up to 15% of patients present with a solitary pulmonary nodule, and up to one third eventually are diagnosed with a primary bronchogenic carcinoma. Marked emphysematous lungs with heterogeneity is ideal, particularly upper lobe predominance in the acquired form or lower lobe in alpha-1-antitrypsin deficiency (A1AT).

Isotope ventilation/perfusion scans should have evidence of apical functionless emphysematous lungs with relatively preserved basal function (or opposite in the case of A1AT). Upper lobe emphysema is associated with a significantly better improvement in FEV_1 than other types of emphysema. The contributions of the lower lobes to total lung function are greater than those of the upper lobes.

Evaluation of cardiac function is mandatory. Although ejection fraction of the left heart is easily obtained with echocardiography, the right side is often more difficult to estimate because of poor images resulting from the hyperinflated lungs beneath the probe. Instead of echocardiography, we prefer to use the MUGA scan with specific instructions to obtain right ejection fraction from the first-pass images. Cardiac catheterization (right) is reserved for those patients whose low (<40%) right heart function on the MUGA may suggest pulmonary hypertension, whereas coronary angiography is indicated in patients with known critical stenosis, previous cardiac history (symptoms, angina, infarct), or pulmonary symptoms out of proportion to the objective pulmonary function. Alternatively, dobutamine-echocardiography may be added before left heart catheterization if the extent of myocardial dysfunction precludes further surgical evaluation.

Two operative approaches exist for LVRS: median sternotomy or video-assisted thoracic surgery (VATS). The operation of choice must be tailored to the needs and characteristics of the individual patient. Compared with the VATS technique (see previous chapter on "Lung Volume Reduction Surgery—Video-Assisted Thoracoscopic Approach"), median sternotomy has the distinct advantage of being able to perform bilateral volume reduction with one incision, thus making it a relatively quick operation. It is associated with a longer hospital stay, although the overall cost is less. There is greater morbidity due to loss of pulmonary mechanics from incisional pain. However, a median sternotomy allows excellent bilateral exposure and flexibility in the operating room. There also is no division of chest wall musculature. Painful intercostal nerve injury can still result from this approach because of pressure from the chest tube insertion sites. Nevertheless, VATS has been gaining in popularity with general increase toward minimally invasive procedures. The VATS procedure does have the advantage of a shorter hospital stay, fewer days with postoperative air leaks, and fewer days on the ventilator.

Table 1 General Objective Contraindications to Lung Volume Reduction Surgery
Age >80 years
FEV_1 <20% of predicted
D_{LCO} <20% of predicted
Systolic pulmonary pressure >50 mm Hg
P_{CO_2} >55 mm Hg or P_{O_2} <45 mm Hg on room air
RV <150% predicted
TLC <100% predicted
<400-feet 6-minute walk

■ CONTRAINDICATIONS FOR MEDIAN STERNOTOMY APPROACH

Less than 10% of patients with emphysema are actually candidates for LVRS. There are a number of contraindications to the traditional median sternotomy approach. If a patient presents with such poor pulmonary status that the morbidity of the procedure outweighs the benefits, that patient is denied surgery. General objective contraindications are listed in Table 1.

The most common reason that patients are denied LVRS is the lack of heterogeneity of emphysematous disease. There are a number of patients who are turned down for comorbid conditions. Age of greater than 80 is a relative contraindication, but such patients are evaluated on a case-by-case basis. Poorly motivated, noncompliant patients and those without adequate social support are not candidates because they will have great difficulty participating in pulmonary rehabilitation programs. Severely obese or cachectic patients are excluded. Patients must have abstained from smoking for at least 6 months before their evaluation—urine cotinines are checked in suspect patients. Patients who had a prior significant myocardial infarction or have another serious comorbid illness with a 5-year survival of less than 50% are not candidates. Although a significant number of patients are steroid dependent, candidates are weaned down to 20 mg of prednisone. Other contraindications include chest wall abnormalities (severe kyphosis, pectus excavatum) and prior major thoracic surgery (sternotomy, thoracotomy with major pulmonary resection, prior pleurodesis).

■ PREOPERATIVE PREPARATION

Patients undergo extensive preoperative preparation before going to the operating room for LVRS via sternotomy. In addition to the radiographic studies discussed previously, routine labs are performed to include assessment of renal and liver function. Patients are evaluated for personal motivation and willingness to work in a vigorous pulmonary rehabilitation program. All patients are required to undergo 6 weeks of pulmonary rehabilitation with the aim of achieving a 60% to 80% maximum predicted heart rate for 30 minutes during aerobic exercise or have the endurance ability to exercise without stopping for 30 minutes.

■ SURGICAL TECHNIQUE

All patients are given a short pulse of steroids (40 mg prednisone/day) for 3 days before surgery. Patients are typically admitted the same day of surgery. An epidural catheter is placed at the bedside after light sedation and local anesthesia. In the rare instance when this is unsuccessful, the operation is cancelled, and the patient is placed in position under fluoroscopy the night before the rescheduled surgery date. A first-generation cephalosporin is administered 30 minutes before the incision. Once in the room, chronically steroid-dependent patients are given a 100-mg bolus of hydrocortisone intravenously, followed by the same dose every 8 hours for 3 doses. Large-bore intravenous and radial arterial lines are placed. Patients are then intubated first with a single-lumen endotracheal tube, and fiberoptic bronchoscopy is performed to clear the airways and look at the anatomy. A sputum sample or bronchial washing is sent for microbiologic examination at the time to help guide postoperative antimicrobial therapy. A double-lumen endotracheal tube is replaced and verified in correct position by bronchoscopy and auscultation.

After the skin incision, the underlying tissues are divided with electrocautery down to the periosteum. To avoid accidental injury to the hyperexpanded lung when dividing the sternum, a tissue plane is first bluntly developed behind the posterior shelf of the sternum in the midline; ventilation is held to drop the lungs away from the anterior chest wall, and the sternum is divided with the bone saw. The side with the most severely diseased lung parenchyma is addressed first; therefore, ventilation is isolated to the contralateral lung. The parietal pleura is gently dissected off the anterior chest wall for the entire length of the incision with Kittners. A sufficient quantity should be freed (approximately 4 cm) so that a fringe of pleura can be approximated when closing.

The pleura is carefully opened, avoiding injury to the underlying lung. Extreme care must be taken to avoid injury to the phrenic nerve. The nerve is most likely to be injured on the medial and superior aspect of each chest cavity. With ventilation to the lung withheld, healthier lung tissue tends to collapse first, leaving the "target" areas hyperinflated on entry into the pleural space. Adhesions are usually encountered from diffuse inflammatory processes and should be taken down carefully to avoid visceral pleural tears that would cause a prolonged air leak. Once the lungs are collapsed, it is our preference to fill the hemithorax with warm saline to elevate the lung toward the incision; this avoids traction injury to the fragile lung to bring it into the field of vision. The lung is carefully palpated for unsuspecting masses and to determine the areas for resection. Based on the findings on the ventilation/perfusion scan and macroscopic findings, the borders of resection are chosen. For the upper lobe, an inverted U-shaped line of resection is used, making this a near-total lobectomy. For lower lobe disease in A1AT deficiency, a more linear technique is used, sparing the superior segment. Approximately 25% of the lung volume is resected.

A linear cutting stapling device is used. The stapler line is buttressed with strips of bovine pericardium or polytetrafluoroethylene (PTFE) inserts. Care should be taken when advancing the stapler arms along the lung tissue because the tips could get hung up and accidentally tear the fragile lung tissue. To help place the stapling arms safely and accurately, the line of resection in the lung tissue is compressed between the second and third fingers or with a long atraumatic clamp. The lung tissue on the specimen side is also incised to decompress the tissue to allow for better visualization.

Once the staple lines are completed, saline solution is then introduced into the chest cavity to assess air leakage. The lung should not be retracted to look at the staple line, as this also could tear the lung tissue. When moderate-to-large air leaks are identified, attempts at closure are performed with suturing, restapling, or placing tissue sealants. Suturing emphysematous lung tissue should be avoided and can often be futile. Mechanical pleurodesis is performed to encourage adhesion formation and early closure of air leaks. An apical pleural tent is developed if there remains significant pleura space. With the lung reexpanded, we also resect a medial segment of the right middle lobe or lingula in a vertical fashion; this helps to prevent accidental injury to the lung tissue while closing the pleura and sternum. One chest tube is placed in the hemithorax posteriorly up to the apex. The pleura is closed with a running 3-0 chromic suture. Attention is then turned to the other side.

The sternum is closed in a standard fashion. Before placing the sternal wires, the double-lumen tube is exchanged for a single lumen to minimize airway irritation. The patient is gently woken to avoid high airway pressures, given nebulizer treatment, and extubated shortly after skin closure in an upright, sitting position.

■ LUNG VOLUME REDUCTION SURGERY AND CORONARY ARTERY BYPASS GRAFTING

A small proportion of patients qualify for LVRS based on pulmonary and radiographic criteria but are deemed ineligible because of significant coronary artery stenosis. These patients are difficult to deny, because although they are somewhat functional and have the potential to obtain vast improvement from LVRS, they have coronary lesions amenable to coronary artery bypass grafting (CABG). They present a difficult challenge in that, conversely, CABG is precluded by the compromised pulmonary disease. In younger and potentially eligible patients, lung transplantation would also be excluded based on the coronary disease.

There have been a number of published reports, including experience at this institution combining LVRS and CABG simultaneously at one operative setting. Operative approach requires a sternotomy if both are considered. In addition to the criteria required for LVRS, these patients are a highly select group requiring coronary lesions amenable to bypass, relatively preserved right and left heart function, and evidence of reversible ischemia.

Preoperative preparation and initial operative approach are as described earlier for LVRS. After sternotomy, the CABG is performed first. It is optimal if this can be done off cardiopulmonary bypass. Great care is taken with the pleura and underlying lung if the internal mammary arteries are used for bypass grafts. Once the CABG is completed and the

LVRS portion started, the bypass conduits, in return, should be left undisturbed or carefully handled. Particular attention to the internal mammary grafts should be paid while performing the upper lobe staple resection.

POSTOPERATIVE CARE

Once extubated in the operating room, patients are observed for approximately 1 hour to ensure that they do not become hypercarbic or hypoxic and that no large air leaks are present. The chest tubes are briefly placed on 10 cm of suction to evacuate residual pleural air, and then on water seal for the duration. If there is a large pneumothorax on postoperative films, the most minimal amount of suction is applied to reexpand the lung.

All patients are given nebulizer treatments at 30-minute intervals for four doses. Intravenous aminophylline is initiated at 0.5 mg/kg for severe bronchospasm. Patients are gently bagged with a facemask if hypercarbia ensues. In addition to the epidural for pain control, intravenous ketorolac is given routinely, and a patient controlled anesthesia pump is given if needed.

All patients spend 1 night in the intensive care unit and then are transferred to a floor or monitored bed the next day. Physical therapy consultation is done immediately, with the intent of ambulation the next day. All patients receive stool softeners, physical therapy and respiratory therapy, orders for early ambulation, chest radiographs as needed, incentive spirometers, and flutter valves. Chest tubes are removed within 24 hours of resolution of air leaks. Follow-up pulmonary function tests are obtained at 3-month intevals during the first year and then at 6-month intervals thereafter.

COMPLICATIONS

Postoperative complications naturally tend to be respiratory in nature. Significant air leaks tend to be the major setback for patients. Suction to the chest tubes is avoided. More than one third of patients require a chest tube for longer than 1 week. Patients with persistent air leaks at 1 week have Heimlich valves attached to the chest tube and are sent home. It is postulated that prolonged air leaks do not originate from the staple line, but rather from other areas of the lung now that airway pressures are redistributed after LVRS. In our experience, only a small percent (5%) require reintubation during their hospital stay for respiratory failure and occasionally progress to tracheostomy.

Infection is the second most common problem, whether it is a pneumonia, empyema, mediastinitis, or wound infection. Sternal dehiscence is occasionally encountered, particularly in these malnourished or diabetic populations, and requires débridement and flap closure by the plastic surgeons. We have had isolated episodes of gastrointestinal bleeding, pulmonary emboli, and cardiac arrhythmias (usually atrial fibrillation and supraventricular tachycardias). The literature notes isolated incidents of bowel perforation. Due to the high-dose steroid requirement, many of these patients mask frank peritoneal signs.

Before the operation, there should be a frank discussion of operative mortality with the patient and family. Mortality rates from larger series range from 0% to 15% (Table 2). Compared with the VATS approach, these numbers are generally higher. Although most commonly attributed to respiratory failure, the other complications described here have also contributed to this mortality rate.

RESULTS

Cooper and Patterson presented data on 20 patients in 1995 on LVRS performed through a median sternotomy. Since then, there have been numerous reports examining the optimal approach: sternotomy versus VATS, unilateral versus bilateral, and one- versus two-staged. LVRS often yields dramatic improvement in spirometry and exercise capability, but significant changes do not usually begin until 3 months postoperatively. At 1 year after surgery, approximately two thirds of patients have improvements in pulmonary function, dyspnea, oxygen dependence, functional status, and quality of life. The end point for most critical evaluations of the benefit of LVRS is to determine symptomatic improvement, namely decreased oxygen use and less dyspnea, not survival. Prolongation of life expectancy may be an added benefit. Table 2 describes a sample of 10 bilateral lung volume reduction series performed over the past several years.

Table 2 Bilateral Lung Volume Reduction Using a Median Sternotomy Approach

LUNG VOLUME REDUCTION SERIES	PATIENTS (n)	PERIOPERATIVE MORTALITY (%)	FEV$_1$ IMPROVEMENT (%)
Cooper, 1996 (Washington University, St. Louis)	150	4.0	51.0
Kaiser, 1998 (University of Pennsylvania)	86	12.8	41.4
Bagley, 1997	55	5.0	27.0
Miller, 1999 (Canadian LVRS Project)	53	9.4	97.0
Date, 1998 (Minami-Okayama Hospital, Japan)	39	0.0	41.0
Hazelrigg, 1998 (Southern Illinois University)	29	6.0	40.0
Daniel, 1996	26	4.0	49.0
Malthaner, 2000 (University of Western Ontario)	24	8.3	36.0
Ko, 1998 (University of California Los Angeles)	19	15.0	20.0
Wisser, 1997 (Vienna, Austria)	15	13.0	40.3

It is hoped that current prospective randomized trials will address a number of questions and controversial issues, including selection criteria, role of pulmonary rehabilitation, and operative approach. The National Emphysema Treatment Trial (NETT) and Canadian Lung Volume Reduction Surgery Trial are examining issues such as the role of pulmonary rehabilitation, optimal surgical selection criteria, differences in operative approaches, how to manage patients without clear target areas, and the short- and long-term costs of these procedures to the health care system. The NETT is a randomized prospective trial by the collaboration of 17 clinical centers using medical therapy versus medical therapy and LVRS for the treatment of patients with severe bilateral emphysema. The primary outcome to be assessed is survival, although additional outcomes to be examined are maximum exercise capacity, pulmonary function, oxygen requirement, distance walked in 6 minutes, quality of life, respiratory symptoms, and health care utilization and costs. The trial is currently closed for enrollment. Interim results have shown an increased mortality of surgery versus medical therapy (16% versus 0%) at 1 month in a select high-risk patient population who present with two of the following criteria: homogeneous distribution of disease, FEV_1 of less than 20% of predicted, and D_{LCO} < 20% of predicted.

■ CONCLUSION

LVRS was developed as a surgical alternative for modest and severe COPD. Initially set out to be a bridge to lung transplantation, it is now a procedure that may obviate the need for transplantation in certain patients, while offering surgical therapy to those who may not qualify for transplantation due to their age. Despite conflicts in the reported literature, LVRS still presents an acceptable alternative in carefully selected patients and should be performed at centers with the expertise and support to manage these high-risk patients.

SUGGESTED READING

Cooper JD, et al: Results of 150 consecutive bilateral lung volume reduction procedures in patients with severe emphysema, *J Thorac Cardiovasc Surg* 112:1319, 1996.

Date H, et al: Bilateral lung volume reduction surgery via median sternotomy for severe pulmonary emphysema, *Ann Thorac Surg* 65:939, 1998.

Koebe HG, et al: Evidence-based medicine: lung volume reduction surgery (LVRS), *Thorac Cardiovasc Surg* 50:315, 2002.

National Emphysema Treatment Trial Research Group: Patients at high risk of death after lung-volume-reduction surgery, *N Engl J Med* 345:1075, 2001.

Roberts JR, et al: Comparison of open and thoracoscopic bilateral volume reduction surgery: complications analysis, *Ann Thorac Surg* 66:1759, 1998.

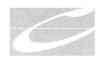

LUNG TRANSPLANTATION

PREOPERATIVE EVALUATION OF THE LUNG TRANSPLANT CANDIDATE

Sean M. Studer

Jonathan B. Orens

Since the first long-term successful lung transplants were performed in the 1980s, the process of identifying appropriate candidates for transplantation and evaluating these patients preoperatively has undergone significant change. Despite this, the goals for selecting appropriate transplant candidates have remained constant: to improve the survival and quality of life of patients with advanced lung disease while appropriately allocating the limited supply of donor organs. This review will address the preoperative assessments for lung transplantation while focusing on the types and severity of respiratory illness that warrant this procedure. The role that each member of a multidisciplinary lung transplant team plays in the evaluation and care of the patient will also be discussed.

■ GENERAL PRINCIPLES OF CANDIDATE SELECTION

The most suitable candidates for lung transplantation generally have advanced and near end-stage lung disease with significant functional limitation, defined as New York Heart Association (NYHA) class III or IV, but are otherwise healthy and meet appropriate age guidelines. The patient must have failed all forms of medical therapy and have a projected life expectancy of less than 2 years due to his or her respiratory illness. Thus, the initial screening for potential lung transplant candidates involves evaluating the patient's age, pulmonary diagnosis, and medical history through discussion with the referring physician and/or review of the medical record. Generally accepted age limits supported by the International Guidelines for Selection of Lung Transplant Candidates are listed in Table 1. In terms of the pulmonary diagnosis, four disease categories account for the majority of patients considered for lung transplantation: (1) chronic obstructive pulmonary disease (COPD) without bronchiectasis; (2) cystic fibrosis (CF) and bronchiectatic lung diseases; (3) fibrotic pulmonary disease; and (4) pulmonary

hypertension with and without congenital heart disease (Table 2). Once the initial screening phase is completed, consultations are scheduled with members of the multidisciplinary lung transplant team and preoperative testing is initiated to assess the severity of lung disease and other comorbid illnesses and to exclude potential contraindications for lung transplantation.

■ MULTIDISCIPLINARY TRANSPLANT TEAM EVALUATION

The lung transplant team is usually composed of the transplant surgeon, pulmonologist, nutritionist, psychologist, physical/occupational therapist, transplant coordinators,

---

Table 1 Age-Limit Guidelines for Lung and Heart-Lung Transplantation

Heart-lung transplants—55 years
Bilateral lung transplants—60 years
Single lung transplants—65 years

Based on the International Guidelines for the Selection of Lung Transplant Candidates.

Table 2 Disease Indications for Lung Transplant

OBSTRUCTIVE LUNG DISEASE WITHOUT BRONCHIECTASIS
Emphysema
Alpha-1 antitrypsin deficiency emphysema
Obliterative bronchiolitis
SUPPURATIVE AND BRONCHIECTATIC LUNG DISEASE
Cystic fibrosis
Bronchiectasis (multiple etiologies)
FIBROTIC LUNG DISEASE
Idiopathic pulmonary fibrosis
Sarcoidosis
Collagen vascular disorders (without significant systemic involvement)
Occupational lung disease
Eosinophilic granulomatosis
Lymphangioleiomyomatosis
Alveolar microlithiasis
Pulmonary alveolar proteinosis
PULMONARY HYPERTENSION
Primary pulmonary hypertension
Eisenmenger's syndrome
Thromboembolic pulmonary hypertension
Pulmonary venoocclusive disease

---

and social worker. At our center, the first consult is scheduled with either the transplant pulmonologist or transplant surgeon to preliminarily assess candidate suitability and to plan for any additional testing beyond the routine regimen. A detailed history and physical examination by the pulmonologist and surgeon are followed by specialized evaluations by other team members. The team meets regularly (weekly at our centers) to discuss any problems that may have arisen for patients remaining in the evaluation process and to decide which patients to place on the transplant waiting list with the United Network for Organ Sharing (UNOS). The listing decision is based on the results of the medical and psychosocial evaluation as discussed later.

■ PREOPERATIVE TESTING FOR LUNG TRANSPLANTATION

Preoperative testing is aimed at evaluating candidate suitability and to help guide the surgical procedure and early postoperative care. Beyond the initial history and physical examination, the evaluation includes extensive testing to evaluate for concomitant disease that may adversely affect the transplant outcome. Diseases affecting the cardiovascular system, kidney, and liver must be excluded. Cardiac evaluation typically includes an assessment of ventricular function, pulmonary artery pressure, and exclusion of ischemic heart disease with tests such as echocardiography, MUGA scanning, dobutamine or Persantine thallium stress testing, and right and left heart catheterization. Renal function is assessed with a 24-hour urine collection to assess creatinine clearance. Liver function is assessed with serum liver function studies, hepatitis screen (hepatitis B and C), and an assessment of synthetic function with serum albumin and prothrombin time. Thoracic computed tomography scans and quantitative ventilation/perfusion scans are useful for determining if asymmetric disease or pleural fibrosis favor a right or left lung in single-lung transplant procedures and the order in which to transplant the lungs in bilateral lung transplant procedures. Additional assessments include bone density measurements, need for immunizations, and an assessment of swallowing function for those with any aspiration risk.

There are both relative and absolute contraindications to lung transplantation (Table 3) based on the presence and severity of comorbid illnesses. For candidates who have no contraindications, follow-up pretransplantation testing is tailored to follow the severity of the underlying lung disease and to determine whether the patient remains a viable candidate for future transplantation.

■ DISEASE-SPECIFIC GUIDELINES

The type of transplant procedure that is offered (single lung, bilateral lung, and combined heart-lung transplant) depends in part on the underlying disease and center-specific criteria. Patients with suppurative lung diseases such as CF and bronchiectasis are chronically colonized with infectious organisms and must receive bilateral lung transplants to prevent infectious complications. There is less agreement

---

Table 3 Contraindications for Lung Transplantation

RELATIVE CONTRAINDICATIONS
Symptomatic osteoporosis
Severe musculoskeletal disease (e.g., kyphoscoliosis)
Poor nutritional status: weight >130% or <70% ideal body weight
Corticosteroid use: >20 mg/day of prednisone
Substance addiction—may be acceptable if abstinent ≥6 months and attending support group
Psychosocial problems—e.g., poorly controlled severe psychoaffective disorder or history of medical nonadherence in absence of psychiatric diagnosis
Invasive mechanical ventilation (noninvasive ventilation is acceptable)
Colonization with atypical mycobacteria or fungi

ABSOLUTE CONTRAINDICATIONS
Human immunodeficiency virus infection
Creatinine clearance <50 mg/ml/min
Cirrhosis of the liver or active hepatitis B or hepatitis C infection
Significant untreatable coronary artery disease or left ventricular dysfunction—may be candidate for heart-lung transplant
Active malignancy within the past 2 to 5 years (depending on malignancy type)—except basal or squamous cell carcinomas of skin, which are acceptable
Other systemic illnesses if there is evidence of end-organ damage that would limit survival
Active substance addiction

Based on the International Guidelines for the Selection of Lung Transplant Candidates.

---

among transplant centers regarding other indications for bilateral versus single transplant. Although data now show a slight survival advantage for two lungs compared with a single lung transplant, two patients can receive a single lung from a set of acceptable cadaveric donor lungs. Thus, there is the potential to help more patients if single lung transplants are performed whenever possible.

The disease-specific International Guidelines for listing patients for lung transplantation are discussed here and summarized in Table 4. These guidelines were developed based on the natural history of these diseases compared with anticipated survival after transplantation.

■ OBSTRUCTIVE AIRWAY DISEASE

COPD is a leading cause of morbidity and mortality and is the most common disease indication for lung transplantation in the United States. Despite the high prevalence of this disease, limited data exist regarding the natural history of severe COPD. This makes decisions regarding the timing for lung transplantation somewhat difficult. Markers such as reduced forced expiratory volume in 1 second (FEV_1), hypoxemia, hypercapnea, and pulmonary hypertension have each been associated with increased mortality in COPD.

The combination of advanced age, low FEV_1, and a low arterial oxygen level have a negative impact on survival.

Table 4 Guidelines for Lung Transplantation

**CHRONIC OBSTRUCTIVE PULMONARY DISEASE AND
ALPHA-1-ANTITRYPSIN DEFICIENCY EMPHYSEMA**
Postbronchodilator FEV_1 <25% of predicted
Resting hypoxemia (PO_2 <55 mm Hg)
Hypercapnia (PCO_2 >55 mm Hg) and/or secondary pulmonary
  hypertension
Deteriorating clinical course requiring long-term O_2 therapy,
  especially associated with hypercapnia
CYSTIC FIBROSIS
Postbronchodilator FEV_1 <30%, or FEV_1 >30% with rapid
  progressive decline
Resting hypoxemia on room air (PO_2 <55 mm Hg)
Hypercapnia (PCO_2 >55 mm Hg)
Clinical course marked by weight loss and increasing frequency
  and severity of exacerbations
IDIOPATHIC PULMONARY FIBROSIS
Symptomatic, progressive disease despite immunosuppressive
  therapy
FVC <60% of predicted
Diffusing capacity <50% of predicted
Early referral of minimally symptomatic patients with any
  abnormality of pulmonary function is encouraged
PRIMARY PULMONARY HYPERTENSION
New York Heart Association functional class III or IV despite
  optimal therapy
Cardiac index <2 L/min/m²
Right atrial pressure >15 mm Hg
Mean pulmonary artery pressure >55 mm Hg

Based on the International Guidelines for the Selection of Lung
Transplant Candidates.

However, supplemental oxygen does improve survival in such COPD patients. Thus, once treated with long-term oxygen, the prognostic value of pulmonary function and arterial blood gas results alone may diminish.

The current UNOS statistics reveal a 1-, 3-, and 5-year posttransplantation survival rate of 80.8%, 62.5%, and 41.8%, respectively, for patients with COPD. Given the relatively limited long-term survival at 5 years after lung transplantation, patients with COPD should undergo this procedure only when their disease is far advanced with a high risk of disease-related mortality. The current recommendation for listing patients with COPD for lung transplantation is when their postbronchodilator FEV_1 is significantly less than 20% to 25% of predicted, $PaCO_2$ is greater than 55 mm Hg, or there is elevated pulmonary artery pressure combined with overall progressive clinical deterioration; these findings potentially identify the group with a high risk for COPD-related mortality. Despite these current recommendations, given the significant variability in survival for patients with COPD, further studies are warranted to better define the subgroup of patients who will best benefit from lung transplantation.

■ IDIOPATHIC PULMONARY FIBROSIS

Idiopathic pulmonary fibrosis (IPF) is an interstitial lung disease process characterized by progressive parenchymal scarring and loss of pulmonary function. Despite aggressive

medical therapy, IPF is associated with poor long-term prognosis. The disease almost universally progresses, and the goal of treatment is to minimize the progression from inflammation to fibrosis. Unfortunately, only about 10% to 30% of patients will demonstrate a clinical response to medical therapy, specifically with high-dose oral corticosteroids or cytotoxic drugs such as cyclophosphamide. Response to therapy can be predicted according to histopathology. Patients with diffuse scarring (usual interstitial pneumonia) carry a worse prognosis than alveolitis without extensive scarring.

Poor outcome is associated with male gender, low predicted forced vital capacity (FVC) and total lung capacity, low predicted diffusing capacity, and diffuse fibrosis on chest radiograph.

The International Guidelines acknowledge the difficulty in predicting the course of disease for patients with IPF and emphasize that this group has the poorest survival rate compared with all other diseases while waiting on the transplant list. The guidelines recommend early referral for any patient with IPF and pulmonary function abnormalities, even though they may be minimally symptomatic. Because this group has the highest mortality rate while awaiting transplantation, they are given a credit of 90 days of waiting time on the list, being the only group to receive such a preference.

Pulmonary fibrosis also occurs in the setting of systemic diseases such as sarcoidosis, collagen vascular diseases, and occupation-related lung disease and as an adverse effect of many drug treatments, including cancer chemotherapy. There are limited data in this group of patients that help to identify who will progress to end-stage lung disease, thus identifying potential candidates for lung transplantation is difficult at disease onset. However, it is suggested that patients with fibrotic lung disease who develop severe lung restriction early, and especially hypoxemia, appear to have a poor disease course. Accordingly, these patients should be considered for lung transplantation. It is important to note that the presence of systemic disease, such as sarcoidosis or collagen vascular disease, if quiescent, is not necessarily a contraindication to lung transplantation at many centers.

■ PULMONARY ARTERIAL HYPERTENSION WITHOUT CONGENITAL HEART DISEASE

For patients with primary pulmonary hypertension (PPH), survival, if left untreated, is around 60% at 2 years, with a median of 2.8 years. Establishing the diagnosis of PPH does not necessarily warrant immediate referral for lung transplant evaluation. Although some centers advocate listing patients shortly after a diagnosis of PPH, others argue that a therapeutic trial with vasodilators and anticoagulation must first be instituted, using results considered for any transplant decision. Patients who respond acutely to vasodilator trial have improved survival with oral calcium channel blockers, anticoagulants, or intravenous prostacyclin. Intravenous prostacyclin also improves hemodynamics and survival in patients who do not show a favorable acute response to vasodilators. Hence, for patients who respond well clinically to prostacyclin, the optimal timing of lung transplantation is not presently known.

For patients who do not stabilize or who deteriorate on medical therapy, transplant referral is indicated. In addition to the hemodynamic profile, it is advisable to consider the patient's functional status, as survival is related to the NYHA functional class. For patients who remain in NYHA classes I and II, median survival is nearly 6 years, whereas the survival for NYHA class III and IV is substantially worse.

Therefore, the optimal time for lung transplantation and the overall clinical and hemodynamic picture must be assessed for each patient, considering functional status, response to medical therapy, and cardiac catheterization findings.

The International Guidelines propose a cardiac index of less than 2 L/min/m^2, a right atrial pressure of more than 15 mm Hg, and a mean pulmonary artery pressure greater than 55 mm Hg as useful markers for failure of optimal pretransplantation medical therapy. Finally, early transplant referral is recommended for patients with pulmonary venoocclusive disease and chronic thromboembolic pulmonary hypertension not amenable to surgical thromboendarterectomy. Both of these diseases are associated with secondary pulmonary hypertension and do not respond well to medical therapy.

■ PULMONARY HYPERTENSION WITH CONGENITAL HEART DISEASE

Both lung transplantation with cardiac repair and combined heart-lung transplantation are offered for pulmonary hypertension secondary to congenital heart disease, or Eisenmenger's syndrome. However, the need for transplantation as a lifesaving measure may not be required for many years after diagnosis, because this group has a better survival for a given level of pulmonary artery pressure compared with other types of pulmonary hypertension. Many patients will respond well to nontransplant surgical or medical management. Selecting patients who may benefit from lung transplantation is based primarily on progression of symptoms such as increasing dyspnea, hemoptysis, dizziness, syncope, chest pain, arrhythmia, cyanosis, or refractory hypoxemia with polycythemia despite optimal medical management.

■ CYSTIC FIBROSIS AND BRONCHIECTASIS

CF is a multisystem disease affecting the lung with chronic suppuration causing bronchiectatic obstructive disease. It is the leading cause of end-stage obstructive lung disease in the first 3 decades of life and the most common indication for double/bilateral lung transplantation in the United States. Due to chronic bacterial colonization of the lungs, bilateral lung transplantation is required for CF and other diseases causing generalized bronchiectasis. Because the waiting period for bilateral versus single lung transplantation may be longer, this must be factored into decisions regarding the appropriate time to list patients with CF. Other factors to consider for patients with CF include body weight, pulmonary function, exercise tolerance, gas exchange, bacterial colonization, and frequency of exacerbations and hospitalizations.

General criteria for referral of patients with CF were developed based on data that documented a 2-year survival of approximately 50% when lung function studies revealed significant reductions of FEV$_1$ and FVC coupled with hypoxemia, hypercapnea, and weight loss. Specifically, an FEV$_1$ less than 30% predicted was associated with a 50% 2-year mortality rate, suggesting this value as a marker for transplant consideration. Other studies confirm these prognostic data, although some reports refute this contention and suggest that reliance on the FEV$_1$ alone prematurely exposes patients to the risk of lung transplantation, resulting in an overall decreased survival. Those who argue against relying solely on FEV$_1$ propose that an individualized comprehensive assessment, including rate of FEV$_1$ decline, oxygen requirement, gender, frequency of hospitalization, bacterial colonization, body mass index, and quality of life, might better serve to guide the timing of lung transplantation.

Diseases other than CF that can cause bronchiectatic lung disease include dysfunctional and immotile cilia syndromes, lung infection, and immunodeficiency syndromes. Data are inadequate to make specific recommendations regarding the timing and candidacy of these patients for lung transplantation.

■ SUMMARY

The success of lung transplantation depends on the selection of suitable candidates based on age, general health considerations, and poor prognosis for survival with medical and nontransplant surgical therapy. The goals of lung transplantation are to prolong life and to improve the patient's quality of life. To optimize these goals, an understanding of patient and disease-specific characteristics that affect survival is crucial. The data regarding the natural history of lung diseases that progress to advanced stage are limited and the relevance of older studies is regularly questioned in light of new therapies that alter disease prognosis. It is a continuing challenge for medical care providers and lung transplant teams to integrate these complex issues and to select patients who will survive the requisite waiting period without being prematurely exposed to the risks associated with transplantation. The appropriate candidate has end-stage lung disease in the absence of other illnesses that may adversely affect posttransplant survival or function. A projected life expectancy of less than 2 years, usually marked by NYHA functional class III or IV, indicates the need for transplantation. With optimal timing and posttransplantation care, lung transplantation patients can receive the maximal benefit that this therapeutic option has to offer.

SUGGESTED READING

Arcasoy SM, Kotloff RM: Lung transplantation (review), *N Engl J Med* 340:1081, 1999.

Hosenpud JD, et al: The registry of the International Society for Heart and Lung Transplantation: eighteenth official report—2001, *J Heart Lung Transplant* 20:805, 2001.

Maurer J, et al: International guidelines for the selection of lung transplant candidates, *J Heart Lung Transplant* 17:703, 1998.

Studer SM, Orens JB: Optimal timing of lung transplantation in end-stage lung disease, *Clin Pulm Med* 7:97, 2000.

Trulock EP: Lung transplantation (review), *Am J Respir Crit Care Med* 155:789, 1997.

LUNG TRANSPLANTATION—SURGICAL OPTIONS AND APPROACHES

Taine T.V. Pechet

Ken C. Stewart

G. Alexander Patterson

Lung transplantation has evolved to become an important therapeutic option for patients with advanced lung disease. Data from the International Society of Heart and Lung Transplantation registry indicate that worldwide activity has reached a plateau of approximately 1300 cases per year. Meanwhile, the number of patients listed for transplantation continues to increase steadily. Lack of suitable donors and chronic graft dysfunction are the most significant barriers to further advances with this clinical endeavor.

The field of lung transplantation has evolved considerably since the first transplant in 1963. Dramatic strides have been made, and the expected 5-year survival now reaches 60%. Much of this success may be attributed to improvements in the pharmacology of immune modulation and advances in donor organ preservation, but major strides have also been made in surgical techniques. The criteria for selecting appropriate candidates for lung transplantation have been covered in "Preoperative Evaluation of the Lung Transplant Candidate." This review focuses on the operative strategies that have evolved during the past two decades and the techniques currently used at Washington University.

■ LUNG TRANSPLANT OPERATIONS

Selection of Operation

Determination of the appropriate transplant operation is dependent on the underlying disease and individual patient factors. Specific patient considerations include disease-related impact on intrathoracic dimensions (e.g., small hemithorax with idiopathic pulmonary fibrosis [IPF], cardiomegaly in pulmonary hypertensive vascular disorders); blood group and size matching; waiting list ranking; location of the donor; and what organs are available for transplantation. Active coordination with the team performing the donor recovery operation is required to minimize graft ischemic time. Anticipated difficulty with recipient pneumonectomy procedures should be considered when coordinating operative schedules.

Current options for lung transplantation include single-lung transplantation (SLT), bilateral sequential single lung (BLT), partitioning of single cadaveric lung for SLT or BLT, living donor lobar transplantation, and combined heart-lung transplantation. This discussion will focus on SLT and BLT only. Double lung transplantation (tracheal anastomosis with complete left atrial cuff and main pulmonary artery [PA] anastomosis) has been replaced with BLT because of ease of performance and reduction in airway anastomotic complications. BLT is mandatory for patients with suppurative lung disease (cystic fibrosis, bronchiectasis) to remove the focus of sepsis and minimize contamination of the allograft. Patients with obstructive, pulmonary hypertensive and fibrotic diseases are candidates for either SLT or BLT. In most cases, BLT is favored particularly in the younger, larger recipient; however, organ allocation, ischemic time, and operative feasibility are important considerations. In addition to a theoretical advantage of improved functional reserve and an opportunity to utilize marginal donors, there are increasing data to suggest improved long-term survival with BLT. In our experience, early gas exchange and long-term survival are superior in the bilateral transplant recipients. ICU management is simplified, and there is a better functional result.

The choice of which lung to transplant in SLT should be guided principally by donor organ availability. Prior theories favoring right-sided grafts, particularly for emphysema, have not been borne out. Recipient characteristics, such as mediastinal deviation, must also be considered. If proceeding with BLT, the choice of which lung to replace first is guided initially by donor factors. Significant trauma or atelectasis in the graft will impair gas exchange during implantation of the second lung. Provided both donor lungs are of equivalent quality, the decision is dictated by the preoperative ventilation/perfusion scan. Replacing the lung with the worst function first provides for improved gas exchange during the period of single lung ventilation and minimizes the chance of requiring cardiopulmonary bypass (CPB). If all other factors remain equal, right lung transplantation is technically less demanding.

Anesthetic Considerations

When possible, preoperative placement of an epidural catheter is placed for analgesia but may be contraindicated if CPB is contemplated. Intubation with a double-lumen endotracheal tube (ETT) provides independent lung ventilation and access for pulmonary toilet. Invasive hemodynamic monitoring with arterial (radial and femoral) and Swan-Ganz catheter placement is mandatory. Transesophageal echocardiography (TEE) is invaluable for intraoperative evaluation of cardiac function. TEE is of particular value in assessing right heart function during PA clamping and to assess response to inotropic and vasoactive medications. Inhaled nitric oxide (NO) and infusible prostaglandin E_1 have been shown to decrease lung allograft reperfusion injury and are frequently used in experienced programs. Broad-spectrum antibiotics are given preoperatively. Patients with suppurative lung conditions receive antibiotics based on preoperative sputum cultures and sensitivities.

Cardiopulmonary Bypass

CPB may be required at any point during the operation. Both recipient factors and surgeon preference predicate the use of CPB during transplantation. CPB is used routinely for pediatric patients undergoing BLT who are too small to accept a double-lumen ETT and for patients undergoing concomitant cardiac defect repair and lung transplantation (e.g., atrial septal defect closure and lung transplantation for pulmonary hypertension secondary to Eisenmenger's syndrome). Although we disagree, some authors suggest the routine use of CPB during conduct of the second recipient pneumonectomy to minimize exposure time of the first allograft to the entire cardiac output.

CPB is used selectively in adults. At Washington University, CPB is instituted in 98% of pediatric patients with cystic fibrosis compared with only 15% of adults. In our experience, the most common indications for institution of CPB are pulmonary hypertension or dysfunction of the first graft during conduct of the second pneumonectomy. The PA is always test clamped and pressures monitored before native lung removal. In addition to pulmonary hypertension, indications to institute CPB are hypercarbia (often the result of poor native lung ventilation resulting from excess secretions), persistent hypoxemia, hemodynamic instability during mediastinal manipulation, and progressive deterioration of right ventricular function. TEE is particularly useful for monitoring right ventricular function and guiding the decision to use CPB.

If CPB is required, access can be obtained without altering the choice of incision. During right SLT or BLT, the ascending aorta and right atrial appendage can be cannulated. We use a 7-mm Terumo-Sarnes (3M, Ann Arbor, MI) aortic and 36/46 dual stage Baxter (Baxter, Middale, UT) venous cannula. During left SLT, the descending aorta and main PA can be accessed. Alternatively, the femoral vessels are accessed. Aprotinin is used in all cases and has been shown to minimize transfusion requirements.

Patient Positioning and Incision

The choice of patient position must allow for safe pneumonectomy and exposure of hilar structures for implantation and facilitate CPB if required. Lung transplantation can be performed through median sternotomy, posterolateral thoracotomy, anterolateral thoracotomy, or bilateral anterior thoracosternotomy or "clamshell" incision. We routinely use the anterolateral approach for SLT or BLT. The patient is placed supine, arms tucked at the side (Figure 1). Our standard incision is an anterolateral skin incision, with division of the fourth interspace intercostal muscles with posterior muscle-sparing extension. The fifth interspace may be used in patients who have hyperinflated chests and relatively inferiorly located hilar structures (preoperative CXR may help guide the selection of incision). This patient position and incision with side-to-side rotation of the operating table afford excellent exposure of each hemithorax.

For bilateral procedures, we use the same incision on the contralateral side. The sternum is not routinely divided so as to avoid wound healing complications and discomfort associated with malunion (Figure 1, inset), while providing adequate hilar visualization and the ability to dissect extensive adhesions. Entering the chest in the fourth interspace with division of the fourth costochondral cartilage permits good visualization in most patients. It is frequently necessary to divide the internal thoracic artery to gain adequate medial access, and the intercostal muscles can be divided internally to the posterior axillary line. A medium Finochietto retractor

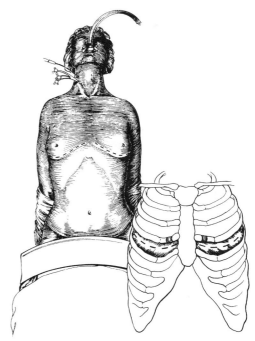

Figure 1
Patient positioning for standard anterolateral thoracotomy. One centimeter of costal cartilage (shaded) is removed for further mobility and exposure. (*Copyright 1999 with permission from W. B. Saunders Company.*)

to distract the ribs and a Balfour retractor at right angles have proved to be the optimal combination of retractors. Rarely, we use selective division of the sternum (clamshell, crossbow, or anterior thoracosternotomy approach) for extended exposure. Even cardiac procedures combined with BLT can frequently be accomplished with bilateral anterolateral thoracotomies.

A decision for alternative incision placement is based on anatomic considerations of significant lung volume loss in one hemithorax, making the anterolateral approach impractical because of rotation and displacement of the mediastinum. Posterolateral incisions can be used in this situation. If a bilateral procedure is anticipated, the procedure through the posterolateral incision is undertaken first, typically followed by repositioning to the supine position for the second, anterolateral incision.

Recipient Pneumonectomy

Ventilation to the lung is stopped, and the tubing is disconnected to facilitate deflation. Many patients have had prior pleural interventions, and an increasing number of emphysema patients have undergone lung volume reduction surgery. It is important during conduct of the recipient pneumonectomy to avoid parenchymal injuries. Large air leaks can impair gas exchange during single lung ventilation. Prior procedures and extensive pleural adhesions can also make preservation of the phrenic nerves more difficult. Care should be taken to preserve the vagus nerves, thereby minimizing impaired gastric function and the risk of postoperative aspiration. Meticulous hemostasis is also critical, particularly in patients likely to require CPB. If time permits, preliminary dissection of the second lung is undertaken before arrival of the donor organs. This minimizes overall ischemic time, as well as time during which the first allograft is exposed to the entire cardiac output. Some recipients, however, will not tolerate single lung ventilation or the manipulation required for lung mobilization, mandating a delay in dissection until the first graft is functioning. When BLT is performed, the lung with the worst perfusion is replaced first, maximizing function of the best native lung during implantation.

Once the PA has been circumferentially mobilized and test clamped, the upper lobe branch is ligated and divided. The main trunk can be divided with a vascular stapler (either endo-GIA or TA-30 with ligation of the distal artery). The PA should be divided at least 1 cm distal to the first branch. The length can be further tailored at the time of anastomosis.

The superior and inferior pulmonary veins are mobilized and the segmental branches ligated and divided. We prefer to maintain as much venous length as possible. Compromising the size of the atrial cuff can be a difficult problem to overcome, and excess length can always be trimmed before performing the anastomosis. After division of the vascular structures, the peribronchial tissue is divided with electrocautery. Large bronchial arteries and the posterior bronchial tissue that often includes the intercostal bronchial artery should be ligated after division of the bronchus. This dissection can be tedious in patients with suppurative lung disease, and hemostasis, particularly in the subcarinal region, is critical. Dissection lateral to the

main stem bronchus must be minimized, and a maximal amount of peribronchial vascularized tissue preserved. The bronchus is divided proximal to the upper lobe branch with a scalpel. If extensive peribronchial inflammation is present, the upper lobe branches can be divided separately and the bronchus trimmed after the lung has been removed. A silk traction suture is placed at the anterior apex of the cartilaginous ring. Small Duvall lung clamps are placed on the pulmonary vessels, and complete mobilization from the pericardium is accomplished with sharp dissection (Figure 2).

Once the recipient pneumonectomy is complete, the hilum is prepared for graft implantation. A complete pericardial release is performed, staying close to the pulmonary veins. If the anterior pericardium on the left side is initially left intact, the left atrial appendage is restrained and does not interfere with the bronchial or PA anastomosis. After the PA has been circumferentially freed of the pericardium, a large Duvall clamp is affixed to the PA stump and retracted superiorly and anteriorly with heavy silk. Two small Duvall clamps are used to retract the superior and inferior vein stumps anteriorly and inferiorly. A silk stitch through the midpoint of the bronchial cartilage will help distract the bronchus from the mediastinum. In the patient with a small chest cavity, it is often helpful to fashion a retractor to maintain caudal positioning of the diaphragm. A wide malleable one, measured and bent, can be fixed between anterior and posterior intercostal spaces for this purpose. A final inspection for hemostasis is performed at this juncture.

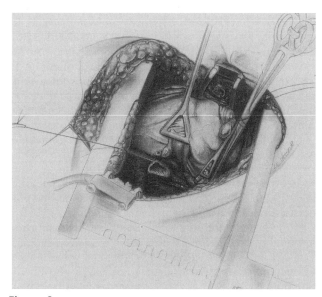

Figure 2
Exposure obtained after recipient pneumonectomy with self-retaining retractors (Finochietto and Balfour) and clamps on pulmonary artery (large Duvall clamp) and pulmonary veins (two small Duvall clamps), and stay suture on bronchus. (*Copyright 1999 with permission from W. B. Saunders Company.*)

Donor Lung Preparation

We favor organ recovery en bloc, including the thoracic aorta and esophagus. After visual and manual inspection of the lungs and minimal preliminary dissection, the PA is cannulated with a Sarnes-Terumo aortic cannula (usually 6.5 mm) directed toward the valve to equally distribute the flush. Immediately before aortic cross-clamping, prostaglandin E_1 is injected directly into the PA and then low potassium dextran (LPD) is flushed antegrade. LPD is superior to Eurocollins in both experimental and human lung transplants. After cardiac explantation, LPD is also flushed retrograde. This provides superior preservation of the bronchial circulation and often flushes the PA of debris and clot. The trachea is then clamped at end-tidal volume to avoid overinflation with resulting pulmonary capillary endothelial injury and pulmonary edema.

The lungs are typically removed en bloc. During transport and preparation, the lungs are kept cool with saline and ice solution surrounding them. The first step in preparing the donor lungs for implantation is to dissect and discard the esophagus and aorta. At all stages, it is crucial to preserve the lymphovascular tissue surrounding the airway and to maintain topical cooling. The posterior wall of the left atrium is then divided in the midpoint, the pericardium divided, and the PA divided at the bifurcation. The left main stem bronchus is detached flush with the carina, leaving the carina with the right lung block. The PA is dissected free of surrounding tissues to expose the first upper lobe branch. The left PA is dissected free from hilar tissues so that the first apical branch is free. On the right, the anterior trunk to the upper lobe is dissected free of mediastinal and hilar tissue. The atrial cuff is prepared by exposing the branches and dividing the investing pericardium to allow increased mobility.

The bronchus should be dissected free of the surrounding lymphatic tissue only to the point of transection. In general, we shorten the bronchus to leave two rings proximal to the upper lobe orifice. This location minimizes the length of the relatively ischemic donor airway (the blood supply to the allograft airway is dependent on retrograde blood flow from the pulmonary circulation). An anastomosis here facilitates placement of an airway stent, should the need arise, that can straddle the anastomosis and maintain patency of the lobar bronchi. The longer the donor main stem bronchus, the greater is the risk of ischemia and necrosis. Swabs of the bronchus are taken for Gram stain, culture, and sensitivities. The airway is cleared of ice and sputum by suctioning with a soft catheter.

Size matching of the donor lungs is of utmost importance. Oversized lung grafts may result in mediastinal compression or shift with possible hemodynamic compromise; significant atelectasis, pulmonary toilet, and subsequent infection are also concerns. There are many options available for managing oversized donors. Often, the chest of a patient with emphysema will accommodate larger lungs than expected. Several techniques for pneumoreduction have also been described; these range from anatomic lobectomy to multiple peripheral wedge resections in a "haircut" fashion using a stapling device. Tissue sealants may be helpful in reducing postoperative air leaks in this setting.

Undersized lungs may present a postoperative pleural space problem with either prolonged air leaks or infection. Overdistention of alveoli may lead to early closure of small airways with resultant air trapping and obstructive physiology. To help minimize this risk, we leave the anterior chest tube open to air during the immediate postoperative period of mechanical ventilation in these patients.

Allograft Implantation

The lung is correctly oriented in the chest and kept cold using topical application of saline slush or a cooling jacket. Allograft warming contributes to postoperative lung injury, and strict adherence to this step reduces the incidence of reperfusion injury. Small chest cavities make this a challenging proposition, but placement of a malleable diaphragmatic retractor greatly aids in this endeavor. We conduct the implantation in a posterior to anterior fashion, beginning with the airway and finishing with the atrial anastomosis.

The airway anastomosis is addressed first. We construct an end-to-end bronchial anastomosis but permit spontaneous intussusception of donor into recipient if there is a size mismatch favoring it. We no longer use telescoped anastomoses because they result in the highest incidence of bronchial stenosis. After the creation of a posterior pericardial layer (see later), the opposing cartilaginous–membranous junctions are approximated with two 4-0 polydioxanone sutures (PDS; Ethicon, Somerville, NJ). These are tied, and one length is used to sew the membranous portion of the airway in a running fashion, and then tied to the opposing corner stitch. The cartilaginous portion of the airway is closed with interrupted 4-0 PDS sutures (either figure of eight or simple stitches). The airway is suctioned clean with a catheter introduced through the ETT lumen, and the sutures are tied. The anterior portion of the peribronchial tissue is secured together with the same suture used on the posterior layer. If the airways are small (a frequent problem on the left side), we will use interrupted simple sutures rather than the figure of eight technique.

The use of omental or muscle flaps to cover the airway anastomosis provides suture line protection, containment of airway fistulas, and vascular inflow, which shortens the time required for donor bronchial neovascularization. This was important during the early days of lung transplant when graft preservation techniques were crude and immunosuppression imprecise. Techniques for direct bronchial artery revascularization have not gained widespread acceptance. The simplest coverage, and the one we favor, is the peribronchial/pericardial tissue flap. Before constructing the airway anastomosis, the peribronchial donor lymphatic tissue is sutured to the posterior recipient peribronchial tissue and free pericardial edge with 4-0 PDS. Then, after completion of the bronchial anastomosis, the running suture is continued anteriorly to completely cover and isolate the suture line.

Next the PA is clamped with a small Satinsky clamp. The clamp is secured to the chest wall with a silk suture to reduce tension on the anastomosis and stabilize the PA. The recipient and donor arteries are cut to a length that will prevent kinking of the vessel. The PA is trimmed, usually proximal to the first branch. The recipient PA can be sized to match the donor PA. Length is also a critical factor, because a donor PA segment that is too long can lead to kinking and obstruction. A 5-0 Prolene (Ethicon) continuous running suture is used to construct the anastomosis in standard vascular fashion. The intersuture distance is kept to a minimum to prevent "pursestringing" and stenosis of the anastomosis as it is tightened and secured. The PA should be deaired before completion of the suture line.

Last, the left atrial anastomosis is fashioned. The pericardium is opened circumferentially, and the recipient left atrium is clamped with a Satinsky clamp that in turn is securely closed with an umbilical tape to prevent unexpected release. With this maneuver, the patient may develop transient hypotension or atrial arrhythmias. If the donor cuff has been trimmed too short on the right, dissection of the interatrial groove may help provide adequate length for clamp placement. Institution of CPB remains another option. After ensuring hemodynamic stability, ligatures are removed from venous stumps, and the atrium is carefully opened longitudinally along a line that bisects the venous branches. The left atrial cuff of the allograft is then anastomosed to the common pulmonary vein or left atrium of the recipient using a running 4-0 Prolene suture. Care is taken to achieve endomyocardial approximation and to exclude any muscle edges from the anastomotic line to prevent possible thrombosis. In addition, one should avoid excessive length of the donor cuff, which may cause kinking and venous obstruction. Before completing the anastomosis, it is imperative to flush the atrium with cold saline to deair. The use of blow-by CO_2 across the field may minimize the risk of intracardiac air.

The highest point of the anastomosis is left open, the allograft is gently inflated through the ETT, and the PA clamp is partially released to flush perfusate and air out of the allograft pulmonary veins. The PA clamp is closed again, and the left atrial clamp is partially released to allow venting of the graft of any intravascular debris or air. After deairing, the suture is tightened, and then tied. The PA is slowly unclamped and the allograft inflated. The anastomoses are examined. Small sponges can be safely placed temporarily around the hilar structures to augment hemostasis. Cauterizing the cut edges of the pericardium on the allograft helps ensure hemostasis.

If the donor atrial cuff has been taken with the heart during procurement, the donor veins will tend to retract into the hilum. In cases of extremely short vein stumps, the veins may be sutured to the perivascular tissue and pericardium in the donor hilum; then the donor pericardium sutured to the recipient atrial cuff. Alternatively, if the donor cuff is short in only one comer, typically the right inferior vein, it may be possible to join the two stumps to provide a common cuff. A common cuff provides superior flow characteristics compared with individual venous anastomosis.

At this point in the operation, 1000 mg of methylprednisolone is administered before reperfusion of the lung, and prostaglandin E_1 should be infusing at 0.02 μg/min. We do not use NO routinely. If the donor lungs were judged of marginal quality or if there is any evidence of immediate reperfusion injury, NO is started. After the atrial suture line has been completed, and before tying the suture, the atria must be carefully deaired and the residual pulmoplege

flushed from the graft. The pericardial edges and all suture lines are carefully policed for hemostasis at this juncture. There have been some data suggesting that a slow, controlled release of the PA clamp may ameliorate reperfusion injury, but we do not routinely use any special techniques.

The chest is closed in a standard fashion. Before approximating the ribs, an anteroapically directed 28 Fr chest tube and an angled 28 Fr tube along the diaphragm are placed. Four figure of eight #2 Prolene pericostal sutures are used, and the chest layers are approximated.

■ RESULTS

Operative and in-hospital mortality and morbidity rates are similar to those of other major thoracic surgical procedures in high-risk patients. In experienced centers, operative mortality is typically less than 5%, and 30-day mortality is less than 5%. Significant improvements in short-term success with this procedure have been accomplished since its inception resulting in 1-year survival rates of 76%. Current 5-year survival rates are approximately 45%. Despite these seemingly disappointing results, most patients enjoy a significant improvement in quality of life and increased survivorship.

Significant contributors to morbidity and mortality include ischemia-reperfusion injury (IRI), infection, and chronic allograft dysfunction. Short- and long-term complications are covered in "Complications Following Lung Transplantation." Clinically significant IRI occurs in 15% of lung transplant recipients, despite advances in preservation techniques and immediate postoperative treatment. This acute lung injury is due to an interaction of activated neutrophils with injured pulmonary vascular endothelium. It is usually apparent within 12 hours of transplantation. IRI is characterized clinically as noncardiogenic pulmonary edema. Increasing ischemic time, elevated storage temperature, high storage F_{IO_2}, and lung hyperinflation during transport worsen the pulmonary endothelial injury. Treatment is initially supportive, with increasing oxygen concentration, positive end-expiratory pressure, sedation and muscle paralysis, aggressive diuresis, and inotropic support. Inhaled NO improves gas exchange and pulmonary hemodynamics in patients with severe IRI. Selective use of extracorporeal membrane oxygenation may be employed in severe situations but will be successful only if applied early in the evolution of the lung injury.

■ SUMMARY

Lung transplantation has emerged as a viable, widely available therapy in the treatment of patients with end-stage pulmonary disease. Excellent results can be achieved with attention to technical detail and appropriate operative strategies. Although a wide range of tactics are available, minimizing ischemic time, maintaining allograft hypothermia, achieving technical perfection in the conduct of vascular anastomosis, and taking a simple approach to the bronchus highlight the areas critical to achieving a successful outcome.

SUGGESTED READING

Egan T: Lung size and impact on transplantation. In Cooper D, et al, editors: *Transplantation and replacement of thoracic organs,* Kluwer Academic Publishers, Hingham, MA, 1996.

Meyers BF, Patterson GA: Bilateral lung transplantation, *Oper Tech Thorac Cardiovasc Surg* 4:162, 1999.

Meyers B, et al: Lung transplantation: a decade of experience, *Ann Surg* 230:362, 1999.

Sundaresan S, et al: Donor lung procurement: assessment and operative technique, *Ann Thorac Surg* 56:1409, 1993.

Trulock EP: Lung transplantation, *Am J Respir Crit Care Med* 155:789, 1997.

COMPLICATIONS FOLLOWING LUNG TRANSPLANTATION

Joseph C. Cleveland, Jr

Martin R. Zamora

Frederick L. Grover

Lung transplantation offers an effective therapeutic option for patients with end-stage pulmonary parenchymal or vascular disease. Evolution of surgical techniques, immunosuppressive medications, and cumulative experience with the management of lung transplant patients has significantly advanced this therapy during the past decade. Complications after lung transplantation, however, remain problematic and contribute significantly to the postoperative mortality and morbidity. The purpose of this chapter is to review the categories of complications after lung transplantation and to address their prevention and management.

Complications after lung transplantation are broadly categorized as follows: perioperative, bronchial or vascular anastomotic complications, acute allograft rejection, obliterative bronchiolitis (OB), complications of immunosuppressive medications, infectious, and nonpulmonary organ system complications. As a general principle, prevention of these complications is often possible with diligent and meticulous preoperative, intraoperative, and postoperative attention to detail.

Appropriate recipient selection and appropriate donor selection remain critical in avoiding complications. The thoracic transplant surgeon should be an integral component of the recipient selection process, and a close working relationship with his or her pulmonary colleagues is vital to ensure appropriate patient selection. The decision to accept a "lung offer" is equally as important, and this decision lies with both the implanting thoracic surgeon and the pulmonary physician. The donor lung is not finally "accepted" until a thoracic surgeon has evaluated the donor with bronchoscopy and visual inspection of the lung. In general, we mandate that both lungs be pristine for bilateral lung transplantation requiring cardiopulmonary bypass, whereas we are willing to accept a normal-appearing contralateral lung for single-lung transplantation when the other lung is damaged (e.g., contusion or aspiration). Due to the risk of severe barotrauma, we have also avoided lungs from donors who have a history of strangulation or hanging. With the appropriate matching of donor and recipient, the first and most serious complication—that of donor/recipient mismatch—can be avoided.

■ PERIOPERATIVE COMPLICATIONS

Although many of the complications outlined in this chapter occur in the perioperative period, there are two that are related to the procedure itself: ischemia-reperfusion injury (IRI) and acute native lung hyperinflation (ANLH), which occurs in the case of single-lung transplantation for emphysema. In the first several hours after lung transplantation, worsening graft function, impaired gas exchange, and pulmonary edema may occur as a manifestation of IRI. Clinically, this entity may mimic vascular compromise, primary graft nonfunction, volume overload, and poor graft preservation. In a minority of cases, this syndrome may progress to severe lung injury such that independent lung ventilation, inhaled nitric oxide (NO), or extracorporeal membrane oxygenation (ECMO) may be necessary. A variety of strategies have been used to reduce IRI, including controlled, progressive reperfusion, antibodies directed against neutrophil adhesion molecules, anticomplement agents, or inhaled NO. Most strategies have shown some efficacy but none are completely preventive.

ANLH occurs after single-lung transplantation for emphysema as the result of the difference in compliance between the overly compliant native lung and the transplanted lung. Positive pressure ventilation may lead to overdistention of the emphysematous lung with resulting barotrauma and cardiovascular instability. ANLH has been reported to occur in up to 42% of procedures and is associated with increased mortality. It has been reported to occur in patients with preoperative forced expiratory volume in 1 second (FEV$_1$) of less than 15%, preoperative pulmonary hypertension, and in the face of severe graft dysfunction. We found that ANLH is indeed common radiographically; however, if recognized, it is rarely associated with severe cardiovascular compromise or mortality. Strategies to prevent ANLH include the use of small tidal volumes, low respiratory rates, and prolonged inspiratory-to-expiratory ratios to allow complete emptying of the emphysematous lung. If there is little evidence of reperfusion injury, early extubation is the preferred method to treat ANLH.

■ AIRWAY COMPLICATIONS

Airway complications after lung transplantation remain prevalent. The initial attempts at single- or en bloc double-lung transplantation were unsuccessful due to disruption of the airway anastomosis. While it is increasingly uncommon to witness bronchial dehiscence with the single or bilateral sequential procedure, bronchial anastomotic complications occur in 5% to 15% of lung transplant patients. Several groups have reported their experiences with airway complications. The complications include stenoses, bronchomalacia, granulation tissue, infection, and dehiscence. Interestingly, in modern series describing airway anastomotic complications, the presence of an airway complication did not adversely affect short-term survival. Airway complications can appear as soon as 7 days after transplantation or several weeks to even years after transplantation. Several hypotheses are offered to explain the incidence of airway complications. Ischemia of the donor bronchus is the most likely reason for anastomotic airway complications. Lung transplantation is the only solid organ transplant in which the systemic arterial blood supply is not reattached at the time of transplantation. Therefore, until collateral bronchial artery revascularization occurs, the donor bronchus remains dependent on pulmonary artery collateral circulation. Bronchial ischemia is accentuated by excessive donor bronchial length and excessive dissection or skeletonizing at the level of the anastomosis.

Other possible causes of airway anastomotic complications include rejection, immunosuppressive medications, infection, or poor organ preservation. Several different adjuncts to bronchial healing have been proposed to aid in bronchial healing. These include shortening the donor bronchus to one or two cartilaginous rings before the take-off of the upper lobe bronchus, and intussusception or "telescoping" the donor bronchus into the recipient bronchus. Reinforcing the anastomosis with vascularized tissue—such as intercostal muscle, omentum, and pericardial fat—is not necessary if the bronchus is left short and not skeletonized.

Treatment of airway complications is directed at the underlying problem. Treatment options include bronchodilation, stenting, laser débridement, or operative revision. Airway stenoses are first managed by bronchoscopy with balloon dilation. If the stenosis persists after repeated dilations, then the patient is a candidate for stent placement. The type of stent placed depends on the specific problem and the length of time the patient will require the stent. Silastic stents are preferred for early postoperative stenoses,

which likely require short-term remedies until such time that adequate healing or scarring occurs. For long-term use, most centers now favor metal stents, as silicone stents are easily dislodged. Similarly, bronchomalacia almost always requires the placement of a metal stent. Excessive granulation tissue can be treated with bronchoscopic laser débridement, and some have used localized radiotherapy with seed implants. Last, airway dehiscence historically was associated with a high mortality. The treatment and outcomes depend to a large degree on the severity of the dehiscence. Mild cases (less than one-fourth the circumference of the airway) may only require pleural drainage, antibiotics, and adequate nutritional supplementation to encourage healing. Larger dehiscences require operative revision.

Although airway anastomotic complications are not uncommon after lung transplantation, attention to meticulous surgical technique—in both procurement and implantation of the lung—will minimize these problems. Our center has stressed the importance of keeping the donor bronchus short, minimizing removal of peribronchial tissue on the recipient bronchus during dissection, and telescoping the donor bronchus. We also follow these patients closely with bronchoscopy during the early postoperative period to assess the anastomosis, remove mucus plugs, and obtain culture samples. Future directions to aid in bronchial anastomotic healing will likely include the use of growth or angiogenic factors.

■ VASCULAR ANASTOMOTIC COMPLICATIONS

Although airway anastomotic complications are fairly common after lung transplantation, both pulmonary arterial and pulmonary venous anastomoses are very uncommon. In our cumulative experience at the University of Colorado, we have had three vascular anastomotic complications in over 200 transplants performed. Our experience is similar to that reported by others in the literature: the incidence of these complications is roughly 1%. Recognition of these complications is more difficult, as the presentation of a vascular anastomotic problem can be subtle.

Pulmonary venous anastomotic complications often present in the early postoperative period and should be suspected clinically when the chest radiograph shows persistent pulmonary edema. This diagnosis may be difficult to differentiate from reperfusion injury, but if the radiograph shows persistent edema and the patient continues to have an unexplained oxygen requirement, a pulmonary arteriogram or transesophageal echocardiography (TEE) should be obtained. Pulmonary arteriography would show a delay in venous emptying if there is a pulmonary venous obstruction. Several authors have noted reliable, accurate imaging of the pulmonary veins with TEE, and this diagnostic option is desirable in that it is rapid and can be obtained at the bedside. However, at our institution, TEE has not proven reliable in definitively imaging this anastomosis. Almost all pulmonary venous obstructions require operative intervention. There are isolated case descriptions of stenting obstructed pulmonary veins with percutaneous techniques, but a frequent cause of the obstruction is excessive donor left atrium.

This excessive donor cuff "buckles" the anastomosis and should be remedied surgically.

Pulmonary arterial anastomotic complications can also present with a variable clinical course. Persistent pulmonary hypertension postoperatively, in the absence of significant graft injury, should warrant a nuclear perfusion scan. If the perfusion scan shows diminished perfusion to the transplanted lung, then a pulmonary arteriogram should be obtained. Therapy for pulmonary arterial stenoses includes balloon angioplasty, operative revision with patch angioplasty, or placement of a pulmonary homograft if the stenosis is at the origin of the main pulmonary artery. Consideration should be given to using cardiopulmonary bypass and intermittent, hypothermic blood perfusion of the lung during the period of pulmonary arterial clamping. Anecdotally, we have revised one pulmonary arterial anastomosis without cardiopulmonary bypass, but others have advocated its use to prevent an ischemic injury to the graft.

■ ACUTE ALLOGRAFT REJECTION

Acute allograft rejection after lung transplantation remains common and problematic. The lung remains vulnerable to a variety of immunologic insults, as it is the only transplanted solid organ that is subsequently exposed to the atmosphere. This exposes it to a variety of exogenous antigens, toxins, viruses, and microbial agents that nonspecifically activate the immune system. In addition, the transplanted lung allograft carries with it a significant number of immune effector cells. Acute rejection not only places the lung allograft at risk in the early posttransplantation period but also is a well-established risk factor for the development of OB or chronic rejection.

Acute allograft rejection can be diagnosed by either clinical or histologic criteria. Some centers report a 75% incidence of acute rejection. Clinically, acute rejection is manifested by dyspnea, low-grade fever, fatigue, a decrease in oxygenation of greater than 10 mm Hg below baseline, exercise desaturation, development of new infiltrates on chest radiograph, and a decrease in FEV_1 of greater than 10% below baseline. Acute rejection can be difficult to distinguish from infection. Bronchoscopy is performed to obtain tissue for histologic diagnosis and to obtain cultures to exclude infectious causes. The Lung Rejection Study Group created a histologic formulation to define acute rejection. The grading of rejection is based on the presence, quantity, and interstitial extension of acute perivascular lymphocytic infiltrates.

Acute allograft rejection is initially treated with high doses of intravenous corticosteroids. Our current protocol administers 10 to 15 mg/kg/day of methylprednisolone for 3 days, with or without a subsequent boost in the oral prednisone dose to 1 mg/kg/day followed by a taper. The maintenance immunosuppressive regimen is also changed: cyclosporine is changed to tacrolimus and azathioprine is changed to mycophenolate mofetil. Newer agents such as rapamycin are coming into clinical practice. Steroid resistant rejection is subsequently treated with cytolytic therapy (ATGAM, thymoglobulin, or OKT3) and/or plasmapheresis for severe forms of steroid-resistant acute rejection. It must be emphasized that evidence supports the hypothesis that acute rejection is a cell-mediated immunologic phenomenon, and conceptually one can then understand the basis for cytolytic therapy. Other modalities for steroid resistant rejection have included photopheresis and total lymphoid irradiation. Controversial issues in the prevention and monitoring of acute rejection are the use of induction immunosuppressive therapy with lympholytics or anti-CD25 antibodies and the use of surveillance bronchoscopy.

■ OBLITERATIVE BRONCHIOLITIS

The most challenging and problematic long-term complication after lung transplantation is OB. This phenomenon currently represents the greatest threat to the long-term survival of the lung allograft and the patient after lung transplantation. OB appears variably (35% at 3 years) and unpredictably after lung transplantation. Clinically, OB may follow a relentlessly progressive course, or there may be long periods of stabilization of pulmonary function interspersed with acute deteriorations. Histologically, OB is characterized by inflammation and bronchiectasis of large airways (bronchioles) with eventual fibrosis of the airway. Both infectious (predominantly viral) and immunologic based mechanisms have evidence to support their primary role in this process, but currently the pathogenesis and molecular mechanisms responsible for this disorder are incompletely characterized. Therapy for OB is disappointing, although high-dose steroids, OKT3 or ATG, photopheresis, and total lymphoid irradiation have been used with limited success. Retransplantation for OB is controversial given the limited number of donor lungs available and the generally poorer results of pulmonary retransplantation. Potential future modalities to treat OB include immune modulating agents such as rapamycin and locally applied antiproliferative agents.

■ INFECTION-RELATED COMPLICATIONS

Infection remains an important cause of morbidity and mortality after lung transplantation. One must include a broad differential diagnosis when a lung transplant patient is believed to harbor an infectious process because bacterial, viral, fungal, and mycobacterial infections are all possible. As a general guideline, the likely infectious agent can be linked to the length of time after transplantation. In the immediate postoperative period, gram-positive and gram-negative bacteria and fungi are the most frequently occurring infectious agents. These typically cause wound or line infections, pneumonia, and intraabdominal or urinary tract infections. *Staphylococcus* and *Streptococcus* species are the most common gram-positive isolates, and *Pseudomonas* species (especially in patients with cystic fibrosis), *Klebsiella*, and *Haemophilus influenzae* are the most common gram-negative pathogens. Cystic fibrosis patients present unique problems as they are frequently colonized with *Pseudomonas* species, including *Burkholderia cepacia*, which is often highly virulent, resistant to multiple antibiotics, and associated with decreased survival after lung transplantation. After the first 2 months posttransplant, cytomegalovirus (CMV) is the most important viral agent causing infection in the lung transplant population. Although it is now an uncommon outcome, early in the collective experience of lung transplantation, severe CMV-associated pneumonitis occurred, resulting in the death of numerous patients. In addition to its acute effects, CMV has been associated with the development of chronic rejection or OB. Therefore, a variety of strategies have been used for the prevention and monitoring of CMV after transplantation. Our CMV prophylactic regimen combines intravenous ganciclovir with CMV hyperimmune globulin (CytoGam). This has resulted in an overall attack rate of 25% in the first year versus the reported 35% to 65% incidence in the lung transplant literature. The ability to measure CMV DNA replication in blood has allowed the rapid diagnosis of CMV and the possibility of preemptive treatment. Other viral infections include herpes simplex viruses 6, 7, and 8, which are treated with acyclovir, and the community-acquired respiratory viruses such as the influenza viruses, parainfluenza, and respiratory syncytial virus, which may be associated with chronic graft failure and are treated with inhaled ribavirin. These viruses can be cultured from nasopharyngeal aspiration or bronchoscopically.

Fungal infections with *Candida albicans* and *Aspergillus* species remain common after lung transplantation. *Candida* species often colonize airways, and they can be difficult to identify as an invasive pathogen, but the presence of *Aspergillus* is generally more worrisome. *Aspergillus* is treated with inhaled or intravenous amphotericin B. We prefer liposomal amphotericin B in these patients to avoid enhanced renal toxicity with calcineurin inhibitors. The native lung can serve as a reservoir for pleural effusion in the setting of a single-lung transplant and may require operative therapy. Other fungal infections are caused by the endemic fungi cryptococcus, histoplasmdes, and coccidiodes.

Mycobacterial infections are fairly uncommon after lung transplantation but may be transmitted by the donor organ. *Nocardia* and *Pneumocystis carinii* infections are also uncommon in the face of trimethoprim-sulfamethoxazole prophylaxis. Late infections, occurring greater than 6 months posttransplant, depend on the degree of immunosuppression and the status of the graft. Patients with chronic graft dysfunction or OB may become colonized with *Pseudomonas* or fungi and are susceptible to viral infections.

■ IMMUNOSUPPRESSIVE, MEDICAL, AND NON–PULMONARY-RELATED COMPLICATIONS

Medical complications of immunosuppression after lung transplantation include hypertension, hyperlipidemia, bone marrow suppression, osteoporosis, renal insufficiency, neurologic or gastrointestinal disorders, and malignancy. Several warrant further discussion here.

Immunosuppression for solid organ transplant is associated with a 6% lifetime risk of developing a malignancy; either de novo or as recurrence of a preexisting malignant condition. For the purposes of this discussion, we will focus on posttransplant lymphoproliferative disorder (PTLD).

Lung transplant patients are at high risk of developing PTLD; with a reported incidence of 4% to 10%. There is a clear relationship between PTLD and the Epstein-Barr virus (EBV). Patients who are seronegative for EBV who subsequently develop primary infection in the face of immunosuppression are at greatest risk of developing PTLD. The lymphoproliferative cells are of B cell origin staining CD20 positive, may be polyclonal or monoclonal, and sometimes appear like immunoblastic lymphomas. The clinical presentation of PTLD in lung transplant patients shows a predilection toward appearance in the allograft and in the central nervous system. Therapy of PTLD is directed at a reduction of immunosuppression, use of antiviral agents, and an anti-CD20 monoclonal antibody. In lymphomas appearing late after transplantation, there may be a role for chemotherapy.

Neurologic complications after lung transplantation occupy a spectrum of disorders ranging from resting tremors to seizures and coma. The majority of these complications are related to the neurotoxicity of the calcineurin inhibitors. Cyclosporine-induced neurotoxicity is suggested on magnetic resonance imaging that reveals characteristic white matter changes representing microvascular injury. These changes are reversible with the discontinuation of cyclosporine. Interestingly, the majority of patients who experience cyclosporine-mediated neurotoxicity have normal cyclosporine levels.

Renal complications after lung transplantation are predominantly caused by calcineurin inhibitors as well. In the immediate perioperative period, it can be difficult to maintain an effective diuresis with the nephrotoxic effects of these agents due to their effect of mediating afferent renal arteriolar vasoconstriction, which in turn decreases glomerular filtration rate. Over time, calcineurin inhibitors cause a chronic form of nephrotoxicity that impairs renal function in all lung transplant patients. Calcium channel blockers are effective in treating the hypertension and delaying the renal insufficiency seen with these agents.

The endocrine complications related to lung transplantation are primarily osteoporosis and the development of diabetes mellitus. Although highly prevalent in this population, the exact cause of the accelerated osteoporosis in this group of patients is not entirely known. It has been associated with the cumulative steroid dose, which is thought to play an integral role in the development of osteoporosis. Use of calcium, vitamin D, and pamidronate is recommended to alleviate this complication. Diabetes mellitus is very common posttransplantation; most likely primarily the result of prolonged steroid use, although tacrolimus has prodiabetogenic properties as well. Treatment is directed at dietary changes, weight loss, and either oral hypoglycemics or insulin.

Gastrointestinal complications occur frequently after lung transplantation and may impart a significant morbidity and mortality on this patient population. We have previously reported our experience with colonic perforation after lung transplantation at the University of Colorado. In our series, 7 of 60 patients experienced colonic perforation, and 2 died (29% mortality). This has affected our approach to recipient evaluation and postoperative management, particularly in the patient with diverticular disease. A screening barium enema is obtained in our recipient evaluation and has confirmed that the prevalence of diverticular disease in this group is very high. The presence of or a history of complicated diverticulitis is considered a contraindication to transplantation in our program. Postoperatively, if clinical suspicion for a perforated diverticulum exists, an abdominal flat plate and computed tomography scan are obtained and prompt exploratory celiotomy is undertaken if there is any suspicion of gastrointestinal tract perforation or active diverticulitis. Keeping narcotics use to a minimum, the use of stool softeners or laxatives, and allowing a normal state of hydration as soon as possible are all important measures in preventing this complication. Since instituting our screening protocol and postoperative management strategies, we have only seen three colonic perforations in 140 procedures. Other gastrointestinal maladies that occur include peptic ulcer disease and gastroparesis. In the cystic fibrosis population, intestinal obstruction is possible due to tenacious secretions that occur in the distal small bowel. In these patients, ensuring adequate hydration and the use of GoLYTELY (polyethylene glycol-electrolyte solution) can prevent this complication.

As lung transplantation is offered to a group of patients with end-stage lung disease, one may expect complications to increase. It is imperative that meticulous preoperative, intraoperative, and postoperative care of these patients occur so that complications can be avoided. The initial unacceptable complication rate with airway anastomoses has been supplanted by the inevitable development of OB as the limiting factor in graft and patient survival. As strides are made to reduce the incidence of OB, significant improvement in lung allograft survival will occur. By avoiding and appropriately treating various post–lung transplantation complications, these patients can return to society as active participants.

SUGGESTED READING

Beaver TM, et al: Colon perforation after lung transplantation, *Ann Thorac Surg* 62:839, 1996.

Boehler A, Estenne M: Obliterative bronchiolitis after lung transplantation, *Curr Opin Pulm Med* 6:133, 2000.

Calhoon JH, et al: Single lung transplantation. Alternative indications and techniques, *J Thorac Cardiovasc Surg* 101:816, 1991.

Chaparro C, Kesten S: Infection in lung transplant recipients, *Clin Chest Med* 18:339, 1997.

Clark SC, et al: Vascular complications of lung transplantation, *Ann Thorac Surg* 61:1079, 1996.

Cooper JD, et al: The International Society for Heart and Lung Transplantation. A working formulation for the standardization of nomenclature and for clinical staging of chronic dysfunction in lung allografts, *J Heart Lung Transplant* 12:713, 1993.

Demeo DL, Ginns LC: Lung transplantation at the turn of the century, *Ann Rev. Med* 52:185, 2001.

Griffith BP, et al: Anastomotic pitfalls in lung transplantation, *J Thorac Cardiovasc Surg* 107:743, 1994.

Maurer JR, Tewari S: Nonpulmonary medical complications in intermediate and long-term survivors, *Clin Chest Med* 18:367, 1997.

Weill D, et al: Acute native lung hyperinflation is not associated with poor outcome after single lung transplant for emphysema, *J Heart Lung Transplant* 18:1080, 1999.

LUNG TRANSPLANTATION IN THE PEDIATRIC PATIENT

Daniel J. Durand

David D. Yuh

Peter J. Mogayzel, Jr

Advances in surgical techniques and immunosuppression have made lung transplantation a viable option for children with end-stage lung disease. Since 1999, over 500 lung transplants have been performed worldwide in patients under age 18. Approximately 75 new cases are performed each year, although this number is unlikely to increase until methods are developed to further maximize the efficiency of procurement or otherwise expand the pool of available organs.

Although children face many of the same problems as adult lung transplant patients, they also present unique challenges. Early reports of higher morbidity and mortality in the young age group have given way to improved results and statistical parity with similar transplants in adults. The requirements of donor and recipient size matching and continued lung growth after transplantation are critical issues. As with adults, the key to success is the presence of a multidisciplinary team with pediatric expertise that can manage children with advanced lung disease, evaluate potential candidates, and care for them postoperatively. This chapter outlines a consensus approach to the performance of lung transplantation and case management in children.

■ INDICATIONS

The indications for lung transplantation in children are similar to those in adults. Transplant candidates must have chronic respiratory failure despite optimal medical therapy, resulting in a significant functional limitation. Children should not have systemic disease or multiple organ dysfunction and should have a projected life expectancy of approximately 2 years. Unfortunately, few studies have investigated objective predictors of mortality in children with advanced lung disease, thereby making transplant referral more problematic for children than for adults. Appropriate timing of transplant evaluation is critical because sicker children do not receive priority on lung transplant waiting lists.

Lung transplants in children are performed for a wide range of pulmonary diseases. The majority of transplants are performed in older children (1 to 10 years old) and adolescents (<17 years old). As shown in Table 1, the reason for transplant differs significantly between age strata within the pediatric population; the leading cause of lung transplant for infants (congenital malformation) is different from that for adolescents (cystic fibrosis [CF]). CF accounts for approximately two thirds of the lung transplants in older children and half of all pediatric transplants. However, transplants in infants and young children are more often performed for congenital cardiopulmonary disease and pulmonary hypertension.

Several clinical indicators have proved useful in predicting the progression of pulmonary disease, most notably measures of lung capacity (forced expiratory volume in 1 second [FEV_1]), pulmonary blood pressure, and hypoxia. To ensure a fair sharing of organs, disease-specific international referral guidelines for lung transplantation have been established for most major respiratory disorders. If the patient is too young for measurements to be obtained or has a rare disorder for which predictive models are unavailable, then other objective criteria are used to determine if and when listing is appropriate. Applying the international guidelines to children has been controversial on occasion because there is evidence that these predictive models may apply poorly to the pediatric population and because transplant waiting times tend to be longer for children than for adults.

Contraindications for pediatric lung transplantation are similar to those for adults (see previous chapters). Transplant centers evaluate each case individually based on institutional experience, but all derive their contraindications from three principal concerns. First, the patient's general level of health must be good enough that he or she is expected to survive the procedure. Second, the patient should be free from any preexisting conditions that preclude recovery. Third, the patient must be willing and able to comply with the strict demands of posttransplant treatment. Compared with the adult situation, more emphasis should be placed on proper social and family support to ensure proper compliance and follow-up.

■ SURGICAL APPROACHES

Bilateral sequential lung transplantation (BLT) is the preferred option for children. It should be the choice for children with CF, which accounts for half of all pediatric transplants performed worldwide. Additionally, BLT provides more pulmonary reserve in infants and small children who may not experience normal lung growth after transplantation. European centers more often perform heart-lung transplantation in children with advanced lung disease. Although this procedure may have surgical advantages, it does necessitate the use of cardiopulmonary bypass (CPB), which can be avoided in BLT for older children and adolescents. Single lung transplants have declined in recent years, although they are still done on rare occasions.

Living lobar transplantation (LLT) is gaining more widespread acceptance. This procedure uses lobes (usually a lower lobe) from two adult living donors to replace the diseased lungs of a child. This procedure has traditionally been reserved for desperately ill children who would not survive the wait for cadaveric lungs. This is an increasingly common predicament for older children, as waiting list times in excess of 2 years are associated with a mortality rate of 30% due to an increasing demand for a static supply of cadaveric organs. Although waiting list times average just 50 days for infants, there are still many deaths due to the rapid progression of the diseases characteristic of this age group. Other advantages associated with LLT include shorter graft ischemic times and potentially improved histocompatibility matching that might translate into improved survival compared to that with cadaveric organs. Although this survival advantage has yet to be conclusively established, LLT remains a viable option for children otherwise destined to die while on the waiting list.

Donor Lung Procurement

Each potential donor is screened according to criteria described in previous chapters for the adult. Typically, fewer than 20% of donor organs are found to be suitable

Table 1 Indications for Pediatric Lung Transplantation

	<1 YEAR OLD	1 TO 10 YEARS OLD	11 TO 17 YEARS OLD
Cystic fibrosis	2	28.9	63.3
Congenital cardiopulmonary disease	36	10.6	3.2
Pulmonary hypertension	11	14.8	10.6
Retransplantation	7	12.7	5.9
Chronic lung disease/ bronchopulmonary dysplasia	0	1.4	1.8
Interstitial pulmonary fibrosis	0	7.7	4.4
Other	44	23.9	10.9

Values are expressed as percentages.
Data adapted from the International Society of Heart and Lung Transplantation Registry (Boucek MM, et al: The Registry of the International Society for Heart and Lung Transplantation: fourth official pediatric report—2000, *J Heart Lung Transplant* 20:39, 2001).

for transplantation. Extraction, preservation, and preparation of the cadaveric organs are similar to those for the adult. Because most transplants in children are BLT, separation is normally performed at the site of the recipient operation.

Recipient Operation

In the small child or infant, CPB is uniformly required because of the lack of a double-lumen endotracheal tube small enough for this patient population. In the larger child or adolescent, a left-sided double-lumen endotracheal tube is preferred to permit selective lung isolation. The native lungs are accessed via a bilateral anterior thoracosternotomy or "clamshell" incision at the fourth intercostal space. Using isolated lung ventilation if possible, each lung is sequentially mobilized by dividing adhesions to the chest wall, mediastinum, and diaphragm and isolating the pulmonary artery and veins. As much dissection should be done off CPB. If there is no double-lumen tube, initiation of CPB should be timed accordingly to arrival of the organs.

The worse functioning lung should be explanted first. If both function equally well, the left is done first because of its increased difficulty. With the lung deflated, the pulmonary artery is first encircled and clamped to determine hemodynamic stability and to determine whether CPB will be necessary. Once the organs have arrived, the artery is clamped and divided, the individual veins divided as far distally as possible, and the main stem transected one ring above the upper lobe bronchus.

After culturing the donor and recipient main bronchi, the lung is placed into the chest and the bronchial anastomosis is performed using a running 4-0 or 5-0 suture line for the membranous portion and interrupted sutures for the cartilaginous portion. Permanent or dissolvable suture may be used; permanent should be avoided to allow for growth of the anastomoses. The right pulmonary artery is clamped centrally and the vessel trimmed to match the donor pulmonary artery. The anastomosis is performed with running the same suture. A side-biting clamp is placed on the recipient left atrium proximal to the pulmonary venous stumps. The ligatures are removed from the stumps of the pulmonary veins, and an incision connecting the openings of the two veins is performed to develop a suitable cuff of left atrium. Donor and recipient atrial cuffs are then anastomosed end-to-end. Before the final suture is secured, the pulmonary artery clamp is released to clear air from the pulmonary vasculature until blood flushes through the atrial suture line. The pulmonary clamp is reapplied, the left atrial clamp is released to allow backbleeding, and the atrial suture line is finally tied. The pulmonary arterial clamp is then removed, and the lung is gently inflated. The other lung is implanted similarly.

If not already on CPB, the remaining lung transplantation is often performed under low-flow partial CPB to avoid imposing full right-sided cardiac output immediately on reperfusion of the first lung. Bypass flow is adjusted to maintain a systolic pressure below 30 mm Hg with an average flow rate of 2 L/min.

The left lung is excised and the donor lung implanted in a similar fashion. The ligamentum arteriosum is usually divided to facilitate proximal placement of the pulmonary arterial clamp. Once normal ventilation and perfusion have been established in both lungs, CPB is discontinued and the vessels decannulated. Two thoracostomy tubes are placed in each thoracic cavity, the sternum is reapproximated with sternal wires, and the thoracotomy incisions are closed in layers. At the termination of the operation, the double-lumen endotracheal tube is removed and the patient is reintubated with a standard single-lumen endotracheal tube. Flexible bronchoscopy is repeated to clear any secretions or blood and to inspect the bronchial anastomoses for patency before the patient is transferred to the intensive care unit.

SLT is performed in a manner analogous to that described for BLT. The right lung is preferred over the left because it is larger. Access is gained via a generous posterolateral thoracotomy. CPB is usually not necessary unless there is the presence of pulmonary hypertension.

Living Lobar Transplant

Living donors are screened according to center-specific ethical criteria in addition to the basic physiologic criteria. These ethical criteria are somewhat controversial and lie beyond the scope of this chapter. Most LLTs are bilateral and require two separate donors. Procurement of the lower right or left lobe is performed through a posterolateral thoracotomy incision through the fourth interspace. Donor lobectomy differs from that performed for infection or cancer in that the condition of the removed lobe is of primary importance. All dissection is performed on the side of the remaining lung to prevent air leaks in the recipient, and adequate cuffs of bronchus, pulmonary vein, and artery are preserved to allow successful transplantation. Prostaglandin E_1 is infused throughout the procurement operation, and the lung is immersed in cold saline, flushed in pulmonoplegic solution, and ventilated immediately on removal from the donor. The recipient operation is performed through a transverse "clamshell" thoracosternotomy. Each lung is mobilized, removed, and replaced with the corresponding donor lobe in a manner similar to that described for whole lungs. CPB is usually necessary for the same reasons described.

■ IMMUNOSUPPRESSION

Immunosuppression is achieved using standard three-drug therapy with cyclosporine/tacrolimus, azathioprine/mycophenolate mofetil, and prednisone. Substantial postoperative clinical monitoring is necessary to maintain appropriate serum dosage levels, to avoid drug interactions, and to detect signs of rejection. For recipients and their families, these clinical complexities translate into a life often interrupted by medical emergencies and false alarms. Even more than most transplant patients, lung recipients trade a terminal illness for a chronic syndrome of immunosuppression with potential life-threatening complications that are discussed later. Beyond these general concerns, there are several issues unique to the pediatric population. For example, the P-450 system undergoes age-related changes that complicate dose titration in children. As a result, older infants and toddlers clear hepatotoxic drugs like cyclosporine faster and require higher weight-adjusted doses. A further consideration is that cyclosporine is fat soluble and is not absorbed efficiently by patients with pancreatic insufficiency that is often seen with CF.

■ COMPLICATIONS

Infection

Respiratory infections are the most common complication after lung transplantation. Lung recipients have a higher rate of infection than do recipients of other solid organ transplants, which can be viewed as a consequence of direct contact between the allograft and the external environment. Pediatric recipients show increased rates of infection due in part to the impact of CF. Recipients with CF retain their native flora within their sinuses and trachea. Furthermore, as the epithelium lining of these structures is still positive for CF, the likelihood of new infections in the immunosuppressed recipient remains high. Infants and toddlers under the age of 3 are also at increased risk because their immune systems are not yet fully developed. A final compounding factor is the increased prevalence of respiratory infections in childhood observed in all populations.

On average, every recipient will have multiple respiratory tract infections during the first year. The majority of infections are caused by bacterial pathogens (i.e., *Pseudomonas, Xanthomonas*), which, although generally well tolerated, can lead to death. Infections caused by viruses (i.e., cytomegalovirus [CMV], respiratory syncytial virus, Epstein-Barr virus [EBV], parainfluenza) and fungi (i.e., *Aspergillus, Candida*) are less frequent but are more likely in children than in adults. Primary infections with CMV, EBV, or adenovirus can have devastating consequences in children after transplantation.

Primary CMV infection and subsequent severe CMV disease occur commonly in children after transplantation. The consequences of these infections, including overwhelming infection, acute rejection, and development of obliterative bronchiolitis, lead to significant morbidity and mortality in children after lung transplantation.

Adenovirus infections are a common cause of lower tract pulmonary infection in young children. Fatal adenovirus infections due to fulminant pneumonia have been described in infants and young children after lung transplantation. In some cases, these infections were derived from the donor. Antibiotics, antivirals, or antifungals are prescribed as needed and delivered intravenously, orally, or via nebulizer.

Over the course of experience, prophylactic protocols consisting of perioperative treatment with antibiotics and antifungals have been developed with the aim of preventing infection. Prophylaxis to prevent primary CMV infection in seronegative recipients is more prolonged and consists of a 4- to 12-week course of ganciclovir. Pretransplant laparoscopic sinus surgery and/or periodic sinus lavage is also used to limit infectious complications in recipients with CF.

Prophylactic considerations sometimes cause modifications to the transplantation procedure itself. For example, CF patients are often placed on CPB so that both lungs can be removed at once, permitting irrigation of the blind trachea by antibiotics with little risk of cross-contamination between the ingoing and outgoing lungs. Alternate forms of intraoperative antibiotic irrigation are also in practice. The degree to which prophylactic concerns impinge on other aspects of the surgical procedure varies based on the needs of the patient and the preferences of the transplant center.

Rejection and Bronchiolitis Obliterans Syndrome

The prevalence of rejection in children is similar to that observed in adults, with recipients averaging multiple episodes of acute rejection over the first three months. Rejection is diagnosed by a pathologist who analyzes transbronchial biopsy specimens and is treated with augmented immunosuppression and pulsed corticosteroid administration. For unresponsive cases of acute rejection and/or chronic rejection, more aggressive forms of immunosuppression, such as lympholytic agents, may be used.

Bronchiolitis obliterans syndrome (BOS) as a sequelae to chronic rejection has been called the Achilles' heel of lung transplantation. Although its time course may vary, BOS is characterized by a progressive narrowing of the bronchioles resulting in a sustained consistent drop in FEV_1 and increasing hypoxia leading to death or retransplantation. Some have conjectured that all recipients will eventually develop BOS, as long-term data show a persistent, unending rise in the incidence of BOS among long-term survivors. This is particularly disturbing because BOS is poorly understood and no therapy has been proved to permanently arrest its progression. Augmented immunosuppression is sometimes successful in delaying or slowing the progression of BOS, but retransplantation is the only present "cure." One cause for hope is that LLT recipients appear to have a much lower incidence of BOS, a result with important implications that are discussed further in the section on outcomes.

Certain factors are associated with increased rates of rejection. Prior CMV disease or frequent viral infections predispose patients to develop chronic rejection and BOS, which may explain why CF patients show a higher incidence of both complications.

Posttransplant Lymphoproliferative Disease

Posttransplant lymphoproliferative disease (PLTD) is a neoplastic process that has been reported in 9% to 28% of pediatric lung transplant recipients. Although reactivation of EBV can lead to PTLD, it is typically associated with primary EBV acquisition. Therefore, children are at a much higher risk of developing PTLD than are adults. PTLD has traditionally been associated with more aggressive immunosuppressive regimens. Cytolytic therapy has been implicated as a risk factor. A recent study has also shown that PTLD is more common in children with CF.

A typical case of PTLD presents at any time at least 3 months after transplantation and is characterized by the development of obstructive pulmonary nodules that contribute to increased respiratory distress. PTLD has been noted at sites outside the graft but with lower frequency. Therapy for PTLD may consist of augmented immunosuppression, ganciclovir, and/or alpha-interferon. Micheals and colleagues at the University of Pittsburgh reported a 70% survival rate for patients developing PTLD, although outcomes vary from center to center due to differences in case definition and patient management.

The mortality rate from PTLD in children is high. The mainstay of treatment is decreasing immunosuppression. Although this therapy can arrest the progression of PTLD, this approach places children at increased risk of acute rejection. More aggressive disease has been treated successfully with chemotherapy and radiation therapy. Recently, several centers have reported successful treatment of a small number of patients with rituximab.

Airway Complications

The incidence of airway complications is higher in children than in adults who have undergone lung transplantation. Anastomotic stenosis has been reported to occur at approximately twice the rate of adult patients. Although bronchomalacia is less common, it presents a more life-threatening problem due to the narrower caliber and more compliant cartilage of the pediatric airway. Conservative management of airway problems is preferred. The use of invasive techniques, such as bronchial stenting, can be problematic due to the lack of small stent sizes and the effects on subsequent airway growth. Surgical approaches typically involve additional procedures to resect the stenosis or revise the anastomosis. In cases of complete anastomotic dehiscence, graft removal or retransplantation often is the only option.

Drug Metabolism

Maintaining appropriate immunosuppressant levels in children can be challenging. The activity of the hepatic CYP3A pathway, which is involved in the metabolism of cyclosporine and tacrolimus, is age dependent. Infants and young children have a faster rate of hepatic clearance of these and other immunosuppressants. These drugs have undesirable side affects, some of which are amplified in CF patients. For example, common neurologic side effects, including seizures, are more frequent among CF patients. Likewise, osteoporosis is greatly exacerbated by prednisone if already present. In addition, they are more likely to develop diabetes as a side effect of hormone therapy. Finally, the cumulative effects of nephrotoxicity and hepatotoxicity develop over time. In the absence of adequate long-term survival data, it has been difficult to determine the validity of this concern.

■ SPECIAL CONSIDERATIONS FOR INFANTS

As mentioned earlier, infants are at increased risk for infection and chronic rejection. In addition, they are especially prone to gastroesophageal reflux disease (GERD) as an early complication. GERD affects approximately half of all infant recipients and can be particularly hazardous if stomach acid is aspirated into the allograft airways. If medical therapy fails to suppress GERD, as is often the case, a Nissen fundoplication is performed.

■ OUTCOMES

The number of pediatric lung transplants performed worldwide has remained relatively stable, at approximately 75 per year. In the United States the survival rate for lung transplant recipients is 95% at 1 month, 83% at 1 year, and 55% at 3 years. Survival rates are highest for the most recent years (1999), indicating that results have improved with experience. Traditionally, infants and younger children tended to have poorer outcomes. However, recent improvements in

survival data suggest that these younger children will have long-term survival rates similar to those of older children.

These data also show that there are few early deaths from postoperative hemorrhage or other surgical complications. Instead, the majority of deaths result from complications related to either medical therapy or the primary disease process. The risk from each possible complication peaks at specific time points during the postoperative period, with acute complications (infection, acute rejection, PTLD) being most dangerous over the first postoperative year and chronic issues (chronic rejection, BOS) posing the greatest threat thereafter.

For those released from the hospital, quality of life is dramatically improved during periods when they are complication free. Most recipients are ambulatory and show improved activity levels and exercise capability. The outward appearance of health and vitality is supported by data indicating that measures of oxygenation and pulmonary function return to normal 3 to 6 months after surgery. There also is evidence to suggest that preanastomotic and postanastomotic tracheal growth in recipients is similar to that seen in the normal pediatric airway. Lungs from younger donors grow with the recipient due to alveolar distention and—in some cases where the donor is below age 8—multiplication. In lungs from older donors, however, growth occurs primarily through an increase in cellular and connective tissue elements that do not contribute to ventilatory capacity.

Chronic rejection and BOS remain the major impediments to long-term survival for lung transplant recipients of all ages. The rates of acute rejection are similar in adults and older children but tend to be lower in infants and younger children. Most children develop some degree of BOS within 3 years of transplantation. Several clinical trials investigating solutions to these and other late complications are currently under way with the hope of improving prospects for long-term survival. The results of the University of Southern California group with LLT are remarkable for their low incidence of BOS (14%) and high survival rates (83%, 78%, and 78% at 1, 3, and 5 years, respectively).

■ SUMMARY

Lung transplantation has evolved into a valuable treatment option for infants and children with end-stage lung disease. In the coming years, improved survival rates will be obtained as more effective immunomodulatory strategies are developed.

SUGGESTED READING

Boucek MM, et al: The Registry of the International Society for Heart and Lung Transplantation: fourth official pediatric report—2000, *J Heart Lung Transplant* 20:39, 2001.

Bridges ND, et al: Lung transplantation in infancy and early childhood, *J Heart Lung Transplant* 15:895, 1996.

Huddleston CB, et al: Lung transplantation in very young infants, *J Thorac Cardiovasc Surg* 118:796, 1999.

Mendeloff EN, et al: Pediatric and adult lung transplantation for cystic fibrosis, *J Thorac Cardiovasc Surg* 115:404, 1998; discussion 413.

Starnes VA, et al: Comparison of outcomes between living donor and cadaveric lung transplantation in children, *Ann Thorac Surg* 68:2279, 1999; discussion 2283.

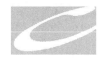

CHEST WALL AND STERNUM

PECTUS EXCAVATUM AND PECTUS CARINATUM

Paul M. Colombani

Anterior chest wall abnormalities are unusual problems seen in children as well as in adults. More than 90% of these abnormalities are pectus excavatum deformities characterized by a concave, sunken, anterior chest wall defect. Approximately, 10% of patients have pectus carinatum, which is a convex, protuberant deformity of the anterior chest wall. More rarely, patients may have Poland's anomaly (anomalous or absent ribs, absent pectoralis major muscle, and limb anomalies). The etiology of these anterior chest wall abnormalities is unclear. There appears to be an overgrowth of the costal cartilages, leading to a depression of the sternum in pectus excavatum and to protuberance and elevation of the sternum in pectus carinatum. These abnormalities may be secondary to an increased elasticity or weakness of connective tissue, including cartilage, since patients with Marfan's syndrome and other connective tissue abnormalities have a relatively high incidence of pectus excavatum (up to 10%). There is a familial incidence of pectus excavatum and a male to female preponderance of 5 to 1. Poland's anomaly probably occurs as a failure of mesodermal migration and development in the anterior chest wall of the fetus. This chapter presents the diagnosis and repair of pectus excavatum as well as pectus carinatum.

Most patients with pectus excavatum deformities present with progressive depression of the sternum through their childhood years and into their teenage pubertal growth spurt. Less commonly patients may develop pectus excavatum at the time of rapid pubertal growth. Pectus carinatum deformities more typically appear during the pubertal growth spurt. They are rarely seen before the age of 12. Patients also may have parasternal discomfort associated with these lesions because of the increased flex of the costal cartilages and costosternal joints.

The management of anterior chest wall abnormalities over the years has been controversial. Patients with pectus excavatum often have exercise intolerance and fatigability. Static pulmonary function test results, however, may not show any significant abnormality. More sophisticated exercise pulmonary function testing on a treadmill may demonstrate significant decrease in exercise tolerance. Echocardiograms may reveal decreased ejection fraction from heart displacement

to the left, which may be an inefficient pumping position. Studies have shown that patients with pectus excavatum have decreased maximal cardiac output with exercise. This completely resolves following repair. For patients with pectus carinatum, no physiologic component appears with the defect.

Patients with pectus excavatum and pectus carinatum have issues with body image. These are developmental malformations that significantly alter body image. The developing child and young adult may have significant psychologic concerns with their body's appearance, and this alone should be an indication for repair.

■ PECTUS EXCAVATUM

Patients with pectus excavatum are evaluated for severity of the defect and for pulmonary and cardiac functional abnormalities. A screening exam for the possibility of a connective tissue disorder may be indicated in some patients. Patients have round shoulders and depressed sternum. In young patients, a protuberant abdomen is seen. Measurement of the pectus defect can be done using a variety of methods. In the past, the distance between the back of the sternum and the anterior spine on lateral chest x-ray was measured. Later, a pectus index was derived from a cross-sectional CT scan at the level of the deepest part of the defect. The width of the chest between the ribs in centimeters is divided by the distance between the back of the sternum and the anterior spine. A pectus index of greater than 3 is significant for a moderately severe pectus excavatum defect. A simple caliper can also be used to measure the deepest part of the defect compared with the chest wall at the midclavicular lines. A moderately severe pectus excavatum defect has a depth of greater than 2.5 cm. This simple measure correlates well with a pectus index greater than 3.0. Prior to repair, patients should also undergo exercise pulmonary function tests and echocardiograms to screen for physiologic abnormalities.

Patients with moderately severe defects with pectus index greater than 3 and/or a depth greater than 2.5 cm should undergo operative repair. Patients with lesser defects or very young patients can be followed expectantly with a yearly exam. The optimal time for repair of a pectus excavatum defect is between the ages of eight and twelve years. Older patients who present as teenagers or adults can undergo repair at any time. We avoid operative repair of pectus excavatum in children younger than 7 years for two reasons. First, there appears to be a higher incidence of damaging the growth areas of the rib cartilages in younger children, resulting in an acquired Jeune's syndrome (i.e., asphyxiating thoracic dystrophy). Second, the very young child is not mature enough to take an active role in deciding to undergo surgery.

The type of operation is also in evolution. Historically, a number of different repairs have been proposed, most of which are modifications of a procedure first published by Ravitch. A precurved, substernal bar to splint the sternum in an anterior position has been utilized with success. This procedure, first developed by Nuss, achieves success without the requirement of cartilage excision. The costal cartilages are bent to a new position, and the sternum is held in place anteriorly by the substernal bar. The bone and cartilage are then allowed to remodel over time, effecting a new position for the sternum.

Ravitch Procedure

The operative goal of the pectus excavatum repair is to elevate the sternum to a neutral, straight position. A modified Ravitch procedure is performed by a number of surgeons around the world. This procedure entails a transverse, inframammary incision over the deepest part of the pectus defect. Subcutaneous flaps are elevated. Pectoralis muscle flaps are created, elevating the muscle off the costal cartilages bilaterally. The downcurved costal cartilages are then removed bilaterally,

which usually includes cartilages 4, 5, 6, and 7. A subperichondrial dissection is used to preserve the perichondrium (Figure 1A).

The sternum is then bluntly dissected off the pleura and pericardium, using the index finger in a sweeping motion. Above the level of the removed costal cartilages, a cuneiform osteotomy is made in the anterior table of the sternum (Figure 1B). This triangle-shaped osteotomy between the 2nd and 3rd rib cartilages allows the sternum to be bent superiorly up to a neutral position. An angled transverse division of the 3rd costal cartilages just below the osteotomy helps elevate the sternum. The sternum can often be elevated to a neutral position without dividing the intercostal muscles on either side.

Dissection and division of the intercostal muscles with electrocautery away from the lateral edge of the sternum may be required to facilitate elevation of the sternum. Care is taken to prevent division of the internal mammary arteries. The third costal cartilages may be used to support the elevated sternum by stepping the cartilage up on itself, using a transverse oblique division (Figure 1C). A transverse

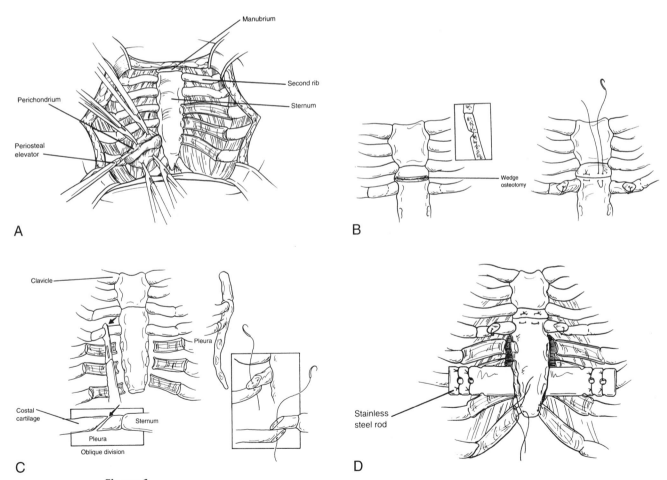

Figure 1
Modified Ravitch repair. Subperiosteal dissection of cartilages 4, 5, 6, and 7 (**A**). Cuneiform (wedge) osteotomy between ribs 2 and 3 to allow elevation of distal sternum (**B**). Tripartite fixation of sternum using step-up of third costal cartilage (**C**). Final placement and anchoring of a substernal Adkins rod (**D**).

retrosternal Adkins strut is then placed, resting on the ribs bilaterally and passing underneath the sternum (Figure 1D).

If the intercostal bundles are not divided, the bar may be placed through a stab wound in the intercostal muscles. The bar is anchored to the ribs using interrupted zero Prolene sutures. A chest tube is placed in the retrosternal position, and a closed suction drain is placed between the reapproximated pectoralis muscle and the subcutaneous flap. With electrocautery, blood loss is negligible. Postoperatively, the patient remains in the hospital 3 to 4 days and is discharged after the drain and chest tube removal.

Postoperative pain is moderate in nature and usually managed with intravenous patient-controlled analgesia. Postoperative complications include pneumothorax, hemothorax, subcutaneous fluid collection, and wound infection. All of these are unusual complications occurring in less than 5% of patients. Patients are released home to limited activity for approximately 6 weeks to allow regrowth of the costal cartilages. The retrosternal bar remains in place for a minimum of 6 months. It can be removed on an outpatient basis. Long-term complications include recurrence, in up to 10% of patients in some series. At the Johns Hopkins Hospital, recurrence is less than 2%.

Nuss Procedure

For schoolage children and adults, including patients with recurrent pectus excavatum, a modified Nuss procedure may be performed. The Nuss procedure entails transverse incisions on the lateral chest wall just above the deepest part of the sternal defect. These incisions are carried down to the pleural space bilaterally. A small stab wound is made at the end of the sternum and xyphoid. A bone hook is placed under the sternum, and the sternum is elevated to a neutral position. A Crawford vascular clamp is passed from left to right through the pleural and retrosternal precardiac space, creating a retrosternal tunnel. A precurved Lorenz bar is passed through that retrosternal tunnel, using umbilical tapes (Figure 2). The bar is turned pivoting on the ribs laterally. The curve

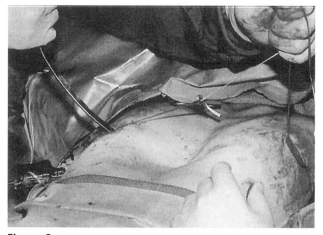

Figure 2
Positioning of a precurved Lorenz bar under the sternum for the Nuss repair.

of the bar elevates the sternum to a neutral position with the lateral part of the arch resting on the ribs bilaterally. In order to fix the bar to prevent movement, a stabilizing clip is slid onto the ends of the bar bilaterally. The bar is bent *in situ*, using bar benders to contour the bar to the chest wall. Bending the end of the bar prevents the clip from sliding off. No. 6 wire sutures anchor the bar to the ribs in two places: where the bar first crosses over the ribs and to a more lateral rib if possible. The wounds are closed, and the pneumothoraces are evacuated with sustained inflation of the lungs. No drain or chest tube is required.

This procedure may be complicated by significant intraoperative bleeding with some reports of penetration of the heart with the Crawford vascular clamp. In order to prevent this problem, we elevate the sternum using a bone hook to allow passage of the clamp from the left side away from the heart. Other surgeons have utilized thoracoscopy to follow the course of the clamp as it passes under the sternum. For recurrent pectus excavatum cases, we have opened the previous incision in the midline to develop the retrosternal plane to facilitiate the bar's passage under the sternum.

Postoperatively, patients have significantly greater pain management issues than those undergoing the Ravitch procedure. Patients remain in the hospital approximately 3 to 4 days to effect adequate intravenous pain control. Younger children may benefit from a thoracic epidural for pain management in the postoperative period. In older children and adults, a thoracic epidural catheter is inadequate for pain control. Sympathetic pleural effusion or hemothorax may occur; wound infection may rarely occur. With the use of surgical wires to fix the bar to the rib cage bilaterally, shifting or moving of the bar with early recurrence of the defect is minimized to less than 2%. The substernal bar remains in place for 2 years to allow for alteration and remodeling of the costal cartilages and sternum. It is then removed on an outpatient basis. To date, most centers performing this procedure have reported excellent results, effecting repair of the sternal defect. The advantage of this operation may be the decrease in postoperative scar formation. The greater scar formation may contribute to postoperative chest restriction. Operative weakening of the anterior chest wall by cutting and removing costal cartilages may contribute to late recurrences. Recurrence rates should be less, and improvement in postoperative pulmonary function may be seen. Long-term results, however, are not available at present.

■ PECTUS CARINATUM

Patients with pectus carinatum are usually teenagers who have developed a convex abnormality of the anterior chest wall, evident on inspection and palpation. No further tests are usually required. Occasionally, a CT scan may be useful to demonstrate more graphically the number of cartilages involved and to rule out a malignant bone or soft tissue tumor. Patients usually have pain and ease of injury associated with the prominence of their anterior chest wall. There are no pulmonary or cardiovascular defects associated with pectus carinatum. Most commonly, the indication for surgery is pain and ease of injury. This is a significant malformation

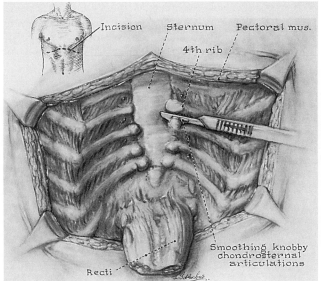

A

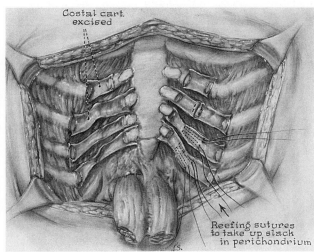

B

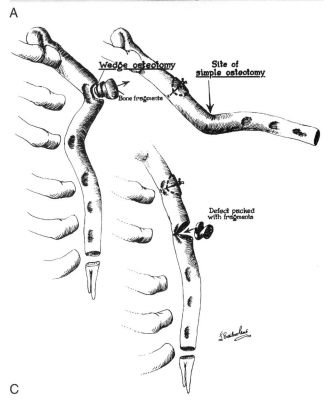

C

Figure 3
Operative principles of pectus carinatum repair. Excision of protuberant nodules (**A**). Subperichondrial resection of protuberant cartilages and reefing of excessively long perichondrial sleeves (**B**). If necessary, an elevated sternum is fractured and depressed to achieve the neutral position (**C**).

affecting body image. These body image concerns are a definite indication for surgical repair. The time of surgery is relatively straightforward. Pectus carinatum deformity should not be repaired before the end of the pubertal growth spurt. Patients who present in their schoolage years or during their teenage growth spurt should be followed expectantly. Anecdotal reports exist of significant recurrences of pectus carinatum defect in patients operated on during these formative periods, requiring reoperation and repair.

The goals of the operation are to restore the normal contour of the anterior chest and to return the sternum to a neutral, straight position if it has been elevated and rotated. The operative technique is similar to the open technique for pectus excavatum repair. A transverse incision is made in the inframammary area usually over the mid portion of the number of cartilages involved. This incision is then carried down through the subcutaneous tissue and muscle to the anterior chest wall. The pectoralis muscle may be elevated through a transverse incision across its dimension, or a midline incision in the muscle may be made. The muscle flaps are made unilaterally or bilaterally as needed. The abnormal cartilages are inspected, excising the protuberant nodules

(Figure 3A)and resecting the cartilage in a subperichondral fashion (Figure 3B).

Once the cartilages are removed, the perichondrial strips may be shortened with reefing stitches. If the sternum is elevated and rotated, anterior osteotomies are created to cause a greenstick fracture of the sternum (Figure 3C). The sternum is then depressed to a neutral position. In order to hold the sternum in a neutral position, blocks from the resected cartilage can be placed in the osteotomy defect to hold the sternum in a depressed position. Often a subpectoral muscle drain is required to remove any blood or fluid that collects in that space.

Postoperatively, the patients remain in the hospital for 3 to 4 days for pain relief and diminished drain output. Following discharge, patients are kept at limited activity until the costal cartilages grow back, which takes approximately 6 weeks. The patients can then return to normal activity. Early complications include wound infection and bleeding; late complications include recurrence of the pectus carinatum defect. Often recurrence arises in the cartilages adjacent to the surgical area and not in the cartilages previously resected.

Anterior chest wall defects may occur with sternal depression (pectus excavatum) or sternal and rib elevation (pectus carinatum). There are well-described operative approaches to effect successful repair with low complication and recurrence rates.

REFERENCES

Croitoru DP, et al: Experience and modification update for the minimally invasive Nuss technique for pectus excavatum repair in 303 patients. *J Pediatr Surg* 37:437-445, 2002.

Haller JA Jr, et al: Use of CT scans in selection of patients for pectus excavatum surgery: A preliminary report. *J Pediatr Surg* 22:904-906, 1987.

Haller JA Jr, et al: Evolving management of pectus excavatum based on a single institutional experience of 664 patients. *Ann Surg* 209:578-582, 1989.

Quigley PM, et al: Cardiorespiratory function before and after corrective surgery in pectus excavatum. *J Pediat* 128:638-643, 1996.

Ravitch MM: *Congenital deformities of the chest wall and their operative correction.* Philadelphia, 1977, WB Saunders.

THORACIC OUTLET SYNDROME

Harold C. Urschel, Jr

Thoracic outlet syndrome (TOS) refers to compression of one or more of the neurovascular structures traversing the superior aperture of the chest. Previously, the name was designated according to the etiologies of compression, such as scalenus anticus, costoclavicular, hyperabduction, cervical rib, or first rib syndromes.

Most compressive factors operate against the first rib and produce a variety of symptoms, depending on which neurovascular structures are compressed. The functional anatomy and pathophysiology of compression in the thoracic outlet and the symptomatology of each of the specific structures compressed are summarized in Figure 1.

■ NERVE COMPRESSION

The symptoms of nerve compression most frequently observed are pain and paresthesias (present in approximately 95% of patients), whereas motor weakness is less common (<10%).

Pain and paresthesias are segmental in 75% of cases, with 90% involving the ulnar nerve distribution.

There may be several points of compression on the peripheral nerves between the cervical spine and hand, in addition to the thoracic outlet. When there are multiple compression sites, less pressure is required at each site to produce symptoms. Thus, a patient may have concomitant TOS, ulnar nerve compression at the elbow, and carpal tunnel syndrome. This phenomenon has been called the "multiple crush" syndrome.

Diagnostic and Objective Tests

A careful history and physical examination are critical for accurate diagnosis. The multiple physical signs of thoracic outlet compression and the classic diagnostic tests have been thoroughly reviewed. Other causes of TOS-like symptoms, such as cardiac or pulmonary disease, must be ruled out. The electromyogram should be normal, ruling out other neuromuscular disorders. The primary objective test for thoracic outlet peripheral nerve compression in our clinic is the nerve conduction velocity (NCV). Reduction in NCV to less than normal (85 m/sec) of either the ulnar or median nerves across the thoracic outlet corroborates the clinical diagnosis.

Management

With an NCV exceeding 60 m/sec, the patient usually improves from conservative physical therapy. Initially, most patients, except those with vascular problems, were treated conservatively with physical therapy. The primary goals of physical therapy are to open up the space between the clavicle

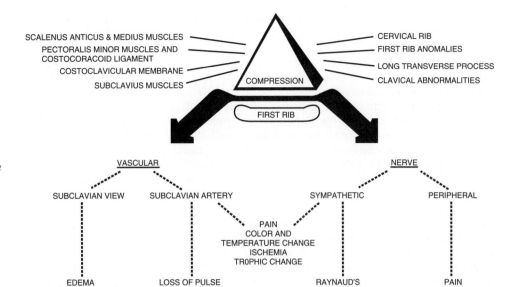

Figure 1
Thoracic outlet syndrome pathophysiology.

and first rib, improve posture, strengthen the shoulder girdle, and loosen the neck muscles. This is accomplished by pectoralis stretching, strengthening the muscles between the shoulder blades, good posture, and active neck exercises, including chin tuck flexion, rotation, lateral bending, and circumduction.

Indications for Surgery

The usual indications for surgery are failure of appropriate conservative therapy to improve symptoms in a patient with a significantly reduced NCV (<60 m/sec) and the elimination of other possible etiologies for the symptoms.

■ ARTERIAL COMPRESSION

The diagnosis is suspected by the history, physical examination, and Doppler studies and is confirmed with arteriography. Therapy for arterial compression depends on its degree of involvement.

An asymptomatic patient with cervical or first rib arterial compression producing poststenotic dilation of the axillary subclavian artery should undergo rib resection, preferably using the transaxillary approach, removing the ribs, both first and cervical, without resecting the artery. The arterial dilation usually returns toward normal after removal of the compression.

Patients with compression from the first or cervical rib producing an aneurysm with or without thrombus should undergo rib resection and aneurysm excision with graft using a supraclavicular and infraclavicular combined approach. Thrombosis of the axillary subclavian artery or distal emboli secondary to TOS compression should be treated with first rib resection, thrombectomy, embolectomy, arterial repair or replacement, and dorsal sympathectomy.

■ SYMPATHETIC COMPRESSION

Compression of the sympathetic nerves in the thoracic outlet may occur alone or in combination with peripheral nerve and blood vessels. The sympathetics are intimately attached to the artery as well as lying adjacent to the bone. They may be compressed or irritated in primary or recurrent TOS.

Pseudoangina

The atypical chest pain is frequently insidious in onset and less commonly involves the neck, shoulder, arm, and hand. It involves the anterior chest wall and parascapular area and is termed "pseudoangina" because it simulates angina pectoris. A group of patients with chest pain simulating angina pectoris, but with normal coronary angiograms, were found to have significant TOS.

Many arterial compressions result in more severe symptoms of sympathetic maintained pain syndrome (SMPS) because of the additive or synergistic sympathetic stimulation. Trauma frequently is associated with SMPS or reflex sympathetic dystrophy (RSD).

For uncomplicated, nontraumatic TOS symptoms, usually first rib resection alone with neurovascular decompression relieves the sympathetic symptoms and dorsal sympathectomy is not required. However, if trauma is significant in the etiology, causalgia or SMPS is often present and concomitant dorsal sympathectomy is routinely required to ameliorate the symptoms. Also, if surgery is required for recurrent TOS symptoms, the relief of accompanying causalgia and SMPS usually requires dorsal sympathectomy. Initially, dorsal sympathectomies were performed at an interval after procedures for traumatic or recurrent TOS, if necessary. However, because they were necessary in so many cases and because of the inconvenience of a second procedure, dorsal sympathectomy is now routinely combined with the initial TOS procedure for either trauma or recurrent cases.

Indications for Surgery

Major indications for dorsal sympathectomy include hyperhidrosis, Raynaud's phenomenon or disease, causalgia, SMPS, reflex sympathetic dystrophy, and vascular insufficiency of the upper extremity. Except for hyperhidrosis, most indications for sympathectomy require the usual diagnostic techniques, including cervical sympathetic block, to assess the relief of symptoms with temporary sympathetic blockade. When Raynaud's phenomenon of a minor to moderate degree is associated with TOS, the simple removal of the first rib with any cervical rib, in addition to stripping the axillary subclavian artery (neurectomy), generally relieves most symptoms after the initial procedure. It is rarely necessary to perform a sympathectomy unless Raynaud's phenomenon is severe, in which case a dorsal sympathectomy is performed with first rib resection. A contraindication to dorsal sympathectomy is venous obstruction (Paget-Schroetter syndrome [PSS] effort thrombosis of the axillary subclavian vein).

The approach most frequently used for TOS and dorsal sympathectomy is the transaxillary approach, for first rib resection. This causes minimal pain and combines two procedures with a low morbidity rate. Video assistance is also used frequently with this approach.

Scalenectomy

Early results in 336 patients were extremely good (310/336). However, the longer-term follow-up was not as satisfactory. Five-year improvement was present in 150 of 336 patients, but at 20 years only 31 of 336 patients were still improved (20 patients were lost to follow-up).

Transaxillary First Rib Resection and Scalenectomy

Transaxillary first rib resection with anterior scalenectomy relieved symptoms of upper plexus (96%) and combined upper and lower plexus (95%) compression as well as it did for lower plexus compression (95%) only.

■ VENOUS COMPRESSION

Paget-Schroetter Syndrome

Effort thrombosis of the axillary subclavian vein (PSS) is usually secondary to unusual, repetitive use of the arm, in addition to the presence of one or more compressive elements in the thoracic outlet. Sir James Paget in 1875 in London and Von Schroetter in 1884 in Vienna independently described this syndrome of thrombosis of the axillary subclavian vein. The word "effort" was added to thrombosis because of the frequent association with exertion producing either direct or indirect compression of the vein. The thrombosis is caused by trauma or repetitive muscular activity (e.g., occupations such as professional weight lifters and athletes, linotype operators, painters, and beauticians). Cold and traumatic factors, such as carrying skis over the shoulder, tend to increase the proclivity for thrombosis. Elements of increased thrombogenicity also increase the incidence of this problem and exacerbate its symptoms on a long-term basis. The diagnosis

is suspected by a careful history, physical examination and Doppler studies, and confirmed with venography.

Indications for Surgery

Intermittent or partial obstruction should be treated by thrombolysis followed by prompt first rib removal through the transaxillary approach, with resection of the costoclavicular ligament medially, the first rib inferiorly, and the scalenus anticus muscle laterally. The clavicle is left in place. The vein is decompressed and all the bands and adhesions are removed.

The availability of thrombolytic agents, combined with prompt surgical decompression of the neurovascular compressive elements in the thoracic outlet, has reduced the morbidity rate and the need for thrombectomy and has produced substantially improved clinical results, including the ability to return to work.

Claviculectomy is occasionally used for decompression, particularly if a fracture of the clavicle has occurred secondary to trauma.

Paget-Schroetter Syndrome

After thrombolysis of the clot, prompt first rib resection with removal of compressive elements is recommended. We have reviewed this technique in 340 patients with PPS. Thrombectomy was necessary in only four extremities, and the long-term results indicate that 205 extremities had good results.

■ RECURRENT THORACIC OUTLET SYNDROME

Recurrent symptoms, primarily neurogenic, should be documented by objective NCVs. When NCVs are depressed in a patient whose symptoms are unrelieved by *prolonged* conservative therapy, a posterior high thoracoplasty muscle-splitting procedure is preferred. Removal of any rib remnants or regenerated fibrocartilage and neurolysis of C7, C8, and T1 nerve roots and the brachial plexus are performed. Dorsal sympathectomy is added to minimize the contribution of causalgia and SMPS.

Depo-Medrol and hyaluronic acid are used to minimize recurrent scar.

Indications for Surgery

The diagnosis and differential diagnosis for recurrence are similar to those for the original procedure. However, the indications for a second procedure are more stringent and longer periods of conservative therapy are usually involved.

The primary technical factor involved in reducing recurrence seems to be complete extirpation of the rib during the initial procedure. If a rib remnant is left (as many surgeons outside of our group seem to prefer), osteocytes and osteoblasts grow from the end of the bone, producing fibrocartilage and regenerated bone, that compress the nerves and blood vessels. The risk of fibrosis may be higher in patients who produce keloid scars, patients in whom hematomas are not drained, or patients who undergo early excessive physical therapy after the first surgical procedure.

Occasionally other approaches have been used for a second procedure.

Surgical Approaches

In the late 1950s and early 1960s, the surgical procedure of choice was the supraclavicular, partial scalenectomy with neurolysis of the brachial plexus when indicated and combined with resection of a cervical rib if present. Because of the 1962 presentation by Clagett, the posterior approach for resection of the first rib was introduced to remove the common denominator for thoracic outlet compression forces. Subsequently, the initial procedure was usually performed through the transaxillary approach because no large muscle division was required and morbidity rates were less. The supraclavicular or infraclavicular approach or the combined approach was employed for arterial lesions. The posterior approach, in our practice, is now reserved for second procedures in patients with recurrent TOS symptoms for removal of rib remnants and regenerated fibrocartilage with neurolysis of C7, C8, and T1 nerve roots and the brachial plexus.

Recurrent Thoracic Outlet Syndrome

Results of 1221 procedures showed a moderately good early effect of a second procedure: 1,092 patients had significant improvement (89%), 93 related fair improvement, and only 36 did not feel better. Late results (5-year follow-up) in 528 extremities that underwent a second procedure revealed 396 (75%) with good results and 132 (25%) with fair to poor recovery. Forty-eight patients (3.1%) required a third surgical procedure.

SUGGESTED READING

Urschel HC Jr, Cooper JD: *Atlas of thoracic surgery,* New York: Churchill-Livingstone, 1995.

Urschel HC Jr, Razzuk MA: Upper plexus thoracic outlet syndrome: outlet therapy, *Ann Thorac Surg* 63:935, 1997.

Urschel HC Jr, Razzuk MA: Neurovascular compression in the thoracic outlet: changing management over 50 years, *Ann Thorac Surg* 67:609, 1998.

Urschel HC Jr, Razzuk MA: Paget-Schroetter syndrome: what is the best management? *Ann Thorac Surg* 69:1663, 2000.

CHEST WALL NEOPLASMS

W. Roy Smythe

■ BACKGROUND

The human chest wall is a bony, ligamentous, and muscular structure that participates in many important physiologic functions. In addition to protecting the underlying thoracic and upper abdominal viscera, the chest wall assists with the process of ventilation and provides an important functional attachment framework for much of the upper extremity and cervical musculature. Anatomically the chest wall is defined arbitrarily. From a surgical standpoint, the chest wall includes from superficial to deep all the overlying musculature (e.g., pectoralis, serratus, latissimus, levators, paraspinals), scapulae, clavicles, ribs and associated external and internal intercostal muscles; the vascular structures and nerves; the internal thoracic musculature; and the endothoracic fascia lined by the mesothelial pleural membrane.

The origin of chest wall neoplasms includes primary malignant and benign tumors of all bony and soft tissue structures as outlined previously. In addition, metastatic tumors and tumors originating in non–chest wall structures with contiguous invasion (i.e., lung, breast, or liver) are noted. As a result of aggressive local control techniques, an association exists between radiation therapy and the induction of chest wall tumors. These neoplasms often occur more than 5 years after completion of radiation therapy and arise most commonly in the ipsilateral pectoral and periclavicular regions of women treated for carcinoma of the breast.

Primary chest wall neoplasms can be noted from infancy to old age, but some reproducible trends are worth mentioning. Children and young adults are more likely to have malignant small round cell tumors (Ewing's sarcoma, primitive neuroectodermal tumor, and Askin's tumor) or rhabdomyosarcoma than older adults, and very elderly patients are more likely to present with plasmacytoma than younger patients. The other primary sarcomas and desmoid tumors are intermediate in age presentation.

■ CLINICAL EVALUATION

Most patients present with an incidental mass noted by the patient or found at physical examination. Malignant lesions are more likely to be painful, and bony tumors, such as chondrosarcoma and osteosarcoma, are more likely to be painful than tumors of soft tissue origin. Rarer symptoms include cough from pleural irritation, paresthesias of dermatomal distribution corresponding to involved intercostal nerves, and shortness of breath from lung compression.

Plain radiographs of the chest often show only a radiopaque mass. An isolated lytic lesion in a rib may indicate plasmacytoma or a metastasis, however, and the flocculent "popcorn" calcifications of chondrosarcoma or the mixed lytic and sclerotic pattern of osteosarcoma sometimes can be recognized. Regardless of plain film findings, however, a high-quality computed tomography (CT) scan of the lower neck, chest, and upper abdomen is the imaging test of choice for chest wall lesions. Parenchymal and bone/mediastinal windows should be studied carefully. Parenchymal windows are important because pulmonary metastases from a chest wall primary sarcoma always should be sought. Mediastinal or bone windows can help delineate the extent of the tumor and at times provide a preliminary diagnosis. A flocculent popcorn calcification pattern in a lobulated mass near the costochondral junction should be considered a chondrosarcoma until proved otherwise, and the mixed osteolysis and sclerosis pattern of osteosarcoma often can be recognized. Primary chest wall lesions form an obtuse angle with the chest wall with convexity directed inward.

Magnetic resonance imaging is not necessary in the routine radiologic evaluation and should be reserved for questions of involvement of vascular and neurologic structures with apical masses (subclavian artery and vein, brachial plexus) or vertebral body and neural foramina involvement for posterior chest wall lesions. Technetium bone scan or positron emission tomography should be performed to rule out systemic extrapulmonary metastases. Cross-sectional imaging of the brain can be reserved for patients experiencing neurologic symptoms because intracranial metastases originating from primary chest wall neoplasms are rare.

To complete a physiologic evaluation, all patients considered for chest wall resection should undergo pulmonary function testing with full spirometry. Quantitative perfusion should be performed in patients potentially requiring pneumonectomy or parenchymal resection with poor pulmonary function. This test also should be performed when anticipating large anterior chest wall resections, which may impede ventilatory mechanics postopertively.

Previous teaching has suggested that incisional biopsies should be performed routinely for all chest wall lesions. The advent of more sophisticated pathologic evaluation techniques and the ability to obtain large-core biopsy specimens of these accessible lesions have placed this recommendation in question, however. Small, single rib lesions can be removed en bloc as a therapeutic excisional biopsy. Most chondrosarcomas can be diagnosed with CT alone, and no biopsy is necessary. Core needle biopsy specimens should be obtained using ultrasound or CT guidance. In addition to careful preoperative imaging, a core biopsy specimen consistent with metastatic disease can abrogate unnecessary operative intervention, unless indicated for palliative reasons (toilet, unremitting pain), and may direct neoadjuvant therapy for high-grade sarcoma. The pathologist should be notified in advance of the procedure so that adequate tissue is obtained and handled appropriately.

If a core biopsy is not successful, a carefully placed incisional biopsy can be performed. The biopsy should be performed with a small incision, preferably placed longitudinally along the axis of the tumor, with consideration for the ability of eventual removal of this area at definitive resection later. The capsule of the mass, if present, should be closed after biopsy, and all efforts should be made to avoid spillage of mass contents into the surrounding tissues or the pleural space. It cannot be emphasized strongly enough that a core biopsy should be attempted in all patients initially because this may avoid larger procedures requiring more involved reconstruction later on due to local spread of tumor into the soft tissues resultant from open biopsy. Since the late 1980s, no patient with a chest wall neoplasm treated at the University of Texas M. D. Anderson Cancer Center has required an incisional biopsy for diagnosis.

Histologic findings consistent with plasmacytoma should prompt an evaluation for systemic multiple myeloma. Because of the high rate of local and distant failure with surgery alone, all high-grade sarcomas and malignant small round cell tumors (with the exception of chondrosarcoma) of the chest wall should be considered for neoadjuvant (preoperative) chemotherapy. This approach is suggested primarily in an effort to treat micrometastatic disease below the resolution of current imaging techniques and to allow in some cases for a technically less difficult resection with tumor response and shrinkage. There are no substantial data to support the use of neoadjuvant radiation therapy in chest wall neoplasms, and the surgeon should be concerned about the ability of the irradiated chest to heal properly at the soft tissue level, accept a prosthetic reconstruction, and resist infection after definitive resection.

■ SURGICAL TREATMENT

The method and safe margin of surgical resection for chest wall lesions have been a source of debate; however, there is no doubt that a complete resection is important. In addition to the issue of local control, many series have suggested that overall survival is affected by completeness of resection, even at the microscopic level. With the chest wall and plastic surgical soft tissue reconstruction options now available, anatomic concerns should not prevent an attempt at a complete resection, unless the patient is deemed physiologically incapable of tolerating the procedure. A suggested margin for high-grade sarcomas is at least 4 cm and one full rib above and below the palpable margin of the lesion. Desmoid tumors, alternatively considered low-grade sarcomas or benign tumors with an unusual proclivity for local recurrence, should be treated in a similar fashion. Resection margins of 2 to 3 cm can be acceptable for lower grade lesions, metastatic tumors, and tumors involving the chest wall by direct extension.

It is strongly suggested that questionable soft tissue margins be submitted for frozen section analysis and bony margins for decalcification and permanent assessment. This recommendation is tempered by the fact, however, that muscle-derived and fibrous tumors may be difficult to discern from surrounding scar or normal connective tissues at frozen section. The submission of bony margins is facilitated by the resection technique described later in this chapter. Adherence to overlying muscular fascia indicates the need for resection of the overlying muscle in question, with the margins dictated earlier, even if frank muscular involvement is not certain. If there is any question of involvement of overlying adipose tissue or skin, especially in the case of previous open procedures for diagnosis or previous resection, these structures should be resected as well. Prophylactic resection of questionably viable overlying soft tissue that has been irradiated or previously operated on is recommended because healthy tissue overlying resected and reconstructed areas is important to structural protection and the prevention of infection of prosthetic material if used.

The surgical approach (positioning, incision) is dictated by the location and nature of the chest wall lesion, the extent of overlying soft tissue involvement, the need for access to the underlying structures of the thoracic cavity, and planned reconstruction techniques. A preoperative assessment by a reconstructive plastic surgeon may assist in the decision-making process; this is strongly encouraged when there is a high likelihood of need for soft tissue transfer. If there is no spine involvement, an epidural catheter is strongly recommended. A double-lumen endotracheal tube should be used to allow deflation of the ipsilateral lung. This deflation may lessen the chance of lung injury during resection, assist with wedge resection of adherent lung, and allow careful palpation of the lung for other lesions. Patients with lateral and posterior chest wall lesions should be placed in the lateral position. If overlying skin and subcutaneous tissues are not involved, a standard posterolateral thoracotomy incision can give access to these areas with appropriate division of overlying chest wall musculature. The intercostal incision should be planned so that the mass can be avoided by at least one intercostal space. For more anterior chest wall lesions involving the sternum or parasternal area, the patient may be positioned supine with a planned sternotomy or "hemiclamshell" access incision.

When the pleural space is entered, the surgeon should palpate the mass and determine appropriate margins of resection. If the chest wall lesion involves overlying soft tissues and skin, which is often the case for cutaneous malignancies, such as squamous cell carcinoma or breast carcinoma with direct invasion, the soft tissues and the mass can be removed en bloc. In these situations, with the mass palpable on the exterior surface of the chest wall proper, a formal thoracotomy or sternotomy may not be required; rather the mass can be removed via margins dictated by palpation of the mass outside the pleural space. When an opening into the pleural space is made, however, the surgeon still should palpate the interior pleural surface to ensure that the margins chosen are appropriate. For high-grade sarcomas, one always should palpate the lung because known or occult pulmonary metastases may be present, and the patient can have them removed on this ipsilateral side at the same setting. Bilateral pulmonary metastases that are deemed resectable are not a contraindication to resection of a chest wall primary lesion. Tumor nodules present on the contralateral side can be removed in a staged fashion after recovery from chest wall resection.

Many techniques can be employed for the resection. Electrocautery has supplanted for many surgeons the use of the periosteal elevator for dissection around the ribs. Judicious use of electrocautery can allow for more reliable division and ligation of the intercostal vessels and lessen postthoracotomy pain resulting from thermal injury to the intercostal nerves.

The superior and inferior margins of the resection are determined, and the periosteal elevator is used to free the intercostal musculature and the neurovascular bundles from the upper and lower ribs proper. When the anterior and posterior planned margins are determined, electrocautery is used to clean the periosteum from a 1.5-cm length of each rib bordering the planned resection. The periosteal elevator is used to separate this rib segment from the underlying pleura, muscle, and neurovascular structures. Using a guillotine or shear rib-cutting device, 1-cm anterior and posterior rib segments are removed and submitted for permanent pathologic examination after decalcification (Figure 1). The pleura can be entered, and the intercostal muscle overlying the neurovascular bundle can be divided with electrocautery. The bundle can be ligated easily in continuity via these openings. If there is any suspicion that soft tissue margins are not adequate, frozen section and permanent tissue evaluation can be obtained. A rare positive finding in the resected bone evaluation can necessitate a reresection if appropriate or guide adjuvant radiation.

There are many options for reconstruction of the bony chest wall defect. Defects less than 4 cm in diameter and not overlying cardiac structures need not be reconstructed if soft tissue coverage is adequate. Larger defects may be left unreconstructed at the posterior apex because the scapula protects the area. It is important to be sure, however, that the scapular tip in the anatomic position will not catch under the rib edge bordering the inferior defect. This can be extremely painful and in some cases necessitate reoperation to alleviate. If this situation appears likely, prosthetic material should be used to cover the defect.

Defects overlying cardiac structures or measuring larger than 4 cm can be reconstructed with polypropylene mesh (Marlex) or polytetrafluoroethylene (PTFE) (Gore-Tex). We prefer polypropylene mesh because it provides a matrix for tissue ingrowth, is less likely to engender an overlying seroma, and even when infected occasionally can be retained. The interstices of the mesh become filled with fibrin within days, and leakage of pleural fluid is rarely a problem. The use of a methyl methacrylate "sandwich," whereby a double sheet of polypropylene mesh is used with a thin layer of methyl methacrylate inserted between, should be considered in larger defects overlying the heart and when chest wall contour is important to maintain adequate lung expansion or for cosmetic concerns (Figure 2). When the methyl methacrylate paste is placed on the mesh, it can be contoured appropriately by placing it over the patient's thigh or flank. Care should be taken to preserve a 1-cm rim of mesh as a "sewing ring" and to provide for some dynamic movement of the reconstructed area.

PTFE is recommended when a chest wall resection accompanies pneumonectomy; however, watertightness is necessary early on to allow the pleural space to fill. The size of the defect (and prosthesis needed) can be measured with a disposable ruler or by placing a dry laparotomy pad over the defect and using the blood outline as a guide.

The polypropylene mesh is sewn tightly to the superior and inferior ribs and to the margins of the anterior and posterior cut rib ends using heavy monofilament suture. To facilitate reliable suture placement and to avoid compression of intercostal nerves, the sutures are placed via 1-mm holes in the ribs created using a high-speed hand-held pneumatic drill. The use of rib punches or perforating towel clamps is

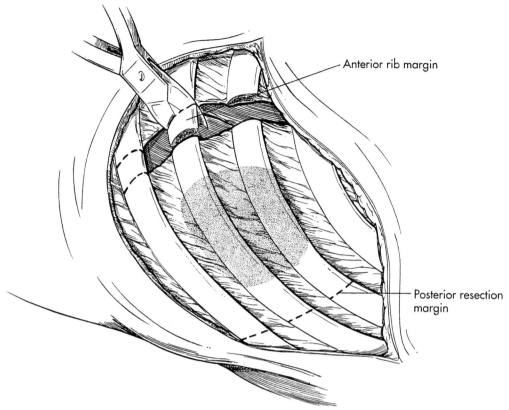

Figure 1
Technique of removal of rib segments in en bloc chest wall resection. *(From Kaiser LR: Chest wall resection. In: Atlas of general thoracic surgery. St Louis, 1997, Mosby.)*

to be avoided because these often fracture the ribs and do not ensure competent suture placement. The sutures are placed with the needles left in place so that they can be inserted through the mesh. Care should be taken to stretch the mesh taught as the sutures are tied to facilitate a sturdy reconstruction. If PTFE is used in the setting of pneumonectomy, the prosthesis is secured in a similar fashion, and the free edge of the material is sewn carefully to surrounding intercostals musculature and other soft tissue with a small monofilament suture to facilitate watertightness.

If overlying chest wall muscle has been removed, closure of skin with attenuated adipose tissue alone over prosthesis should be avoided if possible. The surgeon or a reconstructive surgical colleague should strive to cover the area with a pedicled rotation flap if possible (latissimus, pectoralis, serratus, rectus, or others). If this is not possible, a free flap should be considered. In the case of full-thickness chest wall resection, including skin, a pedicle of free myocutaneous flap can be used or a muscular free flap with skin graft.

Even larger resection defects, if properly reconstructed, should not impair respiratory mechanics to a significant degree. This reconstruction is facilitated greatly by a functioning epidural catheter. Of all resections, large anterior defects are most likely to present difficulties with adequate cough and secretion retention; aggressive pulmonary toilet

and bronchoscopy may be necessary in the immediate postoperative period. Empirical prolonged intubation should be avoided; most patients can be extubated in the operating room after chest wall resection. There is no "stabilization" benefit to elective retention of an endotracheal tube for a short period postoperatively, only the opportunity to develop other intubation-related morbidity.

■ RESULTS

The Mayo Clinic and the University of Texas M. D. Anderson Cancer Center have described survival of approximately 60% at 5 years postresection. In addition to new lesions, surgeons at referral hospitals often may see failed resections with local recurrence. Even in this setting, reresected patients with negative margins in the University of Texas M. D. Anderson series had an equivalent survival to patients treated initially. With careful planning and aggressive surgical resection supported by the reconstructive techniques outlined earlier, patients treated for chest wall neoplasms in most cases should expect prolonged survival and an acceptable functional and cosmetic result. Additional advances based on improvements in systemic treatment for high-grade sarcomas are anticipated.

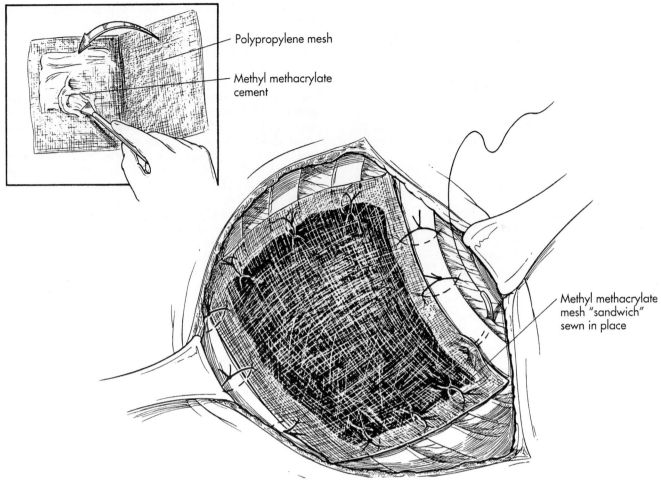

Polypropylene mesh

Methyl methacrylate cement

Methyl methacrylate mesh "sandwich" sewn in place

Figure 2
Addition of rigid prosthesis (methyl methacrylate) to polypropylene mesh for chest wall reconstruction. *(From Kaiser LR: Chest wall resection. In: Atlas of general thoracic surgery. St Louis, 1997, Mosby.)*

SUGGESTED READING

Athanassiadi K, et al: Primary chest wall tumors: early and long-term results of surgical treatment, *Eur J Cardiothorac Surg* 19:589, 2001.

Burt M: Primary malignant tumors of the chest wall, *Chest Surg Clin N Am* 4:137, 1994.

Burt M, et al: Medical tumors of the chest wall, *J Thorac Cardiovasc Surg* 105:89, 1993.

Dang NC, et al: Malignant chest wall tumors in children and young adults, *J Pediatr Surg* 34:1773, 1999.

Pairolero PC, Arnold PG: Thoracic wall defects: surgical management of 205 consecutive patients, *Mayo Clin Proc* 61:557, 1986.

Walsh GL, et al: A single-institutional, multidisciplinary approach to primary sarcoma involving the chest wall requiring full-thickness resections, *J Thorac Cardiovasc Surg* 121:48, 2001.

PROSTHETIC SUBSTITUTES IN CHEST WALL RECONSTRUCTION

Richard H. Lee
Anthony P. Tufaro

Indications for the use of prosthetic substitutes in chest wall reconstruction are not clearly established. Most defects less than 5 cm in diameter require only soft tissue coverage, however. Resections over the dorsoapical and posterior chest wall often do not require rigid support due to stability extended by the overlying scapula. Prosthetic substitutes are indicated most commonly in large defects (>5 cm) along the anterior and lateral aspects of the chest to prevent potential physiologic flail. Since the 1970s, prosthetic substitutes have ranged from rigid stainless steel to semisolid silicone to semipermeable polypropylene mesh. Characteristics of an optimal prosthesis include ease of use, adaptability to size and shape, malleability to contours, durability, inertness to body fluids, resistance to infection, translucency to x-rays, and incorporation by body tissues. Other important factors include the ability to provide an airtight and fluid-tight barrier (although not essential) and to lend rigid stability to the chest wall while not interfering with ventilatory excursion. This chapter focuses on the use of polytetrafluoroethylene (PTFE), polypropylene mesh, and methyl methacrylate in chest wall reconstruction; the pros and cons of each; their long-term results; management of complications; and operative techniques.

■ PROSTHETIC SUBSTITUTES

Polytetrafluoroethylene

PTFE (Gore-Tex; W.L. Gore and Associates, Inc., Flagstaff, AZ) has gained increasing popularity in surgical reconstruction since its development in the 1960s. PTFE has a wide range of applications, including serving as conduits for vascular bypass; soft tissue patch for abdominal wall reconstruction; and more recently soft tissue fillers for depressed scars, wrinkles, and lip and nasal augmentation. The expanded form of polytetrafluoroethylene (e-PTFE) is used for chest wall reconstruction. The material is flexible, durable, easy to conform to various sizes and shapes, and reportedly less susceptible to seroma or infection. e-PTFE is impervious to air and fluid and not incorporated well by the surrounding tissue. Instead a fibrous capsule forms around the patch. The early and long-term results of e-PTFE were studied retrospectively in a large series of patients (n = 197) who underwent chest wall resection and reconstruction using either PTFE or polypropylene mesh (Prolene; Ethicon, Inc., Somerville, NJ). Of patients, 64 underwent reconstruction using Prolene

mesh, and 133 underwent reconstruction using PTFE. Indication for resection included recurrent chest wall malignancy in 33%, primary chest wall malignancy in 31.5%, and contiguous lung or breast carcinoma in 29.4%. A median number of three ribs were resected, and partial sternectomy was performed in 46 patients (23.4%). Postoperative complications occurred in 91 patients (46.2%) with wound seromas in 10 patients with PTFE and 4 patients with Prolene mesh. Only two patients required reexploration and obliteration of the cavity for persistence of the seroma, whereas the rest resolved with conservative measures. Wound infections occurred in nine patients (five patients with Prolene mesh and four with PTFE). Three of the five patients with Prolene mesh had grossly contaminated wounds before resection, and all three patients developed postoperative wound infections necessitating removal of the mesh.

In all patients with postoperatively infected PTFE, the prosthesis was salvaged by débridement and packing. Mean follow-up period was 26 months. Deaths during this period were mostly secondary to recurrent malignancy. At last follow-up or at the time of death, 127 patients (70.9%) had an asymptomatic well-healed chest. On analysis of long-term outcome, preoperative chemotherapy, radiation, steroid use, diabetes, smoking history, chronic obstructive pulmonary disease, and extent of rib or sternal resection were not significantly associated with postoperative complications. The type of prosthesis used did not correlate with postoperative morbidity or mortality. The authors stated, however, that PTFE is preferable to Prolene mesh for its ease of suturing, stretching, and malleability and its ability to provide an airtight and fluid-tight barrier. The authors concluded from their earlier experience that prosthetic substitutes should not be used in contaminated wounds. If a wound infection does occur after prosthetic application in a clean wound, however, the authors recommended leaving the prosthesis in situ with aggressive wound débridement and packing. In their series, none of the salvaged prostheses resulted in the development of late wound infection or draining sinus tract.

In a smaller series of nine patients who underwent chest wall resections for either tumors or radiation ulcers, the results of reconstruction using e-PTFE were studied retrospectively. The defects ranged from 60 to 400 cm², and the resection involved removal of an average of four ribs with a mean skeletal defect of 221 cm². Soft tissue coverage over the e-PTFE involved latissimus dorsi, pectoralis major, and omentum in descending order of frequency. All patients were extubated on postoperative day 2, and none showed evidence of postoperative chest wall instability. Follow-up period was 34 months. Morbidity included a perioperative seroma in one patient and a late infection at 10 months in another patient, necessitating removal of the patch. The authors attributed their low infection rate to meticulous débridement of the wound before reconstruction, back to viable healthy tissue especially in irradiated defects. The authors stated that in grossly contaminated wound beds, reconstruction should be performed in a delayed fashion or without the use of prosthesis.

Polypropylene

Clinical experience with polypropylene mesh has been most extensive in abdominal wall reconstruction and inguinal hernia repair since its development in 1958. Prolene and Marlex (Bard Cardiosurgery, Billerica, MA) are the two most commonly used polypropylene-based mesh. Prolene is a double-stitch knit mesh and is relatively rigid. Marlex is single-stitch knit mesh and is malleable in one direction and rigid in the other. Its proponents claim that polypropylene is easy to sew and to mold to various defect sizes and shapes. Polypropylene is also semipermeable with a relatively large pore size of 75 μ. Macrophages and fibroblasts are able to pass through the mesh, and blood vessels and collagen fibers are able to filter and progress through the pores. This allows polypropylene to be incorporated readily by the surrounding tissue. Kroll et al retrospectively reviewed the data on Marlex mesh used for chest wall support. Included for study were 101 patients who underwent reconstruction with or without stabilization of the chest wall by Marlex mesh. Indications for chest wall resection were recurrent tumor in 41 patients, advanced primary tumor in 34 patients, and radiation necrosis in 9 patients. Chest wall was stabilized with Marlex mesh in 41 patients, 12 of whom also had muscle flap coverage. The remaining patients with Marlex mesh had local tissue realignment. Two patients with Marlex had postoperative wound infections, one of which was attributed to the partial flap necrosis of the overlying muscle flap. Overall complication rate was 25% with problems ranging from flap necrosis and wound dehiscence to pneumopericardium and congestive heart failure. The authors claimed that stabilization with Marlex mesh had a mean duration of ventilator dependence of 0.8 days versus 4.9 days without stabilization. Length of hospital stay also was decreased in patients with stabilization of the chest wall. The margin of these differences markedly increased when separately analyzed for patients with at least four ribs resected or patients who had partial sternectomy. Due to sample size and great patient variability, however, the data did not reach statistical significance. Comparisons made in this study are difficult to interpret because there was no standardization of patients and establishment of specific criteria under which Marlex mesh stabilization was used. The data are reportedly comparable to other studies in which Marlex mesh was used, however, and the authors advocated the use of Marlex mesh in chest wall stabilization as a means to decrease duration of ventilator dependence and length of hospital stay. From their experience, the authors concluded that as long as there is well-vascularized, healthy tissue overlying the mesh, the use of Marlex mesh should be standard in all full-thickness resections of the chest wall if significant instability otherwise would result.

Methyl Methacrylate

Methyl methacrylate in chest wall reconstruction is used in conjunction with mesh. Since its original description, a sandwich of two layers of Marlex mesh with methyl methacrylate in between has gained increasing acceptance due to its ability to provide complete rigid stabilization of the bony chest wall defect. Methyl methacrylate also is easy to mold to the defect size and shape in its prerigid, semisolid state. Care must be used in handling methyl methacrylate in the wound due to its exothermic hardening phase. Temperatures can reach 140°F in situ, causing surrounding tissue necrosis. McCormack described the technique of fashioning the

Marlex mesh initially ex vivo using a pattern made of the defect with a 5-cm sewing rim around the edges. Then the methyl methacrylate is mixed and poured on top of the mesh in its gelatinous phase. A second layer of Marlex is laid on top of the methyl methacrylate, and the composite sandwich is allowed to harden. The finished product is secured with a heavy suture approximating the prefashioned sewing rim to the skeletal defect.

Although rigid stabilization of the chest wall is preferred in the early postoperative period for achieving ventilator independence, the same property in the long-term may have adverse effects with progressive limitation of pulmonary function. Lardinois et al prospectively studied 26 patients who underwent chest wall resections along the anterolateral chest wall with minimal resection of three ribs followed by methyl methacrylate sandwich reconstruction. Indications for resection included primary tumors of the chest wall in nine patients (35%), chest wall metastasis in seven (27%), débridement for chronic infections including radionecrosis in five (19%), and chest wall infiltration of lung cancer in five (19%). All patients had uneventful postoperative extubation without the need for reintubation, although the length of time to ventilator dependence was not reported. Mean hospital stay was 24 days. Two patients (8%) had postoperative infection of their prosthesis at 8 and 12 months from the time of surgery. One of these patients had had resection of the chest wall for chronic pseudomonal osteomyelitis. After a failed trial of conservative therapy of débridement and antibiotics, the prosthetic was removed completely and reconstructed with pedicled omental flap and previously rotated pedicle latissimus dorsi flap. At 6-month follow-up, 73% of patients had resumed unrestricted daily activities with an asymptomatic chest wall. Pulmonary function in patients with methyl methacrylate chest wall fixation was assessed, and dynamic excursion of the chest wall was examined using cine magnetic resonance imaging (MRI) at 6 months postoperatively. There was no statistical difference in preoperative and postoperative forced expiratory volume in 1 second among patients without concurrent lung resection or wedge resection. Cine-MRI showed concordant chest wall movements in 92% of patients during respiratory excursion. Rigidity and limitation of chest wall movement were noted in the remaining 8%. The authors concluded that methyl methacrylate sandwich is useful among patients with large chest wall defects, especially in the anterolateral aspect of the chest. The stiffness of chest wall from methyl methacrylate does not impair pulmonary function.

■ COMPLICATIONS

Common complications encountered with the use of prosthetic substitutes include infection, wound dehiscence, and seroma formation. Infection in the setting of prosthetic hardware can have devastating consequences. Studies suggest, however, that if the prosthetic has well-vascularized healthy tissue coverage, conservative therapy is sufficient for salvaging the prosthetic in most cases of infection or wound dehiscence. Aggressive débridement of devitalized tissue, drainage of fluid collections, frequent dressing changes, and intravenous antibiotics are essential to any successful salvage, however. As stated previously, postoperative infection was treated successfully with conservative management in the study reviewing e-PTFE in chest wall reconstruction. There were no late wound infections and sinus tract formations in cases in which the prosthetic was salvaged with aggressive local wound care alone. In the setting of postoperative infection, the importance of having healthy tissue overlying prosthetic substitutes cannot be overemphasized, especially in cases in which chest wall resection is indicated secondary to chronic osteomyelitis or osteoradionecrosis. The resection must include a margin of healthy bleeding tissue. In cases in which there is underlying ongoing infection, the reconstruction should preclude the use of prosthetic substitutes and should be performed using autogenous tissue only. Rigid stabilization of the chest wall may be performed in a delayed fashion.

There is no general agreement regarding the management of persistent seromas. Some state that seromas usually resolve spontaneously and that serial percutaneous drainage should be discouraged due to the chance of introducing an infection. In these instances, we advocate watchful waiting with a low threshold for drainage of the seroma if infection is suspected.

■ AUTHORS' PREFERRED APPROACH

The authors' preferred prosthetic substitute for chest wall reconstruction is the PTFE soft tissue patch. As previously mentioned, PTFE offers a semirigid, airtight and fluid-tight barrier and is easy to adapt to the size and shape of the defect. PTFE is relatively inert to biologic fluids and is translucent to x-rays. Our experience with salvaging PTFE in the setting of postoperative wound infection with conservative therapy has been positive.

After resection of the chest wall mass by the thoracic surgeons, much time is spent preparing the resultant defect for reconstruction. A rim of tissue is taken additionally around the defect until it is clear that the edges of the defect are healthy and viable. All devitalized soft tissue and bone are débrided sharply with a knife, curet, or rongeur. A meticulous preparation of the defect is essential. In patients who undergo chest wall resection for osteoradionecrosis, it is important to resect all soft and bony tissue damaged by irradiation. After careful hemostasis is obtained, a template of the defect is made using the paper from a pair of surgical gloves. The PTFE patch is introduced into the field and fashioned according to the size and shape of the defect as outlined by the paper template. The patch is secured to the defect with interrupted 0-Gortex sutures. The patch should be on tension as it is sutured to the defect to achieve rigid stabilization of the chest wall. Each bite of the suture must include sturdy soft tissue, ribs, sternum, or even diaphragm in some cases around the defect. The patch must fit the defect without excess, bunching, or irregular border contours. The use of interrupted stitches aids in this effort. We believe that these measures help to prevent postoperative seroma or wound healing problems. After the patch is secured, a muscle flap, usually pedicled latissimus or pectoralis major, is rotated to cover the PTFE patch in its entirety. Even if there is adequate soft tissue for closure using local tissue realignment, we believe the presence of well-vascularized healthy muscle in between skin and the patch is essential. This is especially true in patients who require postoperative irradiation. The introduction of muscle flap over the soft tissue patch usually precludes primary closure of the overlying skin flaps. The muscle should be harvested with a skin island, or a split-thickness skin graft must be applied over the muscle flap. Two 10-mm flat Blake drains (Johnson & Johnson, Summersville, NJ) are placed in between the PTFE patch and the muscle flap.

We also have had success with Marlex mesh. Careful technique avoids infection and wound problems that may prolong time to postoperative irradiation. The Marlex is cut to size by using a glove paper template of the defect. The material is sutured carefully to stable bone or soft tissue with interrupted 2-0 Prolene sutures. The patch should be pulled taut to create semirigid repair. We prefer to cover the Marlex mesh with a muscle flap in almost all cases.

We have used autologous fascia lata grafts for smaller defects of the chest wall with success. The same principles of wide excision and débridement apply. The fascia is contoured to the shape of the defect using a prefabricated paper template. Then the fascia is sutured without excess, bunching, or border irregularities using 2-0 Prolene sutures in an interrupted horizontal mattress fashion. The fascial patch is covered with healthy fasciocutaneous or myocutaneous flaps.

■ SUMMARY OF GENERAL PRINCIPLES

Prosthetic substitutes are used most commonly to reconstruct large bony defects of the anterolateral chest wall. Prevention of physiologic flail by rigid stabilization of the chest wall has been shown to decrease the duration of ventilator dependence. Although many types of prosthetic materials exist, none have been shown clearly to be superior to the other. Certain general principles apply, however, in the use of prosthetic substitutes for chest wall reconstruction. Prosthetic substitutes should not be used in defects with evidence of ongoing preoperative infection. Even in clean wounds, the defect must have an adequate margin of healthy bleeding tissue before application of the prosthetic. Muscle flap coverage is highly recommended in all cases of prosthetic chest wall reconstruction. This increases the likelihood of salvaging the prosthesis if a postoperative infection arises. Lastly, postoperative infection and wound dehiscence can be treated in most cases with aggressive local wound care and intravenous antibiotics.

SUGGESTED READING

Arnold PG, Pairolero PC: Chest-Wall reconstruction: an account of 500 consecutive patients, *Plast Reconstr Surg* 98:804, 1996.

Deschamps C, et al: Early and long-term results of prosthetic chest wall reconstruction, *J Thorac Cardiovasc Surg* 117:588, 1999.

Hyans P, et al: Reconstruction of the chest wall with e-PTFE following major resection, *Ann Plast Surg* 29:321, 1992.

Kroll SS, et al: Risks and benefits of using Marlex mesh in chest wall reconstruction, *Ann Plast Surg* 31:303, 1993.

Lardinois D, et al: Functional assessment of chest wall integrity after methylmethacrylate reconstruction, *Ann Thorac Surg* 69:919, 2000.

MUSCLE FLAPS FOR CHEST WALL RECONSTRUCTION

Geoffrey M. Graeber

■ HISTORICAL CONSIDERATIONS

The use of pedicled muscular and musculocutaneous flaps to close substantial chest wall defects has been rediscovered since the early 1970s. Before that time, some surgeons had described using pedicled muscle flaps to reconstruct chest wall defects. The information they conveyed lay dormant, however, until the current resurgence of interest. Since the 1970s, there have been numerous articles that describe the merits of the use of pedicled muscular and musculocutaneous flaps in chest wall reconstruction. Although the use of free flaps for chest wall reconstruction has been described, their use is infrequent because so many pedicled flaps are readily available.

■ ETIOLOGY

The types of pathology that lead to chest wall defects usually fall into four categories: neoplasms, radiation injuries, infection, and trauma. Usually one of these etiologies is the primary cause of a chest wall lesion; however, radiation damage, infection, and neoplasm all may be present at one time in certain selected circumstances. Resection of the diseased portion of the chest wall commonly leaves a full-thickness defect, which requires reconstruction. Commonly, resection of these defects requires resection of the skeletal structure of the chest wall and the overlying soft tissues. Complete resection of the diseased portion of the chest wall is mandatory for appropriate reconstruction because leaving diseased tissue behind may cause the repair to become infected and break down.

■ CONSIDERATIONS FOR RECONSTRUCTION

Two major factors are important when considering reconstruction for an individual patient. One is that the disease process affecting the chest wall must be resected completely and total reconstruction achieved. Second is that the patient would be able to undergo such a major operative procedure and survive with remaining quality of life. Careful evaluation of potential candidates for chest wall resection and reconstruction includes a thorough preoperative workup that identifies all concomitant medical conditions and addresses their management before, during, and after surgery. Particular emphasis should be placed on evaluating the respiratory system and the amount of reserve present. If the patient has

limited pulmonary reserve, the need for chest wall stabilization increases. Most patients should come out of major chest wall resections and reconstructions without need for ventilatory support; however, some patients still do require ventilation for some time after surgery.

These resections and reconstructions are performed most often by an accomplished team of surgeons consisting of a thoracic surgeon and a plastic/reconstructive surgeon. This experienced team works together to achieve total eradication of the disease processes in the chest wall followed by thorough reconstruction. The goals of the reconstruction should be to preserve chest wall function while achieving maximal cosmetic closure. When pulmonary function is maximized, the patient should have only a small chance of requiring postoperative ventilatory support.

■ SKELETAL RECONSTRUCTION

Although skeletal reconstruction of full-thickness defects of the thorax is controversial, in most instances skeletal stabilization is recommended. In most instances, synthetic mesh or soft tissue patches are used to reconstruct the defect. The impermeable soft tissue patches have the advantage that they isolate the subcutaneous space from the pleural space. Chest tubes are isolated from any subcutaneous drainage system that may be in place. Either one may be removed independent of the other without fear of creating a pneumothorax.

Small chest wall defects generally do not need any skeletal reconstruction. Larger defects (diameter >5 cm) usually are reconstructed using chest wall stabilization. Most surgeons favor the use of a soft tissue patch because it can be contoured to the chest wall. In some instances, rigid materials have been used to stabilize the chest wall; however, these may be complicated by migration and erosion. The most commonly used rigid prostheses consist of a methyl methacrylate sandwich using two layers of polypropylene mesh separated by a solidified complex of methyl methacrylate. This composite graft needs to be formed away from the patient because it is markedly exothermic. In most instances, this composite graft is used in the lateral areas of the chest wall, where there is curvature that needs to be maintained to preserve pulmonary function.

Skeletal stabilization and reconstruction with some sort of material is recommended most for patients who have severe respiratory compromise. In these individuals, the relative rigidity imparted by the soft tissue patch helps maintain and maximize respiratory capabilities. In patients who have respiratory compromise and who require large defects, this type of reconstruction is helpful in assisting the patients to come off the ventilator after surgery. Autogenous tissues, including ribs and fascia lata and preserved animal tissues (e.g., bovine pericardium), are mostly of historical interest currently. A full discussion of chest wall stabilization prostheses may be found in the references.

■ SOFT TISSUE RECONSTRUCTION

Soft tissue reconstruction may be achieved either by the transposition of the omentum or by transposition of pedicled muscular flaps. Muscular and musculocutaneous flaps are preferred in many instances because they can be transposed with ease and may have varying cutaneous islands transposed with them. Muscular flaps alone may be used to close contaminated wounds because muscle is well known to be able to contain infection. Transposition of the omentum may be used when muscular flaps are not available but the omentum lacks structural support. Exposed omentum or muscular flaps may be covered by meshed, split-thickness skin grafts to allow adequate epithelialization.

Transposition of the omentum has two distinct disadvantages in that it requires a ventral hernia in the peritoneal cavity for exit of the pedicle, and infection may follow the omentum into the peritoneal cavity and cause secondary infection there. The use of omentum with muscular or musculocutaneous flaps may be helpful in closing particularly large defects. The omentum may be tailored using creative sectioning of the arterial arcades to fit irregular defects at great distances in the thoracic cavity. Coverage may be obtained by using muscular and musculocutaneous flaps over the omentum. Individual creativity of the surgeons involved is paramount in achieving an excellent structural and cosmetic reconstruction.

■ MUSCLE TRANSPOSITION

Pectoralis Major

The pectoralis major is a pedicled muscular flap that is particularly useful in closing anterior defects and defects of the upper sternum and base of the neck. The pedicled pectoralis major flap, conveyed either as a muscular or as a musculocutaneous flap, is quite robust and is based on the thoracoacromial neurovascular bundle that arises from underneath the lateral third of the clavicle. The secondary blood supply of this muscle is the internal mammary artery and vein, which allow the muscle to be based medially and overturned on itself to help fill midline defects.

Rectus Abdominis Muscle

The rectus abdominis muscle and its musculocutaneous flaps are particularly beneficial in reconstructing anterior and inferolateral defects of the chest wall. These flaps also have been used as a method of reconstruction for the breast. This flap's vascular pedicle is based on the superior epigastric artery and veins because the inferior epigastric artery and veins and all vascular contributions from the intercostals coming in laterally need to be transected to rotate the flap. Any procedure that interrupts the superior epigastric artery and vein (e.g., the harvesting of an internal mammary artery, which is the direct parent of the artery) contraindicates the use of this muscular flap. A few individuals have described rotating this flap based on some of the higher intercostals; however, this may prove to be a dangerous procedure, and the vascular supply may not be adequate to sustain the pedicled flap. The skin island transferred with the rectus is most viable when oriented vertically; however, transverse flaps have been used with varying degrees of success. Transverse skin islands may have compromise of blood flow at the most lateral aspects of the cutaneous portion of the flap.

Latissimus Dorsi Muscle

As a result of its size and location, this muscle is useful in covering posterior, lateral, and anterior defects. Its primary blood supply is the thoracodorsal neurovascular bundle. Its distal blood supply consists of the perforators of the lumbodorsal fascia. Any thoracotomy incision that interrupts the thoracodorsal neurovascular bundle divides the muscle into two territories with respect to its vascular supply. The distal portion of the muscle depends on the lumbodorsal fascia perforators for its blood supply after transection for thoracotomy. The proximal portion of the muscle depends on the thoracodorsal neurovascular bundle. Attempts of mobilization of the entire muscle under these conditions usually results in necrosis of the distal portion of the flap. Integrity of the thoracodorsal neurovascular bundle is mandatory for transposition of the flap and the health of any muscular or cutaneous component of the flap. The harvest site of this large musculocutaneous flap may need to be covered with a meshed, split-thickness skin graft because transposition of such a large flap removes so much tissue from the posterolateral aspect of the thorax that the remaining soft tissues cannot be drawn together successfully.

Serratus Anterior

Serratus anterior muscle relies on the serratus branches of the thoracodorsal neurovascular bundle for its blood supply. Some blood supply also may be derived from the long thoracic artery and vein. In most instances, this muscle is used only as a muscular flap in reconstruction of the chest. It may be used in conjunction with other muscles to fill large defects. Most commonly, the serratus is brought into the chest to cover a bronchopleural fistula or an esophageal injury. In this instance, it is pedicled proximally, and a portion of the second rib is resected to allow the muscle to go into the chest. The muscle is fixed in place to repair the internal thoracic defect. The arc of rotation also allows it to be brought anteriorly to work with other muscles to fill a large anterior defect. Its rotation posteriorly is limited by its pedicle and the surrounding anatomy.

■ RESULTS

Several published series have shown that reconstruction of the chest wall can be conducted safely with excellent long-term results. The morbidity and mortality rates are low. Deterioration of pulmonary function, although it occurs, is relatively infrequent. Most patients are weaned from the ventilator directly after surgery. The necrosis and loss of pedicled muscular and musculocutaneous flaps are relatively rare. Success is achieved best by complete resection of the pathologic process involving the chest wall followed by judicious skeletal stabilization and soft tissue coverage. A thoracic surgeon and plastic surgeon working together to achieve these results have proved to be a successful combination for most teams embarking on these challenging endeavors.

SUGGESTED READING

Arnold PF, Pairolero PC: Chest wall reconstruction: an account of 500 consecutive patients, *Plast Reconstr Surg* 98:804, 1996.

Graeber GM: Surgical techniques for the chest wall and sternum: chest wall resection, chest wall stabilization and soft tissue reconstruction. In Pearson FG, et al, editors: *Thoracic Surgery*, ed 2, New York, 2002, Churchill Livingstone, p 1441.

Graeber GM: Chest wall resection and reconstruction, *Semin Thorac Cardiovasc Surg* 11:251, 1999.

Graeber GM, Langenfeld J: Chest wall resection and reconstruction. In Franco KL, Putnam JB Jr, editors: *Advanced Therapy in Thoracic Surgery,* London, 1998, BC Decker, p 175.

Graeber GM, Seyfer AE: Complications of chest wall resection and the management of flail chest. In Waldhousen JA, Orringer MB, editors: *Complications in cardiothoracic surgery,* St Louis, 1990, Mosby Year Book, p 413.

INFECTIONS OF THE CHEST WALL

John D. Urschel

Infections of the chest wall may be classified into primary and secondary (postoperative, postradiation) infections. Primary chest wall infections, such as actinomycosis and tuberculosis, are encountered regularly in many parts of the world. In industrialized countries, most chest wall infections are complications of surgical procedures, and a few are late complications of radiation therapy. Secondary chest wall infections can be categorized into five major clinical entities: thoracotomy wound infection, sternotomy wound infection, necrotizing soft tissue infection (NSTI), costal chondritis, and radionecrosis of the chest wall. Thoracotomy wounds, similar to other soft tissue wounds, occasionally become infected. Standard management strategies are familiar to all surgeons. The wound is opened, cultured, and packed, and antimicrobial therapy is prescribed. If an empyema is present, it must be drained. Concepts of thoracotomy wound management are sufficiently straightforward that further review in this chapter is not necessary. Sternotomy wound infections, in contrast to thoracotomy infections, are much more morbid, and their management is complex. Associated mediastinitis is often life-threatening. Although the incidence of poststernotomy infection is acceptably low, the sheer number of sternotomies performed on any cardiothoracic service virtually guarantees that all cardiothoracic surgeons have experience recognizing and treating this type of chest wall infection. The treatment of poststernotomy infections is the topic of many reviews and is covered in another chapter; it is not discussed here. This chapter focuses on the last three categories of chest wall infection: NSTI, costal chondritis, and radionecrosis of the chest wall.

■ NECROTIZING SOFT TISSUE INFECTIONS OF THE CHEST WALL

NSTI of the chest wall are rare but highly lethal infections. Classic necrotizing infections due to single organisms, such as *Clostridium perfringens,* can occur, but most infections are polymicrobial. Anaerobes and aerobes act synergistically to invade soft tissue rapidly and elaborate toxins; tissue necrosis and severe systemic sepsis follow. Any thoracic surgical procedure may be complicated by NSTI, but these infections usually occur in the setting of thoracostomy drainage of empyemas and contaminated esophageal operations. Excessive dissection of soft tissues during tube thoracostomy for empyemas may predispose to these infections. The external appearance of the skin or cutaneous wound often initially betrays the magnitude of the necrotizing infection that lies beneath. This fact, along with the mistaken belief that all necrotizing infections produce tissue gas, contributes to diagnostic delay. Postoperative patients exhibiting unexplained septic deterioration and any hint of wound complication should have the wound opened. The presence of necrotic wound tissue is usually obvious. Patients showing signs of septic deterioration after tube thoracostomy should have the dressing removed for proper examination. If the skin is edematous and discolored, a diagnostic 6- or 8-cm incision down to fascia and muscle under local anesthesia is indicated. This incision quickly establishes or refutes the diagnosis of NSTI. Failure to consider the diagnosis of NSTI and failure to diagnose it when the patient is still salvageable are leading causes of treatment failure.

In addition to diagnostic delay, inadequate débridement is another common cause of treatment failure. Débridement must be aggressive. All infected and nonviable tissue must be excised. Incision and drainage strategies are simply not appropriate or acceptable. Associated pleural empyemas should be débrided and the lung decorticated. No attempt should be made to close the wound at the first débridement. Instead the patient is ventilated (severity of illness requires this anyway) and returned to the operating room the next day for examination of the tissues; further débridement usually is needed. Several débridements in the operating room usually are required to control the infectious process adequately. When the wound is healthy and no longer requires débridement, it can be managed in the intensive care unit (ICU).

Hyperbaric oxygen therapy may be beneficial in treating NSTI, especially infections due to clostridial organisms. Initial surgical débridement is therapeutically more important, however, than hyperbaric oxygen therapy; this should be remembered when considering transfer of these critically ill patients to a center with hyperbaric capabilities. In addition to aggressive surgical intervention, patients with NSTI of the chest wall need equally aggressive ICU support. They require intravenous fluid resuscitation, inotropes, correction of coagulation disorders, mechanical ventilation, broad-spectrum antibiotics, and nutritional support. Despite aggressive surgical and ICU management, most patients with NSTIs of the chest wall succumb to the illness.

Patients who survive the initial fulminant phase of the disease face two other formidable problems: weaning from the ventilator and wound closure. Large portions of the chest wall are resected during débridement so that weaning from the ventilator is a slow process. Closure of the wound is even more difficult. Muscle flaps that typically are used to close chest wall defects may have been sacrificed during débridement. Second-line muscle flaps or omental transposition may be needed. An innovative reconstructive surgeon should work with the thoracic surgeon to obtain wound closure. Definitive and complete wound closure may not be possible; part of the wound may have to heal by secondary intention.

■ COSTAL CHONDRITIS

Costal cartilages, in contrast to their osseous counterparts, are essentially avascular structures. Costal cartilages may become infected after any operation that violates the costal perichondrium. Left thoracoabdominal incisions for esophageal surgery, parasternal incisions for minimally invasive cardiac surgery, and pectoralis major flap transposition are some of the most notable predisposing operations. Costal chondritis is an insidious infection that usually appears weeks after a seemingly uneventful operation. Patients are usually already discharged from the hospital when the infection manifests, so it is difficult to obtain accurate incidence data for these postoperative chest wall infections. Costal chondritis can be prevented by avoiding incisions into the perichondrium during mobilization of pectoralis major flaps and by minimizing trauma to costal cartilages during minimally invasive parasternal incisions. If traumatized during surgery, costal cartilages should be resected, but the perichondrium should be preserved. The costal margin is divided intentionally during the course of a left thoracoabdominal incision for esophageal surgery. At my institution, the costal margin is divided sharply with a scalpel during opening, then 1 cm of cartilage is resected subperichondrially from each divided end at the time of closure. The preserved perichondrium is used as a vascularized flap to cover the ends of the cartilage during closure, similar to skin that is fashioned to cover an amputation stump. This flap seems to reduce the risk of postoperative cartilage infection.

Postoperative costal chondritis manifests as wound redness, edema, and drainage of purulent material through wound sinuses. Patients may have a low-grade fever and feel unwell, but it is unusual for them to be acutely ill. For the experienced surgeon, the clinical presentation is immediately recognizable. Inexperienced physicians may prescribe several courses of antibiotics and attempt incision and drainage under local anesthesia before fully appreciating the correct diagnosis of costal chondritis. These simple measures may be successful temporarily, but the drainage and redness eventually recur. Avascular cartilage lies dead in the depths of the wound, and it cannot be cured with antibiotics and minor drainage procedures. Some patients may be so frail from their underlying medical conditions that acceptance of the chronic infection and simple wound care may be advisable. If a permanent cure is desired, formal surgical treatment is needed.

Surgical treatment requires general anesthesia and wide exposure of the affected tissues. Necrotic cartilages should be resected in their entirety, from osseous rib to sternum. One normal cartilage superior and inferior to the diseased cartilages should be resected as well. The perichondrium of these normal cartilages should be preserved, however. Radical excision of osseous structures is not needed. The chest wall is often fairly rigid from the infectious process so that hard tissue (prosthetic material) reconstruction usually is not needed. Soft tissue reconstruction, with omentum or muscle flaps, may be indicated if the surgical defect is large. Skin sinuses are excised, but otherwise skin is preserved for use during closure. Dead space should be eliminated or drained during closure. If all necrotic cartilage is excised, the results are good. If not, the wound is destined to develop recurrent redness and drainage.

■ RADIONECROSIS OF THE CHEST WALL

Chest wall necrosis may occur years after radiotherapy for breast cancer or other malignancies. Radiation causes an obliterative endarteritis with secondary tissue ischemia and necrosis. Minor trauma may lead to progressive tissue loss. Simple débridement of nonviable tissue back to relatively healthy tissue is disappointing; the remaining tissue often promptly necroses. Cartilage, bone, and soft tissue often are affected by the radiation-induced ischemic process, then secondarily infected by bacteria. A foul chronic draining wound results. It causes considerable misery for the patient. Patient fitness (cardiac, pulmonary, and general performance status) and the presence or absence of recurrent malignancy are key issues that influence treatment decisions. The usual workup includes chest wall biopsies, multisystem cancer staging investigations, pulmonary function studies, and computed tomography of the chest. Computed tomography shows the extent of chest wall involvement and any extension into the mediastinum or pleural cavities. Treatment options include conservative management of a chronic nonhealing wound or aggressive resection combined with reconstruction. A conservative approach may be appropriate for frail patients or patients with advanced malignancy. Surgical treatment is ideal for fit patients without recurrent malignancy or patients with a reasonable life expectancy despite recurrent malignancy.

Surgical therapy involves complete resection of nonviable radiated tissue. Necrotic cartilage and osseous sequestra must be vigorously débrided. Incomplete resection is a common cause of recurrent wound failure. Prosthetic material should not be used for reconstruction because the operative field is heavily contaminated. Muscle flaps usually provide enough stability to the chest wall and obviate the need for hard tissue (prosthetic mesh) reconstruction. If the chest wall defect is particularly large, and postoperative chest wall instability is a major concern, absorbable mesh (polyglactin 910 mesh [Vicryl]) can be used. The absorbable mesh provides initial stability to facilitate postoperative pulmonary recovery, but it is hydrolyzed and absorbed approximately 100 days after implantation.

Soft tissue reconstruction is accomplished using a muscle flap, omentum, or both. A contralateral pectoralis major flap, based on its thoracoacromial vascular pedicle, usually is used to reconstruct parasternal chest wall defects. More lateral chest wall defects can be closed with an ipsilateral latissimus dorsi flap, based on its thoracodorsal artery. Muscle flaps have the advantage of creating bulk and stability in the chest wall defect and do not require a laparotomy. The omentum, based on the right gastroepiploic vessels, is well suited for reconstruction of infected radionecrotic chest wall defects. It fits into the irregular contours of the chest wall defect and brings excellent vascularity to the area. The omentum resists infection in these contaminated wounds, and it forms valuable granulation tissue in the event that primary healing partially or completely fails. It is a good bed for skin grafts. The omentum does not have the bulk of muscle flaps, however, and does not contribute to chest wall stability.

■ COMMON THEMES IN THE SURGICAL MANAGEMENT OF INFECTIONS OF THE CHEST WALL

Two important themes are common to the management of the disparate infectious chest wall conditions discussed in this chapter: Diagnostic skill is needed, and incomplete resection of diseased chest wall tissue leads to treatment failure. Surgeons must not lose sight of these two key concepts.

SUGGESTED READING

Arnold PG, Pairolero PC: Reconstruction of the radiation-damaged chest wall, *Surg Clin N Am* 69:1081, 1989.

Urschel JD, et al: Necrotizing soft tissue infections of the chest wall, *Ann Thorac Surg* 64:276, 1997.

Young JE, et al: Costal chondritis after thoracoabdominal esophagectomy, *J Surg Oncol* 80:61, 2002.

THORACOPLASTY

Watts R. Webb
Frank E. Schmidt

■ CONVENTIONAL THORACOPLASTY

Thoracic surgery developed as a specialty through the early attempts to treat pulmonary tuberculosis and its pleural space problems. Early collapse therapy for tuberculosis developed from the realization that nature attempted to heal tuberculosis by collapsing the involved portion of the lung. Early attempts used sandbags and positioning with the diseased side down. Costal excursions were reduced further by intercostal neurectomy and transection of the accessory muscles of respiration, such as the anterior scalene muscle. Later the phrenic nerve was crushed, with pneumothorax and pneumoperitoneum used to create long-term, reversible collapse. Thoracoplasty was developed to achieve a more permanent and greater degree of collapse, particularly in patients unsuitable for lesser attempts.

Thoracoplasty began with de Cerenville in 1885, who resected short lengths of two or more ribs anteriorly to collapse the chest wall over apical disease for tuberculosis. Schede extended this in 1890 by resecting not only multiple ribs, but also the parietal pleura, periosteum, intercostal muscles, and neurovascular bundles primarily for localized empyema. This resection collapsed the chest wall even when the parietal pleura was rigid. It had multiple disadvantages in being mutilating, sacrificing the intercostal nerves, and leaving a poorly protected heart and an unstable chest wall. In 1907, Brauer and Friedrich resected several lengths of the second through the ninth ribs, including the periosteum and intercostal muscles, to mimic collapse obtained by a pneumothorax. This approach produced massive instability of the chest wall, however, and carried a high mortality rate. Goode in 1912 reported good results in treating nontuberculous empyema with short resections of several ribs in the paravertebral gutter. Alexander in 1937 reported the now classic three-stage thoracoplasty, removing the ribs from the vertebral laminae forward. Two to 3 weeks were allowed between stages to permit stiffening of the periosteal beds. Leaving the periosteum in situ allowed new bone formation that ensured long-term collapse of the diseased lung. This approach achieved a 75% to 80% sputum conversion and cavity closure in appropriate patients even before the advent of chemotherapy and was a tremendous step forward.

■ PLOMBAGE THORACOPLASTY

Because the conventional thoracoplasty was debilitating and cosmetically unacceptable, extrapleural paraffin plombage was introduced as a less mutilating form of collapse. Various materials, such as blood, plastic balls, polyvinyl alcohol sponges (Ivalon), or wax, were placed extrapleurally between the ribs and the lung. The periosteum was stripped from the ribs and collapsed with the intercostal muscles and neurovascular bundles; the plombage was placed between the ribs and the periosteum. These operations provided good selective collapse, and an eight-rib or a nine-rib thoracoplasty could be accomplished in one stage. It offered support for an effective cough, freedom from perioperative paradoxical thoracic motion, and minimal deformity of the chest wall. Similarly, pulmonary function was preserved much better by plombage thoracoplasty than the conventional thoracoplasty. Plombage resulted in sputum conversion and control of tuberculosis in more than 60% in one series of patients with few complications. In one series, 150 Ivalon sponges were inserted in 144 consecutive patients. Of these sponges, 85 were used for primary collapse, and the remaining 65 were inserted concomitant with or after pulmonary resections. Only three became infected, and none of these were tuberculous. The infected sponges were removed easily, and the ribs were resected in conversion to a standard thoracoplasty with early healing. Plombage thoracoplasty was abandoned because the osteoplastic thoracoplasty became recognized as a better alternative.

■ OSTEOPLASTIC THORACOPLASTY

In 1954, Bjork described an osteoplastic thoracoplasty that had all the advantages of the plombage thoracoplasty without its disadvantages. Posterior ends of the upper ribs are resected in increasing lengths back to the tip of the transverse processes, which are left intact (Figure 1). A short segment of the first rib could be resected, or preferably the periosteum could be peeled from its inferior surface, preserving a more cosmetic result. The intercostal bundles were divided posteriorly in the original description, but it was found that this often could be avoided. An apicolysis is performed with the apical pleura being reflected down to the aortic arch or the azygos vein or even lower if desired. The periosteum and intercostal muscle and/or pleura are sutured to the mediastinal structures to prevent expansion of the lungs superiorly. The ribs are reflected down, and the posterior ends are affixed with wire to the uppermost intact rib. A seven-rib thoracoplasty can be performed safely even at the time of pulmonary resection because of the immediate complete stability of the chest wall. For most surgeons, this remains the preferred technique when a tailoring thoracoplasty is needed to reduce the size of the hemithorax after an extensive pulmonary resection. This is of particular importance in tuberculosis because all too often reactivation of disease has been observed in an overexpanded lung. Similarly, if the remaining lung is

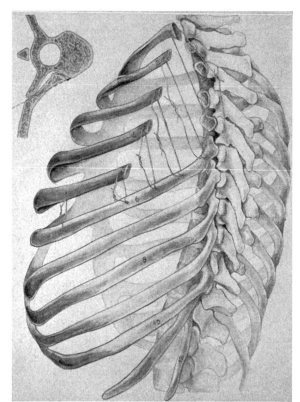

Figure 1
Osteoplastic thoracoplasty as described by Bjork. Increasingly longer segments of the posterior ribs are resected. The ends are wired to the lowest intact rib. The first rib may be left intact, if desired, by stripping the periosteum from its undersurface. (*From Bjork VO:* J Thorac Surg *28:194, 1954.*)

too small or is fibrotic, there may be an unfilled space that is potentially susceptible to infection.

■ THORACOPLASTY FOR EMPYEMA

Use of the conventional thoracoplasty to control an empyema after a pneumonectomy was advocated by Alexander, who noted the following principles for its safe application. All of the procedures should be done in stages limited in extent by the ability of the patient to withstand the operation but rapid enough that immobility does not occur between stages. Also, he advocated resection of the first rib to allow collapse of the apex of the chest cavity. This latter practice is no longer regarded as necessary, however, because periosteal stripping of the undersurface of the first rib allows the apex to collapse and much improve the chest contour. Alexander advocated that the posterior extent of the resection should include portions of the transverse processes. Sloping resection of the anterior portion of the lower ribs would minimize the deformity and help maintain the structural integrity needed for preservation of pulmonary function. Experience showed that this type of thoracoplasty did obliterate the thoracic space and permanently control the empyema. It often closed the bronchopleural fistula or enabled it to be closed more easily by muscle transposition. The overall success rate of thoracoplasty was 73% in one series in eliminating thoracic space problems. This thoracoplasty has disadvantages because of major physical disability and frequently "frozen shoulder" resulting in a poorly functioning arm. Thoracoplasty usually is performed now only when other procedures have failed or cannot be performed.

Empyema, especially with a bronchopleural fistula, may be particularly difficult to eradicate if infection or cavitation remains in the lung. Utley used a one-stage completion pneumonectomy and modified eight-rib thoracoplasty in patients who had fungal cavities in the lung, fungal empyema, and bronchopleural fistulas. He sutured the intercostal bundles to the bronchial stump as reinforcement. Antifungal and antibiotic irrigations were injected postoperatively through the chest tube, which was left in place for 6 to 8 weeks. All healed primarily with good long-term results.

■ SCHEDE THORACOPLASTY

The Schede thoracoplasty involves resection of not only the ribs, but also the intercostal muscles, endothoracic fascia, and parietal pleura so that only the skin and the extrathoracic muscles remain. These are expected to collapse onto the residual lung and obliterate any pleural space. Although this is a mutilating procedure, Horrigas and Snow found that a modified Schede thoracoplasty was effective in 13 patients in closing chronic empyema spaces. Eleven of these patients had bronchopleural fistulas that were closed successfully by the concomitant use of extrathoracic muscle flaps. The Schede and other types of thoracoplasty have virtually been abandoned in the treatment of empyema in favor of use of the Claggett or various other procedures. If there is a viable lung that can be reexpanded, decortication may be much more effective in closing the empyema space. After pneumonectomy or with a nonexpandable lung, chest muscle flaps or the omentum is placed into the pleural space, and these maneuvers along with antibiotic therapy have virtually eliminated the need for thoracoplasty in empyemas.

SUGGESTED READING

Alexander J: *The collapse therapy of pulmonary tuberculosis*, Springfield, IL, 1937, Thomas.

Allen, MB Jr, Webb WR: The use of a plastic sponge (Ivalon) in operative procedures for pulmonary tuberculosis, *J Thorac Surg* 34:21, 1957.

Bjork VO: Thoracoplasty: a new osteoplastic technique, *J Thorac Surg* 28:194, 1954.

Horrigas TP, Snow NJ: Thoracoplasty: current application to the infected pleural space, *Ann Thorac Surg* 50:695, 1990.

Pairolero PC, et al: Postpneumonectomy empyema: the role of intrathoracic muscle transposition, *J Thorac Cardiovasc Surg* 99:958, 1990.

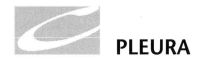

PLEURA

SPONTANEOUS PNEUMOTHORAX

Sean C. Grondin
Willard A. Fry

Etard first introduced the term *pneumothorax* in 1803. It was not until 1819, however, that Laennec described the signs and symptoms associated with this entity. Pneumothorax is an accumulation of air in the pleural space leading to lung collapse. Pneumothoraces are classified based on their etiology or clinical presentation. Although most pneumothoraces can be managed successfully with tube thoracostomy, patients with recurring pneumothoraces should be considered for operative intervention.

■ ETIOLOGY

Primary pneumothoraces occur due to the rupture of the visceral pleura (subpleural blebs) in a patient with no known pulmonary disease. Secondary pneumothoraces occur due to an existing lung condition, trauma, or an iatrogenic injury (Table 1). Primary pneumothoraces are more common than secondary pneumothoraces. A male preponderance of 3:1 is reported, with tall, thin males between the ages of 15 (postpuberty) and 30 most commonly affected. Cigarette smoking increases the risk of primary pneumothorax by a factor of 20.

■ DIAGNOSIS

Most cases of spontaneous pneumothorax present with sudden-onset ipsilateral pleuritic chest pain with some shortness of breath and occur when the patient has been at rest. Physical examination can be deceivingly normal, particularly for a small pneumothorax (<15% of the hemithorax). Patients presenting with larger pneumothoraces may have dyspnea and tachycardia. Findings on respiratory examination may include diminished or absent breath sounds, hyperresonant percussion note, decreased movement of the chest wall, and diminished fremitus on the affected side. A chest radiograph assists in confirming the diagnosis by documenting the presence of a thin visceral pleural line displaced from the chest wall on the upright posterior-anterior chest radiograph. Although a chest radiograph performed during expiration may assist in identifying a small pneumothorax, it is rarely needed. A variety of methods have been devised to estimate the extent of collapse observed in a pneumothorax. Often it is simplest to describe the degree of pneumothorax in terms of the number of centimeters that the lung is down from the apex of the chest cavity, how far down along the lateral wall the lung is retracted, and how far away it is from the lateral border of the chest wall in the midthorax. Occasionally a computed tomography (CT) scan of the chest is helpful in planning surgical intervention.

■ INITIAL TREATMENT

Clinically Stable Patient
Observation
Historically, spontaneous pneumothoraces were treated with observation. Today, observation is reserved for asymptomatic patients who present with a pneumothorax of less than 20%. In such a case, the patient should be observed in the emergency department for 4 to 6 hours and discharged home if a repeat chest radiograph excludes progression of the pneumothorax. On discharge, the patient should be provided with careful instructions for follow-up within 12 to 48 hours, depending on circumstances. A repeat chest radiograph is obtained at the follow-up visit to document resolution of the pneumothorax. If the patient lives a distance away from emergency services or is considered unreliable, it is safest to admit this patient to the hospital for observation and follow-up chest radiographs.

Tube Thoracostomy
Larger pneumothoraces (>20%) usually are treated with prompt reexpansion of the lung by tube thoracostomy. In patients with emphysema or with significant symptoms, a lesser degree of pneumothorax often is treated to reexpand the lung. The size of the chest tube for insertion varies depending on the patient's habitus and the surgeon's preference. Today, chest tubes usually are made of plastic (Argyle tube) with a number scale marking the distance to the first hole on the tube. A tube larger than 20 Fr rarely is required. In many instances, a small 8 Fr pigtail catheter is effective, although care must be taken to ensure the tube does not kink or obstruct. An intravenous or intramuscular narcotic often is given before insertion to relax the patient and assist with analgesia. Normally the tube is placed under generous local anesthesia (1% or 2% lidocaine) in the fourth or fifth intercostal space in the anterior or midaxillary line and is directed toward the apex of the affected hemithorax. The tube is tunneled over the rib to form a subcutaneous tract that can be compressed on removal of the tube. This technique is effective in preventing a hole that may lead to an air leak when a

Table 1 Classification of Pneumothorax

SPONTANEOUS
Primary
    Subpleural bleb rupture
Secondary
    Bullous disease, including chronic obstructive lung disease
    Cystic fibrosis
    Asthma
    Connective tissue diseases, especially Marfan's syndrome
    Interstitial lung diseases, especially eosinophilic granuloma
    Pneumocystis carinii pneumonia
    Pneumonia with lung abscess
    Catamenial
    Metastatic cancer, especially sarcomas
    Lung cancer
    Esophageal perforation
Neonatal
ACQUIRED
Iatrogenic
    Central line placement
    Pacemaker insertion
    Transthoracic needle biopsy
    Transbronchial needle biopsy
    Thoracocentesis
    Chest tube malfunction
    After laparoscopic surgery
Barotrauma
Traumatic
    Blunt trauma
        Motor vehicle accident
        Falls
        Sports related
    Penetrating trauma
        Gunshot wounds
        Stab wounds

tube must remain in place for more than a few days. Insertion of the tube through the chest wall into the pleural space can be accomplished using a clamp, a finger technique, or trocar technique. The Advanced Trauma Life Support course sponsored by the American College of Surgeons recommends the clamp and finger technique. Trocar insertion or pigtail catheter insertion using the Seldinger technique is reserved for experienced surgeons familiar with chest wall anatomy. These latter techniques are usually quicker and more comfortable for the patient.

Catheters or chest tubes can be attached to a variety of chest drainage systems. Typically a Heimlich valve is used for outpatient management, and the water seal device is used for inpatient care. The tube is left in place until the air leak resolves and the lung is fully expanded. If the lung fails to reexpand, the position of the chest tube is reassessed radiographically (chest x-ray or occasionally CT scan), and suction is applied to a water seal device. Reliable patients who are unwilling to be hospitalized may be discharged home from the emergency department with a small-bore catheter attached to a Heimlich valve if the lung has reexpanded after the removal of pleural air. If a Heimlich valve is used, some provision for fluid drainage is required, such as a bronchoscopic mucus trap with some absorbent gauze or a vented urinary drainage bag. These patients usually are seen in follow-up within 48 hours.

In most instances, a primary spontaneous pneumothorax responds to tube thoracostomy. Generally the air leak from the lung seals after 1 to 2 days, and the chest tube can be removed. Patients also are counseled to avoid underwater diving, to avoid isolated travel experiences (e.g., camping trip), and to stop smoking if applicable. Air travel is discouraged for at least 1 week. Patients are informed that there is approximately a 30% chance of recurrence. The risk of recurrence increases to 60% to 70% if a second pneumothorax develops. Given these rates, surgery is recommended for patients with recurrent pneumothoraces.

In some instances, operative intervention is indicated after the first episode of spontaneous pneumothorax as would be the case for a patient with a prior pneumonectomy, a patient with a history of untreated bilateral pneumothoraces, or a patient with occupational hazards such as an airplane pilot or diver. The U.S. Air Force does not allow a pilot to fly until he or she has undergone surgical therapy after a spontaneous pneumothorax.

Needle Aspiration

The role of simple aspiration of a pneumothorax without chest tube placement is controversial. In most cases, simple aspiration is not appropriate for the treatment of spontaneous pneumothoraces because there is commonly an air leak for a short time after tube thoracostomy. Occasionally, surgeons are called to evaluate a patient who has had a pneumothorax for several days (the presence of a small hydrothorax with pneumothorax is a clue that the pneumothorax is a few days old) or a patient whose lung has not reexpanded with observational therapy. In these instances, needle aspiration using the disposable thoracentesis kit can be effective. The kits supply a small-diameter plastic catheter that can be passed over an aspirating needle to minimize the risk of lung injury and a large syringe with a one-way valve.

To perform the aspiration, local anesthetic is injected into the skin and the interspace in the second intercostal space in the midclavicular line. The needle/catheter is inserted gently into the affected hemithorax (above the third rib) until air is aspirated. The catheter is passed over the needle, and the needle is withdrawn. The syringe and one-way valve are attached, and the pleural cavity is aspirated until no further air can be removed.

At this time, the catheter is removed, and a postaspiration chest radiograph is obtained. Some surgeons favor leaving the catheter in place until the chest radiograph is completed. The advantage of this technique is that it allows further aspiration to be performed if the lung is not reexpanded or the option to attach the tube to a Heimlich valve.

Although needle aspiration has gained popularity in the United Kingdom, most surgeons suggest that this technique has limited applicability with success rates of less than 50% reported. Reasons for the failure of this technique include the inability to evacuate the pneumothorax completely, resulting in failure to approximate the visceral and parietal pleurae, and the lack of pleural scarring that can occur after placement of a foreign body, such as a chest tube in the thoracic cavity. In addition, this method does not treat the underlying etiology of the pneumothorax, pleural blebs.

Clinically Unstable Patient

In rare instances, a patient presents with a history consistent with spontaneous pneumothorax and a physical examination showing anxiety, absent breath sounds, tachycardia, cyanosis, hypotension, and deviation of the trachea to the uninvolved side. In this case, a clinical diagnosis of tension pneumothorax should be made without a confirming chest radiograph. Tension pneumothorax occurs when alveolar air enters continuously into the pleural space without evacuation resulting in increased pressure and shift of the mediastinum to the uninvolved side. Prompt decompression of the pleural space by insertion of a needle or chest tube is required to prevent circulatory collapse.

In a trauma patient with multiple injuries, the safest and most conservative treatment of a traumatic pneumothorax is to place a chest tube. This maneuver prevents the possibility of progression of the pneumothorax, eliminating this variable as a cause of respiratory or hemodynamic instability in a trauma patient. Rarely a patient presents with a significant hemothorax associated with the pneumothorax (i.e., hemopneumothorax). If the bleeding persists after chest tube placement (>100 ml/hr), immediate operative intervention is indicated to secure a torn vascular pleural adhesion.

■ PERSISTENT AIR LEAKS

Occasionally the air leak persists for several days after tube thoracostomy. For patients with air leaks that persist for more than 3 days, surgical intervention is recommended to attempt air leak closure, and a pleurodesis is performed to prevent recurrence. In special circumstances in which surgery is contraindicated or the patient refuses surgery, chemical pleurodesis by instillation of a sclerosing agent (e.g., doxycycline or talc slurry) through the chest tube can be used to promote pleural symphysis.

Rarely, there is a massive persistent air leak from the lung after chest tube placement with or without complete reexpansion of the lung. In this setting, immediate operative intervention is indicated to seal a large torn bulla.

■ OPERATION

Indications for surgery after spontaneous pneumothorax include (1) recurrent pneumothorax, (2) persistent air leak or incomplete reexpansion of the lung, (3) massive air leak with incomplete reexpansion of the lung, (4) history of bilateral pneumothoraces either simultaneously or on separate occasions, (5) occupational hazard or possible lack of access to medical care, (6) history of tension pneumothorax or prior pneumonectomy, and (7) hemopneumothorax with persistent bleeding. Historically, operative approaches to treat spontaneous pneumothorax have included thoracotomy (anterior, lateral, or transaxillary) and median sternotomy. In the 1980s, results from muscle-sparing incisions, such as transaxillary thoracotomy, were good. In the 1990s, technologic advances led to the development of video-assisted thoracic surgery (VATS) approaches for pneumothorax. Regardless of the technique selected, the ability of the surgeon to remove the offending bullae and obtain pleural symphysis is key to the success of the procedure.

VATS is performed by a thoracic surgeon in the operating room using double-lumen endotracheal general anesthesia. Patients are positioned in the lateral decubitus position and draped to allow open thoracotomy if necessary. The first thoracoscopic port (5 or 10 mm) is placed through the seventh interspace in the midaxillary line using a direct cutdown technique. The 30-degree thoracoscope is inserted into the hemithorax, and a careful visual inspection of the entire pleural space is performed. Two further ports are placed in the fourth or fifth interspace in the anterior axillary line or in the space between the spine and the medial border of the scapula (i.e., auscultatory triangle). Using lung graspers, the offending bleb is located and removed. Staple bullectomy is the most common approach for eliminating bullae. Other options for bullectomy may include electrocoagulation, laser ablation, or hand sewing depending on institutional experience and expertise using these techniques. If the bleb cannot be located, gentle insufflation of the lung with instillation of sterile saline solution into the thoracic cavity may help to locate the leaking bleb. If no bleb or leak is noted, the apex of the lung is removed using the stapler. The entire lung surface should be inspected to determine whether bullae are present elsewhere in the lung (other than the apex), such as the superior segment of the lower lobe.

For most patients undergoing surgery, intraoperative pleurodesis should be performed using parietal pleural abrasion or resection. Abrasion can be performed using a gauze plug, such as a Kittner dissector, or with the "the scouring pad" from the Bovie electrocautery unit. Apical parietal pleurectomy from the fifth rib superiorly also can be used as an effective technique to obtain pleural symphysis. Generally the intraoperative instillation of a chemical sclerosing agent such as talc is not recommended for young patients with benign disease. One or two chest tubes can be inserted through the VATS port sites and positioned accurately at the chest apex. Postoperatively the chest tubes are kept to suction for at least 24 hours (preferably 48 hours) to promote complete lung reexpansion and pleural symphysis.

Overall the success rate for VATS and transaxillary approaches in the operative management of spontaneous pneumothorax is excellent. The VATS technique is thought to be associated with decreased perioperative pain, shorter hospital stay, and more rapid return to work. Formal cost-effective analyses have not been performed, however. The recurrence rate after the VATS approach is approximately 2% to 5% compared with 1% to 2% for the limited thoracotomy approach. It is hypothesized that the slightly higher recurrence rate associated with the VATS technique is secondary to inadequate exposure of bullae in the chest cavity or to less effective pleural abrasion than may be seen with thoracotomy. In most reported series, the intraoperative conversion rate from VATS to open thoracotomy due to technical difficulties is less than 5% for primary pneumothoraces and 29% for secondary pneumothoraces.

■ SECONDARY PNEUMOTHORACES

Patients with secondary pneumothoraces generally have significant comorbid diseases and are debilitated from a respiratory standpoint and require that treatment be individualized. Treatment should include chemical or surgical pleurodesis in combination with complete lung reexpansion to seal air leaks. Tube thoracostomy alone is associated with a high recurrence rate. Two subgroups of secondary pneumothoraces are worthy of further discussion—patients with acquired immunodeficiency syndrome (AIDS) and patients with pneumothoraces complicating chronic obstructive pulmonary disease.

Since the 1980s, there have been an increasing number of reports describing the association between spontaneous pneumothorax and AIDS. There seems to be a predilection for bilateral pneumothoraces arising from disease at the apex of both lungs. Most commonly, the pneumothorax is secondary to *Pneumocystis carinii* pneumonia; however, pneumothorax also can occur in patients with Kaposi's sarcoma, pneumonia caused by mycobacteria or cytomegalovirus, and necrotizing bacterial pneumonias. Whenever possible, initial management should be conservative with observation alone; however, tube thoracostomy frequently is required to treat large air leaks. CT scan of the chest is useful to evaluate the extent of disease and in planning surgery. Operative intervention with resection of the diseased area and pleurectomy is usually well tolerated.

Pneumothorax secondary to chronic obstructive pulmonary disease is the most common variety of secondary pneumothorax. Typically, this pneumothorax occurs in patients older than age 50 and may be difficult to confirm clinically and radiologically. Chest CT is often necessary to localize the pneumothorax and to distinguish between large bullae and the pneumothorax. Treatment consists of tube thoracostomy, which may need to be continued for a prolonged time compared with that for a primary spontaneous pneumothorax. If the air leak persists more than 14 days, operative intervention or chemical pleurodesis should be considered. Surgical management varies based on the location and extent of disease. Stapling of the bullae and subtotal parietal pleurectomy is our favored approach.

SUGGESTED READING

Baumann MH, et al: Management of spontaneous pneumothorax—an American College of Chest Physicians Delphi Consensus Statement, *Chest* 119:590, 2001.

Beauchamp G: Spontaneous pneumothorax and pneumomediastinum. In Pearson FG, et al, editors: *Thoracic surgery.* New York, 1995, Churchill Livingstone, p 1037.

Harvey J, Prescott RJ: Simple aspiration versus intercostal tube drainage for spontaneous pneumothorax in patients with normal lungs, *BMJ* 309:1338, 1994.

Hatz RA, et al: Long-term results after video-assisted thoracoscopic surgery for first-time and recurrent spontaneous pneumothorax, *Ann Thorac Surg* 70:253, 2000.

Sahn SA, Heffner JE: Spontaneous pneumothorax, *N Engl J Med* 342:868, 2000.

EMPYEMA THORACIS

Robert B. Lee

■ HISTORY

When empyemata are opened by cautery or by knife; and the pus flows pure and white, the patient survives, but if it is mixed with blood; muddy and foul smelling, he will die.
    Hippocrates (460-377 B.C.)

Thoracic surgery in its infancy evolved as techniques were developed to treat complications of intrathoracic infections, particularly empyema thoracis. Hippocrates further described his observations of the clinical and physical findings of empyema thoracis:

Empyema may be recognized by the following symptoms:... the fever is constant, less during the day and greater at night, and copious sweats supervene. There is a desire to cough, and the patient expectorates nothing worth mentioning.

Hippocrates' observations regarding the natural history of empyema were uncanny and remain true today: "In pleuritic afflictions when the disease is not purged off in fourteen days it usually results in empyema." Regarding treatment, he pronounced adequate drainage by intercostal incision or rib resection, followed by packing as the only means for cure. Treatment was virtually unchanged 2000 years later, when Dieffenbach condemned the American surgeon Antony who, on March 3, 1821, resected portions of the fifth and sixth ribs and "all disorganized parenchyma of the lung, [for]... an extensive abscess... about this carious bone." Little changed between that time and 1989, when Lawrence described drainage, rib resection, and thoracoplasty as management techniques for empyema.

The current therapy for management of empyema has progressed and evolved over the past 15 years to include computed tomography (CT)–guided catheter drainage, use of fibrinolytics, diagnostic and therapeutic thoracoscopy, and extrathoracic muscle flap interposition. These advanced techniques as well as thoracotomy with decortication, Eloesser flaps, and other well-established surgical approaches are described.

■ DEFINITIONS AND DETERMINATIONS

Empyema, from the Greek, is defined simply as "pus in the pleural cavity." The precursor of empyema is bacterial pneumonia and subsequent parapneumonic effusion. Other causes of empyema include ruptured lung abscess, bronchogenic carcinoma, esophageal rupture (Boerhaave's syndrome), penetrating or blunt chest trauma, mediastinitis with pleural extension, extension of a subphrenic abscess, infected congenital abnormalities, cervical and thoracic spine infection, and postresection bronchopleural fistula. A common cause of empyema, bronchopleural fistulas, is discussed elsewhere.

The general thoracic surgeon often is involved in the diagnosis and treatment of patients with persistent parapneumonic effusions and subsequent empyema. When the surgeon's involvement is delayed during repeated attempts at "medical management," the sequelae of empyema occur. Parapneumonic effusions occur in 20% to 60% of patients hospitalized for bacterial pneumonia; 5% to 10% of these parapneumonic effusions progress to empyema (approximately 32,000 patients per year in the United States). The mortality rate of empyema is significant: 25% to 75% in the elderly and debilitated.

Pleural fluid first must be determined as exudative or transudative, which is accomplished by examination of pleural fluid obtained by thoracentesis. In the 1970s, Light established differential criteria based on levels of lactate dehydrogenase (LDH) and protein concentrations found in pleural fluid compared with the patient's serum. Light's criteria establish an exudate as having any one of the following characteristics: (1) pleural fluid protein divided by serum protein concentration greater than 0.5, (2) pleural fluid LDH concentration divided by serum LDH concentration greater than 0.6, (3) pleural fluid LDH concentration greater than two thirds of the upper limit of normal serum LDH concentration, and (4) a pH less than 7.0. Parapneumonic effusions are exudative and progress through three stages to an empyema; knowing the stage guides therapy.

The *first or exudative stage,* characterized by relatively low LDH, normal glucose, and normal pH, may be treated successfully by antibiotics. Untreated or inappropriately treated, the *second or fibropurulent stage* evolves with invasion of pleural fluid by bacteria, increased fibrin deposition, cellular debris, and white blood cells with the ultimate formation of limiting fibrin membranes producing loculations. The *third or organization stage* occurs as fibroblasts grow into the exudative fibrin sheet coating the visceral and parietal pleura with an inelastic membrane or pleural "peel" encasing the lung and rendering it functionless. Empyema is established by pus obtained on thoracentesis, glucose concentration less than 60 mg/dl, LDH greater than three times the upper limit of normal, and pH less than 7.0. A meta-analysis was performed of multiple smaller studies evaluating criteria of defining pleural infection and empyema. This study defined pH as the most accurate and sensitive criteria for empyema and need for drainage. This analysis identified a slightly higher pH of 7.21 to 7.29 as the best indicator for drainage as opposed to a pH of 7.0 established by Light in the 1970s. Empyema is determined by analysis of the pleural fluid, and treatment is guided by radiologic assessment.

■ RADIOLOGIC ASSESSMENT AND INTERVENTION

The initial radiographic assessment should include the standard posterior-anterior and lateral projections of a chest radiograph. Pleural fluid is subject to the laws of gravity, collecting in the most dependent area of the involved hemithorax: initially the costophrenic angle, then laterally, anteriorly, and finally superiorly. As much as 75 to 100 ml of pleural fluid may go undetected. As much as 175 to 500 ml is needed to blunt the lateral costophrenic angle. Free-flowing fluid or pus follows the coercion of gravity, making the right and left decubitus film the next essential study. The well-performed, overpenetrated decubitus film can detect 5 ml of fluid, reveal subpulmonic collections, reveal pseudotumors, and identify loculations. The ubiquitous posterior-anterior and lateral chest x-ray can separate the broad air-fluid level of an empyema from the more spherical fluid collection surrounded by lung parenchyma characteristic of lung abscess.

Ultrasonography is widely available in most institutions and frequently employed after the initial chest x-ray. Ultrasound is rapid, portable, and less expensive than CT. This technique can localize small amounts of fluid and loculations; identify and quantify pleural peels; and define solid lesions such as pleural or parenchymal tumors. Using a 3.5- or 5.0-mHz transducer and an intercostal acoustic window, an empyema is characterized as having acoustic homogeneity. Complex or advanced empyemas have debris and floating fronds. An organized empyema has an echogenic pleural peel, and the lung appears immobile or entrapped. Diagnostic thoracentesis, catheter drainage, or tube thoracostomy can be guided by ultrasound.

CT of the chest became clinically applicable in 1975 and widely available by the early 1980s. During the subsequent 20 years, CT has become the radiographic technique most frequently relied on for characterization of an empyema and for treatment. Present helical CT scanners have scan rates of 1 second, reliably reproducing cross-sectional images of the thorax, readily showing the anatomic separation between lung parenchyma, pleural space, and chest wall. Intravenous contrast material is necessary to define pulmonary blood vessels and enhance the parietal pleura. Exudative effusions (empyema) have abnormally high Hounsfield units (−20 HU) compared with transudative effusions (−100 HU). Differentiating empyema, lung abscess, transudative pleural fluid, and subdiaphragmatic fluid (ascites) is often difficult without CT. Lung abscesses generally are seen as air-fluid spherical lesions forming acute angles with the lung parenchyma. The lung appears destroyed rather than compressed. There is an abrupt cutoff of vessels and bronchi. Empyemas appear laterally, pushing or compressing lung parenchyma, vessels, and bronchi. The shape is not uniform, and angles with the pleura are acute. Lateral lung abscesses or abscesses in the basilar segments of the lung near the diaphragm may be difficult to distinguish from the pleural location of an empyema.

Magnetic resonance imaging has been used to image the pleural space and offers the advantage of coronal, sagittal, and axial planes. This modality is more expensive and cumbersome, adds little information beyond CT, and rarely is used.

MEDICAL MANAGEMENT

Medical management of empyema is a misnomer. Medical management or conservative noninterventional therapy is rarely effective and often contraindicated for management of empyema. Thoracentesis and culture sensitivity–based antibiotic therapy are appropriate and generally successful for stage I parapneumonic effusions but not stage II effusions or stage III empyema. Drainage of the pleural space by radiologically guided catheters or surgical drainage must be employed for successful management of empyema.

Thoracentesis not only may be diagnostic as previously discussed, but also occasionally therapeutic. When the amount of pleural fluid is small to moderate, free flowing (not loculated), and fluent, the initial "diagnostic" thoracentesis using a vacuum bottle may clear the pleural space completely and become a therapeutic drainage procedure. If the fluid does not reaccumulate, no further intervention is required. If the fluid reaccumulates and the initial analysis of the fluid has defined an empyema, however, a drainage procedure should be initiated.

Historically, tube thoracostomy using a large-bore chest tube (32 Fr to 38 Fr) was the initial intervention when empyema was established. These chest tubes were converted to an "empyema tube" at 14 to 21 days when pleural symphysis had occurred. The tube was withdrawn slowly over several weeks. Patients often were discharged with the tube connected to a drainage bag. When the initial drainage by chest tube was unsuccessful or the empyema loculated, open surgical drainage was performed. An empyema tube rarely is used today and has infrequent indications.

Image-guided catheter placement should be the initial method of drainage unless lung entrapment has been proved. This is effectively accomplished by placement of one or more flexible polyethylene pigtail catheters (8 Fr to 14 Fr) using CT guidance. After catheter placement, fibrinolytics are administered until the pleural space is cleared radiographically and the patient's clinical condition is improved. Streptokinase initially was used by Tillet and Sherry in 1949. Subsequently, urokinase was used and found to be more efficacious (90% to 92%) compared with streptokinase (66%) and less likely to cause a febrile or allergic reaction. Most authors report using 250,000 U of streptokinase on 3 consecutive days. We have used 100,000 U of urokinase in 100 ml of normal saline in similar fashion. The U.S. Food and Drug Administration (FDA) recalled urokinase from most institutions in 1999 for apparent quality control issues, making it no longer available. I am currently using tissue plasminogen activator (Activase) for fibrinolysis. Tissue plasminogen activator, 10 mg, is diluted in 50 ml of normal saline and injected into the catheter on 3 consecutive days. Results have been similar to urokinase. This is not an FDA-approved use for this drug, so it cannot be recommended. No prospective randomized trials have been done to evaluate fibrinolytic therapy with tissue plasminogen activator.

Urokinase first was used by transcatheter delivery for management of loculated intrathoracic effusion in 1989. Clinical trials comparing streptokinase with placebo, comparing different doses of streptokinase, and comparing different amounts of saline for diluting the streptokinase have been performed using tube thoracostomy as the standard for drainage. Most studies show increased drainage and clearance of chest x-ray findings using fibrinolytics but lack sophistication to make statistically based conclusions. Only one study by Bouros et al was conducted in a prospective, randomized, double-blinded fashion. The study compared 250,000 U of streptokinase with 100,000 U of urokinase, delivered in similar fashion in matched patient populations. Drainage amounts were similar, urokinase was more expensive, and length of stay was similar. Fever was more common in the streptokinase group (28%). No study has compared streptokinase, urokinase, and tissue plasminogen activator.

SURGICAL MANAGEMENT

Success rates with image-guided catheter placement and fibrinolytics approach 70% to 80% for early stage III parapneumonic effusion (empyema) when the appropriate dosage of drug is given repeatedly until the chest x-ray clears or the clinical condition improves. Of these patients, 20% to 30% require a surgical drainage procedure. These patients often can be identified early in their course by findings on chest CT, such as multiple loculations and contrast enhancement of the parietal pleura suggesting a "peel or rind."

Thoracoscopy should be the next therapeutic maneuver after attempted fibrinolysis. Some authors argue that thoracic early in the management of the fibrinopurulent stage of empyema is more effective. Initially performed in 1910 for lysis of pleural adhesions in a tuberculous empyema by Jacobaeus, this technique has become remarkably safe and effective since the introduction of charged coupled device ("Chip") cameras for video assistance. Video-assisted thoracic surgery (VATS) has become an extension of the thoracic surgeon's physical examination. VATS affords the advantage of being able to visualize the infected pleural space and determine if complete drainage of all empyema fluid and disruption of all adhesions and loculations can be accomplished. If not, decortication is indicated to free the entrapped lung. Performed early before collagen deposition on the visceral pleura and entrapment of the lung, VATS can be used to disrupt fibrinous adhesions, completely drain all infected fluid, débride the parietal and visceral pleura, and accurately place large-bore chest tubes under direct vision. VATS must accomplish two therapeutic goals to be successful: (1) establish a unified pleural space and (2) ensure total reexpansion of the lung parenchyma with obliteration of the pleural cavity. Wait et al at Parkland Memorial Hospital, Dallas, Texas, performed a randomized trial on 20 patients comparing VATS and standard tube thoracostomy with streptokinase fibrinolysis (250,000 U streptokinase in 100 ml of normal saline repeated over 3 days). The VATS group had significantly less chest tube drainage, fever, and intensive care unit and hospital days and a higher success rate. Although this is a small group of patients, it supports the concept of early intervention using VATS.

I perform VATS within 48 to 72 hours (three treatments) after fibrinolytic therapy if fibrinolysis has failed to clear the pleural space effectively and reexpand the lung. VATS has been described using various techniques, under local anesthesia, in the awake patient, using flexible or rigid scopes, and with and without single-lung ventilation. A 0-degree or

30-degree lens and Chip camera using port access and single-lung ventilation of the contralateral side is the technique most widely accepted and used. When a double-lumen endotracheal tube is positioned correctly, the patient is placed in the lateral decubitus position with affected side up. I use the tube thoracostomy site for my camera port when present. When a chest tube is not present, a site in the midaxillary line along the fifth or sixth intercostal space may be used, in line with the thoracotomy incision should this be necessary.

On examination of the pleural space, a determination is made as to (1) whether all fluid can be drained and (2) the extent of lung entrapment. When the lung is not entrapped, débridement, irrigation, and disruption of all adhesions and loculations can be accomplished through a second appropriately placed port using a sponge forceps and suction-irrigating device. Two 32 Fr chest tubes are placed using video assistance and left to suction drainage for 3 to 5 days. Success depends on whether the lung is entrapped by a thick visceral peel (chronic organized phase of empyema). Only the fibrinopurulent, multiloculated stage of empyema is amenable to thorascopic management. If the lung is found to be entrapped, conversion to thoracotomy for decortication is advised. Decortication using VATS is frequently frustrating and often results in parenchymal lung injury and bleeding.

Decortication via a thoracotomy should be performed when the third or fibrotic stage of empyema is suggested by CT scan that reveals visceral pleural enhancement without fibrin septation in multiple areas of loculation. Entrapment should be suspected when this has occurred and when the pleural process is known to have been ongoing for greater than 10 to 14 days. I almost always attempt to use the videoscope to perform an initial evaluation, then convert to a 10- to 15-cm vertical incision in the midaxillary line for a muscle-sparing thoracotomy and decortication when lung entrapment is found. Using this incision, a complete pleurectomy-decortication can be performed quickly and effectively. The videoscope can be used through the incision to access the hard-to-reach areas better, such as the diaphragmatic sulcus; place chest tubes; and ensure full reexpansion of the lung parenchyma. The first objective of this operation is to remove all purulent fluid, fibrinous debris, and thickened parietal pleura from the pleural space. When partial or complete pleurectomy is required to accomplish this, complete hemostasis must occur, or a resulting hemithorax may occur, defeating the initial purpose. The second, more difficult, but most critical task is to resect the visceral pleural peel. A plane of separation between the peel and visceral pleura must be established; this is accomplished with knife, scissors, sharp-pointed clamp, or even bluntly with a Kittner dissector. When the proper plane is established, the peel is stripped completely from the entire lung surface. The lung must be freed entirely from the rib cage, mediastinum, and diaphragm. All of the fibrotic visceral peel must be removed, even within the lung fissures. The costophrenic angle should be reestablished. Complete and total reexpansion of all lung parenchyma must be accomplished to ensure success. Decortication is achieved most easily through the sixth intercostal space, which allows better access to the diaphragm and costophrenic angle. This is a major operation and physiologically challenging to a compromised or debilitated patient. When the operative morbidity or mortality seems prohibitive, a lesser open drainage procedure may be considered.

The Eloesser flap or procedure originally was described by Eloesser in 1935 as a drainage procedure for tuberculous empyema. He described forming a U-shaped flap of skin and subcutaneous tissue and sewing it into the most dependent portion of the empyema cavity after resecting a portion of the underlying two or three ribs and attached intercostal muscles. With the flap acting as a tubeless, one-way valve, air is allowed to egress against less resistance than air entering. The lung is allowed to reexpand and obliterate the cavity. This procedure is most effective when a unilocular empyema is present and located inferiorly or laterally. The procedure can be accomplished under local anesthesia with intravenous sedation in a high-risk surgical patient with an empyema. Miller and others at Emory University reported a 90% success rate in 84 patients (1974-1998) using the inverted-U modified Eloesser flap.

■ CONCLUSION

The heterogeneity of empyema thoracis, the underlying primary disease process, and the patient's physiologic status make no single therapy a universal first intervention. The diagnosis of pus in the pleural space must be made and the pace and progression of the disease process recognized to avoid sequelae. Optimal therapy and cost containment require selection of the most appropriate initial intervention. Thourani, Miller, and I reviewed our experience with 77 empyema thoracis patients at Emory University and Crawford Long Hospitals in Atlanta, Georgia (1990-1997). The treatment modalities previously discussed were employed. Of the effusions, 65% were parapneumonic, and 68% were multiloculated. There were 35% of effusions that failed primary intervention (image-directed catheter or tube thoracostomy [CT] and antibiotics), subsequently requiring surgical intervention. We found that 94% of cases requiring decortication as a primary or delayed intervention had a multiloculated effusion. Seventy-eight percent of the image-directed catheter failures were in patients with multiloculations. Early surgical decortication in patients with multiple loculations was more effective and resulted in decreased length of stay (5 days) and decreased cost (approximately $20,000 per patient).

Findings of this study have led me to adopt and recommend the following: (1) Thoracic surgeons should be involved early in the treatment planning of a patient with empyema thoracis, the goal being complete drainage of the pleural space and reexpansion of the lung parenchyma; (2) early stage empyema (before the fibrinopurulent stage) that is unilocular is treated most effectively by image-directed catheters and fibrinolytic therapy; and (3) a multiloculated empyema, an empyema in the fibrinopurulent stage with an established visceral peel, and an empyema that has not cleared within 48 to 72 hours of treatment with an image-directed catheter and fibrinolytics should be treated by surgical intervention. The physiologically sound patient with empyema thoracis should be considered for early decortication.

SUGGESTED READING

Bouros D, et al: Fibrinolytics in the treatment of a parapneumonic effusions: Monaldi, *Arch Chest Dis* 54:258, 1999.

Lee RB: Radiologic evaluation and intervention for empyema thoracis, *Chest Clin North Am* 6:439, 1996.

Light RW, Rodriguez RM: Management of parapneumonic effusions, *Clin Chest Med* 19:373, 1998.

Thourani VH, et al: Evaluation of treatment modalities for thoracic empyema: a cost-effectiveness analysis, *Ann Thorac Surg* 66:1121, 1998.

Wait MA, et al: A randomized trial of empyema therapy, *Chest* 111:1548, 1997.

PLEURAL EFFUSIONS

David M. McMullan
Garrett L. Walsh

The diagnostic evaluation and management of a pleural effusion is a common problem confronting thoracic surgeons. Approximately 3.5 ml/kg of pleural fluid is produced and reabsorbed on a daily basis; however, the pleural space normally contains only 0.1 to 0.3 ml/kg of fluid. An imbalance between fluid production and absorption leads to the net accumulation of pleural fluid. Progressive extrinsic compression of the lung parenchyma produces the hallmark symptom of dyspnea. Although the volume of excessive pleural fluid necessary to produce symptoms is determined by the rate of fluid accumulation and the patient's underlying pulmonary function, symptoms generally do not occur until at least 300 to 500 ml have accumulated. In addition to dyspnea, patients may manifest symptoms (e.g., fever, cough, or pleuritic pain) associated with the underlying cause of effusion.

Pleural effusions classically are characterized as either transudative or exudative depending on the underlying etiologic process and resulting fluid composition (Table 1). Transudative effusions are caused by altered osmotic or hydrostatic forces that produce excess fluid with composition similar to serum. The treatment of transudative effusions should focus on the systemic cause. Exudative effusions develop from alterations in the pleura or its lymphatic drainage, and appropriate diagnostic studies should be ordered to determine the underlying cause. Malignant effusions result either from primary pleural malignancies (i.e., mesotheliomas) or from metastatic, pleural-based disease (typically lymphomas or carcinomas of the lung, breast, or ovary). Chylous effusions may develop after traumatic disruption of the thoracic duct with ongoing chyle leak or malignant involvement of mediastinal nodes with secondary obstruction to lymphatic flow.

■ EVALUATION

The initial evaluation of patients suspected of having a pleural effusion includes a detailed history and physical examination followed by an upright posterior-anterior and lateral chest radiograph. Effusions of 175 ml may be detected on the upright chest radiograph through blunting of the costophrenic margin. Lateral decubitus films may show effusions of 100 ml and may aid in determining whether the fluid is free flowing or loculated.

Diagnostic pleural fluid aspiration should be performed in all patients with newly diagnosed effusions of unknown etiology. Symptomatic patients and patients in whom an infectious source is suspected should have the fluid removed for diagnostic and therapeutic reasons.

Thoracentesis may be performed at the bedside when the effusion is noted to layer on the chest x-ray. The patient is placed in the seated position with the upper body leaning slightly forward. The fluid level is determined by review of the radiograph and by chest percussion. A point is selected

Table 1 Etiology of Pleural Effusion
TRANSUDATIVE
Congestive heart failure
Cirrhosis
Pulmonary embolism
Myxedema
Uremia
EXUDATIVE
Malignancy (metastatic, mesothelioma)
Pneumonia (bacterial, tuberculous, fungal, viral, parasitic)
Collagen vascular disorders (rheumatoid arthritis, SLE, Sjögren's syndrome)
Drug-induced (amiodarone, bromocriptine, dantrolene, nitrofurantoin)
Postpericardiotomy (Dressler's) syndrome
Wegener's granulomatosis
Asbestosis
Pancreatitis
Intraabdominal abscess
Esophageal perforation
Pulmonary infarction
Chylous (trauma, lymphoma)

SLE, systemic lupus erythematosus.

two intercostal spaces inferior to this fluid level along the scapular line. Attempts to aspirate fluid anterior to the axillary line can result in injury to abdominal organs and mediastinal structures, including the heart. A clear understanding of the three-dimensional anatomy of the chest and how it can be altered by various disease states is essential. Using sterile technique, a skin wheal is created with 1% lidocaine (Xylocaine), and a 22-gauge needle is used to create a lidocaine tract and localize the pleural fluid. A 16-gauge to 18-gauge angiocatheter is introduced into the pleural space, and fluid is aspirated under gentle negative pressure. Inspiration-induced pneumothorax may be prevented by using a three-way stopcock.

The initial character of the fluid should be noted (clear, straw-colored, bloody, milky, or purulent), and the fluid should be sent for analysis (Table 2). If malignancy is suspected (often bloody in nature), all of the remaining fluid should be sent for cytologic analysis. If the exfoliated malignant cells are scarce, a large volume of fluid often is required to create the centrifuged cell block for pathologic examination. Heparin (5000 to 10,000 U) may be added to the bottle if the fluid is grossly bloody.

Although enough fluid should be withdrawn to provide symptomatic relief, rapid removal of only 1.0 to 1.5 liters may induce reexpansion pulmonary edema, which can be fatal, in some patients. If the patient starts to cough, drainage should be interrupted for several minutes before continuing. If the patient coughs again, further drainage should be aborted.

A postprocedure chest radiograph should be obtained to rule out an apical pneumothorax and to evaluate the degree of reexpansion of the lung. The radiographic finding of what appears to be a large basal "pneumothorax" may signify an entrapped lung. Placement of a chest tube in this setting results in persistent high-volume fluid drainage and is of no benefit to the patient. Inability of the lung to expand completely after the initial thoracentesis poses a much more difficult problem for the surgeon to manage. Complete evacuation of the pleural effusion permits better visualization of the obscured lung parenchyma and other intrathoracic pathologies that might be contributing to the effusion.

Aspiration of small or loculated fluid collections should be performed using computed tomography (CT)–guided or ultrasound-guided techniques to prevent inadvertent organ injury. CT almost always provides important additional diagnostic information, including anatomic pathology within the chest and upper abdomen. CT more clearly differentiates a suspected loculated effusion detected by plain chest films

from consolidated pulmonary parenchyma, an elevated hemidiaphragm, or a pleural mass.

When pleural disease or malignancy is suspected, an open or closed pleural biopsy can be a useful diagnostic adjunct. The diagnostic sensitivity of thoracentesis with cytology is only 62% in cases of malignant effusions. Although diagnostic sensitivity increases to 74% with the addition of a closed pleural biopsy, diagnostic thoracoscopy alone yields a definitive diagnosis in 95% of cases. We recommend the use of diagnostic thoracoscopy when aspiration cytology is nondiagnostic. Although thoracoscopy may be performed under local anesthesia in a conscious, spontaneously breathing patient, we prefer to perform this diagnostic study in the operating room under general anesthesia. This permits a more thorough examination of all pleural and pulmonary surfaces, lysis of adhesions, generous biopsy specimens of any visualized pathology under direct vision, and expansion of the lung under positive pressure. After the procedure, a chest tube is left in place until drainage is nonbloody and less than 150 ml/day.

■ TREATMENT

Transudates

The underlying cause, the duration of disease, and the patient's symptoms determine the clinical management of pleural effusions. The principal therapy for a transudative pleural effusion is directed at identifying and treating the systemic illness, which often can result in complete resolution of the pleural effusion. In terminally ill patients who are refractory to medical management (e.g., patients with end-stage congestive heart failure, renal failure, or cirrhosis), chemical pleurodesis to control the pleural effusion can provide symptomatic benefit.

Exudates

Acute exudative pleural effusions occasionally may resolve after complete evacuation during the initial diagnostic thoracentesis. More typically, however, the effusion reaccumulates, and symptoms recur. Therapy should be directed at controlling the underlying problem (e.g., pneumonia, subphrenic abscess, or pancreatitis) and, if symptoms dictate, providing continuous drainage of the pleural space.

Drainage Techniques

Repeated therapeutic thoracentesis is discouraged because of the increased risk of lung injury, bacterial contamination of the pleural effusion, and possible creation of loculated pockets from resulting pleural adhesions. Provided that the lung is not entrapped (often seen in late empyemas), tube thoracostomy generally provides adequate drainage and permits full lung expansion and pleural symphysis. In general, a 32 Fr chest tube should be inserted in the sixth to eighth intercostal space at the midaxillary line and directed superiorly and posteriorly if the fluid is free flowing. The tube should be removed when there is no evidence of effusion on chest radiograph and the pleural drainage is less than 150 ml/day. CT-guided thoracostomy is helpful when multiple loculations are present or when routine chest tube thoracostomy has failed to drain all fluid completely.

Table 2 Pleural Fluid Analysis

Total and differential cell count
Gram stain
Culture (bacterial, fungal, mycobacterial)
Total protein
Lactate dehydrogenase
Glucose
Amylase
pH
Cytology

Pleural effusions of infectious etiology may be sterile or may contain microorganisms. Although noncomplicated parapneumonic effusions may be observed, complicated parapneumonic effusions (defined by pleural fluid pH <7.2, glucose <40 mg/dl, LDH >1000 IU/liter, and the absence of organisms) should undergo closed tube drainage because of the increased incidence of subsequent empyema. Empyema (defined by the presence of gross pus or organisms on Gram stain or culture) must be treated by closed drainage of the pleural space with a large (32 Fr to 40 Fr) chest tube, selected by the consistency of the fluid. When loculations are present, ultrasound guidance for surgical placement of a chest tube may be helpful. If this is not feasible, CT-guided drainage can be useful, although the small caliber of catheters typically placed by interventional radiologists may compromise adequate pleural drainage. Intrapleural instillation of fibrinolytics through these catheters may be employed to break down adhesions and fibrinous debris, which would facilitate drainage and complete the reexpansion of the underlying lung. Streptokinase (250,000 U) is dissolved in 100 ml of sterile saline and instilled through the chest tube. After 3 hours, the tube is unclamped, and closed pleural drainage is continued. Daily treatments for 1 week are necessary to lyse the fibrinous debris adequately and evacuate the pleural space.

Video-Assisted Thoracic Surgery

Advancements in optics and instrumentation for minimally invasive surgical techniques in the 1990s have permitted a more aggressive and proactive approach to patients with pleural effusions. These techniques, which now can be performed with 5-mm ports, may be employed as a component of the initial diagnostic evaluation of the pleural cavity to disrupt loculations, lavage the hemithorax, and expand the lung under positive-pressure ventilation. Early use of video-assisted thoracic surgery (VATS) techniques for the evaluation and management of effusions would eliminate the unnecessary costs and prolonged hospitalization associated with fibrinolytic therapy and prevent later complications, such as an entrapped lung with a secondary empyema cavity.

Patients who present with 4 to 5 weeks of symptoms (late empyema) may require initial drainage of the empyema cavity followed by open pulmonary decortication when the fibrinous peel has matured. Premature decortication results in excessive parenchymal injury to the lung and significant air leaks that may be difficult to control.

Malignant Effusions

Malignancy accounts for almost half of all pleural effusions. As the average survival time for patients who present with malignant effusions is 4 to 6 months, the goal of therapy is strictly palliation. Early pleural sclerotherapy is encouraged for all dyspneic patients who previously have shown symptomatic improvement after therapeutic thoracentesis and who have an estimated life expectancy of less than a few months. In patients who develop rapid symptom recurrence in which the lung fully expands after an initial, successful diagnostic or therapeutic thoracentesis, we would proceed directly to one of three sclerotherapy techniques. When the patient requires hospitalization for other concurrent medical problems, a

chest tube or VATS procedure should be performed. If the patient's primary symptoms are related to the effusion and family support is available, a Denver Pleurx (Surgimedics, Denver Biomaterials, Inc., Denver, CO) catheter would be our treatment of choice for outpatient management. Patients with small cell lung cancer, breast cancer, or lymphoma who have mild-to-moderate symptoms and whose tumors are likely to respond to systemic therapy are good candidates for chemotherapy before sclerosis. Malignant pleural effusions caused by these tumors may resolve after systemic chemotherapy, obviating the need for pleurodesis.

Pleurodesis Techniques

Pleurodesis must be considered for patients with recurrent, noninfectious pleural effusions. The mechanism of pleurodesis centers on producing diffuse pleuritis leading to fibrogenesis and pleuropleural adhesions. This may be achieved by either mechanical or chemical techniques, depending on the clinical circumstance. Several pleural sclerosing agents are currently available, and each has a different therapeutic profile. Talc is the least expensive sclerosing agent and is available in an aerosolized form for insufflation during thoracotomy or thoracoscopy or as a powder to be instilled into the pleural space through a draining thoracostomy tube on the ward. Talc powder may be sterilized by dry heat, ethylene oxide or γ-irradiation before being mixed as a slurry with sterile saline.

Talc pleurodesis treats recurrent pleural effusions with greater than 90% efficacy regardless of the route of administration. The major drawbacks of talc pleurodesis are self-limited pleuritic pain and fever and—in rare instances—acute respiratory distress syndrome, pneumonitis, and respiratory failure.

Talc poudrage is performed using a manual insufflator during thoracoscopy or using a commercially available aerosolized delivery system, such as that available through Axion Corporation, Aubagne, France. When present, loculations must be disrupted to ensure wide, even distribution of talc. A closed pleural drain is inserted and placed to suction. The tube may be removed when daily drainage is less than 150 ml.

Closed pleurodesis using other sclerosing agents (e.g., bleomycin, 60 IU, and doxycycline, 500 mg) may be done through a chest tube placed on the ward. Disadvantages of these agents include lower efficacy than talc (doxycycline 80% to 85%, bleomycin 50% to 70%) and side effects from partial systemic absorption of these agents. These side effects may include nausea and anecdotal reports of complete hair loss after bleomycin use. Although cost analysis comparing these methods suggests that bleomycin is the most cost-effective sclerosing agent, these analyses do not include talc-based closed pleurodesis. Eliminating the additional costs associated with poudrage presumably would show a distinct cost advantage for closed talc pleurodesis.

Denver Pleurx Catheter

The Denver Pleurx catheter system (Figure 1) is a 15.5 Fr flexible silicone rubber catheter with a felt cuff and a valved access port. It is connected to a self-contained vacuum collection bottle. It may be inserted in the ambulatory setting under local anesthesia. The catheter is inserted over a wire in

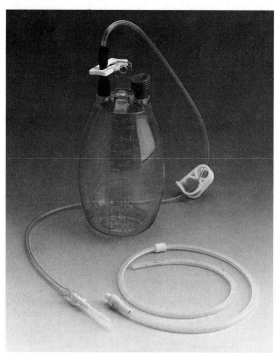

Figure 1
Denver Pleurx catheter. A Dacron felt cuff is positioned in subcutaneous tunnel. One-way valve and cap are shown. This self-contained, disposable vacuum bottle is for home drainage of pleural effusions. *(Photo courtesy of Surgimedics, Denver Biomaterials, Inc., Denver, CO.)*

the fourth to sixth intercostal space at the anterior axillary line using the Seldinger technique. A small incision is made at the insertion site, and the external end of the catheter is tunneled under the skin to exit through a separate incision

5 to 8 cm away. The catheter may be used immediately. Patients drain pleural fluid at home every day initially, then every 2 to 3 days depending on the volume of fluid produced. The overall efficacy of this method is greater than 90%. In addition, almost half of patients undergoing ambulatory intermittent Pleurx catheter drainage can exhibit spontaneous pleurodesis. This is likely a result of the pleural reaction to a foreign body. The catheters can be removed in the outpatient clinic after a simple cutdown on the Dacron cuff in the subcutaneous tunnel. Risks of the catheter include occasional pleuritic chest pain if fluid is drained too quickly (this can be regulated by the vacuum drainage system), empyema (the catheter has remained in for >6 months in some patients), and development of pleural loculations.

Persistently high-volume chest tube drainage for more than 3 or 4 days after a VATS procedure or chest tube pleurodesis is considered a failure of these techniques. Reintroduction of the sclerosis agent is usually unsuccessful. We recommend inserting a Denver Pleurx catheter in these patients to permit their immediate discharge from the hospital rather than subjecting them to a prolonged chest tube drainage trial and lengthy hospital stay.

SUGGESTED READING

American Thoracic Society: Management of malignant pleural effusions, *Am J Respir Crit Care Med* 162:1987, 2000.

Ferrer J, Roldan J: Clinical management of the patient with pleural effusion, *Eur J Radiol* 34:76, 2000.

Miserocchi G: Physiology and pathophysiology of pleural fluid turnover, *Eur Respir J* 10:219, 1997.

Putnam JB Jr, et al: A randomized comparison of indwelling pleural catheter and doxycycline pleurodesis in the management of malignant pleural effusions, *Cancer* 86:1992, 1999.

Rodriguez-Panadero F, Antony VB: Pleurodesis: state of the art, *Eur Respir J* 10:1648, 1997.

FIBROTHORAX AND DECORTICATION OF THE LUNG

Thomas J. Watson

The pleural space is normally a potential cavity bordered by the visceral and parietal pleurae. A variety of pathologic conditions may cause fibrous thickening of these pleural membranes, leading to their fusion or entrapment of the underlying pulmonary parenchyma. *Decortication* refers to the process of peeling this restrictive fibrous layer from the pleura, promoting lung reexpansion and improving thoracic excursion. As opposed to thoracoplasty, which collapses the rigid thorax to obliterate pleural space disease, decortication allows for the disentrapment of lung parenchyma, even when chronically involved, to bring about resolution of pleural pathology, improve pulmonary function, and increase chest wall dynamics.

■ PATHOGENESIS

Any pleural fluid left undrained, regardless of cause, has the potential to initiate an inflammatory response with fibrin deposition on the visceral and parietal pleural surfaces (Table 1).

Table 1 Common Causes of Fibrothorax

Empyema thoracis
Retained hemothorax
Tuberculosis
Chronic pneumothorax
Pleural effusions
    Transudative
    Exudative
    Chylous
    Pancreatic

The severity of such a reaction depends on the initiating cause. Chronic transudative effusion may lead to a thin, translucent membrane, whereas empyema thoracis and hemothorax tend to cause a thick, irregular, fibrous peel. The parietal reaction is typically thicker than the visceral one. The fibrous layer develops over the lung, chest wall, diaphragm, and mediastinal surfaces.

The pulmonary parenchyma generally is unaffected by the pleural reaction per se, unless the pleural disease was initiated by an underlying lung infection, inflammatory process, or trauma. The peel that forms over the lung is discrete from the underlying visceral pleura and generally can be separated from it in the process of decortication. The goal of surgical therapy is removal of the encasing fibrotic membrane without damaging the normal pleura or, more importantly, the underlying pulmonary parenchyma.

■ DIAGNOSIS AND EVALUATION

The clinical presentation of a fibrothorax depends on the underlying cause, its severity and extent, and whether appropriate therapy was initiated. Because most fibrothoraces are secondary to parapneumonic empyema or traumatic hemothorax, associated parenchymal damage is common and may contribute substantially to the symptom complex. No inciting cause may be elicited in 50% of cases.

The most common presenting symptom of fibrothorax is dyspnea on exertion. Other common complaints include chest pain, pressure, or tightness; fever; malaise; and cough. The onset of these symptoms may be insidious without an obvious antecedent respiratory infection or acute traumatic event. Physical examination may reveal diminished breath sounds on the affected side with dullness to percussion. Deep inspiration shows decreased chest wall excursion with relative fixation of the hemidiaphragm.

Chest radiography is the mainstay of diagnostic testing for chronic empyema and fibrothorax. Milder cases show pleural-based radiodensities involving the lower hemithorax and diaphragmatic surface with obliteration of the costophrenic angle. Discrete loculations may occur more superiorly as well. In more severe cases, most of the pleural space can be involved with encasement of the entire lung. Closer inspection of the structures surrounding the lung may reveal narrowing of the intercostal spaces, elevation of the ipsilateral hemidiaphragm, and shift of the mediastinum toward the fibrothorax. Pleural calcification can occur in more chronic

cases and provides an accurate assessment of the thickness of the pleural rind.

Computed tomography (CT) scans provide a more detailed evaluation of the extent of pleural disease and associated parenchymal pathology, which can be difficult to differentiate on plain chest radiographs. Specifically, densities seen on chest x-ray in large part may represent parenchymal consolidation, especially in the earlier stages of disease, with a relatively small pleural component. Similarly the CT scan may show an underlying carcinoma, fibrosis, atelectasis, or bronchiectasis that was missed on conventional chest x-ray and may affect the outcome of decortication. Finally, CT may help determine the chronicity of the pleural pathology, the degree of fluid component to the process, the extent of loculations, and the thickness of the visceral pleural membrane.

When a patient is considered for surgery, physiologic testing can provide an assessment of the degree of respiratory compromise and a baseline against which to compare the outcome of intervention. Conventional pulmonary function testing with spirometry, lung volumes, and diffusion capacity for carbon monoxide show a restrictive ventilatory defect with diminished lung volumes (total lung capacity and vital capacity) and expiratory flows (forced expiratory volume in 1 second). If the lung parenchyma is not diseased, the diffusion capacity of the lungs corrected for the reduced volumes is normal, indicative of extrapulmonary chest wall restriction. Fibrothorax may cause a more severe impairment in respiratory function than might be anticipated from radiographic findings. Similarly, pleural restriction may compromise lung function more than parenchymal consolidation.

■ INDICATIONS AND CONTRAINDICATIONS

The timing of intervention for pleural effusion, infection, or hemothorax is crucial to the outcome and determines the appropriate therapy. When effusions are thin, simple aspiration may suffice. Purulent collections and acute hemothoraces generally mandate closed tube thoracostomy with underwater seal drainage. Fibrinopurulent, loculated empyema and clotted hemothorax may be managed successfully with thoracoscopic irrigation, débridement, and evacuation. If these processes are not resolved at this stage, however, fibrin deposition ensues with resultant fibrothorax.

Decortication of the lung is indicated for patients with symptomatic extrapulmonary restriction due to fibrothorax. Decortication becomes necessary if malignant pleural disease is excluded, and less invasive measures have failed to drain the pleural space, reexpand the lung, or control pleural infection. In tuberculosis, decortication is indicated if long-term antituberculous therapy has failed to bring about resolution of pleural disease and thoracentesis does not eliminate an associated pleural effusion. Because decortication generally requires a thoracotomy, the degree of symptoms and respiratory compromise must be weighed carefully against the patient's comorbidities and the inherent risks of surgical intervention. Many patients being evaluated for surgical therapy have significant acute or chronic pulmonary disease that can affect their candidacy for decortication and the timing of operation.

In general, the longer surgical intervention is delayed, the more mature the pleural peel becomes. For this reason, traditional teaching has been to wait a period of approximately 4 to 6 weeks before operating on patients with fibrosing empyema thoracis or organizing hemothorax. This time allows for an easier plane of dissection between the fibrous rind and the underlying visceral pleura. A delay also allows any underlying parenchymal infectious consolidation to resolve, as otherwise lung reexpansion does not always follow successful decortication.

In practice, the recommendation to postpone surgical therapy is not always feasible. The onset of disease may be difficult to ascertain from historical information, and the pleural rind may be mature at the time of presentation to the surgeon. The patient may be hospitalized with acute symptoms and may be unwilling to delay definitive therapy. Unresolved pleural infection may need to be addressed in an urgent fashion. The costs of a prolonged hospitalization must be considered, and the treating physicians may feel pressure to discharge the patient as expeditiously as possible. Finally, excessive delays may lead to more extensive fibrosis with obliteration of the plane between the fibrous peel and visceral pleura, making decortication difficult and hazardous. It has been our practice to recommend decortication when CT shows the absence of any serious parenchymal consolidation or fibrosis, such that pulmonary reexpansion can be anticipated when the restrictive fibrous membrane is removed. Decortication is contraindicated in the setting of serious comorbidities, such that the patient is not a candidate for thoracotomy; chronic debility; and ongoing parenchymal disease, especially when secondary to associated bronchial obstruction.

■ OPERATIVE TECHNIQUES

Bronchoscopy always is indicated at the time of surgery to rule out an associated endobronchial obstruction from tumor, foreign body, or broncholith that might impede expansion of entrapped lung. Single-lung ventilation is established with the use of a double-lumen endotracheal tube or single-lumen tube with or without a bronchial blocker. This ventilation strategy allows a variety of intraoperative manipulations to aid in the process of decortication, such as intermittent positive-pressure ventilation of the involved side alternating with lung collapse.

The patient is placed in the lateral decubitus position, providing access to the preferred operative approach, the posterolateral thoracotomy. We generally divide the latissimus dorsi and spare the serratus anterior muscle. The pleural cavity is entered through the fifth, sixth, or seventh intercostal space, depending on the location of the pleural pathology. Generally the fibrotic process is most dense within the inferior aspect of the hemithorax and along the hemidiaphragmatic surface, making the sixth or seventh interspace preferable. A portion or the entirety of one or two ribs may be resected to allow access because the chest wall typically is rigid and contracted, making exposure difficult. Often, by freeing the thickened parietal pleura from the chest wall before placing a rib retractor, however, rib resection can be avoided.

The thickened parietal membrane is incised, and the pleural cavity is entered. Although violating the empyema cavity has the potential to contaminate the thoracotomy wound, it is generally unavoidable. Clinically significant postoperative wound infections are uncommon, however, if perioperative antibiotics are administered and complete lung expansion is achieved with obliteration of the pleural space. If the lung is densely fused to the chest wall by the fibrotic process, entry may be gained into the pleural space closer to the mediastinum, where the adhesions typically are less dense. The intrapleural fluid and fibrinopurulent debris are evacuated with suction and forceps. Cultures are taken for microbiologic analysis, including acid-fast and fungal smears and cultures, when indicated.

Pulmonary decortication starts by incising the fibrous peel that encases the lung. Depending on the inciting cause and the severity of disease, several layers may be penetrated before the thin visceral pleura is reached. Ideally, dissection continues just superficial to the pleura, stripping the rind in continuous sheets. A variety of techniques can be used to separate the peel from the pleura, including sharp dissection with a knife or scissors, blunt dissection with a suction tip or Kittner dissector, and stripping using DeBakey or Russian forceps. The lung may be intermittently ventilated to show the correct tissue plane, the extent of any ongoing restriction, and the adequacy of the decortication at bringing about complete lung expansion. Most of the dissection is performed best with the lung collapsed, to minimize damage to the visceral pleura and underlying lung parenchyma. The difficulty of stripping the different lung surfaces may be variable and unpredictable. In regions where a tissue plane is difficult to detect, patches of the fibrotic rind may be left on the lung. Areas of lung parenchyma that are superficially denuded of pleura generally can be left alone because air leaks resolve with spontaneous ventilation, especially if the lung is fully expanded, and the parenchyma apposes the chest wall. More extensive parenchymal injury leading to bleeding and large air leaks must be controlled with cautery or suture.

The extent of parietal pleurectomy has been the subject of considerable controversy. The advantage of freeing the chest wall, diaphragm, and mediastinum of the restrictive peel is the improvement of chest ventilatory dynamics that can be expected. The counterargument has been the potential for increased blood loss, operative time, and damage to neighboring structures. Likewise, complete pulmonary expansion may facilitate subsequent resolution of thick parietal membranes. Our practice has been to add at least a partial, if not complete, parietal pleurectomy if it can be done expeditiously, safely, and conservatively. The plane of dissection along the chest wall is generally between the parietal pleura and endothoracic fascia. Bleeding is managed with manual pressure and electrocautery. Care must be taken in regions that are difficult to visualize because the control of bleeding may be a challenge. A dental mirror can aid in viewing areas not seen under direct vision. As the mediastinum is approached, the surgeon must be continually vigilant as to the location of the esophagus, major vascular structures, pericardium, nerves (phrenic, vagus, brachial plexus, and sympathetic chain) and diaphragm. Damage to any of these structures can have devastating consequences.

If there is associated parenchymal pathology to be addressed, lung resection may be necessary at the time of decortication. Depending on the extent of resection, complete filling of the residual pleural space may be an issue. If adequate lung expansion is not provided by decortication, a small tailoring thoracoplasty or parietal wall collapse without rib resection ("pleural tent") can be added. A variety of muscle flaps also may be used to obliterate pleural space and obviate the need for thoracoplasty.

The involved lung is inflated fully under positive pressure on completion of the procedure. The pleural space is drained with at least two chest tubes, given the likelihood of some postoperative air leak, the possibility of ongoing bleeding, and the potential for areas of incomplete lung expansion. Positioning of the tubes depends on the particular outcome of decortication, although at least one tube generally should be placed inferiorly to drain the costophrenic sulcus. The double-lumen endotracheal tube may be changed back to a single-lumen tube at the termination of the procedure if bronchoscopy is necessary to suction excessive airway secretions or purulence. The chest tubes are left to suction via an underwater seal drainage system.

■ OUTCOMES

Operative mortality reported in most series is low (<5%), which reflects careful patient selection. Common postoperative complications include hemorrhage, prolonged air leaks, and residual empyema. With appropriate attention to operative technique, however, including control of bleeding and lung parenchymal damage and achieving adequate lung expansion, the incidence of these adverse outcomes should be minimized. Proper patient selection is crucial to ascertain that underlying lung pathology is managed adequately preoperatively or intraoperatively, allowing for maximum return of lung volume and function. Several authors have noted that the absence of underlying lung disease is the best predictor of improved pulmonary function after decortication. Although patients with diseases of a shorter duration might be expected to achieve a better operative result, even chronically entrapped lungs of many years' duration can expand fully after decortication, attesting to the relative sparing of the visceral pleura and parenchyma by the fibrotic process. Operative injury to the phrenic nerve, esophagus, or diaphragm can bring about postoperative complications with suboptimal, or even catastrophic, outcomes. Decortication, with the associated thoracotomy, is a major surgical undertaking with the potential for postthoracotomy pain and the loss of some degree of chest wall and upper extremity function.

■ CONCLUSIONS

Despite improvements in imaging techniques and the ability of physicians to intervene early in the course of pleural space diseases, patients still present to thoracic surgeons with the sequelae of chronic empyema, retained hemothorax, and eventually fibrothorax. The disease processes leading to fibrothorax may present insidiously, such that the patient does not seek medical attention until the sequelae of fibrothorax are already firmly established or may go unrecognized by the treating physician. Despite the desire to avoid a major surgical undertaking, less invasive medical or surgical therapies are doomed to fail in the setting of a lung that is chronically entrapped by a restrictive pleural rind. Symptomatic improvement can be anticipated only after surgical intervention designed to remove this encasing membrane from the lung parenchyma, chest wall, and diaphragm. In properly selected patients, surgical decortication can be performed with low mortality; acceptable morbidity; and resultant improvements in pleural sepsis, respiratory dynamics, and symptoms. With appropriate attention to operative technique, even lungs that have been chronically entrapped can be decorticated successfully and restored to premorbid level of function, assuming underlying pulmonary parenchymal pathology has been managed.

SUGGESTED READING

Deslauriers J, Perrault LP: Fibrothorax and decortication. In Pearson FG, et al, editors: *Thoracic surgery*, New York, 1995, Churchill-Livingstone, p 1107.

Rice TW: Fibrothorax and decortication of the lung. In Shields TW, et al, editors: *General thoracic surgery*, Philadelphia, 2000, Lippincott Williams & Wilkins, p 729.

Samson PC, Burford TH: Total pulmonary decortication: its evolution and present concepts of indications and operative technique, *J Thorac Surg* 16:127, 1947.

Wright GW, et al: Physiologic observations concerning decortication of the lung, *J Thorac Surg* 18:372, 1949.

POSTPNEUMONECTOMY EMPYEMA AND BRONCHOPLEURAL FISTULA

Jean Deslauriers

Philippe Demers

Postpneumonectomy bronchopleural fistulas (BPF) are uncommon but life-threatening events. As a result of improvements in surgical techniques, the prevalence of BPF has declined markedly since the 1970s to a current level of less than 5%. When it occurs, however, BPF remains associated with reported mortalities of 30% to 50%. Empyemas without BPF are seldom seen, and although patients may have a prolonged course of management with multiple interventions, this complication rarely in itself is associated with death.

■ ETIOLOGY

Several risk factors have been associated with the development of postpneumonectomy BPF (Table 1). Because the most important aspect in the management of postpneumonectomy BPF is their prevention, every effort should be made to identify clearly all predisposing factors, especially factors relating to preoperative management and technical conduct of the operation. It is well known that there is a higher risk of BPF in older patients and in patients with diabetes mellitus, hypoalbuminemia, and prolonged steroid therapy. If these conditions cannot be controlled adequately preoperatively, the bronchus is at risk of dehiscence. Prophylactic reinforcement of the bronchial stump with pericardium, pericardial fat, or intercostal muscle has been shown to reduce the risk of BPF in such cases.

The influence of induction therapies is controversial, although several reports have shown increased incidence of BPF in patients who have received more than 45 cGy of radiation therapy preoperatively. Because these bronchi are at much higher risk of dehiscence, coverage of the stump with large transposed intrathoracic muscles or omentum is recommended. In one report, the operative mortality associated with right pneumonectomy was close to 25% when the operation was done in the context of induction chemotherapy.

In patients who have obstructive pneumonia secondary to lung cancer, the infection ideally should be controlled before surgery. The same principle applies to patients undergoing pneumonectomy for tuberculosis; the incidence of BPF can be 20% in such cases. Patients with bronchiectasis are not at risk for BPF because they already have an increased vascular supply to the bronchus due to bronchial artery hyperplasia associated with this pathology.

The development of postpneumonectomy BPF is associated with several intraoperative factors, one of which is the

Table 1 Predisposing Risk Factors for Postpneumonectomy Bronchopleural Fistula and Empyema

PREOPERATIVE FACTORS
Age (>70 years)
Chronic obstructive pulmonary disease (predicted FEV_1 <0.8 liter)
Comorbidities (diabetes mellitus, collagen vascular disease)
Malnutrition (low serum albumin)
Prolonged steroid therapy
Induction therapies (chemotherapy, radiation therapy)
Pulmonary infection
Pneumonectomy through an empyema cavity

INTRAOPERATIVE FACTORS
Right pneumonectomy (versus left)
Extended pneumonectomy or completion pneumonectomy
Higher stage tumors
Extensive nodal dissection (devascularization and devitalization of bronchial stump)
Unhealthy bronchus (ossification of bronchial cartilage, endobronchial mucosal disease)
Inadequate bronchial closure (with tension or poor mucosal approximation)
Residual cancer in bronchial margin
Inexperienced operator
Long bronchial stump
Contamination of pleural space during pneumonectomy

POSTOPERATIVE FACTORS
Need for mechanical ventilation
Hemothorax or empyema

FEV_1, forced expiratory volume in 1 second.

inexperience of the operator who may not be familiar with the local anatomy or surgical principles involved in healthy bronchial closure. Most authors have reported a higher incidence of BPF after right pneumonectomy; this is not surprising because the right main bronchus vascular supply usually is provided by only one bronchial artery (versus two for the left main bronchus), making it more susceptible to devascularization during extensive nodal dissection. In addition, the left main bronchus retracts underneath the aortic arch after pneumonectomy and is protected better by mediastinal tissues. Whether there is a higher incidence of BPF in manually sutured bronchi than in stapled bronchi is unclear from the literature. The technique of bronchial closure is probably not important so long as the bronchus has not been devitalized, there is no tension at the sutured or stapled line, and there is good mucosal approximation.

In all cases, the bronchus must be closed near the carina to avoid excessively long stumps and pooling of secretions. Although residual malignancy in the bronchial resection margin impairs healing and increases the incidence of BPF, it is sometimes advisable to accept a positive resection line rather than increase the operative mortality by extending the resection to the lower end of the trachea.

Other intraoperative factors that have been shown to increase the potential risks for BPF development include surgery for higher stage tumors with more extensive mediastinal node dissections, pneumonectomy through an already infected pleural space, and contamination of the space during the operation. This last-mentioned factor is always a high possibility when pneumonectomy is done for benign disease, and sometimes contamination can be avoided by extrapleural dissection. It is important that these intraoperative risk factors be recognized and that bronchi at risk be covered with vascularized tissues. The benefits of routine coverage of low-risk bronchi are not clear, however, despite the fact that most surgeons tend to cover all right main bronchi with local tissues, such as pleura, pericardium, or mediastinal fat.

Perhaps the most significant risk factor for bronchial dehiscence is the need for postoperative mechanical ventilation. In several multivariate analyses, this factor was an independent predictor of BPF development. Postoperative mechanical ventilation is sometimes unavoidable. If mechanical ventilation is necessary, the tip of the intratracheal tube must be as far as possible from the sutured bronchus, and suctioning must be gentle. High peak pressures and positive end-expiratory pressure levels must be avoided. Although the use of high-frequency ventilation has been recommended for this purpose, this mode of ventilation can be applied successfully only to a few individuals. In most cases of BPF occurring in patients being mechanically ventilated, it is a terminal event for which nothing much can be done.

■ TREATMENT

In patients with suspected BPF, early diagnosis is paramount because the sooner it is made, the better the prognosis. Early dehiscence (within 2 weeks) usually is associated with increased dyspnea, expectoration of serosanguineous fluid, increased subcutaneous emphysema, and bulging of the thoracotomy incision. Serial x-rays often show a decreasing air-fluid level and mediastinal shift toward the remaining lung. In those cases, bronchoscopy is a crucial part of the evaluation because it usually documents the dehiscence and its exact site and size. It also documents the quality of the endobronchial mucosa and the length of the involved main bronchus. If the BPF is not seen, indirect signs, such as the presence of fibrin or bubbling within the bronchus, can be helpful. Occasionally, water-sealed drainage of the pleural space reveals an air leak.

Late occurring BPF or empyemas without fistulas (up to 3 months postoperatively) may be difficult to diagnose. Bronchoscopy and thoracentesis in cases of empyema are important parts of the evaluation when these diagnoses are suspected.

Although the management of an acute postpneumonectomy BPF remains a major problem, immediate drainage of the pleural space is often lifesaving because it may prevent flooding of the contralateral lung by what already has accumulated within the pneumonectomy space. The size of the BPF does not correlate with the importance of aspiration. When the patient's clinical condition has been stabilized, the next step in management is to attempt closure of the BPF. If the fistula is small (i.e., <2 to 3 mm), several authors have reported successful endobronchial closure through local bronchoscopic application of fibrin sealants. If this can be accomplished, videothoracoscopy may be used to evacuate the space completely, remove all necrotic tissue, and insert two thoracostomy tubes that later will be used for continuous irrigation of the hemithorax.

If the BPF is large (>3 mm), direct reclosure of the bronchial stump through repeat thoracotomy should be performed as soon as possible. In instances in which gross disruption of the bronchus has occurred, the reclosed stump should be reinforced with intercostal or pectoralis major muscles. Occasionally, one also can use a flap of diaphragm or the omentum to cover the stump. The omentum, which is brought through the diaphragm, is particularly useful because of its extendibility, good adherence to inflammatory surfaces, ability for neovascularization, and immunologic properties. When this is accomplished, two chest tubes are left to irrigate further and attempt to sterilize the space, or an open thoracic window is created. When the bronchial stump is too short for reclosure, the transposed muscle flap or omentum is sutured circumferentially around the defect to obtain an airtight closure. When the chest cavity is cleaned, the tubes are removed, or the patient is taken back to the operating room for chest wall reclosure if he or she has an open thoracic window.

Early empyemas without BPF are uncommon, and they are managed best by videothoracoscopic débridement of the space, tube irrigation, and systemic antibiotics. With this regimen, most infected spaces can be sterilized, avoiding the need for an open thoracic window or thoracoplasty. When the space has been sterilized, as documented by two or three negative cultures, it is filled with the débridement antibiotic solution, and the tubes are removed. In all of these patients, special emphasis must be placed on maintaining adequate nutrition during the recovery period.

Treatment strategies for late occurring BPF (>4 weeks postoperatively) are different because the risks of aspiration in the remaining lung are low. Initial tube drainage is important, and occasionally, small BPF close spontaneously, especially in cases in which the fistula is secondary to an empyema. Drainage also can be accomplished by fenestration when the space and fistula site can be inspected and débrided on a daily basis. Large BPF usually require surgical reclosure, which is accomplished best by a transpericardial approach via a median sternotomy (Figure 1). The main advantages of this approach are the uninfected operative field and the well-defined anatomy. When doing this procedure, the bronchus must be fully redivided, rather than stapled in continuity, and the closure must be reinforced with vascularized pericardium, mobilized thymus, or omentum, which is obtained easily through an extension of the sternotomy. Occasionally the BPF can be closed via a cervical approach using a videomediastinoscope (Figure 2). Ultimately the residual empyema cavity can be sterilized by tube irrigation or open fenestration.

An alternative method is to drain the hemithorax initially by way of an open thoracic window. When the cavity appears healthy, the patient is returned to the operating room for muscle or omental transposition to achieve fistula closure and space obliteration.

Controversy remains regarding the role of thoracoplasty with or without added myoplasty to achieve space obliteration and fistula closure. In our experience, these procedures are well tolerated, and for most patients, they achieve the desired goals.

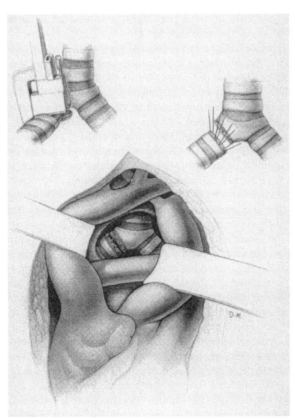

Figure 1
Chronic right main bronchus fistula treated by division and reclosure of the proximal and distal stumps. *(From Ginsberg RJ, et al: Ann Thorac Surg 47:232, 1989; with permission.)*

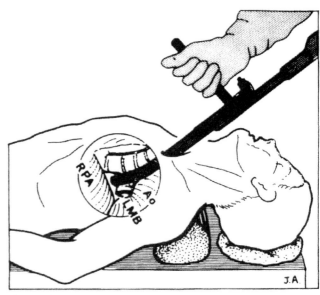

Figure 2
Closure of BPF through cervicotomy. *(From Azorin JF, et al: Presse Med 25:805, 1996; with permission.)*

■ SUMMARY

In all patients with postpneumonectomy BPF, definitive surgery should be considered only when the medical and nutritional status of the patient have been optimized; when the cavity is cleaned and healthy; when the BPF has been carefully categorized (site, size, quality of mucosa, length of stump) by bronchoscopy and CT scan; when the patient no longer requires or is unlikely to require mechanical ventilation; and when the patient has no evidence of recurring carcinoma. Although mortality and morbidity remain high in these patients, careful understanding of the complication and systematic and aggressive management can be successful in some cases. Prevention is the most important consideration.

SUGGESTED READING

Deschamps C, et al: Empyema and bronchopleural fistula after pneumonectomy: factors affecting incidence, *Ann Thorac Surg* 72:243, 2001.

Ginsberg RJ, et al: Closure of chronic postpneumonectomy fistula using the trans-sternal transpericardial approach, *Ann Thorac Surg* 47:231, 1989.

Grégoire R, et al: Thoracoplasty: its forgotten role in the management of non tuberculous postpneumonectomy empyema, *Can J Surg* 30:343, 1987.

Hollaus PH, et al: Video-thoracoscopic debridement of the postpneumonectomy space in empyema, *Eur J Cardiothorac Surg* 16:283, 1999.

Regnard JF, et al: Open window thoracostomy followed by intrathoracic flap transposition in the treatment of empyema complicating pulmonary resection, *J Thorac Cardiovasc Surg* 120:270, 2000.

CHYLOTHORAX

Robert M. Cortina
David W. Johnstone

■ DEFINITION AND DIAGNOSIS

Chylothorax is the presence of lymph in the pleural space. Chylothorax may be caused by congenital or primary lymphatic disease but usually is due to intrathoracic malignancies with intrinsic or extrinsic obstruction, iatrogenic injury, and blunt or penetrating trauma. Postoperative chylothorax may complicate surgical procedures anywhere along the path of the thoracic duct between the diaphragm and the neck.

The initial symptom of intrathoracic chyle accumulation is dyspnea resulting from compressive atelectasis of the lung. Prolonged drainage leads to dehydration, malnutrition, and immunologic compromise due to loss of fluid, fats, protein, and T lymphocytes. Before the advent of thoracic duct ligation, the mortality of postoperative and traumatic chylothorax was nearly 50%.

Although chyle can be clear in the fasting state, it becomes milky after oral intake that includes fats. Biochemical and microscopic examination of the effusion confirm the diagnosis. The concentration of triglycerides is higher than that of plasma; fluid with a triglyceride level of more than 110 mg/dl has a 99% chance of being chylous compared with a 5% chance when less than 50 mg/dl. The presence of chylomicrons in the fluid is specific for the diagnosis of chylothorax. Prompt diagnosis is essential to effective therapy because of the severity of complications from prolonged chylous drainage.

■ MEDICAL MANAGEMENT

Conservative (nonsurgical) management of chylothorax may be appropriate as an initial strategy, particularly in the first few days after surgery or trauma or in cases of malignant chylothoraces that may respond to treatment of the underlying neoplasm (particularly lymphoma). The components of initial management are drainage of the pleural space, reduction of chyle flow, maintenance of hydration, and provision of adequate nutrition.

Evacuation of the pleural space is achieved most commonly by tube thoracostomy. This provides lung reexpansion, continuous drainage, and accurate measurement of chyle flow. Close attention must be paid to tube patency, position, and changes in drainage because prolonged drainage can lead to tube obstruction or loculation away from other portions of the pleural space. Chyle is bacteriostatic, and infection from the indwelling tube is unlikely.

In 1934, Hepner stated that chylous fistulas close by obliteration of the adjacent pleural space rather than healing of the lymphatic vessels themselves. To accelerate pleural symphysis, various chemical sclerosants have been applied to the pleural space, including antibiotics (tetracycline, doxycycline), antineoplastic agents (bleomycin), biologic modifiers (OK-432, interferon, and interleukins), and talc. Chemical pleurodesis may be most appropriate for patients with malignant chylothoraces, in whom direct closure of the leak is impossible, but we have had a low success rate in this setting.

Maintenance of nutrition, prevention of dehydration, and reduction of chyle flow are closely related. Large losses of fluid, electrolytes, protein, fat, fat-soluble vitamins, and lymphocytes may result in severe metabolic and immunologic derangement. A reduction in enteral intake and specifically in the dietary intake of long-chain fatty acids is associated with a significant reduction in lymphatic flow. The substitution of dietary fat with medium-chain triglycerides is practiced widely, predicated on the preferential uptake of medium-chain triglycerides by the portal circulation. These diets have had variable degrees of success. The reason may be that intestinal triglycerides derive from endogenous and exogenous sources and that any oral intake increases chyle production. When a fat-free, nonelemental diet was compared with total parenteral nutrition (TPN), the closure rate of chylous fistulas favored TPN. Many authors prefer complete bowel rest and TPN as the optimal means of nutritional support to reduce chyle production.

Traumatic chylothoraces that close with conservative management do so within 2 weeks in most cases. When the chest drainage is low, the pleural space is evacuated, and the lung is expanded, oral intake can be resumed. When the patient is eating a normal diet with no evidence of persistent chyle leak, the chest tube can be removed.

When chylothorax is secondary to lymphatic obstruction by tumor, treatment of the primary condition with radiotherapy and/or chemotherapy may control the chyle fistulas either by producing local fibrosis or by relieving lymphatic obstruction. Pleuroperitoneal shunting may be appropriate in these patients because nutritional losses are minimized while dyspnea is relieved. Success has been reported to be 75% to 90% in treating pediatric chylothoraces and 80% in adults. The procedure is associated with minimal discomfort, but the subcutaneous chamber must be compressed several hundred times per day to shunt an adequate volume. In debilitated cancer patients, this is not a useful solution. Intermittent external drainage with either thoracentesis or a semipermanent catheter may be a reasonable palliative alternative.

Other methods of conservative management include positive-pressure ventilation, inhaled nitric oxide at 20 ppm, and percutaneous embolization of the thoracic duct. The institution of positive-pressure ventilation and/or nitric oxide reportedly has resulted in a marked reduction in chest tube drainage and has stopped the chyle leak. It is believed that systemic venous hypertension may be a significant contributing factor to a persistent chyle leak. Nitric oxide, a predominately pulmonary arterial vasodilator, may decrease systemic venous pressures by augmenting forward flow through the right side of the heart.

Percutaneous transabdominal duct catheterization and embolization can be a safe and effective alternative treatment for persistent chylothorax and may be warranted in patients too frail to undergo duct ligation. Patients with previous major abdominal surgery involving retroperitoneal organs may not be suitable for this intervention because they may have occlusion of the major retroperitoneal lymphatic ducts and cisterna chyli.

■ SURGICAL MANAGEMENT

Before Lampson's report of transpleural thoracic duct ligation in 1948, repeated thoracentesis and oral nutritional support commonly were employed. Mortality from traumatic chylothorax was greater than 50%, and nontraumatic chylothorax was usually fatal. After the introduction of thoracic duct ligation, the mortality rate improved to 10%.

There is general consensus that failed conservative management warrants surgical intervention. There is less agreement on clinical parameters necessitating surgical intervention. In 1971, Selle et al proposed the following parameters for surgical intervention. Idiopathic chylothorax in neonates and nontraumatic chylothorax should be managed nonoperatively. Indications for thoracic duct ligation in traumatic chylothorax are an average daily loss of greater than 1500 ml/day in adults or greater than 100 ml/year of age in children over 5 days, persistent leak for more than 2 weeks despite conservative management, and nutritional or metabolic complications. In 1981, Strausser et al recommended operative therapy for nontraumatic chylothorax as well. In their report, only 3 of 13 patients responded to nonoperative therapy, whereas 3 of 4 patients who had transthoracic duct ligation had permanent relief of their chylothorax.

Lymphangiography provides useful information regarding the lymphatic anatomy and fistula site, but it is laborious. We generally have reserved lymphangiography for refractory chylothoraces that have failed initial surgical closure. Other methods used to locate the leak include preoperative subcutaneous injection of 1% Evans blue dye in the thigh or enteral administration of a fat source, such as cream or olive oil. Methylene blue may be added to the fat source to highlight the site of the fistula.

The surgical options for control of chylothorax are direct ligation of the thoracic duct, mass ligation of the thoracic duct with and without thoracotomy, thoracoscopic ligation of the thoracic duct, pleurectomy, application of fibrin glue, and placement of a pleuroperitoneal shunt. If the chyle leak can be identified, direct ligation with nonabsorbable ligatures should be performed on either side of the leak. If the leak cannot be identified, extensive dissection should be avoided. Mass ligation of all tissue between the aorta, spine, esophagus, and pericardium is performed most easily above the diaphragmatic hiatus via the right pleural space. This ligation traditionally has been performed via a right thoracotomy through the sixth or seventh interspace. Parietal pleurectomy may promote pleural symphysis and should be considered when control of the duct is uncertain. Pulmonary decortication may be necessary if the lung is entrapped in a benign peel.

Since its introduction in the early 1990s, thoracoscopic ligation of the thoracic duct has become a therapeutic option. There are few reported series but multiple successful case reports. Enteral administration of 50 ml of heavy cream is given shortly before surgery. Thoracoscopy is performed under general anesthesia using single-lung ventilation. A trocar is placed in the right sixth or seventh intercostal space in the midaxillary line. A 30-degree scope is inserted, and the pleural space is evaluated. A second port in the right eighth posterior intercostal space is used for dissection and division of the inferior pulmonary ligament. A third port is placed in the anterior axillary line superiorly for retraction of the lung. The pleura is incised above the diaphragm. If the duct can be identified easily, it is dissected free. A small segment usually is taken for pathologic confirmation, then both ends are doubly clipped. If the thoracic duct cannot be identified easily, mass ligation of all tissue in the position previously described is performed using clips. Chest drainage is established. The chest drain is removed when chyle drainage has ceased with the patient on a normal diet.

Chylothorax complicates esophagectomy in 2% to 4% of transthoracic approaches and 10% of transhiatal resections. A recognized intraoperative thoracic duct injury should be closed immediately. Most postoperative chylothoraces in this setting do not heal with conservative management. Early surgical closure of the duct is optimal. Thoracoscopic closure of the duct has been reported, but the gastric conduit can make exposure difficult, and a low thoracotomy is often the best approach.

Chylothorax after pulmonary resection is unusual. An initial course of conservative management is prudent after lobectomy if the lung is fully expanded. If a large residual pleural space remains after bilobectomy or pneumonectomy, we recommend early surgical closure of the duct. Pleuroperitoneal shunts may be appropriate in some patients with obligatory pleural spaces.

■ SUMMARY

Chylothorax may be iatrogenic, traumatic, or spontaneous due to congenital or acquired disorders. Early recognition is crucial to preventing serious complications of chronic lymphatic loss. Initial drainage, combined with measures to reduce chyle flow and maintain nutrition, may resolve the condition. For cases that do not show prompt response, particularly in the postoperative or trauma setting, early surgical ligation of the thoracic duct should be performed with the expectation of prompt resolution. Thoracoscopy offers a minimally invasive approach and warrants consideration by experienced surgeons. Other alternatives require consideration of the underlying etiology, consideration of the patient's medical condition and prognosis, and an understanding of the limitations of these approaches.

SUGGESTED READING

Bessone LN, et al: Chylothorax: collective review, *Ann Thorac Surg* 12:527, 1971.

Johnstone DW, Feins RH: Chylothorax, *Chest Surg Clin N Am* 4:617, 1994.

Kent RB, Pinson TW: Thoracoscopic ligation of the thoracic duct, *Surg Endosc* 7:52, 1993.

Lampson RS: Traumatic chylothorax: a review of the literature and report of a case treated by mediastinal ligation of the thoracic duct, *J Thorac Surg* 17:778, 1948.

LOCALIZED FIBROUS TUMORS OF THE PLEURA

Paul A. Kirschner

David S. Mendelson

Localized fibrous tumors of the pleura (LFTP) arise from the submesothelial connective tissue of the pleura. They are distinct from tumors derived from the surface mesothelium, which are called *diffuse malignant mesothelioma*. The term *mesothelioma* sometimes is applied incorrectly to LFTP.

■ ETIOLOGY

The etiology of LFTP is unknown. It is not related to asbestos exposure, as is the case with diffuse malignant mesothelioma.

■ PATHOLOGY

LFTP is essentially a connective tissue tumor of the spindle cell variety. It presents as a localized nodule or solid mass. Most cases (>75%) arise from the visceral pleura, about 15% to 20% stem from the parietal pleura, and a few arise from the mediastinum. Rarely, LFTP may present as an intrapulmonary mass due to "inverted growth" from the visceral pleura.

LFTP are slow-growing tumors and range in size from a few centimeters to a huge mass occupying the entire pleural cavity. They may weigh 2 kg or more. They compress but usually do not invade vital structures, such as airways, lung tissue, or great vessels. Despite their foreboding appearance on x-ray, they are usually completely resectable.

Visceral pleural LFTP often are attached to the underlying lung by a narrow pedicle, which sometimes arises deep in the fissure. Parietal LFTP have a much broader apposition to the subcostal chest wall. It is rare for them to invade ribs or chest wall, but rib deformities may be seen in long-standing tumors.

Large lesions may have a bosselated rather than smooth surface and are covered by large, thin-walled, fragile "venous lakes," which are prone to bleed furiously at the slightest surgical manipulation. When mobilization of the mass is complete, the arterial supply usually does not present a problem in hemostasis.

Occasionally, LFTP are accompanied by serous or rarely bloody pleural effusions. They only rarely, if ever, contain malignant cells, however, and do not preclude successful resective surgery. Parietal pleural hyaline plaques, commonly seen in patients exposed to asbestos, are not seen in LFTP.

Microscopically, LFTP display the spectrum of connective soft tissue tumors ranging from a benign appearance with an orderly arrangement of fibroblasts and collagenous tissue and little pleomorphism to a wildly malignant appearance with a disorderly and richly cellular pattern including frequent mitotic figures and areas of necrosis. Such extreme appearance may warrant the diagnosis of fibrosarcoma. In any single case, it is difficult to prognosticate, however, which tumors will recur based on microscopy alone.

Recurrent tumors may mimic their primary gross appearance, may recur locally, and often still may be amenable to reresection. Local recurrence may appear 10 or more years after resection of the primary tumor.

■ IMMUNOHISTOCHEMISTRY

Sometimes microscopic differentiation cannot be made between LFTP and the fibrosarcomatous variant of diffuse malignant mesothelioma. Immunohistochemistry displays positive staining for vimentin and CD 34 and negative staining for cytokeratin and carcinoembryonic antigen, indicating a mesenchymal rather than an epithelial origin. DNA studies indicate a diploid population with a low proliferative rate, reflecting the less aggressive behavior of LFTP.

■ IMAGING

The imaging appearance of LFTP reflects their gross anatomic structure. Small lesions, 3 to 4 cm in diameter, are nonspecific and appear like a solitary pulmonary nodule. Larger tumors present as solid masses with a rounded contour and can measure 25 cm or more in diameter. Because of their great weight and narrow long pedicle, they tend to hang down into the bottom of the pleural cavity. In so doing, they obscure the normal diaphragmatic contour, and their convex upper margin can simulate an elevated hemidiaphragm. Over time, as these tumors enlarge upward, this convex contour invokes the comparison with a "rising sun" or "sunrise."

Special imaging techniques such as computed tomography and magnetic resonance imaging reveal a heterogeneous appearance due to areas of liquefaction, necrosis, and hemorrhage. Sometimes scattered deposits of calcium may be seen.

Rarely a nonadherent tumor on a long slender pedicle may be observed to move about in the chest with changes in bodily position. This movement may be accompanied by curious subjective symptoms of a heavy object moving about in the chest.

■ CLINICAL PRESENTATION

LFTP present in a variety of ways. Small lesions simulating solitary pulmonary nodules may be detected on routine screening x-rays. With enlargement, they encroach on functioning lung tissue, producing progressive symptoms of shortness of breath. Bronchial symptoms are rare because LFTP do not invade the airways. Chest discomfort has been alluded to. Extrinsic venous compression producing superior vena cava syndrome may occur with large tumors. This is not a contraindication to operation because it may be relieved by resection.

Of particular interest is the occurrence of two paraneoplastic syndromes—hypertrophic pulmonary osteoarthropathy with clubbing and hypoglycemia (Doege-Potter syndrome). Hypertrophic pulmonary osteoarthropathy and clubbing occurs in LFTP proportionately more than in lung cancer. It frequently is misdiagnosed as arthritis. Hypoglycemia (Doege-Potter syndrome) is characterized clinically by mania, confusion, and coma due to lowered blood glucose. This phenomenon is due to the secretion by the tumor of insulin-like growth factor II and is a feature of several other different connective tissue tumors, not strictly confined to LFTP.

Both of these paraneoplastic syndromes usually occur with large tumors and subside after resection. In one instance, the hypoglycemia appeared only with the second large recurrence of the primary tumor and responded favorably to a third operation. Either of these syndromes may reappear with local recurrence of the primary tumor.

■ SURGERY

The surgical treatment of LFTP is usually straightforward. Preoperative needle biopsy is not essential because even if negative it does not alter the method of treatment.

Pedunculated tumors are removed easily by clamp and ligature of the stalk. Even huge tumors occupying practically the entire hemithorax and measuring 26 cm in diameter can be removed without requiring any pulmonary resection. The surgeon should be alerted to the possible occurrence of reexpansion pulmonary edema in the removal of giant lesions. Thoracoscopy and video-assisted thoracic surgery are beginning to be used as a primary definitive approach as

exemplified by Cardillo et al, who removed 39 of 49 tumors with clean resective margins.

Postoperative follow-up should be for the lifetime of the patient. Recurrences have been noted 10 or more years after the primary operation and still may be amenable to reresection. Neither chemotherapy nor radiotherapy plays a significant role as adjuvant treatment.

■ SUMMARY

LFTP are uncommon tumors of the pleura that arise from the submesothelial connective tissue of the pleura. They often mistakenly are regarded as or referred to as *mesotheliomas*. LFTP are part of a group of connective tissue tumors of the spindle cell variety that occur in soft tissues throughout the body and the pleura. They are slow-growing, relatively noninvasive, localized lesions that sometimes can attain huge size and still remain resectable. They may present with one of two paraneoplastic syndromes—hypertrophic pulmonary osteoarthropathy and hypoglycemia (Doege-Potter syndrome)—both of which respond favorably to resection. LFTP have no relation to asbestos.

SUGGESTED READING

Briselli M, et al: Solitary fibrous tumors of the pleura: eight new cases and review of 360 cases in the literature, *Cancer* 47:2678, 1981.

Cardillo G, et al: Localized (solitary) fibrous tumors of the pleura: an analysis of 55 patients, *Ann Thorac Surg* 70:1808, 2000.

Clagett OT, et al: Localized fibrous mesothelioma of the pleura, *J Thorac Surg* 24:213, 1952.

Klemperer P, Rabin CB: Primary neoplasms of the pleura, *Arch Pathol* 11:383, 1931.

Mendelson DS, et al: Localized fibrous pleural mesothelioma, *Clin Imaging* 15:105, 1991.

MALIGNANT MESOTHELIOMA

Harvey I. Pass

The role of surgery in managing diffuse pleural mesothelioma is controversial. Overwhelming pessimism for surgical options persists in most centers that do not deal routinely with the disease because the combination of effusive disease and bulky tumor renders complete surgical eradication virtually impossible. The disappointing long-term overall survival results, the historically high morbidity and mortality rates, and the propensity for local recurrences have forced many centers to abandon radical operations except for the rare localized situation.

■ INDICATIONS FOR SURGICAL MANAGEMENT

Surgery plays a role in the management of malignant pleural mesothelioma (MPM) for diagnosis, for palliative therapy, or as part of a multimodal therapeutic plan. Basically, operative intervention in mesothelioma is for primary effusion control, for cytoreduction before multimodal therapy, or to deliver and monitor innovative intrapleural therapies. The procedures include thoracoscopy, pleurectomy/decortication, and extrapleural pneumonectomy (EPP). The indications for each of these operations depend on the extent of disease, performance and functional status of the patient, and philosophy of the treating institution.

Effusion Control

In general, the indications for palliative surgery in MPM include the control or prevention of effusion that results in disabling dyspnea. The most efficacious and least invasive of the surgical procedures to accomplish effusion control is thoracoscopy with talc pleurodesis. Asbestos-free, sterile talc, 2 to 5 g, can be insufflated over the lung and the parietal surfaces; success rates in effusion control with talc, used either via thoracoscopy or via slurry, approach 90%. Failures of these techniques usually are associated with entrapped lung, a large solid tumor mass, a long history of effusion with multiple thoracenteses leading to loculations, or age older than 70 years. The median survival for patients with mesothelioma having talc pleurodesis ranges from 6.8 to 9.4 months.

Effusion control via palliative surgery occasionally is performed after lesser procedures (including sclerotherapy) have failed due to the inability of the lung to expand and the patient continues to have dyspnea. Generally the procedure of choice for palliation is a pleurectomy with or without decortication of the underlying lung. The use of EPP for palliative intent is described only rarely in the literature, and due to its morbidity and mortality some surgeons state that EPP should never be used for palliative purposes.

■ CYTOREDUCTION SURGERY

Staging

All of the staging systems for mesothelioma are surgical/pathologically based. The few patients with mesothelioma are placed in surgical-based protocols; most patients at the time of diagnosis never have a truly accurate stage. The Union Internationale Contre Cancre (UICC) proposed a TNM staging system that has evolved into the presently described International Mesothelioma Interest Group (IMIG) staging system. The IMIG staging system has been available only more recently, but it has been validated in two large surgical series of mesothelioma. Sugarbaker et al proposed the alternative but complementary Brigham staging system based on tumor, resectability, and nodal status. The bulk of disease volume reflecting T status itself may predict stage and prognosis for mesothelioma.

Three-dimensional computed tomography (CT) reconstructions of preresection and postresection solid tumor in 48 patients with mesothelioma were prospectively performed, and the disease was staged postoperatively according to the new IMIG staging. Tumor volumes associated with negative nodes were significantly smaller than volumes with positive nodes, and progressively higher stage was associated with higher median preoperative volume of tumor. Patients with preoperative tumor volumes greater than 52 ml had shorter progression-free intervals than patients with tumor volumes 51 ml or less.

Surgical Evaluation

The preferred approach for early stage mesothelioma remains to be defined. For patients who are unable to fulfill functional criteria for entry into an aggressive treatment program (see later) or who desire palliation therapy only, pleurodesis is an acceptable option. More patients with mesothelioma should have an informed discussion at the primary care level, however, to know exactly what "standard" or innovative strategies are available to them. Most patients seeking treatment for mesothelioma are middle-aged to older adults with a long latency period between asbestos exposure and tumor development. If surgical intervention is to be considered, a detailed physiologic and functional workup directed chiefly at the cardiopulmonary axis must be performed.

Pulmonary Evaluation

Poor underlying pulmonary function in patients with MPM usually reflects the burden of asbestos exposure, concomitant smoking history (70% of the patients have had a heavy tobacco intake), degree of lung trapped by tumor or fluid, and patient age. Patients with a forced expiratory volume in 1 second (FEV_1) of greater than 2 liters/sec usually are able to withstand a pneumonectomy. In general, an FEV_1 of less than 1 liter/sec, a Po_2 less than 55 torr, and a Pco_2 greater than 45 torr are relative contraindications to performance of EPP. If the patient presents with an FEV_1 of less than 2 liters/sec or if the predicted FEV_1 is less than 1.2 liters/sec after pneumonectomy, quantitative ventilation-perfusion scanning should be performed.

Cardiac Evaluation

Operations for MPM are associated with profound blood loss and potentially significant cardiac demands. The patient should be screened carefully for a history of hypertension, angina, and previous myocardial infarction, and routine electrocardiograms should reveal no signs of previous injury. Any patient having a myocardial infarction within the past 3 months or having an arrhythmia requiring medication should not be considered for EPP. Patients without objective evidence of cardiac injury who have a history of chest pain compatible with angina or remote myocardial infarction should have stress thallium screening to investigate reversible perfusion defects indicative of myocardium at risk. In general, patients with an ejection fraction of less than 45% are not considered to be candidates for EPP. This also may have an impact on their enrollment in innovative multimodality programs using potentially cardiotoxic drugs. Patients with reversible defects may be considered for angioplasty before operative intervention for their disease and may be better candidates if a multimodality approach is being contemplated.

Other Preoperative Evaluation

Preoperative medications must be scrutinized carefully, specifically any nonsteroidal antiinflammatory drugs that could affect platelet function. If patients are to participate in multimodality programs that use drugs with potential renal toxicity (i.e., cisplatin), a preoperative creatinine clearance should be performed.

Candidates for Surgery

The question then becomes "who is a surgical candidate in MPM?" In the United States, patients with presumed stage I disease who have a good performance status are considered candidates for surgical-based multimodal schemes. Given the above-described problems with mesothelioma staging, however, how do we know preoperatively what stage the patient is? Nodal status is highlighted as an independent predictor of survival in mesothelioma; should we be performing mediastinoscopy or mediastinotomy for mesothelioma as we do with lung cancer? In light of the data that only 30% to 40% of nodes involved from resected patients are in the upper mediastinum, routine mediastinal staging before thoracotomy for mesothelioma would give a significant number of false-negative results due to level variation. It is also unclear whether the prognostic importance of mediastinal nodal involvement in mesothelioma is equal to or greater than the prognostic importance of the nodes within the visceral envelope of the lung, and these N1 nodes within the lung may reflect disease at a later time in the natural history of the disease. In the absence of routine thoracoscopic sampling of multiple nodal stations in mesothelioma before definitive resection, mediastinoscopy may be justified in patients with obvious (i.e., >1.5 cm) nodal involvement in levels 7, 4R, 4, 5, or 6L or in patients with a suspicion for contralateral nodal involvement on presentation. It is possible that fluorodeoxyglucose positron emission tomography will help at least to define patients with higher stage mesothelioma in the future.

Other sites of concern for satisfactory debulking independent of lymph node basins include the diaphragm proper and the diaphragmatic sulci. Because mesothelioma tends to originate in the lower region of the chest, the degree or bulk of involved areas may represent a caudad-cephalad spectrum, with the highest regions having the least involvement. Careful inspection of a CT scan or magnetic resonance imaging (MRI) may suggest subdiaphragmatic involvement by direct extension. Laparoscopic investigation of this area to exclude peritoneal involvement is mandatory in patients presenting with bulky disease in the sulci or who have a worrisome MRI scan.

Operative Approach

Some investigators believe that EPP offers the best chance for complete surgical extirpation of mesothelioma. Most diffuse MPMs cannot be surgically removed en bloc with truly negative histologic margins because many of the patients have had a previous biopsy, and there is invasion of the endothoracic fascia and intercostal muscles at that site or pleural effusion that, although cytologically negative, may be breached, leading to local permeation of tumor cells either into the residual cavity or into the abdomen. Nevertheless, it is encouraging that in one of the larger series of EPP performed for mesothelioma, 66 of 183 patients were defined as having negative resection margins after EPP. Patients with this finding who had epithelial mesothelioma were found to have 2-year and 5-year survival rates of 68% and 46%, if the node dissection did not reveal tumor.

Nevertheless, if negative margins are the exception, is it justifiable to spare functioning lung if the visceral pleura is minimally involved by performing a parietal pleurectomy instead of EPP? Minimal visceral pleural disease is an undefined entity. There are no criteria for how many sites should be involved, the size of these involved sites, or whether involvement of the fissure is worse than nonfissural involvement. Individual surgeons with expertise in the management of mesothelioma have different philosophies about the use of pleurectomy in this situation, and some make the decision regarding the type of operation in an individual patient at the time of the exploration.

There is no doubt that EPP is a more extensive dissection and may serve to remove more bulk disease than a pleurectomy, chiefly in the diaphragmatic and visceral pleural surfaces. Some surgeons include diaphragmatic resection and pericardial resection with pleurectomy, however, to accomplish removal of "all gross disease." For EPP, it is almost a necessity to include pericardiotomy during the resection because the maneuver aids in the exposure of the vessels and allows intrapericardial control to prevent a surgical catastrophe. The presence of irregular, bulky disease that on CT infiltrates into the fissures probably dictates the necessity for EPP; a large effusion with minimal bulk disease may call for pleurectomy decortication. The philosophy of the surgeon regarding the operation may affect his choice: Some surgeons reserve EPP for patients with bulk disease that precludes simple pleurectomy, whereas others believe that the greatest chance for complete gross excision would be via EPP performed in the patient with minimal disease. This important factor, preoperative quantitative bulk of disease, not only may influence the choice or resection, but also may be an important preoperative prognostic factor in any patient with MPM, as previously described.

At this time, there are no data to suggest which operation "stage for stage" is superior for malignant pleural mesothelioma; patients should be well counseled regarding the possibilities before having surgical exploration. Rusch and Pass confirmed that there seemed to be no survival difference in their series between patients who received EPP and patients who received pleurectomy decortication. The discussion regarding the type of resection may be influenced by analysis of the regional lung function by quantitative lung perfusion. The final decision as to whether pleurectomy and decortication or EPP is to be performed, given the aforementioned caveats, becomes an intraoperative decision, unless a protocol calls specifically for one operation or the other.

■ PLEURECTOMY

Morbidity and Mortality

When performed routinely, pleurectomy for MPM is associated with few major complications. In the series that specified postoperative morbidity, the most common complication was prolonged air leak (i.e., >7 days), occurring in 10% of patients. On average, the chest tubes can be removed in approximately 5.5 days with greater than 50% of the patients having the chest tube removed within 4 days. Pneumonia and respiratory insufficiency may occur and usually is related to the burden of disease and preoperative functional status. Empyema is a rare occurrence (2%) and is managed by prolonged chest tube drainage and antibiotics. Hemorrhage requiring reexploration is rare (i.e., <1%).

Earlier studies in patients requiring pleurectomy (but not having mesothelioma) had an in-hospital or operative mortality of 10% to 18% in the 1960s. The modern-day mortality from pleurectomy has decreased and generally is considered to be 1.5% to 2% with death either from respiratory insufficiency or from hemorrhage.

Short-Term and Long-Term Results

Pleurectomy and decortication are effective in controlling malignant pleural effusion. Law reported effusion control in 88% of patients having decortication for mesothelioma. In 63 patients having partial decortication and pleurectomy, Ruffie et al reported 86% control of effusion. Brancatisano et al reported a 98% control of effusion after pleurectomy in 50 cases of pleural mesothelioma.

Many of the published series using pleurectomy for palliative management added therapies postoperatively in an uncontrolled, institution-related fashion. Most series had no sampling of the mediastinal nodes, let alone a mediastinal dissection. Nevertheless, the overall median survival for patients having pleurectomy alone is approximately 13 months. Patients who receive pleurectomy and decortication alone usually have early effusive disease with minimal bulk tumor. If these patients have epithelial mesothelioma and are not found to have nodal involvement, survival rates can be significantly longer than the rates stated previously.

■ EXTRAPLEURAL PNEUMONECTOMY

Radical EPP classically has been described for a pure epithelial stage I tumor that is technically resectable and encapsulated by the parietal pleura. Because of sampling error, it is impossible to clarify with 100% certainty whether the tumor is a pure epithelial type or mixed tumor based on the preoperative or intraoperative biopsy specimen.

In reality, there are few patients who qualify for exploration for EPP. In Butchart's review, 29 of 46 (63%) patients were eligible for EPP, and in a series of EPPs performed at Rush–Presbyterian–St. Luke's Hospital in Chicago, 33 of 56 (59%) patients over a 27-year period had EPP. Sugarbaker reported 50% of the patients seen at his institution are not eligible for EPP and adjuvant therapy. These series do not define why one patient may have a pleurectomy while another may have EPP; some institutions simply have never adopted EPP as feasible for treatment of MPM. One of the more enlightening studies to comment on eligibility for EPP was the Lung Cancer Study Group malignant mesothelioma pilot study from 1985 through 1988. To be eligible for entry into the study, the patient was required to have disease limited to the hemithorax by radiographic evaluation, a residual FEV_1 after resection of at least 1 liter/sec, and no significant cardiovascular illness—clearly more lenient criteria than those that limited eligibility due to age, histologic type, or presumed stage. Even with these "relaxed" criteria, only 20 of the 83 evaluated patients had an EPP. The reasons that EPP could not be performed were chiefly extent of disease not allowing complete gross resection (54%), inadequate respiratory reserve (33%), stage IV disease (11%), and concurrent medical illness (10%).

Morbidity and Mortality

As a result of its magnitude, EPP has significantly greater morbidity than pleurectomy. The major complication rate ranges from 20% to 40%; arrhythmia requiring medical management is the most common complication. The rate for bronchopleural fistula is greater with right-sided EPPs, with an overall fistula rate of 3% to 20%. Bronchopleural fistula can be treated for the most part with open thoracostomy drainage with or without muscle flap interposition.

The mortality rates after EPP were unacceptably high in the 1970s, with 31% reported by Butchart. Since then, however, there has been a steady decline in the operative mortality for EPP to consistent rates less than 10% in series of 20 of more patients. Mortality occurs chiefly in older patients from respiratory failure, myocardial infarction, or pulmonary embolus. Rusch reported a perioperative mortality of 5% after EPP, and Sugarbaker et al reported a perioperative mortality of 3.8%. Similar mortality rates have been reported from the series from the National Cancer Institute.

Short-Term and Long-Term Results
Recurrence After Extrapleural Pneumonectomy

EPP is associated with distant sites of recurrence compared with sites of recurrence in patients having biopsy only or pleurectomy and decortication, and the local control for EPP is superior to that of the other modalities. Pass et al also found a higher proportion of first sites of local recurrence seen in the pleurectomy population compared with the patients having EPP. In Sugarbaker's series of patients, Baldini et al reported that the sites of first recurrence were local in 35% of patients, abdominal in 26%, the contralateral thorax in 17%, and other distant sites in 8%.

Survival

Long-term survival rates after EPP remain disappointing, with median survivals ranging from 9.3 to 17 months for most series. Rusch and Venkatraman reported a median survival of 10 months in their series, and the median survival of MPM patients having EPP (all types of histologies) in the National Cancer Institute series was 9.4 months. Most patients were pathologic stage II or III in these two series. More recently, Grondin and Sugarbaker reported a 17-month median survival for all patients in a series heavily weighted with stage I, epithelial patients (52 of 183), whose 2-year and 5-year survivals were 68% and 46%. In the series by Rusch, the 2-year and 5-year survivals of stage I patients (16 of 131) were 65% and 30%.

■ SURGERY AS PART OF A MULTIMODALITY APPROACH

Surgery is only one part of the aggressive treatment for mesothelioma. The adjuvant and intraoperative treatments have included intrapleural chemotherapy, photodynamic therapy, hyperthermic chemoperfusion, gene therapy, adjuvant radiation therapy, immunochemotherapy, and combination chemotherapy with or without radiation. More recently, there has been an interest in the feasibility of induction chemotherapy in selected patients with gemcitabine and cisplatin (Yang, personal communication). The multitude and variety of trials bespeak overall results that are not significantly different among the protocols. Novel agents based on molecular phenotyping of the tumor that target specific signal transduction pathways are needed.

SUGGESTED READING

Baldini EH, et al: Patterns of failure after trimodality therapy for malignant pleural mesothelioma, *Ann Thorac Surg* 63:334, 1997.

Grondin SC, Sugarbaker DJ: Pleuropneumonectomy in the treatment of malignant pleural mesothelioma, *Chest* 116:450S, 1999.

Pass HI, et al: Surgically debulked malignant pleural mesothelioma: results and prognostic factors, *Ann Surg Oncol* 4:215, 1997.

Pass HI, et al: Preoperative tumor volume is associated with outcome in malignant pleural mesothelioma, *J Thorac Cardiovasc Surg* 115:310, 1998.

Rusch VW, Venkatraman ES: Important prognostic factors in patients with malignant pleural mesothelioma, managed surgically, *Ann Thorac Surg* 68:1799, 1999.

PLEURECTOMY FOR DIFFUSE MESOTHELIOMA

Sean C. Grondin
Michael J. Liptay

Diffuse malignant pleural mesothelioma (MPM) is an aggressive malignancy arising from the serosal layer of the pleura that affects 2000 to 3000 Americans yearly. A male predominance of 3:1 is reported with most patients developing MPM being older than age 55. MPM is causally related to asbestos exposure and exhibits a long latency period between exposure and disease. Other agents, such as simian virus 40 (SV40), have been identified as potentially responsible for the development of MPM in patients with no history of asbestos exposure.

The initial presentation of MPM is variable given the wide range of symptoms associated with the disease and its rate of progression. Commonly, patients report dyspnea and chest pain; however, nonspecific complaints, such as night sweats or fever, weight loss, malaise, and cough, also may be described. In advanced stages, a chest or abdominal wall mass, ascites, cachexia, or evidence of small bowel obstruction may be observed. Although distant metastases are uncommon at the time of presentation, at least 50% of all patients with MPM have evidence of systemic disease at the time of autopsy.

If by patient history and clinical examination a diagnosis of MPM is suspected, a thorough radiologic evaluation using chest radiographs, computed tomography, and magnetic resonance imaging of the chest should be performed. Chest radiographs are useful in showing pleural thickening, pleural effusion, and parenchymal fibrosis. Scans of the chest improve the evaluation of tumor infiltration into the chest wall, diaphragm, lung fissures, and mediastinal structures and the presence of mediastinal adenopathy. Positron emission tomography has been shown to be effective in determining resectability of MPM.

Many procedures are available to secure a pathologic diagnosis of MPM. Although thoracocentesis and closed pleural biopsy are valuable in the initial evaluation of patients presenting with a pleural effusion or pleural thickening, the role of minimally invasive techniques, such as pleuroscopy and video-assisted thoracic surgery (VATS), should be emphasized. These techniques allow for better visualization of the tumor, which improves the adequacy of tissue sampling. Placement of biopsy incisions during minimally invasive procedures must be strategic to allow for resection of these sites should the patient be deemed a candidate for resection. In cases in which computed tomography is equivocal, transdiaphragmatic involvement can be assessed by laparoscopy.

Despite improvements in tissue biopsy techniques and refinements in histologic stains, electron microscopy, and immunohistochemistry, confirming the diagnosis of MPM may be difficult and require the assistance of an expert pathologist. Specifically, distinguishing among various subtypes of mesothelioma and other types of neoplasms, such as adenocarcinoma or benign mesothelial hyperplasia, often presents a challenge. Microscopically, MPM is classified into three pathologic subtypes—epithelial, sarcomatoid, and mixed. Epithelial histology is reported in 50% of cases, with sarcomatoid histology associated with a poorer prognosis. Currently, there is no widely accepted staging system of MPM. Although the Butchart staging system has been used historically to stage MPM, the International Mesothelioma Interest Group and Brigham staging systems have been used more recently.

Life expectancy for untreated patients with MPM is usually less than 1 year from the time of diagnosis. Despite advances in standard treatment modalities, such as surgery, chemotherapy, and radiotherapy, MPM remains difficult to treat. To date, nonrandomized data from selected patients suggest improved long-term survival with multimodality therapy using extrapleural pneumonectomy (EPP) with chemotherapy and radiotherapy. Innovative therapeutic modalities, such as gene therapy and intraoperative heated chemotherapy, currently are being investigated as means to improve long-term survival for patients with MPM.

SURGERY

When the diagnosis of MPM has been confirmed, a thorough evaluation is required to determine if surgery is appropriate. Resectability is determined by the clinical, radiologic, and pathologic stage of disease. Operability of the patient is determined by the individual's ability to withstand surgery. Potential surgical candidates should undergo a pulmonary and a cardiac evaluation using pulmonary function studies and cardiac stress tests. Echocardiography also may be helpful in determining the patient's baseline cardiac function and in ruling out transpericardial spread or effusion. If lung resection is being contemplated, a ventilation-perfusion scan may be necessary to assess postoperative predicted lung function.

Surgical options for patients with MPM include VATS with talc poudrage, parietal pleurectomy, pleurectomy/decortication, and EPP. VATS with talc pleurodesis is effective for inoperable patients who have free-flowing symptomatic effusions. Parietal pleurectomy involves removal of the parietal pleura to obtain a durable pleurodesis and is appropriate for symptomatic patients whose medical conditions preclude a more aggressive resection and who have multiloculated effusions or recurrent effusions after VATS. Pleurectomy/decortication and EPP are performed with a curative intent in patients with acceptable cardiopulmonary function and medical comorbidities who show no evidence of mediastinal, chest wall, or abdominal involvement. The role of pleurectomy/decortication versus EPP in the surgical treatment of MPM is controversial. Aspects of this controversy relate to the adequacy of tumor resection, the morbidity and mortality associated with each procedure, and the impact of each approach on the feasibility of adjuvant therapy. Both procedures are technically demanding and should be performed in centers experienced in the treatment of MPM.

Pleurectomy/decortication involves the removal of all gross parietal and visceral pleural disease without resection of the underlying lung. EPP involves en bloc removal of the pleura, lung, ipsilateral diaphragm, and pericardium. In patients with advanced disease, EPP may permit a more complete resection of gross tumor when confluent bulky tumor encases the lung and infiltrates the fissures.

Given the extent of resection with EPP, careful preoperative selection criteria must be met for patients to be eligible. These criteria include an ejection fraction greater than 45%, predicted postoperative forced expiratory volume in 1 second greater than 1 liter, P_{CO_2} less than 45 torr, and room air P_{O_2} greater than 65 torr. Historically, EPP has been associated with a high mortality (30%). More recent reports from experienced centers suggest, however, that with better patient selection and improvements in operative techniques and perioperative management, mortality (4% to 6%) can be reduced substantially. In contrast to EPP, pleurectomy/decortication has been associated consistently with low mortality (<5%).

With respect to adjuvant therapy, EPP and pleurectomy/decortication have advantages and disadvantages. EPP allows higher doses of postoperative radiotherapy to be given without the concern of developing radiation-induced pneumonitis. In contrast, pleurectomy/decortication may allow cisplatin-based adjuvant chemotherapy regimens to be better tolerated.

TECHNIQUE OF PLEURECTOMY/DECORTICATION

Patients deemed suitable for surgery should be assessed preoperatively by an experienced thoracic anesthetist. At the time of operation, a left-sided double-lumen tube and appropriate venous access and arterial line monitoring are necessary. An epidural catheter, Foley catheter, pneumatic stockings, and prophylactic antibiotics also are used routinely. Placement of a nasogastric tube assists in identifying the esophagus intraoperatively.

The patient is positioned in the lateral decubitus position, and a posterolateral thoracotomy incision is made. The incision is extended anteriorly to the costal margin. The sixth rib is removed to allow access to the extrapleural plane. Occasionally a counterincision is necessary in the 10th intercostal space to provide access to the diaphragm.

When the extrapleural plane between the endothoracic fascia and parietal pleura is visualized, a combination of blunt and sharp dissection is used to develop a plane toward the apex of the chest superiorly and the diaphragm inferiorly. Dissection is continued anteriorly to the pericardium. In an effort to prevent injury to the posterior mediastinal structures, the posterior dissection toward the spine is reserved until adequate exposure has been obtained anteriorly. Hemostasis is achieved using electrocautery and packing of each section of the chest.

On the right side, the dissection proceeds to the brachial triangle with exposure of the subclavian and internal mammary vessels. The parietal pleura subsequently is mobilized off of the superior vena cava and azygos vein posterosuperiorly. The right main stem bronchus is identified, and the subcarinal node packet is removed. Placement of the nasogastric tube to identify the esophagus facilitates the inferior-posterior dissection. If the mediastinal pleura cannot be removed easily from the pericardium, pericardium and anterior pleura may be resected en bloc later in the procedure.

Next the plane between the palpable tumor and the diaphragm is identified in the posterior costophrenic angle, allowing the tumor to be mobilized anteromedially using blunt dissection. In advanced disease, a full-thickness resection of the diaphragm may be necessary. Every attempt should be made to leave the peritoneum intact in an effort to prevent abdominal seeding.

When the diaphragmatic portion of the tumor is completely mobilized, the pleura is dissected off of the pericardium. If the tumor is adherent to the pericardium, the pericardium is resected. If necessary, reconstruction of the diaphragm and pericardium is performed with Gore-Tex (W. L. Gore, Phoenix, AZ) at the end of the decortication. The pericardial patch should be fenestrated to allow free drainage of pericardial fluid into the pleural space and to prevent cardiac tamponade.

When the parietal pleural dissection is complete, the decortication portion of the procedure is begun. The degree to which the tumor can be resected away from the visceral pleura is variable. After opening the parietal pleural envelope, a combination of electrocautery and blunt dissection is employed. Removal of tumor from the fissures may be difficult. As the decortication is completed, air leaks from the raw surface of the lung frequently are observed. These leaks normally settle within the first 2 to 3 days postoperatively if good expansion of the lung is obtained. Typically, estimated blood loss is 1500 to 3000 ml.

The postoperative management of the pleurectomy/decortication patient begins with ensuring adequate analgesia in a monitored thoracic step-down unit. Arterial line and oximetry is routine along with close monitoring of fluid intake and output. Thoracic epidurals (maintained for 3 to 5 days), chest physiotherapy, and early mobilization are important means by which to decrease the risk of atelectasis and pneumonia.

■ CLINICAL RESULTS AND MULTIMODALITY THERAPY

The value of pleurectomy/decortication versus EPP remains controversial. In experienced hands, pleurectomy/decortication can be performed safely with effective palliation of symptoms. Surgery-related morbidity and mortality for pleurectomy/decortication is 6% to 29% and 1% to 10%. Limited data suggest that selected patients with early disease and favorable histology may have longer survival after EPP.

Given the high rate of local recurrence observed in patients who have had surgery for MPM, investigators have attempted to optimize local control using a variety of modalities. The results using adjuvant radiotherapy or chemotherapy have been disappointing. These poor outcomes likely reflect the relative resistance of MPM to radiation and currently available chemotherapeutic agents. Similarly, intrapleural therapies using chemotherapy or photodynamic therapy have not shown a significant benefit. Studies are under way to evaluate the role of new therapeutic interventions such as gene therapy in the treatment of MPM.

SUGGESTED READING

Allen KB, et al: Malignant pleural mesothelioma: extrapleural pneumonectomy and pleurectomy, *Chest Surg Clin N Am* 4:113, 1994.

Grondin SG, Sugarbaker DJ: Malignant mesothelioma of the pleural space, *Oncology* 13:919, 1999.

Ho L, et al: Malignant pleural mesothelioma, *Cancer Treat Res* 105:27, 2001.

Roberts J: Surgical treatment of mesothelioma: pleurectomy, *Chest* 116:446S, 1999.

Rusch VW: Pleurectomy/decortication in the setting of multimodality treatment for diffuse malignant pleural mesothelioma, *Semin Thorac Cardiovasc Surg* 9:367, 1997.

EXTRAPLEURAL PNEUMONECTOMY FOR DIFFUSE MALIGNANT PLEURAL MESOTHELIOMA

Lambros S. Zellos

David J. Sugarbaker

Diffuse malignant pleural mesothelioma (DMPM) remains a rare malignancy despite an increased incidence over the years. Currently, 2000 to 3000 cases are estimated to occur annually. Although the main etiology is still asbestos exposure, other factors, such as exposure to simian virus 40, are being explored. Most physicians are unfamiliar with this disease and the challenge it presents in diagnosis, staging, and treatment. The natural history, median survival of 4 to 12 months, lack of randomized studies, and modest impact of aggressive protocols on overall survival have resulted in ongoing controversy regarding the optimal treatment strategy.

■ APPROACH TO TREATMENT

Extrapleural pneumonectomy (EPP) and pleurectomy/decortication (P/D) have been implemented for cytoreduction in patients with DMPM. Proponents of EPP suggest that it achieves superior cytoreduction than P/D because it removes the lung and the tumor that has infiltrated the lung fissures. Additionally, because the lung is removed, radiation can be targeted optimally at areas with positive margins or lymph nodes, and higher total doses can be delivered than with the lung present. Proponents of P/D point to the historically higher mortality rates with EPP for DMPM and to the lack of survival prolongation with EPP over P/D when EPP has been used as a single modality. In modern series of DMPM patients treated with EPP and adjuvant chemoradiation, EPP was conducted with markedly decreased mortality and improved survival in the subset of patients with early stage disease compared with historical studies of P/D with adjuvant therapy.

Staging Systems

The purpose of a staging system is to determine extent of disease, stratify survival, and direct therapy. Numerous staging systems have been proposed, but none are universally accepted. The most commonly used are the Butchart staging system and the TNM system of the International Mesothelioma Interest Group (Table 1). These staging systems fail to stratify patient survival by stage, however. Based on a series of 183 DMPM patients who were treated with EPP and adjuvant chemoradiation, the revised Brigham/Dana-Farber Cancer Institute (DFCI) Staging System was proposed by Sugarbaker et al in 1998. This system is based on resectability,

nodal status (intrapleural versus extrapleural, i.e., N2 nodes), and extent of disease into the diaphragm and pericardium (Table 2). Although the other systems fail to stratify survival by stage, in this report, the overall median patient survival with triple-modality therapy was 25, 20, and 16 months for Brigham/DFCI system's stage I, II, and III disease. For patients with epithelial histology and Brigham/ DFCI stage I disease, median survival was 51 months.

■ APPROACH TO EVALUATION

Diagnostic Workup

The typical patient is a man (3:1 male-to-female ratio) older than age 50 who presents with symptoms of dyspnea, cough,

---

Table 1 International Mesothelioma Interest Group Staging System for Diffuse Malignant Pleural Mesothelioma

T—TUMOR	T1a	Tumor limited to the ipsilateral parietal pleura, including mediastinal and diaphragmatic pleura No involvement of the visceral pleura
	T1b	Tumor involving the ipsilateral parietal pleura, including mediastinal and diaphragmatic pleura Scattered foci of tumor also involving the visceral pleura
	T2	Tumor involving each of the ipsilateral pleural surfaces (parietal, mediastinal, diaphragmatic, and visceral pleura) with at least one of the following features: Involvement of diaphragmatic muscle Confluent visceral pleural tumor (including the fissures) or extension of tumor from visceral pleura into the underlying pulmonary parenchyma
	T3	Tumor involving all of the ipsilateral pleural surfaces (parietal, mediastinal, diaphragmatic, and visceral pleura) with at least one of the following features: Involvement of the endothoracic fascia Extension into the mediastinal fat Solitary, completely resectable focus of tumor extending into the soft tissues of the chest wall
	T4	Tumor involving all of the ipsilateral pleural surfaces (parietal, mediastinal, diaphragmatic, and visceral) with at least one of the following features: Diffuse extension or multifocal masses of tumor in the chest wall, with or without associated rib destruction Direct transdiaphragmatic extension of tumor to the peritoneum Direct extension of tumor to the contralateral pleura Direct extension of tumor to one or more mediastinal organs Direct extension of tumor into the spine Tumor extending through to the internal surface of the pericardium, with or without a pericardial effusion, or tumor involving the myocardium
N—LYMPH NODES	NX	Regional lymph nodes cannot be assessed
	N0	No regional lymph node metastases
	N1	Metastases in the ipsilateral bronchopulmonary or hilar lymph nodes
	N2	Metastases in the subcarinal or ipsilateral mediastinal lymph nodes, including the ipsilateral internal mammary nodes
	N3	Metastases in the contralateral mediastinal, contralateral internal mammary, ipsilateral, or contralateral supraclavicular lymph nodes
M—METASTASES	MX	Presence of distant metastases cannot be assessed
	M0	No distant metastasis
	M1	Distant metastasis present
	STAGE	**DESCRIPTION**
	Ia	T1aN0M0
	Ib	T1bN0M0
	II	T2N0M0
	III	Any T3M0 Any N1M0 Any N2M0
	IV	Any T4 Any N3 Any M1

From Rusch VW: Chest 108:1122, 1995.

Table 2 Revised* Staging System for Malignant Pleural Mesothelioma†

I	Disease completely resected within the capsule of the parietal pleura without adenopathy: ipsilateral pleura, lung, pericardium, diaphragm, or chest wall disease limited to previous biopsy sites
II	All of stage I with positive resection margins and/or intrapleural adenopathy
III	Local extension of disease into chest wall or mediastinum; heart, or through diaphragm, peritoneum; or with extrapleural lymph node involvement
IV	Distant metastatic disease

*From Sugarbaker DJ, et al: J Thorac Cardiovasc Surg 117:54, 1999.
†Butchart stage II and III patients are combined into stage III. Stage I represents resectable patients with negative nodes. Stage II patients are resectable but have positive nodal status.

and chest pain due to the presence of a pleural effusion that is unilateral in 95% of patients. DMPM develops at a median 32 years after asbestos exposure.

Evaluation begins with a thorough history and physical examination. It is important to assess the patient's functional status to determine whether surgery is appropriate and which cytoreductive procedure should be used. A standardized method, such as the Karnofsky performance scale, is useful. Because these patients have multiple thoracenteses for diagnosis and drainage of the effusion, it common to develop multiple chest wall masses at the incision sites within a short time. Evidence is sought for extrathoracic disease, such as abdominal masses, ascites, or bowel obstruction. Although thrombocytosis has been shown in some studies to be a negative prognostic factor, laboratory tests are not especially useful except as part of the usual workup of patients who will undergo a surgical procedure.

Extent of the disease is assessed best with a chest computed tomography scan and magnetic resonance imaging (MRI). Resectability is determined based on the absence of distant disease; absence of extension into mediastinal structures such as heart, esophagus, or major vessels; absence of extensive chest wall involvement; and lack of intraperitoneal extension. Fluorodeoxyglucose positron emission tomography is becoming increasingly useful to detect distant occult disease and has been found to be sensitive. Two-dimensional echocardiography has the dual role of assessing cardiac function and determining resectability by assessing pericardial involvement.

Diagnosis still may be in doubt at initial presentation. The inexperience of the pathologist and the difficulty in differentiating DMPM from sarcoma and adenocarcinoma along with insufficient tissue sample supplied with thoracentesis contribute to the diagnostic difficulties. The surgeon

may need to perform a video-assisted thoracic surgery (VATS) procedure for palliation and to obtain sufficient tissue for immunohistochemical and electron microscopy studies. VATS can disrupt loculations and provide excellent palliation and more than adequate samples for the various studies. Because seeding of the VATS incision with tumor cells and eventual development of chest wall masses is inevitable, strategic placement of the VATS incisions along a future thoracotomy incision is crucial.

When the diagnosis has been established and the workup completed, patients who meet the selection criteria (Table 3) are offered EPP. For patients who have questionable resectability because of borderline functional status based on Karnofsky's scale or predicted postoperative forced expiratory volume in 1 second and because MRI findings suggest the resection margins could be positive, mediastinoscopy can assist further by assessing N2 nodes. Positive N2 nodes are a negative prognostic factor, and although they do not preclude EPP, in the presence of additional clinical or radiologic findings they may delineate better whether an aggressive resection should be carried out.

■ TECHNIQUE

The operation is conducted with a dedicated thoracic anesthesia team that is experienced in the intraoperative management of pneumonectomy patients. Standard management includes a double-lumen endotracheal tube, thoracic epidural, nasogastric tube to decompress the stomach and aid in palpation of the esophagus during dissection, arterial and central venous lines, and continuous oximetry.

In cases in which transdiaphragmatic involvement cannot be ruled out with preoperative MRI, laparoscopy before

Table 3 Patient Selection Criteria

Karnofsky performance	>70
Renal function	Creatinine <2 mg/dl
Liver function	AST <80 IU/liter, total bilirubin <1.9 mg/dl, PT <15
Pulmonary function	Postoperative FEV_1 >0.8 liter as per PFTs and quantitative ventilation-perfusion scans
Cardiac function	Grossly normal cardiac function as per ECG and echocardiogram (EF preferably >45%)
Extent of disease	Limited to ipsilateral hemithorax with no transdiaphragmatic, transpericardial, or extensive chest wall involvement

AST, aspartate aminotransferase; FEV_1, forced expiratory volume in 1 second; PFTs, pulmonary function tests; ECG, electrocardiogram; EF, ejection fraction; PT, prothrombin time.

thoracotomy can resolve this issue. Unless laparoscopy is required, the patient is placed on the operating table in standard thoracotomy position.

Right Extrapleural Pneumonectomy

The entire right EPP procedure is carried out through a single incision along the bed of the sixth rib that extends from the costovertebral junction to 2 cm lateral to the costochondral junction. Excision of the sixth rib after periosteal stripping provides improved exposure. After the rib is excised, incision of the posterior periosteum is carried out, and anterior extrapleural dissection is performed using blunt and sharp techniques, advancing toward the apex of the thorax and toward the diaphragm. When the anterior dissection is completed and exposure is adequate, the posterior dissection is conducted using similar methods. At the apex, care should be taken not to avulse the subclavian vessels because the parietal pleura tends to thin out in this region. Anteriorly, attention should be paid to the internal mammary vessels that could be avulsed easily. During posterosuperior dissection, attention should be paid to the azygos vein as well.

The extrapleural dissection is continued until the superior vena cava, azygos vein, right upper lobe, and right main stem bronchus are exposed. At this point, the surgeon has to determine resectability by assessing pericardial involvement by opening the pericardium and palpating the pericardial space. Posteriorly, esophageal or aortic involvement is assessed by palpation. Palpation of the nasogastric tube aids in avoiding esophageal injury.

When unresectability has been ruled out, diaphragmatic resection is carried out. Resection begins with dissection of the pleural envelope off the diaphragm so that continuity of the pleural envelope is maintained. The diaphragm is incised first at its lateral margin, then circumferentially toward the anterior border of the pericardium. Using blunt technique, the diaphragm is dissected off the peritoneum. Dissection along the esophageal and caval hiatus is carried out with caution. The pericardium is incised fully to provide exposure to the inferior vena cava (Figure 1), and palpation of the nasogastric tube helps in avoiding injury.

Completion of the pericardial incision is followed by division of the pulmonary artery and veins. To guide safe placement of the stapler around the vessel that is to be divided, a soft catheter is placed on one end of the endostapler. The pulmonary artery is divided in this fashion intrapericardially. When the vessels are divided, the posterior resection of the pericardium is completed. The right main bronchus is divided as close to the carina as possible. A mediastinal node dissection is performed routinely for staging purposes. Additionally, multiple sections are taken from the pericardium, chest wall, diaphragm, and bronchus and sent to the pathologist for margins.

The pericardial and diaphragmatic defects are reconstructed with a Gore-Tex patch (W.L. Gore, Flagstaff, AZ) (Figure 2). The pericardium is reconstructed on the right side to avoid cardiac herniation and death. The patch should be fenestrated to allow blood to evacuate and avoid tamponade. Tension should be avoided because the patch may rupture, and tamponade physiology may develop if the patch is too tight. The pericardium is reconstructed with a 1-mm patch, whereas the diaphragm is reconstructed with a 2-mm patch.

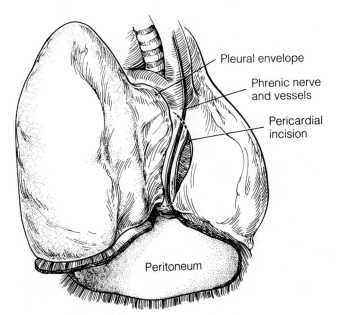

Figure 1
The pericardium is opened anteriorly medial to the phrenic nerve and hilar vessels. *(From Sugarbaker DJ, et al:* Ann Thorac Surg *54:941, 1992.)*

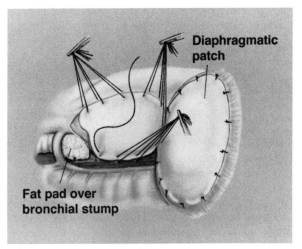

Figure 2
The pericardium and diaphragm are reconstructed and a fat pad placed over the bronchial stump. *(From Garcia JP, et al: In Kaiser LR, et al, editors:* Mastery of cardiothoracic surgery. *Philadelphia, 1997, Lippincott-Raven, p 230.)*

Running polypropylene suture is used for both reconstructions. The diaphragmatic patch is sutured to the posterior diaphragmatic remnants, the anterior chest wall, and the medial hiatal musculature. Areas with gross disease are marked with clips for postoperative radiation.

A 12-Fr, red rubber catheter is introduced in the pleural space through the wound and is used postoperatively to add or remove air from the residual pleural space to avoid excessive mediastinal shift after pneumonectomy. When the procedure is completed and before the patient is extubated,

750 ml of air is removed in women and 1000 ml in men. Additional air can be removed or added if the postoperative chest x-ray shows mediastinal deviation. If a hemothorax is present, a chest tube is placed to monitor drainage and is left on water seal. An argon beam coagulator is useful in achieving hemostasis and avoiding hemothorax.

Left Extrapleural Pneumonectomy

The technique of left EPP is similar to right EPP, but there are a few differences. Although the dissection is generally easier, attention needs to be paid during dissection in the preaortic plane. Avulsion of intercostal vessels or aortic injury can occur. The esophagus can be injured during dissection at the base of the diaphragm.

Because the left main pulmonary artery is quite short, extrapericardial extrapleural division is done to avoid encroachment on the right pulmonary artery. The pulmonary veins can be ligated intrapericardially and the left main bronchus should be divided as close as possible to the trachea.

Pericardial reconstruction is performed routinely during either left or right EPP. If a small pericardial defect is present, a reconstruction should be carried out to reduce the risk of left ventricular herniation and strangulation.

■ POSTOPERATIVE MANAGEMENT

Postoperative management of EPP patients focuses on prevention of pulmonary complications by implementing adequate pain control with thoracic epidural, aggressive chest physiotherapy, fluid restriction, and avoidance of risk factors for aspiration. Thoracic epidural catheters are used for 3 to 5 days depending on the individual patient's needs. Fluid restriction of 1 liter/day similarly is implemented for 3 to 5 days. Diuretics are used as needed. Subcutaneous heparin and pneumatic stockings are used for deep vein thrombosis prophylaxis. Daily chest x-rays are obtained to assess mediastinal shift and as needed for desaturation episodes. Low threshold for bronchoscopy should exist because mucous plugs are not well tolerated. Vocal cord paralysis can occur, and a low threshold for endoscopy is needed. Cord medialization should be carried out to reduce the risks of complications, such as aspiration. The return of gastric function should be evident before advancing the patient's diet. Contralateral infiltrates are treated with intravenous antibiotics because pneumonia is not tolerated in patients with one lung.

Excessive mediastinal shift can be treated with aspiration of air. Rarely a small catheter may need to be placed in the residual pleural space for repeated aspirations. If cardiac arrest occurs, standard cardiopulmonary resuscitation techniques in postpneumonectomy patients are inadequate; when the airway is secured, the chest should be opened and open cardiac massage instituted. Also, cardiac arrest due to tamponade from pericardial clot, too tight a patch, or cardiac torsion from a dehisced patch can be treated effectively.

Complications that may not be evident in the immediate postoperative period include empyema, bronchopleural fistula, and post-EPP constrictive physiology. The treatment of empyema and bronchopleural fistula is similar. The presence of infection necessitates the removal of the prosthetic material.

Post-EPP constrictive physiology has been seen after left-sided EPP, during the first postoperative year. Patients develop symptoms and physiology similar to constrictive pericarditis and pericardial effusion. Although resolution of the effusion and constrictive physiology can occur, cardiac decortication may be needed. Approximately half of patients who require reoperation have tumor recurrence. If complaints of dyspnea, chest pain, and fatigue are reported when such symptoms had not been reported previously, an echocardiogram should be obtained.

■ RESULTS

Although mortality of 30% has been reported for EPP for mesothelioma, there has been a significant decrease in the operative mortality reported in modern series. The largest series from the Brigham and Women's Hospital reported an operative mortality of 3.8%. In that series 183 patients underwent EPP from 1980 to1997. Median hospital stay was 9 days with a 50.5% minor and major morbidity rate. Atrial fibrillation accounted for most of the morbidity (37% of patients developed atrial fibrillation). Prolonged intubation was seen in 7.1% of patients, and 5.5% had vocal cord paralysis. Technical complications, such as bleeding and patch failure, occurred in 6.6% of patients. Median survival was 17 months. These patients also underwent adjuvant chemoradiotherapy (platinum-based chemotherapy with radiation to the ipsilateral hemithorax up to 54 Gy depending on margins and node status). The subset of patients with negative nodes and margins (stage I of Revised Brigham/DFCI Staging System) and epithelial histology had a median survival of 51 months.

The patterns of failure after EPP and adjuvant chemoradiotherapy are primarily locoregional. Ipsilateral chest is the most common site followed by peritoneal, contralateral chest recurrence, and distant metastases. Although overall median survival may not differ significantly from patients treated with P/D and adjuvant therapy, the subset of patients with early stage disease, epithelial histology, and adequate functional status to tolerate aggressive cytoreduction benefits the most from EPP and adjuvant chemoradiotherapy.

SUGGESTED READING

Baldini EH, et al: Patterns of failure after trimodality therapy for malignant pleural mesothelioma, *Ann Thorac Surg* 63:334, 1997.

Herndon JE, et al: Factors predictive of survival among 337 patients with mesothelioma treated between 1984 and 1994 by the Cancer and Leukemia Group B, *Chest* 113:723, 1998.

Rusch VW: The International Mesothelioma Interest Group: a proposed new international TNM staging system for malignant pleural mesothelioma, *Chest* 108:1122, 1995.

Schneider DB, et al: Positron emission tomography with f18-fluorodeoxyglucose in the staging and preoperative evaluation of malignant pleural mesothelioma, *J Thorac Cardiovasc Surg* 120:128, 2000.

Sugarbaker DJ, et al: Resection margins, extrapleural nodal status, and cell type determine postoperative long-term survival in trimodality therapy of malignant pleural mesothelioma: results in 183 patients, *J Thorac Cardiovasc Surg* 117:54, 1999.

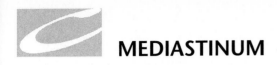

MEDIASTINUM

MYASTHENIA GRAVIS AND THYMOMA

Duc Thinh Pham
Frank C. Detterbeck

■ MYASTHENIA GRAVIS

Clinical Features and Medical Management

Myasthenia gravis is an autoimmune disease, characterized by exertional voluntary muscle weakness, caused by antibodies to the acetylcholine receptor complex of the motor end plate. The age of onset can vary from the teens to the 60s, with a bimodal distribution peaking during the teens in women and the 50s in men. Overall the disease is more common in women by nearly a 2:1 ratio.

The onset of symptoms can be slow and insidious, or it can be fairly precipitous. The modified Osserman scale is the most widely used system for classification of symptoms and severity of disease (Table 1). Although most patients experience generalized muscular weakness, 15% have symptoms confined to extraocular muscles (class I). The clinical course of the disease in individual patients varies. Approximately one third of patients have spontaneous remissions, one third have a stable course, and one third have acute exacerbations of symptoms that can lead to life-threatening respiratory failure.

Medical treatment for myasthenia gravis involves the use of anticholinesterase agents; immunosuppressive medications, such as steroids, azathioprine, and cyclosporine; and plasmapheresis, each alone or in combination. Overall, clinical improvement ranges from 80% to 95% with medical treatment alone. The drug-free remission rates are low with medical management alone, however, and most patients require long-term medication.

Role of Thymectomy

In 1910, Sauerbruch first noted clinical improvement in myasthenia gravis after thymectomy. The frequency of drug-free remissions after thymectomy has allowed this modality of treatment to become widely accepted. Overall, 80% to 90% of patients have improvement by at least one Osserman classification, and 50% to 70% of patients have a drug-free remission after thymectomy. The exact relationship between the thymus and myasthenia gravis has not been clearly elucidated, however, and no randomized study has been conducted comparing thymectomy with medical management in myasthenia gravis.

At our institution, thymectomy is recommended for patients with class II or greater disease, for patients with class I disease that is refractory to medical therapy, and for patients with a thymoma. This is consistent with the indications for thymectomy used by most other institutions, although some institutions recommend thymectomy for patients with class I disease who require medications continuously.

Preoperative Assessment and Anesthetic Management

Before surgical treatment of myasthenia gravis, a careful evaluation of concomitant disease should be undertaken. A thymoma is present in 10% to 20% of patients with myasthenia gravis. A computed tomography scan of the chest is usually obtained as part of the initial evaluation of patients with myasthenia gravis. In our experience, a normal chest radiograph is sufficient for preoperative planning, however, because a thymoma that is too small to be visible on a chest x-ray does not alter the operative approach. Approximately 10% of patients with myasthenia gravis have other associated autoimmune or endocrine disorders. Evidence of these conditions specifically should be sought and the conditions treated appropriately before thymectomy to avoid postoperative complications. Hypothyroidism can be missed easily because the symptoms can be similar to myasthenia gravis. Systemic lupus has been described in association with myasthenia gravis and can have significant cardiac, pulmonary, renal, musculoskeletal, and nervous system effects. Arrhythmias and conduction defects have been described in patients with myasthenia gravis, possibly due to associated myositis.

It is important that the patient's medical treatment of myasthenia gravis has been optimized before thymectomy to avoid postoperative respiratory compromise. Pulmonary function tests, especially forced vital capacity and negative inspiratory force, can be valuable in the evaluation of the patient's response to medical treatment. At our institution,

Table 1 Modified Osserman Classification for Myasthenia Gravis	
CLASS	**DISTRIBUTION OF SYMPTOMS**
I	Ocular
II	Mild generalized weakness, usually with ocular muscle weakness
III	Predominantly bulbar involvement, usually with mild generalized weakness
IV	Moderate generalized weakness
V	Severe generalized weakness

plasmapheresis is used preoperatively in most patients with generalized symptoms. Plasmapheresis is preferred to high doses of steroids or other immunosuppressive drugs. Patients receiving steroids are given stress dose coverage the evening before and the day of surgery, then are weaned off as quickly as possible postoperatively.

Intraoperatively, neuromuscular blocking agents should be avoided. Inhaled anesthetic agents, such as isoflurane or halothane, usually provide sufficient muscle relaxation. If muscle blockage is required, several issues need to be considered. Patients with active myasthenia gravis can be resistant to succinylcholine or have a delayed and shortened response to the drug. Nondepolarizing agents should be used in one fifth to one tenth the usual dose, and a short-acting drug is recommended. Volatile inhalational agents and short-acting narcotics are the anesthetic agents of choice. Using the preoperative preparation and anesthetic management just outlined, 67% of patients were extubated in the operating room, 84% within 1 hour, and 96% within 10 hours in our experience since 1977. We do not routinely observe patients in an intensive care unit (ICU) unless respiratory compromise is present on discharge from the postanesthetic recovery room.

Surgical Technique

Various surgical approaches and techniques for thymectomy have been advocated, including a transsternal, a transcervical, and, more recently, a video-assisted thoracic surgery (VATS) approach. The extent of thymectomy performed also varies from removal of only the thymus gland proper, to an extensive thymectomy involving the thymus and much of the anterior mediastinal fatty tissues, to a radical ("maximal") thymectomy that involves skeletonization of the mediastinal vessels and essential structures. The radical approach is founded on anatomic studies that have shown small clumps of thymic cells to be dispersed widely throughout the anterior mediastinal fat.

At the University of North Carolina, we advocate the transsternal approach with removal of the thymus and perithymic fatty tissue. This approach is straightforward, provides excellent exposure, and causes no more patient discomfort than bilateral VATS. It is easily taught and has reproducible results. It does not require a change in approach if a thymoma is discovered. It has low morbidity with equally good short-term and long-term results compared with less extensive or more extensive resections.

After a median sternotomy, the pericardial fat pad is divided at the level of the diaphragm, and the fatty tissue around the lower pole of the thymus is dissected bluntly from the pericardium and the pleura. This dissection continues laterally to 1 cm from each phrenic nerve and cephalad to the top of the manubrium. Opening the pleura assists in visualization of the phrenic nerve. Care is taken to leave no fat on the pericardium or the innominate vein except around the phrenic nerves. The superior poles of the thymus are identified easily and are resected completely en bloc with the rest of the thymus, taking care not to violate the capsule of the thymus, but without excision of additional fatty tissue from the lower cervical area. The tissue posterior to the innominate vein (between the carotid arteries and trachea) is not removed. Unless parenchymal lung injury has occurred, a chest tube is not routinely left in place. A positive-pressure breath during closure of the fascia is sufficient to remove air from the chest.

Occasionally a small thymoma may be discovered on palpation of the thymus that was not noted on preoperative evaluation. If the thymoma is small and free of adjacent tissue, the operative approach is not altered. If there is any suspicion that adjacent structures might be invaded, however, these are resected en bloc with the thymus.

The transcervical thymectomy involves a small collar incision. After mobilization of the upper poles of the gland, the sternum is retracted anteriorly, and the lower poles are dissected using a combination of direct vision and blunt dissection. Although the morbidity of the incision is less than that of a sternotomy, it is technically more difficult and risks leaving small rests of thymic tissue behind in unresected anterior mediastinal fat; this approach is used in only a few centers. The maximal thymectomy, done through a median sternotomy, extends from the thyroid gland to the diaphragm and from phrenic nerve to phrenic nerve, skeletonizing all structures in between by removing all mediastinal fat.

Postoperative Management

Postoperative care is generally uneventful. In our experience, most patients can be extubated immediately as stated previously, and all patients can be extubated within 24 hours. In the past, patients routinely were monitored in the ICU for 1 day. Because of the low rate of patients with respiratory compromise, however, most patients now are sent to a regular floor, albeit one that has experience with patients who have myasthenia gravis. The negative inspiratory force and forced vital capacity are measured in the recovery room and routinely every 8 hours for the first few postoperative days. Occasionally, adjustments in the pharmacologic treatment of myasthenia gravis must be made. With early intervention and careful monitoring of these pulmonary parameters, potential problems can be avoided without transferring the patient to an ICU. Potassium and magnesium levels are measured daily and kept within normal range.

Patients who are on steroids are given stress-dose hydrocortisone preoperatively and postoperatively, then weaned off steroids rapidly. Immunosuppressive medicines are maintained initially, then discontinued after discharge. Anticholinesterase drugs are withheld postoperatively unless symptoms indicate. Narcotics (primarily morphine and oxycodone) are used liberally for pain. Most patients are discharged on postoperative day 3 or 4.

Results

We reported the results of 100 consecutive thymectomies for myasthenia gravis performed at the University of North Carolina Hospitals between 1977 and 1993. No perioperative mortality occurred. The mean hospital stay for this group of patients was 6.3 days (range, 3 to 18 days), and the mean ICU stay was 1.2 days (range, 1 to 4 days). Since 1993, patients no longer routinely stay in the ICU, and most patients are discharged on postoperative day 3 or 4. Most patients were extubated in the operating room, and all patients were extubated within 24 hours. No patients had respiratory difficulty requiring reintubation, and there was no incidence of phrenic nerve injury. Overall, minor complications occurred in 17% of patients, and 4% experienced major complications, which included a wound infection requiring a pectoralis major flap, pericardial effusion requiring readmission, reoperation for a retained chest tube, and cardiac arrest on induction of anesthesia that resolved without further sequelae. Minor complications consisted mostly of pleural effusions, superficial wound infections, and pneumothoraces.

Symptoms at most recent follow-up were improved by at least one level on the modified Osserman scale in 78% of all patients compared with the preoperative maximal disease severity (Figure 1), when medical management of myasthenia had been optimized with intensive therapy. There was no correlation between the rate of improvement and the initial disease severity, age of the patient, or pathology of the thymus. Long-term drug-free remission was more common, however, in patients with class I, II, and III disease versus class IV and V disease (69% versus 29%, $p = .001$). The clinical improvements after thymectomy are not immediate; symptoms continue to decrease over the course of 5 to 10 years. Drug-free remission is achieved in approximately 50% of patients, with decreases in prednisone and pyridostigmine (Mestinon) dosages by 60%. These results are comparable to results reported in the literature for transcervical, maximal, and VATS approaches to thymectomy.

■ THYMOMA

Clinical Features
Thymomas and lymphomas constitute most tumors in the anterior mediastinum. Usually it is easy to distinguish these tumors on the basis of computed tomography appearance and clinical presentation. About 50% of patients with a thymoma have myasthenia gravis, and many patients with lymphoma have fevers, night sweats, weight loss, and evidence of a more rapidly progressive tumor. If there is any doubt about the diagnosis, a biopsy (either open or by needle) should be performed. Common dogma claims that violation of the capsule is undesirable, but there is no evidence that this affects the prognosis. Thymomas are seen in patients ranging from age 10 to older than age 80 but are most common between the ages of 30 and 50. There is an equal distribution across gender. Patients are often asymptomatic but may present with chest pain, cough, or dyspnea.

Although thymomas are generally indolent tumors, they have the ability to be locally invasive and recur at local or distant sites and can be malignant despite their nonaggressive appearance. Even small, apparently encapsulated thymomas have been known to metastasize, making the term *benign thymoma*, which sometimes is used for these tumors, inappropriate. Thymomas are predominantly locally invasive; metastases occur most commonly as pleural or pericardial nodules, although distant metastases to liver, bones, and other sites are seen occasionally. The Masaoka staging system (Table 2) reflects this behavior and is used widely for thymomas. The surgeon is usually in the best position to judge macroscopic invasion of a thymoma into the mediastinal fat or other organs. Evidence of microscopic invasion as determined by the pathologist is also important, however, and is reflected in the staging classification.

Various classification systems based on histologic appearance have been used for thymomas, but the clinical utility of any of these systems is controversial. Thymomas may have a spindle cell, lymphocytic, epithelial, or mixed appearance. Most often the cells themselves do not have a malignant appearance, but an undifferentiated type with frequent mitotic figures, known as *thymic carcinoma,* is seen occasionally. A classification of thymomas into cortical, medullary, or mixed types has gained in popularity. The cortical tumors have a worse prognosis, but this is related primarily to the fact that these tumors generally are seen in a more advanced stage.

In 1999, the World Health Organization proposed a new classification scheme (types A, AB, B1, B2, B3, and C); however, the prognostic value of this system remains unclear beyond a worse prognosis for thymic carcinoma (type C).

Treatment
Surgical resection is the mainstay of treatment for thymomas, including stage III and IVa thymomas. Resection of even a small stage I thymoma should involve removal of the entire thymus and the tumor because the subsequent development of myasthenia gravis or a second focus of tumor in the thymus has been seen in the experience of most major centers.

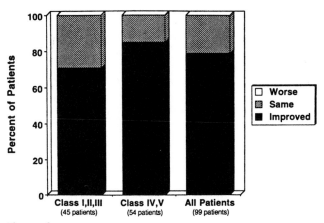

Figure 1
Most recent disease severity compared with preoperative maximal disease severity in 100 consecutive thymectomies for myasthenia gravis at the University of North Carolina. The patients are stratified by worst disease severity (modified Osserman scale). No patient had worse symptoms. Differences are not statistically significant. *(From Scott W, Detterbeck F: Semin Thorac Cardiovasc Surg 11:54, 1999.)*

Table 2 Masaoka Staging System for Thymoma	
STAGE	**DESCRIPTION**
I	Macroscopically completely encapsulated, no microscopic invasion
IIa	Macroscopic invasion into surrounding fatty tissue or mediastinal pleura
IIb	Microscopic invasion into the capsule
III	Macroscopic invasion into neighboring organs (lung, pericardium, great vessels)
IVa	Pleural or pericardial implants
IVb	Distant (extrathoracic) metastasis

The standard surgical approach generally should be a median sternotomy. If there is any suspicion of invasion of a thymoma into adjacent structures, these should be resected en bloc with the tumor and the thymus gland. This may require resection of lung, pericardium, innominate vein, phrenic nerve, portions of the superior vena cava, or even the aorta. Although it is unappealing to resect the phrenic nerve in patients with myasthenia, unilateral resection is usually well tolerated and is preferable to leaving gross tumor behind. The value of subtotal resection, even with adjuvant radiotherapy, is controversial at best, and every effort should be made to achieve a complete resection.

Stage I thymomas are treated adequately with a complete resection alone. Postoperative radiotherapy is recommended by most of the larger centers for stage II and stage III thymomas, even when a complete resection with negative margins has been achieved. The bulk of available data does not support a reduction in the recurrence rate, however, or improvement in survival with adjuvant radiotherapy. The optimal treatment of stage IV thymomas is unclear. Aggressive treatment with surgical resection, usually with adjuvant radiotherapy and sometimes chemotherapy, has been reported to result in long-term survival.

Thymomas are moderately responsive to radiotherapy and chemotherapy. A prospective phase II study involving preoperative chemoradiotherapy in 65 patients with stage II, III, and IVa thymomas has suggested that this approach results in significantly better 5- and 8-year survival compared with surgery alone in historical controls. Because thymoma is an indolent tumor, however, it is generally necessary to analyze 10-year data. Only about half of the deaths are due to the thymoma, and it is probably best to consider recurrence rates to judge the effectiveness of treatment. Although preoperative treatment is promising, longer follow-up is needed before this approach is defined clearly as the standard of care.

Patients with a history of thymoma should be followed carefully for at least 10 years. Most series report a median time to recurrence of 3 to 5 years, but recurrences are reported occasionally by most large centers after more than 10 years. Several centers have reported long-term survival when a recurrence is treated with another resection. Although there is selection bias in the patients undergoing resection, the available data are fairly convincing that this is the treatment of choice whenever feasible.

There is more recent but limited evidence that some unresectable thymomas have a high uptake with octreotide. One series showed an overall response rate of 37%. There may be a role for somatostatin analogues for recurrent or malignant thymomas refractory to standard therapies. Prospective trials are ongoing.

■ RESULTS

The reported 5- and 10-year survival rates after resection of a thymoma are about 90% and 80% for stage I, 90% and 70% for stage II, 65% and 50% for stage III, and 60% and 35% for stage IVa. Many of the deaths, particularly for patients with stage I and II thymomas, are not due to the tumor, however. The reported data for stage III and IVa thymomas come from surgical series and likely represent only a select subset of these patients. Several series have reported multivariate analysis of factors associated with survival. The stage of disease is a most consistent factor, as is the completeness of resection. The histologic subtype, age, gender, presence of myasthenia gravis, and whether postoperative radiation therapy was given have not been found to be independent prognostic factors in these studies.

SUGGESTED READING

Buddle JM, et al: Predictors of outcome in thymectomy for myasthenia gravis, *Ann Thorac Surg* 72:197, 2001.

Detterbeck FC, et al: One hundred consecutive thymectomies for myasthenia gravis, *Ann Thorac Surg* 62:242, 1996.

Krucylak PE, Naunheim KS: Preoperative preparation and anesthetic management of patients with myasthenia gravis, *Semin Thorac Cardiovasc Surg* 11:47, 1999.

Regnard J, et al: Prognostic factors and long-term results after thymoma resection: a series of 307 patients, *J Thorac Cardiovasc Surg* 112:376, 1996.

Shrager JB, et al: Transcervical thymectomy for myasthenia gravis achieves results comparable to thymectomy by sternotomy, *Ann Thorac Surg* 74:320, 2002.

SUBSTERNAL GOITER

V. Seenu Reddy
John R. Roberts

Substernal goiter represents 10% of mediastinal masses in most surgical series and is encountered commonly in clinical practice. Diagnosis and surgical therapy are not always straightforward, however, and must be tailored for each patient.

■ HISTORY

The history of the study of substernal goiters is responsible for much of the early study of the mediastinum. Haller first described substernal extension of goiters into the mediastinum in the mid-18th century. In 1820, Klein was the first to remove a substernal goiter. Billroth formalized the techniques of resection and published a large series in 1869. Kocher subsequently reported 1000 thyroidectomies in 1901, in which he described techniques for removing substernal goiters. Along with the surgical therapy of mediastinal parathyroids and myasthenia gravis, the early treatment of substernal goiters is responsible for the development of mediastinal surgery at a time when surgery on any part of the chest was considered anathema.

■ ANATOMY

The anterior-superior compartment is the largest mediastinal compartment and can contain the greatest variety of pathologies, including substernal goiters. It extends from the manubrium and the first ribs to the diaphragm. Its posterior border is defined by the anterior aspect of the pericardium inferiorly and curves posteriorly to include the arch of the aorta and great vessels. Structures contained within this compartment include the ascending aorta, the superior vena cava, the azygos vein, the thymus gland, lymph nodes, fat, connective tissue, transverse aorta, and great vessels. Substernal goiters arise as an extension of a cervical gland into the mediastinum, rather than growth of a mediastinal gland, as the neurovascular supply for nearly all substernal goiters arises from the neck.

■ PRESENTATION

Substernal goiter is one of many lesions found as a mass in the anterior mediastinum. Because there is no predominance of any one lesion, a systematic approach to evaluation and therapy is necessary. Substernal goiters present most often in asymptomatic women with a palpable cervical goiter.

A 3:1 female-to-male preponderance is typical. Common symptoms (Table 1), other than a neck mass, include symptoms secondary to compression, such as dysphagia, dyspnea, or pain.

Davis found that 20% of cervical goiters extend into the mediastinum, most of which extend into the anterior mediastinum, typically projecting toward the patient's left. More rarely, a substernal goiter may extend into the right posterior mediastinum, toward the right paratracheal groove. Primary mediastinal goiters lacking a cervical component are even rarer but must be considered in patients with anterior mediastinal masses without an enlarged cervical thyroid.

The incidence of malignancy in substernal goiters ranges from 2.5% to 17%. Many of these malignancies are early cancers that may have not been detected otherwise in the patient's lifetime and may not be clinically significant.

■ IMAGING

Basic imaging of a substernal goiter includes a chest radiograph and a computed tomography (CT) scan, which shows continuity between the cervical and mediastinal components of the enlarged thyroid. These goiters appear heterogeneous due to hemorrhage, cysts, or variable iodine concentration. The masses are multilobulated and encapsulated. Calcifications commonly are seen. Mediastinal goiters can cause vascular engorgement or occasionally superior vena caval obstruction, which can be appreciated on preoperative imaging. On intravenously contrast-enhanced CT scans, these goiters typically exhibit intense, sustained enhancement. Functional scanning using either iodine-123 or iodine-131 can be diagnostic if functioning thyroid tissue is present within the cervical and mediastinal components of the gland.

Malignancy
Table 2 reviews the largest series of resected substernal goiters. The incidence of malignancy ranged from 2.5% to 22%, with most of them incidental malignancies.

Surgical Management
Symptomatic substernal goiters should be resected. In addition, patients who have potentially symptomatic goiters (i.e., there is clear radiologic evidence of compression of adjacent structures) benefit from resection. Most substernal goiters can be approached through the standard transverse cervical incision, but occasionally a limited upper sternotomy

Table 1 Symptoms and Associated Clinical Syndromes in Patients with Substernal Goiter

SYMPTOM	CLINICAL SYNDROME
Cough	Airway narrowing, compression
Dyspnea	Airway compromise, pericardial compression
Dysphagia	Esophageal narrowing/obstruction, esophageal motor dysfunction
Hoarseness	Vocal cord paralysis
Facial swelling	Superior vena cava syndrome

Table 2 Resection of Substernal Thyroids

AUTHOR (YEAR)	NO. PATIENTS	COMPLICATIONS*		INCIDENCE OF MALIGNANCY	ADDITIONAL INCISIONS†
		MAJOR	MINOR		
Allol (1983)	50	1 (2%)	10%	8 (16%)	?
Sanders (1992)	52	3 (6%)	20%	11 (21.2%)	?
Netterville (1998)	23	1 (4%)	12%	4 (17%)	0%
Arici (2001)	52	12%	6%	6 (12%)	4%
Hedayati (2002)	116	3%	49%	25 (22%)	2%
Dedivitis (1999)	32	12%	1%	?	6.25%
Rodriguez (1999)	72	3%	0%	3 (4%)	9%
Vadasz (1998)	175	9%	26%	10 (5.8%)	24%
Hsu (1996)	234	2%	13.2%	16 (7%)	1.7%

*Major complications were those that prolonged hospital stay, whereas minor complications did not.
†Additional incisions included either sternotomies or thoracotomies.

through the manubrium is required for adequate exposure for total resection. Rarely, full sternotomy or thoracotomy is needed. In the review of series in Table 2, the need for additional incisions ranged from 0 to 24%.

Kocher, in 1901, described many of the basic techniques employed when resecting retrosternal goiters. The patient should be positioned on a shoulder roll with the head elevated and extended on the operating table. The initial incision should consist of a transverse cervical or "collar" incision. Care should be taken to avoid making the incision too caudal. A large goiter with a substernal component is likely to require the division of strap muscles, often bilaterally. The division of strap muscles increases the exposure and facilitates the dissection of the lateral and inferior portions of the gland.

As with standard thyroidectomies, the superior poles of the gland should be mobilized, and the superior blood supply should be identified and ligated. When the superior thyroid vessels have been ligated, and the external branch of the superior laryngeal nerve has been identified, the superior poles can be mobilized adequately. Next, additional blood supply to the gland, such as middle thyroid veins, should be ligated, allowing for additional lateral mobilization of the gland.

When the gland has been mobilized along the superior and lateral aspects by division of the attachments, the superior parathyroid glands and recurrent laryngeal nerve at its point of entry into the larynx should be identified positively and protected. Digital or blunt dissection, combined with occasional sharp dissection, can be used to free the thyroid gland from the posterior sternum and gradually deliver the retrosternal component of the gland into the cervical incision. In most cases, the thyroid gland should be able to be mobilized fully and delivered into the incision at this stage of the procedure.

In cases in which the gland is still unable to be delivered into the cervical incision, additional retrosternal dissection may be required. With superior elevation by retraction of the manubrium, the surgeon's finger can be used to dissect bluntly any remaining inferior attachments. Visible vessels should be clipped or ligated.

Mortality approached zero in most series. Major complications ranged from 0 to 12%. Paralysis of recurrent laryngeal nerves, hypoparathyroidism, and bleeding were the most common complaints.

■ SUMMARY

Surgical therapy is the best therapy for most patients with substernal goiter. It should be considered in all patients with significant symptoms and in patients with evidence of compression of structures on CT scan. CT is the most useful modality because other imaging does not always identify substernal thyroid tissue. Most resections can be done through the neck because the vascular supply almost always descends from cervical structures. Perioperative mortality should approach zero.

SUGGESTED READING

Allol MD, Thompson NW: Rationale for the operative management of substernal goiters, *Surgery* 94:969, 1983.

Hedayati N, McHenry CR: The clinical presentation and operative management of nodular and diffuse substernal thyroid disease, *Am Surg* 68:245, 2002.

Hsu B, et al: Recurrent substernal nodular goiter: incidence and management, *Surgery* 120:1072, 1996.

Sanders LE, et al: Mediastinal goiters: the need for an aggressive approach, *Arch Surg* 127:609, 1992.

Vadasz P, Kotsis L: Surgical aspects of 175 mediastinal goiters, *Eur J Cardiothorac Surg* 14:393, 1998.

ANTERIOR MEDIASTINAL MASSES

David R. Jones

The thoracic surgeon frequently is asked to evaluate and treat patients with anterior mediastinal masses. The role of the thoracic surgeon depends on the working clinical diagnosis. If lymphoma is suspected, all that is necessary is to obtain adequate tissue for diagnosis. Alternatively the surgeon may plan to resect the mass completely if it is a substernal goiter or other anterior mediastinal tumor. An understanding of the various diagnostic modalities and technical approaches to these tumors is important.

The anterior-superior mediastinal compartment extends superiorly from the thoracic inlet to the diaphragm inferiorly and anteriorly from the sternum to the anterior surface of the pericardium and is bounded laterally by the phrenic nerves. Structures contained within this region include the thymus, the brachiocephalic vessels, the anterior wall of the superior vena cava (SVC), lymph nodes, and a moderate amount of adipose tissue. There are numerous case reports of uncommon tumors of the anterior mediastinum, but the primary tumors and cysts of the region include thymomas (discussed elsewhere), germ cell tumors, lymphoma, lipomas, hemangiomas, teratomas, mesothelial cysts, and substernal goiters.

■ DIAGNOSIS

The initial evaluation begins with a directed history and physical examination. Approximately 50% of patients have symptoms of fever, chills, night sweats, or weight loss ("B symptoms") if they have lymphoma. The absence of these symptoms does not rule out the diagnosis of lymphoma, however. Patients also may complain of dull chest pain, a new cough, a substernal pressure or fullness sensation, hoarseness, occasional palpations, dyspnea with exertion, and rarely dysphagia. If there is partial obstruction of either the tracheobronchial tree or the esophagus, patients may have recurrent respiratory tract infections. Most of the symptoms secondary to anterior mediastinal tumors relate to compression or irritation of structures contained within or adjacent to the anterior mediastinal compartment.

Many patients have nothing specific on physical examination related to the anterior mediastinal mass. If present, examination findings generally are related to the size and invasiveness of the mass. If the mass is significantly compressing the SVC, signs of SVC obstruction, such as jugular venous distention and enlarged superficial veins on the anterior chest wall, may be present. The patient also may have audible expiratory wheezing if the mass is obstructing the trachea or main stem bronchi. A complete neck examination should be performed, including the thyroid and both supraclavicular fossae.

Finally, although occurring in only 5% of cases, a testicular examination should be performed in all men with an anterior mediastinal mass to rule out metastatic disease from a primary testicular germ cell tumor. Similarly the absence of gynecomastia should be documented. Accordingly, in this population of patients, serum markers of β-human chorionic gonadotropin and α-fetoprotein also should be checked. Table 1 outlines common serologic findings for these tumor markers for mediastinal germ cell tumors.

■ RADIOGRAPHIC EXAMINATION

Radiographic assessment of anterior mediastinal masses begins with a posteroanterior and lateral chest x-ray. The anterior mediastinal mass is identified as an obliteration of the retrosternal air space on the lateral chest x-ray. On the posteroanterior chest x-ray, there may be a loss of the right paratracheal stripe with or without a silhouette sign.

A computed tomography (CT) scan of the chest generally is performed next. Although there are no pathognomonic radiographic findings for anterior mediastinal tumors, certain constellations of findings suggest specific diagnoses, as follows:

Lymphoma: Lymphoma within the mediastinum as the only repository of disease occurs in only 5% of the cases. These tumors may invade contiguous structures, chest wall, and lung. They are often heterogeneous in nature and rarely have any cystic component. In addition, pleural or pericardial effusions may be evident.
Teratoma: Most teratomas have well-defined margins that are smooth or lobulated. Most have a heterogeneous attenuation with soft tissue fluid, fat, and calcium components. In others, there may be a fat-fluid level seen on CT.
Seminoma: Seminoma is the most frequent mediastinal germ cell neoplasm after teratoma and is identified on CT as a bulky mass, which projects into one or both sides of the anterior mediastinum. These lesions typically have a homogeneous attenuation on CT and enhance only slightly after intravenous contrast administration. They rarely invade contiguous structures and have infrequent calcifications.

Table 1 Tumor Markers in Various Germ Cell Tumors

GERM CELL TUMOR	AFP	β-HCG
Embryonal carcinoma	+	−
Embryonal carcinoma with ST	+	+
Choriocarcinoma	−	+
Yolk sac tumor	+	+
Teratoma	−	−
Teratoma with embryonal carcinoma	+	−
Seminoma	−	−
Seminoma with ST	−	−

AFP, α-fetoprotein; β-HCG, β-human chorionic gonadotropin; ST, syncytiotrophoblasts.

Adapted from Kohman LJ, Powers CN: Tumors and masses: biologic markers. In Pearson FG, et al, editors: *Thoracic surgery,* New York, 1995, Churchill-Livingstone, p 1411; with permission.

Nonseminomatous tumors: These tumors are generally inhomogeneous, are large, and have areas of necrosis and hemorrhage contained within. They frequently compress or invade adjacent structures, resulting in symptoms or signs of obstruction.

Substernal goiter: Characteristic CT features of a substernal goiter include continuity with a cervical thyroid, focal calcification, and a prolonged enhancement after intravenous contrast administration. Focal nonenhancing areas within the thyroid gland are a result of a hemorrhage or cyst formation.

Magnetic resonance imaging is used rarely except when the patient is allergic to intravenous contrast material or if there is concern about involvement of the mass with the brachiocephalic vessels or SVC. The use of positron emission tomography to diagnosis anterior mediastinal masses has been described in small series of patients; its clinical role in diagnosing and managing these tumors is unclear.

■ TISSUE DIAGNOSIS

A tissue diagnosis of anterior mediastinal tumors is particularly important if one has a high index of suspicion that the mass may be a lymphoma or germ cell tumor. These tumors are treated best by chemotherapy or radiotherapy and not surgery initially. We advocate CT-guided core needle biopsy as the primary method of obtaining a tissue diagnosis for these patients. Our experience and that of others strongly favor a core biopsy in contrast to fine needle aspiration. With on-site cytopathology and an experienced radiologist, approximately 90% of mediastinal masses will have a tissue diagnosis made using this technique. If this approach fails or is not technically feasible, an anterior mediastinotomy (Chamberlain procedure) or thoracoscopy is recommended to make the diagnosis. Both of these procedures can be done with low morbidity and in many cases are performed as an outpatient procedure or 23-hour admission.

If the anterior mediastinal mass is well circumscribed, does not appear to invade adjacent structures, and can be excised completely, the tissue diagnosis is best obtained at the time of surgery. There is little role for mediastinoscopy in the diagnosis of anterior mediastinal tumors because this technique primarily allows access to the middle mediastinum but not to the anterior mediastinum. Occasionally, however, lymphoma may involve subcarinal or paratracheal lymph nodes, which are accessible by mediastinoscopy.

Although infrequent, a satisfactory amount of tumor to confirm the diagnosis may not be possible despite performing a core needle biopsy (Figure 1) or a Chamberlain procedure. Under these circumstances, it may be necessary to perform a sternotomy or thoracotomy to obtain enough tissue to make the diagnosis. This situation most commonly occurs in patients with nodular sclerosing Hodgkin's disease, who have a significant fibrotic component to their tumors.

■ INDICATIONS FOR SURGERY

Indications for surgery for an anterior mediastinal tumor include symptoms or signs directly related to the tumor

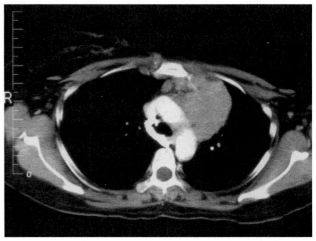

Figure 1
Computed tomography scan shows a large homogeneous anterior mediastinal mass anterior to the aortic arch. Despite two core needle biopsies, the diagnosis remained in question. A left Chamberlain procedure was performed, which confirmed the diagnosis of nodular sclerosing Hodgkin's lymphoma. The patient had a complete response to combination chemotherapy and radiation.

and the need to establish a tissue diagnosis. As previously mentioned, the presence of an anterior mediastinal mass is not an absolute indication for surgery because many of these tumors can be diagnosed with a less invasive procedure.

Surgical indications for anterior mediastinal germ cell tumors deserve further comment. For the patient with a known mediastinal seminoma, there is little, if any, role for surgery. Most of these tumors respond to cisplatin-based chemotherapy with response rates of 80% to 90% and 5-year survival rates of 70% to 85%. For cases of local recurrence or persistent disease after treatment with chemotherapy, radiation is frequently curative.

Similarly, there is little role for surgery for mediastinal nonseminomatous malignant germ cell tumors. These tumors frequently are large and infiltrative, and surgery plays no role as a primary treatment modality. These tumors should be treated primarily with cisplatin-based combination chemotherapy; 5-year survival rates are 40% to 90% depending on the volume of disease. There is, however, a role for surgery in a patient who has undergone combination chemotherapy and has a residual mediastinal mass with normal serum tumor marker levels. These patients should undergo resection for residual mediastinal tumor. The pathology is likely to be either a benign teratoma or tumor necrosis in the resected specimen. If patients are found to have residual tumor in the specimen, salvage chemotherapy should be employed.

It is controversial as to whether surgery should be employed for patients with persistently elevated serum tumor markers and a mass on CT after chemotherapy. Studies have suggested surgery may have a role in these patients. If the patients have a normalization of serum tumor markers after resection, these patients seem to have a more favorable prognosis compared with patients with persistent elevation of markers despite surgical resection.

■ SURGERY

Surgery for any mediastinal mass begins with a thoughtful anesthetic plan effectively communicated between the surgeon and the anesthesiologist. Because some of these tumors may be quite large, their compression of the tracheobronchial tree can become life-threatening. The surgeon should be in the operating room as these patients are being induced. In patients with large anterior mediastinal masses, we recommend performing an awake intubation using fiberoptic bronchoscopy with the endotracheal tube jacketed over the scope. After intubation, the patient may undergo general anesthesia, and the operation can proceed in a safe manner. Rapid induction of anesthesia without primary control of the airway may result in a significant loss of motor tone, and patients can develop respiratory distress rapidly, which can be difficult to manage even when an airway is secured. Alternatively, if only a tissue biopsy is required, a small thoracotomy (e.g., a Chamberlain procedure) can be done under local anesthesia with the patient spontaneously breathing through a laryngeal mask airway.

After safe induction of anesthesia, resection of most of these tumors can be approached either through a median sternotomy or with video-assisted thoracic surgery (VATS). We prefer to approach large tumors or tumors with radiographic or clinical evidence of invasion into adjacent structures through a sternotomy. Only small tumors are approached using VATS techniques. For the occasional VATS procedure, we prefer to have a left-sided endotracheal tube inserted such that selective left lung ventilation may be employed. The right lung is allowed to deflate, and the thoracoscopy ports and utility incision (if necessary) are placed in the right anterolateral chest wall. This right-sided approach permits the surgeon to have a larger operating field because the right hemithorax is generally larger than the left. Alternatively, if the mass is predominately in the left hemithorax, a left-sided approach is reasonable.

If the patient has a substernal thyroid, a collar incision in the neck generally suffices to remove the tumor. Occasionally, with larger tumors, it may be necessary to perform a partial upper sternal split to remove the tumor safely. Technical caveats for removal of these tumors include attention to the blood supply, which can arise from the aortic arch and from tributaries from the innominate vein. Failure to appreciate the arterial and venous supply to these large substernal thyroid tumors can result in bleeding that is difficult to control from a collar incision alone. One also should be thoughtful about identifying both recurrent laryngeal nerves before extensive posterolateral dissection. As the substernal thyroid mass increases in size over time, these nerves frequently are displaced from their normal anatomic position and are at risk for injury during subsequent removal of the tumor. Sharp dissection instead of electrocautery is recommended wherever the recurrent laryngeal nerve is near.

On opening the incision, the location, extent, and invasiveness of the mass are ascertained. Both pleural spaces are opened to identify the phrenic nerves. The tumor's relationships to the SVC, innominate vein, pericardium, phrenic nerves, and great vessels all need to be assessed and calculated into decisions regarding the extent of resection required to remove the tumor completely. The tumor also may involve lung parenchyma of the upper or middle lobes. A generous wedge excision of the involved lung should suffice to obtain an adequate tumor margin. Should the tumor invade a portion of the pericardium, it should be removed with grossly clear margins. It is rare that the pericardial defect needs reconstruction with prosthetic material. If the tumor involves one of the phrenic nerves, it may be taken to achieve an adequate margin and an R0 resection. If both phrenic nerves are involved by tumor, only one of the nerves should be taken and the other spared. Division of both nerves may result in significant respiratory difficulty and the need for a permanent tracheostomy.

Invasion of the tumor into the innominate vein is uncommon, but should it occur, the vein may be taken with impunity. If the SVC is involved with tumor, and this is the only area preventing an R0 resection, the surgeon should consider resection of the SVC. In most cases, a tangential excision of the SVC wall is adequate. Before SVC occlusion, care should be taken to identify the phrenic nerve and if necessary dissect it off of the SVC first. A partial occluding vascular clamp is applied, the tumor is excised tangentially, and the defect is closed either primarily or with a pericardial patch. Tumor involvement of the SVC does not mandate resection of the ipsilateral phrenic nerve. If a patient requires only tangential excision of the SVC, systemic heparin is not administered routinely. Alternatively, if the tumor involves greater than 50% of the SVC circumference, it is likely that complete resection of the SVC is necessary to obtain an R0 resection. Heparin (7500 U) is administered intravenously, the SVC is mobilized, the azygos vein is divided, and proximal and distal control is obtained. Vascular clamps are applied, and the involved portion of the SVC is resected. A ringed no. 12 to 16 polytetrafluoroethylene graft is used to reconstruct the SVC. The average SVC system clamp time generally is 30 to 45 minutes. Cardiopulmonary bypass is not required for uncomplicated caval resections. Postoperatively the patient is placed on aspirin and coumadin for anticoagulation. The coumadin can be discontinued 3 to 6 months postoperatively.

After resection of the tumor, the margins are assessed grossly, and if adjuvant radiation is considered, the resection margins are marked with metallic clips to facilitate future radiation planning. Both pleural spaces are inspected for any tumor involvement, and pleural catheters are inserted into both spaces. Depending on the magnitude of resection, a mediastinal drainage catheter also may be inserted.

Postoperative complications are uncommon after surgery for anterior mediastinal tumor removal. Complications that can occur involve inadvertent injury to either the phrenic or the recurrent laryngeal nerves on both sides, development of a mediastinal hematoma, chylothorax, atrial dysrhythmias, pneumonia, and sternal wound infections. With attention to detail, good surgical technique, adequate postoperative pain control, and early mobilization, most patients do well postoperatively.

SUGGESTED READING

Kesler KA, et al: Primary mediastinal nonseminomatous germ cell tumors: the influence of post-chemotherapy pathology on long-term survival after surgery, *J Thorac Cardiovasc Surg* 118:692, 1999.

Petersdorf SH, Wood DE: Lymphoproliferative disorders presenting as mediastinal neoplasms, *Semin Thorac Cardiovas Surg* 12:290, 2000.

Protopapas Z, Westcott JL: Transthoracic hilar and mediastinal biopsy, *Radiol Clin North Am* 38:281, 2000.

MIDDLE MEDIASTINAL MASSES

George L. Zorn III
Jonathan C. Nesbitt

The mediastinum is an anatomic division of the thorax extending from the thoracic inlet to the diaphragm between the left and right pleural cavities; included within are vital elements of the circulatory, respiratory, digestive, and nervous systems. Division of the mediastinum into anterior, middle, and posterior sections facilitates directed diagnostic and therapeutic strategies. The middle mediastinum is composed primarily of the heart and great vessels, but also contains the pulmonary trunk, phrenic nerves, trachea, and paratracheal lymph nodes. It is the site of several congenital lesions and is a region that can be affected as a consequence of pulmonary and systemic diseases. Table 1 lists the most common middle mediastinal masses in decreasing order of frequency. Many of these diseases involve contiguous compartments of the mediastinum.

■ CLINICAL FEATURES

Currently the most common stimulus for evaluation of a mediastinal mass is a fortuitous finding on a routine radiograph. A careful history can elucidate symptoms, however, in 65% of patients. The most common symptoms are chest pain, fever, cough, and dyspnea. Symptoms related to local invasion, such as superior vena cava syndrome, Horner's syndrome, hoarseness, and severe pain, are more likely caused by a malignancy, although benign processes also can present this way.

Systemic symptoms from ectopic hormone or antibody production are less likely with masses of the middle mediastinum than with anterior or posterior mediastinal masses. Lymphomas are prominent in the differential diagnosis for middle mediastinal masses, however, and usually have systemic symptoms, such as fever, chills, weight loss, and anorexia.

■ DIAGNOSIS

Diagnostic evaluation of a patient with a middle mediastinal mass follows a careful history and physical examination that can help direct further evaluation. Goals of study include (1) differentiation between primary mediastinal masses and masses secondary to systemic disease, (2) detection of compression or invasion of major structures (great vessels, trachea, esophagus, spine) that determines resectability, and (3) identification of significant patient comorbidities that help to determine operative risk.

Posteroanterior and lateral chest radiographs are standard screening tools that locate the mediastinal abnormality.

Computed tomography (CT) with oral and intravenous contrast material is standard and helps to define further the lesion's location, size, extent of invasion, and degree of vascularity. Concurrent abnormalities also can be evaluated. Rarely, angiography is required to define the vascular anatomy in relation to a middle mediastinal mass. Magnetic resonance imaging is useful for evaluating vascular structures or masses, neurogenic tumors, and cystic lesions. Cysts commonly have low signal intensity on T1-weighted images (Figure 1A) but bright signal intensity on T2-weighted images (Figure 1B). Echocardiography, particularly transesophageal echocardiography, is useful to evaluate masses that involve the pericardium or great vessels and to differentiate cystic from solid masses. If noninvasive methods suggest lymphoma confined to the mediastinum, transesophageal echocardiography or CT can be used to help guide percutaneous biopsy techniques. Mediastinoscopy is the most common diagnostic procedure for middle mediastinal pathology. It is used to evaluate lesions in the paratracheal and subcarinal region and can provide a therapeutic benefit to selected patients who require drainage of cystic abnormalities.

■ MANAGEMENT

Congenital Foregut Cysts

Congenital foregut cysts account for 15% to 20% of mediastinal masses. They originate from sequestrations of the ventral foregut, the antecedent of the esophagus and tracheobronchial tree. They are spherical, homogeneous, unilocular lesions that occur equally in men and women. Most cysts are asymptomatic because of their small size and failure to compress surrounding structures. With increasing size, even these benign cysts can cause compression of the adjacent airway or esophagus, however, or can become infected with resultant mediastinitis.

Bronchogenic cysts are the most common congenital foregut cysts, comprising 60% of all cysts. These cysts may develop in the mediastinum or within the lung parenchyma, but most often they originate near the carina. They are lined with respiratory epithelium and contain a milky white or brown mucoid material. Direct communication with the tracheobronchial tree is rare, although superimposed infection can lead to erosion into the airway.

Surgical excision is recommended in all patients to provide definitive pathologic diagnosis, to prevent future complications, and to alleviate symptoms. Malignant degeneration is rare but has been reported. Bronchoscopic aspiration and

Table 1 Most Common Middle Mediastinal Masses*
Foregut duplication cysts
Pericardial cysts
Lymphoma
Metastatic lymphadenopathy
Benign lymphadenopathy
Vascular dilation
Castleman's disease
Tracheal malignancy

*In decreasing order of frequency.

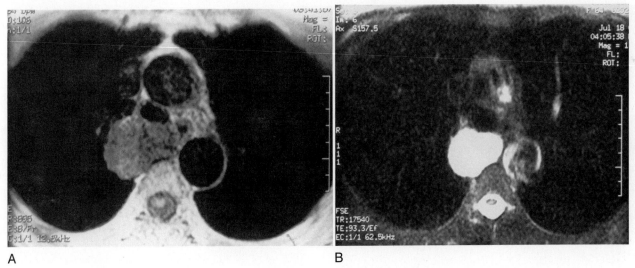

Figure 1
Magnetic resonance imaging of a mediastinal cyst on T1-weighted **(A)** and T2-weighted **(B)** images.

mediastinoscopic or percutaneous drainage have been performed in high-risk surgical patients. These techniques do not retrieve cyst wall tissue for analysis, and recurrence is likely. Infectious complications have been reported with simple drainage alone. We recommend that aspiration be reserved only for patients unable to tolerate a surgical procedure with the goal of short-term palliation of symptoms only.

Resection traditionally is accomplished through a standard posterolateral thoracotomy, allowing complete resection of the cyst wall, while protecting surrounding structures. The complication rate is low with this procedure. Video-assisted thoracic surgery (VATS) is used in selected patients with small, noninfected lesions. Intraoperative decompression of the lesion is safe and facilitates exposure. For patients with large, inflamed, or chronically infected cysts, VATS excision is difficult because of dense adhesions. An open procedure is best in this circumstance.

Pericardial Cysts

Pericardial cysts are the second most common mediastinal mass and make up one third of all primary cysts of the mediastinum. These cysts arise from the mesenchymal lacunae failing to fuse normally to form the pericardial sac. They most commonly occur at the cardiophrenic angles, 70% on the right and 22% on the left. The remaining 8% are found in other sites on the pericardium.

There is a characteristic radiographic appearance to these masses. Classically, they appear as unilocular cysts at the right cardiophrenic angle with smooth borders and a Hounsfield number of almost zero by CT (Figure 2). They rarely cause symptoms secondary to compression. Lesions showing these characteristics have been managed with simple aspiration or observation. Surgical excision is performed occasionally, primarily for diagnostic purposes, although therapeutic excision is used on occasion. A lateral thoracotomy has been the standard procedure for resection of pericardial cysts. In the 1990s, VATS emerged as the most popular technique for

management, however, because of its definitive result in a minimally invasive setting.

Lymphoma

Although the mediastinum often is involved in patients with lymphoma at some point in the course of their disease, it is rarely the only site of disease. Only 5% to 10% of patients with lymphoma present with disease localized only to the mediastinum. Characteristically, these tumors occur in the anterior-superior mediastinum or in the hilar region of the middle mediastinum.

Hodgkin's disease (HD) and non-Hodgkin's lymphomas (NHL) are separate diseases with unique and sometimes overlapping features. Although HD represents only 25% to 30% of all lymphomas, it is the most common mediastinal lymphoma, involving 70% of patients with mediastinal disease. Nodular HD is the most common subtype and is found most often in the anterior mediastinum, specifically the thymus. The other types of HD affect primarily the mediastinal nodes and typically do not manifest as an isolated mediastinal mass. NHL also typically localizes mediastinal disease to the anterior mediastinum but can present with isolated middle mediastinum adenopathy.

Surgical excision of lymphoma is usually not possible, and the primary role for the surgeon in the care of these patients is to provide tissue for diagnosis and to assist in appropriate pathologic staging. Fine needle aspiration biopsy (FNAB) is often insufficient for tissue diagnosis. Mediastinoscopy, mediastinotomy, thoracoscopy, and even thoracotomy all are appropriate options to obtain sufficient tissue for diagnosis.

The management of HD is determined by the stage of the disease and the relevant prognostic factors for the patient and the tumor. Treatment consists of radiation therapy for early stage disease and chemotherapy for late stage disease. NHL typically is treated with combined radiation and chemotherapy.

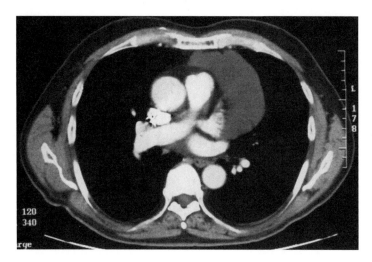

Figure 2
Typical computed tomography scan of a pericardial cyst.

Metastatic Lymphadenopathy

Although it is not considered a definitive mediastinal mass, lymphadenopathy within the middle mediastinum can present as a masslike process and always raises the suspicion of metastatic disease. Metastatic disease to mediastinal or hilar lymph nodes is usually secondary to lung cancer. Other malignancies that spread to mediastinal lymph nodes include tumors that have a propensity to extend into the abdominal or thoracic lymph node system and to the thoracic duct tributaries. These include esophageal carcinoma, gastrointestinal malignancies, renal cell carcinoma, and germ cell carcinoma. Breast carcinoma and melanoma can spread to the lung or pleural cavity and from there can metastasize to mediastinal lymph nodes.

The management of patients with lymphadenopathy is purely diagnostic and not therapeutic. When a diagnosis is obtained, treatment directed toward the primary illness is determined. Positron emission tomography is a useful modality for heightening the suspicion for metastatic lesions in a patient with a known malignancy in the face of CT-identified lymphadenopathy. Cytologic analysis of the disease can be obtained by transthoracic FNAB or bronchoscopically guided FNAB. Mediastinoscopy is the optimal approach for direct tissue biopsy. Anterior mediastinotomy or VATS procedures are used in selected patients.

Benign Lymphadenopathy

Benign mediastinal lymphadenopathy also can appear as a mediastinal mass and occurs secondary to a variety of idiopathic or infectious causes. Lymphadenopathy commonly is seen in association with sarcoidosis, a multisystem disorder of unknown etiology characterized by the presence of noncaseating granulomas in the lymph nodes and in multiple organs. Patients with pulmonary infections often develop secondary mediastinal lymphadenitis. Inflamed lymph nodes can remain enlarged even after resolution of the primary pulmonary infection. This persistent or enduring adenopathy is seen frequently in association with fungal and mycobacterial infections, most commonly histoplasmosis and tuberculosis. Dense calcium deposition, noted on radiographs, occurs as a response to the inflammatory process and suggests benignity. Organisms can be identified by special stain or culture of biopsied material.

Bronchoscopy often is performed as an initial diagnostic modality. Transbronchial FNAB can produce enough tissue for cytologic analysis and culture. Diagnosis commonly is made, however, by tissue biopsy at mediastinoscopy.

Vascular Dilations

Pulmonary venous aneurysms are rare lesions that typically present as asymptomatic masses found on routine chest radiographs. The natural history of these lesions is poorly described, although it appears that lesions associated with trauma or surgical manipulation progressively enlarge, suggesting a propensity for rupture. Transesophageal echocardiography is the definitive study to define the anatomy and associated pathology. CT scans are usually sufficient for diagnosis and surveillance. If the aneurysm is symptomatic (embolic phenomena, compression of adjacent structures) or enlarging by serial studies, resection with possible cardiopulmonary bypass is the preferred route. Asymptomatic lesions without antecedent trauma or surgical instrumentation are managed with close surveillance that includes serial transthoracic echocardiograms or CT scans.

POSTERIOR MEDIASTINAL MASSES

Brendan J. Collins
Stephen C. Yang

Owing to the embryologic complexity of the mediastinum, a variety of pathologic lesions may be encountered, including thymic neoplasms, germ cell tumors, lymphomas, neurogenic tumors, and cysts. Any diagnostic approach to a suspect mediastinal mass must begin with a thorough history and physical examination, with particular attention to aerodigestive, circulatory, and neurologic symptoms. A posteroanterior and lateral chest radiograph is an appropriate initial intervention, and chest computed tomography (CT) or chest magnetic resonance imaging (MRI) often facilitates anatomic localization with respect to the anterior, middle, or posterior mediastinum. This chapter focuses on tumors of the posterior mediastinum.

The commonly accepted boundaries of the posterior mediastinum include the ribs and vertebrae posteriorly, the posterior surface of the heart anteriorly, and the diaphragm inferiorly. Contents of this space include the esophagus, descending aorta, thoracic duct, azygos vein, vagus nerves, sympathetic chain and its ganglia, and segmental nerve roots. For all mediastinal lesions, those involving the posterior mediastinum occur in approximately 40% of pediatric cases and 20% of adult cases. Neurogenic tumors are the most common masses encountered in the posterior mediastinum. They comprise 25% to 35% of all mediastinal neoplasms and occur more commonly in children. Neurogenic neoplasms are usually asymptomatic and are benign roughly 75% of the time. They typically arise in the costovertebral sulcus, originating from the sympathetic chain or from one of the rami of an intercostal nerve. All are derived from the embryonic neural crest and can be classified as arising from peripheral nerves, sympathetic ganglia, or parasympathetic ganglia, the latter two being more common in children.

Most tumors of the posterior mediastinum can be accessed via a posterolateral thoracotomy incision. Absolute contraindications to resection include myocardial involvement, invasion of the great vessels, or a long tracheal segment.

■ TUMORS OF NERVE SHEATH ORIGIN

Peripheral nerve tumors, such as schwannomas (neurilemomas) and neurofibromas, are the most common mediastinal neurogenic tumors. Both have a peak incidence in the 20s and 30s, are usually benign, and may arise from any thoracic nerve. Schwannomas represent 75% of nerve sheath tumors and consist of cells proliferating in the endoneurium, with the perineurium encapsulating a heterogeneous mass that frequently contains areas of cystic degeneration. In contrast, neurofibromas are usually noncapsulated and homogeneous. The patient with a posterior mediastinal schwannoma or neurofibroma is usually asymptomatic, although paresthesias from nerve compression or intraspinal tumor extension may occur. Both tumors occasionally can become large and produce benign pressure erosion that can be manifest by deformities of ribs, thoracic vertebrae, or neural foramina. Approximately 10% proliferate through an intervertebral foramen into the spinal canal; 30% to 40% of these tumors can be asymptomatic. This specific tumor type is known as a *dumbbell tumor* based on its characteristic shape. Any suspicious posterior mediastinal mass should be evaluated by chest CT and MRI if there is suspected intraspinal extension. The treatment of dumbbell tumors requires a combined neurosurgical and thoracic approach, as discussed subsequently.

Tumors of nerve sheath origin are benign in 90% of cases. The malignant variety consists of rare spindle cell sarcomas that usually are seen in patients with neurofibromatosis/von Recklinghausen's disease. Malignant nerve sheath tumors typically arise from a preexisting neurofibroma or rarely from a schwannoma. The incidence of malignant degeneration of a benign neurofibroma is roughly 5% in patients with neurofibromatosis. These tumors are usually locally invasive and may have distant metastases. Malignant nerve sheath tumors also can arise sporadically in a previously irradiated field.

Treatment

Schwannomas and neurofibromas can be enucleated or, rarely, excised with an adjacent nerve structure when involved. Recurrence is rare. Tumors arising from the vagus or phrenic nerves usually can be excised with nerve preservation. Dumbbell tumors also can occur and likewise require a combined thoracic and neurosurgical approach. When intraspinal extension is observed in the lower half of the thorax, preoperative angiographic localization of the spinal artery may be necessary for intraoperative protection. Tumor removal can be accomplished through a single incision via a posterior approach. The incision begins midline above the intraspinal extension of tumor, proceeding below the inferiormost aspect of the tumor, then extending ipsilaterally to the mid axillary line. Ipsilateral hemilaminectomy is carried out to enable visualization and mobilization of the intraspinal aspect of the tumor. The pleural space can be entered posteriorly from the same incision, with or without partial rib resection. This approach usually allows the tumor to be removed in toto, and the intercostal nerve root usually can be spared.

For malignant nerve sheath tumors that often are locally invasive, radical excision with wide margins is the premise. When complete excision is not feasible, resection with postoperative radiation therapy may palliate symptoms of cord compression or local tumor involvement. Recurrence is frequent despite aggressive resection, with survival rarely beyond 1 year.

■ TUMORS OF THE AUTONOMIC NERVOUS SYSTEM

Tumors of sympathetic ganglia include benign ganglioneuromas, malignant ganglioneuroblastomas, and highly malignant neuroblastomas, the last-mentioned being more common in children. These autonomic nerve tumors, particularly neuroblastomas, may produce catecholamines and can produce symptoms of diarrhea, sweating, flushing, and abdominal distention. The catecholamine metabolites vanillylmandelic acid and homovanillic acid may be detectable in the patient's urine. Autonomic nerve tumors also have a propensity for intraspinal extension, and similarly preoperative CT or MRI should be evaluated carefully for this possibility. The benign ganglioneuromas usually are encapsulated and can be removed by simple excision. Ganglioneuroblastomas and neuroblastomas are often densely adherent to surrounding vital structures, and total removal is usually not possible. Adjuvant radiation and chemotherapy usually is indicated.

■ TUMORS OF THE PARAGANGLIONIC SYSTEM

Approximately 10% to 15% of pheochromocytomas are located above the diaphragm, a small percentage of which are paragangliomas found in the posterior mediastinum. These lesions tend to occur in middle-aged men and may be benign or malignant, active or inactive (chemodectomas), sporadic or familial, and associated with other syndromes such as Zollinger-Ellison syndrome or Carney's triad (paragangliomas, gastric epithelioid leiomyosarcomas, and pulmonary chondromas). Pheochromocytomas occurring in the posterior mediastinum have a greater propensity for malignancy than their adrenal counterparts. The malignancy of this tumor is based not on histology, but on its potential for metastasis. These tumors also produce catecholamines, although usually less than adrenal pheochromocytomas. Roughly 50% of patients with posterior mediastinal paragangliomas present with symptoms related to excess catecholamines, such as hypertension, flushing, and pulmonary edema. The diagnosis of a pheochromocytoma can be difficult but can be facilitated by detecting vanillylmandelic acid and homovanillic acid in urine or elevated serum norepinephrine levels. A serum norepinephrine level greater than 2000 pg/ml is virtually diagnostic. Because mediastinal pheochromocytomas generally produce low levels of catecholamines, a clonidine suppression test can differentiate cases that are not as definitive.

Treatment
Paragangliomas that occur in the posterior mediastinum are often localized by CT, MRI, MIBG-I[131] scanning, or selective venous sampling. Surgical resection is the definitive standard of care. Because of the effects of excess catecholamines, careful preoperative preparation and intraoperative monitoring are necessary. Simultaneous β-blockade and α-blockade is necessary because isolated β-blockade can precipitate a hypertensive crisis or pulmonary edema via unopposed α-receptor stimulation. These patients also are often volume depleted, and preoperative volume resuscitation is necessary. Pheochromocytomas are often vascular and may be difficult to remove via a video-assisted thoracic surgery (VATS) approach. When resected, patients should be monitored closely for recurrence, which can be achieved by monthly blood pressure checks for 1 year and thereafter every 6 months.

Patients also should have plasma catecholamines measured yearly for 5 years. Five-year mortality rates approaching 50% have been reported for malignant pheochromocytomas. Tumor recurrence is managed best by debulking followed by some combination of adjuvant chemotherapy, radiation, or MIBG-I[131] therapy, although these therapies still are under investigation. Prognosis is excellent for benign lesions; however, other benign paragangliomas may recur in different anatomic locations.

Paragangliomas that do not contain chromaffin are inactive variants of paragangliomas and are known as *chemodectomas*. These lesions are found most commonly in adolescents. Chemodectomas tend to occur near the aortic body in the middle mediastinum, arising from chemoreceptor tissue around the aortic arch, vagus, and aorticosympathetics. They can be difficult to visualize radiographically due to these locations and are often difficult to resect because of their close association with the heart and great vessels. Surgical resection is the treatment of choice, best accomplished via a median sternotomy. Similar to their functional counterparts, chemodectomas can be vascular, and removal requires careful hemostasis. Preoperative embolization may help reduce intraoperative blood loss.

■ FOREGUT CYSTS

Because of the similar embryologic origins in the mediastinum, congenital foregut cysts should be entertained in the differential diagnosis of a posterior mediastinal mass. These cysts are classified not by their location, but by the type of epithelium lining the cyst. They include bronchogenic and enterogenic cysts. Bronchogenic cysts encompass 50% to 60% of all mediastinal cysts, are more common in the middle mediastinum, and usually become symptomatic by the 30s. Enterogenic cysts include esophageal duplication and neuroenteric cysts, which usually become symptomatic in early childhood. Bronchogenic and enterogenic cysts occur in equal frequency in both sexes, and symptoms usually result from compression of the esophagus or tracheobronchial tree or spinal cord compression due to intraspinal extension of a neuroenteric cyst. Foregut cysts occasionally can enlarge rapidly due to cyst hemorrhage or excessive production of epithelial secretions. Rarely, they also have been observed to undergo malignant transformation in the epithelial lining.

Symptomatic or enlarging foregut cysts are treated best with complete surgical excision. These cysts are occasionally densely adherent to vital structures in the posterior mediastinum, however, and deepithelialization or VATS needle drainage may be the only safe alternative. Recurrence is extremely rare after complete excision.

■ VATS MANAGEMENT OF POSTERIOR MEDIASTINAL TUMORS

With the wide availability of VATS, several multicenter retrospective analyses have shown the feasibility of this technique in the management of neurogenic tumors of the thorax. Contraindications to the VATS approach include intraspinal extension, spinal artery involvement, and mass size greater than 6 cm when located in the thoracic sulcus or a low paravertebral position. Preoperative considerations (MRI, angiography) are the same as for the open approach. Most series report a low conversion rate to open thoracotomy, usually due to bleeding, large lesion size, patient body habitus, poor exposure, or rib attachments. In general, the minimally invasive technique is associated with shorter hospital stays, shorter chest tube duration, and less postoperative pain.

SUGGESTED READING

Bacha EA, et al: Surgery for invasive primary mediastinal tumors, *Ann Thorac Surg* 66:234, 1998.

Demmy TL, et al: Multicenter VATS experience with mediastinal tumors, *Ann Thorac Surg* 66:187, 1998.

Gale AW, et al: Neurogenic tumors of the mediastinum, *Ann Thorac Surg* 17:434, 1974.

Sandur S, et al: Thoracic involvement with pheochromocytoma, *Chest* 115:511, 1999.

MEDIASTINITIS

Riyad Karmy-Jones
Eric Vallières

■ DESCENDING NECROTIZING MEDIASTINITIS

Descending necrotizing mediastinitis (DNM) is a rare, acute, most often virulent polymicrobial infection of the mediastinum originating as an oropharyngeal or a cervical level infection that descends into the mediastinum via the contiguous cervicomediastinal fascial planes and compartments. DNM has a mortality of 30% to 40%; mortality is related directly to delays in posing the diagnosis and a lack of aggressive surgical management.

The downward migration of the cervicopharyngeal infection into the mediastinum is promoted by the presence of anatomic fascial planes and spaces that communicate directly in between the cervical and mediastinal compartments. The three resulting deep spaces are the pretracheal space, the retrovisceral space, and the prevertebral space (Figure 1). Gravity, respiratory movements, and negative inspiratory intrathoracic pressure also are thought to facilitate migration. As a result of these anatomic connections, DNM potentially can be complicated by infections involving the pleural spaces, lung, pericardial sac, and subphrenic space.

Evaluation

Plain chest radiographs may be deceptive even in the presence of well-established DNM. A contrast-enhanced computed tomography (CT) scan of the neck and chest should be obtained early in every patient presenting with a deep cervical infection. CT findings of DNM may range from the subtle loss of normal mediastinal fat planes, to the presence of mediastinal soft tissue infiltration with or without fluid collections or gas bubbles, to the identification of established mediastinal abscesses. By CT, one also must evaluate the pleural spaces, the pericardial sac, and the subphrenic compartment.

Management

The treatment of patients with DNM involves in most cases a multidisciplinary surgical team consisting of head and neck, oral and maxillofacial, and thoracic surgeons. This team is particularly important when planning operative approaches because it may be crucial to preserve chest wall muscles for eventual neck reconstruction. After prompt initiation of empirical broad-spectrum intravenous antibiotics, early aggressive drainage and débridement at all levels involved is indicated. Considering the high mortality of DNM, it is probably prudent to err on the side of being "too aggressive" initially. At the cervical level, one must treat the initiating focus of infection and establish wide open drainage and débridement of all deep cervical spaces. Although in the past most clinicians considered the establishment of a tracheostomy mandatory in every patient with DNM, a more selective use of tracheostomies has been advocated in more recent series.

The type of thoracic approach to use in these patients is debated. Estrera et al concluded in 1983 that transcervical drainage of the superior mediastinum sufficed if the mediastinal process was limited to "above the level of the T4 vertebra." Wheatley et al believed, however, that transcervical mediastinal drainage is inadequate in 80% of these cases. In a literature review in 1997, Corsten et al calculated a mortality rate of 47% from several published series in which transcervical drainage alone was used versus 19% in which an open transthoracic approach additionally was performed. More recent and larger published studies also concluded in favor of combining a cervical with a thoracic approach to débride all affected fields aggressively.

Although some surgeons have described the use of sternotomy, clamshell incisions, or video-assisted thoracic surgery (VATS) to access the mediastinum and occasionally to explore both pleural spaces simultaneously, we believe that the

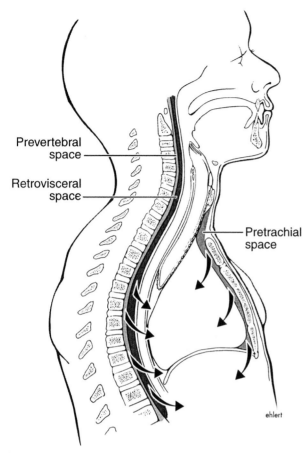

Figure 1
The three deep spaces of the neck and their communication with the chest. *(From Freeman RK, et al: Descending necrotizing mediastinitis: an analysis of the effects of serial surgical debridement on patients' mortality,* J Thorac Cardiovasc Surg 119:260, 2000.)

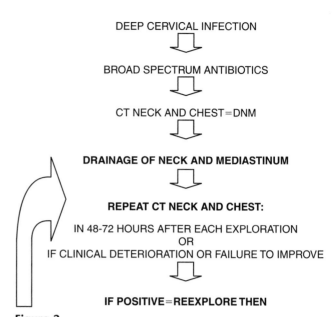

Figure 2
Algorithm suggested for aggressive management and follow-up of patients with descending necrotizing mediastinitis (DNM). CT, computed tomography.

best approach to access, evacuate, débride, and drain all mediastinal compartments is a standard posterolateral thoracotomy. A contralateral thoracotomy may be necessary to evacuate completely all of the compartments involved. Irrigation systems may allow further mechanical washout of the mediastinum.

In addition to aggressive surgical drainage and débridement, close follow-up of these patients is recommended. A policy of routine second-look operation in 48 to 72 hours after initial drainage follows such an aggressive plan of intervention in patients with DNM. In situations in which the patient fails to improve or when there is clinical deterioration despite initial or repeat explorations, repeat contrast-enhanced cervicothoracic upper abdominal imaging by CT should be performed to look for undrained foci of mediastinal debris or the interval development of sepsis in adjacent compartments. Freeman et al recommended routine follow-up cervicothoracic CT 48 to 72 hours after each exploration even when the condition appears stable or improved. In their series, 59% of such surveillance CT scans led to reexploration. With this management approach and follow-up strategy (Figure 2),

Freeman et al reported zero mortality in a consecutive series of 10 patients.

■ ACUTE MEDIASTINITIS AFTER STERNOTOMY

Mediastinal infection after sternotomy for cardiac surgery occurs in 0.5% to 3% of cases. Mortality is 20% to 40% related to erosion of cardiac structures with catastrophic hemorrhage, sepsis, progressive heart failure, or multiple organ failure. The primary pathogens are *Staphylococcus aureus* and *Staphylococcus epidermidis*. Risk factors include prolonged cardiopulmonary bypass, low preoperative ejection fraction, renal failure, reoperation for bleed, the presence of diabetes, obesity, and chronic pulmonary disease. The use of bilateral internal mammary arteries for grafts also has been implicated but not universally accepted. The diagnosis usually is suggested by the development of sternal instability, manifested by a palpable "click," often with serosanguineous drainage and systemic signs of infection. Drainage may occur from a superficial wound infection alone and, if confirmed by exploration, can be treated by simple wound care and drainage. Patients who have early sternal instability but no obvious signs of infection should be treated aggressively as if mediastinal infection exists. Patients with systemic signs of infection but without obvious wound changes (including drainage or instability) should not be reexplored routinely. Noninvasive tests are usually not helpful in the acute postoperative setting. Needle aspiration of the retrosternal space may confirm infection but if negative does not rule out mediastinitis. The optimal approach is expectant management and close surveillance with the understanding that if mediastinitis is present, it will become clinically apparent, and appropriate interventions can be made at that time.

Early experience with open drainage, dressing changes, and anticipating healing by granulation showed unacceptable mortality and failure rates. This approach now is reserved for patients with severe sepsis and mediastinal purulence as a temporizing measure before definitive closure with muscle or omental flaps. Subsequently a variety of operative strategies have been described, depending on the depth of invasion and whether or not the bony sternum is involved and has adequate vascular supply (Table 1). Currently, there are two general approaches. Primary débridement and reclosure seems to be effective in most patients when the sternum is viable without gross necrosis, when no significant potential space exists along the sternal edges, and when there are no systemic signs of sepsis. This approach can be accompanied postoperatively by constant irrigation with antimicrobials or povidone-iodine (Betadine) solutions. More recently, it has been suggested that high-pressure suction drainage without irrigation is associated with greater primary success and shorter length of stay. This avoids the morbidity associated with flap closure, including abdominal wall weakness, hernias, and possibly shoulder girdle dysfunction. Alternatively, in many series, immediate muscle flap closure also has an associated high success rate with decrease in overall morbidity and length of stay. This is the treatment of choice in patients who have necrotic or grossly infected sternums, have fibrosis of the mediastinum such that closing the sternum would leave an obvious potential space, or have failed more conservative approaches. Regardless of the method chosen, 6 to 8 weeks of antibiotic therapy is required postoperatively.

■ ACUTE MEDIASTINITIS COMPLICATING STERNAL FRACTURE

Mediastinal infection after trauma commonly is associated with penetrating injuries to the tracheobronchial tree or esophagus, with subsequent contamination, usually in the posterior mediastinum. Anterior mediastinal abscess, with or without sternal fracture, is a rarer event, however. Bony injuries to the chest wall can be associated with significant hematoma formation, which may act as a site for secondary infection (osteomyelitis) by hematogenous spread of bacteria, particularly *Staphylococcus*. Clinical manifestations include the development of sternal click in a previously stable sternum, fevers, and leukocytosis. In contrast to the postoperative cardiac patient, sternal fractures are usually transverse and the pericardium is closed, and the risks of death are comparatively reduced. Severe infections, associated with large retrosternal collections and significant sepsis, may require radical débridement and use of muscle flaps. Simpler approaches, including drainage, rewiring the sternum, and use of irrigation system under the skin and sternal flaps, usually are sufficient, however.

■ CHRONIC MEDIASTINITIS

Chronic fibrosing (or sclerosing) mediastinitis is an unusual and slow process that is often relentlessly progressive. Symptoms are related to compression of the trachea, esophagus, superior vena cava, or pulmonary artery and veins. Although malignancy must be considered, the cause usually is thought to be benign, idiopathic, or a consequence of histoplasmosis (Table 2). Pathologically the process is similar to hypertrophic wound healing, probably representing a vigorous autoimmune reaction to histoplasmosis. It has been suggested that treating with antifungal agents may exacerbate the inflammatory response. Because most patients come from areas where histoplasmosis is endogenous, serologic tests do not add to the diagnostic management. Urschel et al in 1990 noted, however, that ketoconazole, particularly in the setting of a persistently elevated *Histoplasma* complement fixation level, seemed to result in a diminished degree of mediastinal fibrosis. Radiologically a localized form is more common (82%), appears to be associated more often with histoplasmosis, and is not responsive to steroid therapy. The primary goal of surgical intervention is diagnosis, which usually, even in the setting of superior vena cava syndrome, requires mediastinoscopy, anterior mediastinotomy, or VATS mediastinal sampling. Palliation of superior vena cava syndrome can be achieved by spiral vein graft between the internal jugular vein and right atrial

---

Table 1 Surgical Approaches to Mediastinitis After Cardiac Surgery

Primary débridement and closure
Sternal irrigation with
    Normal saline
    0.5%-1.0% povidone-iodine (Betadine)
    Antibiotics
Delayed primary closure of the superficial subcutaneous wound
    (if sternum intact)
Omental flap
Muscle flap
    Pectoralis major
    Rectus abdominis
    Latissimus dorsi

Table 2 Differential Diagnosis of Chronic Fibrosing Mediastinitis

MALIGNANCY
Small cell lung cancer
Non–small cell lung cancer
Lymphoma
Thymic cancer
BENIGN
Infectious
(histoplasmosis, tuberculosis)
Autoimmune
Sarcoidosis
Riedel's struma
Postradiation fibrosis

appendage, but more recently endovascular stent grafts have been used. Stents also have been described as palliative measures for tracheobronchial, esophageal, and pulmonary artery obstruction.

SUGGESTED READING

Braxton JH, et al: Mediastinitis and long-term survival after coronary artery bypass graft surgery: Northern New England cardiovascular disease surgery group, *Ann Thorac Surg* 70:2004, 2000.

Cuschieri J, et al: Anterior mediastinal abscess after closed sternal fracture, *J Trauma* 47:551, 1999.

Freeman RK, et al: Descending necrotizing mediastinitis: an analysis of the effects of serial surgical debridement on patients' mortality, *J Thorac Cardiovasc Surg* 119:260, 2000.

Garret HE, Roper CL: Surgical intervention in histoplasmosis, *Ann Thorac Surg* 42:711, 1986.

Marty-Ané CH, Berthet JP, Alric P, et al: Management of descending necrotizing mediastinitis: an aggressive treatment for an aggressive disease, *Ann Thorac Surg* 68:212, 1999.

Wheatley MJ, et al: Descending necrotizing mediastinitis: transcervical drainage is not enough, *Ann Thorac Surg* 49:780, 1990.

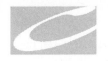

ESOPHAGEAL NEOPLASIA

BENIGN TUMORS OF THE ESOPHAGUS

Stephen M. Cattaneo II
Stephen C. Yang

Benign esophageal neoplasms are rare, constituting approximately 1% of all esophageal tumors. They usually cause nonspecific gastrointestinal symptoms with dysphagia being the most common. These tumors are typically slow growing, and many are asymptomatic until they achieve considerable size. Although they rarely undergo malignant change, benign neoplasms should be treated promptly to avoid developing irreversible swallowing difficulties. In most cases, surgical resection is curative and associated with only minimal morbidity. Although various classification schemes exist for these tumors, only the more commonly encountered neoplasms are described in detail.

■ LEIOMYOMAS

Leiomyomas are the most common benign esophageal tumors, comprising about 75% of these uncommon lesions. They are frequently small, asymptomatic tumors arising from smooth muscle fibers in the esophageal wall. When symptomatic, they cause dysphagia, pain, and other diverse digestive complaints. They are more common in men and usually are diagnosed in the 20s to 60s. Most of these tumors originate in the lower two thirds of the esophagus because esophageal smooth muscle predominates below the cervical level. Less than 3% are multiple.

Often these lesions are discovered incidentally. Barium esophagography classically shows a smooth, concave submucosal defect with sharp borders and no delay of barium passage. Endoscopic ultrasound and computed tomography may help define further the extent of these intramural lesions. Esophagoscopy should be performed to evaluate the character of the overlying mucosa. Typically, leiomyomas are mobile with overlying normal mucosa bulging into the esophageal lumen. Ulceration of the mucosa suggests sarcomatous degeneration of the tumor. Endoscopic biopsy is not warranted because subsequent submucosal inflammation may complicate eventual extramural enucleation.

Treatment decisions are based on size and symptoms. Although some authors recommend following small, asymptomatic leiomyomas by serial evaluations, all should be removed eventually to confirm the diagnosis and to preempt the possibility of malignant degeneration. Surgical excision is definitely warranted if these lesions are symptomatic or larger than 5 cm. A right-sided thoracotomy provides adequate exposure to middle third tumors, whereas lower third lesions necessitate a left-sided approach. Rare upper thoracic leiomyomas can be accessed by a transcervical approach with the option of an upper sternal split for tumors extending into the thoracic inlet.

The esophagus is encircled, and the tumor is located by palpation. After splitting the outer longitudinal muscle in the direction of the fibers, the tumor can be dissected away from the submucosa and adjacent muscle. Because these lesions typically are well encapsulated, enucleation usually can be achieved without entering the esophageal lumen. The integrity of the mucosa can be assessed by insufflation through a flexible scope (left in place after initial endoscopy) or a nasogastric tube with the distal tip positioned proximal to the gastroesophageal junction. Sizable extramucosal defects can be left without complication. If adequate removal necessitates mucosal resection, closure can be achieved with a low likelihood of stricture by resecting the mucosa in a longitudinal fashion and reapproximating in the same direction with absorbable suture. Short segment esophagectomy with end-to-end anastomosis may be necessary when these neoplasms are circumferential or affect the esophagogastric junction. Involvement of the latter may require a partial fundoplication. Reinforcement of any suture line or defect can be accomplished by covering the area with tissue, such as pleura or pericardial fat.

Leiomyomas occasionally can be removed by enucleation via video-assisted thoracic surgery (VATS). Flexible esophagoscopy is required simultaneously to avoid penetration into the esophageal lumen and to test the integrity of the mucosa.

When completely excised, leiomyomas almost never recur. Postoperative morbidity is low and most commonly related to esophageal stricture after mucosal resection.

■ INTRALUMINAL POLYPS

Polyps consisting primarily of fibrous and adipose tissue are much less common than leiomyomas, but these lesions can cause devastating complications. These fibrolipomas almost always originate in the cervical esophagus attached via a stalk near the level of the cricoid cartilage adjacent to the cricopharyngeus muscle. More common in older men, these polyps can achieve considerable size, sometimes longer than 20 cm, as peristaltic contractions pull on the polyp resulting in progressive lengthening of the pedicle. If symptomatic, patients most commonly experience dysphagia with the lesions often discovered by regurgitation of the pedicled tumor into the mouth. This method of presentation can be sensational, but regurgitation may result in laryngeal and upper airway obstruction with resultant asphyxiation. Less commonly, hematemesis or melena may occur if mucosal ulceration develops in polyps extending to the esophagogastric junction.

Although definitive diagnosis typically can be made only on surgical removal, diagnostic studies are useful in evaluating the characteristics and location of the lesion and planning the operative approach. Barium esophagography in most cases shows a smooth, intraluminal defect with rounding of the lower border. Occasionally the origin of the stalk also can be visualized. A large polyp may result in a dilated proximal esophagus, however, suggestive of achalasia. Manometry or other studies may be necessary to distinguish the two entities.

Esophagoscopy commonly shows an intraluminal mass easily displaced by the scope. Occasionally, false-negative examinations result if the overlying mucosa is intact and appears normal. Direct visualization may be helpful in determining the exact level of attachment of the stalk. Endoscopic biopsy can be difficult and may be complicated by perforation because these polyps are mobile. Computed tomography and magnetic resonance imaging are useful for larger masses and may provide information about the size of the mass and origin of the stalk.

Early surgical intervention is essential due to the risk of asphyxiation and potential for malignancy. Malignant, polypoid esophageal lesions, including carcinosarcoma, pseudosarcoma, and squamous cell carcinoma, can appear similar to benign fibrolipomatous polyps on diagnostic studies, so removal is necessary to exclude malignancy.

Surgical route is determined by the location and characteristics of the polypoid tumor in a similar manner to that discussed previously for leiomyomas. Options include a transoral approach or a cervical or transthoracic esophagotomy. Small, cervical polyps with relatively avascular stalks can be removed endoscopically with electrocoagulation of the stalk. A large cervical polyp can be excised via a lateral cervical longitudinal esophagotomy just distal to the upper esophageal sphincter. Large or intrathoracic polyps require an open approach. A polyp originating significantly below the thoracic inlet necessitates a thoracotomy with an esophagotomy opposite the site of attachment for adequate visualization. Additionally, highly vascular lesions require open excision so that the stalk can be ligated properly.

All approaches typically produce excellent results with only rare recurrences. Significant morbidity is rare, although patients who have a dilated esophagus preoperatively may experience mild, persistent dysphagia after the polyp is removed until return of normal esophageal size and function.

◼ HEMANGIOMAS

Hemangiomas are extremely rare, constituting only 2% to 3% of benign esophageal tumors. These lesions can occur throughout the esophagus, with half arising in the upper third.

Most symptomatic patients complain of dysphagia, but they also may experience hematemesis or melena due to periodic bleeding from the hemangioma.

Several diagnostic studies provide useful information. Barium esophagography typically identifies a well-circumscribed or lobulated intramural filling defect. Esophagoscopy can be diagnostic by showing normal mucosa overlying a reddish or bluish intramural lesion. Biopsy is not recommended due to potentially significant bleeding, despite the fact that the characteristic histology is diagnostic. Endoscopic ultrasound may be helpful for delineating tumor location and depth with a subsequent impact on resection options.

Hemangiomas discovered incidentally can be followed via serial endoscopies. If a hemangioma bleeds, however, treatment is essential. Multiple options exist, including endoscopic removal, endoscopic injection sclerotherapy, combined esophagoscopy and control via VATS, partial esophagectomy, and radiation therapy. Pedicled lesions located in mucosal or submucosal layers that are smaller than 2.5 cm can be treated adequately via endoscopic coagulation. Due to significant hemorrhagic and perforation risks, larger lesions with broad pedicles or intramuscular origins require complete open resection. Similar to other benign lesions, operative approach is dictated by tumor location within the esophagus. Local resection with standard closure is adequate because hemangiomas do not metastasize to lymph nodes or distant organs. During acute bleeding episodes, resection is necessary, as no reports exist of successful endoscopic injection sclerotherapy in these situations.

◼ GRANULAR CELL MYOBLASTOMAS

Granular cell myoblastomas, typically benign lesions now commonly referred to as *granular cell tumors,* are exceedingly uncommon. They likely are derived from Schwann cells, and 4% can be malignant. Although commonly found in the distal third of the esophagus, granular cell tumors can occur anywhere throughout the organ. As these lesions increase in size, they can cause symptoms of dysphagia or epigastric pain. Radiographic and endoscopic findings are similar to findings for leiomyomas.

Granular cell tumors assume a variety of shapes, including nodular, plaquelike, and polypoid. Consequently, various surgical options exist. Endoscopic removal, enucleation, and local resection all have been used successfully. Resection should be performed in symptomatic patients or if malignancy is suspected. In some instances, conservative management via serial examination is adequate.

◼ OTHER BENIGN TUMORS

Adenomas, papillomas, fibromas, fibromyomas, neurofibromas, carcinoid tumors, melanotic schwannomas, and inflammatory fibroid polyps are so rare that no consensus for management exists. These lesions are mentioned only for completeness.

SUGGESTED READING

Araki K, et al: Esophageal hemangioma: a case report and review of the literature, *Hepatogastroenterology* 46:3148, 1999.

Koyuncu M, et al: Giant polypoid tumor of the esophagus, *Auris Nasus Larynx* 27:363, 2000.

Postlethwait RW, Lowe JE: Benign tumors and cysts of the esophagus. In Orringer MB, Zuidema GD, editors: *Shackelford's surgery of the alimentary tract*, vol 1, *The esophagus*, ed 4. Philadelphia, 1996, WB Saunders, p 369.

Pross M, et al: Thoracoscopic enucleation of benign tumors of the esophagus under simultaneous flexible esophagoscopy, *Surg Endosc* 14:1146, 2000.

Vrabec AP, Colley AT: Giant intraluminal polyps of the esophagus, *Ann Otol Rhinol Laryngol* 92:344, 1983.

CARCINOMA OF THE CERVICAL ESOPHAGUS

Jonathan Trites
Alan G. Casson

Less than 10% of all primary esophageal tumors involve the cervical esophagus, and they are almost exclusively squamous cell carcinomas. The cervical esophagus, which measures only 3 to 5 cm in length, extends from the cricoid cartilage to the thoracic inlet (suprasternal notch) and is in close proximity to several vital structures. Direct invasion of the airway or adjacent neurovascular structures generally has limited surgical resection of cervical esophageal cancers, which traditionally have been treated with radiotherapy. The cervical esophagus also may be invaded directly by primary tumors of the larynx, hypopharynx, thyroid, and trachea.

Despite an aggressive tumor biology and advanced tumor stage at presentation, selected patients with cervical esophageal cancer or tumors of the head and neck invading the esophagus may benefit from surgery, in terms of both palliation and survival. Optimal management now generally is achieved using a multidisciplinary approach, employing the expertise of radiation and medical oncologists, speech therapists, nutritionists, nurses, and social workers, in addition to various surgical specialists, including otolaryngology, general thoracic surgery, and plastic and reconstructive surgery.

■ DIAGNOSIS AND STAGING

A thorough history and physical examination is performed initially to diagnose and assess symptoms related to the local effects of the primary tumor, possible metastatic sites, and the general physiologic status of the patient. Symptoms of esophageal obstruction inevitably include dysphagia, or change in swallowing. Airway or pulmonary symptoms occasionally may predominate. Physical examination may show a neck mass, cervical lymphadenopathy, or signs of metastatic or comorbid disease. Objective studies of the upper aerodigestive tract are essential to establish a tissue diagnosis, for staging, and to plan further treatment. These studies include a dynamic contrast swallowing study (dilute barium); rigid and/or flexible endoscopy (laryngoscopy, bronchoscopy, esophagogastroscopy) with biopsy; and computed tomography of the neck, chest, and upper abdomen. Additional imaging to evaluate potential distant metastases (or second primary tumors) should be based on clinical suspicion rather than performed routinely. Because many patients have significant associated disease, particular attention should be paid to assessment of nutritional and fluid and electrolyte status, in addition to cardiorespiratory and thyroid function.

Interest in multimodality therapy, particularly induction chemotherapy or chemoradiotherapy, through multicenter cooperative clinical trials, mandates accurate tumor staging if valid comparisons are to be made between participating centers and between therapeutic modalities. To date, a totally satisfactory staging system has not been developed for cervical esophageal cancers, however.

■ MANAGEMENT

Progressive dysphagia, severe dehydration, malnutrition, chronic aspiration with pulmonary sepsis, and upper airway obstruction are the sequelae of untreated cervical esophageal carcinoma. Tracheostomy and gastrostomy alone are associated with extremely poor quality of life and should be avoided. Selected patients (generally poor performance with limited life expectancy) may benefit from placement of endoluminal stents. Despite technical advances in the development of self-expanding covered wire stents, which may be readily placed radiologically or endoscopically, large proximal tumors still may be technically difficult or impossible to stent in a satisfactory manner. Other complications of stent placement include bleeding, perforation, migration, and obstruction, against the background of tumor progression. Techniques to dilate the airway and esophagus and laser ablation of endoluminal disease are only of temporary benefit and should be used in conjunction with more definitive therapy.

External beam radiation therapy traditionally has been used to palliate cervical esophageal cancer. Although improved palliation is reported using radical (versus palliative) doses, local edema, mucositis, and fibrosis may result in increased dysphagia. Consideration should be given to early placement of surgical feeding tubes (jejunostomy) for fluid and nutritional support, which may be removed easily on completion of radiation therapy, when swallowing is restored. Long-term complications of radiation therapy include esophageal stricture (which may be particularly difficult to manage, especially if associated with gastroesophageal reflux) and the development of tracheoesophageal fistula. Strategies to improve radiation therapy outcomes include use of brachytherapy, hyperfractionation schedules, and concurrent chemotherapy, particularly the administration of radiosensitizing agents. Currently available chemotherapeutic agents (single or combination) have limited efficacy in esophageal malignancy.

To date, relatively few studies have critically evaluated outcomes (including quality of life) of various treatment modalities for these uncommon tumors. For selected patients with localized, early stage, or recurrent cervical esophageal tumors, surgical resection, comprising pharyngolaryngoesophagectomy (with radical neck dissection or exenteration) and one-stage reconstruction of the upper gastrointestinal tract (stomach or free jejunum), has been used successfully to palliate and "cure" this disease. Although current surgical mortality rates for this major surgical resection are low (now generally <5%), postoperative morbidity is significant, even in centers with considerable experience in managing these patients. Current controversies relate to patient selection and the role of induction (preoperative) therapy.

■ SURGICAL APPROACH

Preoperative

Careful attention should be directed to the general medical condition of the patient in preparation for general anesthesia, particularly cardiorespiratory function. Hypothyroidism should be treated, especially in patients who have received previous radiation therapy. Stopping cigarette smoking for at least 2 weeks before surgery is recommended because this significantly reduces secretions and improves perioperative respiratory function. Although cessation of tobacco and alcohol intake, both well-established risk factors for squamous cell carcinomas of the upper aerodigestive tract, is advisable, the effects of withdrawal may become apparent. Preoperative nutritional support is advocated by some surgeons but is unlikely to reverse the catabolic state. Rather, attention should be directed to correction of fluid and electrolyte anomalies.

Table 1 summarizes several key surgical management issues that are helpful in planning the operative approach. The extent of resection generally is based on preoperative staging. The technique of reconstruction of the upper gastrointestinal tract must be planned in advance. If a free jejunal interposition graft is planned, this requires microvascular anastomosis; reconstruction with colon requires a thorough mechanical bowel preparation. Preoperative mesenteric angiography to define colonic vascular anatomy is useful in planning which segment to interpose. The final assessment

---

Table 1 Surgical Management Issues to Consider When Planning Resection and Reconstruction for Cervical Esophageal Carcinoma

Extent of esophageal resection
　Partial versus total (transhiatal/thoracoscopic/transthoracic)
Preservation of the larynx
Status of the neck
　Unilateral or bilateral lymphadenectomy
　Cervical exenteration
Superior mediastinum
　Transsternal exposure
　Mediastinal tracheostomy
Thyroid/parathyroid function
　Preservation versus reimplantation
Reconstruction of the upper gastrointestinal tract
　Gastric transposition (whole stomach versus greater curve
　　gastric tube)
　Free jejunal interposition (with microvascular anastomosis)
　Colon (isoperistaltic; descending/transverse versus ascending)
　Tubed skin-free flap (e.g., forearm)
Placement of feeding jejunostomy

---

of colon viability is made operatively, however. Prophylactic antibiotics are administered intravenously to all patients on induction of anesthesia.

Finally, it is important to have a full and a realistic discussion of expected outcomes and potential complications with the patient and family. Informed consent must be obtained from the patient before surgery.

Operative

In the presence of airway invasion, it is essential for the surgeon and anesthesiologist to discuss how the airway should be secured. It may be necessary for the surgeon to perform a tracheostomy or rigid/flexible bronchoscopy to place the endotracheal tube. After general anesthesia, it is often advisable to repeat selected endoscopic procedures (laryngoscopy, bronchoscopy, esophagogastroscopy), especially if there has been a delay after initial diagnosis, to ensure there has been no interval change in the tumor and to reevaluate upper aerodigestive tract anatomy. Patient positioning is generally supine. Draping should permit access to the neck, chest, and abdomen.

The neck is explored initially through a (collar) neck incision. Limited lesions involving only the cervical esophagus are uncommon. The difficulty is usually the extent of proximal resection required (1) to obtain a clear proximal resection margin and (2) to avoid injury to adjacent structures, particularly the recurrent laryngeal nerves, larynx, and posterior membranous trachea. Although en bloc sleeve resection of the trachea with primary end-to end anastomosis (preserving laryngeal function) is reported, this is appropriate for few patients in practice. Despite extensive submucosal spread, distal resection margins for cervical esophageal carcinomas are rarely difficult to obtain, and even 3 to 4 cm below macroscopic tumor (with negative histology on frozen section) would be appropriate. Distal extension of tumor through the thoracic inlet may require a partial (upper) median sternotomy. Further exposure of the upper thoracic esophagus (above the tracheal bifurcation) may be obtained by extending the sternotomy across the right anterior chest wall in the third or fourth interspace. If the tumor extends to or below the thoracic inlet, resection of the entire thoracic esophagus generally is performed using a transhiatal approach. The rationale for total esophagectomy is primarily to facilitate reconstruction (gastric transposition), to avoid an intrathoracic anastomosis, and to resect all esophageal squamous mucosa that may be at risk for second primary carcinomas or skip lesions.

For most patients with cervical esophageal carcinoma, it is technically impossible to salvage a functional larynx. In addition to resection of the cervical esophagus, adequate proximal and lateral resection margins can be obtained only with en bloc resection of the entire larynx, proximal trachea, and lower pharynx. Partial laryngectomy is inappropriate for cervical esophageal carcinoma.

Carcinomas secondarily involving the cervical esophagus (by direct invasion) generally require more extensive surgery. These include tumors invading the posterior cricoid, tumors involving the apex of the pyriform sinus, tumors presenting with vocal cord paralysis, and tumors presenting with localized tracheal stomal recurrence after previous laryngectomy.

Surgical management of regional lymph nodes must be considered in all patients with cervical esophageal cancer because the incidence of cervical nodal metastasis at the time of presentation ranges from 60% to 75%, with 10% to 25% of patients presenting with bilateral neck disease. Most squamous cell carcinomas requiring laryngopharyngo-esophagectomy warrant concurrent bilateral neck dissections. For the N0 neck, lymphadenectomy is performed at levels II, III, IV (high, mid, and low parajugular), and VI (central) and the paratracheal nodes, which represent the first echelon drainage basin for the cervical esophagus. Overt neck disease is managed with a radical or modified radical neck dissection of levels I through VI. Many of these tumors are managed best with a "cervical exenteration," which involves en bloc resection of all tissue between the carotids, superior to the innominate artery, and superficial to the prevertebral fascia.

Techniques for primary reconstruction of the upper gastrointestinal tract depend on the extent of esophageal resection. Reconstruction after total esophagectomy is preferably by gastric transposition, which remains the most satisfactory substitute for the esophagus in terms of swallowing and gastrointestinal function. The technique for mobilizing the stomach is technically straightforward and has been well described. Care must be taken to minimize handling of the stomach and to preserve the right gastroepiploic artery and corresponding venous drainage. A relatively narrow isoperistaltic tube is created from the greater curvature of the stomach, by resecting the lesser curvature and esophagogastric junction. This is preferable to use of the whole stomach. A generous Kocher maneuver to mobilize the second part of duodenum, including the proximal third part to the superior mesenteric vessels, is essential. Sufficient length of stomach to reach the oropharynx can be obtained for most patients, even for patients who have had previous antireflux surgery (fundoplication). The most direct route to the neck is to place the gastric tube in the esophageal bed (orthotopic position). The tip of the gastric tube is anastomosed to the pharynx, generally using a single layer of interrupted absorbable sutures. The anastomosis should be tension-free but should not be anchored to the adjacent prevertebral fascia (or anterior longitudinal ligament).

Free jejunal interposition grafts have been used with increasing frequency since the 1990s. Their success reflects advances in microvascular surgery. Provided that a clear distal esophageal resection margin is obtained, the advantage of this approach is that the mediastinal dissection is avoided. When performed by experienced surgeons, results (mortality, morbidity, anastomotic leak, graft viability, stricture, long-term swallowing) are generally comparable to gastric transposition, although operative time is longer. Alternative free tissue transfer approaches for esophageal reconstruction include use of a tubed fasciocutaneous flap, avoiding laparotomy. The radial forearm free flap provides sufficient surface area of skin and subcutaneous tissue that is highly pliable and well suited to reconstruct a tubed viscus. Although stricture rates are less frequent for mucosa-lined flaps, speech rehabilitation is superior for those lined by skin.

Pedicled myocutaneous flaps (deltopectoral, latissimus dorsi, pectoralis major) were used historically for delayed (staged) closure of pharyngoesophageal defects. In current practice, they rarely are used for primary reconstruction, but they have a place in the surgical armamentarium for managing postoperative complications. Finally, it is recommended that a surgical feeding tube, preferably a jejunostomy, be placed.

Postoperative

Careful attention to postoperative management is essential to minimize the morbidity associated with this procedure. A short period of respiratory support (<12 hours) is often useful, especially if operating time is prolonged. Because the patient has a permanent tracheostoma, access to the airway presents little difficulty. All patients receive chest physiotherapy and are ambulated early to reduce further potential respiratory complications. Enteral feeding usually is started within 24 hours postoperatively, using the feeding jejunostomy. A nasogastric tube is kept on low suction to minimize reflux to the anastomosis and to decompress the interposed gastric conduit. A contrast study, initially water-soluble followed by barium, is obtained on the fifth to seventh postoperative day. If no anastomotic leak is seen, the nasogastric tube is removed, and the patient is started on clear liquids by mouth. If the patient develops signs of sepsis at any stage during the postoperative course, investigations are initiated immediately to determine its etiology. In addition to the usual sites of postoperative infection, it is essential to evaluate the viability of interposed conduit (careful endoscopy) and anastomosis (contrast study). At the time of discharge from the hospital, the patient should be able to manage several small meals of semisolid food daily. The patient is discharged with the feeding tube clamped, and this is removed at the first postoperative follow-up visit.

■ RESULTS

Large series data are limited because these are infrequent procedures. Morbidity and mortality generally are related to the reason for resection, the extent of surgical extirpation and reconstruction, and the use of preoperative radiation. Squamous cell carcinoma is the histology in nearly 90% of all cases, arising from the cervical esophagus, hypopharynx, or larynx. Primary tumors of the thyroid or trachea account for the rest. Using the stomach as the conduit to restore gastrointestinal continuity is possible in 95% of the cases; the colon or a jejunal free flap is required for the rest. The anastomosis is particularly susceptible to leaks or disruption if there is a history of radiation to the cervical area, with an estimated incidence of 30%; this almost always resolves with open drainage alone. Iatrogenic hypothyroidism and hypoparathyroidism also are significant depending on the extent of resection and preoperative radiation use. Along with the increased complication rate is a prolonged length of hospital stay, with half of all patients requiring hospitalization for 3 to 8 weeks. Although operative mortality is comparable to standard esophagectomy of the intrathoracic esophagus,

1-year survival of 60% is much less, usually due to recurrence of the primary tumor. Long-term survival is associated with general satisfaction of dysphagia and respiratory symptoms, however.

SUGGESTED READING

Bardini R, et al: Therapeutic options for cancer of the hypopharynx and cervical esophagus, *Ann Chir Gynaecol* 84:202, 1995.

Goldberg M, et al: Transhiatal esophagectomy with gastric transposition for pharyngolaryngeal malignant disease, *J Thorac Cardiovasc Surg* 97:327, 1989.

Grillo HC, Mathiesen DJ: Cervical exenteration, *Ann Thorac Surg* 49:401, 1990.

Reece GP, et al: Morbidity and functional outcome of free jejunal transfer reconstruction for circumferential defects of the pharynx and cervical esophagus, *Plast Reconstr Surg* 96:1307, 1995.

UPPER THORACIC ESOPHAGEAL CANCER

Carolyn E. Reed

■ BACKGROUND

Cancer of the esophagus is an uncommon malignancy in the United States (6 cases per 100,000 per year), but worldwide it is one of the 10 most common solid tumors. Squamous cell cancer dominates in non-Western countries. There has been a dramatic shift in histology in Western countries, however, with the incidence of esophageal adenocarcinoma in the United States increasing more rapidly than any other cancer. The etiology of this steady rise in white men is thought to be related to chronic gastroesophageal reflux and the development of columnar-lined esophagus. The risk factor of Barrett's esophagus and the institution of endoscopic surveillance programs allow the potential to identify esophageal adenocarcinoma in early stages, when surgical management can be most effective.

Of patients with esophageal cancer, 50% or more present with advanced locoregional or distant disease. Palliative options include many endoluminal therapies to relieve dysphagia, such as esophageal stenting, photodynamic therapy, and laser ablation. Radiotherapy has been the gold standard for palliation, but it has a delay in treatment effect and risk of

stricture formation. Self-expanding metallic stents are presently the most popular palliative method in the United States. There is a high technical success rate, but these devices require careful follow-up because the reintervention rate for a variety of complications is high.

The surgical options for a patient with esophageal cancer involve many issues, including proper staging, surgical approach, extent of resection, the role of adjuvant therapy, and increasing emphasis on quality-of-life issues. Esophageal resection results in a significant surgical insult to the patient. Improvements in surgical technique and perioperative management have decreased mortality to less than 10% (2% in some series), but morbidity remains high (20% to 40%).

■ STAGING

The staging of esophageal cancer has been imprecise, and the adequacy of the present TNM system has been questioned. With the rising incidence of distal and gastroesophageal junction (GEJ) adenocarcinomas, the inclusion versus exclusion of patients for surgery with M1a (celiac nodal) disease is an important issue.

Computed tomography (CT) has been the most frequently used staging tool. CT can show distant metastases or obvious locally unresectable disease in 50% of patients. CT underestimates stage in greater than 40% of patients, however. It cannot differentiate adequately the depth of tumor invasion and has an accuracy of detecting regional lymph node disease of only 55% to 60%.

Endoscopic ultrasound (EUS) is presently the most accurate noninvasive method to assess tumor (T) status and should be considered a standard staging tool. In experienced hands, dilation of obstructing lesions before EUS results in successful completion of EUS staging in greater than 90% of cases. The ability of EUS to detect regional lymph nodes is much increased over CT. Celiac axis lymph nodes are accessible by EUS-guided fine needle aspiration. EUS/fine needle aspiration allows potential assessment of response to induction therapy. Residual M1a disease predicts poor survival.

Thoracoscopic/laparoscopic staging has been proposed as a more accurate method for lymph node assessment in esophageal cancer. Several studies have shown the feasibility and high accuracy in identifying positive lymph nodes. The final role of thoracoscopic/laparoscopic staging remains to be proven, however.

Positron emission tomography can detect unsuspected distant metastases in 10% to 20% of patients. The role of positron emission tomography for detecting nodal disease is less clear because peritumoral lymph nodes often are obscured by tumor uptake.

■ SURGICAL APPROACH

Surgical approaches for esophagectomy include Ivor-Lewis (abdominal–right thoracic), three-field or McKeown (right thoracic-abdominal-cervical), transhiatal (abdominal-cervical), left thoracic, and left thoracoabdominal. Choice of approach depends on tumor characteristics and location, surgeon's preference, and overall surgical philosophy. The right or left transthoracic approach is used for lower third and GEJ tumors and anastomosis is in the upper thorax. For middle third or higher lesions, a three-field approach or transhiatal approach allows anastomosis in the neck. Because a transhiatal approach avoids thoracotomy, the purported advantages are the minimizing of respiratory complications and the easy management of anastomotic complications. Disadvantages are the inability to perform a complete node dissection and the inability always to visualize the tumor. A transthoracic technique allows direct visualization and dissection of periesophageal and nodal tissue. Disadvantages include the increased morbidity of anastomotic leak and cardiopulmonary insult secondary to a thoracotomy. The two most popular surgical approaches in the United States are the Ivor-Lewis and transhiatal, both of which are discussed in more detail. Despite continuing controversy, retrospective and prospective series have shown no difference in mortality or morbidity. Some series have shown less pulmonary morbidity with the transhiatal approach. No contemporary study has shown any difference in long-term survival outcome.

Ivor-Lewis Technique

After an upper abdominal incision, the left triangular ligament is incised, and the esophagus at the hiatus is assessed for tumor resectability. A Penrose drain is used to encircle the esophagus. If there are no intraabdominal contraindications, the stomach is mobilized, preserving the right gastroepiploic artery (omentum divided at least 2 cm away from the vessels) and right gastric artery. Short gastric arteries are divided (using 2-0 silk ties or harmonic scalpel). When the greater curvature of the stomach is mobilized to the hiatus, the gastrohepatic ligament is divided. Exposure of the left gastric vessels is easiest through the lesser sac with the stomach retracted upward.

A celiac node dissection is performed, and lymphoareolar tissue is swept upward to be included en bloc with the specimen. The celiac axis is marked with a stitch for pathologic examination. A generous Kocher maneuver is performed. A pyloroplasty or pyloromyotomy is performed to avoid problems with gastric emptying secondary to vagotomy. The hiatus is widened, and dissection of the esophagus is extended into the lower thorax. This greatly facilitates final dissection at this level from the chest. An area at the fourth level of the left gastric vascular arcade (necessary to include lesser curvature lymph nodes) is cleared on the lesser curvature in preparation for stapling of the stomach. A soft jejunostomy tube is placed routinely, and the abdomen is closed.

The patient is placed in the left lateral decubitus position, and the chest is entered through the fifth intercostal space. The azygos vein is ligated and divided. The esophagus is dissected in the retrotracheal region and encircled with a Penrose drain used for traction. The pleura is incised over the esophagus from the divided azygos vein superiorly to the thoracic inlet. Inferior to the vein, the pleura is incised along the spine (avoiding injury to the thoracic duct) and along the right bronchus and pericardium. The inferior pulmonary ligament is incised. The esophagus is circumferentially dissected with its periesophageal tissues and lymph nodes (including the subcarinal packet) between the aorta posteriorly and the trachea and pericardium anteriorly. The esophagus is transected above the azygos vein, allowing 7 to 10 cm of margin above tumor. The stomach is guided into the chest and tubularized by excising the proximal two thirds of the lesser curvature. The stapler is applied from the fundus down and from the lesser curvature up so that a V-shaped wedge of stomach beyond the GEJ is removed (at least 5 cm from tumor).

There are several choices of anastomotic suturing. If using a stapling technique, the side-to-side esophagogastrostomy using an Endo-GIA is favored and creates a large anastomosis with a minimal leak rate (Figures 1 and 2).

Transhiatal Esophagectomy

The abdominal portion proceeds as outlined for the Ivor-Lewis technique. The cervical dissection is performed through an incision along the anterior border of the left sternocleidomastoid muscle. This muscle and the carotid sheath are retracted laterally, the omohyoid muscle is cut, and dissection is carried down to the prevertebral fascia. Blunt dissection is performed posterior to the esophagus along the prevertebral fascia. The recurrent laryngeal nerve is identified and preserved in the tracheoesophageal groove. The cervical esophagus is encircled carefully with a blunt dissector, and a small Penrose drain is used for traction during mediastinal dissection.

The mediastinal dissection is performed from above and below along the posterior and anterior surfaces of the esophagus with a finger or sponge-on-a-stick (peanut dissector better from the cervical end). With the hiatus widened and good retraction, the mediastinal dissection from below can proceed under direct vision until almost the carina. Thoracoscopic instruments are helpful here. Fingers are used to rake the lateral attachments that cannot be visualized in the small distance between the carina and mobilized cervical esophagus.

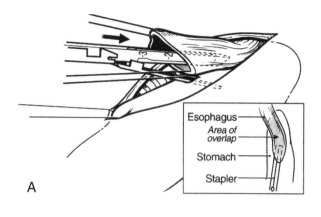

A

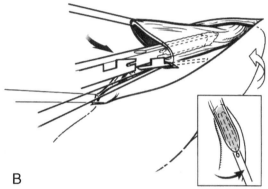

B

Figure 1
A, An Endo-GIA staple cartridge is inserted into the esophagus and stomach. **B,** The stapler is advanced and rotated. *(From Orringer MB, et al:* J Thorac Cardiovasc Surg *119:279, 2000.)*

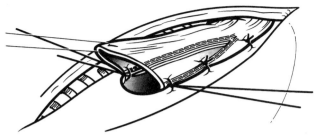

Figure 2
After firing the stapler, a long side-to-side anastomosis is created. Suspension seromuscular sutures between the adjacent esophagus and stomach have been placed before firing. The gastrotomy and remaining open esophagus are then closed. *(From Orringer MB, et al:* J Thorac Cardiovasc Surg *119:280, 2000.)*

The tubularized stomach is delivered to the neck, either by an endoscopy bag placed on suction or guided and pushed through the posterior mediastinum with gentle traction on a sutured Penrose drain, until the fundus can be grasped with a Babcock clamp in the cervical wound. Extensive traction at the point of anastomosis must be avoided. It is recommended that prevertebral tacking sutures not be placed to avoid complications. Either a hand-sewn or stapled anastomosis is performed.

Other Approaches
Three-field esophagectomy combines aspects of the thoracic, abdominal, and cervical portions of the previously outlined procedures. It allows for complete nodal dissection. The left thoracic approach can be used for distal third and GEJ tumors. It is carried out through a left seventh intercostal space and a semilunar diaphragmatic incision 2 to 4 cm from the costal margin. The disadvantages of this approach include the inability to perform a generous Kocher maneuver and a gastric emptying procedure, the difficulty performing a jejunostomy, and the limitation of proximal extension if tumor is found at the margin.

Surgeons have investigated a minimally invasive approach to esophagectomy. Video-assisted thoracic surgery potentially avoids the risks of thoracotomy, yet allows mobilization of the thoracic esophagus and lymph node sampling under direct visual control. Laparoscopic mobilization of the stomach and subsequent open cervical anastomosis complete the approach. Minimally invasive esophagectomy has been shown to be technically feasible and safe in centers with extensive laparoscopic/thoracoscopic experience.

■ EXTENT OF LYMPHADENECTOMY

The extent of lymph node dissection is an ongoing controversy (i.e., improved survival versus only improved staging). Some thoracic surgeons have favored a radical en bloc esophagectomy that encompasses complete mediastinal and upper abdominal lymph node dissections potentially to enhance survival in a few patients with nodal metastases. The Japanese have extended dissection to lymph nodes in the neck and thoracic inlet (a three-field lymphadenectomy). They have shown a 20% to 30% incidence of cervical lymph node metastases in patients undergoing three-field lymphadenectomy, and this has been confirmed by a U.S. group for adenocarcinoma. Some Japanese surgeons have shown improved survival with three-field compared with two-field lymphadenectomy. It seems, however, that survival benefit is not appreciable for early or advanced (more than five positive lymph nodes or T4) esophageal cancer. This aggressive approach requires considerable surgical skill and must be weighed against increased morbidity. Extended lymphadenectomy has a marked impact on postoperative respiratory function with increased tracheal bronchorrhea and subsequent need for mechanical ventilation and recurrent laryngeal nerve injury.

■ ADJUVANT THERAPY

Results of surgery alone for esophageal cancer depend on stage. The basic biology of this cancer when the patient presents with symptoms and the anatomic realities make a resection for cure difficult to achieve, however. The 5-year survival for stage III disease is about 10% to 15% in most series. This lack of success with surgery alone has led to the investigation of preoperative and postoperative adjuvant therapies.

Postoperative adjuvant therapy allows for treatment based on precise pathologic findings. The rationale for neoadjuvant or induction therapy has been to (1) improve local control and enhance tumor resectability, (2) assess tumor response, (3) treat micrometastases when chemotherapy is used, and (4) treat the patient when potential toxicity can be tolerated better.

Preoperative Radiation Therapy

Five randomized studies comparing preoperative radiotherapy followed by resection to surgery alone failed to show any survival benefit. These studies are old, staging was poor, and the delivery techniques are outmoded. A meta-analysis updating these five trials showed an absolute survival benefit of 4% at 5 years, but this did not reach statistical significance. At present, preoperative radiotherapy cannot be recommended.

Induction Chemotherapy

Several phase III studies have been completed, with the largest being the U.S. intergroup trial reported by Kelsen. Although the studies show the feasibility of this approach, survival benefit has not been shown. There may be a variety of reasons for this finding, but a low pathologic complete response rate (<10%) may be the major factor. As in stage III (N2) non–small cell lung cancer, improved survival is seen when significant down-staging occurs. In the U.S. study, induction chemotherapy did decrease the distant failure rate but not local failure. Almost all studies have used 5-fluorouracil and cisplatin as induction agents. Newer drugs (taxanes and camptothecins) have yet to be studied adequately.

Induction Chemoradiotherapy

Phase II studies with induction chemotherapy and concurrent radiotherapy (40 to 50 Gy) have shown higher pathologic complete response rates (20% to 40%). Phase III studies have shown contradictory results. The Walsh study from Ireland reported on 105 patients with adenocarcinoma randomized to induction chemoradiotherapy (cisplatin/5-fluorouracil/40 Gy) versus surgery alone with a striking improvement in survival favoring the combined modality arm.

The long-term follow-up of the Michigan trial (induction triple-drug chemotherapy and hyperfractionated radiotherapy versus surgery alone) failed to show superiority for the investigational arm. A European study enrolling only patients with squamous cell carcinoma also failed to show a survival advantage for induction chemoradiation. Further studies need to be done. The U.S. intergroup trial was closed secondary to lack of accrual. Standard community practice has embraced the chemoradiation induction approach, but the data fail to support its use as routine. Future studies need to address uniform staging practices, selection bias, inclusion of M1a patients (positive celiac lymph nodes), and the statistical power of the study.

Postoperative Adjuvant Therapy

Although a lower rate of local recurrence has been shown in some studies using postoperative adjuvant radiotherapy, there has been no benefit to overall survival. The use of chemotherapy as postoperative adjuvant therapy targeting occult micrometastases has been studied best by the Japanese and is restricted to squamous cell carcinoma. These studies have failed to show significant benefit even with lymph node stratification.

■ NONSURGICAL TREATMENT FOR STAGE I THROUGH III ESOPHAGEAL CANCER

For patients who are potentially resectable (stages I through III) but are medically unfit, who refuse surgery, or who are treated by physicians with a nonsurgical bias, options include radiotherapy alone or chemoradiotherapy. Various studies have established the superiority of the combined approach. The Herskovic trial randomizing patients to chemotherapy (cisplatin/5-fluorouracil) and radiotherapy (50 Gy) versus radiotherapy alone (64 Gy) showed that the use of combined chemoradiotherapy improved local control and had a lower risk of distant failure. Five-year survival was 26% in the combined arm, but no patient treated with radiotherapy alone was alive at 5 years. Combined chemoradiotherapy was associated with significant severe and life-threatening acute toxicities, however. The use of three-dimensional treatment planning and conformal therapy, the implementation of intensity-modulated radiotherapy, and continued investigation of differing fractionation schedules will bring new information to this therapeutic option.

■ COMPLICATIONS OF SURGERY AND QUALITY OF LIFE

Esophageal surgery is a morbid procedure. Anastomotic leak affects quality of life and can lead to stricture formation. Although easily managed in the neck by simple open drainage, thoracic leaks lead to sepsis and high risk of death. Leaks are related to surgical technique and tension. The catastrophic complication of gastric tip necrosis must be identified early and treated aggressively (takedown of remnant to the abdomen) to salvage the patient. Any early sign of dysphagia should be treated by bedside Maloney bougienage because development of fibrotic strictures may require numerous dilations. Chylothorax requires early intervention to avoid nutritional consequences and prolonged hospitalization. Reoperation with thoracic duct ligation is recommended early (5 to 7 days) or after talc slurry via chest thoracostomy has failed. Cardiac arrhythmias are common but usually of atrial etiology and easily controlled. Pulmonary complications are the leading cause of morbidity in most series, and hospital-acquired pneumonia is highly lethal. The patient's baseline pulmonary function, nutritional status, use of induction therapy, thoracotomy, and extent of lymphadenectomy all may play a role.

Quality of life after esophagectomy is affected by post-thoracotomy pain, recurrent laryngeal nerve injury, altered gastric motility, and the presence of anastomotic stricture. Esophagectomy patients require careful follow-up for management and provider psychosocial support. Use of the stomach as a conduit results in altered gastric function in all patients. Routine measures (elevation of head of bed on blocks, decreased drinking of fluids with meals, small frequent meals, and abstinence from oral intake about 2 hours before bedtime) suffice in most patients. Reflux, delayed gastric emptying, and the dumping syndrome may require more aggressive medical management, however, and willingness to try a variety of agents. The use of oral erythromycin (750 mg twice a day), a motilin-receptor agonist, has shown efficacy in improving gastric emptying.

■ FUTURE ISSUES

The role of surgery in esophageal cancer will continue to evolve. The value of new staging techniques, the ability to detect responders versus nonresponders to induction therapy, and the role of molecular stratification need clarification. The true prevalence of Barrett's esophagus and easier, more cost-effective screening to identify the early stages of carcinogenesis await development. Continued modification of palliative techniques to increase the quality of life of patients with advanced disease is needed.

SUGGESTED READING

Ellis FH, et al: Esophagogastrectomy for carcinoma of the esophagus and cardia: a comparison of findings and results after standard resection in three consecutive eight-year intervals with improved staging criteria, *J Thorac Cardiovasc Surg* 113:836, 1997.

Kelsen DP, et al: Chemotherapy followed by surgery compared with surgery alone for localized esophageal cancer, *N Engl J Med* 339:1979, 1998.

Krasna MJ: Esophageal cancer, *Chest Surg Clin N Am* 10:441, 2000.

Orringer MB, et al: Transhiatal esophagectomy: clinical experience and refinements, *Ann Surg* 230:392, 1999.

Reed CE: Surgical management of esophageal carcinoma, *Oncologist* 4:95, 1999.

Urba SG, et al: Randomized trial of preoperative chemoradiation versus surgery alone in patients with locoregional esophageal carcinoma, *J Clin Oncol* 19:305, 2001.

Walsh TN, et al: A comparison of multimodality therapy and surgery for esophageal adenocarcinoma, *N Engl J Med* 335:462, 1996.

CANCER OF THE GASTROESOPHAGEAL JUNCTION

Richard F. Heitmiller

Elaine E. Tseng

Cancer of the gastroesophageal junction (GEJ) is adenocarcinoma. Since the late 1980s, there has been a dramatic increase in the prevalence of esophagogastric adenocarcinoma in the United States. Currently at Johns Hopkins, esophageal adenocarcinoma (including tumors at the GEJ) is more common than squamous cell carcinoma by a factor of 3:1 (Figure 1). Not all esophageal adenocarcinoma involves the GEJ. Esophageal adenocarcinoma invariably involves the lower third of the esophagus, however, near the GEJ, and the clinical characteristics, staging workup, and treatment options are similar for the two groups (esophageal adenocarcinoma with and without GEJ involvement). Whether or not esophagogastric adenocarcinoma is a distinct clinical entity with unique pathogenesis, pattern of nodal metastatic spread, and prognosis is unresolved. This chapter summarizes the current data related to these tumors.

■ PATHOGENESIS

The reason for the increase in prevalence of esophageal adenocarcinoma is not known with certainty. Clinical and molecular genetic evidence support a unified model of tumor pathogenesis. Adenocarcinoma arises from Barrett's mucosa through an intermediate step involving mucosal dysplasia in a process mediated by gastroesophageal reflux (GER). Whether the pathogenesis of esophageal, esophagogastric, and gastric adenocarcinoma is the same is not proved. Patients with esophageal and esophagogastric tumors have similar clinical characteristics, which are distinctly different from gastric tumors; this suggests that esophageal and esophagogastric tumors share a similar pathogenesis, which is different than gastric tumors.

■ CLINICAL CHARACTERISTICS

The clinical characteristics of patients with esophageal or GEJ adenocarcinoma are remarkably consistent. Esophageal adenocarcinoma is a disease of white men (87%), 57 to 66 years old (mean age 60), with a history of GER. A history of cigarette smoking and alcohol consumption is elicited in approximately 50% of patients. Barrett's mucosa is identified in 63% of patients undergoing esophagectomy for adenocarcinoma. Many believe that all cases of adenocarcinoma arise from Barrett's esophagus, and when Barrett's mucosa is not identified, it was replaced by tumor. The clinical characteristics of patients with and without Barrett's esophagus are similar.

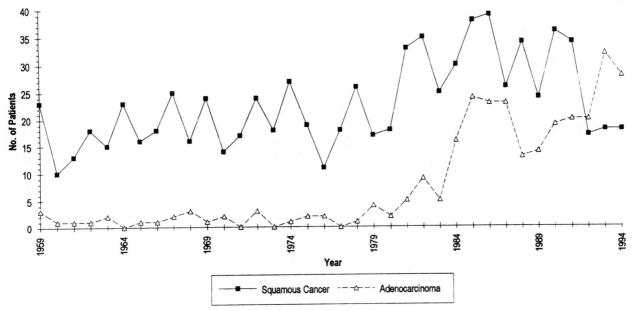

Figure 1
Prevalence of esophageal cancer by cell type at the Johns Hopkins Hospital, 1959-1994.

In contrast, patients with gastric adenocarcinoma are much less likely to be white men (30%), with a 2.1:1 male-to-female ratio. The data suggest a trend toward greater age with increasing gastric involvement with a mean age at presentation of 65 years for gastric cancer. The prevalence of Barrett's esophagus is 2%, considerably less than esophageal and esophagogastric tumors.

The clinical characteristics of junctional tumors are harder to characterize. If the characteristics of patients with esophageal and gastric tumors form two ends of the clinical spectrum, the data suggest that patients with junctional tumors have intermediate demographics with a mean age of 60 years, a male-to-female ratio of 5.4:1, and a prevalence of Barrett's esophagus of 10%.

■ CLASSIFICATION

Our practice has been to classify esophagogastric tumors as primary gastric versus esophageal. We group patients with distal esophageal and true gastric cardia adenocarcinoma together and stage and treat them in the same manner. We do this based on clinical experience. The pathogenesis, clinical characteristics, response to treatment, and outcome of these patients is similar. The validity of this approach is reflected by the fact that the most recent revision of the American Joint Commission for Cancer (AJCC) acknowledges that adenocarcinomas of the GEJ are to be staged as esophageal tumors.

This practice is by no means universally accepted. In 1987, Siewert et al proposed a new classification of tumors of the GEJ with the goal of standardizing classification, treatment, and outcome for these tumors. Whether or not the etiology of esophagogastric tumors may be similar, there clearly are differing patterns of regional lymphatic tumor spread based on specific tumor location. Authors who embrace this classification advocate different surgical approaches based on specific esophagogastric tumor location to encompass the appropriate regional lymph nodes in an en bloc fashion. This classification system is included in this chapter.

Tumors are classified by topographic or anatomic findings. Tumors are considered esophagogastric if they are centered within 5 cm (in either direction) of the GEJ. From a therapeutic and prognostic standpoint, tumors are classified into three types as shown in Figure 2. Type 1 tumors are true distal esophageal tumors centered within 5 cm of the GEJ with associated Barrett's esophagus. Type 2 tumors are true cancers of the cardia. They are located within 1 cm proximal to and 2 cm distal to the GEJ. These tumors also are known as *junctional cancers*. Type 3 tumors are subcardial tumors. Their center begins greater than 2 cm distal to the GEJ. Type 3 tumors involve the GEJ and distal esophagus secondarily by upward invasion. The clinical relevance of this classification relates to the pattern of lymph node metastases for each tumor type. Type 1 tumors show a "standard" pattern of esophageal cancer nodal metastasis to the paraesophageal nodes from the neck to the celiac axis. Type 3 tumors show a standard pattern of gastric cancer nodal metastasis to the lesser curvature, celiac axis, posterior gastric, splenic hilum, distal greater curvature, and omental nodes. Type 2 tumors show a pattern of nodal metastasis to the distal paraesophageal, proximal gastric, and celiac lymph nodes. Understanding this pattern of nodal spread of tumor is important in planning the appropriate surgical approach for patients with these tumors. The distribution of type 1, 2, and 3 tumors is reported to be 36%, 27%, and 37%.

■ DIAGNOSIS

The typical patient with gastroesophageal adenocarcinoma is a white man approximately 60 years old who presents

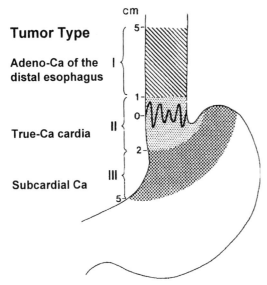

Figure 2
Classification of gastroesophageal tumors according to tumor location.

with progressive solid food dysphagia. Some patients may complain of epigastric burning pain, hiccups, or a change (worsening or improvement) in GER symptoms. Less frequently, patients present with occult anemia and Hemoccult-positive stools and are diagnosed with a GEJ tumor on endoscopic workup. A few patients may be asymptomatic. Persistent, severe, epigastric or mid back pain is an ominous finding, which suggests extensive local tumor invasion. New-onset headache/dizziness or bone/joint pain should raise the suspicion of brain and bone metastases.

If esophagogastric tumor is suspected on clinical grounds, a contrast esophagogram is the next best test. In addition to screening for the junctional tumor, this study screens for associated esophagogastric pathology and gives an excellent anatomic "overview" in planning surgical therapy. The classic radiologic finding for these tumors is a fixed, irregular, circumferential narrowing of the esophagogastric lumen resulting in a so-called apple-core lesion. Other radiographic findings that may be encountered with smaller tumors are noncircumferential polypoid lesions and focal mucosal ulcerations or irregularities.

Even if the radiographic findings are classic for carcinoma, esophagoscopy is necessary to establish the diagnosis pathologically. Endoscopic biopsy in combination with brushings for cytology yields the diagnosis of cancer in greater than 90% of cases. In addition to obtaining cells or tissue for diagnosis, the endoscopists should determine the exact location and length of the tumor and any associated pathology, such as Barrett's mucosa.

■ STAGING AND PREOPERATIVE EVALUATION

There are two objectives in the preoperative staging workup. The first objective is to define the location of the tumor at the

GEJ—to determine if the tumor is esophageal, junctional, or true gastric. This seemingly simple determination can be difficult. It is important, however, because treatment options, surgical approach, and outcome vary depending on whether a tumor is primary esophageal (including true cardia tumors) or gastric. Our approach is to begin by asking the gastroenterologist to determine the extent of the tumor and to judge its point of origin at the time of initial endoscopic diagnosis. To do so, the endoscopist needs to traverse the tumor and evaluate the stomach, including retroflexed views of the gastric cardia. A tight malignant stricture can make this evaluation difficult or impossible. Endoscopic ultrasound (EUS) is the most effective means of determining the size and depth of penetration, or T stage, of esophageal tumors. EUS also differentiates primary tumor versus regional adenopathy. It is assumed that the primary tumor mass is deepest at the point where it originated. EUS localizes this point, permitting accurate tumor classification.

Diagnostic laparoscopy is the final step in specifying tumor location. It may not be possible to see the proximal extent of the tumor from the abdominal side of the esophageal hiatus; however, the extent of gastric involvement with tumor is seen clearly. In addition, differentiation between tumor and regional adenopathy is made during this procedure. Pathologic confirmation of visual findings is performed routinely. In our experience, chest and abdominal computed tomography (CT) has proved to be of limited help at determining tumor origin. Regional adenopathy involving the proximal lesser curve of the stomach frequently, and incorrectly, is interpreted as gastric extension by the primary tumor. By CT, extent of gastric invasion by tumor is determined best in a stomach that has been distended with oral contrast material. Frequently, this is not possible for patients with tight malignant strictures.

The second objective in preoperative evaluation is to determine the specific TNM stage of the tumor. The AJCC staging classification is presented in Table 1. The best initial staging test for patients with esophagogastric cancer is CT of the chest and abdomen. CT scans are readily available, quick, and well tolerated by patients. CT images the tumor, tumor-mediastinal interface, regional lymph nodes, celiac lymph nodes, and solid organs (liver and lung) at risk for harboring metastatic disease. CT accurately detects vertebral or mediastinal soft tissue tumor invasion (T4 tumors) and lung and liver metastases (M1 disease). CT is notably inaccurate in differentiating between T1, T2, and T3 tumors and in determining the presence or absence of nodal metastases (N status). Chest and abdominal CT is an excellent initial staging test to detect advanced staged disease for which palliative therapy only is indicated. Magnetic resonance imaging staging of esophageal tumors, similar to CT, is most accurate at detecting T4 tumors and M1 disease but is poor at determining earlier staged disease. It offers no specific advantage over CT, is more costly, takes longer, and has poorer patient tolerance.

T stage, or depth of tumor invasion, is determined best by EUS. EUS is recommended for all lesions in which a previous CT scan has ruled out T4 and M1 disease. In experienced hands, the depth of tumor invasion into the esophageal wall can be determined with an accuracy of 89%. The accuracy of EUS also depends on the experience of the operator.

Table 1 American Joint Commission for Cancer TNM Staging for Esophageal Cancer

PRIMARY TUMOR (T)

TX	Primary tumor cannot be assessed
T0	No evidence of primary tumor
Tis	Carcinoma in situ
T1	Tumor invades lamina propria or submucosa
T2	Tumor invades muscularis propria
T3	Tumor invades adventitia
T4	Tumor invades adjacent structures

REGIONAL LYMPH NODES (N)

Cervical esophagus (cervical and supraclavicular nodes)

Nx	Regional lymph nodes cannot be assessed
N0	No regional lymph node metastasis
N1	Regional lymph node metastasis

Thoracic esophagus (nodes in the thorax, not those in cervical supraclavicular or abdominal areas)

N0	No nodal involvement
N1	Nodal involvement

DISTANT METASTASIS (M)

MX	Distant metastasis cannot be assessed
M0	No evidence of distant metastasis
M1	Distant metastasis present

STAGE GROUPING

Stage 0	Tis	N0	M0
Stage I	T1	N0	M0
Stage IIA	T2	N0	M0
	T3	N0	M0
Stage IIB	T1	N1	M0
	T2	N1	M0
Stage III	T3	N1	M0
	T4	Any N	M0
Stage IV	Any T	Any N	M1

In approximately 25% of patients, the examination is incomplete or cannot be performed for technical reasons, most commonly from the inability to pass the endoscope beyond the obstructing tumor. Accuracy of determining T stage ranges from approximately 60% for T1 tumors to 98% for T4 tumors. Overstaging and understaging occurs in 6% and 5%. Regional lymph node size, shape, and internal echogenicity are the criteria used to determine the probability of nodal metastatic disease. In addition, numerous studies have shown a direct correlation between the depth of tumor invasion and the probability of nodal metastasis. Using T stage, nodal size, and appearance, accuracy rates of assessing nodal involvement of 81% have been reported (sensitivity of 95%, specificity of 50%). More recently, real-time ultrasound-guided transesophageal biopsy techniques permit cytologic confirmation of nodal metastatic disease in many cases.

The role of diagnostic laparoscopy in determining tumor classification based on location has been discussed previously. Regional lymph nodes for esophagogastric tumors are accessible for visual inspection and biopsy during laparoscopy. Laparoscopy is the most effective method to confirm pathologically regional nodal (N stage) staging. Additional benefits of laparoscopic staging include screening for small foci of metastatic disease (e.g., liver surface) and the potential for placing enteral feeding tubes. In our experience, regional lymph nodes that appeared benign by CT were found to contain metastatic disease in 27% of patients. Diagnostic laparoscopy changed treatment planning in 17% of patients. Finally, laparoscopy has been shown to be more accurate at determining regional lymph node status than CT, EUS, and positron emission tomography (PET).

PET is a new staging modality whose role in the pretreatment workup of patients with esophagogastric tumors is currently under investigation. PET has been shown to be effective at detecting the presence of distant metastatic disease with a sensitivity, specificity, and overall accuracy of 88%, 93%, and 91%. Most studies show that CT and PET have similar accuracy at imaging the primary tumor and determining regional lymph node involvement. As stated earlier, we have shown that PET is less sensitive than laparoscopy at determining N status. PET and CT are considered complementary screening tests to detect metastatic disease with a combined accuracy superior to that of either test alone.

Bone metastases, more common in adenocarcinoma than squamous cell tumors, are nonetheless infrequent sites of early metastatic disease in patients with esophageal cancers. Routine screening bone scan staging for all esophageal cancer patients is not recommended. A bone scan should be obtained to evaluate patients who have suspicious symptoms, radiographic findings, or elevated alkaline phosphatase.

■ TREATMENT

Treatment options are based on classification of tumor location and TNM staging. In this chapter, treatment options that include surgery are emphasized.

Esophagogastric (Distal Esophageal, True Cardia) Tumors

We consider tumors of the distal esophagus, GEJ, and true gastric cardia collectively as a single clinical entity and treat these patients as if they have esophageal tumors. Surgery is recommended for patients with stage 1 adenocarcinoma unless there are coexisting medical issues that would make the risk of surgery prohibitive. The surgical procedure is esophagogastrectomy with regional lymphadenectomy. There are many incisional approaches to perform this surgery, including Ivor-Lewis, three-incision, transhiatal, and left thoracoabdominal. Some authors have advocated extended lymphatic dissection as part of the standard surgical resection. No data show a clear survival advantage in the surgical management of patients with esophageal cancer *based on surgical approach.* Many surgical esophagectomy techniques, such as the Ivor-Lewis and three-incision approaches, have been employed and are acceptable. For stage 1 tumors of the distal esophagus and gastric cardia, we prefer the transhiatal approach with cervical esophagogastric esophageal reconstruction.

For stage 2 and 3 tumors, our bias has been to offer patients combination therapy using preoperative chemoradiotherapy followed by esophagectomy. Although unproved, data suggest that this approach improves survival specifically for patients with stage 2 and 3 tumors. Ideally, treatment with chemoradiotherapy followed by surgery should be implemented in the setting of an approved study protocol until its efficacy can be established. Depending on tumor location, either a transhiatal or a three-incision esophagogastrectomy is employed to remove the tumor, establish a clear surgical margin, and remove the regional lymph nodes. Patients with unresectable tumors or metastatic disease (stage 4) are treated best with palliative therapy because patient survival is often short, and quality-of-life issues are immediate and paramount. Earlier studies to evaluate the efficacy of palliative surgical resections or substernal bypass showed that the risks of surgery for this group of patients exceeded the benefits.

Gastric (Subcardial) Tumors

These tumors originate in the stomach. If there is esophageal involvement, it is by upward tumor migration, usually confined to the distal esophagus. Nodal metastases occur in a pattern consistent with primary gastric tumors. Surgery is recommended for stage 1 through 3 tumors and involves gastrectomy, distal esophagectomy, gastric regional nodal dissection, and reconstruction. Surgical variables include the type of incision to use, the extent of stomach and lymph node resection, and the method for esophagogastric reconstruction. Much of the time, this surgery can be performed through a midline laparotomy. If the tumor is bulky, shows posterior invasion, or has prominent upward extension into the esophagus, a left thoracoabdominal incision is preferable. For small, early stage tumors, partial gastrectomy has been advocated. Most authors advocate total gastrectomy to ensure a wide surgical margin and to facilitate complete lymph node dissection. Wide lymphatic dissection is beneficial; however, we do not routinely perform a splenectomy unless there is direct tumor invasion or clear nodal metastatic disease in the splenic hilum. Reconstructive options include isoperistaltic jejunal or colon (we prefer jejunal) interposition in patients undergoing subtotal gastrectomy. After total gastrectomy, most authors favor Roux-en-Y esophagojejunal reconstruction. We routinely place a feeding jejunostomy tube at the time of surgery.

■ RESULTS

Esophagogastric and True Cardia Tumors

Morbidity and mortality after esophagogastrectomy has been well documented. Regardless of specific surgical approach, mortality rates of 0% to 5% are reported. Complication rates of 30% or greater are common if major and minor complications are included. Esophageal anastomotic leak rates of 0% to 5% generally are cited. Pneumonia is reported in 3% to 20% of cases. We have shown previously that implementation of a standardized patient care plan for the care of esophagectomy patients decreases length of hospital stay and cost without altering results. Our experience has been that the addition of preoperative chemoradiotherapy does not increase postsurgical morbidity, mortality, and length of hospital stay.

In our experience, 75% of patients had stage 2 or 3 tumors on presentation. Postesophagectomy survival is related to stage, and survival results are summarized in Table 2. Cumulative postsurgical survival (all stages) is approximately 20% regardless of specific surgical technique used. The addition of preoperative chemoradiotherapy increases cumulative postoperative survival to approximately 36%. Postsurgical survival continues to be related to the posttreatment stage. Tumors can be down-staged with improved survival. The best survival results are obtained when no residual viable tumor (complete pathologic response) is identified in the resection specimen. In these patients, the projected 5-year survival is 56%.

Gastric Tumors

Mortality rates after gastrectomy vary from 1.8% to 14%. Five-year survival rates vary from 0% to 12% for palliative resections (incomplete resection or nodal involvement) to 15% to 75% for curative resections. Factors traditionally reported that affect survival include tumor stage, location, extent of resection, and presence or absence of nodal metastases. We previously have documented that increased hospital volume decreases surgical mortality after gastrectomy.

Table 2 Postesophagectomy Survival by Stage	
AJCC STAGE	**5-YEAR SURVIVAL (%)**
1	70-80
2	30-35
3	10-15
4	0

AJCC, American Joint Commission for Cancer.

Cumulative Survival

In a series of more than 1000 esophagogastric adenocarcinomas, Siewert et al showed cumulative 5-year and 10-year survival rates of 32.3% and 24.3%. Factors associated with survival include ability to perform a curative resection, presence or absence of nodal metastatic disease, and specific tumor location. Survival with type 1 (esophageal) and 2 (true cardia) tumors was similar and superior to that for type 3 (subcardia) tumors in a statistically significant fashion.

■ SUMMARY

The prevalence of adenocarcinoma of the esophagus and GEJ is increasing. The pathogenesis of esophageal adenocarcinoma from Barrett's mucosa has been established based on clinical and molecular genetic data. At this time, it is not clear whether there is a single etiology for junctional adenocarcinoma and whether that etiology is the same as for esophageal adenocarcinoma. The clinical characteristics of patients with esophageal and gastric adenocarcinoma are distinctly different. The demographics of patients with junctional tumors are intermediate between these two groups. Gastroesophageal tumors have been classified clinically into esophageal (type 1), true cardia (type 2), and subcardia-gastric (type 3), reflecting the differences in demographics, possible etiology, pattern or nodal metastatic spread, and outcome. Surgical therapy, alone or in combination with chemotherapy and radiation, should include primary tumor resection and appropriate regional nodal dissection.

SUGGESTED READING

Fein M, et al: Application of the new classification for cancer of the cardia, *Surgery* 124:707, 1998.

Hamilton SR, et al: Prevalence and characteristics of Barrett esophagus in patients with adenocarcinoma of the esophagus or esophagogastric junction, *Hum Pathol* 19:942, 1988.

Husemann B: Cardia carcinoma considered as a distinct clinical entity, *Br J Surg* 76:136, 1989.

Siewert JR, et al: Adenocarcinoma of the esophagogastric junction, *Ann Surg* 232:353, 2000.

Siewert JR, Stein HJ: Carcinoma of the cardia: carcinoma of the gastroesophageal junction—classification, pathology and extent of resection, *Dis Esophagus* 9:173, 1996.

RADIOTHERAPY FOR ESOPHAGEAL CANCER

Lawrence Kleinberg

Radiotherapy is important in the definitive and palliative therapy of esophageal cancer. It is used as an alternative to surgery for potentially curative therapy, usually in combination with chemotherapy because randomized trials have indicated that long-term survival is substantially improved with a combined approach. Radiotherapy alone as an adjuvant to surgery, either preoperatively or postoperatively, has not been shown to be beneficial despite numerous randomized trials. Combined chemoradiotherapy, usually given preoperatively, is under study and frequently offered as a standard management option. External beam radiation therapy and brachytherapy can be useful in palliation of swallowing difficulties resulting from advanced disease. The role of radiation therapy in each of these situations is summarized in this chapter.

■ PRIMARY RADIOTHERAPY

Historically, radiation alone has been the standard alternative to surgical therapy. This approach provides palliation for swallowing difficulties and pain and temporary control of local disease, but a small chance for long-term control or cure. Generally, a dose of 50 to 60 Gy over 5 to 6 weeks is given to the esophageal tumor along with an extensive proximal and distal margin to allow for submucosal spread. The main toxicities of this treatment generally include transient esophagitis (resulting in weight loss despite narcotics), skin erythema, and fatigue. More severe side effects, such as pneumonitis and permanent symptomatic damage to the esophagus, are rare. Stricture in the area of treated tumor may occur, and a thorough evaluation is warranted before presuming recurrent tumor in a patient with persistent swallowing difficulties. Rupture of the esophagus is a rare toxicity. The survival data with primary radiotherapy have been disappointing. Although single institutional trials have reported 5-year survivals of 5% to 10%, two large U.S. randomized trials found no 3-year survivors with radiation alone.

Definitive radiotherapy given in combination with concurrent chemotherapy has resulted in improved long-term survival compared with radiation alone. A landmark multiinstitutional trial done by the Radiation Therapy Oncology Group (RTOG) compared esophageal cancer patients treated with 64 Gy of radiotherapy alone with patients treated with

50 Gy of radiotherapy given concurrently with two cycles of cisplatin (75 mg/m^2) and 5-fluorouracil (1000 mg/m^2/day) for 4 days, followed by an additional two cycles. With the addition of chemotherapy, 3-year and 5-year survival improved to 30% and 27% from 0%. An update of this study showed an 8-year survival of 22% with no cancer-related deaths after 5 years. Following therapy, 53% had local failure or persistent local disease, whereas 22% had distant failure initially. Outcome was similar for patients with adenocarcinoma and squamous cell carcinoma, although the former group was smaller. Other trials have confirmed a benefit of combining chemotherapy with radiation so that this approach is now standard for patients who are medical candidates for aggressive therapy. Initial reports of an RTOG randomized trial escalating the dose of radiotherapy given with chemotherapy (cisplatin and 5-fluorouracil) have not confirmed a benefit to increasing the radiotherapy dose beyond 50 Gy.

The toxicities of combined chemoradiotherapy are worse than with radiotherapy alone. The incidence of severe esophagitis is higher. Esophagitis may result in substantial weight loss despite narcotic therapy for pain control; a gastrostomy tube may be needed. Systemic chemotherapy has toxicities that depend on the regimen selected.

■ ADJUVANT RADIOTHERAPY

Radiotherapy also has been advocated as an adjunct to surgery, given either preoperatively or postoperatively. The rationale for adding radiotherapy to surgery is the need to improve control of local disease. A U.S. intergroup randomized trial that accrued patients from 1990 to 1995 had a control arm of 227 patients with localized esophageal cancer treated with surgery alone. Of these patients initially thought to have resectable disease, 59% were able to undergo a total resection with negative margins. Of this group, recurrence occurred initially in 29%; there was an overall 58% failure to control local disease. This trial provides a rationale for adding treatments designed to improve local control to surgery. The role of radiotherapy, generally combined with chemotherapy, for this purpose remains controversial, however.

■ PREOPERATIVE (NEOADJUVANT) RADIOTHERAPY

Preoperative radiation alone has been evaluated in five randomized trials. No benefit was seen except for one trial in which many of the patients also received chemotherapy. Preoperative radiotherapy alone is not generally appropriate.

Preoperative combined chemotherapy and radiotherapy may improve survival outcome. Generally, a lower dose of radiation is used to reduce the chances of surgical complications. A typical dose is approximately 45 Gy given over 5 weeks, although other regimens using higher doses have been shown to be safe in clinical trials.

Preoperative chemotherapy has been tested in three randomized trials with mixed results. In the 1996 trial reported by Walsh, 113 patients with adenocarcinoma of the esophagus were randomized to surgery alone or surgery with preoperative chemotherapy and concurrent radiotherapy (40 Gy in 15 fractions). The chemotherapy was 5-fluorouracil (15 mg/kg) for 5 days and cisplatin (75 mg/m^2) starting the first day of radiotherapy and given again after the completion of radiotherapy. The pathologic complete response rate to this preoperative therapy was 25%, and median survival was improved from 11 months to 16 months ($p = .01$, with 3-year survival improving from 6% to 32%). This trial has been questioned because of its unexpectedly poor results with surgery alone. In 2001, Urba reported the results of a randomized trial using a more aggressive regimen with cisplatin (20 mg/m^2/day) for 5 days, vinblastine (1 mg/m^2/day) for 4 days repeated for two cycles, and 5-fluorouracil (300 mg/m^2/day) for 21 days during radiotherapy. The radiation was given at 1.5 Gy twice a day, an intensified approach to treatment delivery. The median survival was similar in both arms, and 3-year survival was improved from 16% to 30%, a difference that was not significant in this relatively small trial. An additional trial conducted in France showed no benefit in outcome but involved less intensive chemotherapy, a usual radiotherapy regimen, and a chemotherapy regimen not always given with concurrent radiotherapy. Although the results from these trials are mixed, regimens based on this approach frequently are used in the standard management of esophageal cancer.

At the Johns Hopkins Medical Institutions, we have treated 92 patients with stage II through IVA esophageal cancer (65 adenocarcinomas and 27 squamous cell carcinomas) on two sequential protocols of preoperative chemoradiotherapy. In trial A (1989-1994), 50 patients were treated with 44 Gy of radiation (2 Gy/day) combined with concurrent 5-fluorouracil (300 mg/m^2/day) protracted infusion days 1 to 30 and cisplatin (26 mg/m^2) on days 1 to 5 and 26 to 30. In trial B (1995-1997, 42 patients), the chemotherapy dosages during radiotherapy were reduced to 225 mg/m^2/day for 5-fluorouracil protracted infusion and 20 mg/m^2/day for cisplatin on days 1 to 5 and 16 to 30; three cycles of paclitaxel (135 mg/m^2) and cisplatin (75 mg/m^2) were given postoperatively. Surgery generally occurred 4 to 6 weeks after completion of the planned preoperative therapy. Transhiatal resection was performed whenever possible.

Of patients, 93% (86 of 92) underwent surgery (one refused, two preoperative deaths, three developed metastatic disease), and 87% (80 of 92) were completely resected with negative margins (three had positive margins, three had distant metastasis discovered at surgery). The pathologic complete response rate was 33% (30 of 92). With a median follow-up of 63.5 months, the median survival and disease-specific survival of all enrolled patients is currently 35 months and 59 months. Five-year survival and disease-specific survival are 40% and 49%. Patients with a pathologic complete response had a 67% survival at 5 years (median not reached), whereas the remainder of the patients had 5-year survivals of 26% (median 21 months) ($p < .001$). The pattern of initial failure was locoregional alone in 6% (5 of 90), locoregional plus distant in 3% (3 of 90), and distant alone in 47% (42 of 90). There were no differences in survival or response rate between patients with adenocarcinoma and squamous cell carcinoma. The promising 5-year survival results suggest that these regimens of intensive neoadjuvant therapy may improve the overall cure rate. Although pathologic complete response of local disease is associated with long-term survival, isolated local failure is uncommon, indicating that efforts to improve the therapeutic outcome should focus on optimizing systemic therapy rather than intensifying the local radiotherapy.

■ POSTOPERATIVE (ADJUVANT) RADIOTHERAPY

Postoperative radiotherapy has been evaluated in two randomized trials without showing significant benefit. Postoperative radiation still is warranted in situations in which there are positive margins or known residual disease. In general, postoperative radiotherapy should be combined with chemotherapy because the efficacy of this approach in other clinical settings is greater. There have been no large-scale studies of postoperative chemoradiotherapy.

■ PALLIATIVE RADIOTHERAPY

Radiotherapy is useful for the palliation of swallowing difficulties. External beam radiation treatments can improve swallowing function in approximately 50% to 75% of patients. The palliation and duration of control may be higher when the radiation is combined with chemotherapy, and this approach should be used in patients with a significant chance of living 3 months or longer. To provide durable palliation, relatively high doses of approximately 50 Gy are used. Relief is not immediate, and median time to maximal improvement is about 4 weeks, although response can take significantly longer in some patients.

In the past, radiotherapy was not used in the setting of tracheoesophageal fistula for fear of widening the fistula. It seems that those fears are unfounded and that radiotherapy with or without chemotherapy may be useful. Although the prognosis for patients treated in that situation remains poor, several retrospective studies now show that radiotherapy can be of palliative value in that situation.

Radiotherapy can be given by brachytherapy. In brachytherapy, a radioactive source is inserted directly into the esophagus, usually via endoscopy. The advantage to this approach is that treatment can be given directly to the area that needs it without going through normal tissues. This can allow additional treatments to be given after normal tissues have reached the tolerance of external beam radiation therapy or allow recurrent tumor to be treated after prior radiation. The main disadvantage is that the effective dose penetrates only to a depth of approximately 1 cm, much smaller than most tumors. The most appropriate role for this approach may be in patients with recurrent symptoms after external beam radiation therapy.

■ COMPLICATIONS

Common short-term side effects include local skin changes, such as erythema, irritation, and darkening; fatigue; decreased blood cell count; temporary hair loss in the treated area; and esophagitis. Uncommon short-term side effects include shortness of breath from pneumonitis, nausea, and vomiting. Common long-term side effects include minor to moderate difficulties or discomfort with swallowing. Stricture may occur in the treated area and is a potential cause of delayed dysphagia. Uncommon long-term side effects include fistulization with the airway and shortness of breath from lung fibrosis, radiation-induced malignancy, and spinal cord injury.

SUGGESTED READING

Cooper JS, et al: Chemoradiotherapy of locally advanced esophageal cancer: long-term follow-up of a prospective randomized trial (RTOG 85-01). Radiation Therapy Oncology Group, *JAMA* 281:1623, 1999.

Forastiere AA, et al: Intensive chemoradiation followed by esophagectomy for squamous cell and adenocarcinoma of the esophagus, *Cancer J Sci Am* 3:144, 1997.

Heath EI, et al: Phase II evaluation of preoperative chemoradiation and postoperative adjuvant chemotherapy for squamous cell and adenocarcinoma of the esophagus, *J Clin Oncol* 18:868, 2000.

Urba SG, et al: Randomized trial of preoperative chemoradiation versus surgery alone in patients with locoregional esophageal carcinoma, *J Clin Oncol* 19:305, 2001.

Walsh TN, et al: A comparison of multimodal therapy and surgery for esophageal adenocarcinoma, *N Engl J Med* 335:462, 1996.

NEOADJUVANT THERAPY FOR ESOPHAGEAL CANCER

Bapsi Chak

Arlene A. Forastiere

Since the 1980s, there has been a decrease in the age-adjusted incidence of squamous cell carcinoma of the esophagus and a 350-fold increase in the incidence of adenocarcinoma of the distal esophagus and gastroesophageal junction. Although the risk factors for the development of squamous cell carcinoma have been identified (smoking, alcohol, diet), they are less clear for adenocarcinoma of the esophagus. Smoking remains a risk factor, but there seems to be less of an association with alcohol. Chronic gastroesophageal reflux disease and associated Barrett's dysplasia, obesity, and tobacco use have been shown to be predisposing factors in the development of adenocarcinoma of the esophagus.

Two approaches are considered standard of care for the management of locally advanced esophageal cancer: (1) surgery alone and (2) primary chemoradiotherapy. Although there are no randomized trials comparing these two treatment options, the overall 5-year survival with either approach is approximately 20%. Current trials have focused on adding chemotherapy with or without radiation to surgery to reduce distant and local failure and to improve overall survival.

The introduction of chemotherapy and radiotherapy before surgical resection has made pretreatment clinical staging an important aspect of care. All patients with esophageal cancer should be staged with high-resolution computed tomography of the chest, abdomen, and pelvis and esophageal endoscopic ultrasound. An experienced endoscopist performing endoscopic ultrasound can determine T stage with 80% to 90% accuracy and N stage with approximately 70% accuracy. Laparoscopic staging is recommended for distal esophageal cancers to exclude peritoneal spread and small liver metastases. Studies have shown that laparoscopy leads to a change in treatment in 15% to 20% of patients. Positron emission tomography is a new staging modality that also is useful for detecting distant metastases and nodal involvement.

Most patients in the United States present with stage IIB, III, or IV disease. Patients with stage IIB and III disease who have undergone resection have a 5-year survival rate of approximately 20%. These figures have not changed despite more recent improvements in postoperative care and patient selection, indicating the need for alternative therapies. Since the 1980s, cisplatin-based chemotherapy regimens have been identified that can reduce tumor volume by 50% or more in approximately half of patients with newly diagnosed, untreated disease. In addition, most of the cytotoxic agents with antitumor activity against esophageal cancer also enhance radiation effects. These findings have led to numerous trials evaluating the effect on survival and pattern of failure of administering chemotherapy alone or concurrent with radiotherapy before esophagectomy and using chemoradiotherapy alone as definitive treatment in settings where nonsurgical treatment is warranted.

■ COMBINED MODALITY APPROACHES TO SURGICAL MANAGEMENT

Preoperative Radiation

Radiation has been given before surgery in an attempt to improve local control. There have been many randomized trials of preoperative radiation followed by surgery compared with surgery alone, but only one, which included a subset of patients receiving chemoradiotherapy, has shown a survival benefit. Virtually all patients enrolled in these studies have had squamous cell carcinoma. The studies have been criticized for using varied dose and fractionation schedules and an inadequate time interval between completion of radiation and surgery. In general, at least 4 to 6 weeks are required for the maximum therapeutic effect of radiation. In some studies, patients have undergone surgery within 1 to 2 weeks after completing radiation, however. A meta-analysis of randomized trials enrolling 1147 patients showed that preoperative radiation afforded an overall reduction in risk of death of 11% and an absolute survival benefit of 3% at 2 years and 4% at 5 years. These results were not statistically superior to surgery alone, and preoperative radiotherapy alone is not standard of care and has no role in patients for whom surgery is indicated.

Preoperative Chemotherapy

Another strategy to address distant and local failure is the use of preoperative chemotherapy to down-stage patients and facilitate surgical resection, improve local control, and eradicate micrometastatic disease. Studies show that chemotherapy administered before surgery is feasible and does not increase operative mortality or morbidity. Cisplatin-based combinations result in 50% or greater regression of tumor in half of patients, whereas no residual tumor in the resection specimen (pathologic complete response) occurs in about 5% of patients. The most frequently used regimen consists of two or three 5-day courses of cisplatin and 5-fluorouracil (5-FU) given every 3 weeks before esophagectomy. For squamous histology, response rates range between 42% and 66%, with less than 10% pathologic complete response; curative resection rates range from 40% to 80%, and median survival rates range from 18 to 28 months. There is one report of preoperative cisplatin and 5-FU for adenocarcinoma of the esophagus and gastroesophageal junction. A 37% response rate and an actuarial 4-year survival rate of 42% were observed in 16 patients.

Trials designed specifically for patients with adenocarcinoma of the distal esophagus or gastroesophageal junction have evaluated etoposide, 5-FU, and cisplatin and etoposide, doxorubicin, and cisplatin. Response rates were similar, ranging from 49% to 55% after two or three cycles. Curative resection rates varied from 65% to 90% and survival from 12.5 to 23 months. Regimens that include doxorubicin and etoposide are used commonly to treat gastric cancer. The activity of these single agents in patients with adenocarcinoma of the esophagus is unknown. These combinations seem to have antitumor activity that is comparable to cisplatin and 5-FU, but toxicity is greater. These observations from uncontrolled trials in the 1980s suggested that preoperative chemotherapy might provide a survival advantage compared with surgery alone and led to many prospective randomized trials within and outside of the United States.

Seven randomized trials of preoperative chemotherapy compared with immediate surgery have been published, and the results are conflicting. The largest and most recent multicenter trials include adenocarcinomas and squamous cell cancers and were conducted in the United States and in Great Britain. The U.S. G-I Intergroup compared (1) three cycles of cisplatin and 5-FU followed by surgery, then two additional cycles of cisplatin and 5-FU with (2) immediate surgery. More than 400 patients were randomized, and of these, 55% had adenocarcinoma of the esophagus or gastroesophageal junction. No survival differences were observed between the two treatment groups or between histologies; 2-year survival rates were 35% and 37%. The Medical Research Counsel (MRC) in Great Britain randomized 802 patients to two cycles of cisplatin and 5-FU before surgery or to immediate surgery. Of patients, 65% had adenocarcinoma histology. In a preliminary abstract, the 2-year survival rate reported was significantly improved (43% versus 34%) for patients in the chemotherapy group. The MRC and U.S. Intergroup trials reported survival rates for the surgery control arms that were nearly the same, 34% and 37%. It is unclear why the results of these two trials are discordant with respect to benefit from chemotherapy. Until the complete report of the MRC trial is published, however, preoperative chemotherapy, at least in the United States, is considered investigational and has no role in the routine management of patients with esophageal cancer. Preoperative chemotherapy should be administered only in the context of an approved clinical trial. Studies of newer chemotherapy regimens are in progress.

Preoperative Chemoradiotherapy

It can be hypothesized that esophagectomy after maximal tumor clearance by chemotherapy plus radiation therapy could contribute to local control of disease, improve quality of life, and improve survival. This approach takes advantage of radiation sensitization from cisplatin and 5-FU. Many nonrandomized studies have been carried out to test this hypothesis with results that suggest benefit over surgery alone.

In general, these trials report pathologic complete response in 25% to 30% of patients with associated long-term survival for this subset. About two thirds of patients are down-staged after preoperative chemoradiotherapy. Median survival rates exceed 2 years, and 3-year and 5-year survival rates are in the 30% to 40% range. This compares favorably with historic series of surgery alone with 5-year survival rates of 15% to 20%.

Three randomized trials compared chemoradiotherapy followed by surgery with immediate surgery (Table 1). Urba et al at the University of Michigan tested a preoperative regimen of continuous infusion 5-FU and cisplatin plus twice-a-day hyperfractionated radiation (total dose 45 Gy) followed by transhiatal esophagectomy. This relatively small randomized trial (100 patients) primarily enrolling patients with adenocarcinoma showed a nonsignificant survival advantage for the combined modality treatment group compared with surgery alone (30% versus 16% at 3 years, $p = .15$) and a significant decrease in local failure rate in the combined treatment group. No difference was observed in the percentage of patients developing distant metastases. There was a significant survival advantage for patients who achieved a pathologic complete response with a median survival of 49.7 months compared with patients with residual disease in the resected specimen who had a median survival of only 12 months. Had this trial been powered to show a more modest difference, requiring a larger sample size, a significant difference in overall survival may have emerged.

A second randomized trial conducted by Walsh et al in Ireland was limited to patients with adenocarcinoma of the esophagus and gastroesophageal junction. A total of 113 patients were randomized to receive preoperative cisplatin and 5-FU with radiotherapy (40 Gy) or to undergo immediate surgery. The preoperative regimen was well tolerated with only a 15% incidence of grade 3 toxicity. Operative mortality was comparable between the two groups (9% and 4%). At a median follow-up of 18 months, there was a significant improvement in median survival (16 versus 11 months, $p = .01$) and 3-year survival (32% versus 6%, $p = .01$) for patients receiving preoperative chemoradiotherapy compared with immediate surgery. The trial has been criticized for nonuniform staging of patients and the poor survival rate of the surgery controls. The surgical control arm had a 3-year survival of only 6%, which is much lower than the 23% 3-year survival rate from the surgery control arm of the U.S. G-I Intergroup trial, which provides contemporary data from a multicenter trial.

Table 1 Randomized Studies of Preoperative Chemoradiation

SERIES	HISTOLOGY	TREATMENT*	NO.	CR	MEDIAN SURVIVAL (MO)	3-YR SURVIVAL (%)
Urba	Adeno +	Surgery	50		17.6	16
	Squamous	Preop chemotherapy + 45 Gy	50	28	16.9	30
Walsh	Adeno	Surgery	55		11	6
		Preop chemotherapy + 40 Gy	58	25	16	32[†]
Bosset	Squamous	Surgery	139		18.6	36
		Preop chemotherapy + 37 Gy	142	26	18.6	36

*Cisplatin/fluorouracil–based chemotherapy.
†Difference statistically significant.
CR, complete response.

Although there were few early stage tumors in the surgical arm, the number of early stage patients in the chemoradiotherapy arm is unknown because preoperative staging was based only on clinical examination, chest radiography, abdominal ultrasound, and upper endoscopy. Computed tomography scans were performed only on patients with equivocal findings on chest radiograph or abdominal ultrasound. This may have resulted in an imbalance of advanced stage patients in the surgery control arm. Finally, the radiation dose and techniques used in this study are those commonly applied today. Conventional preoperative radiation doses are 1.8 to 2.0 Gy per fraction to total doses of 4500 to 5040 cGy. Walsh et al used 267 cGy per fraction, which adds to normal tissue toxicity. The use of multiple fields, computerized treatment planning, and customized blocks may have allowed higher doses to be delivered to the tumor while sparing surrounding normal tissue.

A third randomized trial from the European Organization for Research and Treatment of Cancer (EORTC) enrolled 297 patients with stage I and II squamous cell carcinoma of the esophagus. This trial, reported by Bossett et al, administered two doses of cisplatin (80 mg/m^2 per dose) with split-course radiotherapy preoperatively. Disease-free survival (40% versus 28%) was significantly improved, death due to esophageal cancer was reduced, and there was a higher frequency of curative resection in the chemoradiotherapy group. Overall survival was the same, however, 36% for both treatment groups, and the rate of postoperative complications was significantly higher in patients receiving preoperative chemoradiotherapy. The 36% 3-year survival rate for the surgery controls was likely due to the more favorable population enrolled in this trial compared with the trials of Urba and Walsh because this study was limited to stage I and II disease. This study used split-course radiation and a high dose per fraction. Radiobiologic principles would predict increased normal tissue toxicity and worse tumor control. This may explain in part the lack of survival benefit.

The role of preoperative chemoradiotherapy is controversial due to the conflicting results of these randomized trials. To address this, in 1998, the U.S. Intergroup mounted what was to be a definitive study (CALGB 9781). Patients were randomized to receive immediate surgery or two cycles of cisplatin and 5-FU with concurrent radiotherapy (50 Gy) followed by surgery. The trial was adequately powered to show differences in survival in patient cohorts with adenocarcinoma and squamous cell carcinoma. After 2 years, the trial was closed, however, due to poor accrual. It is unlikely that a similar study of this magnitude could be mounted again.

The cumulative data from limited institutional experiences and randomized comparisons suggest that triple modality therapy can improve survival over that achievable with surgery alone. All of the randomized trials have limitations as noted, however, and an adequately powered multicenter trial using standard radiation technique and chemotherapy failed to accrue patients. Preoperative chemoradiotherapy has become common practice in the United States despite the absence of unequivocal supporting data from well-controlled, adequately powered randomized trials. Several studies indicate that patients achieving pathologic complete response have a better survival outcome. Methods that may improve pathologic complete response rates are an area of active investigation. Patients with esophageal cancer should be referred for enrollment in clinical trials.

■ POSTOPERATIVE ADJUVANT CHEMOTHERAPY OR CHEMORADIOTHERAPY

The role of postoperative adjuvant chemotherapy or chemoradiotherapy needs further study. Adjuvant chemotherapy is appealing as a therapy for occult micrometastatic disease after surgery. The Japanese have conducted several prospective randomized trials of adjuvant chemotherapy in patients with resected squamous cell carcinoma, stratifying for nodal involvement. A more recent trial evaluated two cycles of cisplatin and 5-FU. No difference in survival was found comparing adjuvant treatment with observation after surgery. Adjuvant chemotherapy in responders to preoperative combined modality approaches also has appeal but is feasible in only about half of patients in which this strategy has been tested in phase II and III studies. In the previously described U.S. Intergroup trial, the investigational treatment arm of neoadjuvant chemotherapy followed by surgery then two additional cycles of postoperative chemotherapy attempted to give adjuvant chemotherapy to initial chemotherapy responders. Only 52% of patients were able to receive at least one cycle, however, and only 38% were able to receive both cycles of postoperative chemotherapy. These therapies are experimental and should be administered only in the context of a formal research protocol. The only controlled trial data available evaluating chemoradiotherapy after surgery are in gastric cancer.

Postoperative Adjuvant Chemoradiotherapy: Adenocarcinoma of the Gastroesophageal Junction and Cardia

There are efforts currently to stratify large trials by histology. To date, no survival differences have been reported from combined modality trials enrolling squamous carcinoma and adenocarcinoma histologies of esophageal origin, although we believe that adjuvant therapies need to be studied systematically in both histologies. One trial of adjuvant chemoradiotherapy in resected gastric cancer included a subset of patients with primary tumors located at the gastroesophageal junction and cardia.

Reported in preliminary abstract form, Intergroup trial 0116 is a randomized study of postoperative 5-FU, leucovorin, and radiation compared with observation in patients with resected adenocarcinoma of the stomach and gastroesophageal junction. A statistically significant increase in 3-year survival (52% versus 41%, $p = .03$) was reported. This is the first study to show an advantage to adjuvant therapy in this setting. This is primarily a study of gastric adenocarcinoma with 20% of the enrolled patients having tumors of the gastric cardia or gastroesophageal junction. The pattern of failure of gastric cancer is different from proximal lesions of the cardia, gastroesophageal junction, and distal esophagus. The predominant site of first failure (80%) is locoregional for the former versus distant metastases as the site of first failure for 80% of the latter. Although the results of INT0116 may be used to justify postoperative chemoradiotherapy for node-positive, completely resected cardia and gastroesophageal junction adenocarcinoma, benefit may be marginal for this subsite, and toxicity may be significant. Postoperative therapy can be offered to patients who have recovered well from surgery, have an excellent performance status, and are at high risk for recurrence.

■ NONSURGICAL MANAGEMENT

Radiation

Historically, radiation alone was used to treat medically inoperable patients with esophageal cancer. Today, radiation as the sole treatment modality is used primarily for symptom palliation, whereas the standard of care for the nonsurgical management of localized esophageal cancer is concurrent chemoradiotherapy. For patients who are unable to tolerate surgery or chemotherapy due to comorbid medical conditions, radical radiation may be used. Five-year survivals of 10% to 21% are reported. Doses for radical radiotherapy alone are 6000 to 6500 cGy, using multiple fields. In patients with known distant metastases, radiation alone can be used to palliate symptoms of pain, bleeding, and dysphagia. Palliative treatment regimens vary from 30 Gy in 2 weeks for extremely poor performance patients to 60 Gy in 6 weeks for more durable palliation in patients with excellent performance.

Concurrent Chemoradiotherapy

Table 2 shows the results of five randomized studies of chemoradiotherapy compared with radiotherapy alone. These studies consisted primarily of squamous cell carcinoma of the mid esophagus. No studies have evaluated this approach adequately in adenocarcinoma of the esophagus. Nonsurgical treatment approaches for adenocarcinoma are extrapolated from data based on trials of squamous cell carcinoma.

A landmark trial was Intergroup study RTOG 85-01 in which patients with locally advanced esophageal cancer were randomized to chemoradiotherapy or radiotherapy alone. Chemotherapy consisted of 5-FU (1000 mg/m^2/24 hours × 4 days) and cisplatin (75 mg/m^2, day 1) and was given on the first day of weeks 1, 5, 8, and 11. Radiation therapy (5000 cGy/ 25 fractions) was begun concurrently with day 1 of chemotherapy. Four cycles of chemotherapy were given, two during radiotherapy and two after radiotherapy. The control arm consisted of radiation alone, 6400 cGy in 32 fractions. Only 50% of patients were able to complete all four cycles of chemotherapy.

Patients receiving concurrent chemoradiotherapy had a significant improvement in median survival (14 months versus 9 months) and 5-year survival (26% versus 0%, $p < .0001$). The incidence of local failure (defined as persistent disease or recurrence) at 1 year was significantly decreased in the combined modality arm (45% versus 68%, $p = .0123$). Although randomization was discontinued early due to the positive results, an additional 69 patients treated with the same chemoradiotherapy regimen had similar results (3-year survival 30%).

Based on these studies, the standard of care for the nonsurgical management of esophageal cancer is concurrent chemoradiotherapy. Radiation alone is reserved for patients whose performance status or organ dysfunction precludes the use of chemotherapy. Despite a survival benefit, there was an unacceptably high local failure rate (45%) in RTOG 85-01. Other approaches have been investigated, including intensification of chemotherapy or radiation or both, but to date, these strategies have increased toxicity but not survival or local control.

■ NEWER AGENTS IN COMBINED MODALITY TRIALS

In addition to improving the results of standard chemoradiotherapy by intensifying chemotherapy or radiation or both, another approach has been to combine radiation therapy with some of the newer chemotherapeutic agents, such as

Table 2 Randomized Trials of Primary Chemoradiotherapy versus Radiotherapy Alone

TRIAL	TREATMENT	NO.	LOCAL FAILURE (%)	MEDIAN SURVIVAL (MO)	SURVIVAL (%)
Herskovic*	RT	62	68	9	0 (5-yr)
(RTOG)	RT + CDDP/5-FU	61	47	14§	27§
Smith*	RT	69		9	7 (5-yr)
(ECOG)	RT + 5-FU/mito	59		15§	9
Aranjo†	RT	31	84	6	
(NCI Brazil)	RT + CDDP/mito/5-FU	28	61	16	
Roussel‡	RT	111	66	8	10 (4-yr)
(EORTC)	RT + CDDP	110	59	10	8
Slabber‡	RT	36		5	
(Pretoria)	RT + CDDP/5-FU	34		6	

*Resectability not specified.
†Stage II only (1982 American Joint Commission for Cancer).
‡Unresectable.
§Difference statistically significant.
RTOG, Radiation Therapy Oncology Group; ECOG, Eastern Cooperative Oncology Group; NCI, National Cancer Institute; EORTC, European Organization for Research and Treatment of Cancer; RT, radiotherapy; CDDP, cis-diaminedichloroplatinum; 5-FU, 5-flourouracil; mito, mitomycin C.

paclitaxel, UFT, oxaliplatin, and CPT-11, which also are known to be potent radiation sensitizers. These agents have been used in primary chemoradiotherapy protocols and in the preoperative setting. The taxane paclitaxel has been studied the longest. Although pathologic complete response rates have been encouraging, ranging from 11% to 41%, paclitaxel combination regimens have not been tested in a randomized fashion against the more standard cisplatin and 5-FU–based therapies. Comparisons with institutional historic controls of similarly staged patient cohorts treated with cisplatin and 5-FU show no advantage in overall survival for the newer taxane-based regimens.

■ CONCLUSIONS

In the 1980s and 1990s, chemotherapy regimens with substantial antitumor activity against esophageal squamous cell carcinoma and adenocarcinoma have been developed. Randomized controlled trials have shown a significant survival advantage for concurrent chemoradiotherapy used as definitive treatment for patients treated nonsurgically compared with radiotherapy alone. This is now standard of care. For patients treated surgically, it appears from the accumulated literature that neoadjuvant or preoperative chemoradiotherapy may provide a survival advantage, particularly for patients down-staged to pathologic complete response status, but the results of controlled trials to date are conflicting.

We encourage all patients to be enrolled in clinical trials testing neoadjuvant strategies. No trials have compared directly chemoradiotherapy with preoperative chemoradiotherapy followed by surgery or compared chemoradiotherapy with surgery as a single modality. These trials are needed but would be difficult to mount. Current standard of care for patients with resectable disease is surgery but with an expectation of poor survival rates averaging 15% to 20% at 5 years. Investigational cytotoxic agents, radiosensitizers, and molecularly targeted therapeutics now in development offer hope for achieving much larger gains in survival when combined with surgery and radiation in future trials.

SUGGESTED READING

Bosset JF, et al: Chemoradiotherapy followed by surgery compared with surgery alone in squamous-cell cancer of the esophagus, *N Engl J Med* 337:161, 1997.

Forastiere AA, et al: Intensive chemoradiation followed by esophagectomy for squamous cell and adenocarcinoma of the esophagus, *Cancer J Sci Am* 3:144, 1997.

Kelsen DP, et al: Chemotherapy followed by surgery compared with surgery alone for localized esophageal cancer, *N Engl J Med* 339:1979, 1998.

Urba SG, et al: Randomized trial of preoperative chemoradiation versus surgery alone in patients with locoregional esophageal carcinoma, *J Clin Oncol* 19:305, 2001.

Walsh TN, et al: A comparison of multimodal therapy and surgery for esophageal adenocarcinoma, *N Engl J Med* 335:462, 1996.

LYMPH NODE DISSECTION IN ESOPHAGEAL CANCER

Wayne Hofstetter
Stephen G. Swisher

The extent and indication for lymph node dissection is a controversial issue for many cancers. With increasing specialization, each field has addressed this issue on an organ-specific basis, and esophageal cancer surgeons continue to be on the front lines of this debate. At present, no definitive randomized trials exist to resolve this question on an evidence-based platform. The integration of esophageal cancer management into multimodality treatment may have an impact on the extent to which radical lymph node dissections are performed. This chapter describes the technical aspects of various types of lymphadenectomies (radical and nonradical) currently being performed for esophageal cancer.

■ INDICATIONS

The choice of the approach and the extent of esophageal resection and lymphadenectomy depend on the surgeon's and patient's preferences and the extent and location of disease. The most commonly encountered esophageal neoplasms in North America are mid to distal esophageal adenocarcinomas, representing a shift away from squamous cell histology. The surgeon can approach these lesions from a transthoracic or transhiatal route as long as fixation of the tumor is not an issue. Surgeons who prefer more extensive lymphadenectomies can adjust their procedure according to the stage and comorbidities of the patient, often selecting the better performance and earlier staged patients for more extensive radical lymph node dissections. Proponents of a radical lymph node dissection believe that the benefits include advantages in staging, local control, and survival. Proponents of nonradical lymph node resections quote a lack of evidence to support more extensive lymph node dissections and argue that these operations may be associated with higher morbidity and mortality, especially when combined with neoadjuvant or adjuvant therapy or when performed in lower performance status patients.

■ TECHNIQUES

Several popular techniques of esophageal lymph node dissections differ in the approach and extent of lymph nodes resected. These procedures can be divided into radical and nonradical lymph node dissections. Radical lymph node dissections include esophagectomies with three-field or two-field lymph node dissections (Table 1). Nonradical lymph node dissections remove lymph nodes from similar fields of dissection but are less aggressive about the number and extent of lymph nodes removed and the surrounding tissue and organs resected.

Radical Lymph Node Dissection
Most radical lymph node dissections use three incision fields (neck, chest, and abdomen) but differ in the extent of lymph nodes and organs resected from each of these areas (Table 2).

Two-Field Radical Lymph Node Dissection
The two-field en bloc esophagectomy is performed through a right thoracotomy, abdominal incision, and left cervicotomy. The major difference from other techniques is that a more radical thoracic dissection is performed, and reconstruction of the resected esophagus often uses a colon interposition. The underlying goal is total clearance of metastatic deposits from vascular and lymphatic areas surrounding the tumor.

The initial incision is usually a standard right thoracotomy performed through the fifth intercostal space through which the chest is explored. A double-lumen endotracheal tube is used to facilitate the exposure during the esophageal and lymph node dissections. An incision is made in the pleura lateral to the azygos vein. Dissection proceeds to the contralateral pleura, including the azygos vein, segmental intercostal veins, and all soft tissue including the esophagus along three fourths of the length of the intrathoracic esophagus. At the conclusion of the thoracic dissection, all tissue anteriorly from the posterior hilum and pericardium, posteriorly to the

chest wall, superiorly up to the azygos arch, and inferiorly to the hiatus is removed. Medial dissection extends to the contralateral pleura along the plane of the right and left main stem bronchus. The aorta is left bare with the intercostal arteries intact. Above the level of the azygos arch, the esophagus is mobilized to the thoracic inlet along the muscular wall to avoid injury to vital structures. The thoracic duct is identified and ligated at the hiatus. Lymph nodes from levels 3P (posterior mediastinal), 7 (subcarinal), 8M/L (middle and lower paraesophageal), and 9 (inferior pulmonary ligament) are resected en bloc with the specimen. Paratracheal nodes (2, 4, and 10) are dissected separately.

In the abdomen, the resection includes a complete resection of all lymph-bearing tissue from the hiatus along the lesser curve to the vena cava (level 16, 17), then a resection along the named vessels of the celiac axis, porta hepatis to the splenic hilum (levels 18 through 20). The left gastric artery is sacrificed as close to the celiac axis as possible, and all lymphatic tissue along the left gastric artery is resected. Splenectomy, which previously was included as part of the en bloc resection, is now omitted as a routine, although an omentectomy often is performed. Reconstruction of the esophagus is performed with the colon or the stomach.

The cranial surfaces of the celiac plexus, hepatic, and splenic arteries are completely dissected of all lymph-bearing tissue (levels 16 through 20). The lymph-bearing tissue in the retroperitoneum along the medial edge of the inferior vena cava down to the pancreas and to the left crus also is included in the resection. If colon is being used as a conduit, a proximal two thirds gastrectomy is performed, including all the lymph nodes around the stomach. If the stomach is used, the lesser curvature and cardia lymph tissue (levels 16 and 17) are included in the resected portion of the stomach as it is fashioned into a tubular conduit.

The final incision is a left transverse cervicotomy, which is used to mobilize the remainder of the esophagus and perform the reconstruction with the neoesophagus conduit (stomach or colon). A central lymph node dissection is performed, although a formal bilateral cervicothoracic lymph node dissection as in the radical three-field resection (Japanese en bloc esophagectomy) usually is not performed. The esophagus is transected in the neck, and the entire specimen is brought into the abdomen and removed. Reconstruction is performed by bringing the colon or stomach into the neck for an anastomosis to the remaining cervical esophagus.

Three-Field Radical Lymph Node Dissection
A three-field (extended or radical) lymph node dissection (Japanese en bloc esophagectomy) is similar to the two-field dissection but includes a thorough dissection of the cervical lymph nodes, where tumor deposits can exist as skip metastases (occult or clinical disease). The operation proceeds as in the two-field en bloc resection with the addition of a cervicothoracic, bilateral recurrent nerve, internal jugular, and supraclavicular lymphadenectomy. Some Japanese surgeons have added an "extended" resection taking the upper mediastinal lymph node stations (levels 2R/L and 3P) as well, including the nodes at the aortopulmonary window (levels 5 and 6).

The extended resection in the chest proceeds through a right posterolateral thoracotomy in the fifth interspace.

Table 1 Radical and Nonradical Lymph Node Dissections

RADICAL LYMPH NODE DISSECTION
Two-field dissection (chest, abdomen)
   En bloc esophagectomy
Three-field dissection (chest, abdomen, neck)
   Japanese en bloc esophagectomy
NONRADICAL LYMPH NODE DISSECTION
Two-field dissection (chest, abdomen)
   Right transthoracic (Ivor-Lewis)
   Left transthoracic
Three-field dissection (chest, abdomen, neck)
   Total esophagectomy
   Transhiatal (no chest incision)
   Vagal-sparing esophagectomy

Table 2 Lymph Node Stations for Esophageal Cancer

STATION/DESCRIPTION*	LOCATION
1/Supraclavicular	Above suprasternal notch and clavicles
2R/Right upper paratracheal nodes	Between intersection of caudal margin of innominate artery with trachea and the apex of the lung
2L/Left upper paratracheal nodes	Between top of aortic arch and apex of the lung
3P/Posterior mediastinal nodes	Upper paraesophageal nodes, above tracheal bifurcation
4R/Right lower paratracheal nodes	Between intersection of caudal margin of innominate artery with trachea and cephalic border of azygos vein
4L/Left lower paratracheal nodes	Between top of aortic arch and carina
5/Aortopulmonary nodes	Subaortic and paraaortic nodes lateral to the ligamentum arteriosum
6/Anterior mediastinal nodes	Anterior to ascending aorta or innominate artery
7/Subcarinal nodes	Caudal to the carina of the trachea
8M/Middle paraesophageal lymph nodes	From the tracheal bifurcation to the caudal margin of the inferior pulmonary vein
8L/Lower paraesophageal lymph nodes	From the caudal margin of the inferior pulmonary vein to the esophagogastric junction
9/Pulmonary ligament nodes	Within the inferior pulmonary ligament
10R/Right tracheobronchial nodes	From cephalic border of azygos vein to origin of right upper lobe bronchus
10L/Left tracheobronchial nodes	Between carina and left upper lobe bronchus
15/Diaphragmatic nodes	Lying on the dome of the diaphragm and adjacent to or behind its crura
16/Paracardial nodes	Immediately adjacent to the gastroesophageal junction
17/Left gastric nodes	Along the course of the left gastric artery
18/Common hepatic nodes	Along the course of the common hepatic artery
19/Splenic nodes	Along the course of the splenic artery
20/Celiac nodes	At the base of the celiac artery

*Intrapulmonary stations 11 (interlobar), 12 (lobar), 13 (segmental), and 14 (subsegmental) have been excluded.

The arch of the azygos vein is resected, the brachiocephalic and right subclavian arteries are exposed, and lymph nodes along the right recurrent nerve and the right paratracheal area (2R) are removed. After esophageal transection, lymph nodes along the left recurrent nerve and in the left paratracheal areas (2L) are removed. The infraaortic, infracarinal, and paraesophageal lymph nodes (levels 3P, 7, and 8M) are removed with the esophagus, which allows exposure of the left pulmonary artery and hilar lymph nodes (level 4L). As with a standard two-field en bloc resection, the thoracic duct also is removed. After closure of the chest, a T-shaped neck incision is performed, and the sternomastoid and strap muscles are divided off the clavicular heads. The cervical nodes (internal jugular nodes below the cricoid, supraclavicular nodes, and cervical paraesophageal nodes) are cleared bilaterally. Both inferior thyroid arteries are ligated, and the paraesophageal nodes, including the recurrent nerve nodes in the cervicothoracic junction, are removed. This more radical procedure involves a higher rate of recurrent laryngeal nerve paresis because of the extensive dissection along the nerves in the neck and upper thorax but allows a thorough removal of all lymph nodes in the cervical region.

Nonradical Lymph Node Dissection
Two-Field Nonradical Lymph Node Dissection
The traditional two-field nonradical esophagectomy involves either a thoracoabdominal approach or the now preferred separate fifth interspace thoracotomy (right or left) combined with a transabdominal lymph node resection and mobilization of the conduit (neoesophagus). Regional nodal and lymphatic tissue around the left gastric artery, lesser curvature, and paraesophageal area usually are included in the

resection (levels 16 and 17), although deep celiac (level 20), common hepatic (level 18), and splenic (level 19) arteries usually are not removed unless involved with disease. In the thorax, subcarinal, inferior pulmonary ligament, and paraesophageal and paratracheal lymph nodes usually are removed (levels 4 and 7 through 10). Although the fields of dissection are similar to the more radical operations, the amount of surrounding tissue and lymph nodes removed is less, which may result in decreased operative times, hospital stays, and morbidity. Reconstruction of the esophagus usually is performed with the stomach, unless this conduit cannot be used, in which case colon or jejunum can be used. The anastomosis is performed in the chest (two-field, nonradical, right or left transthoracic) or the neck (three-field, nonradical, total esophagectomy), in which case a cervical incision is added, and the upper thoracic esophagus is removed. Lymph nodes are not typically removed from the upper thorax in nonradical lymph node dissections in an attempt to avoid injuries to the recurrent laryngeal and phrenic nerves.

Three-Field Nonradical Lymph Node Dissection
The transhiatal esophagectomy involves an abdominal and neck incision without a thoracic incision, although the thoracic field is entered and dissected from the abdomen (three-field, nonradical, chest, abdomen, and neck). This procedure can be performed on patients with mid to distal tumors not invading surrounding structures. The mid thoracic portion of the esophagus (from the arch of the aorta to the carina) is dissected by tactile technique and is performed close to the esophageal wall to avoid injury to vital structures. Contrary to intuition, most of the lower esophageal dissection can be done under direct vision from the abdomen by enlarging the

hiatus and using an appropriately placed retractor. Lymph nodes in the thoracic inlet and outlet can be sampled, and most surgeons perform a partial dissection up to the level of the inferior pulmonary ligament or the carina. Cervical lymph nodes are resected if they appear clinically involved through the cervical incision. Most of the intrathoracic lymph nodes (apart from levels 2 through 6 and 10 through 14) can be removed, although not as completely as with a thoracotomy incision. Lymphadenectomy in the abdomen is similar to other nonradical procedures and includes the paraesophageal, lesser curvature, left gastric, and superficial celiac nodes (levels 16, 17, and 20). Formal dissection of lymph nodes from the porta hepatis to the splenic hilum, including the deep celiac axis nodes, is not usually performed unless clinically involved (levels 18 through 20).

Vagal-Sparing Esophagectomy

Another procedure that is reserved for a select group of patients is the nonradical vagal-sparing esophagectomy. This esophagectomy is performed by stripping the esophagus from the mediastinum while sparing the vagal nerves. Three fields are entered (neck, chest, and abdomen), but lymph nodes are not usually removed during this surgery. The stomach and pylorus remain intact, and a colon interposition is used to reconstruct the resected esophagus. Most surgeons believe this operation is appropriate only for patients with high-grade dysplasia or early mucosal lesions because it does not allow an extensive oncologic resection. Because preoperative staging currently has limitations in correctly assessing the primary tumor, much of the assessment must be performed at the time of surgery. Any evidence of deeper invasion at the time of surgery should prompt a wider resection with a more traditional radical or nonradical lymphadenectomy. Advocates of this procedure believe the operation allows similar survivals in early stage patients and leads to improved functional outcomes with less dumping and nutritional sequelae. Randomized comparisons have not yet been performed, however, and the procedure remains experimental.

■ RESULTS

The esophageal surgeon should be familiar with the lymphatic drainage of the esophagus as it relates to esophageal neoplasms. Proponents of the radical lymph node resections in esophageal cancer have paved the way to understanding the lymphatic drainage patterns of metastases to local and regional lymph nodes. Most importantly, these investigators have found that there is a significant incidence of local and regional lymph node involvement and skip metastases even in lesions that previously were considered early disease. The oncologic benefit of the more extensive and potentially morbid radical lymph node dissections still has not been determined. Although many nonrandomized single-institution series have been published claiming improved long-term survival and decreased local recurrence with radical lymph node dissections, no meaningful randomized studies have been performed to date in esophageal cancer. Additionally, of concern is the fact that in gastric cancer randomized trials have shown increased morbidity and no improved survival when radical lymph node dissections were performed. At present, the type of lymph node dissection performed for esophageal cancer remains controversial and depends on the practicing surgeon's and patient's preferences.

SUGGESTED READING

Baba M, et al: Long-term results of subtotal esophagectomy with three-field lymphadenopathy for carcinoma of the thoracic esophagus, *Ann Surg* 219:310, 1994.

Bonekamp JJ, et al: Extended lymph-node dissection for gastric cancer, *N Engl J Med* 340:908, 1999.

Hagen JA, et al: Superiority of extended en bloc esophagogastrectomy for carcinoma of the lower esophagus and cardia, *J Thorac Cardiovasc Surg* 106:850, 1993.

Hosch SB, et al: Esophageal cancer: the mode of lymphatic tumor cell spread and its prognostic significance, *J Clin Oncol* 19:1970, 2001.

Rice TR: Superficial oesophageal carcinoma: is there a need for three-field lymphadenectomy? *Lancet* 354:792, 1999.

PALLIATIVE SURGICAL PROCEDURES FOR ESOPHAGEAL CARCINOMA

Ozuru Ukoha
William H. Warren

The symptoms of esophageal carcinoma, as with other solid malignancies, present so late in the course of the tumor that only a few patients are candidates for surgical resection with curative intent. Even among these patients undergoing a "complete" resection, most experience recurrence locally and/or distantly, providing at best a 5-year survival of only 20%. One may argue logically that, with the exception of patients whose carcinoma was detected incidentally or as part of a screening process, esophagogastrectomy is itself in most patients only a palliative surgical procedure. Many surgeons would perform an esophagogastrectomy in the face of celiac or small, solitary liver metastases if the patient were a good surgical risk because this resection of the esophagus and reconstruction in many cases provides the best palliation. The role of esophagogastrectomy in the management of esophageal carcinoma is discussed in another chapter.

This chapter focuses on surgical procedures and other treatment options designed to palliate the patient. Palliation, by definition, means focusing and limiting the treatment plan to the amelioration of symptoms. In common parlance, the term *palliation* infers that either the patient is not a good candidate to undergo a curative treatment modality or the tumor is beyond the limits of resectability. Although there are several options, not all are readily available at all institutions, and the treatment choice should be influenced, at least in part, by the status of the patient, the location of the tumor, and the chief complaint (i.e., whether the patient has or is likely to develop aspiration pneumonia, an esophago-tracheal fistula, or incapacitating reflux symptoms). It is also true that, with few exceptions, these treatment modalities are not mutually exclusive, and often combinations are used.

Ideal palliation should be safe, efficacious, well tolerated, easy to learn and apply, and cost-effective. There is a temptation, particularly in this group of terminal, malnourished, and generally miserable patients, to do little or nothing. This nihilistic approach is seldom justified, however, and most patients given the opportunity would accept reasonable surgical risk for palliation of their symptoms. Simple placement of a feeding gastrostomy tube usually requires a laparotomy and does not address the issue of salivary retention and the high incidence of aspiration pneumonia.

■ ESOPHAGEAL BYPASS

When carcinoma of the esophagus has invaded local structures (classically middle third tumors fixed to the tracheobronchial tree or lower third tumors fixed to the aorta or pericardium) such that it is technically unresectable, but the patient is a reasonable candidate for major surgery, some authors have advocated a surgical bypass procedure. This procedure reestablishes continuity of the upper gastrointestinal tract, allowing oral alimentation, while leaving the tumor in place. Patients considered for these procedures must have maintained their nutritional status and have cleared their airway contamination to the degree that they present an acceptable operative risk. Such a scenario is uncommon.

Over the years, many operative procedures have been described, and each has its advocates. Generally, these procedures can be discussed according to the route of bypass (retrosternal, presternal, or posterior mediastinal) and bypassing conduit (stomach, colon, or jejunum). In patients with carcinomas in the middle third of the esophagus, the most popular bypass procedure is a retrosternal bypass using a gastric conduit. The retrosternal route is preferred because it is shorter than the presternal (with less tension on the conduit), while avoiding proximity to the tumor (with the possibility of local invasion by the tumor or injury by radiotherapy). The stomach is the preferred organ because it has a reliable blood supply and requires only a single anastomosis. We prefer to place this anastomosis in the neck because this minimizes the consequences of an anastomotic leak. Some authors have cautioned, however, that if the whole stomach is used in an isoperistaltic fashion, the leak rate is high. One reason may be extrinsic compression at the thoracic inlet compromising the blood supply. If this is assessed to be the case, resection of the medial third of the clavicle and the first rib is indicated.

In these procedures in which the tumor-bearing portion of the esophagus is detached, the isolated and obstructed length of esophagus has the potential of distending with mucosal secretions. This risk of developing such an esophagocele is minimized by radiating the isolated segment. Nevertheless, the risk is such that the excluded segment of esophagus must be drained through the neck with a Mallencot drain for at least 1 month. If after this time interval the esophageal segment distends with secretions, a tract will have been established.

Other authors have advocated fashioning longer gastric conduits from the greater curvature using isoperistaltic or reversed (i.e., antiperistaltic) tubes. Advantages of constructing these gastric tubes from the greater curvature as opposed to using the entire stomach are simplicity and timeliness of the procedure. These conduits generally are believed to have a higher incidence of anastomotic leaks, however, presumably due to compromised blood supply. All of the above-mentioned techniques can reestablish satisfactory swallowing and allow the patient to undergo palliative radiotherapy. The perioperative mortality is generally 20%, the anastomotic leak is greater than 20%, and the median survival in these select patients is only 6 months.

A special circumstance arises with unresectable carcinomas of the esophagogastric junction. Tumors in this location may be fixed to the hiatus and extend along the lesser curvature such that mobilization of the stomach is impossible. In this situation, the tumor can be bypassed using the gastric fundus.

Colonic interposition is indicated when use of the stomach is contraindicated by previous surgery or extensive gastric involvement. Any segment of the colon can be used, but interposition of the descending colon based on the left colic artery is preferred due to the more reliable blood supply. Use of the jejunum as a conduit for interposition is the least desirable because it is unable to reach to the neck and has a more tenuous blood supply. Intrathoracic bypass using a Roux-en-Y jejunal loop can be used to advantage, however, when extensively infiltrating carcinomas of the esophagogastric junction require bypass of the distal esophagus and the stomach.

Most patients with unresectable esophageal carcinomas are not candidates for esophageal bypass procedures due to prohibitive operative risk factors. In the past, some have attempted to palliate the symptoms of obstruction by simple intermittent dilation. Although their symptoms can be palliated, relief is usually short-lived, and future dilations become progressively more frequent and technically challenging.

Most clinicians believe that when the esophageal passage is reopened, additional therapy should be employed to maintain patency. Esophageal intubation, direct ablation of the obstructing tumor (using neodymium:yttrium-aluminum-garnet (Nd:YAG) photoablation, bipolar electrocautery, or cryoablation), and photodynamic therapy all have been employed to accomplish this, and each has its advocates.

■ ESOPHAGEAL INTUBATION

Prosthetic intubation of the esophagus has been performed for more than 60 years with many modifications in the design of the stents and insertion techniques. Today, several products are available, but almost all are inserted through the mouth without need for a laparotomy. Attractive features of this method of palliation include low cost, ease of insertion, prompt palliation of obstructive symptoms, short hospital stay, and generally good early results.

The two categories of esophageal stents are best discussed according to their composition. Plastic stents (Celestin; Wilson-Cook, Wilson-Cook Medical, Winston-Salem, NC; Atkinson, Keymed/Olympus, New York, NY; Montgomery; Hood Laboratories, Pembroke, MA) all require predilation of the strictured esophagus to allow positioning. With the exception of the Montgomery-Hood stent, these prostheses are available in only one or two diameters and are held in place by the esophageal stricture. Inability to dilate the esophagus to a predetermined diameter precludes placement, whereas overdilation favors migration, which is seen to occur in 12% of cases. Perforation of the esophagus at the time of placement (6%) and obstruction of the stent by tumor overgrowth or food impaction (4% to 10%) are other complications. Ideal malignant strictures for plastic prostheses are short and straight and are at least 2 cm below the upper esophageal sphincter and 4 cm above the esophagogastric junction. Among the plastic prostheses, the exception to these limitations is the Montgomery-Hood stent.

Self-expanding metal stents (SEMS) (Wallstent, Ultraflex, Microvasive/Boston Scientific, Natick, MA; Gianturco-Z, Wilson-Cook, Winston-Salem, NC; Esophacoil-Instent, Intra Therapeutics, Eden Prairie, MN) have enjoyed popularity due to their ease of insertion, flexibility to accommodate a tortuous passage, and variable diameter. Overall, operative mortality with simple obstruction (as opposed to cases complicated with a respiratory tract fistula) has been 1%.

Disadvantages include the cost of the prosthesis and the fact that SEMS, in contrast to plastic stents, once deployed cannot be removed or repositioned in the event of poor initial placement or subsequent migration.

Although the perforation rate can be 3% without dilation, palliation still is limited because the radial force of the stents alone is insufficient to dilate the stricture. Most clinicians dilate the stricture either before placing the stent or when the stent is in place using a balloon. Uncovered SEMS have a lower migration rate than plastic prostheses but allow tumor ingrowth through the interstices, which eventually causes repeat obstruction. Covered SEMS minimize the risk of tumor ingrowth but have a migration rate comparable to plastic stents. In addition, all stents bridging the esophagogastric junction precipitate gastroesophageal reflux. In addition, placement of stents within 2 cm of the cricopharyngeus causes pain and a choking sensation, limiting their use. Especially in these last two clinical scenarios, alternative strategies should be considered.

■ DIRECT TUMOR ABLATIVE TECHNIQUES

Although there are many techniques to ablate esophageal carcinomas directly, the most popular method currently has been the Nd:YAG laser. This technique usually is applied using a fiberoptic bundle through a flexible esophagoscope after the stricture has been dilated sufficiently to allow for passage of the scope into the stomach. The tumor is photoablated at 80 to 100 W as the scope is withdrawn across the stricture to avoid extensive gas bloating and to accomplish palliation in a single session. Precision of aiming and depth of ablation have been advantages over a variety of alternative techniques, including intralesional injection of chemotherapeutic agents, electrocautery, and cryoablation.

Direct tumor ablation ideally is suited for exophytic endoesophageal tumors but alone does not palliate patients with significant extrinsic compression. Although the initial palliation of dysphagia is thought to be better than after prosthetic intubation, predictably tumor regrowth requires repeat treatments at 6- to 12-week intervals. We prefer to stent all obstructing esophageal lesions with the exception of proximal and distal lesions.

■ PHOTODYNAMIC THERAPY

The more recent Food and Drug Administration approval of photodynamic therapy as a standard therapy for palliating obstructing esophageal carcinomas has stimulated further interest in this therapeutic modality. Patients are administered an intravenous dose of a photosensitizing agent (porfimer sodium), which is selectively retained in malignant cells. The agent is photoactivated 48 hours later by 630 nm by a pumped argon dye laser. The activated drug causes cell death to a tissue depth of 1 cm. Subsequently the necrotic tumor is sloughed to the gastrointestinal tract or débrided using a flexible esophagoscope. Attractive features include safety and duration of palliation longer than Nd:YAG therapy alone. Palliation without prior dilation is slower in onset, however, than after placement of an endoprosthesis. The treatment is expensive, and the patient is unable to be exposed to direct sunlight for 6 weeks owing to risk of severe sunburn.

■ ESOPHAGOTRACHEAL FISTULA

Of all the aforementioned therapeutic modalities, only esophageal bypass surgery or placement of a prosthesis (either plastic or covered SEMS) effectively excludes esophagotracheal fistula. Chronic aspiration usually precludes the former option. Although some authors have advocated placement of the stent in the airway, diversion of the secretions is more secure, the procedure is accomplished more easily, and accompanying obstructive symptoms are better palliated by placement of the stent in the esophagus.

■ CARCINOMAS INVOLVING PROXIMAL 3 CM OF ESOPHAGUS

Unresectable tumors in the proximal 3 cm of the esophagus present a special clinical problem because the involvement of one or both recurrent laryngeal nerves makes the risk of aspiration pneumonitis especially high. Stents in this area can be uncomfortable because the flange causes a choking sensation or because there is impingement against an osteophyte of the cervical spine. Tumor overgrowth into the

proximal funnel of the stent also is common, causing recurrent dysphagia. The most easily tolerated stent in this location is the Montgomery-Hood salivary bypass stent. Alternatively, Nd:YAG laser photoablation and/or photodynamic therapy is a more appealing modality especially in this area, but clinical experience is limited.

SUGGESTED READING

Conlan AA, et al: Retrosternal gastric bypass for inoperable esophageal cancer: a report of 71 patients, *Ann Thorac Surg* 36:396, 1983.

Heier SK, et al: Photodynamic therapy for obstructing esophageal cancer: light dosimetry and randomized comparison with Nd:YAG laser therapy, *Gastroenterology* 109:63, 1995.

Popovsky J: Esophagogastrectomy in continuity for carcinoma of the esophagus: its use for unresectable tumors of the lower third of the esophagus and cardia, *Arch Surg* 115:637, 1980.

Reed CE: Endoscopic palliation of esophageal carcinoma, *Chest Surg Clin N Am* 4:155, 1994.

Warren WH: Palliation of dysphagia, *Chest Surg Clin N Am* 10:605, 2000.

Warren WH, et al: Clinical experience with Montgomery salivary bypass stents in the esophagus, *Ann Thorac Surg* 57:1102, 1994.

LASERS, STENTS, AND PHOTODYNAMIC THERAPY IN ESOPHAGEAL CANCER

Sanjay Jagannath
Marcia Irene Canto

T he estimated 5-year survival of esophageal cancer is only 5% to 10%, and currently it is the fifth leading cause of cancer death worldwide. The prevalence of esophageal cancer in the United States is rising at an alarming rate. Despite curative intentions, a large proportion of patients treated surgically eventually develop recurrence of malignancy. Given that the morbidity (20% to 60%) and mortality (10% to 33%) of palliative surgery is high and without any survival advantage, these approaches have largely been replaced by nonsurgical techniques.

Malignant dysphagia is difficulty swallowing due to malignancy and often results from a partially or completely occluded esophageal lumen (intraesophageal or extraesophageal tumor) or occasionally from tumor encroachment on esophageal

innervation. The goals of treatment in the management of malignant dysphagia are (1) to maintain esophageal luminal patency, (2) to minimize hospitalization, (3) to obtain adequate pain relief, and (4) to eliminate reflux and regurgitation. Table 1 lists the currently available endoscopic palliative techniques for the management of malignant dysphagia. Choosing the appropriate technique depends on the patient's clinical factors, physician's experience, and tumor characteristics. This chapter discusses the current role of lasers, stents, and photodynamic therapy (PDT) in the management of malignant dysphagia.

Table 1 Endoscopic Modalities for Management of Malignant Dysphagia

Chemical injection therapy (e.g., alcohol)
Chemotherapy
Dilation
Enteral feeding (e.g., percutaneous endoscopic gastrostomy)
Photodynamic therapy
Radiotherapy (external beam radiotherapy, brachytherapy)
Self-expanding metal stents
Thermal ablation
    Laser therapy (Nd:YAG or diode)
    Bipolar cautery ablation probe
    Argon plasma coagulator

■ LASER THERAPY

Laser therapy has been used for decades in the palliative management of malignant dysphagia, and it is a well-accepted form of treatment for esophageal and gastric cardia tumors. The greatest experience is with the neodymium:yttrium-aluminum-garnet (Nd:YAG) laser, which uses light at a wavelength of 1064 nm.

Factors that influence the success of laser therapy include the degree of obstruction, the length of the tumor (<5 cm), its circumferential extension, the course of the residual lumen, and the nutritional status of the patient. Malignant dysphagia due to exophytic lesions, short segment tumors, or noncircumferential or discrete strictures is particularly amenable to laser treatment. Laser treatment has been shown to be superior to dilation and other methods of thermal destruction, and it is well suited for the management of proximal esophageal lesions in which stent placement may not be feasible.

The overall success rate of laser therapy varies from 62% to 93%. Advantages for laser therapy include the prompt relief of dysphagia, the long duration of dysphagia relief (2 to 4 months), and the low complication rate. A distinct disadvantage is that multiple laser treatment sessions often are required to palliate fully the dysphagia symptom (two to three sessions). The dysphagia-free interval can be prolonged further when combined with percutaneous or intracavitary radiotherapy. Complications include tracheoesophageal fistula formation (0.7% to 6.3%), bleeding, and perforation (1% to 5.8%), with a method-related 30-day mortality of 1% to 5%. The relatively high perforation rate is likely due to the preliminary step of dilation of the malignancy rather than laser treatment itself. The mean survival after successful palliation is 12 to 22 weeks and is comparable to other treatment modalities for malignant dysphagia.

■ ESOPHAGEAL STENTS

For decades, semirigid plastic esophageal stents commonly were used for the management of malignant dysphagia. These plastic stents contained a fixed internal diameter that was often less than 12 mm, and placement required aggressive presenting dilation, resulting in a relatively high esophageal perforation rate of 8% to 12.5%. Given the small internal diameter, successful deployment of plastic stents did not always guarantee a clinical improvement in dysphagia.

The advent of self-expanding metal stents (SEMS) in the 1990s was an important development in the management of malignant esophageal strictures (Table 2). SEMS are composed of tightly wound wire coils or mesh that is wrapped around a small delivery device, making endoscopic placement simple and often obviating the need for aggressive dilation. On deployment of the SEMS, the radial expansive force allows the stent to expand to its final diameter and shape. The wire coils/mesh embedded in the esophageal mucosa or submucosa trigger a mild inflammatory response. Placement of SEMS is usually atraumatic, and dysphagia is relieved immediately.

A variety of commercially manufactured SEMS are available, and they differ in their physical properties (Table 3).

Table 2 Advantages of Self-Expanding Metal Stents
Easily placed through the endoscopic channel (a small-diameter delivery system)
Greater internal diameter compared with plastic stents (expand 18-25 mm in internal diameter)
Available in a variety of lengths (4 cm, 6 cm, 9 cm)
Lower risk of perforation compared with plastic stents
Insertion through a tight stricture without need for endoscopic dilation
Potential as a single therapeutic procedure that functions for the remainder of the patient's life

Being aware of these properties allows the physician to choose the most appropriate stent based on the characteristics of the malignant stricture. Certain stents are covered with a thin silicone lining, which helps to prevent tumor ingrowth and to manage tracheoesophageal fistulas.

No comparative trials evaluating the safety and efficacy of the various SEMS exist. Successful stent deployment is reported in 90% to 100% of patients with primary or secondary esophageal obstruction and in 67% to 100% of patients with tracheoesophageal fistulas. Double SEMS can be used in advanced extrinsic esophageal or bronchial tumors with stenoses of the esophagus and the respiratory tract.

Indications and Contraindications

An esophageal stent is indicated when dilation becomes ineffective or too risky or when the frequency of dilation is too great to justify the risk of perforation. Table 4 lists lesions most amenable to SEMS placement. Relative contraindications are soft or noncircumferential stenoses or markedly angulated strictures that may prevent adequate anchoring of the SEMS.

Complications

Early minor complications include chest pain, stent misplacement (minimized by choosing a stent 4 cm longer than the length of the stricture), and migration. The incidence varies widely from 0% to 40%, but the higher complication rates are likely related to using stents with suboptimal radial expansion. Early major complications include perforation and bleeding, which are observed in 6% of patients. Life-threatening long-term complications include gastrointestinal bleeding, perforation, and development of a tracheoesophageal fistula. The incidence varies from 4% to 7%, but in patients with a prior history of chemotherapy or radiotherapy, there is a statistically significant increased rate of life-threatening complications and an associated increase in mortality rate. This increased risk is not related to the patient's age, the length of the stricture, the grade of dysphagia, or a prior history of surgery. Presumably, tissue integrity was compromised with the administration of chemotherapy or radiation therapy, and this predisposes SEMS patients to a higher risk of life-threatening complications. Tumor ingrowth is a late complication (incidence 10% to 60% in uncovered wall stents) that has been reduced with the advent of silicone-covered or polyurethane-covered SEMS, but at the cost of increased stent migration (16% migration rate for

Table 3 Properties of Selected Self-Expanding Metal Stents

	WALL STENT*	ULTRAFLEX*	Z-STENT†
Material	Elgiloy	Nitinol	Stainless steel
Radial force	Very strong	Moderate	Mild
Internal diameter (mm)	19	18-23	18
Covered	Yes	Yes	Yes
% Shortening	30	30-40	0-10
Fistula closure	Yes	Yes	Yes

*Microvasive/Boston Scientific Inc., Natick, MA.
†Wilson-Cook Medical Inc., Winston-Salem, NC.

Table 4 Lesions Amenable to Esophageal Stenting

Long, circumferential stenoses
Rapidly growing tumors
Extraluminal neoplasms resulting in compression of the
    esophageal lumen
Recurrent stenosis due to
    Chemoradiotherapy
    Laser photocoagulation
    Surgery
Tracheoesophageal fistula

uncovered SEMS versus 4% for covered SEMS). Treatment options for management of tumor ingrowth include laser therapy, injection therapy, electrocoagulation, PDT, argon plasma coagulation, and placing an overlapping second SEMS. Management should be tailored to the individual case.

■ PHOTODYNAMIC THERAPY

PDT is a nonthermal ablative technique resulting in local necrosis of malignant esophageal tissue. A photosensitive chemical (hematoporphyrin, porfimer sodium [Photofrin]) is administered to the patient intravenously 48 to 72 hours before drug activation. Porfimer sodium has a relative specificity for malignant tissue and is activated by the direct application of light. At the time of the procedure, an optical fiber with a linear diffuser tip is positioned intraluminally within the tumor segment. A laser generates a monochromatic beam, which activates porfimer sodium and generates cytotoxic singlet oxygen radicals. These radicals result in rapid vascular stasis and hemorrhage and induce an acute inflammatory reaction followed by direct and anoxia-induced tumor necrosis.

The localized effect of PDT is based on several factors: the relative specificity of a photosensitizer for malignant tissue, the directed application of light, the transmission depth of the wavelength of light, and the oxygen content of the tissue. The remaining tissue heals well, and because there is no cumulative toxicity, PDT can be repeated as needed without interfering with or precluding other forms of therapy. Approximately 48 hours after the first light treatment session, a second endoscopy is performed to assess the degree of necrosis, to measure the luminal diameter, and to débride

residual tumor. Any remaining visible tumor is treated again in the same manner without reinjection of porfimer sodium.

Indications

PDT is indicated for malignant esophageal strictures. Most PDT patients have failed, refused, or are ineligible for surgery or systemic therapy due to stage IV disease or associated comorbidity. Tumor characteristics amenable to PDT include length greater than 8 to 10 cm; circumferential lesions; tumor location in the upper third of the esophagus or at the gastroesophageal junction; and flat, recurrent anastomotic tumors.

Clinical contraindications to PDT include known porphyria (or hypersensitivity to porphyrins), tumor infiltration into the respiratory tract, and the presence of a tracheoesophageal fistula. Relative contraindications include symptomatic pleural or pericardial effusions and unstable arrhythmias.

Adverse Effects

The adverse effects of PDT are shown in Table 5. Patients may develop transient substernal or epigastric pain, odynophagia, or worsening dysphagia. Fever, leukocytosis, and asymptomatic pleural effusions may be present and often resolve promptly without intervention.

Porfimer sodium is retained primarily by the reticuloendothelial system of the liver, spleen, and kidney and is distributed into the skin. Given that the longest half-life of porfimer sodium is 36 days, skin photosensitivity can occur for 3 months after injection. Patients are cautioned to avoid direct sunlight, strong fluorescent or incandescent light, strong residential indoor lights, and radiant heat for at least 30 days. Skin photosensitivity can vary from mild erythema and pruritus, to severe erythema and edema, to blisters with skin desquamation. Topical sunscreens are *not* beneficial because they block ultraviolet light, not the offending infrared light.

■ CLINICAL TRIALS

Comparative studies of laser therapy and PDT have been performed to evaluate their efficacy in managing malignant dysphagia. PDT has a remarkable ability to reduce tumor bulk. Studies showed that PDT and Nd:YAG laser therapy were equivalent in improving dysphagia at 1 week; however, at 1 month, PDT-treated patients exhibited significantly greater improvements in dietary performance and Karnofsky

Table 5 Adverse Effects of Photodynamic Therapy

SYMPTOMS	SIGNS
Odynophagia	Fever
Dysphagia	Leukocytosis
Epigastric/substernal pain	Pleural effusion
	Skin photosensitivity

performance status. The number of endoscopic sessions required to treat the lesion completely was not significantly different for the two modalities, but the duration of response was longer with PDT-treated patients (84 days versus 53 days, $p = .0008$).

A large, multicenter trial showed that 45% of patients treated with PDT or laser had complete or partial luminal response at 1 week, and at 1 month, this response was statistically higher for PDT patients (32% versus 20%, $p < .05$). Palliation of dysphagia was equivalent with both therapies, with almost 50% achieving one or more grades of improvement in dysphagia and half of these responders being able to swallow normally. The time to palliative failure was 34 days for PDT and 42 days for Nd:YAG laser therapy, and the median survival with both modalities was 4.5 months.

PDT is excellent for the management of tumor ingrowth through uncovered metal stents and tumor overgrowth in covered stents. The mean dysphagia-free interval has been reported to be 92 days. The nonthermal nature of PDT obviates concerns about damaging the metal frame or plastic coverings of stents as observed with Nd:YAG laser, monopolar electrocoagulation, and argon plasma coagulation. PDT treatment is less painful, and successful ablation often is accomplished in fewer sessions than required by other modalities.

Stenting now is performed primarily only with SEMS. A randomized trial showed that early complications were significantly less frequent in the metal stent group compared with the plastic stent group. In contrast, delayed morbidity with expandable stents is large, with complications such as dislocation, hemorrhage, perforation, and chronic severe thoracic pain. Studies raise concern over an increased morbidity in patients previously treated by chemoradiation. Covered metal stents are ideal for closure of a tracheoesophageal fistula and can be placed in the respiratory tract with double stenting of the esophagus and the trachea to improve fistula control.

Due to a lack of controlled trials, selection of SEMS for palliation of malignant dysphagia is based on the physical properties of the stents, the clinical results, the individual anatomy, and personal experiences. The risk of stent migration is high in patients with gastric cardia stenoses, noncircumferential tumor growths, and soft or necrotic lesions. Tumor or granulation infiltration is expected in most patients with intrinsic tumors who receive uncovered stents, and covered devices usually are preferred. Sealing of tracheoesophageal respiratory fistulas or perforation of the esophagus can be accomplished with covered SEMS. In certain clinical scenarios, the ability to remove a stent can be important in patients with a difficult anatomy and a high risk of migration or misplacement. Plastic stents are easy to reposition or to remove, whereas SEMS traditionally are considered permanent once deployed, especially when the filaments of the mesh are embedded in esophageal tissue.

■ CONCLUSION

The overall prognosis of esophageal cancer remains poor, but the spectrum of available therapeutic modalities for improvement in quality of life after treatment is greater. Options such as laser therapy, PDT, and stenting are complementary, and it is important to understand the advantages, disadvantages, and indications for each type of modality. Without further controlled studies, the current decisions on which modality is most appropriate rely on the clinical scenario, patient comorbidities, tumor characteristics, and physician's experience.

SUGGESTED READING

Lightdale CJ: The role of photodynamic therapy in the management of advanced esophageal cancer, *Gastrointest Endosc Clin N Am* 10:397, 2000.

Nelson D: The Wallstent I and II for malignant esophageal obstruction, *Gastrointest Endosc Clin N Am* 9:403, 1999.

Saidi RF, Marcon NE: Nonthermal ablation of malignant esophageal strictures: photodynamic therapy, endoscopic intratumoral injections, and novel modalities, *Gastrointest Endosc Clin N Am* 8:465, 1998.

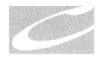

ESOPHAGEAL REPLACEMENT

IVOR-LEWIS ESOPHAGECTOMY

Jeffrey L. Port
Nasser Altorki

Historically the Ivor-Lewis esophagectomy was a two-staged procedure. A laparotomy was performed with gastric mobilization, followed 1 week later by thoracotomy, esophagectomy, and esophagogastric anastomosis. This was a radical deviation from the standard of blunt esophagectomy, cervical esophagostomy, gastrostomy, and later skin tube reconstruction. The evolved one-stage Ivor-Lewis procedure has become the benchmark procedure by which all approaches currently are measured.

■ INDICATIONS AND CONTRAINDICATIONS

A variety of surgical approaches exist for esophageal resection. The choice of which type of resection is most suitable takes several factors into consideration, including the tumor's location, the patient's condition and body habitus, previous operations, prior irradiation, the replacement conduit organ, limits of node dissection, and the surgeon's preference. Controversy abounds in regard to the best management of middle and lower third tumors. Traditionally, these tumors have been resected by an Ivor-Lewis approach or combined laparotomy and right thoracotomy. Indications for an Ivor-Lewis esophagectomy, other than carcinoma, include high-grade dysplasia, caustic esophageal injury, and esophagectomy after previously failed antireflux procedures. The Ivor-Lewis esophagectomy is not indicated in patients with proximal carcinomas and may be difficult in a patient with a previous right thoracotomy.

■ PREOPERATIVE PREPARATION

Preoperative evaluation should be aimed at establishing a histologic diagnosis, establishing extent of local and distant disease, and assessing the patient's physiologic status. Radiologic evaluation should include an upper gastrointestinal series. The esophagogram documents the location and length of the lesion and may suggest extraesophageal extension. Esophagoscopy should be performed routinely by the surgeon to document the precise location of the tumor and the presence of associated findings, such as Barrett's esophagus. Bronchoscopic examination also is mandatory in all proximal and middle tumors. A computed tomography scan of the chest and abdomen, although routinely obtained, is of limited value in determining the extent of mural penetration or nodal involvement. Its principal value is in the detection of visceral metastases. Endoscopic ultrasound, although not mandatory, quickly has become established as an invaluable tool in evaluating the depth of tumor penetration and involvement of regional lymph nodes. In our opinion, it is essential for all patients being considered for neoadjuvant therapy. Thoracoscopy and laparoscopy for the staging of local and distant lymph nodes, the identification of serosal and peritoneal implants, and the identification of liver metastases also has been reported; however, their role remains unclear. All esophageal cancer patients must have a careful assessment of pulmonary and cardiac status before resection. Many patients when questioned are current smokers who must be counseled to abstain at least 2 weeks before resection.

■ ANESTHETIC MANAGEMENT

All patients undergoing an Ivor-Lewis procedure should have an epidural catheter placed for postoperative pain control. In addition, a double-lumen endotracheal tube allows for single-lung ventilation and assists in the thoracic dissection. A radial arterial line preferably in the left arm for continuous blood pressure monitoring is recommended. Two large-bore peripheral intravenous catheters should be inserted, and urinary output should be monitored with a Foley catheter.

■ SURGICAL MANAGEMENT

The patient is positioned first in a supine manner for laparotomy, and a limited upper midline incision is performed. Full abdominal exploration ensues with special attention paid to evidence of tumor dissemination in the form of peritoneal and serosal implants, liver metastases, and celiac nodal disease and to assess local resectability of the tumor. Barring evidence of unresectability, the incision is extended. An abdominal self-retaining retractor (e.g., Omni, Buchwalder, or Goligher) is useful. The left lobe of the liver can be retracted cephalad or the triangular ligament divided and the lateral segment of the left lobe retracted to the right.

The lesser sac is entered safely away from the right gastroepiploic artery, and the greater omentum is divided along the greater curvature. The short gastric vessels are sequentially ligated and divided as close to the spleen as possible so as not to interrupt the epiploic arcade. One also must take care that stomach wall is not included in the ligature to avoid gastric necrosis. Through the lesser sac, the peritoneum is incised along the top of the pancreas, and all lymphatic tissue overlying the crura is taken in the specimen. With the stomach retracted upward, the left gastric vessels are ligated individually. Following this, the gastrohepatic ligament is opened, and the right gastric artery is preserved. Next the hiatus and distal esophagus are dissected, and the hiatus is widened. A Penrose drain is placed around the esophagus for traction. A Kocher maneuver is performed, and a pyloromyotomy is constructed. Much of the dissection of the distal esophagus can be performed bluntly through the abdomen. This dissection can be performed under direct vision up to the

level of the inferior pulmonary ligament. Before completion of the abdominal portion of the Ivor-Lewis procedure, a 16 Fr jejunostomy tube is placed. The abdomen is closed, and the patient is repositioned in the left lateral decubitus position for a right thoracotomy.

A posterolateral thoracotomy is performed through the fifth interspace, and the serratus muscle is spared. The right lung is selectively deflated and retracted anteriorly. First the azygos vein is transected with an endoscopic linear vascular stapler, and the pleura overlying the esophagus is opened sharply anterior to the azygos vein. The esophagus is dissected circumferentially and looped with an umbilical tape. The dissection is carried cephalad separating the esophagus from its tracheal and prevertebral attachments (Figure 1).

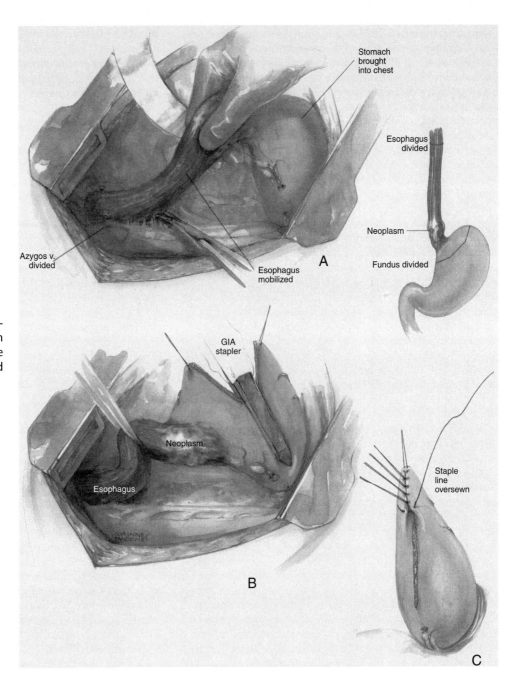

Figure 1
Intrathoracic dissection encompassing all tissue between the aorta and pericardium. The stomach is tubularized and the staple line oversewn.

Dissection of the esophagus proceeds inferiorly encompassing all tissue between the aorta and pericardium, including all periesophageal and subcarinal nodes. The esophagus should be transected at least 5 cm above the tumor with frozen section examination of the proximal resection margin.

The stomach is pulled into the chest, and the stomach is divided and tubularized with two to three firings of the linear GIA stapler. This staple line should be reinforced with interrupted 3-0 silk Lembert sutures. The esophagogastrectomy can be performed in a variety of ways, including the use of an EEA surgical stapler passed through a gastrostomy with no less than a 25-mm stapler. Alternatively a hand-sewn anastomosis can be created using continuous 3-0 PDS suture, interrupted at two or three points to avoid a purse-string effect (Figure 2). A nasogastric tube is positioned in the intrathoracic stomach. It is imperative to return any redundant stomach back into the abdomen to ensure proper gastric emptying. The edges of the gastric tube are sutured to the edge of the hiatus to prevent visceral herniation. The pleural cavity is drained with one 28 Fr chest tube placed in a paraspinous position.

■ POSTOPERATIVE MANAGEMENT

In the past, mechanical ventilation was maintained until the following postoperative day. Currently, with improved pulmonary physiotherapy and epidural pain control, patients are extubated immediately after surgery. Patients are encouraged to be out of bed and to ambulate with assistance the following day. The nasogastric tube often is removed by day 3, and jejunostomy feeding is begun the same day. A postoperative barium swallow is obtained by day 6, and if the anastomosis is intact, the patient's diet is advanced and the chest tube removed. Patients are discharged when they tolerate a soft diet, often still requiring supplemental jejunostomy feeds at night. Eventually the jejunostomy tube is removed 4 weeks after operation.

■ RESULTS

Modern-day results of the Ivor-Lewis procedure have shown that the technique can be performed safely with a low mortality and morbidity. In a report from the Massachusetts

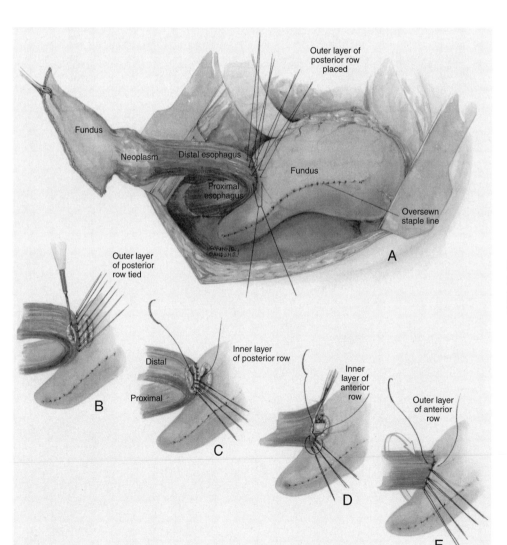

Figure 2
Hand-sewn anastomosis with placement of the nasogastric tube across the anastomosis.

General Hospital where 100 patients underwent an Ivor-Lewis esophagectomy, mortality was only 2.9%, and there were no anastomotic leaks. Dilation for postoperative stricture was required in five patients.

The concern over an intrathoracic leak undoubtedly has contributed to the popularity of the transhiatal esophagectomy, in which the anastomosis is created in the neck. In most retrospective reviews, there is a higher incidence of anastomotic leak in the cervical position with a less devastating effect compared with intrathoracic leaks. Similarly, although respiratory insufficiency and atelectasis may be higher in the transthoracic approach, pneumonia rates are similar. Also, chylothorax, recurrent nerve palsy, and tracheal tears are more common after transhiatal esophagectomy. Overall, most reports have failed to show the superiority of one procedure over the other.

■ MANAGEMENT OF COMPLICATIONS

Anastomotic Leaks

An asymptomatic leak that is detected on a routine barium swallow and appears to drain back into the esophageal lumen usually heals without intervention. Larger uncontained leaks require adequate drainage, however, by an interventional radiology pigtail catheter, chest tube, or open drainage. Any signs of sepsis in conjunction with a leak that is not drained adequately require thoracotomy and drainage of the chest and mediastinum and potentially decortication of the lung. Endoscopy is useful to determine the viability of the stomach and size of the leak. Small, well-drained leaks often heal if the lung is well expanded and there is no local sepsis. If there is extensive necrosis, however, often the safest plan is resection of the conduit and diverting cervical esophagostomy.

Anastomotic Stricture

In many reports, one third of patients develop a stricture at the anastomosis by 3 months after surgery. Dilation of this stricture can be accomplished by several means. We prefer endoscopic dilation with wire-guided Savory dilators.

Delayed Gastric Emptying

Clinically significant delayed gastric emptying is uncommon. Causes of delayed gastric emptying include the lack of a pyloric drainage procedure, obstruction at a tight hiatus, and a redundant intrathoracic stomach. Endoscopies and balloon dilation of the pylorus can be tried along with the addition of promotility agents, such as metoclopramide and erythromycin. If conservative management fails, the patient may require reoperation and an adequate drainage procedure.

Reflux

Reflux is a common problem after gastric pull-up. The level of severity seems to vary with the level of the anastomosis, with those above the azygos vein having a lower incidence than similarly constructed anastomoses below the vein. These symptoms are improved by smaller frequent feedings, avoidance of liquids with meals, and remaining upright after meals. Also, placement of a wedge for sleeping can palliate symptoms.

SUGGESTED READING

Allen MS: Ivor-Lewis esophagectomy, *Semin Thorac Cardiovasc Surg* 4:320, 1992.

Bains MS: Ivor-Lewis esophagectomy, *Chest Surg Clin N Am* 5:515, 1995.

Lewis I: Surgical treatment of carcinoma of the oesophagus, *Br J Surg* 34:18, 1946.

Mathisen DJ: Transthoracic esophagectomy: a safe approach to carcinoma of the esophagus, *Ann Thorac Surg* 45:137, 1988.

TRANSHIATAL ESOPHAGECTOMY

Mark Iannettoni
Andrew Chang

$\mathbf{V}$irtually every patient who is a candidate for esophageal resection is regarded as a candidate for transhiatal esophagectomy without thoracotomy. In our experience, nearly 75% of patients have undergone transhiatal esophagectomy for intrathoracic malignancies primarily involving the middle to lower third of the esophagus. Indications for transhiatal esophagectomy among patients with benign disease include esophageal neuromotor dysfunction, esophageal stricture, and Barrett's mucosa with high-grade dysplasia. More than 50% of patients referred with benign disease undergoing transhiatal esophagectomy have undergone one or more prior esophageal or periesophageal procedures, including most commonly previous antireflux repair, esophagomyotomy, repair of perforation, and vagotomy.

For patients with esophageal carcinoma, the basic evaluation includes a barium swallow examination, endoscopy, and a computed tomography (CT) scan of the chest and upper abdomen. Esophageal endoscopic ultrasound allows greater precision in the preoperative assessment of tumor invasion and regional lymph node metastases. Biopsy confirmation of distant (M1a, b) disease (e.g., hepatic, supraclavicular, or celiac lymph node involvement), suggested by the staging CT scan or endoscopic ultrasound, precludes the patient from esophagectomy. Positron emission tomography offers another novel means for showing occult metastatic disease.

The CT scan has not proved to be a reliable indicator of resectable disease. Contiguity of the esophageal tumor and the aorta or prevertebral fascia is not synonymous with invasion. Tracheobronchial invasion by upper or middle third esophageal tumors, confirmed by preoperative bronchoscopy, is an absolute contraindication to transhiatal esophagectomy. At exploration, palpation of the esophagus through the diaphragmatic hiatus allows the surgeon to determine whether the transhiatal approach is unsafe and transthoracic esophageal resection is necessary. Periesophageal fibrosis after prior mediastinal irradiation or severe intrathoracic adhesions arising from previous esophageal operations can result in palpable mediastinal periesophageal fixation to the aorta, the pericardium, or the tracheobronchial tree, which portends catastrophe should efforts persist to continue transhiatal esophageal resection.

■ PREOPERATIVE PREPARATION

Most of our patients undergoing transhiatal esophagectomy are admitted on the day of operation. We advocate vigorous preoperative pulmonary physiotherapy, consisting of regular use of incentive spirometry, a regimen of daily ambulation of 1 to 2 miles when possible, and absolute discontinuation of smoking for a minimum of 2 weeks preoperatively. With early postoperative ambulation and thoracic epidural analgesia, patients routinely are extubated in the operating room and do not require intensive care monitoring. Preoperative nutritional support is instituted with liquid diet supplements and a nasoenteric feeding tube, particularly in patients with high-grade esophageal obstruction. A preoperative percutaneous gastrostomy or jejunostomy feeding tube should be avoided, although satisfactory gastric mobilization can be obtained in patients with previously placed percutaneous gastrostomy tubes. Patients with prior gastric resection or with a history of ulcer disease or caustic ingestion undergo barium enema examination to assess the colon as an esophageal substitute should colonic interposition be required.

■ OPERATIVE TECHNIQUE

Transhiatal esophagectomy with a cervical esophagogastric anastomosis proceeds in four phases: (1) abdominal, (2) cervical esophageal mobilization, (3) transhiatal mediastinal dissection, and (4) cervical esophagogastric anastomosis. An intraarterial radial catheter is routine for continuous assessment of blood pressure, particularly during the mediastinal dissection, in which the heart can be displaced. Two large-bore peripheral intravenous lines should be maintained for rapid infusion, if necessary. With our current average intraoperative blood loss of less than 500 ml, however, we no longer require crossmatched blood for transfusion routinely. Central venous access is not required, and the left neck and upper chest should be kept free of intravenous lines. A double-lumen endotracheal tube is not used routinely in patients undergoing transhiatal esophagectomy. Routine thoracic epidural analgesia for postoperative pain management facilitates early extubation and provides better postoperative pulmonary hygiene.

The entire abdominal portion of the operation is performed through a supraumbilical incision. The triangular ligament of the liver is divided, and a table-mounted, self-retaining retractor is positioned to retract the left hepatic lobe and facilitate exposure of the upper abdomen. It is ascertained quickly whether the stomach is essentially normal, and the right gastroepiploic artery is identified early and protected. This is particularly important in patients with a history of prior abdominal surgery, in whom the need to divide adhesions may jeopardize the gastric blood supply.

Mobilization of the stomach begins at the midpoint of the greater curvature, where the right gastroepiploic artery terminates as it enters the stomach or anastomoses with small branches of the left gastroepiploic artery. Separation of the greater omentum from the right gastroepiploic artery is carried distally to the pylorus at least 1.5 to 2 cm inferior to the vessel to minimize the chance of injury to this artery, with care taken to avoid injury to the origin of the right gastroepiploic artery from the gastroduodenal artery. The left gastroepiploic and short gastric vessels are divided and ligated along the high greater curvature of the stomach, which avoids splenic trauma and gastric necrosis from ligation of these vessels too near the gastric wall. When the greater curvature of the stomach is mobilized, the peritoneum overlying the esophageal hiatus is incised, and the distal esophagus is encircled with a 1-inch Penrose drain.

Proceeding downward along the lesser curvature of the stomach, the gastrohepatic omentum along the high lesser curvature is incised, and the left gastric artery and vein are isolated, ligated, and divided. When the esophagectomy is being performed for carcinoma, the celiac axis lymph nodes are resected and submitted separately to the pathologist for staging purposes. When possible, the left gastric artery is divided near its origin from the celiac axis, but if there is a large celiac axis lymph node mass secondary to metastatic disease, cure is not possible, and unless these lymph nodes are relatively easily resectable, they should be biopsied, but not completely excised to decrease the risk of uncontrolled hemorrhage. The right gastric artery is protected as the remainder of the gastrohepatic omentum is divided inferiorly along the lesser curvature. After the stomach has been mobilized, a generous Kocher maneuver is performed to provide sufficient duodenal mobility that the pylorus can be displaced to the level of the xiphoid process in the midline. A pyloromyotomy is performed to avoid the possibility of delayed gastric emptying after the vagotomy that accompanies the esophagectomy.

The distal 5 to 10 cm of esophagus is mobilized from the posterior mediastinum into the abdomen by retracting the esophagogastric junction downward with the encircling Penrose drain, while dissecting upward into the mediastinum with the opposite hand. The mobility of the esophagus within the posterior mediastinum is assessed at this time. When operating for carcinoma, the tumor is grasped, and the esophagus is "rocked" from side to side to ascertain that it is not fixed to the prevertebral fascia, aorta, or adjacent mediastinal structures. If there is no marked fixation of the esophagus, which would preclude a transhiatal resection, the mediastinal dissection is temporarily discontinued. A 14 Fr rubber jejunostomy feeding tube is inserted 4 to 6 inches beyond the ligament of Treitz but is not brought out through the abdominal wall until the transhiatal esophagectomy is completed.

The cervical phase of the operation is performed through an oblique incision that parallels the anterior border of the left sternocleidomastoid muscle and extends from the suprasternal notch to the level of the cricoid cartilage. The platysma and omohyoid fascial layer are incised, the sternocleidomastoid muscle and carotid sheath and its contents are retracted laterally, and the larynx and trachea are retracted medially. No retractor should be placed in the tracheoesophageal groove during the cervical portions of this operation because injury to the recurrent laryngeal nerve can result not only in hoarseness, but also in episodes of aspiration due to impaired swallowing. The middle thyroid vein usually is ligated and divided, and the inferior thyroid artery may be ligated and divided as well. This vessel is an important landmark for the cricopharyngeus muscle, which is the superior extent of the esophageal dissection. Tumors requiring resection above these points are fraught with problems of aspiration and deglutination. Should resection be required above this point, a laryngopharyngoesophagectomy usually is required. This situation should have been evaluated preoperatively. In patients with a "bull neck" habitus or patients in whom cervical osteoarthritis prevents extension of the neck, there may be an inadequate length of cervical esophagus available for the anastomosis. In these cases, addition of a partial upper sternal split provides the prerequisite access to the high retrosternal esophagus. This procedure usually is not required, however.

The dissection proceeds directly posterior to the prevertebral fascia, which is followed by blunt finger dissection into the superior mediastinum. Dissection in the tracheoesophageal groove and injury to the left recurrent laryngeal nerve are avoided as the esophagus is retracted posteriorly away from the trachea, and by gentle blunt dissection anteriorly and along the right lateral esophageal wall, the cervical esophagus gradually is encircled with a Penrose drain. This drain is retracted superiorly as blunt dissection of the upper thoracic esophagus from the superior mediastinum is carried out. The volar aspects of the fingers are kept against the esophagus in the midline, and care is taken not to tear the posterior membranous trachea. By using this technique, the upper thoracic esophagus is mobilized almost to the level of the carina through the neck incision.

The transhiatal dissection of the esophagus is carried out in an orderly, sequential fashion. One hand in the abdomen is inserted through the diaphragmatic hiatus posterior to the esophagus as a "half sponge on a stick" is inserted into the superior mediastinum through the cervical incision along the prevertebral fascia. The esophagus is swept away from the prevertebral fascia from above until the sponge stick makes contact with the hand inserted through the diaphragmatic hiatus. Blood is evacuated from the posterior mediastinum by means of a 28 Fr Argyle Saratoga sump catheter (Tyco Healthcare, Mansfield, MA) inserted from the cervical incision downward into the mediastinum.

After completion of the posterior esophageal dissection, the anterior dissection is begun. The Penrose drain encircling the esophagogastric junction is retracted inferiorly as the surgeon's hand is inserted palm down against the anterior esophagus and is advanced into the mediastinum. The esophagus is mobilized progressively away from the posterior aspect of the pericardium and the carina. The hand must be kept posterior to minimize cardiac displacement and hypotension. Simultaneous dissection through the abdominal and cervical incisions along the anterior surface of the esophagus divides the typically filmy attachments to the posterior trachea.

With the anterior and posterior esophageal dissection now complete, the remaining lateral esophageal attachments now must be divided. The cervical esophagus is tensed gently by placing upward traction on its encircling Penrose drain. The lateral upper esophageal attachments are dissected gently away from the upper thoracic esophagus as it is delivered progressively into the neck wound. Now with downward traction on the Penrose drain encircling the esophagogastric junction, one hand is inserted palm downward through the diaphragmatic hiatus anterior to the esophagus and is advanced into the superior mediastinum behind the trachea until the completely circumferentially mobilized upper esophagus and its intact lateral attachments are palpated. The remaining periesophageal attachments and smaller vagal nerve branches are brought into direct view with a downward raking motion of the hand, and a retractor is placed into the hiatus and larger branches are ligated and divided, while smaller, filmy adhesions can be controlled with electrocautery or the harmonic scalpel. Larger vagal branches frequently are palpated along the distal esophagus, identified, ligated, and divided under direct vision. At times, subcarinal or subaortic periesophageal adhesions or fibrosis prevents complete mobilization of a 1- to 2-cm segment of mid esophagus. It may be necessary to compress this tissue firmly between the index finger and thumb, fracturing it. Alternatively, access to the upper thoracic esophagus to the level of the carina may be achieved by means of a partial upper sternal split so that the remaining periesophageal attachments can be divided under direct vision.

When the entire intrathoracic esophagus has been mobilized, an 8- to 10-cm length is delivered into the cervical wound, and the esophagus is divided with the gastrointestinal anastomosis (GIA) surgical stapler (US Surgical Co, Norwalk, CT). (When resecting the esophagus for benign disease, particularly that involving the distal half, the esophagus should be divided in the neck to leave a generous length of cervical and upper thoracic esophagus. In the event that there is any difficulty with the stomach reaching to the neck, a partial upper sternal split can be made, and the extra remaining length of upper esophagus then easily reaches to the gastric fundus.) After dividing the cervical esophagus, the stomach and thoracic esophagus are drawn out of the abdomen.

With the esophagus now removed, narrow deep retractors are placed in the diaphragmatic hiatus to allow direct inspection of the posterior mediastinum and the mediastinal pleura. If entry into either chest cavity has occurred during the esophageal dissection, a 32 Fr chest tube is inserted into the appropriate chest. The stomach and attached esophagus are placed on the anterior abdominal wall. The gastric fundus is retracted superiorly, and the lesser curvature of the stomach is cleaned of adjacent fat by dividing the vessels and fat at the level of the second vascular arcade ("crow's foot") from the cardia. The GIA stapler is used to divide the stomach beginning at this point. When the partial proximal gastrectomy has been completed, the esophagus and attached upper stomach are removed from the field. The stomach is divided typically 4 to 6 cm below palpable tumor. The gastric staple suture line is oversewn with a running 4-0 polypropylene Lembert stitch.

The point along the greatest curvature of the stomach that reaches most cephalad is identified. By gentle manipulation of the stomach through the diaphragmatic hiatus, the stomach is advanced gradually into the posterior mediastinum until the fundus appears in the cervical wound above the level of the clavicles. The gastric fundus is grasped gently and guided upward, while the other hand inserted into the mediastinum from the abdomen continually pushes the stomach upward, avoiding traction on the gastric conduit. Care must be taken to avoid torsion of the stomach during its positioning in the posterior mediastinum. In most patients, after mobilizing the gastric fundus so that its apex is several centimeters above the level of the clavicles, the pylorus comes to rest within 1 to 3 cm of the diaphragmatic hiatus in the abdomen.

Before performing the cervical anastomosis, the abdominal phase of the operation is concluded. The diaphragmatic hiatus is narrowed with interrupted 0 silk sutures so that it admits three fingers easily alongside the stomach. The edges of the diaphragmatic hiatus are tacked to the anterior gastric wall with one or two 3-0 silk sutures to prevent subsequent herniation of intraabdominal viscera into the chest. The pyloromyotomy is covered by adjacent omentum, which is covered by the previously retracted left hepatic lobe, which is returned to its normal location. The feeding jejunostomy tube is brought out through a separate left upper quadrant stab wound. After closing the abdominal wound, the last major portion of the operation, the cervical esophagogastric anastomosis, is performed.

Attention is returned to the neck incision, where the end of the remaining esophagus is retracted superiorly, and the anterior wall of the stomach behind the level of the clavicle is grasped gently with a Babcock clamp and drawn upward. A seromuscular traction suture in the anterior gastric wall elevates the stomach out of the depth of the incision and helps to maintain exposure of the stomach as the anastomosis is constructed. A needle-tipped electrocautery is used to create a 1.5-cm vertical gastrotomy, approximately 3 to 4 cm below the apex of the stomach, and submucosal bleeding points are coagulated sequentially. The required length of esophagus needed to fashion a tension-free anastomosis is estimated carefully, and excess esophagus is divided and submitted for histologic examination by beveling the end of the esophagus with a new knife blade so that the anterior edge is 1 to 1.5 cm longer than the posterior. The cervical esophagus must not be cut too short because when the gastric traction suture is removed and the upper stomach retracts back into the superior mediastinum, some additional esophageal length is needed to prevent tension on the anastomosis. Leaving the cervical esophagus too long can result in an inadequate cancer resection, however, leaving Barrett's mucosa or frank tumor behind. More importantly, a cervical esophagus that is too long can result in poor postoperative swallowing due to a tortuous conduit.

Two stay sutures facilitate alignment of the esophagus and stomach for the subsequent anastomosis. An Auto-Suture Endo GIA II 30-3.5 stapler (U.S. Surgical, Norwalk, CT) is inserted into the stomach and esophagus. Proper alignment of the posterior esophageal and anterior gastric walls is crucial as the stapler jaws are approximated (see Figure 1 in chapter on "Upper Thoracic Esophageal Cancer"). Before firing the cartridge, absorbable lateral suspension sutures are placed between the anterior gastric wall and adjacent posterior esophageal wall. To avoid further injury to the gastric tip and possible inadvertent seeding of an intervertebral disk, we no longer anchor the gastric fundus to the cervical prevertebral fascia. A 3-cm side-to-side anastomosis is created with the stapler. A 16 Fr nasogastric tube is inserted by the anesthetist and guided across the anastomosis into the intrathoracic stomach for postoperative gastric decompression. The opened edges of the esophagogastrostomy are approximated with two layers of interrupted absorbable suture. Singh et al reported their total mechanical stapled cervical esophagogastric anastomosis, using the Endo GIA stapler to close the esophagogastrostomy. Metallic clips are placed on either side of the final suture line to assist in future radiographic assessment. A small rubber drain is placed into the base of the wound near the anastomosis, the divided strap muscles and platysma are reapproximated loosely with interrupted absorbable sutures, and the skin is closed with a subcuticular suture. A portable chest radiograph, obtained in the operating room before extubation, establishes that the lungs are fully expanded, that there is no hemothorax or pneumothorax, and that the nasogastric and chest tubes are in proper position. Marked deviation of the nasogastric tube to either side should alert the surgeon to the possibility of a mediastinal hematoma.

■ TRANSHIATAL ESOPHAGECTOMY FOR CARCINOMA OF THE ESOPHAGOGASTRIC JUNCTION

The technique of transhiatal esophagectomy described earlier is applicable in most patients with carcinoma localized to the cardia and proximal stomach. The traditional proximal hemigastrectomy performed for such tumors "wastes" valuable stomach, which can be used for esophageal replacement; contributes little to the patient's longevity; and commits the surgeon to an intrathoracic esophageal anastomosis. In most cases, it is possible to divide the stomach 4 to 6 cm distal to palpable tumor, preserving the entire greater curvature of the gastric fundus. The narrowed remaining gastric "tube" functions well as an esophageal substitute.

When carrying out a transhiatal esophagectomy and proximal partial gastrectomy for tumors of the esophagogastric junction, the cervical esophagus should not be divided until the surgeon is satisfied that there will be adequate remaining stomach to reach to the neck. If after the cervical esophagus is divided and the thoracic esophagus is removed the esophagogastric junction tumor is found to involve so much stomach that a proximal hemigastrectomy is required to remove it, there will be insufficient remaining gastric length to reach to the neck. If the colon is not prepared, the patient is left with a cervical esophagostomy and a feeding tube, a dismal outcome of an esophageal operation intended to relieve dysphagia.

POSTOPERATIVE CARE

On average, patient hospitalization after an uncomplicated transhiatal esophagectomy has been 7 days, after postoperative barium swallow examination has shown that (1) the anastomosis is intact, (2) intrathoracic stomach empties well, and (3) pyloromyotomy provides adequate drainage. Typically, patients are extubated immediately after operation and transferred to monitored care without an intensive care unit admission. Early ambulation and pulmonary physiotherapy, aided by postoperative epidural analgesia, is encouraged. The nasogastric tube is removed 3 days after operation, and jejunostomy feedings are initiated at that time. During the first postoperative week, the diet is advanced gradually to a mechanical (pureed) diet with concomitant reduction and eventually discontinuation of jejunostomy feedings. Patients are discharged with instructions to supplement their oral intake with nightly jejunostomy feedings if they experience postoperative anorexia. The feeding tube typically is removed 4 weeks after operation.

RECOMMENDATIONS

Initial experience with transhiatal esophagectomy has focused on particular techniques of esophagectomy (e.g., to minimize intraoperative blood loss and to limit injury to the left recurrent laryngeal nerve and subsequent postoperative hoarseness and aspiration). More recently, we have sought to reduce the incidence of anastomotic leak and other complications associated with the cervical esophagogastric anastomosis. In particular, we have limited trauma to the gastric conduit during its mobilization and manipulation through the mediastinum. Historically, our incidence of cervical esophagogastric anastomotic leakage using manual suture techniques has varied between 10% and 15%. Nearly 50% of these patients develop anastomotic stricture as fibrosis with anastomotic healing occurs. In contrast, we and others have shown that the side-to-side stapled cervical anastomosis can reduce the incidence of anastomotic leak to less than 5%.

SUGGESTED READING

Iannettoni MD, et al: Catastrophic complications of the cervical esophagogastric anastomosis, *J Thorac Cardiovasc Surg* 110:1493, 1995.

Orringer MB: Current status of transhiatal esophagectomy, *Adv Surg* 34:193, 2000.

Orringer MB, et al: Eliminating the cervical esophagogastric anastomotic leak with a side-to-side stapled anastomosis, *J Thorac Cardiovasc Surg* 119:277, 2000.

Orringer MB, et al: Transhiatal esophagectomy: clinical experience and refinements, *Ann Surg* 230:392, 1999.

Singh D, et al: Experience and technique of stapled mechanical cervical esophagogastric anastomosis, *Ann Thorac Surg* 7:419, 2001.

LEFT THORACOABDOMINAL ESOPHAGOGASTRECTOMY

Cameron D. Wright
Earle W. Wilkins, Jr.

Many incisional approaches to esophagectomy may be simplified into left, right, and midline (transhiatal). Typically an experienced esophageal surgeon has a strong bias toward performing one particular approach, usually based on the approach used during training. There are benefits and limitations to each approach, leading the thoughtful surgeon to tailor the approach to the patient at hand. Three left-sided operations commonly are described: (1) an exclusive thoracotomy approach, in which the abdominal dissection is done through a diaphragmatic incision; (2) a thoracoabdominal incision in combination with a left neck incision for a cervical esophagogastrectomy; and (3) the standard thoracoabdominal esophagogastrectomy with intrathoracic esophagogastrostomy. The disadvantages of the last-mentioned approach include the need for costal arch division, a perception of more postoperative pulmonary complications, the limitation of length of esophagus resected, the poor visualization of the middle third of the esophagus due to the presence of the aortic arch, and perhaps an increased tendency for troublesome gastroesophageal reflux. The advantages of a thoracoabdominal approach include the unparalleled access to the stomach and lower esophagus and the single incision that allows access to the entire operative field at once and an expeditious operation. With the shift in esophageal cancer away from squamous cell cancer to adenocarcinoma that typically involves the lower third of the esophagus, the approach involving left thoracoabdominal esophagectomy deserves consideration. The lymph node spread of Barrett's adenocarcinoma is concentrated mostly in the lower chest and upper abdominal area, which are exposed best through a thoracoabdominal incision.

ANESTHESIA

An epidural catheter always is placed preoperatively by the anesthesiologist, and its postoperative use has reduced greatly the risk of postoperative pulmonary complications. The catheter typically is removed on the third to fifth postoperative day. A double-lumen endotracheal tube always is used to allow selective lung isolation to facilitate the dissection in the left chest. Central lines typically are not used because blood loss is usually minimal. Cefazolin and metronidazole are administered intravenously before the skin incision. A nasogastric tube is placed after induction of anesthesia but is not taped in place until after the esophageal anastomosis has been performed. The conduct of anesthesia is planned to allow extubation at the end of the operation. The patient is positioned in a right lateral decubitus position with the shoulders in full lateral position and the hips turned about 60 degrees up.

ENDOSCOPY

Before the incision is made, a careful endoscopic assessment of the upper gastrointestinal tract is done by the operating surgeon (even if a gastroenterologist has performed this in the preceding weeks). The operating surgeon needs to know (1) the specific location of the tumor and its length (from the incisors in centimeters and from the cardia in centimeters), (2) the cephalad extent of Barrett's mucosa above the tumor, (3) the cephalad extent of radiation changes, (4) whether there is any extension of the tumor into the stomach (or other stomach pathology), and (5) the ease of passage of the endoscope through the pylorus and whether there is evidence of old duodenal ulcer disease. The gastroenterologist rarely provides such specific information to the operating surgeon. This information is gathered best by the operating surgeon immediately before the operation and occasionally leads to a change in operative approach of the patient.

INCISIONAL APPROACH

The standard incision for a lower third tumor is an oblique one, starting at the linea alba about equidistant between the xiphoid and umbilicus extending across the left upper quadrant to cross the costal arch and finish at the tip of the scapula. The abdomen typically is opened and explored first. If conditions are favorable for resection, the rest of the incision is opened. The interspace opened usually is chosen based on what level the expected anastomosis will be at (usually from the sixth to the eighth rib). In general, it is better to be on the high side because superb access to the anastomosis greatly facilitates the operation. The chest is entered on top of the chosen rib, and the rib is cut and shingled posteriorly to allow wide opening of the incision. Rib resection rarely is needed. The costal arch is divided next, usually with a scalpel, and a piece of cartilage from either end of the divided arch is removed to prevent the ends from rubbing one another when they are reapproximated. The diaphragm is divided 8 to 10 cm along the periphery of the chest wall to avoid injury to any major branches of the phrenic nerve. Then chest and abdominal retractors are placed. If subsequent findings dictate a supraaortic anastomosis, a higher interspace thoracotomy is needed and is surprisingly well tolerated.

The incision needs to be extended around and above the scapula as for a standard posterolateral thoracotomy. Usually the fourth interspace is chosen for the second thoracotomy level. If a cervical anastomosis is planned with a left thoracoabdominal approach, this can be performed without a position change if the left arm is prepared into the field, allowing it to be retracted up for access to the chest and inferiorly for access to the left neck.

EXPLORATION

As noted, the abdomen is explored first through a limited incision to look for evidence of metastatic disease. Fixed, matted celiac nodes; liver metastases; and omental or peritoneal metastatic deposits portend a limited survival, which rarely makes resection worthwhile. Actively bleeding patients should be resected if technically (not oncologically) resectable. Obstruction is well palliated with endoscopically placed stents so that resection in the face of metastases rarely is performed. After the full incision is opened, the chest also is explored, paying careful attention to the lung, pleura, pericardium, lymph nodes, and aorta.

DISSECTION

When a metastatic or grossly unresectable lesion has been eliminated, the dissection and preparation of the gastric conduit take place. The mediastinal dissection always is done first if there is any question as to whether the tumor is resectable because of local invasion (usually aortic invasion). If the tumor is known to be confined to the muscular wall, either the abdominal dissection or the mediastinal dissection can be done first. The mediastinal dissection includes four key components: (1) division of the mediastinal pleura and exposure of the esophagus below the aortic arch; (2) encirclement of the proximal esophagus and division of the vagus nerves; (3) dissection of the esophagus and periesophageal fat from the aorta, pericardium, and right pleura with division of segmental esophageal arteries; and (4) entry into the abdomen usually by taking a cuff of diaphragm at the gastroesophageal junction.

The resection is begun in the mediastinum, freeing the esophagus and its draining lymph nodes in continuity. The pulmonary ligament is divided close to the lung to permit removal of its nodes. The dissection is carried out medially along the back of the pericardium and the inferior pulmonary vein up to the level of the left main bronchus. The esophagus is encircled with first the fingers and then a Penrose tape, at a point well away from tumor. This permits gentle traction and facilitates dissection of mediastinal nodes and fat with the esophagus. Two to five direct aortic arterial branches to the esophagus are ligated immediately against the adventitial aortic wall. The tumor itself is freed last. Tumor is left behind if there is definite aortic invasion. The vagus nerves are divided on the wall of the esophagus just below the aortic arch. The thoracic duct seldom is seen from the left thoracotomy incision and is not removed or ligated routinely. If it is encountered, it may be ligated with impunity just above its entry into the mediastinum through the aortic hiatus.

The abdominal dissection includes four key components: (1) separation of the greater omentum with preservation of the gastroepiploic arcade, (2) removal of the left gastric lymph nodes with division of the left gastric artery as it arises from the celiac axis, (3) pyloromyotomy, and (4) transection of the stomach.

The lesser omental sac is entered at a convenient level, and the omentum is divided from pylorus to spleen. Use of the stomach to replace the esophagus hinges on preservation of the right gastroepiploic and the right gastric arteries. The omental gastroepiploic branches are divided 5 to 10 mm from the arcade, allowing accurate ligature without compromise of the arcade itself. Cautery coagulation is avoided because of the threat of thrombosis of the arcade. Greater curvature dissection is carried to the esophageal hiatus by division of the gastrosplenic or so-called short gastric vessels and with them the left gastroepiploic artery as it arises from the splenic artery.

The approach to the left gastric lymph nodes is facilitated by division of the gastrohepatic omentum well away from the stomach wall, placing an encircling Penrose tape for traction. Access is from behind the stomach. Care is taken with division of the uniformly present branches of the splenic artery to the back of the proximal gastric wall. With upward traction on the stomach, the left gastric artery and vein are identified, doubly ligated at their origins, and divided. All adjacent tissue, including nodes along the celiac axis itself, is swept toward the stomach.

The need for a gastric drainage procedure has never been settled scientifically. Because of an inevitable vagotomy effect resulting frequently in diminished gastric motility, a pyloromyotomy has been performed routinely and arbitrarily. A pyloroplasty is not used because of the enhanced possibility of alkaline reflux. Pyloroplasty (a two-layered Heineke-Mikulicz type) is carried out only if substantial peptic ulcer scarring compromises the pyloric channel or if duodenal entry occurs during myotomy. The duodenum is mobilized with a Kocher maneuver to facilitate the drainage procedure and the mobility of the stomach into the thorax.

Points are chosen and marked with sutures on the lesser and the greater curvatures. On the lesser side, this is usually just distal to the left gastric, node-containing tissue; on the greater side, it is at the upper extent of the gastroepiploic arcade. These points should be at a minimum of 5 cm from the gastric extent of gross tumor. The stomach is divided with a long 100-mm GIA stapler, and the staple line is inverted with interrupted 4-0 silk Lembert sutures.

■ ADEQUACY OF RESECTION

In all cases except perhaps in the purely palliative procedure in which gross disease is known to have been left behind, the resection margin should be checked carefully. This checking is done by the surgeon with direct inspection and the pathologist with frozen section. The latter is particularly necessary in the esophageal margin in cases of adenocarcinoma, in which submucosal extension of tumor or the presence of Barrett's epithelium is common. When this extension is found, an additional resection of the esophagus must be carried out, often with the need for a supraaortic anastomosis.

This added dissection is facilitated by resection of a higher rib, typically the fourth, through a paravertebral extension of the same incision. When the esophagus is exposed above the aortic arch, the thoracic duct is at particular risk for injury and usually must be ligated. For this extended procedure, the stomach is brought through the posterior mediastinum to the right of or behind the aortic arch before supraaortic anastomosis.

■ ANASTOMOSIS

Basic Principles
The integrity of an esophagogastrostomy anastomosis after resection of an esophageal carcinoma is predicated on the observation of a set of specific principles. Careful concurrence with the details involved in these principles ensures a successful anastomosis.

Blood Supply
Maintenance of an adequate arterial supply and of venous drainage of the gastric segment is mandatory and is the most important essential. The right gastric and right gastroepiploic arteries with their respective arcades are both necessary for viability of the stomach. Venous return rarely is discussed, but its interruption could result in venous infarction. The esophagus is not dissected out of its proximal bed more than is necessary to perform the anastomosis, usually no more than 2 cm.

Atraumatic Tissue Handling
Clamps are not applied to the edges of portions of esophagus and stomach to be anastomosed. Cautery is not used. The placement of sutures is guided by holding the previous stitch rather than by grasping with even the most atraumatic of tissue forceps.

Inversion of Tissue
The esophagus is void of an outer mesothelial layer, such as the peritoneum covering the abdominal viscera. Its strongest layer is its mucosa: It must be completely inverted and covered by esophageal muscle as the anastomosis is completed.

Gastric Decompression
Egress for gastric contents under pressure must be provided, especially in the event that gastric amotility results in retention. For this reason, a nasogastric tube is left in place after operation. Vomiting exerts undue force against the suture line and must be avoided.

A two-layer sutured anastomosis always is carried out. The general thoracic resident must learn this technique during training. The use of the mechanical stapler, although it produces a satisfactory anastomosis, does not save real time. Based on thorough review of literature statistics, the one-layer anastomosis results in an unnecessarily high rate of leakage. The particular suture material is perhaps the least important detail. Use of interrupted sutures is important, however, in providing capillary flow to the healing and sealing edges and in permitting an adequate anastomotic orifice. Purse-string sutures are avoided. Fine silk is easily handled, is inexpensive, and provides no untoward foreign body complication.

An end-to-side anastomosis is preferred. This anastomosis is accomplished, after inversion closure of the transection line of the stomach, by excising a circular button of stomach from its anterior surface. The exact placement of this button must be precise: no closer than 2 cm to the gastric turn-in and near the greater curve, where maximal length is obtained and where arterial inflow is the greatest. A posterior row of 4-0 silk mattress sutures is placed first through muscle of the esophagus and the combined serosa and muscle wall of the stomach. Appropriate placement of these four to six sutures is ensured before they are tied; when they are tied, the stomach is brought up to the esophagus, with the finger securing the knot placed above the anastomosis. Approximating only the posterior third of the circumference of the anastomosis with this row facilitates exposure of the mucosal layer. This second layer, also of 4-0 silk, approximates the mucosa of the stomach to the mucosa of the esophagus. Interrupted technique in simple inverting fashion is used; these sutures are tied as they are placed, permitting gentle upward traction to expose the proper placement of the ensuing suture. The posterior layer is carried out from both directions around to the anterior aspect, taking particular care to invert this layer with knots tied on the inside. The nasogastric tube is threaded through the anastomosis after the posterior mucosal layer is about half complete. The final suture in this layer is a Connell's mattress suture. The outer anterior row is completed in its residual two thirds with interrupted mattress sutures, again lifting the stomach upward to the esophagus. If there is omentum available, it is sutured over the anterior suture line.

This anastomosis, so placed in end-to-side fashion, has gastric serosal coverage supporting its posterior aspect. It provides a mucosal flap-valve that helps to minimize postoperative reflux.

■ JEJUNOSTOMY

A jejunostomy is performed routinely just before closure to allow early postoperative feeding and to facilitate early discharge from the hospital. A 14 Fr latex whistle-tip catheter is placed into the upper jejunum about 15 cm distal to the ligament of Treitz. Several 4-0 silk sutures are used to Witzel the catheter, then it is tacked to the anterior abdominal wall inferior to the incision.

■ INCISION CLOSURE

The chest and abdomen are irrigated with warm saline before closure. A chest drain is inserted and placed in the posterior gutter. Heavy interrupted sutures (typically 0 silk) are used to close the diaphragm. The chest is closed with heavy no. 2 polyglactin 910 (Vicryl) pericostal sutures, then in layers with running sutures. The costal arch is not tightly reapproximated so that the two cut ends do not rub on each other and cause pain. It is important to obliterate the space beneath the costal arch by reapproximating the diaphragm

to the costal arch in this area. The stomach is tacked to the margin of the diaphragmatic hiatus to prevent intraabdominal contents from herniating. The abdominal fascia is closed in two layers of heavy running nonabsorbable monofilament sutures.

■ POSTOPERATIVE CARE

The patient is extubated in the operating room and nursed with the head of the bed elevated to 45 degrees to help prevent aspiration. Fluid management is important in the first 48 hours, and typically there is a large third space requirement. Patients are mobilized on the first postoperative day. Pain usually is eliminated by the epidural infusion. If shoulder pain is problematic, intravenous ketorolac usually is used. Elemental jejunostomy tube feedings are started on postoperative day 2 and increased to goal by postoperative day 5. The nasogastric tube is removed after the patient has a bowel movement and any ileus has resolved, usually postoperative day 4 or 5. The chest tube is removed as soon as the drainage diminishes to less than 50 ml in an 8-hour period, usually postoperative day 4 or 5. A diatrizoate meglumine (Gastrografin) swallow typically is done on postoperative day 6 or 7 to ensure the integrity of the anastomosis. A liquid diet is begun thereafter. The tube feedings are changed to a typical nonelemental formula and cycled to be given at nighttime only. Patients usually are discharged on postoperative day 9 with instructions to begin a soft solid diet within 1 week. The jejunostomy tube usually is removed on the first postoperative visit.

■ RESULTS

Several comparative series and two small, randomized series show no difference in overall morbidity, pulmonary complications, or operative mortality between transhiatal and transthoracic esophagectomies. Long-term survival is also no different between the two approaches. Our group reported a consecutive case series of 64 left thoracoabdominal esophagectomies with no anastomotic leaks and only a 2% mortality. This approach allows an elegant operation to be done under direct vision with excellent exposure.

SUGGESTED READING

Altorki NK: Three-field lymphadenectomy for esophageal cancer, *Chest Surg Clinic N Am* 10:553, 2000.

Heitmiller RF: The left thoracoabdominal incision, *Ann Thorac Surg* 46:250, 1988.

Heitmiller RF: Results of standard left thoracoabdominal esophagogastrectomy, *Semin Thorac Cardiovasc Surg* 4:314, 1992.

Mathisen DJ, et al: Transthoracic esophagogastrectomy: a safe approach to carcinoma of the esophagus, *Ann Thorac Surg* 45:137, 1988.

Sonett JR: Esophagectomy: the role of the intrathoracic anastomosis, *Chest Surg Clin N Am* 10:519, 2000.

ESOPHAGEAL RECONSTRUCTION—COLONIC INTERPOSITION

Claude Deschamps

In most situations, the stomach remains the conduit of choice for esophageal replacement in adults. A colon or small bowel interposition is favored in instances in which the stomach is inadequate or absent. This is most likely to be the case in patients who have undergone distal gastrectomy in the past or who presently require complete removal of the esophagus and the stomach. When a short segmental resection of the distal esophagus is performed, usually in benign disease, reconstruction with colon serves the dual purpose of preserving gastric function and acting as an effective barrier to reflux. In all cases, the ultimate goal is to restore the function of swallowing as close to normal as possible, with minimal morbidity and mortality.

■ PREOPERATIVE PREPARATION

When a colon interposition is likely, a colonoscopy is performed in advance to detect any significant colonic lesion that would preclude using the colon, such as carcinoma, extensive diverticulosis, or inflammation. A barium enema can replace colonoscopy if the latter is incomplete or impossible. Angiogram of the abdominal aorta and its visceral branches is reserved for patients older than age 50, patients with a history of previous abdominal vascular or colonic surgery, and patients at risk for vascular lesions from systemic diseases such as diabetes or hyperlipidemia. The patient is admitted the day before surgery for a mechanical bowel preparation, which includes 2 liters of an isosmotic solution (GoLYTELY) and enemas as needed. On call to the operating room, 1 g of intravenous cefazolin (Ancef) is given, to be continued for 48 hours postoperatively.

■ POSITION OF THE PATIENT AND CHOICE OF INCISION

For a transhiatal esophagectomy or a delayed reconstruction after esophageal diversion, the patient is in the dorsal decubitus position, with the abdomen and neck prepared and draped simultaneously. The abdomen is entered through an upper midline laparotomy, and the cervical esophagus is approached with an oblique incision, anterior to the left sternocleidomastoid muscle. The conduit is placed in the posterior mediastinum whenever possible because it is the shortest route. The substernal route is chosen when the posterior mediastinum is obliterated or in the rare instances in which residual tumor would become a significant threat to the conduit. When a substernal tunnel is used, the thoracic inlet is enlarged by removing the left half of the manubrium, head of the clavicle, and median portion of the first rib. The manubrium is divided with a vertical saw (Hall Micro 100 Sagittal Saw; Zimmer, Warsaw, IN), and a Gigli saw is used for the clavicle and rib. This avoids compression of the conduit and facilitates execution of the anastomosis. When neither the substernal nor the posterior mediastinal route is available, a transpleural route is created by making an opening in the anterior portion of the left or the right diaphragm and delivering the transplant through the enlarged thoracic inlet. The subcutaneous route is not a desirable route, being the longest and least cosmetic alternative.

A left thoracoabdominal approach is favored when a limited distal esophageal resection is performed. The patient is in the lateral decubitus position at a 45-degree angle. The replacement conduit is passed through the hiatus, and the anastomosis is performed in the posterior mediastinum. This incision allows adequate exposure for gastric resection if necessary and access to the small bowel and left and transverse colon for reconstruction. In addition, by preparing the left arm in the field, one gains simultaneous access to the left neck if needed. For a carcinoma of the cardia extending up in the distal esophagus or whenever the upper anastomosis is to be performed in the upper chest, an upper midline laparotomy followed by a right thoracotomy approach is preferred.

■ CHOICE AND PREPARATION OF CONDUIT

In cases in which the proximal anastomosis is in the neck, the left colon is the best choice of conduit. It also is most suitable when a subtotal esophagectomy is performed and reconstruction involves a right thoracic approach with the proximal anastomosis high in the chest. The size of the left colon, thickness of its wall, and favorable blood supply make it a better choice over the right colon. For a short segmental resection of the distal esophagus, either a short left or a transverse colon is the most appropriate replacement conduit. A right colon interposition is done in patients in need of a long interposition when the left or transverse colon is inadequate. All conduits are placed preferably in the isoperistaltic position.

Colon

The descending colon is mobilized to the midline by incising the lateral peritoneal fascia. The incision is extended upward to free the splenic flexure by incising the phrenocolic and splenocolic ligaments, carefully preserving the spleen, tail of the pancreas, and left adrenal gland. When freeing the descending colon, care is taken to avoid injury to its vulnerable venous supply, left kidney, and ureter. The greater omentum is lifted upward and separated from the transverse colon and is left attached to the stomach. The transverse and left descending colon is inspected, and its blood supply is evaluated by palpation and transillumination of the mesentery by gently holding up the colon. Intraoperative Doppler examination can be useful in rare situations, but a positive signal on a pulseless artery is worrisome, and an alternate conduit probably should be sought if pulse is not restored after topical application of 1% lidocaine.

The marginal artery of Drummond, the middle colic artery with its right and left branches, and the left colic artery with its ascending and descending branches are identified. The middle colic arterial trunk lies to the right of the ligament of Treitz in the base of the transverse mesocolon. The left colic artery is the first main branch of the inferior mesenteric artery and can be found easily by following the latter distally. The length of the transplant required is measured with an umbilical tape from the epigastric area to the presumed site of the proximal anastomosis. It is suggested at this time to overestimate by 5 cm the required length to avoid the devastating problem of tension on the anastomosis or insufficient length. If there is no obvious anomaly in the blood supply or intrinsic pathology of the colon, conduit length is verified by applying the umbilical tape against the wall of the colon. Determination is made whether a short or a long conduit is required. The appropriate vascular pedicles are isolated carefully by incising the overlying peritoneum, and the branches that are to be ligated are occluded using atraumatic bulldog vascular clamps.

Marking stitches are placed proximally and distally on the bowel at the intended levels of transection. The right and transverse colon is mobilized, carefully preserving the vascular supply, right kidney and ureter, gonadal vessels, and inferior vena cava. After this, evaluation and confirmation of viability of the conduit is performed by examining the bowel and feeling for the presence of pulsation in the pedicle. Intravenous fluorescein (1 to 2 g) may be helpful to determine viability in borderline situations. The needed bowel length is verified again. The bowel is transected using a linear-cutting stapler, and the mesentery, including the marginal artery, is divided and ligated along the dotted line as shown in Figure 1.

A short colon interposition is based on the left colic artery. It also can be based essentially on the ascending branch of the left colic artery, and one has to ensure this branch is in continuity with the marginal artery. The venous drainage is as important to the survival of the graft as the arterial supply and should be preserved during the dissection. The descending colon is divided between the ascending branch and the descending branch of the left colic artery. It also can be divided distal to the descending branch if additional length is needed. The proximal colon is divided distal to the middle colic artery, slightly to the left of the splenic flexure (Figure 1A). A long colon interposition is based on the left colic artery. The descending colon is divided distal to both branches of the left colic artery, and the transverse colon is divided between the two branches of the middle colic artery. If additional length is needed, the middle colic artery is divided at its origin, and the transverse colon can be divided more proximally (Figure 1B). When a long right colon interposition is required, it is based on the middle colic artery so that it remains in the isoperistaltic position and requires division of the right colic and ileocolic arteries, provided that the marginal artery is uninterrupted (Figure 1C).

Disadvantages include multiple potential variations in the blood supply, bulkiness of the cecum, and vulnerability of the proximal portion of the conduit to ischemia. The appendix routinely is removed, and the terminal ileum occasionally has to be included in the conduit to reach up into the neck. In this last instance, the most distal ileal branch of the superior mesenteric artery should be ligated, collateral permitting.

A transverse colon interposition is based on the middle colic artery and can be used for a short or a long conduit as long as the marginal artery is intact.

The final decision on the choice of conduit is based on many factors, including but not limited to required length, pattern of blood supply, and local anatomy. Alternatives to the aforementioned choices include conduits based on different vascular pedicles and placed in the antiperistaltic position.

After mobilization, the conduit is placed through the lesser sac, in a retrogastric position, then through the hiatus for the posterior mediastinal route. A variety of techniques have been described to facilitate the passage of the conduit in the posterior mediastinum using plastic bowel bags. I find this rarely necessary. Three 3-0 silk sutures are tied at the proximal end of the graft. A long vascular clamp is introduced carefully through the cervical incision, and under direct vision through the hiatus, the sutures are grasped by the clamp and gently pulled upward while the surgeon's hand guides the conduit through the posterior mediastinum, avoiding torsion in the process. This maneuver also is applicable when the substernal route is chosen. The conduit should be stretched gently to avoid redundancy, and one should plan for approximately 10 cm of intraabdominal colon as an efficient barrier to reflux. The colon is anchored carefully to the hiatus with multiple 3-0 silk sutures to avoid torsion and herniation, and the hiatus is closed simultaneously. The proximal esophagocolic anastomosis is performed first, end-to-end, in one layer, using inverting 3-0 absorbable monofilament polyglyconate (Maxon) sutures after resecting the staple line on the transplant. All knots are tied in the inside except the last one, which is a Connell's stitch. The distal cologastric anastomosis is constructed using the same technique. If the stomach is intact, the anastomosis is positioned posteriorly, at the level of the gastric body. This position is facilitated by lifting the greater curvature upward and cephalad with Babcock clamps, partially rotating the stomach on itself and delivering the posterior wall in the field for an easier anastomosis. If a partial gastrectomy had been performed previously, the anastomosis is done end-to-side with the residual gastric antrum. In all cases, a pyloromyotomy or pyloroplasty is performed. Colocolic continuity is reestablished with an end-to-end anastomosis, two layers, with 2-0 chromic and 3-0 silk sutures.

In the situation in which a right thoracotomy is necessary, the graft is delivered in the right chest through the hiatus before abdominal closure and anchored securely to the hiatus as described previously. One has to plan for the appropriate length of conduit before the turn to a right thoracotomy position and should overestimate slightly rather than face the consequence of a short conduit. A feeding jejunostomy routinely is inserted at the end of the procedure to resume nutrition early postoperatively. At all times, great care should be taken to avoid tension and torsion on the vascular pedicle.

■ RESULTS

Results of large series comparing the use of stomach versus colon for esophageal replacement in a nonrandomized fashion show no significant difference in functional outcome,

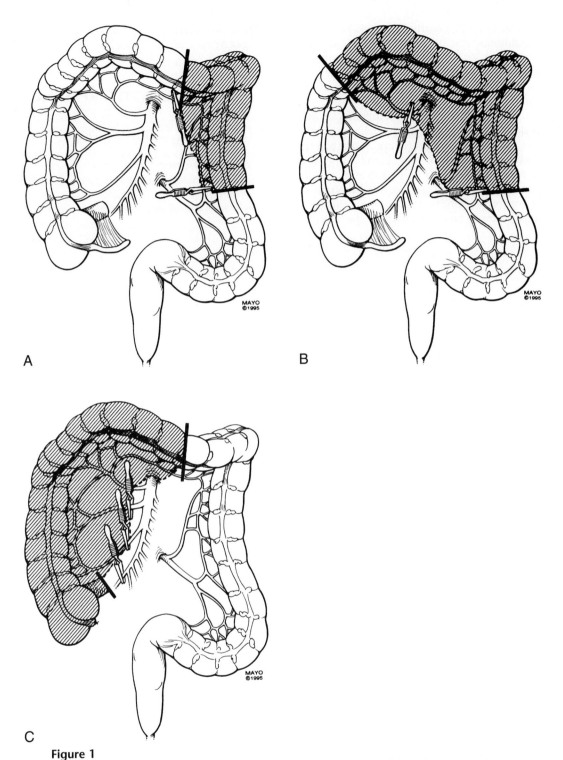

Figure 1
A, A short colon interposition is based on the colic artery. Bulldog clamps are shown occluding the marginal artery proximally and distally. The mesentery is incised along the dotted line. The dark lines show the intended levels of bowel transection. **B,** A long colon interposition is based on the left colic artery. Bulldog clamps are shown occluding the origin of the middle colic artery proximally and the distal marginal artery distally. The mesentery is incised along the dotted line. The dark lines show the intended levels of bowel transection. **C,** A right colon interposition is based on the middle colic artery. Bulldog clamps are shown occluding the right colic and ileocolic branches and the most distal branch of the superior mesenteric artery in the case where the distal ileus is included. The mesentery is incised along the dotted lines. The dark lines show the intended levels of bowel transection.

morbidity, or mortality. Overall morbidity ranges from 15% to 65%, with anastomotic stricture being the most common complication, averaging 20%. The incidence of anastomotic leak, graft ischemia, or loss is approximately 7%. Other less common short-term and long-term findings include aspiration, gastric stasis, colonic redundancy and tortuosity, anastomotic ulcers, bile reflux, and gastroesophageal reflux into the residual esophagus. Some authors believe that the need for dilation of an anastomotic stricture is less than for gastric tube conduits because of the better blood supply. The long-term reoperation rate varies from 15% to 30%, usually due to the development of colon redundancy. Resection of the redundant portion and primary anastomosis usually is required; however, care is taken to preserve the vascular pedicle. Mortality rates are less than 5%, no different than for gastric pull-up procedures.

SUGGESTED READING

Cerfolio RJ, et al: Esophageal replacement by colon interposition, *Ann Thorac Surg* 59:1382, 1995.

DeMeester SR: Colon interposition following esophagectomy, *Dis Esoph* 14:169, 2001.

Deschamps C: Use of colon and jejunum as possible esophageal replacements, *Chest Surg Clin N Am* 5:555, 1995.

Wain JC: Long segment colon interposition, *Semin Thorac Cardiovasc Surg* 4:336,1992.

ESOPHAGEAL RECONSTRUCTION—JEJUNAL SEGMENT INTERPOSITION AND FREE GRAFT

Henning A. Gaissert

In comparing conduits for esophageal replacement, jejunum commonly is ranked after stomach and colon. This order is probably an acknowledgment of the limited experience with small bowel and has some justification because jejunum is selected preferably for reconstruction after partial, rather than total, esophageal resection. The reason for this preference is the finite length of the mesenteric pedicle, which hinders mobilization of the jejunum on its own blood supply from the abdomen to the neck except in particular circumstances. In the appropriate situation, however, jejunum provides durable and entirely satisfactory swallowing function.

There are three indications for small bowel interposition: (1) reconstruction of distal esophagus and esophagogastric junction for undilatable stricture or unremitting reflux disease with a pedicled graft; (2) replacement after circumferential resection of pharynx, larynx, and cervical esophagus with a free graft; and (3) total esophageal replacement with or without vascular augmentation when other options, such as stomach or colon, are unavailable. Contraindications to its use are short gut syndrome and inflammatory bowel disease.

Jejunal interposition is a complex operation; it follows that the decision to proceed should not be made unless in benign disease esophageal function is destroyed and in malignant disease a simpler option, such as a gastric tube, is not available. Because of its complexity, an interposition should be deferred in emergency interventions. Preoperative arteriography usually is not required because the superior mesenteric artery and its branches rarely have important arteriosclerotic disease. The surgeon must be familiar, however, with the anatomy of the jejunum; more than in acquired disease, anatomic variation of its vasculature matters for this type of conduit. The first one or two arcades below the ligament of Treitz are usually short and should be avoided for either interposition or free graft. Jejunal vascular arcades below this level may be interrupted or have insufficient collateralization as Barlow has shown and prevent consideration of an interposition or reduce available length. The surgeon has to pay close attention in the operating room using transillumination and test clamping before committing to isolating small bowel.

■ SHORT SEGMENT INTERPOSITION

Merendino and Dillard in the United States and Brain in England were among the first to report resection of the esophagogastric junction and replacement with jejunum. Animal models showed the resistance to peptic mucosal disease in the interposed segment even when histamine administration led to ulceration of the duodenum. The indications for this operation are strictures due to acid or bile reflux disease that do not respond to dilation, symptomatic gastroesophageal reflux disease after previously unsuccessful fundoplication, and reconstruction after resection for esophageal malignancy when stomach is not available (i.e., after previous gastrectomy).

Operative Approach

The surgeon should seek exposure of the lower esophagus and the upper abdomen. A left thoracoabdominal incision is the ideal approach. The esophagus is resected—for localized strictures, this is a short resection—and the cardia is oversewn.

A suitable segment of jejunum is identified by transillumination of the mesentery to show the location and length of vascular arcades (Figure 1). The jejunal arcades to be divided are clamped with soft bulldog clamps to ascertain adequate arterial supply and venous drainage. The proximal jejunum is divided, and as many jejunal vessels are ligated close to the superior mesenteric artery as needed for a sufficient long segment. The greater curvature and posterior wall of the stomach are mobilized, and the jejunal segment is brought up through the transverse mesocolon, where the pedicle is placed behind the stomach and into the mediastinum. Routing the pedicle anterior to colon or stomach introduces undesired tension. The absence of any tension and the torsion-free orientation of the pedicle behind colon and stomach are crucial to avoiding venous congestion. Esophagus and jejunum are connected end-to-side in two layers with an outer layer of horizontal mattress 4-0 silk and an inner layer of full-thickness simple sutures of the same material, tying the knots on the luminal side. Minimal jejunal length is left proximal to the anastomosis to avoid development of a pouch. A straight course of the intestine without redundancy is crucial to long-term success. The anastomosis to the stomach is constructed high on the posterior wall. Finally, abdominal jejunojejunal continuity is restored. A nasogastric tube is placed into the stomach, and a feeding tube is inserted into the jejunum below the lowest anastomosis. A contrast swallow is obtained 6 or 7 days after operation and before removing the nasogastric tube. The diet is advanced gradually.

Early reports described pitfalls related to the course of the vascular pedicle and the jejunum. An antecolic jejunal pedicle shortens available length and compromises blood supply. Implantation of the jejunum into the stomach low on the antrum or in an angled position (i.e., from posterior mediastinum into anterior fundus) leads to obstruction and may require revision).

■ FREE JEJUNAL GRAFT

Circumferential resections for carcinomas or strictures of the hypopharynx, larynx, and cervical esophagus often exhaust the reconstructive capacities of local tissue, particularly in the radiated neck, and demand replacement with nonirradiated intestine. Although stomach may be mobilized to the cricoid level, and colon reaches as far as to the base of the tongue, a free jejunal graft is the preferred conduit for most head and neck surgeons. The free graft avoids mediastinal dissection and limits the abdominal procedure. Surgeons experienced in microvascular tissue transfer master the disadvantage of greater complexity due to three intestinal and two vascular anastomoses with limited graft loss (5% to 10%) and mortality (approximately 5%). The ability to obtain a disease-free margin at the thoracic esophagus through a purely cervical approach is limited; cervical esophageal carcinomas or caustic strictures are in general not suitable for cervical resection alone. Prior radiation of the neck is not a contraindication but may render exposure of donor vessels difficult.

Operative Approach

During cervical dissection, suitable donor vessels are identified; these are branches of the external carotid artery, such as facial, lingual, and superior thyroid vessels, or the transverse cervical artery and vein. If these vessels are unavailable, common carotid artery and internal jugular vein on either side of the recipient are selected. Via laparotomy, a jejunal segment is retrieved on a long vascular pedicle. Trial clamping may help to ensure that the entire length of isolated bowel maintains good color and peristalsis. The jejunal artery and vein are divided close to their origin and are flushed with heparinized saline when resection is complete and recipient vessels are prepared. About 20 cm of bowel are taken,

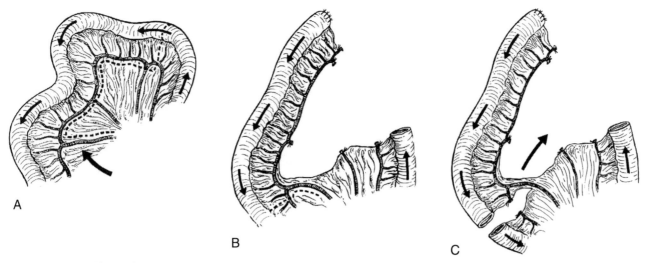

A   B   C

Figure 1
A-C, Preparation of the jejunal segment. Note the high ligation of the jejunal vessels almost flush with the arcade. This maneuver straightens the intestine, but its success requires an uninterrupted arcade of adequate size ascertained by trial clamping. The direction of peristalsis is marked, in this case by closure of the cephalic end of the bowel. *(From Wright C, Cuschieri A: Ann Surg 205:54, 1987, with permission.)*

anticipating further tailoring to a final length of 10 to 15 cm. The direction of peristalsis is marked. A jejunojejunostomy is performed, and a tube jejunostomy is created distal to the anastomosis to allow postoperative feeding.

In the neck, the cephalic or the caudal intestinal anastomosis is performed first to stabilize the segment, checking again for an isoperistaltic course (Figure 2). The cephalic anastomosis may be created end-to-side or end-to-end, whereas an end-to-end technique is preferred on the caudal side. Vascular anastomoses are performed with 8-0 or 9-0 nylon under the microscope. Color and peristalsis of the free graft are expected to return within minutes. The second intestinal anastomosis is completed with attention to avoiding redundancy, and a sump suction tube is passed from the nasopharynx into the esophagus. The neck flaps are closed, leaving a small portion of the small bowel exposed for visual assessment of viability. Seven days after operation, a contrast swallow is obtained to exclude a leak, and the diet is advanced.

■ LONG SEGMENT INTERPOSITION

Few series have reported meaningful numbers for interposition of long jejunal segments, defined as those reaching to the neck on the native pedicle. These reports have emphasized two alternative techniques: staging of the interposition or the microsurgical recruitment of thoracic blood supply. The paucity of reports reinforces the view that both procedures are the primary choice for reconstruction only in the hands of the most experienced surgeon.

Ring et al reported a staged procedure with construction of a cervical jejunostomy and leaving the jejunum in continuity below the diaphragm at the first stage. Esophagojejunal and jejunogastric anastomoses are constructed during a second stage 1 week later. All of their reported 32 patients were children, there were no deaths and no graft loss, and all tolerated a regular diet. These authors described careful, extensive mobilization of the pedicle with division of selected jejunal arcades.

Successful anastomosis of jejunal vessels to internal thoracic artery and vein first was reported by Longmire. Heitmiller et al reported a similar technique that allows single-stage, long segment interposition with microvascular augmentation from internal thoracic vessels. A substernal course is chosen to bring jejunum and pedicle in proximity to these vessels. The aim of this technique is a reduction of ischemic complications; its disadvantage is a greater technical complexity.

■ LONG-TERM FUNCTION

The interposed jejunum as a pedicled or free graft has excellent long-term function. Deterioration of swallowing over time is uncommon and probably related more to the operative technique than to the length of time after operation or the type of interposition. Important features of the original operation

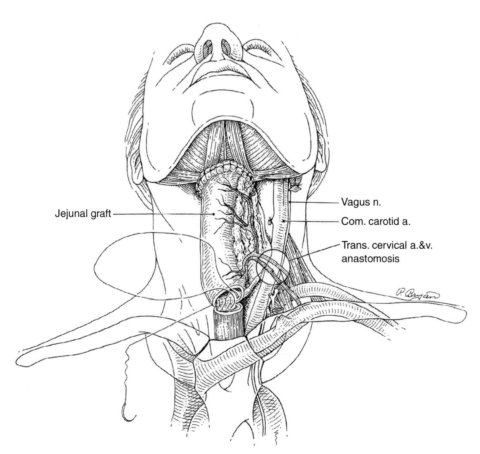

Jejunal graft

Vagus n.

Com. carotid a.

Trans. cervical a.&v. anastomosis

Figure 2
The free jejunal graft interposed between hypopharynx and cervical esophagus with vascular anastomosis to the transverse cervical vessels. *(From Miller JI, Lee RB: Semin Thorac Cardiovasc Surg 4:286, 1992, with permission.)*

are a straight, nonredundant course; avoidance of graft angulation; and creation of unobstructed intestinal anastomoses.

SUGGESTED READING

Barlow TE: Variations in the blood supply of the upper jejunum, *Br J Surg* 43:473, 1955.

Coleman JJ 3rd, et al: Ten years experience with the free jejunal autograft, *Am J Surg* 154:394, 1987.

Foker JE, et al: Technique of jejunal interposition for esophageal replacement, *J Thorac Cardiovasc Surg* 83:928, 1982.

Gaissert HA, et al: Short-segment intestinal interposition of the distal esophagus, *J Thorac Cardiovasc Surg* 106:860, 1993.

Heitmiller RF, et al: Long-segment substernal jejunal esophageal replacement with internal mammary vascular augmentation, *Dis Esophagus* 13:240, 2000.

ESOPHAGEAL RECONSTRUCTION—REVERSED AND NONREVERSED GASTRIC TUBES

Stanley C. Fell
Manoel Ximenes-Netto

A tube constructed from the greater curvature of the stomach vascularized by the gastroepiploic arcade, for anatomic and physiologic reasons, may be the ideal method for esophageal replacement. In adults, preexisting colonic disease or prior colon resection prohibits the use of a colon conduit. Anomalous arterial patterns or a poor marginal artery makes colon interposition hazardous. In contrast, the stomach has an excellent arterial supply in a predictable pattern. The gastroepiploic arcade, which is situated peripheral to the greater curvature of the stomach and has a greater arc, straightens and lengthens when the gastric tube is created and does not limit the length of the conduit. The colon and jejunum, with their fan-shaped mesenteries, are longer than their vascular arcades and tend to be redundant when interposed between the esophagus and stomach. These mesenteries are subject to tension and torsion, in contrast to the gastroepiploic vessels, which are applied closely to the stomach.

Colon interposition, even if it is not redundant when first performed, dilates and becomes redundant years later with attendant problems of stasis and poor emptying. This phenomenon has not been noted with the gastric tube.

Prior gastrostomy is not a contraindication to the construction of a gastric tube. It is to great advantage because the stomach may be dilated when large amounts (1000 to 1500 ml)

of a liquid diet are offered every 3 to 4 hours while awake. In 2 to 3 months, the stomach is enlarged so that there is abundant stomach available for esophageal replacement. If this form of reconstruction is anticipated and prior gastrostomy is required, it should be performed toward the lesser curvature of the stomach. The location of the gastrostomy is of little consequence, provided that the stomach is dilated as described. Prior gastric resection and outlet obstruction are usually contraindications to the application of the gastric tube for esophageal reconstruction.

■ OPERATIVE TECHNIQUE

Reversed Gastric Tube

Laparotomy is performed through a midline incision that extends from the xiphoid to below the umbilicus. A self-retaining retractor is inserted, and the stomach and omentum are drawn into the operative field. The vascular arcade and the greater curvature are inspected and palpated. A decision is made in regard to which gastroepiploic artery will vascularize the tube. A reversed gastric tube (RGT) is based on the left gastroepiploic artery; a nonreversed gastric tube (NRGT) is based on the right gastroepiploic artery.

The greater omentum is dissected from the transverse colon and both hepatic and splenic flexures, avoiding injury to the middle colic artery. The resultant omental flap is left attached to the gastric tube, to be elevated into the neck and wrapped about the cervical anastomosis to protect against anastomotic leak (Figures 1 and 2). At the level of the spleen, the gastroepiploic artery is no longer present on the greater curvature, and only short gastric arteries need to be isolated individually and divided, usually with the endovascular-stapling device. Although splenectomy was an integral part of the operative procedure as originally described, it is not required unless there is an irreparable splenic laceration. When the stomach is dilated by means of a previous gastrostomy, the greater curvature does not come near the hilum of the spleen, making splenectomy unnecessary. The gastrophrenic attachments are divided, and the stomach is freed from its avascular adhesions to the pancreas, mobilizing the entire greater curvature and fundus.

To prepare the RGT, the right gastroepiploic artery is ligated and divided approximately 4 cm from the pylorus (see Figure 1).

Supported by the Feldesman Fund for Thoracic Surgery at the Albert Einstein College of Medicine, Bronx, NY.

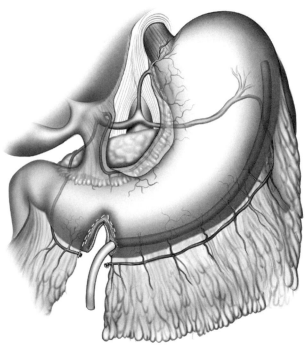

Figure 1
The reversed gastric tube is constructed over the catheter starting 4 cm proximal to the pylorus. *(From Fell SC, Ximenes-Netto M: Gastric tubes, reversed and nonreversed. In Pearson FG, editor:* Esophageal surgery, *ed 2, Philadelphia, Churchill-Livingstone, 2002.)*

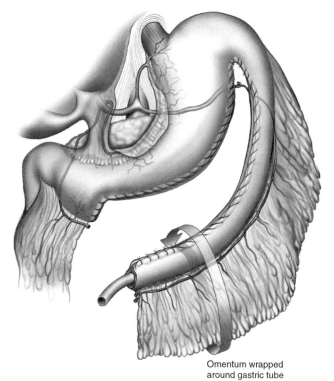

Omentum wrapped
around gastric tube

Figure 2
The omentum, preserved to buttress the cervical anastomosis, is wrapped about the tube to facilitate its transposition to the neck. *(From Fell SC, Ximenes-Netto M: Gastric tubes, reversed and nonreversed. In Pearson FG, editor:* Esophageal surgery, *ed 2, Philadelphia, Churchill-Livingstone, 2002.)*

This area of the antrum must be sufficiently wide to allow emptying of the gastric remnant. A linear stapling instrument is placed at that point at a right angle to the greater curvature. In adults, a 2.5-cm double row of staples is fired. The distal staple line is oversewn with a continuous 3-0 polypropylene suture. Several of the staples are removed from proximally to the fundus. In children, a 20 Fr to 26 Fr catheter is used, depending on the age of the child.

The RGT is constructed with multiple applications of a linear stapling instrument in loose proximity to the catheter to avoid tension on the staple line. A 2.5-cm diameter tube with length sufficient to reach the cervical esophagus is created. Usually four applications of the stapling device are required to construct the tube.

The staple line of the newly formed curvature of the stomach is oversewn with a continuous 3-0 polypropylene suture. The staple line of the RGT is similarly oversewn (see Figure 2). Interrupted sutures are used at an angle where the tube joins the stomach. Keeping the tube stretched to its full length on the catheter ensures that it is not shortened by the application of the suture. The continuous suture is completed 5 cm from the end of the tube. At this point, interrupted sutures are again used. This allows the excision of redundant tube if necessary. The tube may be placed on the anterior chest wall to verify that its length is sufficient for the cervical anastomosis.

In cases of caustic stricture, we have transected the esophagogastric junction closing both defects by staple lines

and oversewing. This maneuver allows the fundus to be positioned anteriorly, effecting a 30% to 40% increase in tube length for anastomosis to the pharynx. In our experience, decompression of the distal esophagus via external tube drainage or anastomosis to the jejunum has not been necessary because the esophageal mucosa has been effectively destroyed by the initial injury.

The omentum is inspected. If any has been devascularized, it should be excised. The remaining omentum is wrapped about the tube to facilitate its transportation to the neck. This is accomplished by shielding the tube and catheter in a plastic sleeve. The tube may be transposed via the substernal, transthoracic, or transhiatal route as circumstances dictated. Three possibilities exist regarding the cervical anastomosis of the RGT, which depend on the location of the cervical anastomosis of the RGT and the extent of fibrosis that resulted from caustic injury. The anastomosis may be performed above the hyoid bone, through it after its removal, or below. When the anastomosis is done to the pharynx, we have used the Montgomery T-tube as a stent; the tube is left in place for as least 3 months. The higher the anastomosis, the more frequently leak and stricture occur. The cervical anastomosis is wrapped with omentum. Closed suction drainage of the cervical incision is not necessary, and the wound is closed loosely. If a leak develops, one or two sutures are removed to facilitate drainage.

A feeding jejunostomy is constructed, and internal nutrition is started on postoperative day 3. An oral contrast study is performed on postoperative day 7. If the contrast study is satisfactory, a soft diet is begun.

Nonreversed Gastric Tube

Initially an extensive Kocher maneuver is performed to free the duodenum and the head of the pancreas so that the pylorus approaches the midline. The greater omentum and vasa brevia are managed as previously described, and the gastric fundus is freed from its diaphragmatic attachments and the pancreas. The prepyloric region is examined for an area that is sufficiently wide to allow for construction of a tube 2.5 cm in diameter, with at least an equal amount for the remaining antrum. At that point, the anterior and posterior walls of the stomach are opened by cautery. A 25-mm circular stapling instrument is inserted with the anvil applied to the posterior wall of the stomach (Figure 3A). The linear stapler is inserted through a defect created by the circular stapler. The tube is not constructed over a catheter. Its width must be appraised carefully before each application of the stapling device. It is helpful to mark the line of staple application on the anterior wall of the stomach with needle tip cautery at low power setting. The final application of the stapling instrument is an oblique one in the fundus area. The staple closure of the stomach and the tube are reinforced by a continuous polypropylene suture as previously described (Figure 3B). Interrupted sutures are used at the fundic end so that any excess tube may be excised if necessary.

■ RESULTS

Anastomotic leak and stricture have been common occurrences in cases of gastric tube esophagoplasty, just as they are after transhiatal interposition of the entire stomach to the neck. A 10% to 15% leak rate has been reported in patents undergoing transhiatal esophagectomy. Leaks do not result in stricture, and the reverse is also true. Ximenes-Netto et al reported a 10% (8 cases) fistula rate in 80 RGTs, but only 3 cases required reoperation.

The gastric tube that is constructed is a vagotomized structure. Peristalsis has not been noted in the gastric tube. It is erroneous to term the RGT as *antiperistaltic* and the NRGT as *peristaltic*; both tubes serve only as conduits. The RGT has a theoretical advantage. It has mucus-secreting antral mucosa anastomosed to the esophagus, whereas the NRGT has acid-secreting fundic tissue at the suture line. Nevertheless, no long-term clinical differences have been found between the two procedures.

The gastric tube has advantages over other conduits in addition to the anatomic reasons previously mentioned.

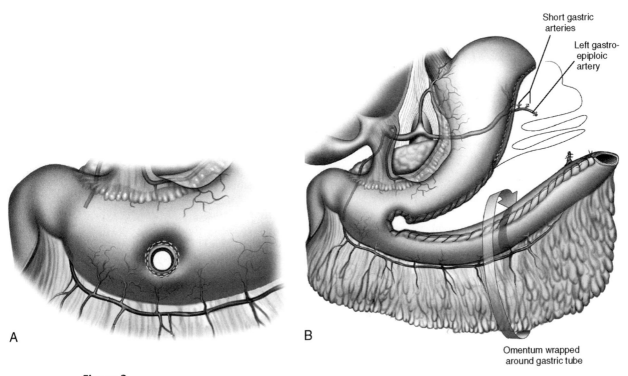

A

B

Short gastric arteries

Left gastro-epiploic artery

Omentum wrapped around gastric tube

Figure 3
A, Preparation of the nonreversed gastric tube. The circular stapler creates the defect required for the insertion of the stapler. **B,** Omental wrap of the nonreversed gastric tube before cervical transportation. *(From Fell SC, Ximenes-Netto M: Gastric tubes, reversed and nonreversed. In Pearson FG, editor:* Esophageal surgery, *ed 2, Philadelphia, Churchill-Livingstone, 2002.)*

The diameter of the tube is similar to that of an esophagus and occupies less space in the thorax and neck than does the colon or whole stomach. Reflux may occur in all conduits, but it is better tolerated in the gastric tube than in the colon, which may develop ulceration. Colon interposition requires three enteric suture lines; the gastric tube has only one. Gastric tube interposition is technically easier to perform, takes less operating time, and does not require colonoscopy, angiography, or bowel preparation.

The major deficiency of the gastric tube esophagoplasty is the relatively frequent occurrence of anastomotic leak or stricture. These complications, reported by all who use this method of reconstruction, suggest that impaired vascularity of the gastric tube is the cause, no matter whether the tube is reversed or nonreversed.

Lieberman-Meffert et al showed that the right gastroepiploic artery is the exclusive conduit of blood to the tube and that the right gastric artery makes an inconsequential contribution. The branches of the left gastroepiploic artery vascularize the midportion of the tube, and there is only a weak connection between the right and left gastroepiploic arteries. The arterial supply of the upper 20% of the gastric tube (fundus) is through arterioles and capillaries. Arterial communication between the right and left gastroepiploic arteries is by means of retrograde flow if either of these vessels is divided. The arterial supply of the fundus is also retrograde after division of the vasa brevia.

If the gastric tube is to be placed substernally, the thoracic inlet should be widened by a resection of the sternal attachments of the strap muscles and the sternocleidomastoid muscle if necessary. This maneuver prevents compression of the arterial supply and venous drainage of the tube.

SUGGESTED READING

Fell SC, Ximenes-Netto M: Gastric tubes, reversed and nonreversed. In Pearson FG, editor: *Esophageal surgery*, ed 2, Philadelphia, Churchill-Livingstone, 2002.

Lieberman-Meffert D, et al: Vascular anatomy of the gastric tube used for esophageal reconstruction, *Ann Thorac Surg* 54:1110, 1992.

Ximenes-Netto M, et al: The reversed gastric tube revisited a useful replacement for benign disease, *S Am J Thorac Surg* 5:22, 1998.

COMPLICATIONS OF ESOPHAGEAL RESECTION

Stephen C. Yang

Rates of morbidity and mortality after esophageal resection have decreased mainly due to improvements in surgical technique, perioperative care, and standardized postoperative clinical care pathways. Although surgical referrals now often are made to high-volume centers, one can never be fully prepared for complications after esophageal resection.

Overall morbidity and mortality rates after esophagectomy vary but average around 15% and 3%, respectively, in experienced hands. These figures do not differ significantly between the operative approaches used or whether the procedure was done for benign or malignant disease. The most common cause of death results from respiratory complications. Risk factors common to most complications include anatomic considerations, patient age, length and complexity of the operation, preoperative neoadjuvant therapy, and experience of the operating surgeon. Complications after esophagectomy are presented in terms of intraoperative, postoperative, and functional morbidities, omitting general problems indirectly associated with surgery (e.g., myocardial infarction, pulmonary embolus).

■ INTRAOPERATIVE COMPLICATIONS

Bleeding

With careful dissection, massive bleeding during routine esophagectomy should not occur. Average blood loss should be less than 500 ml with either a transthoracic (Ivor Lewis or McKeown three-incision) esophagectomy (TTE) or transhiatal esophagectomy (THE) approach. Hemostasis is a more important issue with THE because most of the esophageal dissection is done blindly. In either case, a plan should be formulated before every case should uncontrollable bleeding occur. One should never compromise operative exposure based on the planned procedure.

With TTE, nearly all the dissection is done under direct visualization without much difficulty. Meticulous hemostasis should be attained with TTE and THE while mobilizing the stomach and duodenum, particularly around the spleen and celiac axis. The sterile field should be wide enough so that access to the upper mediastinum and both pleural cavities can be obtained in the emergent setting.

If further access is needed to the lower third of the esophagus during a THE, the abdominal incision can be extended to a left thoracoabdominal exposure or by closing the abdomen and carrying out a formal low left thoracotomy. Catastrophic bleeding can occur during blunt dissection of the upper esophagus from the aortic and bronchial arterial branches and from the azygos vein. In these situations, if hemostasis cannot be obtained from packing, ligation, or cautery, direct control is gained via a partial upper sternal split.

Tracheobronchial Injury

Tears to the membranous portion of the trachea or main stem bronchus can occur during mobilization of the upper half of the esophagus by either TTE or THE. Bronchoscopy should be performed routinely after induction of anesthesia if tumor proximity to the airway is a concern. If full thickness of the airway is involved, generally chance for cure is low. In these situations, tumor should be left attached to avoid an airway injury. Large defects (>1 cm) in the airway require buttressing with a vascularized tissue pedicle, such as intercostal muscle, parietal pleura, mediastinal fat, or pericardium; smaller holes can be closed directly with absorbable suture, but also should be reinforced with a tissue pedicle to avoid fistulization with adjacent structures (esophagus, aorta).

During THE, subtle observations suggest an airway injury has occurred. These observations include increasing inability to ventilate the patient, loss of returned tidal volume, decreased peak airway pressure, persistent air bubbles from the mediastinum, and the odor of anesthetic fumes. If an airway injury is suspected, the endotracheal tube should be deflated, advanced past the tear, and reinflated. With distal tracheal or right main stem bronchial tears, tube placement should be guided into the left main stem bronchus by the surgeon's hand passing up through the esophageal hiatus. When the airway is controlled and the patient is stable, the rest of the esophagectomy can be completed, and repair of the airway injury can be approached via the right chest after gastrointestinal continuity has been restored.

Hydropneumothorax

The parietal pleura borders with the esophagus intimately. Entry into the pleural spaces can be unavoidable during THE, especially if tumor involves the mediastinal pleura. If violation of the contralateral pleura is recognized during the course of TTE, attempts should be made to repair the defect; if this is not possible, the area should be packed off to prevent spillage of blood and fluid into that pleural space. When the operation is completed, a chest tube is placed into that pleural space. Violation of one or rarely both pleural spaces occurs in more than half of patients undergoing THE. This situation should be recognized early so that appropriate chest tube placement is performed at the closure of the procedure.

Recurrent Laryngeal Nerve Injury

Damage to the recurrent laryngeal nerve is never evident until the patient recovers sufficiently to show hoarseness or aspiration problems. Injuries invariably occur during mobilization of the cervical esophagus. Self-retaining metal retractors, extensive cautery use, and grasping extraesophageal tissue in the tracheoesophageal groove all are maneuvers that induce injury and should be avoided. Gentle retraction of the trachea and thyroid tissue is best achieved with either the surgical assistant's finger or a small malleable retractor. Traction injuries are usually self-limiting and take several months to resolve; however, if earlier resolution is required

for airway protection, cord medialization procedures have been used with excellent results.

Cardiac Complications

During THE, blunt dissection through the esophageal hiatus and posterior mediastinum usually compresses the left atrium and results in systemic hypotension. Less commonly, this same maneuver causes other cardiac arrhythmias, such as premature ventricular contractions, bradycardia, and supraventricular ectopy. These complications can be prevented with adequate filling pressures and normalization of electrolytes, although most are self-limiting and recover quickly after the surgeon's hand is withdrawn. Electrocardioversion paddles always should be readily available because malignant arrhythmias do occur rarely and should be acted on quickly with standard cardiac resuscitation protocols.

■ POSTOPERATIVE COMPLICATIONS

Anastomotic Leaks

Disruption of an intrathoracic anastomosis with subsequent mediastinitis and sepsis is a frequent cause of death after esophagectomy for benign and malignant disease, accounting for 40% of operative-related causes. This remains the primary reason why some surgeons prefer a THE approach with a cervical anastomosis. Anastomotic leaks occur infrequently, ranging from 0% to 12% in larger series.

Defense remains the best offense in avoiding anastomotic complications. Oral hygiene should be inspected during the initial clinic visit, addressing carious teeth and infected gums well in advance of surgery. Whether a manual or stapled anastomosis is performed, a precise technique should be done tension-free with intact vascularization to the conduit (stomach or bowel) remnant, while limiting mobilization of the proximal esophageal segment. The method of approximation does not influence leak problems; equivalent results have been obtained using staples or sutures, absorbable or nonabsorbable sutures, one-layer or two-layer anastomosis, and running or interrupted sutures.

Proper preparation of the esophageal replacement conduit and preservation of adequate vascular supply is hallmark and influences anastomotic healing. In preparing the gastric tube remnant, the right gastroepiploic and, if possible, the right gastric arteries should be left intact. The short and left gastric vessels are divided sequentially. In preparing the gastric line of resection, it is important to preserve the fundus rather than the cardia of the stomach, which maintains maximal length of the gastric tube. Left colonic interposition grafts require adequate collateralization through the marginal artery off the middle colic branch. Other operative maneuvers also maintain arterial and venous integrity. The conduit should be delivered up into the chest or cervical region in proper alignment to avoid twisting. At the time of closure, the esophageal hiatus should be large enough to permit passage of at least two fingertips around the conduit. Postoperatively a nasogastric tube is kept in place to avoid excessive distention of the gastric or bowel pull-up segment, and hypotension and low-output states should be corrected to preserve splanchnic blood flow.

Cervical leaks, though they prolong hospital stay, are rare causes of death. Leaks most commonly occur between postoperative days 5 and 10 and are manifested by fever, leukocytosis, crepitance, or increased wound drainage or erythema. When the diagnosis is suspected, the cervical incision should be opened widely and drained; this should be done in the operating room for patient comfort and to assess adequately the degree of disruption and contamination. Often, computed tomography (CT) scan of the neck and chest is performed before open drainage to determine the extent of contamination. Attempts should never be made to mobilize the anastomosis or to repair the defect. The wound is opened in its entirety and packed gently with dry gauze. Infrequently, mediastinal contamination occurs, which usually can be treated with local measures and closed suction drainage. In the face of sepsis or conduit necrosis, diverting cervical esophagostomy is required. Nearly all cervical leaks close with conservative wound management; however, one third develop a stricture requiring repeat dilation. Rarely, thoracotomy is needed for wider drainage of the mediastinum or pleura. A feeding jejunostomy (16-gauge red rubber catheter) always is placed at the time of the original esophageal resection not only for immediate postoperative nutrition, but also as the alternative means of nutrition should these complications occur.

Thoracic anastomotic leaks present more difficult circumstances than their cervical counterparts, with associated mortality rates of 50%. These leaks commonly present after postoperative day 7, usually with unexplained fever, leukocytosis, or sepsis. A prompt diatrizoate meglumine (Gastrografin) swallow examination should be performed and followed by urgent chest reexploration if free or uncontained leaks are found. Alternatively, a contrast-enhanced CT scan can provide the same information. At the time of reoperation, it is useful to perform a limited endoscopic examination of the anastomosis with a pediatric flexible esophagoscope to assess the degree of disruption and amount of mucosal necrosis. The findings may help guide the best approach to repair.

All reexplorations are performed through their original incisions. Minimal disruptions with healthy mucosal edges can be reclosed carefully and, more importantly, buttressed with a well-vascularized tissue pedicle, such as thickened pleura, intercostal muscle, or pericardial fat. Care must be taken to minimize dissection around the anastomosis. More commonly, patients are septic and have larger areas of anastomotic disruption or tissue necrosis. In these situations, local repair ultimately leads to an unfavorable result. The anastomosis is taken down, the edges are débrided, and an end cervical diverting esophagostomy is created, with the gastric remnant débrided, closed, and returned back to the abdomen. Wide drainage of the anastomosis and the mediastinum is necessary in all cases of anastomotic leaks. Reconstruction is done several months later after the patient fully recovers.

Silent Radiologic Leaks

An asymptomatic anastomotic leak is a common finding detected on routine postoperative Gastrografin examinations. We typically perform a cine esophagram on postoperative day 5 to 7. Small (<1 cm) contained leaks that drain back into the lumen of the esophagus usually are not clinically significant. These leaks are treated conservatively, with oral feedings withheld an additional 5 to 7 days before the radiographic examination is repeated. A nasogastric tube (usually removed on postoperative day 4) is not reinserted.

Larger leaks, although they may be contained, should be drained operatively. These pose a potential disaster because they can lie in close proximity to the membranous wall of the trachea or to the aorta and can cause erosion into these structures by local infection.

Delayed Hemorrhage

Reexploration for delayed postoperative hemorrhage rarely occurs and is usually a result of persistent bleeding from esophageal aortic branches in the chest or from short gastric vessels or unrecognized splenic injuries in the abdomen. Delayed splenic rupture can occur 1 week after surgery. Achalasia patients undergoing resection for megaesophagus represent a subpopulation at increased risk for bleeding. Due to the hypertrophied muscle associated with the disease process, an enriched blood supply is present; meticulous attention to hemostasis should be addressed at the time of initial resection.

Conduit Necrosis

Necrosis of the gastric or bowel conduit used for esophageal reconstruction is a rare complication after esophagectomy but is fatal in 50% of cases. The clinical presentation is not subtle, usually with associated sepsis, acidosis, leukocytosis, hyperthermia, and respiratory failure. The diagnosis is given a high degree of clinical suspicion especially if these signs are present within the first 5 days after surgery. It can be confirmed by CT scan or Gastrografin swallow; if these tests prove to be negative, and the presence of necrosis is still in question, a gentle endoscopy with a pediatric flexible scope should be diagnostic. Treatment is similar to a large anastomotic disruption, in which an end cervical esophagostomy is created, and the conduit is débrided and closed, and if appropriately viable, returned back to the abdomen. Enteral nutrition is resumed through a jejunostomy tube, and reconstruction is performed after months of recuperation.

Conduit Obstruction

Mechanical obstruction of the esophageal substitute graft after esophagectomy usually occurs from a failure to enlarge the diaphragmatic esophageal hiatus adequately. It can occur in the early postoperative period, but differentiation from a functional obstruction is difficult. An esophagogram should identify the site and degree of obstruction. This problem is avoided by opening the hiatus large enough at the time of initial surgery to permit passage of the surgeon's entire hand and forearm into the posterior mediastinum. If the obstruction is found in the postoperative period, however, reoperation through the abdominal approach should be performed promptly to correct the defect.

Placement of the esophageal replacement graft in the retrosternal position poses other specific obstructive complications. An inadequate retrosternal neohiatal opening can create an obstruction at this point, necessitating reoperation. Proximally the clavicular head can narrow the anterior aspect of the thoracic inlet, by projecting posteriorly and further compressing the conduit. To avoid this problem, the medial aspect of the left clavicle, first rib, and adjacent manubrium should be resected at the time of the original esophagectomy.

Respiratory Complications

Atelectasis, pneumonia, and respiratory failure account for the leading causes of morbidity and mortality after esophageal resection and reconstruction. These complications are seen more commonly in patients undergoing a combined thoracic and abdominal approach and in part support the rationale for a THE approach to minimize morbidity and mortality after esophagectomy. Larger published series now report definite risk factors that increase the chances for respiratory complications, including advanced age, chronic obstructive pulmonary disease, malnutrition, history of severe reflux, neoadjuvant therapy, and operative blood loss greater than 1000 ml.

Regardless of the operative approach, early intervention should be directed toward these factors in the preoperative period. Although preoperative nutrition has never been shown to benefit patients undergoing esophagectomy, enteral nutrition is particularly useful in the subpopulation of patients undergoing neoadjuvant therapy. Abstinence from cigarette smoking and participation in pulmonary rehabilitation help optimize pulmonary hygiene and function.

Epidural or intrathecal analgesia is offered to the patient before induction of anesthesia and should be insisted on if TTE is done or if the patient has compromised pulmonary function. Perioperatively, appropriate prophylactic broad-spectrum antibiotics are administered. Intermittent nasogastric decompression with the head of the bed elevated minimizes the risk of tracheobronchial aspiration. Although the timing of extubation is controversial, ventilatory assistance is continued at least through the night of the operation until the patient shows satisfactory gag reflex and pulmonary mechanics. The rationale behind overnight intubation is threefold: (1) The presence of unrecognized recurrent laryngeal nerve injury can cause immediate impaired swallowing and aspiration; (2) a reflex bronchorrhea can occur after mobilization of the upper esophagus away from the trachea; and (3) an overdistended esophageal conduit (stomach, colon, jejunum) with retained secretions, owing to a malfunctioning nasogastric tube or distal obstruction, may result in regurgitation and aspiration.

Postextubation care should consist of early ambulation, chest physiotherapy, incentive spirometry, and humidified supplemental oxygen. Patients with signs of a pneumonic process should be given appropriate antibiotics to cover anaerobic and gram-negative organisms. If pulmonary complications persist, early flexible bronchoscopy is advocated not only to sample properly and identify infectious organisms, but also to aid in pulmonary toilet and to exclude tracheobronchial injuries.

Respiratory failure seems to occur more commonly with TTE compared with THE, although this have never been proved in a controlled study. Tracheostomy is indicated if ventilator dependency is required for more than 1 week. Early cricothyroidotomy may be used alternatively if a cervical incision is in the way and later converted to a standard tracheostomy.

Chylothorax

Because of its intimacy with the esophagus, the thoracic duct can be injured at any level in the thorax during esophagectomy. The reported incidence is 1% to 3%, with nearly equal frequency between TTE and THE. Although death is rare from this complication, mortality approaches 50%, particularly in debilitated patients with total esophageal obstruction undergoing esophageal resection. Increased risks for this complication include tumor adherence to soft tissues posteriorly, prior intrathoracic surgery, and preoperative radiation therapy.

Chyle leaks are difficult to see during the course of the operation because patients have fasted. Because there is no harm in ligating the thoracic duct, it should be done if the possibility of an injury exists. During TTE, I prefer routinely to oversew the duct in the right prevertebral area just above the esophageal hiatus before chest closure. The duct is more difficult to visualize during THE; however, after the esophagus is removed, the posterior mediastinum can be visualized through the esophageal hiatus up to the level of the carina, and any suspicious tissue leaking chyle should be ligated.

In the early postoperative period, a diagnosis of a chylothorax usually presents around postoperative day 5, when excessive serous chest tube output is noted (>800 ml/24 hr). In the patient undergoing THE when neither pleural space was entered, the clinical picture is heralded by acute respiratory distress and hypotension from the accumulation of chyle in the pleural space that is under tension. The diagnosis usually is made easily by feeding the patient cream through the jejunostomy tube and observing that the serous chest tube drainage turns opaque. Sophisticated studies on the pleural fluid, such as measuring a high triglyceride level (>110 ml/dl) or high lymphocyte count, although confirming the diagnosis, are often not necessary.

An aggressive approach to the treatment of this problem is advocated because most chyle leaks after esophagectomy do not close spontaneously with conservative management. It is important not to delay treatment because nutritional and immunologic depletion rapidly ensues, leading to early shock or sepsis. Lower morbidity and mortality rates and shorter hospital stays have been reported using this approach of early intervention. When the diagnosis is made, enteral feeding should be stopped and total parenteral nutrition started. In preparing the patient for surgery to control the leak, drainage can decrease to less than 200 ml/24 hours, indicating a potential response to nonoperative therapy. Most continue to drain beyond this amount, however, and surgery is expedited in patients with outputs greater than 1000 ml/24 hours.

Exposure to the thoracic duct is gained through the prior thoracotomy or a low right thoracotomy if THE was performed previously. After thorough irrigation of the chest cavity, the site of injury is located clearly if cream is given again through the jejunostomy tube several hours before surgery. Applying external pressure to the anterior abdominal wall increases the flow of chyle into the thorax. The duct is ligated above and below the tear. Alternatively, video-assisted thoracic surgery can be used to identify and control the site of injury.

Bowel Herniation

Herniation of abdominal viscera into the chest through an enlarged esophageal hiatus can occur after esophagectomy and conduit replacement. This is a rare complication and should not occur if precautions are taken at the time of the initial operation. Usually the esophageal diaphragmatic hiatus is closed to the point so that it allows easy passage of two fingers around the esophageal conduit. In addition, three or four interrupted sutures are placed between the conduit and the hiatal musculature to prevent herniation cephalad.

This complication can occur acutely within the first week of surgery. Although most cases are usually asymptomatic and are found on a routine postoperative chest film, some patients may exhibit signs and symptoms of bowel obstruction or ischemia. Plain radiographs of the chest usually show an extraneous and unusual bowel gas pattern in the chest and mediastinum. CT scans or contrast studies may be needed when the diagnosis is in doubt. Visceral herniations are found more commonly years after esophagectomy. Similar to chronic traumatic diaphragmatic hernia, patients present with vague lower thoracic or upper abdominal cramping pain, with associated nausea and vomiting.

Surgical repair is advocated in all cases to avoid the potential complications of obstruction, strangulation, and perforation. A bowel preparation is required only in the chronic situation. Reduction of the evisceration can be accomplished via the abdomen in nearly all cases. As described earlier, the esophageal hiatus should be closed comfortably and anchored to the esophageal substitute.

Anastomotic Stricture

Strictures after esophagectomy at the anastomotic site occur regardless of the type of conduit replacement (stomach or bowel), type of anastomosis (suture or staple), or type of approach (TTE or THE). Documented stricture rates range from 5% to 42%. Most experienced surgeons find that resecting a 1- to 2-cm "button" of stomach at the anastomosis site helps to minimize the chance of late stenosis. The incidence of an anastomotic stricture increases if the esophageal pathology resulted from lye ingestion, there was a postoperative anastomotic leak, small stapling devices (25 to 27 mm) were used, excessive suture material was used, or the anastomosis was performed in an irradiated field. Most strictures are managed successfully with esophageal bougienage and do not require surgical revision. In addition, early dilation is recommended after a patient has recovered from an anastomotic leak to ensure that the anastomosis is patent and to prevent a tight stenosis from developing.

Initial dilation should be performed by flexible esophagoscopy to inspect the degree, length, and nature of the stricture. Most can be dilated with soft tapered Maloney dilators, using a 46 Fr or larger size until no further resistance is obtained. Tight or angulated strictures should be dilated, however, over a wire or with balloon dilators under fluoroscopic guidance. Placement of the esophageal substitute proximally along the native esophageal bed in the posterior mediastinum helps to minimize these angulation problems. Multiple dilations over several weeks usually are required to prevent stricture recurrence. Treatments usually are stopped after 6 months of stability and are resumed only if dysphagia develops.

More caution should be used in dilating an anastomosis in which bowel (colon, jejunum) is used as the replacement conduit rather than the stomach because of the thin-walled nature of the former and subsequent higher propensity for perforation. As a result, some authors have suggested that surgical revision should be considered earlier over dilation in the presence of esophagocolonic or esophagojejunal anastomoses.

A small group of patients with cervical anastomoses have strictures that are chronic and resistant to nonoperative therapy and may be candidates for surgical intervention. These include not only high-risk patients mentioned earlier, but also patients who continue to require repeat dilation for more than 12 months after surgery and patients who develop an anastomotic leak with a chronic cutaneous fistula. A variety of strictureplasty techniques using various myocutaneous tissue flaps have been reported to manage these complications. A sternocleidomastoid myocutaneous flap has been described in a small series of patients. Owing to the random blood supply, a flap necrosis rate of 50% has been reported. The latissimus dorsi flap also has been used successfully, based on the excellent blood supply from the thoracodorsal artery; this approach requires a separate operative positioning of the patient. Similarly a free tissue transfer flap from the radial forearm is popular, but it is technically challenging and requires microimplantation of the radial artery and vein.

At this institution, we have applied the use of a pectoralis myocutaneous flap (PMF) for the management of select patients with cervical esophageal anastomotic complications. The PMF has been well established for head and neck reconstruction and is an ideal structure to widen the stricture based on the flap's mobility, skin paddle for epithelial replacement, and well-vascularized muscular tissue. Briefly the skin pedicle of the PMF is designed in an elliptical shape overlying the medial and inferior aspect of the pectoralis major muscle. An oblique incision is made to the ipsilateral axilla, and the exposed pectoralis muscle is raised to the level of the clavicle, preserving the thoracoacromial vascular pedicle. When the cervical stricture is exposed and the lumen opened proximally and distally, the PMF is tunneled toward the cervical field and inverted. The skin paddle is sewn in place to patch the mucosal defect, and the accompanying pectoralis muscle secondarily reinforces the repair (Figure 1).

■ FUNCTIONAL COMPLICATIONS

Dysphagia

Approximately 5% of patients experience persistent symptoms of dysphagia 1 year after surgery that is not attributed to anastomotic strictures or mechanical obstruction. Dilation is continued through this time, despite the fact that the dilators pass easily through the anastomosis without resistance. Cine esophagograms confirm that the dysphagia is due to a functional cause rather than a mechanical obstruction. Although the underlying problem likely has a neurogenic basis, treatment is mainly supportive.

Regurgitation

Occasional regurgitation of ingested food is seen in 30% of patients with a cervical anastomosis. Regurgitation occurs particularly after the patient eats a large meal and assumes a recumbent position. The classic symptoms of gastroesophageal reflux are not encountered, but a small subset develop pulmonary complications secondary to aspiration. Supportive care is the mainstay of therapy.

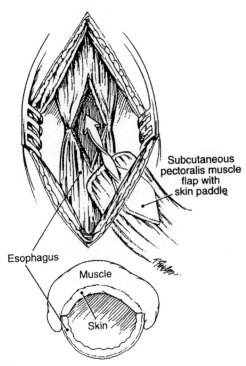

Figure 1
Technique of rotation and positioning the pectoralis myocutaneous flap for the surgical treatment of chronic and refractory anastomotic strictures. *(From Heitmiller R, et al:* J Thorac Cardiovasc Surg *115:1250, 1998.)*

Delayed Conduit Emptying

Retention of swallowed food and secretions in the esophageal substitute conduit is a complication that is poorly understood with few treatment options. Symptoms can appear in the immediate postoperative period. Retention is seen more often with colonic than with gastric reconstruction because of the more thick-walled stomach. Sluggish flow is usually a late result from redundancy of the intrathoracic portion of the conduit just above the hemidiaphragm. This can be avoided by maintaining structural integrity of both pleural envelopes during THE, which would provide a straight alignment of the conduit in the posterior mediastinum. If the TTE approach is used, this same concept can be achieved by anchoring the conduit to the surrounding transected pleura adjacent to the lung and spine.

Another significant factor causing delayed emptying is an inadequate myotomy of the pylorus. Controversy exists whether the pylorus should be divided and if so by what technique. Some authors report, however, that only 15% of patients develop obstruction at the pylorus if it is preserved during esophagectomy. Nevertheless, most surgeons advise that either pyloromyotomy or pyloroplasty be performed because morbidity is minimal with this short maneuver. Pyloromyotomy is preferred in most cases when the pylorus is normal. I prefer also to suture on a Graham patch of omentum over the myotomy site (in case an unsuspected mucosal injury is made) and mark it with radiopaque clips for easy identification on plain radiographs. Pyloroplasty should be used, however, in situations in which this portion of the duodenum is extensively scarred or if the mucosa is inadvertently violated during attempts at pyloromyotomy.

Medical treatment of delayed emptying is primarily pharmacologic, in addition to the usual dietary precautions. All narcotics are stopped to help restore intestinal motility; this poses a problem for the patient in the immediate postoperative period who still is experiencing significant incisional discomfort. A trial of promotility agents, such as metoclopramide and/or erythromycin, is begun simultaneously, but efficacy has been mixed. If narrowing of the pylorus still is suspected, upper endoscopy followed by balloon dilation should be performed.

Dumping Syndrome

The dumping syndrome can present even before discharge following esophagectomy. Of patients, 20% experience some degree of this problem. Most patients with an intrathoracic stomach also experience early satiety. Treatment is directed at two general maneuvers. First, dietary measures can be controlled by eating smaller, more frequent meals; by drinking liquids after meals to avoid gastric distention; and by avoiding foods high in carbohydrates. Second, antidiarrheal agents are used liberally, such as kaolin/pectin, codeine compounds, and tincture of opium. Most symptoms diminish over 6 to 12 months with conservative management.

SUGGESTED READING

Boyle MJ, et al: Transhiatal versus transthoracic esophagectomy: complication and survival rates, *Am Surg* 65:1137, 1999.

Iannettoni MD, et al: Catastrophic complications of the cervical esophagogastric anastomosis, *J Thorac Cardiovasc Surg* 110:1493, 1995.

Karl RC, et al: Factors affecting morbidity, mortality, and survival in patients undergoing Ivor-Lewis esophagogastrectomy, *Ann Surg* 231:635, 2000.

Merigliano S, et al: Chylothorax complicating esophagectomy for cancer: a plea for early thoracic duct ligation, *J Thorac Cardiovasc Surg* 119:453, 2000.

Urschel JD: Esophagogastrostomy anastomotic leaks complicating esophagectomy: a review, *Am J Surg* 169:634, 1995.

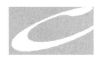

PREOPERATIVE EVALUATION OF GASTROESOPHAGEAL REFLUX DISEASE

N. S. Balaji

Jeffrey H. Peters

Surgical therapy for gastroesophageal reflux disease (GERD) has undergone considerable evolution. The advent of a minimally invasive surgical approach coupled with excellent long-term control of symptoms has made surgery an increasingly adopted alternative. Given this fact, careful evaluation of patients before offering a surgical option is more important than ever. Inadequate or inappropriate preoperative evaluation is a major cause of poor outcomes after antireflux surgery. A thorough understanding of the underlying pathophysiology is fundamental to the successful treatment of GERD. Evaluation starts with a detailed and structured elucidation of the patient's symptoms and continues with the use of appropriate investigations to characterize the anatomic and physiologic derangements of the disease. The objectives of preoperative evaluation are as follows:

1. Objective confirmation of GERD
2. Assessing the severity of GERD (Barrett's esophagus, short esophagus, stricture, large hiatal hernia, abnormal acid exposure)
3. Assessing the risk for progressive disease and the development of complications
4. Predicting the probability of response to surgical therapy
5. Deciding the most appropriate antireflux procedure
6. Planning the operative approach for the procedure (laparoscopic, transabdominal, transthoracic)

■ SYMPTOM ASSESSMENT

A careful, detailed, and structured assessment of the patient's symptoms is crucial to the decision making regarding surgery. After all, symptomatic improvement is the final arbiter of success. As such, it should not be left to the referring gastroenterologist. It becomes evident quickly that GERD is a functional disorder often accompanied by non–reflux-related gastrointestinal and respiratory symptoms that do not improve or may be worsened by antireflux surgery. Symptoms consistent with irritable bowel syndrome, such as alternating diarrhea and constipation, bloating, and crampy abdominal pain should be sought and detailed separately from GERD symptoms. Likewise, symptoms suggestive of gastric pathology, including nausea, early satiety, epigastric abdominal pain, anorexia, and weight loss, are important. It is increasingly recognized that oral symptoms, such as mouth and tongue burning and sore throat, rarely improve with antireflux surgery.

The patient's perception of what each symptom means should be explored in an effort to avoid misinterpretation. Of equal importance is to classify the symptoms as primary or secondary for prioritization of therapy and to allow an estimate of the probability of relief of each of the particular symptoms. The response to acid-suppressing medications predicts success and symptom relief after surgery. In contrast to the widely held belief that failure of medical therapy is an indication for surgery, a good response to proton-pump inhibitors is desirable because it predicts that the symptoms are actually due to reflux of gastric contents.

GERD-related symptoms can be divided into typical symptoms of heartburn, regurgitation, and dysphagia and atypical symptoms of cough, hoarseness, asthma, aspiration, and chest pain. Because there are fewer mechanisms for their generation, typical symptoms are more likely to be secondary to increased esophageal acid exposure than are atypical symptoms.

The relationship of atypical symptoms such as cough, hoarseness, wheezing, or sore throat to heartburn or regurgitation should be established. Other more common factors that may contribute to respiratory symptoms also should be investigated. The patient must be informed of the relative diminished probability of success of surgery when atypical symptoms are the primary symptoms. Of note is the comparative longer time taken for the respiratory symptoms to improve after surgery.

■ DIAGNOSTIC STUDIES

The initial diagnostic evaluation should include the following:

1. Videoesophagography
2. Upper gastrointestinal endoscopy
3. Stationary esophageal manometry
4. 24-Hour esophageal pH monitoring (distal or proximal or both)

These four tests allow the surgeon to determine the presence of gastroesophageal reflux in an objective fashion; the underlying reasons for its presence, such as hiatal hernia or a deficient lower esophageal sphincter (LES); and its severity, including the presence or absence of complications. Although it has been argued that one or more of these studies are superfluous, experience constantly reminds us that they are complementary and that all add useful information before antireflux surgery. Further investigations, in particular gastric emptying studies and pancreaticobiliary testing, are added depending on the findings of these four tests.

Videoesophagography

Radiographic assessment of the anatomy and function of the esophagus and stomach is one of the most important parts of the preoperative evaluation. Carefully performed videoesophagography not only provides information about the underlying anatomic defects, such as the presence or absence of stricture and the size and reducibility of a hiatal hernia, but also it is one of the few ways to assess actual bolus transport. A standardized protocol is advised so as to ascertain different aspects of esophagogastric function during different phases of the study.

Anatomic variables, such as esophageal contour (e.g., dilated, narrowed, corkscrew), the presence of obstructive lesions (e.g., webs, diverticula, strictures, tumor), and the presence or absence of a hiatal hernia and its characteristics (e.g., size, type, reducibility) if present, are readily delineated. The anatomy of the cricopharyngeal region and the stomach also are ascertained.

Functional information includes an assessment of esophageal motility patterns, effectiveness of bolus transport, and swallow effectiveness in the cricopharyngeal segment and a subjective impression of the adequacy of gastric emptying. Radiographic gastroesophageal reflux occasionally is seen. If present, particularly if spontaneous, it is a reasonable indicator of reflux; however, its absence does not signify the absence of clinically important reflux. Roughly 40% of patients with classic symptoms of GERD have spontaneous reflux observed by the radiologist (i.e., reflux of barium from the stomach into the esophagus with the patient in the upright position). Videotaping the study greatly aids the evaluation, providing the surgeon with a real-time assessment of the aforementioned information.

Given routine review before antireflux surgery, the value of videoesophagography becomes increasingly clear. A hiatal hernia is present in greater than 80% of patients with gastroesophageal reflux. Hiatal hernias are shown best when the patient is in the prone position, which causes increased abdominal pressure and promotes distention of the hernia above the diaphragm. The presence of a hiatal hernia is an important component of the underlying pathophysiology of gastroesophageal reflux. Other relevant findings include a large (>5 cm) or irreducible hernia, suggesting the presence of a shortened esophagus; a tight crural "collar" that inhibits barium transit into the stomach, suggesting a possible cause of dysphagia; and the presence of a paraesophageal hernia, which is likely to influence the surgeon's decision regarding the operative approach.

The assessment of peristalsis on videoesophagography often adds to, or complements, the information obtained by esophageal manometry studies. This is in part because the video barium study can be done upright and supine and with liquid and solid bolus material, which is not true of a stationary motility examination. Videoesophagography is

particularly valuable with subtle motility abnormalities. During normal swallowing, a stripping wave (primary peristalsis) is generated, which completely clears the bolus. Residual material can stimulate a secondary peristaltic wave, but usually a second pharyngeal swallow is required. Motility disorders with disorganized or simultaneous esophageal contraction have "tertiary waves" and provide a segmented appearance to the barium column; this often is referred to as *beading* or *corkscrew*. In dysphagic patients, barium-impregnated marshmallow, bread, or hamburger is a useful adjunct, which can discern a functional esophageal transport disturbance not evident on the liquid barium study. The functional effectiveness of bolus transport is likely to have a bearing on the choice of operative procedure (total versus partial wraps) based on complementary evidence from the manometry studies, although the evidence for this rationale increasingly is disputed.

Upper Gastrointestinal Endoscopy and Biopsy

Direct visualization of the pharynx, larynx, esophagus, and stomach gives objective evidence of the presence or absence of complications secondary to reflux disease, such as esophagitis, stricture, or columnar lined esophagus. Grading of esophagitis as degrees from I through V is known to correlate well with the severity of the disease (Table 1). It also provides anatomic correlates, such as the presence of a large hernia, intrathoracic stomach, or twisted previous fundoplication, that may influence decision making on operative strategies. Therapeutic interventions in the form of dilation of strictures can be performed at the time of diagnostic endoscopy if necessary. Retained food material or bile in the esophagus and stomach may serve as gross indicators of motility disorders of the respective organs and may pave the way for more detailed investigations (second tier) if appropriate.

Biopsy evaluation of the distal esophagus, cardia, and stomach is an important component in the assessment of the disease. Biopsy specimens are taken routinely from the gastric antrum, squamocolumnar junction, and esophageal body 2 to 3 cm above the squamocolumnar junction. Additional biopsy specimens are obtained based on clinical findings. Four quadrant biopsy specimens at 2-cm intervals should be taken in the presence of a columnar lined esophagus. Carditis, manifest as inflamed, cardiac-type mucosa at the gastroesophageal junction, is believed to be an early marker of GERD. The etiology of intestinal metaplasia of the cardia in the absence of an endoscopically visible columnar

Table 1 Grades of Esophagitis: New Savary-Miller, 1990	
Grade I	Single erosion oval or linear
Grade II	Multiple linear erosions on more than one longitudinal fold
Grade III	Circumferential erosive lesions
Grade IV	Ulcer, stricture, or short esophagus with or without grades I-III
Grade V	Columnar lined esophagus with or without grades I-IV

Modified from Ollyo JB, et al: *Gastroenterology* 89:A100, 1990.

lined esophagus is controversial with evidence in favor of a reflux-related phenomenon.

Ambulatory pH Monitoring

Because of its invasive nature, the lack of availability in many hospitals, and the supposed benefits of other objective measures such as the presence of esophagitis or Barrett's esophagus, 24-hour ambulatory pH monitoring often is neglected before antireflux surgery. This is true despite evidence that shows it is the most important predictor of outcome after laparoscopic fundoplication (see later).

One of the key goals before taking a patient to the operating room is to connect the patient's complaints to gastroesophageal reflux. Antireflux surgery reliably and reproducibly prevents the return of gastric contents into the esophagus but does little else. If the symptoms that drove the patient to seek surgical treatment are not secondary to reflux, there is no benefit. One has a patient who not only is no better, but also often unusually focused on normally trivial side effects, such as bloating and flatulence. The best way to prevent this scenario is to use 24-hour pH monitoring to prove the presence of pathologic esophageal acid exposure before surgery. The study not only provides for an objective diagnosis, but also provides other useful information. By quantifying the time that esophageal mucosa is exposed to gastric juice, it gives the clinician a perspective on where the patient stands in the spectrum of disease severity, an important piece of information before making the decision for surgery, which cannot be gained from symptoms alone. It is well documented that symptom severity does not correlate with the severity of the underlying disease. pH monitoring also measures the ability of the esophagus to clear refluxed acid and correlates esophageal acid exposure with the patient's symptoms. It is the only way to express quantitatively the overall degree and pattern of esophageal acid exposure, both of which may affect the decision for surgery. Patients with nocturnal or bipositional reflux have a higher prevalence of complications and failure of long-term medical control. pH monitoring is considered by many to be the gold standard for the diagnosis of GERD because it has the highest sensitivity and specificity of all tests currently available.

Ambulatory pH monitoring is the gold standard for the assessment of pathologic esophageal acid exposure. Present technology includes the transnasal placement of an antimony or glass pH electrode 5 cm above the manometrically determined upper border of the LES. Given that normal values were established at this level and this level only, placement of the pH probe via endoscopic or pH measurement is not sufficient and leads to inaccurate results. All acid-suppressant medications are discontinued before the procedure (proton-pump inhibitors 2 weeks prior and H_2 blockers and prokinetics 48 hours prior). The patient is sent home with set instructions and a diary to record any symptoms during the 24-hour period. The test is completed after a minimum of 21 hours, and data obtained are analyzed.

The following six variables are analyzed to arrive at a composite score (Table 2):

1. Frequency of reflux episodes
2. Percentage of total time spent in an acid environment with a pH less than 4

Table 2 Normal Values for Esophageal Exposure to pH Less than 4 (n = 50)

COMPONENT	MEAN	STANDARD DEVIATION	95TH PERCENTILE
Total time pH < 4	1.51	1.36	4.45
Upright time pH < 4	2.34	2.34	8.42
Supine time pH < 4	0.63	1.0	3.45
No. episodes	19.00	12.76	46.9
No. > 5 minutes	0.84	1.18	3.45
Longest episode	6.74	7.85	19.8

From DeMeester TR, Stein HJ: In Moody FG, et al, editors: *Surgical treatment of digestive disease*, ed 2, Chicago, 1989, Year Book Medical Publishers, p 68.

3. Percentage of upright time spent in an acid environment with a pH less than 4
4. Percentage of supine time spent in an acid environment with a pH less than 4
5. Longest reflux episode
6. Number of reflux episodes longer than 5 minutes

Four of these are measures of the frequency and severity of reflux (1 through 4), and two are measures of the ability of the esophagus to clear acid (5 and 6). The composite score gives a qualitative and quantitative assessment of the exposure of the distal esophagus to an acid environment and has been shown to correlate well with the competency of the gastroesophageal barrier. An abnormal pH value has been shown to be the most important predictor of successful outcome after laparoscopic Nissen fundoplication.

Dual-channel pH studies provide important information about the proximal extent of the acid reflux that may be useful in the assessment of patients with respiratory symptoms. Normal values have been established with proximal channel placement either 20 cm above the LES (15 cm from the distal channel) (single catheter assembly) or 1 cm distal to the lower border of the upper esophageal sphincter (two-catheter study). The probes are placed after ascertaining the position of the upper esophageal sphincter and lower esophageal high-pressure zone (LEHPZ) after standard esophageal manometry.

In healthy volunteers with probe placement 20 cm above the LES, acid exposure of proximal esophagus is less than 1.3% of the total time pH is less than 4, and acid exposure is 0% in the supine position. Other reliable markers of proximal reflux are mirror-image reflux events occurring in concordance with a distal reflux and greater than seven proximal reflux events outside the meal period.

Prediction of Response to Surgical Therapy

A multivariate analysis of the factors that predict successful outcome after laparoscopic Nissen fundoplication was published. Consecutive patients undergoing laparoscopic Nissen fundoplication (n = 199) were studied, and a variety of demographic, anatomic, clinical, and physiologic factors were analyzed. The three most important predictors of successful clinical outcome in order of importance were an abnormal pH score, a typical primary symptom, and a complete or partial (>50%) response to medical therapy. When all three were present, the patient was 90 times more likely to have relief of symptoms than when they were not.

Stationary Esophageal Manometry

The primary aims of esophageal manometry before antireflux surgery are to:

1. Exclude an alternative diagnosis, such as a primary motility disorder
2. Allow accurate placement of the pH probe
3. Stratify the severity of disease via an assessment of the presence or absence of an incompetent LES or ineffective esophageal motility
4. Gauge the risk of postoperative dysphagia

Manometry can be done using either water-perfused or solid-state catheter systems. The study is divided into three parts, including an assessment of the LES, esophageal body, and cricopharyngeal segment. The catheter is placed transnasally, and the length and resting pressure of the LEHPZ are evaluated with a stationary pull-through method (Table 3). The transition from the abdominal to the thoracic pressure environment is noted as the respiratory inversion point, which anatomically corresponds to the insertion of the phrenoesophageal membrane. This is visualized as a change in the pressure variations with respiration from an abdominal (positive with inspiration) to a thoracic (negative with inspiration) pattern. This change is followed by the assessment of the capacity of the LEHPZ to relax to 5-ml swallows of water. The esophageal body function is evaluated by placing three to five measuring segments within the body and noting the intraluminal pressure changes to 10 swallows of 5 ml of water. The amplitudes, progression, and morphology of the waves are noted, and a global assessment of the body function is made based on the capacity to clear liquid bolus.

The upper esophageal sphincter and the pharynx are assessed for their resting, contraction, and relaxation characteristics based on a pull-through maneuver and noting the response to dry and wet swallows. Although this part of manometry is of limited value in assessment of GERD, valuable information can be obtained in differentiating causes of dysphagia (transfer versus transport).

■ SECOND-TIER DIAGNOSTIC STUDIES

In most patients, the investigations discussed previously (videoesophagography, upper gastrointestinal endoscopy with biopsies, stationary esophageal manometry, and ambulatory pH measurement) identify the underlying cause of the patient's symptoms and enable surgical decision making.

A subgroup of patients may warrant further investigations, however, to elucidate the underlying pathophysiology. These patients include the following:

1. Patients with typical or atypical symptoms of GERD and the first tier of investigations are normal
2. Patients with equivocal findings that may or may not explain the symptoms experienced
3. Patients with results from the above-mentioned investigations that do not tally with one another
4. Patients with gastric or pharyngeal symptoms, such as nasal regurgitation, nausea, anorexia, and vomiting

Under these circumstances, the patient's symptoms should be reassessed carefully, the diagnostic tests checked to ensure they were performed and interpreted correctly, and further studies selected as needed. Common errors include (1) a pH probe placed in the wrong position; (2) achlorhydria secondary to atrophic gastritis or continued acid-suppressant medications; (3) mischaracterization of the LES in a patient with a stricture or a hiatal hernia; and (4) misinterpretation of a body study in a patient who continuously swallows, which makes deglutitive inhibition appear like ineffective motility. Studies that may help identify additional pathology or lead to a better understanding of the patient's disease pathophysiology include (1) radioisotope gastric emptying studies, (2) 24-hour esophageal bile monitoring, (3) 24-hour gastric pH monitoring, (4) 24-hour gastric bile monitoring, and (5) 24-hour esophageal impedance and pH monitoring.

24-Hour Esophageal Bile Monitoring

The role of the duodenogastric refluxate in contributing to the injury of the esophageal mucosa and intestinal metaplasia of the columnar lined esophagus is well established. It also has been shown that esophageal exposure to bile is an independent prognostic variable in the development of Barrett's esophagus. Esophageal bile measurement is not done routinely in all patients presenting for evaluation of possible GERD, however, because of the high specificity and sensitivity of the 24-hour pH monitoring for acid reflux and the greater likelihood of bile reflux occurring in association with acid reflux. Bile monitoring may be of value in patients with indirect evidence of GERD (e.g., esophagitis, incompetent sphincter, large hiatal hernias) and a normal pH score, in patients with Barrett's esophagus, or in patients with previous upper gastrointestinal surgery.

Bilirubin is detected on the basis of its specific light absorption properties at a wavelength of 453 nm. The study involves the transnasal placement of a spectrophotometric probe 5 cm above the upper border of the manometrically determined LEHPZ. The probe is connected to an external

Table 3 Normal Manometric Values of the Distal Esophageal Sphincter (n = 50)

PARAMETER	MEDIAN VALUE	2.5TH PERCENTILE	97.5TH PERCENTILE
Pressure (mm Hg)	13	5.8	27.7
Overall length (cm)	3.6	2.1	5.6
Abdominal length (cm)	2	0.9	4.7

Modified from Johnson LF, Demeester TR: *J Clin Gastroenterol* 8(Suppl 1):52, 1986.

data logger that detects the absorbance characteristics of the environment at the level of the probe from which a quantitative assessment is made of bile exposure. The normal values are based on the absorbance level, which is chosen in different centers based on a common graph.

Tests of Gastroduodenal Function

Associated gastric pathology is often a contributing factor in the pathogenesis of GERD. It has been shown that the receptive relaxation and accommodation of the fundic reservoir of the stomach often is deranged in patients with GERD. Delayed gastric emptying can contribute to increased and prolonged gastric distention, which places the LEHPZ at a mechanical disadvantage. Identifying these potentially contributing factors in subsets of patients helps in choosing optimal therapy and in predicting successful outcome after surgery.

■ USING RISK ASSESSMENT IN SELECTING THERAPY

The choice of treatment for GERD in present-day practice ideally should take into account the underlying severity of disease and the patient's risk for complications of end-stage reflux disease. This is particularly true given the rising incidence of Barrett's esophagus and adenocarcinoma of the gastric cardia.

Studies on the natural history of GERD have shown that although most patients have limited disease and respond well to lifestyle modifications and medical therapy, a substantial proportion (22% to 50%) progress to complications of GERD. This group should be identified early and offered antireflux surgery. The following factors when identified during the workup of patients help to identify patients at risk:

1. Anatomic and physiologic markers of severe disease, such as a defective LES, poor contractility of the esophageal body, large hiatal hernias, and bile reflux
2. Severe erosive esophagitis on presentation or the development of esophagitis or peptic strictures during the course of medical therapy
3. Barrett's esophagus
4. Young age, particularly patients with the above-listed characteristics
5. Progressive respiratory symptoms, aspiration, or pneumonia

SUGGESTED READING

Campos GM, et al: Multivariate analysis of factors predicting outcome after laparoscopic Nissen fundoplication, *J Gastrointest Surg* 3:292, 1999.

DeMeester TR, et al: Chronic respiratory symptoms and occult gastro-esophageal reflux: a prospective clinical study and results of surgical therapy, *Ann Surg* 211:337, 1990.

DeMeester TR, et al: Technique, indications, and clinical use of 24 hour esophageal pH monitoring, *J Thorac Cardiovasc Surg* 79:656, 1980.

Dobhan R, Castell DO: Normal and abnormal proximal esophageal acid exposure: results of ambulatory dual-probe pH monitoring, *Am J Gastroenterol* 88:25, 1993.

Peters JH, et al: Clinical and physiologic comparison of laparoscopic and open Nissen fundoplication, *J Am Coll Surg* 180:385, 1995.

THE HILL PROCEDURE FOR GASTROESOPHAGEAL REFLUX

Ralph W. Aye

The Hill repair is performed less commonly than the Nissen fundoplication for the surgical management of gastro-esophageal reflux disease. It has many distinct advantages, however, over the Nissen and other repairs and is worth the effort required to master it. These advantages include the following:

1. The most anatomically accurate and complete reconstruction of the antireflux barrier of any of the repairs
2. An extremely low incidence of gas bloat and long-term dysphagia
3. No wrap per se and no chance for slippage of the wrap
4. The ability to control and adjust final lower esophageal sphincter (LES) pressure
5. Suitability for patients with nonprimary motility disorders, such as low peristaltic amplitude or propagation
6. No need for an esophageal lengthening procedure, even in cases of so-called short esophagus
7. Suitability for complex reoperative cases or after partial gastrectomy
8. Proven durability
9. No need to take the short gastric vessels

The Hill repair reconstructs all components of the antireflux barrier, which include adequate length of intraabdominal esophagus; the angle of His; hiatal closure; normal LES pressure; posterior fixation of the gastroesophageal junction (GEJ) (its normal anatomic point of fixation); and, most importantly, correct reconfiguration of the gastroesophageal valve (GEV). The GEV has been overlooked in its importance in preventing reflux because of emphasis on the LES, but it plays a dominant antireflux role during marked changes in intraabdominal and intragastric pressure, while the LES does the discriminatory work. The Hill repair more accurately reconstructs the valve compared with any other repair.

Perceived barriers to performing the Hill repair include questions about the concept behind the repair, the need for manometrics, and concerns about the ability of others to replicate Hill's results. The fundamental concept behind the Hill repair is downward/medial traction on, and posterior fixation of, the anterior and posterior aspects of the collar-sling musculature, which wraps around and over the greater curvature aspect of the GEJ. By pulling down on this sling, as in pulling down the ends of a horseshoe, the valve is recreated, and the angle of His is reestablished. In addition, posterior fixation to the preaortic fascia gives the valve a buttress against which to work. LES pressure is restored. Secure fixation keeps the GEJ from migrating.

The technique for intraoperative manometrics has been simplified and is discussed during the description of the procedure. Manometry can be performed easily in any modern operating room with minimal additional equipment. Although the Hill repair can be performed without manometrics, results are optimized with its use.

The Hill repair has been performed successfully at many centers throughout the world, with excellent results. Further evidence of this is found in the outcome of a completed multiinstitutional study, discussed at the end of this chapter.

■ INDICATIONS AND PATIENT SELECTION

Most patients with gastroesophageal reflux can be managed medically. Proper patient selection is crucial to obtaining satisfactory results. There is virtually no indication for urgent or emergent surgery except in cases of impending strangulation of an intrathoracic stomach. Factors to consider are symptom profile, the presence of complications, and results of objective testing.

Symptom Profile
Classic reflux pain is high epigastric or substernal burning discomfort radiating upward or through to the back, relieved with medication and worsened by foods and position. A sense of fluid regurgitation or frank fluid to the mouth are typical of more advanced disease but can be due to obstruction from achalasia or neoplasm. Bloating is not typical and may be a sign of biliary disease or gastric outlet obstruction. Pulmonary symptoms, including cough, wheezing, laryngeal symptoms, or sinusitis, are relatively common and may or may not be caused by reflux. For the patient with pure pulmonary symptoms suspected to be due to reflux or for whom pulmonary symptoms are the primary reason to consider surgery, other causes must be ruled out because only two thirds of these patients respond to surgery.

Complications
Complications include peptic stricture, bleeding, recurrent aspiration, Barrett's metaplasia, and the presence of a paraesophageal component to a hiatal hernia. Stricture and bleeding often resolve on medical therapy, but failure to respond completely is a strong relative indication for surgery, as is a history consistent with aspiration, which can lead to recurrent pneumonia and pulmonary fibrosis. In cases of dense peptic stricture requiring dilation, several months of aggressive medical therapy should be followed by repeat endoscopy and dilation before surgery, to obtain as much resolution and patency as possible before repair. Barrett's metaplasia is a sign of advanced gastroesophageal reflux disease and is considered a complication of the disease, but in the absence of convincing proof that surgery reduces the risk of cancer in this group, it is hard to recommend surgery based purely on its presence. Many Barrett's patients have other strong reasons to consider surgery, however. A paraesophageal hernia, whether type II or type III, is often asymptomatic, but it should be repaired if there are no strong contraindications.

Objective Testing
The minimum workup before surgery includes a careful history, upper endoscopy with grading of the GEV, and esophageal manometry. A 24-hour pH study is not required for patients with documented esophagitis and classic symptoms responding well to medication, but even in this group it can be helpful to determine to what extent symptoms are entirely due to reflux. pH monitoring is necessary for patients with a confusing symptom complex and conflicting results of other studies. A barium swallow is helpful to delineate the anatomy for large hiatal hernias. Gastric emptying scintigraphy is added if a generalized motility disorder is suspected or in cases of profound regurgitation. Minor delays in gastric emptying are common with gastroesophageal reflux disease and are not a contraindication to repair, but a severe delay should prompt concern. Ultrasound or computed tomography scan is considered if gallstones are suspected and to help resolve other concerns in the workup.

Indications for Repair
Indications for surgery in patients with well-documented gastroesophageal reflux disease, in order of importance, include the presence of complications, as discussed previously; poor tolerance for medication; poor symptomatic control on medical therapy with evidence that symptoms are due to reflux; desire to discontinue medication, particularly for patients younger than age 50; and the cost of medication.

Contraindications to Repair
Patients should be on appropriate medical therapy for at least 2 months before repair, to assess response to medical therapy and to subdue inflammatory changes. Contraindications include those to general anesthesia and an upper midline incision; uncontrolled peptic stricture due to inadequate medical therapy; and because most antireflux surgery is performed laparoscopically today, inadequate skill by the surgeon to perform a complex laparoscopic procedure. Distal esophageal amplitude less than 30 mm Hg or significantly disordered peristalsis results in greater short-term but not long-term dysphagia and requires careful patient counseling. Poor peristalsis is not a contraindication to Hill repair, however, unless it is nearly or totally absent. Even in that case, the repair can be performed more loosely with intraoperative manometric control, a fact that highlights one of the advantages of the Hill repair.

Counseling Before Surgery

The patient is informed about relative risks and benefits of ongoing medical versus surgical management. Dysphagia for solids is common during the first 4 to 6 weeks postoperatively and in rare cases can be profound, although it always improves. The patient must be prepared for this. Bloating and flatulence also are common during the first few months. These symptoms are rarely limiting and usually improve with time.

■ SURGICAL TECHNIQUE— LAPAROSCOPIC APPROACH

Because almost all primary and some reoperative repairs now are done laparoscopically, this approach is covered in detail. The patient is positioned in low dorsal lithotomy with the right arm tucked, the surgeon between the legs, the assistant on the patient's left, and the camera operator on the right (Figure 1). Before beginning the repair, the manometric equipment is prepared. The catheter is a single-channel, water-perfused modified nasogastric tube with a pressure port 12 cm from the tip (Island Scientific, Bainbridge Island, WA). The manometric catheter is placed through a clear 43 Fr dilator (Cook Medical, Winston-Salem, NC) with the pressure port 7 cm beyond the tapered tip of the dilator and taped together. This arrangement is passed through the esophagus to 30 cm at the beginning of the case by the surgeon or an experienced anesthesiologist, permitting gastric suctioning. When calibration is needed, the system is advanced until the dilator is positioned across the GEJ, followed by pulling back across the GEJ for manometrics. If a formal manometric

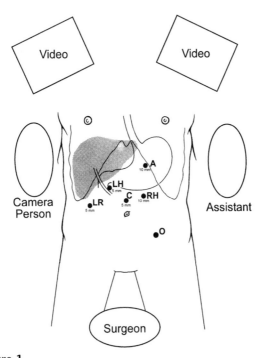

Figure 1
Trochar placement and room configuration for laparoscopic Hill repair. A, assistant; RH, right hand; C, camera; LH, left hand; LR, liver retractor; O, optional.

system is not available, an arterial monitor is adequate, although sluggish, and it may be necessary to go slowly across the high-pressure zone to avoid missing the peak pressure.

Five trochars are used, as shown in Figure 1. A sixth optional port for downward traction may be added in the left lower quadrant for patients with difficult exposure. It is important to use a trochar system with a valve that will not tear excessively with repeated needle insertions and that will remain competent with extracorporeal tying. U.S. Surgical, Ethicon, and Applied Medical products all have functioned satisfactorily in our experience. A high-flow insufflator also is important, preferably coupled with the use of bifurcated insufflation tubing. The left lobe of the liver is lifted with a 5-mm retractor (Thompson, catalogue no. 89-6112) and fixed to a self-retaining, table-mounted system.

Dissection is performed with electrocautery scissors, using clips where appropriate. The ultrasonic dissector is reserved for large complex hernias or very obese patients. The gastro-hepatic ligament is opened to its full length. The hiatus is dissected out beginning in the middle anteriorly, taking care to begin above the fatty tissue overlying the GEJ (the anterior phrenoesophageal bundle). Care also must be taken to avoid going too deeply and injuring the esophagus or anterior vagus nerve. From this point, dissection continues along the left crus, and the fundus superior to the spleen is freed as exposure permits. The short gastric vessels are not routinely taken. There is an arterial branch from the phrenic artery to the posterior aspect of the GEJ, which should be avoided. Access to this artery is much easier from below.

The esophagus is freed from the right crus beginning inferiorly just above the fatty tissue overlying the celiac artery then working superiorly along the well-defined anterior edge of the crus. This line of dissection now can be continued across the anterior aspect of the esophagus, taking any remaining attachments not divided previously.

Next, attention is directed to developing the retroesophageal space. With a closed grasper behind the esophagus, the assistant retracts the GEJ anteriorly and to the left, exposing the space, and blunt dissection develops the space just lateral to the left crus and the left aspect of the preaortic fascia. (The preaortic fascia is a dense connective tissue lying deep to the fusion of the right and left crura and extending inferiorly to the celiac axis, where its inferior edge forms the median arcuate ligament.) Most of this space opens up nicely with blunt dissection. From this point, dissection of the posterior fundus is aided by identifying the posterior vagus nerve and posterior phrenoesophageal bundle. As the assistant grasps the tissue between the vagus nerves and retracts to the left and superiorly, fatty tissue overlying the posterior fundus is retracted anteriorly and to the right. The posterior vagus nerve lies in the groove created by this maneuver and should be exposed carefully. The fatty tissue immediately posterior to the vagus is the posterior phrenoesophageal bundle and now may be given to the assistant to retract anteriorly and to the left. The veil of tissue overlying the fundus may be divided, exposing and freeing the fundus. There are few vessels in this tissue except at the superior aspect, where an arterial branch from the phrenic, described earlier, may need to be clipped and divided.

The anterior vagus nerve is identified by pulling down on the medial aspect of the anterior phrenoesophageal bundle.

It is important to identify this nerve as an important land-mark for subsequent suture placement and to avoid injury to the nerve.

Suture used throughout the repair is an 0-Ethibond green and white, 48 inches in length (Ethicon Endosurgery, cata-logue no. 22970D8684). The hiatus is closed posteriorly. Usually two sutures are sufficient. For larger hernias, two modifications are advisable: (1) polytetrafluoroethylene (Teflon) pledgets add further reinforcement, and (2) some of the repair may need to be completed anteriorly because too much angula-tion of the esophagus may be created from excess posterior closure and posterior fixation of the GEJ to the preaortic fascia. The superior aspect of the posterior fundus is fixed to the left crus and left aspect of the preaortic fascia using two or three sutures, taking care not to injure the underlying aorta or the phrenic artery.

Next, four repair sutures are placed and left untied. This is the most crucial part of the repair, and exact placement is important (Figure 2). The first suture is introduced through the right-hand work port. There are three maneuvers. The first is placement through the anterior bundle, from inferior to superior, exiting immediately to the left of the anterior vagus nerve. Grasping the bundle with the left hand and maneu-vering the tissue over the needle facilitates this. This bite must go deep enough to grab the collar sling musculature. The second maneuver is placement through the posterior bundle. The assistant retracts the tissue between the vagus nerves anteriorly and to the left, exposing the posterior vagus nerve. The surgeon grasps and manipulates the posterior bundle with the left hand. Beginning just posterior to the posterior vagus, the same suture now is passed through the bundle, as inferiorly as possible, while still grabbing a good bite of the stomach wall immediately underlying. To do this successfully,

the needle is nearly upside down at the time of entry. The third maneuver is placement through the preaortic fascia. The assistant retracts the GEJ to the left and simultaneously pushes it inferiorly. The same suture is passed through the preaortic tissue as inferiorly as possible but where muscle fibers are present, immediately superior to the fatty tissue overlying the celiac axis. The aorta lies 5 to 10 mm beneath and may be avoided by lifting the tissue upward with the left hand and driving the needle from left to right, rather than too deeply. Finally, this suture is brought out again through the right-hand port, buttressing it with a grasper where it exits the tissue.

This same process is repeated with three more sutures, advancing each one 2 to 3 mm farther up the two bundles and the preaortic fascia. With excess advance, the repair is too snug, whereas with inadequate advance the repair may be too loose. The uppermost suture should enter the anterior bundle at approximately the left lateral border of the esoph-agus. It should enter the posterior bundle at its upper extent without going behind the esophagus. The third and fourth sutures are introduced and withdrawn through the assistant port. Colors are alternated. Care should be given to the angle of entry of the sutures through the ports, to prevent crossing.

With all repair sutures placed but not tied, the 43 Fr dilator is advanced carefully and positioned across the GEJ, and the top two sutures (i.e., those through the assistant port) are tied sequentially with a single half-hitch and clamped just above the knot by the surgeon. The left-hand instrument clamps the upper knot, whereas the right-hand instrument clamps the lower knot. Manometric measurements are taken by withdrawing the system until the pressure port is 5 cm below the repair, zeroing out background pressure at this point, and withdrawing at a rate of 1 cm/sec. This should be

Figure 2
Proper placement of repair sutures after closure of hiatus and fixation of posterior fundus to the left aspect of preaortic fascia. *(Reprinted with permission of the illustrator, Corinne Sandone. © 2001.)*

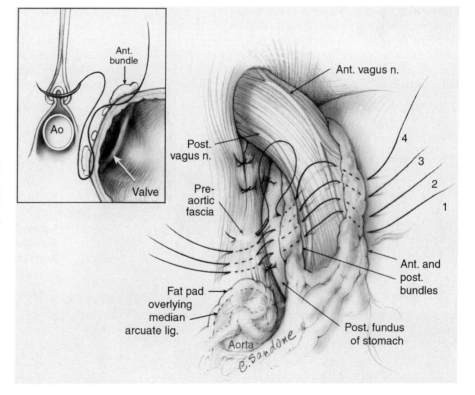

done more slowly with an arterial monitor and during crossing of the high-pressure zone to avoid missing the peak. The ideal pressure is 30 to 40 mm Hg. Sutures may be tightened or loosened at this time as needed. The first pressure increase is the repair, whereas an additional spike representing the diaphragm may be seen just above this. Finally, the dilator is positioned across the GEJ again, and all sutures are tied permanently before final manometrics.

The anterior hiatus often is reinforced with one or two sutures. The fundus is sutured to the anterior rim of the hiatus along right and left crura to prevent herniation and to accentuate the valve. The 10-mm ports are closed with a heavy absorbable suture. While this closure and skin closure are accomplished, flexible upper endoscopy is performed by the surgeon to assess resistance to passage of the scope across the repair and to assess the valve configuration (Figure 3). This is an invaluable tool to aid the surgeon in refining technique and occasionally prevents a disastrous outcome.

■ RECOVERY

A postoperative nasogastric tube is not used routinely. Nausea is treated aggressively. Diet and activity start immediately as tolerated. The patient is instructed to take a soft-to-pureed diet, avoiding meats and carbonated or ice-cold beverages. Discharge is usually within 36 hours. Dilation for dysphagia is rarely of value initially but can be considered after 6 to 8 weeks; it should not exceed a 51 Fr dilator. Acid blockers are used during the first few weeks, then may be discontinued. Heavy lifting should be avoided for 6 weeks.

■ OPEN REPAIR

The patient is positioned supine with the right arm tucked. An upper midline incision is used, extending to the upper aspect of the xiphoid, often excising it. Retraction is facilitated with a self-retaining "upper hand" type of retractor. The left lobe of the liver is mobilized and retracted to the right, often held in place with a wide malleable retractor.

From this point, the repair is essentially identical to the laparoscopic repair. The preaortic fascia can be lifted off the aorta through the esophageal hiatus before closing the hiatus, and it can be lifted up further with a Babcock clamp. Similarly, Babcock clamps on the anterior and posterior phrenoesophageal bundles facilitate placement of repair sutures. The manometric system and its use are identical. Recovery in the hospital and for return to work is a bit longer, but otherwise the recovery issues are the same.

■ PARAESOPHAGEAL HERNIA

Type II and type III hiatal hernias can be quite complex and are an order of magnitude more difficult in their technical demands. An ultrasonic scalpel is used for dissection. The hernia sac is excised, taking care to protect the mediastinal structures and vagus nerves. The landmarks for repair are not as clear, but experience with standard repairs provides the necessary anatomic perspective. There is a tendency to begin the repair stitches too low on the phrenoesophageal bundles, owing to redundancy and vagus nerve distraction away from the wall of the esophagus. It is important to perform a buttressed repair of the hiatus (we prefer Teflon felt pledgets), and a diaphragmatic relaxing incision may be helpful, to prevent the relatively high anatomic recurrence rate that has been reported with Nissen fundoplication for paraesophageal hernias. The Hill repair is well suited to these cases, particularly because an esophageal lengthening procedure is never required.

■ RESULTS

Our postoperative rating system is as follows: excellent—no significant symptoms; good—heartburn requiring occasional medication; fair—significant heartburn, requiring medication on a regular basis; poor—unimproved or worse. A multiinstitutional study of the open Hill repair included 2253 cases from our center, University of Virginia, University of Kansas, Massachusetts General Hospital, and Queens University. This included 1784 primary repairs and 469 reoperations.

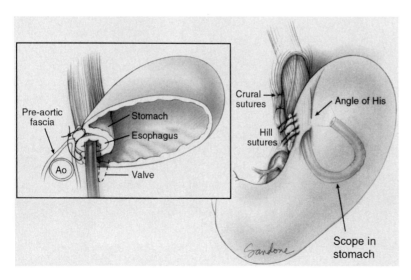

Figure 3
Completed repair with intraoperative endoscopy to evaluate valve configuration. *(Courtesy of Blair Jobe, MD.)*

Good to excellent results were obtained consistently in 90% to 92% of patients over 12 years. This study shows that the Hill repair can be performed elsewhere with equally good results.

We have performed more than 600 laparoscopic repairs. There have been no deaths, and morbidity has been remarkably low. In follow-up testing of 24 patients, LES pressure was increased from a mean of 10.7 mm Hg preoperatively to 25.0 mm Hg postoperatively, and 24-hour pH normalized in 21 of 23 patients. In the entire series, 1-year good to excellent results were 92% to 94%. In a 5-year follow-up of the first 200 patients, 92% remain satisfied with their operation.

■ SUMMARY

The Hill repair is the most comprehensive of all antireflux operations. It has an excellent track record and many advantages over other repairs. Its strengths are particularly notable in cases of disordered motility, paraesophageal hernia with or without short esophagus, and redo surgery.

SUGGESTED READING

Aye RW, et al: Early results with the laparoscopic Hill repair, *Am J Surg* 167:542, 1994.

Aye RW, et al: Laparoscopic Hill repair in patients with abnormal motility, *Am J Surg* 173:379, 1997.

Hill LD, Kraemer SJM: Does modern technology belong in gastro-intestinal surgery? A step from subjective perception to objective information, *World J Surg* 16:341, 1992.

Hill LD, et al: The gastroesophageal flap valve: in vitro and in vivo observations, *Gastrointest Endosc* 44:541, 1996.

Low DE, Hill LD: Fifteen to 20-year results following the Hill anti-reflux operation, *Thorac Cardiovasc Surg* 98:444, 1989.

BELSEY MARK IV REPAIR FOR GASTROESOPHAGEAL REFLUX

Robert J. Keenan
Jason J. Lamb

The Belsey Mark IV fundoplication provides an effective antireflux mechanism in the treatment of symptomatic gastroesophageal reflux that is refractory to medical therapy. It incorporates a transthoracic approach and was first reported in 1952. In 1971, Pearson et al reported their experience with a modified procedure, the Collis-Belsey. In this operation, a Collis gastroplasty was performed before the Belsey fundoplication to create a tension-free wrap. With or without the Collis modification, the essential features of this procedure are to restore a 3- to 4-cm length of intraabdominal functional esophagus, to create an anterolateral 270-degree fundoplication to increase lower esophageal sphincter tone, and to anchor the wrap to the musculature of the diaphragm to prevent recurrent hiatal herniation.

■ INDICATIONS

The original indication for the Belsey operation was for patients in whom a transthoracic approach was desirable. Patients included those with significant esophageal shortening, patients in whom mobilization of the esophagus to the aortic arch was needed, patients with previous upper abdominal surgery, obese patients, and patients with concomitant thoracic pathology.

With the advancement of minimally invasive surgery, most patients today undergo laparoscopic Nissen or Toupet fundoplications for control of gastroesophageal reflux disease. Excellent results have been reported with these procedures, and modifications have been incorporated to allow for the addition of a transthoracic or transabdominal Collis gastroplasty in cases of severe esophageal shortening. The Belsey Mark IV repair is an excellent choice in patients with previous esophageal surgery, patients with previous failed fundoplication, patients with an esophageal stricture, or patients who have other indications for left thoracic exploration. The partial wrap of the Belsey Mark IV fundoplication provides control of reflux without a large elevation of lower esophageal pressure as seen in other fundoplications. It is an excellent option for patients with impaired esophageal motility, such as patients with scleroderma or severe reflux esophagitis. A partial fundoplication also often is added to an esophageal myotomy for motility disorders, such as achalasia or diffuse esophageal spasm, to prevent postoperative reflux. The unmodified Belsey Mark IV repair is described next.

■ TECHNIQUE

With the patient in a right lateral decubitus position, the Belsey Mark IV repair is performed through a left lateral thoracotomy in the sixth intercostal space. Typically a short segment of the posterior seventh rib is excised to avoid an uncontrolled fracture during retraction. The temptation to use a lower intercostal approach should be avoided because it leads to more difficulty in mobilization of the mid to upper esophagus, and the incision is often more painful.

Initial adequate mobilization of the esophagus is essential and is performed from the hiatus to the aortic arch. Care should be taken to include the periesophageal tissue, including both vagus nerves with particular caution proximally as they join the esophageal wall. The left vagus nerve is at particular risk as it courses over the inferior pulmonary vein. A tape or Penrose drain passed around the esophagus and surrounding tissue aids in this dissection. During the mobilization, feeding esophageal arteries, originating from the descending aorta, should be divided with care to avoid adventitial hematomas. Ischemia to the esophagus is not a concern because the submucosal blood supply is rich. Every effort should be made to maintain the integrity of the right parietal pleura to avoid pooling of blood and fluids in the right chest.

The hiatal dissection is performed with upward traction on the esophagus, exposing the phrenoesophageal membrane and peritoneum that are divided circumferentially around the hiatus to allow the stomach to be delivered into the left chest. To aid in this dissection, the lesser sac must be entered, and a thick band of upper gastrohepatic tissue must be divided posteriorly. Found within this band is the phrenoesophageal or Belsey's artery, which is a communicating vessel connecting the ascending branch of the left gastric artery and the inferior phrenic artery. Failure to divide Belsey's artery carefully may result in unrecognized and possibly devastating intraabdominal hemorrhage. The anterior esophagogastric fat pad and connective tissues at the gastroesophageal junction are removed with care to protect the vagus nerves.

In a fashion similar to other fundoplications, a posterior buttress to reapproximate the crura is a vital component of the Belsey Mark IV repair. The two limbs of the right crus are identified and fully dissected to the level of the aorta. Care must be taken with the right posterior tissues because they are more fragile and easily torn than the left anterior muscle. Traction on the central tendon with an Allis or Babcock forceps can aid in the identification of tissue planes. Interrupted no. 1 silk sutures on an atraumatic needle are passed through the right (posterior) and left (anterior) halves of the right crus starting just anterior to the aorta and continuing anteriorly at 1-cm intervals. The distance between stitches is slightly greater on the right to account for the slightly longer length of the right side of the crus. Typically, three or four sutures are placed, but more may need to be incorporated into an excessively wide hiatus. These are left untied until return of the fundoplication to the abdomen.

An anterolateral 270-degree fundoplication is performed with two separate rows of three interrupted, mattressed 3-0 silk sutures. The first of these rows is placed vertically with an atraumatic needle 2 cm distal to the gastroesophageal junction in the seromuscular wall of the stomach, then vertically through the muscular and submucosal layers of the distal esophagus 2 cm proximal to the gastroesophageal junction. The stitch is reversed in mattress fashion back through the esophagus and stomach. The row is begun with the first stitch laterally, the second suture placed in the midline, and the last medially near the right vagus nerve. Manual rotation of the esophagus assists in the proper placement of the stitches. The row is tied carefully to provide apposition without strangulation over approximately 270 degrees. It is crucial to achieve a three quarters wrap; anything less provides suboptimal reflux control.

The second row of sutures is performed in a manner similar to the first (Figure 1) but also incorporates anchoring stitches to the diaphragm. With the aid of a retractor to protect the intraabdominal contents, the lateral suture is passed from the superior aspect of the diaphragm through the junction of the central tendon and muscular hiatal ring. The suture is brought back up through the hiatus and passed through the seromuscular stomach layer approximately 4 cm from the gastroesophageal junction and the esophageal muscle layer 4 cm above the junction. It is reversed again in mattress fashion back through the esophagus and stomach, passed through the hiatus and back up through the diaphragm. The remaining two sutures are placed in the corresponding positions to those in the first row to encompass the 270-degree circumference. These sutures are not tied until reduction of the repair below the diaphragm.

The reconstructed gastroesophageal junction now is replaced manually into the abdominal cavity. Care must be taken to avoid trapping abdominal contents between the wrap and the diaphragm. The second row of sutures is tied again gently. The importance of these sutures cannot be underestimated because they are the key to success of the fundoplication. With a proper reconstruction, an infradiaphragmatic 4-cm lower esophageal sphincter zone now exists, partially

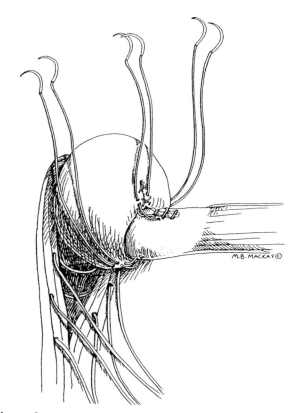

Figure 1
The technique of fundoplication showing placement of the second row of sutures. Crural repair sutures have been placed posterior to the wrap and are left untied until the fundoplication has been reduced below the diaphragm. (*From Pearson FG*: Textbook of esophageal surgery, *New York, 1995, Churchill Livingstone; with permission.*)

surrounded by the fundic wrap with an additional 1-cm muscular ring proximally at the hiatus when the posterior right crural repair is completed. When fully mobilized, the reconstruction should lie comfortably below the hiatus without tension. Any retraction back into the thoracic cavity suggests esophageal foreshortening, which increases the risk of recurrence. If in doubt, the wrap should be taken down and a Collis gastroplasty performed to lengthen the esophagus.

The previously placed right crural posterior buttress sutures now are tied securely starting with the most posterior stitch and carried anteriorly. Care must be taken not to overtighten the hiatus, which could lead to postoperative dysphagia. At completion, the hiatus should allow passage of an index finger easily posterior to the esophagus.

Before closure, an intercostal thoracostomy tube is placed in an apical position and put to suction. The thoracotomy is closed in the usual fashion. No nasogastric tube is necessary except for reoperative cases. In these situations, a postoperative water-soluble contrast medium followed by thin barium swallow test is performed immediately after postoperative recovery and before the patient's transfer to the nursing floor. If the swallow is negative for a leak, the nasogastric tube can be removed, and the patient can be started on liquids and advanced to a soft diet as tolerated.

■ RESULTS

When performed by experienced esophageal surgeons, the Belsey Mark IV fundoplication is well tolerated, is associated with low morbidity, and has a perioperative mortality of less than 1%. Literature reports of mortality vary between 0% and 3%. Postoperative thoracotomy pain is managed with either an epidural infusion or patient-controlled analgesia. Pain usually resolves within 2 to 3 months. The partial fundoplication is associated with less dysphagia and gas bloat than with complete fundoplication, such as the Nissen repair. Mild dysphagia may be seen immediately postoperatively, however, and is usually transient due to localized tissue edema at the site of repair. Patients must be warned to advance their diet slowly, to chew their food well, to take small bites, and to avoid breads and certain meats for several weeks. In most cases, the dysphagia resolves spontaneously, although esophageal dilation may be indicated in rare situations. In such cases, dilation should be avoided in the first week after operation. Severe dysphagia is uncommon with the Belsey Mark IV and is usually the result of a technical problem, most commonly the result of an overtight crural closure. This problem usually responds to dilation but rarely may require reoperation. Mild gastric distention may be seen, although severe gas bloat is uncommon and most likely the result of injury to the vagus nerves. It usually is treated with simethicone and metoclopramide improving symptoms in most cases. Esophageal leak is uncommon and seen in less than 1% of repairs. Most often the leak is contained within the wrap and is probably the result of sutures being overtightened or passed through the full thickness of the wall of the stomach or esophagus. Contained leaks may be treated with antibiotics and expectant observation, but larger or uncontrolled leaks should be treated operatively with drainage or revision at the time of diagnosis. Complications such as wound infection, recurrent pleural effusion, and empyema are uncommon and seen in less than 5% of cases.

Long-term reflux control (>5 years) is achieved in approximately 85% of patients with varying rates reported depending on the experience of the surgeon. Fenton et al reported control of reflux in 95% of a large series of complicated and uncomplicated repairs. Factors that affect failure rates are technical errors, a foreshortened or thick-walled esophagus, or recurrence of hiatal hernia. Of these, the most common problem is a failure to recognize the foreshortened esophagus. Tension on the sutures causes them to pull out. The experienced surgeon recognizes the presence of the foreshortened esophagus and adds a Collis gastroplasty to the Belsey repair. Symptomatic, recurrent reflux in these situations occurs in 10% to 15% of patients, mainly within the early postoperative course, although some may occur years after initial repair. This situation stresses the importance of long-term follow-up. Appropriate workup, including esophagogastroduodenoscopy with biopsy as indicated, esophageal pH probe testing, esophageal manometry, and barium swallow radiographs for documentation of failure, must be performed before any consideration of reoperative surgery. We and others have seen patients placed back on proton-pump inhibitors and other medications for subjective reasons without any documentation of return of objective signs of reflux. Approximately half (5% to 8%) of patients with recurrent reflux return to surgery for revision or correction. Technical failures, such as breakdown of the repair or inadequate circumference of fundoplication, usually are found and can be corrected by an experienced surgeon with a second Belsey Mark IV repair. Esophageal shortening is corrected by addition of a Collis lengthening procedure at reoperation. Extensive esophageal damage secondary to peptic stricture or fibrosis may require esophagectomy.

■ CONCLUSION

The transthoracic Belsey Mark IV repair for symptomatic reflux disease is a safe and effective method of surgical control. It offers excellent exposure to the distal esophagus and is particularly useful in patients who have undergone previous upper abdominal surgery. If the repair is seen to be under tension after adequate mobilization of the esophagus, a lengthening procedure must be added to reduce the risk of postoperative failure.

SUGGESTED READING

Fenton KN, et al: Belsey Mark IV antireflux procedure for complicated gastroesophageal reflux disease, *Ann Thorac Surg* 64:790, 1997.

Orringer MB, et al: Long term results of the Mark IV operation for hiatal hernia and analyses of recurrences and their treatment, *J Thorac Cardiovasc Surg* 63:25, 1972.

Pearson FG, et al: Gastroplasty and Belsey hiatus hernia repair, *J Thorac Cardiovasc Surg* 61:50, 1971.

NISSEN FUNDOPLICATION

Riivo Ilves

Gastroesophageal reflux (GERD) is the most common upper gastrointestinal ailment in modern society. Half of the population experience symptoms at some time in their life. The investigation and treatment of this condition are expensive and attract considerable attention. Many patients with occasional and typical symptoms may be treated medically without further investigation. Patients with more severe, long-standing, or atypical symptoms require more investigations, including contrast radiography, upper gastrointestinal endoscopy, 24-hour pH monitoring, and esophageal manometry studies. The extent of investigation is determined by how satisfied the physician is in establishing the diagnosis and its severity.

■ INDICATIONS FOR SURGERY

I have always divided the indications for surgery for GERD into three groups: (1) absolute, (2) relatively absolute, and (3) absolutely relative. Among the absolute indications are complete obstruction, perforation, and massive bleeding. Relatively absolute indications include severe and intractable esophagitis, peptic stricture, continued occult blood loss, and intrathoracic stomach. The largest group of patients fit the absolutely relative indications category. These patients may have inadequate symptom control on medical therapy or may not wish to continue medical therapy for potentially a lifetime.

Most patients fall into the relatively absolute category. Often the surgeon influences the patient in the direction of surgery. In the 1990s, major reputable centers did only a small fraction of the operations that now are done at many community hospitals throughout the world. Despite the claim that indications have not changed, the fact that endoscopic surgery is less risky has promoted this surge in antireflux operations. The complications and most risks are just as frequent in endoscopic surgery as in open surgery, however. Some complications, such as perforation or complete obstruction, are seen rarely in open surgery but are more frequent with endoscopic procedures, particularly on the "learning curve."

■ CHOICE OF OPERATION

Over at least 50 years, many named antireflux operations have been proposed and touted. Some operations have been abandoned. Many others still are performed and have indications in specific circumstances related to esophageal motor disorders or anatomic considerations, such as shortened esophagus. The ideal antireflux operation should (1) provide relief of symptoms of GERD, (2) have no side effects, (3) be reproducible, and (4) be teachable to other surgeons and residents.

In my opinion, the transabdominal Nissen fundoplication most reliably meets these criteria. It is best at providing symptom control. The transabdominal approach avoids the long-term and short-term increased pain often associated with thoracotomy. When the Nissen fundoplication is done properly, side effects are short-lasting and minimal. The operation is technically straightforward and can be performed reproducibly and taught well to others.

■ SURGICAL TECHNIQUE

My technique for the open Nissen fundoplication is described here. In some hands, the endoscopic operation adheres to the same principles and produces the same end product. In that case, I have no problem with the endoscopic approach, but the indications and results should be comparable.

Operation

The incision is an upper midline one from the xiphoid to the umbilicus. I resect the falciform ligament from the umbilicus to the liver. The left triangular ligament of the liver is mobilized beginning from left lateral and moving centrally. In so doing, care should be taken with the phrenic vein on the undersurface of the diaphragm. Also, centrally the hepatic veins are at risk with too-aggressive mobilization. I prefer to use a Bookwalter retractor, but an upper hand retractor and Balfour also can be used. The left lateral lobe of the liver is folded back and retracted to the right with a malleable blade. I begin my dissection by entering the lesser sac through an almost always avascular area in the gastrohepatic ligament. The right crus is visualized, and dissection of the gastrohepatic ligament cephalad is continued with a combination of electrocautery or the harmonic scalpel. Usually the hepatic branch of the vagus nerve and accompanying artery are taken. Occasionally, there may be a particularly large left hepatic arterial branch, which should be preserved.

When the hiatus is reached, dissection is carried out anteriorly through the peritoneum and phrenoesophageal ligament anterior to the esophagus. A Babcock clamp is placed on the edge of the diaphragm at the anterior hiatus, and finger dissection frees the anterior and right sides of the esophagus from the hiatus. The left side of the hiatus is dissected next with care paid to adhesions to the spleen and an occasional ascending phrenic artery. When the left crus is freed, blunt dissection posterior to the esophagus allows two fingers to encircle the esophagus. A 0.5-inch Penrose drain is passed between the fingers and pulled through. A clamp holds the Penrose drain, allowing it to be used as an esophageal retractor. The esophagus is mobilized into the mediastinum using mostly blunt finger dissection. This allows an adequate segment of esophagus to be brought tension-free below the diaphragm. I keep the vagus nerves with the esophagus. They are less likely to be traumatized there, and rarely, if the vagi are lifted off, one may develop severe distal esophageal motor dysfunction resembling esophageal spasm.

Good results and fewer postoperative symptoms require extensive mobilization of the short gastric arteries. I begin well down on the greater curve of the stomach and work cephalad toward the hiatus. The short gastric arteries are taken as close to the stomach as possible. The harmonic scalpel is used for this, and if double placement of the instrument is used, even the largest vessel encountered does not need to be manually tied. As one works cephalad, the vessels become shorter, and the gastric fundus becomes more intimate with the spleen. Starting from the distal greater curvature gives better exposure and control of these vessels.

Despite great care, occasionally the spleen sustains capsular tears. The bleeding from these usually can be managed conservatively using hemostatic agents and gentle pressure from a sponge pack. In my experience, the spleen has never had to be removed during a hiatal hernia repair.

When the fundus is mobilized completely, it is passed behind the esophagus with the surgeon's right hand. The knuckle of fundus is grasped to the right of the esophagus using a long Babcock clamp. More fundus is pulled around, and looseness of the wrap is checked. If the wrap feels too tight, more lower short gastric vessels are taken until a "floppy" wrap is achieved.

The fundus is reduced back to its original position, and closure of the hiatus is begun. Both limbs of the crus are grasped by Babcock clamps. The esophagus is retracted anteriorly and to the left so that the left crus can be visualized from the right of the esophagus. This crus is grasped by another Babcock clamp to the right of the esophagus, and the Babcock clamp previously on that crus is released. Both crura now are visualized to the right of the esophagus.

Occasionally the left crus cannot be visualized from the right. In this case, a crural stitch can be placed in the left crus, and the needle and stitch can be passed behind the esophagus to the right with a large curved clamp. This stitch can be used to pull the crus to the right, allowing grasping with a Babcock clamp.

Closure of the hiatus is done with large, nonabsorbable sutures. My own preference is no. 1 silk. Pledgets of polytetrafluoroethylene (Teflon) or Gore-Tex may be used, particularly in redo operations in which dissection has stripped peritoneum or muscle from the crus. The crural stitches are placed beginning distally, just above the crural decussation, or median arcuate ligament. The stitches are placed deep but not too deeply. If the lower stitches are deep, bowstringing of the stitch might cause aortic erosion, and too deep a stitch on the right could injure the vena cava or hepatic veins. The sutures are placed in an interrupted manner and not tied until all are placed. The ends of the sutures are held together with clamps, using in sequence Crile, Kelly, and Kocher clamps and repeating if necessary for a particularly large hiatus. Occasionally, with a large intrathoracic stomach, posterior closure alone is not sufficient. In such a case, crural sutures anterior to the esophagus also may be employed. The tightness of hiatal closure is subjective. If too tight, it may produce unrelenting, undilatable dysphagia. If too loose, herniation of the entire wrap or some other viscus may occur. My teaching and practice have been closure to a tightness accepting the index finger to the first knuckle between the esophagus and posterior closure. When all of the hiatal closure sutures have been placed, they are tied in order from distal to cephalad.

The fundoplication is now performed. The fundus is passed again around the esophagus, anterior to the hiatal closure. It is grasped with a Babcock clamp, and a generous amount of fundus is pulled around. Another Babcock clamp is used to grasp the widest part of the fundus remaining on the left. These widest points are used to create the wrap, ensuring it will be floppy. The wrap performed this way is so loose that

a bougie is unnecessary. Sizing with a bougie alone, regardless of caliber, may allow too tight a wrap, with all the side effects that produces.

I use two double-ended 2-0 nonabsorbable sutures for my wrap. Pledgets may be used if desired, using pledgeted sutures and a separate pledget on the other side. The sutures are placed in a horizontal mattress fashion, beginning superiorly. The suture passes through the gastric fundus on the left, the esophageal submucosa 1 cm below the diaphragm, then through the fundal knuckle on the right. The second arm is passed the same way, 1 cm below, then both needles through a free pledget, if so desired. A second double-armed suture is placed similarly 1 cm below the first. It is imperative that the sutures include the esophagus. If they do not, a "slipped" Nissen may result. Alternatively, if misidentified, a slipped Nissen can be created by wrapping fundus around the stomach. The upper suture is tied, rocking the suture ends to tighten the suture before tying. The lower suture is tied, leaving one needle uncut. If it will go without undue tension, this suture is passed through the crural closure or median arcuate ligament. I add one more suture between the top of the wrap and the diaphragm anterolaterally on the left.

A nasogastric tube is used for most repairs, but a gastrostomy tube also is placed when there is repair of a large intrathoracic stomach. I perform the latter because the stomach is so mobile in many such patients that it might torque in the abdomen. Abdominal closure is the same as that for a standard midline incision.

■ RESULTS

As with most reconstructive operations, the reporting of results in the literature can be subjective. How and by whom patients are questioned may determine answers given. Also, if one wanted to do more rigorous testing, many patients would object to the expense and inconvenience of studies such as a barium swallow or 24-hour pH monitoring. With this in mind, initially there is relief of GERD symptoms in all properly selected patients. With time, however, there is a falling off in satisfaction, leaving long-term good to excellent results in 80% to 85% of people.

Initially the most common side effects are early satiety and bloating, excess belching or flatulence, inability to belch or vomit, and dysphagia. These symptoms improve or disappear in 3 months to 1 year, with improvement in gastric motility, reduction of swelling in the surgical area, and less aerophagia. There are long-term side effects and complications that may require further surgery. Most patients are satisfied, however, free of GERD and side effects.

SUGGESTED READING

Grande L, et al: Value of Nissen fundoplication, *Surg Endosc* 9:869, 1995.

Hill LD, et al: Reoperation for disruption and recurrence after Nissen fundoplication, *Arch Surg* 114:542, 1979.

Luostarinen M: Nissen fundoplication for reflux esophagitis, *Ann Surg* 217:329, 1993.

Pearson FG, et al: Massive hiatal hernia with incarceration: a report of 53 cases, *Ann Thorac Surg* 35:45, 1983.

Schauer PR, et al: Mechanisms of gastric and esophageal perforations during laparoscopic Nissen fundoplication, *Ann Surg* 223:43, 1996.

THE COLLIS GASTROPLASTY FOR GASTROESOPHAGEAL REFLUX

Victor F. Trastek

Antonio L. Visbal

■ PATHOGENESIS

The evolution of repair of diaphragmatic hiatal hernia began with reduction of the hernia and closing of the crura. It soon was realized that symptoms associated with gastroesophageal reflux were not consistently relieved. Increased knowledge of the pathophysiology of gastroesophageal reflux disease (GERD) led to the development of an antireflux valve, including the Nissen fundoplication, the Belsey vertical partial fundoplication, and the Hill repair. Scarring due to severe GERD, previous procedures, or large diaphragmatic hiatal hernia may lead, however, to a short esophagus and place a repair under tension, increasing the risk of recurrence.

The objectives of gastroplasty repair include an esophageal lengthening maneuver (Collis gastroplasty), construction of an antireflux valve, and closure of the hiatal defect. Lengthening of the esophagus allows relocation of the gastroesophageal junction to its original place at the hiatus level and decreases tension on the repair. In 1957, Collis described the use of gastric tissue to form a connecting tube between the lower end of the short esophagus and the main body of the stomach by dividing the proximal stomach along the lesser curvature to make a "neoesophagus." Preliminary results published in 1957 and later in 1961 suggested lower morbidity and mortality than with esophagogastrectomy. In 1973, Pearson, by laboratory and clinical experience, showed reduction of GERD symptoms when a vertical partial fundoplication was added to the gastroplasty (cut Collis-Belsey). In 1974, Bingham modified the cut gastrotomy portion of the repair with an uncut staple line and a 360-degree stomach wrap over the connecting tube (uncut Collis-Nissen). Demos in 1983 and Phieler in 1984 reported results with larger series that showed better relief of symptoms associated with GERD. Although the uncut Collis procedure adds less length than the cut Collis, both maneuvers avoid placement of stitches in an inflamed outer esophageal wall during the antireflux procedure.

■ INDICATIONS

Acquired shortening of the esophagus is usually due to long-standing severe peptic esophagitis. During a barium study, a short esophagus is suggested by loss of the angle of His and the irreducibility of a sliding hernia even in the upright position. Esophagoscopy may show shortening of the distance to the cardia, peptic strictures, confluent ulceration, and Barrett's esophagus more than 3 cm. Esophageal length below the fifth percentile of normal determined by manometry, as suggested by DeMeester's group, also may alert the surgeon to the possibility of a short esophagus. The presence of esophageal stricture either alone or in combination with hiatal hernia of 5 cm or more may be a strong predictor of esophageal shortening. During operation, the most important suggestion of a short esophagus is the inability to reduce the gastroesophageal junction below the hiatus when the hernial sac has been resected and the esophagus and stomach have been mobilized.

Gastroplasty also may be indicated for the treatment of large diaphragmatic hiatal hernia or intrathoracic stomach. Most such cases represent advanced degrees of sliding hiatal hernias with intrathoracic displacement of the esophagogastric junction. Unanticipated cicatricial changes may be present in the distal esophagus from reflux esophagitis, resulting in acquired short esophagus. Pearson's group reported using cut Collis gastroplasty because of short esophagus in 80% of 94 patients with a large diaphragmatic hiatal hernia.

The poor outcome after an antireflux procedure is associated most commonly with persistent or recurrent reflux resulting from anatomic recurrence of a hiatal hernia, a perigastric fundoplication, or an incompetent repair or disruption of the repair. Collis gastroplasty is indicated in reoperation for GERD if the scarring process has damaged the tissue involved in previous repair, resulting in a short esophagus. Deschamps et al reported using a cut Collis gastroplasty in 17% of patients during redo antireflux procedures.

■ TECHNIQUES

The goals of the procedure include full mobilization of the lower esophagus and proximal stomach, creation of an antireflux valve, and reduction of the diaphragmatic hernia with closure of the hiatus.

Cut Collis Gastroplasty

Collis advocated a thoracoabdominal incision, but the procedure now is done through a left thoracotomy. The thoracic route allows adequate mobilization of the esophagus, dissection of the hernia sac, and division of the phrenoesophageal membrane and short gastric vessels, achieving mobilization of the gastroesophageal junction. The stomach is reduced into the abdomen to check for shortening. Collis originally applied two Parker-Kerr clamps parallel to the lesser curve; the stomach was incised between the clamps, and the free cuff was sewn up before the clamps were removed. Currently the gastroplasty is performed by applying a 4.5- or 5-cm linear stapling device parallel to the lesser curvature, and a 50 Fr to 54 Fr Maloney bougie is introduced perorally (Figure 1A). A running polypropylene (Prolene) 3-0 suture reinforces the staple line (Figure 1B). A Belsey or Nissen fundoplication is added for reflux control. The repair is reduced below the hiatus, and the crura are reapproximated.

Uncut Collis Gastroplasty

With a 50 Fr to 54 Fr dilator in place, the fundus is elevated superiorly, and a TA-30 stapler (3M Company, St. Paul, MN),

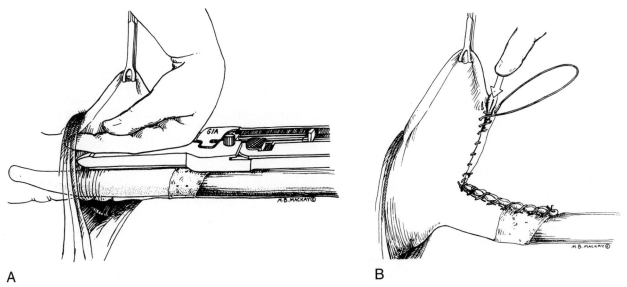

A

B

Figure 1
A, A 4.5- or 5-cm linear stapling device is applied parallel to the dilator at the angle of His to create the gastric tube. **B,** A running polypropylene (Prolene) 3-0 suture reinforces the staple line. *(From Pearson FG: In Pearson FG, et al, editors:* Esophageal surgery, *New York, 1995, Churchill Livingstone, p 339.)*

without insertion of the pin, is applied to the stomach parallel to the dilator at the angle of His (Figure 2A). The staple line creates a 3-cm neoesophagus out of the stomach. The gastric fundus is wrapped posteriorly around the neoesophagus to form a fundoplication (Figure 2B). The width of the fundoplication is 1.5 to 2 cm to minimize dysphagia. When tied, the wrap should allow one fingerbreadth along the side of the dilator without tension. Care is taken to locate and protect both vagus nerves within the fundal wrap in their normal position. Then the wrap is reduced, and the crura are reapproximated.

The cut Collis gastroplasty has been performed laparoscopically or thoracoscopically on patients with a short esophagus. The results have been good symptomatic relief from GERD, minimal operative morbidity, and faster return to the presurgical standard of living.

■ POSTOPERATIVE CARE

Postoperative care is similar to that used for any antireflux procedure performed by thoracotomy. The patient is given a

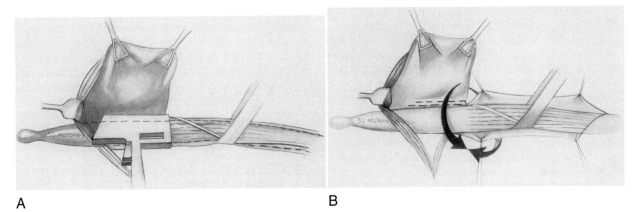

A

B

Figure 2
A, Without insertion of the pin, a TA-30 stapler is applied parallel to the dilator at the angle of His. **B,** The gastric fundus is wrapped posteriorly around the neoesophagus to form a fundoplication of 1.5 to 2 cm in width. *(Modified from Trastek VF, Payne WS: In Jamieson GG, Debas HT, editors:* Rob and Smith's operative surgery: surgery of the upper gastrointestinal tract, *ed 5, New York, 1994, Chapman & Hall, p 327. By permission of Edward Arnold Limited.)*

clear liquid diet 48 hours after operation, and this is advanced during the next 2 to 3 days as tolerated. If there is any concern about the integrity of the repair, a diatrizoate meglumine (Gastrografin) swallow study is performed the morning after the procedure. Chest tubes are removed when drainage has been reduced. We encourage the use of epidural analgesia during the first 60 to 72 hours after operation for better pain control, pulmonary care, and early mobilization. Total hospitalization is usually 6 days.

■ RESULT OF TREATMENT

Results of the cut Collis gastroplasty with fundoplication for GERD have been described extensively in the literature. Henderson reported subjective outcome of the cut Collis gastroplasty and Nissen fundoplication for intractable GERD in 500 consecutive patients. Clinical results were excellent in 93.4% of patients at an average follow-up of 38.4 months. Results were poor in seven patients (1.4%), and they required reoperation—two (0.4%) for hernia recurrence and five (1%) for severe dysphagia. Severe dysphagia was present in 10 of the first 200 patients. The wrap length was reduced to 1 cm, and the number of patients with severe dysphagia decreased to 5 of the last 300 patients. There was no mortality, and the operative morbidity rate was 3.6%. The rate of leak from the gastroplasty was 1%.

Orringer et al described subjective and objective results of the cut Collis-Nissen procedure for GERD in 261 patients with an average follow-up of 43.8 months. No symptoms were found in 75% of the patients, 11% had mild reflux (no treatment required), 9% had moderate reflux (controlled by medical therapy), and 5% had severe reflux (uncontrolled by medication or reoperation was needed). Mild dysphagia requiring no dilation was present in 25% of patients, moderate dysphagia requiring occasional dilation was present in 8%, and severe dysphagia requiring regular dilation or reoperation was present in 9%. Objectively the average high-pressure zone increased from 4.0 ± 5.1 mm Hg preoperatively to 11.5 ± 3.6 mm Hg at 1 year and was 10.7 ± 2.9 mm Hg at 48 months. A pH reflux study was positive in 9% of patients. Of patients, 26 (10%) required reoperation because of reflux or dysphagia, as follows: esophagectomy in 20 (transhiatal in 18, transthoracic in 1, and distal with short segment colon interposition in 1), redo Collis-Nissen in 3, repair of paraesophageal hiatal hernia in 2, and division of scar tissue at the hiatus in 1. The reported operative mortality rate in 353 patients after the cut Collis-Nissen operation was 1.1%, and the morbidity was 7.9%. The leak rate was 1.6% (two patients had leaking from the gastroplasty and four from the distal esophagus). There was better subjective control of reflux and reduction of postoperative dysphagia by decreasing the wrap length from 6 to 3 cm in the last 63 patients.

Subjective results of the Collis-Belsey procedure for GERD were reported by Pearson et al for 75 patients with a median follow-up of 72 months. Results were excellent (no symptoms) in 80% of the patients, good (inconsequential symptoms requiring no therapy) in 13%, and fair (reflux requiring medical therapy) in 4%. The mortality rate was 2%, and the morbidity rate was 19%. Four patients had leaking from the gastroplasty.

Paris et al compared 35 patients who had the cut Collis-Belsey procedure with 43 patients who had the cut Collis-Nissen procedure and described early subjective and objective outcomes for treatment of GERD. At an average follow-up of 60 months, 77% of the patients reported no reflux, and 23% had reflux after the cut Collis-Belsey operation. Manometry in 32 patients showed an increase of the mean high-pressure zone from 11.2 ± 8.19 mm Hg preoperatively to 17.31 ± 10.5 mm Hg postoperatively, and it decreased to 13.69 ± 7.24 mm Hg at 12 to 24 months. A pH reflux study was positive in 11% of patients in the early postoperative period and in 23% at 1 year. Five patients (14%) required reoperation for recurrence of symptoms. In the cut Collis-Nissen group, 89% of the patients reported no reflux, and 11% had reflux at an average follow-up of 36 months. Manometry in 44 patients showed an increase in the mean high-pressure zone from 9.36 ± 4.8 mm Hg preoperatively to 17.70 ± 7.53 mm Hg postoperatively, and this decreased to only 16.46 ± 7.99 mm Hg at 12 to 24 months. No patient had positive results of an early postoperative pH reflux study, and 3% had positive results at 1 year. Three patients (6.5%) required reoperation (colon interposition) for nondilatable reflux stricture.

Results of uncut Collis gastroplasty and fundoplication also have been described. Early objective outcomes of the uncut Collis-Nissen procedure for GERD were described by Pera et al in 27 consecutive patients with a mean follow-up of 22 months. Endoscopic surveillance showed reduction in the mean length of Barrett's esophagus from 6.16 cm to 4.7 cm, esophageal ulcer healing in 100% of patients, and recurrence in 7%. By manometry, the high-pressure zone increased from 20.9 mm Hg preoperatively to 27.2 mm Hg postoperatively, and the lower esophageal gradient increased from 8.3 mm Hg to 14.6 mm Hg. Esophageal acid exposure decreased from 8% preoperatively to 1.7% postoperatively in 24-hour pH studies. Slow esophageal emptying was reported by 22% of the patients, 11% had occasional episodes of dysphagia, but no patient required dilation. There was no operative mortality, and the morbidity rate was 19%. There were no reported leaks.

Trastek et al described subjective long-term results of the uncut Collis-Nissen procedure in 100 patients with a median follow-up of 100 months. Results were excellent (no symptoms) in 59% of the patients, good (mild reflux and no treatment required) in 25%, fair (moderate reflux controlled by medical therapy or dilation) in 8%, and poor (severe reflux not controlled by medication or worse postoperatively or reoperation needed) in 7%. Dysphagia was present in 6%, recurrence of reflux symptoms in 5%, and hernia in 3%. The operative mortality rate was 2%, the morbidity rate was 23%, and there were no leaks.

■ CONCERNS ABOUT CREATION OF A NEOESOPHAGUS WITH A GASTRIC TUBE

Concern that the gastroplasty creates an aperistaltic neoesophagus lined with acid-secreting mucosa, with its potential complications, is valid. The gastroplasty tube, whether cut or uncut, is functionally amotile and does seem to offer some resistance to swallowing. Long-term studies have described a low incidence of complications in association with these particular issues, however.

■ FINAL RECOMMENDATIONS

The perfect operation for GERD has yet to be devised. Gastroplasty should be added without hesitation to an antireflux procedure if, after adequate mobilization, the repair would result in tension on the fundoplication. Failure to recognize and manage a shortened esophagus is associated with an increased risk of hernia recurrence and failure. Which type of fundoplication is added to the gastroplasty depends on the patient's condition and on the surgeon's preference. Nissen and Belsey fundoplications have been used with similar success. A cut or uncut Collis gastroplasty, in addition to a fundoplication, needs to be included in the surgeon's armamentarium for patients with acquired short esophagus, large diaphragmatic hiatal hernia, or redo antireflux procedure. This procedure has withstood the test of time, with its low mortality rate, acceptable morbidity rate, and satisfactory long-term results.

SUGGESTED READING

Bingham JA: Evolution and early results of constructing an anti-reflux valve in the stomach, *Proc R Soc Med* 67:4, 1974.

Collis LJ: An operation for hiatus hernia with short esophagus, *Thorax* 12:181, 1957.

Deschamps C, et al: Long-term results after reoperation for failed antireflux procedures, *J Thorac Cardiovasc Surg* 113:545, 1997.

Gastal OL, et al: Short esophagus: analysis of predictors and clinical implications, *Arch Surg* 134:633, 1999.

Henderson RD, Marryatt G: Total fundoplication gastroplasty: long-term follow-up in 500 patients, *J Thorac Cardiovasc Surg* 85:81, 1983.

Maziak DE, et al: Massive hiatus hernia: evaluation and surgical management, *J Thorac Cardiovasc Surg* 115:53, 1998.

Paris F, et al: Gastroplasty with partial or total plication for gastroesophageal reflux: manometric and pH-metric postoperative studies, *Ann Thorac Surg* 33:540, 1982.

Pera M, et al: Uncut Collis-Nissen gastroplasty: early functional results, *Ann Thorac Surg* 60:915, 1995.

Stirling MC, Orringer MB: Continued assessment of the combined Collis-Nissen operation, *Ann Thorac Surg* 47:224, 1989.

Trastek VF, et al: Uncut Collis-Nissen fundoplication: learning curve and long-term results, *Ann Thorac Surg* 66:1739, 1998.

LAPAROSCOPIC TECHNIQUES FOR GASTROESOPHAGEAL REFLUX

Chandrakanth Are
Mark A. Talamini

Gastroesophageal reflux disease (GERD) is a common disorder, affecting an estimated 61 million Americans with symptoms of heartburn and indigestion. Initially, hiatal hernia was assumed to be essential for GERD to exist. It is now clear that breakdown of mechanical reflux competence, poor esophageal body motility, and delayed gastric emptying all play a significant role. Alkaline reflux also seems to play a role. Although short periods of reflux are normal, reflux is considered pathologic when esophageal refluxate exposure exceeds normal levels.

■ PATHOPHYSIOLOGY

GERD can be due to a defect in the lower esophageal sphincter (LES), the esophageal body, the gastric reservoir, or a combination of these. A defective LES accounts for 60% of GERD and is the anomaly that responds most poorly to medical management and benefits the most from antireflux surgery. The LES normally remains closed to prevent reflux by providing a pressure barrier between the positive-pressure environment of the stomach in the abdominal cavity and the negative-pressure environment of the esophagus in the chest. Several features of the LES, such as resting pressure, intraabdominal length, and total length of the sphincter, are important in preventing reflux. The intrinsic pressure of the LES, the pressure of the intraabdominal environment, and the compression of the crura determine the resting pressure of the LES. Esophageal intraabdominal length is defined as the distance from the distal border of the esophagus to the respiratory inversion point (where positive deflections with inspiration change to negative deflections, i.e., transition between the abdomen and the chest). Total esophageal length is defined as the distance between the proximal and distal esophageal borders. If a defect exists in one or two components of the LES, normal esophageal body function can compensate, avoiding pathologic reflux. Loss of all three features almost always leads to pathologic reflux, however.

The esophageal body prevents reflux by clearing acid through peristalsis (volume clearance) or by salivary neutralization (chemical clearance). Most acid is cleared by peristalsis, with small residual amounts neutralized by saliva. Gastric reservoir function can be affected adversely by gastric dilation, increased intragastric pressure, increased gastric acid production, or persistent gastric reservoir. Excessive gastric dilation can cause a reduction of intraabdominal length of the LES, producing reflux. In the presence of a normal LES, reflux can be caused by abnormal esophageal body function or by abnormal gastric reservoir function. Pinpointing the abnormal components of the sphincter complex when reflux exists is important in determining the potential role of antireflux surgery.

CLINICAL FEATURES

Heartburn, in the form of substernal burning chest pain occurring 30 to 60 minutes after meals, is the most common symptom of GERD. Bland regurgitated material usually arises from the esophagus, whereas bitter regurgitation suggests duodenal gastric reflux. GERD also can present as asthma, isolated episodes of pneumonia, or hoarseness due to laryngeal irritation. Dysphagia in patients with GERD might reflect an underlying motility disorder caused by esophagitis, stricture formation, or tumor. Reflux disease accounts for 20% to 50% of angina-like chest pain when findings are negative on coronary artery angiography.

COMPLICATIONS

Patients can develop complications due to persistent LES failure, residual defects of esophageal body function, associated hiatal hernia, and presence of alkaline reflux along with acid reflux. Complications are more likely to occur if alkaline and acid reflux are present than if acid reflux is present alone. The major potential complications of reflux disease are esophagitis, esophageal ulceration, stricture, Barrett's esophagus, and short esophagus. Esophagitis is diagnosed endoscopically by the presence of macroscopic mucosal erosions with characteristic neutrophil infiltration. Ulceration usually occurs at the squamocolumnar junction and commonly is associated with Barrett's esophagus. Reflux-related strictures are circumferential, occur in the distal esophagus, and lead to symptoms of dysphagia. Barrett's esophagus occurs in 7% to 10% of GERD patients. The diagnostic feature of Barrett's esophagus is the presence of specialized columnar epithelium with characteristics of intestinal metaplasia identified by the presence of goblet cells. On gross endoscopy, it appears as velvety, orange-red mucosa lining the esophagus. Changes noted in segments less than 2 cm in length are referred to as *short segment Barrett's esophagus*. When present, Barrett's epithelium persists despite medical therapy or antireflux surgery, although more recently strategies for ablation of Barrett's esophagus have emerged. The risk of Barrett's esophagus lies in its potential for malignant transformation. Some authors conjecture that the increase in incidence of adenocarcinoma in recent decades is related to the increased incidence of Barrett's esophagus. Short esophagus is associated with shortening of esophageal longitudinal muscle, hiatal herniation, and periesophageal inflammation.

DIAGNOSIS

Initial diagnostic studies should include barium swallow and upper gastrointestinal endoscopy. These studies detect structural defects, such as stricture, hiatal hernia, or tumor. Videoesophagography or cine esophagography can detect short esophagus and provides a real-time record of swallowing function. Endoscopy directly observes the esophageal mucosa and can gauge the severity of esophagitis and the presence of Barrett's esophagus or the presence of a mass lesion. These tests should be followed by direct assessment of system function (i.e., motility and acid production).

Stationary manometry is performed initially to (1) assess the state of the LES; (2) rule out primary motility disorders of the proximal esophagus, which may be contraindications to laparoscopic Nissen fundoplication (LNF); and (3) detect esophageal body disorders. It also locates the LES, guiding the eventual placement of a pH probe for 24-hour pH monitoring and for assessment of the upper esophageal sphincter. Manometric findings of an LES resting pressure of 6 mm Hg or less, a total LES length of less than 2 cm, or an intraabdominal esophageal length of less than 1 cm are associated with reflux. Ambulatory (24-hour) esophageal manometry has the advantage of recording esophageal function during a patient's normal activities.

For measuring esophageal acid exposure, 24-hour pH monitoring has replaced other techniques. It is recommended for all patients with symptoms persisting beyond 12 weeks of therapy. Prior manometry guides placement of a pH probe at a point 5 cm above the upper border of the LES. H_2 blockers, prokinetics, and proton-pump inhibitors should be discontinued before the test (2 weeks for proton-pump inhibitors, 48 hours for other agents). Reflux episodes are recorded when esophageal pH is less than 4. Some systems also can detect alkaline duodenal gastric reflux (pH >7), which may play a role in the patient's disease. Other tests used to assess esophageal function include dual esophageal pH monitoring, standard acid reflux test, and esophageal bile probe. The Bernstein test, which subjectively measures patient symptoms when the distal esophagus is exposed to acid, rarely is used today.

Gastric emptying is assessed directly by measuring how long it takes for solid or liquid meals containing barium or radioactive tracer to leave the stomach. Poor gastric emptying can contribute to reflux and can be a harbinger of bloating problems after antireflux surgery. This array of tests should be used to document that reflux exists and that the reflux is the likely cause of the patient's symptoms. Taken together, they also are useful in predicting the likelihood of success after an antireflux procedure.

TREATMENT

The aim of surgery is to relieve symptoms of reflux along with the social, dietary, and physical restrictions or the inconvenience of prolonged drug regimens associated with medical management.

Operative Indications
Indications for operation are as follows:

1. Symptoms despite appropriate medical management
2. Presence of complications of GERD, such as ulcers or stricture
3. Presence of respiratory symptoms, such as asthma, pneumonia, and aspiration in association with reflux disease

Results are not as consistent in the presence of respiratory symptoms alone. The option of surgery should be offered as a cost-effective alternative to prolonged medical treatment even in the absence of complications.

Prerequisites

Prerequisites for surgery include the following:

1. Upper endoscopy is performed to evaluate the mucosa. The presence of GERD is assessed by 24-hour pH monitoring.
2. A firm diagnosis of GERD is determined by 24-hour pH monitoring, esophagitis on endoscopy, or clear reflux by radiographic contrast study.
3. The possibility of esophageal or gastric motility dysfunction should be evaluated before proceeding with antireflux surgery.
4. Detection of short esophagus before surgery can be helpful in operative planning.

Technique
Laparoscopic Nissen Fundoplication

Originally described by the Swiss surgeon Nissen in 1955, the 360-degree gastric wrap has been shown to provide relief in most patients with reflux symptoms. The first successful performance of LNF, in Belgium by Dallemagne in 1991, produced a paradigm shift of preference toward surgery over long-term medical management. The main principles of the procedure are (1) restoring intraabdominal esophageal length, (2) increasing resting LES pressure to levels greater than resting intragastric pressure, (3) using the fundus for the wrap, (4) ensuring that the propulsive power of the esophagus can overcome the resistance of the reconstructed valve, and (5) accentuating the esophagofundic angle of His. These objectives are accomplished by following these steps: (1) adequate fundic mobilization, (2) crural dissection and preservation of both vagal trunks, (3) circumferential dissection of the esophagus, (4) crural approximation, and (5) creation of a loose wrap with the anterior and posterior walls of the fundus over the lower esophagus.

The patient is placed supine on a beanbag in a modified lithotomy position with the knees slightly flexed and the head of the table elevated 30 to 45 degrees. The beanbag is aspirated to prevent the patient from slipping during extremes of tilt (reverse Trendelenburg) during the procedure. Excessive flexion of the hips should be avoided to prevent interference with instrument mobility. The stomach and bladder are decompressed with a nasogastric tube and a Foley catheter.

The abdominal cavity is accessed by the closed or open technique. We prefer using the Veress needle to establish pneumoperitoneum with a working pressure of 12 mm Hg. The Veress needle puncture is made through a small skin stab wound just above the umbilicus. The telescope port is placed about 16 cm below the xiphoid, and 3 cm to the left of midline. The four other ports are placed under direct laparoscopic vision using the 30-degree telescope. The right-sided trocar is roughly midway between the right costal margin and the umbilicus, positioned in a spot where the liver retractor can reach and be effective in elevating the lateral left lobe of the liver. We favor a 5-mm liver retractor placed through the trocar in the right abdomen, which is advanced into the port in a floppy configuration but forms into a triangle through tightening when inside the abdomen. The left lower trocar is usually most effective near or just medial to the anterior axillary line one or two fingerbreadths below the costal margin. This site is the easiest through which to retract the stomach

and eventually the gastroesophageal junction. The two operating ports are placed fairly high along the right and left costal margin, often with the right-sided port higher than the left. The right-sided trocar is most convenient when it enters the peritoneal cavity at the left edge, where the falciform ligament meets the inner peritoneum. The insertion of ports in this fashion places the xiphoid in the middle of the operating field, below which lies the gastroesophageal junction. Placing the operating ports on either side of the camera permits triangulation, allowing the surgeon to operate straight ahead and avoiding "video mirror images" and difficulty associated with instruments being in direct line with the camera. Ideally, ports should be 8 cm apart from one another to avoid interference between instruments, but this is not always possible in small individuals. The right-sided instruments may have to be manipulated around the falciform ligament that hangs low in many patients.

We favor beginning the operation along the short gastric vessels, just as most surgeons begin the open operation. The stomach is grasped about midway along the greater curve, and the branches between the gastroepiploic vessels and the stomach are divided one by one, gaining access into the lesser sac. As the dissection moves cephalad, the vasa brevia are divided, which allows the spleen to fall away into the left upper quadrant. The anatomic objective of this dissection is the clear identification of the left crus of the diaphragm and the clearance of the spleen away from the gastroesophageal junction. If the anatomy is clear, some of the retroesophageal space can be opened from the left side, making the later dissection easier. If a hiatal hernia exists, the stomach must be retracted into the abdomen for this step, and a hernia sac if present can be dissected off the left crus.

The next step is to expose the esophageal hiatus. A fan-shaped retractor is placed in the perixiphoid port to lift the left lateral segment of the liver toward the anterior abdominal wall. A Babcock clamp is placed through the left flank port to retract the stomach inferiorly and to the left, providing a good view of the hiatus. The hiatal dissection begins with the key step of identifying the right crura. This is accomplished by incising the thin tissue of the hepatogastric ligament (lesser omentum) overlying the caudate lobe. The hepatic branch of anterior vagal nerve and a potential replaced left hepatic artery arising from the left gastric artery (said to occur in 25% of patients) traverse this tissue. If a large vessel is visualized in this tissue, it is best to preserve it. If the operation cannot be carried out laparoscopically because this vessel is in the way, the procedure should be converted to an open operation. When the gastrohepatic omentum is opened, the lateral aspect of the right crus is identified to the (patient's) left of the caudate lobe of the liver. The peritoneum over the right crus is incised to gain access onto the medial aspect of the crus and the mediastinum. By gently lifting the posterior esophagus with a blunt instrument, the right crus can be dissected away carefully until a retroesophageal space is created. Blunt dissection, carried out by gently moving tissues away from the lateral and posterior esophagus, allows clear identification of the right side of the esophagus and posterior vagus nerve. This dissection eventually breaks through posteriorly to the space created around the left crus; the esophagus then can be encircled with an umbilical tape or Penrose drain.

The next major step is mobilization of the esophagus, the goal being to create a sufficient length of intraabdominal esophagus around which to wrap the fundus. At this point, the right, posterior, and left aspects of the esophagus have been dissected from the surrounding tissues, leaving the anterior esophagus as the primary target for mobilizing the remaining esophagus. The posterior vagus nerve already has been dissected, and the anterior nerve lies within the tissue anterior to the esophagus. Using the retraction sling around the esophagus as countertraction, the anterior tissue is teased gently and dissected away from the esophagus, on up into the mediastinum. The anterior vagus usually lies right on the esophagus itself. When this tissue is dissected, the tissue on all sides of the esophagus is dissected to mobilize a sufficient length of esophagus for the wrap.

Holding the esophagus anteriorly and to the left with the Penrose drain, the crura now are approximated from behind with enough sutures to close around the esophagus containing an appropriately sized dilator. The surgeon must be careful regarding the aorta, which lies between the crus of the diaphragm and can be close, particularly in instances of large hiatal hernias. The phrenic artery also can ambush the surgeon because its course near the edge of the crus is variable. We favor braided polytetrafluoroethylene (Teflon) for all sutures because it is permanent and ties easily. We also favor placing the sutures with standard laparoscopic needle holders and tying them with a combination of an extracorporeal slipknot and intracorporeal square knot.

The posterior fundus is grasped from behind the esophagus and pulled to the right side of the abdomen, and the anterior fundus is pulled in front of the esophagus, while the gastroesophageal junction is retained well into the abdomen by retraction on the sling retractor. Care must be taken that the fundus is not twisted. This can be tested with a "shoeshine" maneuver in which the anterior and posterior fundus are pulled back and forth about the esophagus to judge the potential suture location and the conformation of the potential fundoplication. The location of the sutures to create the fundoplication is important. If they are placed too high on the fundus, the gastroesophageal junction can become constricted; if too low, an extra "pouch" of fundus is created above the wrap. The ideal length of the wrap should be about 4 cm, and this usually requires three sutures each 1 cm apart. After suturing, the wrap and its underlying esophagus should lie completely in the abdomen without tension or twists. The bougie is replaced with a nasogastric tube passed under laparoscopic vision, which should pass smoothly.

The abdominal cavity is irrigated thoroughly and aspirated dry. To ensure hemostasis, all ports are removed under direct vision. The port sites are irrigated, closed (if ≥10 mm), and injected with 0.5% bupivacaine. Mild dysphagia is common during the first 2 postoperative weeks due to traumatic edema. Patients are advised to remain on a soft diet, avoid carbonated beverages and heavy lifting, and eat five to six small meals a day rather than three large ones. Intramural hematoma at the site of fundoplication can cause dysphagia that subsides after 4 to 6 weeks. Any dysphagia after this period needs to be investigated.

Tips
1. Only the fundus, which can relax in synchrony with the LES after swallowing, should be used for creating the wrap. The fundic muscle has been shown to share many of the physiologic characteristics of the LES. Care should be taken to avoid including the upper body of the stomach (which does not exhibit receptive relaxation with swallowing).
2. It is important to attempt to preserve the vagi because they are responsible for the receptive relaxation of the LES and the fundus after swallowing.
3. The fundus should be completely mobilized. A twisted fundus or a fundus under tension increases the risk of dysphagia. The ideal situation exists when the anterior and posterior lips of the fundus encircle the lower part of the esophagus, meeting anterior or to the right of the mobilized esophagus.
4. The fundus must be placed around the lower esophagus. In patients with hiatal hernia, the tubular-appearing upper stomach can be mistaken for esophagus. Creating a wrap around this can lead to dysphagia and recurrent heartburn. This situation can be prevented by identifying the gastroesophageal fat pad, keeping the dissection above the level of the hepatic branch of anterior vagal nerve, and placing the fundoplication between the esophagus and the posterior vagus nerve.
5. After drawing the fundus through the posterior esophageal window, the surgeon must let go of the fundus. If the fundus recoils around the esophagus or develops a bluish discoloration, it can produce ischemia or a tight wrap. This indicates that further mobilization of the fundus is required. The ability to slide a 10-mm Babcock clamp under the wrap with ease indicates a loose fundoplication.
6. The crura must be closed to prevent herniation of the entire wrap. This must be done even in the absence of preoperative hiatal hernia due to the opening of the hiatus from the dissection necessary to accomplish the wrap.
7. The operating ports should not be placed too medially because this may interfere with the camera and make dissection difficult.

Laparoscopic Nissen-Rossetti Procedure
In 1965, Rosetti modified the original fundoplication by using only the anterior wall of the fundus to create a 360-degree wrap. Studies have shown that this can produce a one-way valve and replace a deficient LES in the same way as the complete fundus. The advantage of the laparoscopic Nissen-Rossetti procedure is that one can avoid the division of lateral (short gastric) attachments of the stomach. Although the incidence of postoperative dysphagia may be higher, some surgeons routinely perform the Rosetti modification laparoscopically. The rest of the procedure is similar to the conventional LNF.

Laparoscopic Toupet Fundoplication
In the laparoscopic Toupet fundoplication, the fundus is brought behind the esophagus as a 270-degree posterior fundoplication. This type of fundoplication is beneficial in patients with esophageal motility disorders in which a 360-degree wrap can lead to dysphagia. An added advantage is that full mobilization of the fundus is not necessary because less fundus is required for the wrap. It is also the antireflux procedure of choice after laparoscopic Heller myotomy for achalasia. The port placement and esophageal dissection are similar to Nissen fundoplication. The crura are sutured together if there is a large defect. The posterior fundic wrap is sutured

Table 1 Results of Laparoscopic Nissen Fundoplication

STUDY	NO. PATIENTS	PROCEDURE	NO. PATIENTS/ LENGTH OF FOLLOW-UP	MORTALITY (%)	MORBIDITY (%)	SUCCESS RATE (%)	DYSPHAGIA (%)
Hinder et al, 1994	198	LNF	198/6-32 mo	0.2	5	97	NS
Cadiere et al, 1997	274	LNF	154/2.5 yr	0	3.2	91	1
Dallemagne et al, 1998	550	LNF	127/2 yr	0	2.3	92	2.1
Constantine et al, 1998	362	LNF	100/6 mo-6 yr	0	1.9	>90	0.5
Kiviluoto et al, 1998	200	LNF	200/26 mo	0	5	87	NS
Peters et al, 1998	100	LNF	100/21 mo	0	4	96	2
Bammer et al, 2001	171	LNF	171/6.4 yr	0	NS	>90	27
Lafullarde et al, 2001	178	LNF	166/6 yr	0	NS	90	3.9

LNF, laparoscopic Nissen fundopliction; NS, not stated.

to the crura to prevent the wrap from slipping into the chest. The fundus is sutured to the right and left sides of the abdominal esophagus to create a 270-degree posterior wrap.

Laparoscopic Hill Repair

The laparoscopic Hill repair is based on securing the posterior aspect of the cardia to the preaortic fascia and plicating the lesser curvature. Plication of the lesser curvature presumably produces elongation of the intraabdominal segment of the esophagus. The dissection is less extensive because it does not involve creation of a window or fundoplication. The disadvantages are that the sutures must be placed correctly in the preaortic fascia, and it is more difficult to perform laparoscopically.

Special Situations

Special situations that may arise include the following:

1. Patients with primary esophageal motility disorder can have worsening of symptoms after a 360-degree wrap and may benefit from a partial fundoplication (Toupet).
2. Stricturing due to chronic reflux produces a shortened esophagus that can prevent creation of a tension-free wrap. These patients may require an esophageal lengthening procedure along with the antireflux procedure.
3. Obesity is only a relative contraindication, but these patients may require longer instruments and extra ports. Surgeons increasingly are performing the procedure laparoscopically regardless of the body habitus.

■ RESULTS

Several studies have shown that LNF is associated with a greater than 90% success rate (Table 1). Similarly, studies comparing the laparoscopic approach with open fundoplication have proved the efficacy of LNF. In addition, the laparoscopic approach has the benefit of reducing postoperative pain and hospital stay. Modifications of LNF are being

performed increasingly to reduce the incidence of postoperative dysphagia. Toupet fundoplication (180 to 270 degrees) has been shown to offer comparable results with reduced postoperative dysphagia. Nissen-Rossetti modification procedures initially were associated with a high rate of dysphagia. Leggett et al showed that the Rossetti modification can be performed with a similar incidence of dysphagia.

■ CONCLUSION

The reluctance on the part of internists and patients to refer and seek surgery for GERD was in some part due to the morbidity associated with open Nissen fundoplication. The laparoscopic approach to fundoplication has eliminated these drawbacks, while offering similar results and several other added benefits. Laparoscopic antireflux surgery is a proven and viable treatment strategy for reflux disease refractory to drug therapy. It also can be an effective alternative to prolonged medical treatment in the absence of complications. LNF currently is the gold standard surgical procedure for reflux disease. The procedure of choice depends on the patient's underlying abnormality and individual surgeon's preference.

SUGGESTED READING

Campos GM, et al: Multivariate analysis of factors predicting outcome after laparoscopic Nissen fundoplication, *J Gastrointest Surg* 3:292, 1999.

Carlson MA, Frantzides CT: Complications and results of primary minimally invasive antireflux procedures: a review of 10,735 reported cases, *J Am Coll Surg* 193:428, 2001.

Hagen JA, Peters JH: Minimally invasive approaches to antireflux surgery, *Semin Thorac Cardiovasc Surg* 12:157, 2000.

Hinder RA: Surgical therapy for GERD: selection of procedures, short- and long-term results, *J Clin Gastroenterol* 30(3 Suppl):S48, 2000.

Ritter MP, et al: Outcome after laparoscopic fundoplication is not dependent on a structurally defective lower esophageal sphincter, *J Gastrointest Surg* 2:567, 1998.

Talamini MA, et al: Increased mediastinal pressure and decreased cardiac output during laparoscopic Nissen fundoplication, *Surgery* 122:345, 1997.

THE FAILED ANTIREFLUX OPERATION

Alex G. Little

■ PREOPERATIVE CONSIDERATIONS

Antireflux operations fail for one of two possible reasons. The first is when an inappropriate antireflux procedure is performed based on an erroneous preoperative diagnosis of gastroesophageal reflux disease (GERD). An example is when chest pain due to esophageal contractions or retention esophagitis is misinterpreted as heartburn, and an antireflux procedure is done for a motility disorder, such as achalasia. This type of failure emphasizes the need for establishment of a secure diagnosis before an operation for GERD. Esophageal function tests, including motility and pH monitoring, should be performed and the results used when the clinical diagnosis is equivocal.

This chapter focuses on the second type of failure of antireflux surgery, which is that due to inadequate performance of an operation that never relieves the patient's symptoms and/or when the operation, after early success, subsequently fails. In either case, these patients present with dysphagia or recurrent GERD symptoms of heartburn and/or regurgitation. Indications for reoperation are based on the severity of the patient's symptoms. Mild to moderate heartburn can be treated initially with a medical regimen including proton-pump inhibitor medication. Management of mild dysphagia due to an excessively tight wrap or to an iatrogenic stricture can be initiated with a limited number of dilations. When these approaches are sufficient and the patient is content, reoperation is not mandatory.

When symptoms are severe and reduce the patient's quality of life and medical therapy is not sufficient, reoperation is reasonable. These patients do not have normal anatomy. They possess an iatrogenically disturbed cardia. Improvement over time is unlikely. With a mechanically defective gastroesophageal junction fixed in place with postoperative scarring, the patient is at high risk for continued exposure to reflux and its sequelae, including esophagitis, stricture, and the possibility of pulmonary aspiration. If initial conservative management is unsuccessful, persistence is not in the best interest of the patient. In addition, all patients whose symptom complex includes regurgitation are at risk for pulmonary aspiration, and these patients should be considered candidates for early reoperative intervention to prevent this dire event.

Evaluation of every patient being considered for reoperation should be compulsively thorough. This evaluation should include a careful history of the patient's symptoms and review of the original operative report. This review predicts anatomic findings, which facilitates the planning for and performance of a reoperation. An upper gastrointestinal x-ray series and esophagogastroduodenoscopy are necessary to delineate anatomy, such as the presence or absence of a hiatal hernia, and to assess mucosal integrity. Esophageal function tests are helpful in these patients because they determine the adequacy of esophageal motility, determine the status of the lower esophageal sphincter, and quantitate reflux.

The most common anatomic findings in patients requiring reoperative antireflux surgery are a completely or partially disrupted wrap with or without a concomitant sliding or paraesophageal hiatal hernia. Variations include the finding of a seemingly misplaced and/or slipped wrap, which is around the proximal stomach rather than the distal esophagus. Rarely, after one but more frequently after multiple prior operations, actual leaks and tissue loss are encountered.

■ OPERATIVE MANAGEMENT

When reoperation is appropriate, the spectrum of operative approach alternatives includes a left thoracotomy, an open laparotomy, and a laparoscopic approach. The most conservative approach is a left thoracotomy. This approach provides initial exposure to the distal esophagus through an unoperated field, which eases the dissection and esophageal mobilization. If dissection of the esophageal hiatus to free up the previous fundoplication and stomach is difficult because of adhesions to the diaphragm, access to the intraabdominal esophagus and other upper abdominal structures can be gained via a peripheral incision in the left diaphragm (Figure 1). This technique preserves diaphragmatic function by avoiding the phrenic nerve branches and eliminates the painful (to the patient) necessity of transecting the costal cartilages as required by a thoracoabdominal incision. If at the conclusion

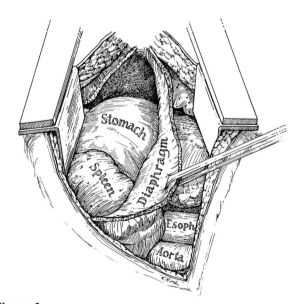

Figure 1
View from the perspective of a left thoracotomy. An incision is made in the diaphragm, starting centrally at the pericardial fat pad, extended peripherally and located 2 to 3 cm from the chest wall. Excellent exposure of the left upper quadrant is provided, and diaphragmatic function is preserved.

of mobilization of the esophagus and stomach, a Collis lengthening gastroplasty is necessary to achieve a tension-free reduction of the distal esophagus into the abdomen, a thoracotomy is the preferred exposure for this maneuver.

An open laparotomy is reasonable for some patients. Although a laparotomy is in general less painful for a patient than a thoracotomy, this approach for reoperation necessitates the tedium and actual risk of dissecting in a previously operated and scarred field, in which injury to the esophagus, stomach, or spleen is possible. In addition, an inflamed esophagus that is shortened and no longer pliable is difficult to reduce below the diaphragm for a tension-free repair. Longitudinal tension on the esophagus may disrupt the repair and/or lead to reherniation. This situation presents a challenge because the performance of a Collis gastroplasty to eliminate tension on the esophagus, although possible, is more difficult and complicated from this orientation than from a left thoracotomy.

It is possible to consider a laparoscopic approach to these patients. Initial entry into the abdomen has to be with an open Hasson technique to minimize the risk of injury to bowel that may be adherent to the abdominal wall. My concerns about this approach are identical to those for an open laparotomy. It is my opinion from personal and reported experiences that a laparoscopic approach is much more likely to be successful in the early postoperative period and when the surgeon has reason to suspect that a minimum amount of dissection was carried out at the first operation. When some time has elapsed and/or the first operation was not a "minimalist procedure," I believe a thoracotomy is the preferable alternative for most patients for the stated reasons.

At reoperation, regardless of the surgical approach, the steps of the procedure are similar. The esophagus and gastric fundus need to be dissected fully and sharply from the diaphragmatic hiatus itself and mobilized from the posterior mediastinum and from the retroperitoneum. From the abdomen, after dissection of the left lobe of the liver from the stomach and hiatus, this dissection usually is initiated medial to the right pillar of the esophageal hiatus. If the short gastric vessels have not been divided, this should be carried out at this stage of the operation. If these vessels have been divided previously, the fundus and greater curvature should be released sharply from all adhesions to the lesser sac. At this point when mobilization has been achieved, the surgeon should address the previous antireflux operation. If an intact wrap is in place, the stitches should be divided and the wrap dissected free from the esophagus and/or stomach until the fundus is released completely. The goal is to restore normal anatomy to the extent possible. If at this point the esophagus is viable and preoperative esophageal motility testing has shown preserved esophageal peristalsis, the esophageal hiatus is closed, and a standard three-stitch Nissen fundoplication is performed with a large esophageal dilator, such as a 50 Fr (or larger) Maloney bougie, in place to ensure that the wrap is loose around the esophagus.

If the esophagus is severely inflamed and inelastic, a Collis gastroplasty should be performed, followed by a loose Nissen fundoplication around the neoesophagus. Performing a new antireflux procedure with the esophagus stretched into the abdomen under tension results in vertical tension on the distal esophagus, drawing it toward the mediastinum. This tension is likely to predispose to hiatal herniation and/or wrap disruption and result in a second failure. Finally, if the scarring is severe, if there is a chronic esophageal or gastric leak with actual tissue disruption, or if esophageal motility testing shows loss of effective esophageal contractile function, the surgeon must consider distal esophagectomy and replacement with either colon or a small bowel. This scenario is uncommon, but the need should be suspected when the patient has undergone multiple prior operations. As attractive as esophageal preservation is, retention of a nonviable or nonfunctioning esophagus would not benefit the patient. An appropriately performed distal esophageal resection and a colon interposition through a left thoracotomy gives the patient the best opportunity for a high quality of life under these circumstances.

■ RESULTS

It has been shown consistently that for most patients undergoing reoperation, particularly if only one antireflux operation has been performed previously, the results are nearly as good as they are for initial operations. Most reports of reoperation document an 80% to 85% long-term control of reflux symptoms of heartburn and regurgitation. When reoperation is necessitated by stricture and/or tissue disruption, the results are less satisfactory. This situation is more likely to be seen in patients with multiple than single prior antireflux operations who, in addition to or instead of heartburn and regurgitation, experience dysphagia. In these patients, only approximately 60% can expect an excellent to good outcome after reoperation. Many remain symptomatic. This is not an acceptable outcome for patients with benign disease, and although there are not many patients in this category, it does emphasize the need for surgical flexibility and the occasional use of resection and replacement of severely diseased esophagus with healthy colon or jejunum at reoperation.

SUGGESTED READING

Gadenstatter M, et al: Esophagectomy for unsuccessful antireflux operations, *J Thorac Cardiovasc Surg* 115:296, 1998.

Horgan S, et al: Failed antireflux surgery, *Arch Surg* 134:809, 1999.

Hunter JG, et al: Laparoscopic fundoplication failures, *Ann Surg* 230:595, 1999.

Little AG, et al: Reoperation for failed antireflux operations, *J Thorac Cardiovasc Surg* 91:511, 1986.

Yau P, et al: Early reoperation following laparoscopic antireflux surgery, *Am J Surg* 179:172, 2000.

PARAESOPHAGEAL HERNIA

Jonathan Limpert

Keith S. Naunheim

■ CLASSIFICATION

Paraesophageal hernia, or hiatal hernia, is defined as herniation, or protrusion, of abdominal contents through the esophageal hiatus into the thoracic cavity. These hernias generally are classified into four types, the most common of which is the sliding, or type I, hiatal hernia. In this type, the gastroesophageal junction moves cephalad, as the stomach follows, through the esophageal hiatus due to weakening of the phrenoesophageal ligament. Frequently associated with loss of tone of the lower esophageal sphincter, type I hiatal hernias have clinical significance when responsible for gastroesophageal reflux and esophagitis. The paraesophageal, or type II, hiatal hernia is uncommon and accounts for 2% or less of all hiatal hernias and is distinguished by the protrusion of the gastric fundus into the mediastinum paralleling the esophagus, although the gastroesophageal junction remains in its normal location. A type III hernia, the most common paraesophageal hernia, is a combination of types I and II: a sliding and rolling hernia in which the gastroesophageal junction and the fundus or greater curvature herniated into the chest. It has been suggested that this defect occurs after the presence of a type II hernia for many years, which eventually enlarges the esophageal hiatus so that the gastroesophageal junction no longer lies below the diaphragm. With progressive enlargement of the hiatus, organs other than the stomach may traverse the hiatal opening to form a type IV hernia. The transverse colon and omentum are most commonly involved, but spleen and small bowel also may herniate.

■ CLINICAL PRESENTATION

Many type II hernias are asymptomatic and are discovered when the patient undergoes radiologic examination of the chest for other reasons. As with any true anatomic hernia, however, the potential complications include bleeding, incarceration, volvulus, obstruction, strangulation, and perforation. Patients who present with these symptoms are usually elderly.

Some patients may describe postprandial discomfort, such as substernal fullness or pressure, which has been present for years and can be mistaken for angina. This discomfort may result from an intrathoracic gastric segment that becomes dilated by food and swallowed air. Although a hernia may be large, many patients become accustomed to and tolerate these gas-bloat symptoms well. If a patient has associated chronic bleeding from gastritis or ulcers, this may lead to an iron deficiency anemia and present with fatigue and exertional dyspnea. A large type III or type IV hiatal hernia, which occupies a significant portion of the thoracic cavity, also may cause respiratory symptoms, such as postprandial dyspnea with a sense of suffocation.

Occasionally, patients present with gastric volvulus and resultant obstruction. Most patients give a long history of such postprandial complaints, although many have never had the pain evaluated. Symptoms include chest pain or pressure accompanied by nausea, retching, and dysphagia. These patients frequently are diagnosed as having myocardial ischemia. If a volvulus is allowed to progress, the patient may present with an incarceration and strangulation of the entrapped mediastinal organs.

■ DIAGNOSIS

Asymptomatic patients are diagnosed by the presence of a retrocardiac air-bubble or air-fluid level on a chest radiograph. When a hiatal hernia is suspected, a barium study of the upper gastrointestinal tract is the diagnostic study of choice with the pathognomonic finding defined as an "upside-down" stomach in the chest.

Acutely symptomatic patients may be diagnosed in a variety of fashions. In acute gastrointestinal hemorrhage or in patients with reflux symptoms, the diagnosis may be made by endoscopy. Patients with obstructive symptoms most often are diagnosed with an upper gastrointestinal barium study that shows the hernia. Occasionally an incidental diagnosis of paraesophageal hernia is made during a chest computed tomography scan performed for respiratory symptoms.

■ THERAPY

The presence of a paraesophageal hernia traditionally has been considered an indication for surgery since the report of Skinner and Belsey, who noted a 29% mortality rate in 21 patients followed conservatively. Although patients may have transient resolution of symptoms under medical management, the mortality rate far exceeds the less than 2% operative mortality documented for surgical repair. In patients presenting with obstruction, hemorrhage, or perforation, nasogastric tube decompression should be initiated promptly. As a result of the twisting inherent in gastric volvulus, however, it may not be possible to advance a tube into the stomach. In either case, urgent operative intervention is indicated.

■ OPERATIVE APPROACHES

Although a paraesophageal hernia universally is recognized as a surgical indication, there is still controversy about which operation to perform and by which approach. A repair can be performed through a laparotomy, a thoracotomy, or a transthoracic laparoscopic approach. The operative principles of hernia repair should remain inviolate for each approach: reduction of the hernia, resection of the intrathoracic sac, and closure of the hiatal defect. In addition, it is necessary to fix the stomach within the abdominal cavity employing either a gastrostomy or a fundoplication. It also is important to ensure that the lower esophageal sphincter (the distal 2 to 4 cm of esophagus) remain in the abdominal cavity without tension. In cases in which foreshortening of the esophagus has occurred, this requires an esophageal lengthening procedure, such as a Collis gastroplasty.

Authors who advocate a left thoracotomy approach point out the ease of intrathoracic dissection of the hernia contents and sac. Morbidly obese patients and patients with multiple prior abdominal surgeries or prior esophageal operations may be approached better transthoracically due to the ease of dissection of the esophagus and exposure of the hiatal arch. Thoracotomy proponents note that in patients with type III defects, one can perform a thorough mobilization of the esophagus up to the aortic arch, obviating the need for an esophageal lengthening procedure in some patients. Disadvantages of this approach include increased morbidity and discomfort, as manifested by increased incidence of respiratory complications (i.e., pneumonia), longer hospital length of stay, and increased analgesia requirement compared with a transabdominal approach. Although a fundoplication can be done easily via thoracotomy, performance of a gastroplasty or gastrostomy would necessitate either a concomitant laparotomy or a diaphragmatic incision and closure.

Supporters of a laparotomy approach (usually an upper midline incision) note the ease of performing the procedure through the abdomen and believe that the intraabdominal gastric fixation via fundoplication or gastrostomy is accomplished more easily transabdominally. Patients with type III hernias and patients with a foreshortened esophagus may be more difficult to manage via this approach, although transhiatal dissection of the esophagus through an enlarged hiatus occasionally allows the experienced surgeon to mobilize an adequate length of esophagus.

The laparoscopic repair of paraesophageal hernias was introduced in 1992 by Congreve and is now the mainstay of surgical therapy for this condition at many institutions. This approach has been well shown to have a decrease in morbidity, hospital length of stay, analgesia requirements, need for intensive care, and time to resumption of oral intake. The procedure is performed in the dorsal lithotomy position with the patient in reverse Trendelenburg position. The surgeon performs the procedure either from the patient's right side or between the legs. Trocar placement is variable among individuals, and most surgeons employ five sites. The left lateral segment of the liver is retracted, and the herniated organs (mostly the stomach) are reduced into the abdomen using a hand-over-hand technique. The gastrosplenic ligament, short gastric vessels, and gastrohepatic ligament are divided, ultimately exposing the right crus of the diaphragm. The hernia sac is divided at the hiatus, gentle traction is applied, and the sac is dissected bluntly out of the thoracic cavity and resected. The esophagus is mobilized circumferentially as far up in the mediastinum as possible, taking care to preserve the vagal nerves. One must be certain that

3 to 4 cm of esophagus lies beneath the hiatus without tension after mobilization. If shortening is present, as evidenced by inability to maintain the gastroesophageal junction in an infradiaphragmatic position, a Collis gastroplasty may be required. When an adequate length of esophagus or neoesophagus lies without tension in the abdomen, the surgeon must decide whether or not to perform an antireflux procedure. If the patient has shown significant signs of gastroesophageal reflux preoperatively by clinical history, endoscopic findings, or pH monitoring, a fundoplication is indicated. If the presence of gastroesophageal reflux has been ruled out using these techniques, however, many surgeons would proceed simply with intraabdominal gastric fixation, most commonly using a gastrostomy. This is a controversial point, however, and some authors recommend performance of a fundoplication in all such patients. If a fundoplication is to be performed, it is helpful to have a preoperative esophageal manometry, which should be performed in all but urgent or emergency patients. Normal manometry suggests that either partial or complete (360-degree) fundoplication can be performed safely in the patient. Significant esophageal dysmotility as evidenced by poor peristalsis or multiple simultaneous contractions should alert the surgeon, however, to consider a partial fundoplication to minimize the risk of significant postoperative complications (i.e., regurgitation). Several authors have reported relatively large series of paraesophageal hernia repairs with high success rates for the laparoscopic treatment of paraesophageal hernia with operative mortality of less than 2%, hospital length of stay varying from 2 to 3 days, and a rate of recurrence of 8% or less with follow-up lasting 19 months. Schauer et al directly compared open and laparoscopic repairs and noted that there is a significantly lower incidence of major and minor complications, presumably due to the elevated level of cardiopulmonary compromise associated with an open technique. Gastroesophageal perforation is a significant complication associated with a laparoscopic approach, however. The incidence of perforation has been reported to be 5% and is associated with extensive dissection, bougie placements, and redo operations.

■ CONCLUSIONS

Paraesophageal hernias should be repaired when recognized. Gastric volvulus with obstructive symptoms constitute a surgical emergency. Although the overall incidence of these hernias is small, the death rate is greater than 50% in the face of severe complications, such as hemorrhage, perforation, or gangrene. Although medical management may provide symptom relief, most would agree that correction of the underlying anatomic defect is indicated. The laparotomy and thoracotomy approaches continue to be acceptable methods of treatment for the repair of these defects. With continuing education of the surgical community and the progressively increasing expertise in laparoscopic surgery, it seems likely that within the next decade, laparoscopy will become the approach of choice for the treatment of this potentially fatal disorder.

SUGGESTED READING

Luketich JD, et al: Laparoscopic repair of giant paraesophageal hernia: 100 consecutive cases, *Ann Surg* 232:608, 2000.

Maziak DE, et al: Massive hiatus hernia: evaluation and surgical management, *J Thorac Cardiovasc Surg* 115:53, 1998.

Schauer PR, et al: Comparison of laparoscopic versus open repair of paraesophageal hernia, *Am J Surg* 176:659, 1998.

Swanstrom LL, et al: Esophageal motility and outcomes following laparoscopic paraesophageal hernia repair and fundoplication, *Am J Surg* 157:359, 1999.

Wiechman RJ, et al: Laparoscopic management of giant paraesophageal hernia, *Ann Thorac Surg* 71:1080, 2001.

BENIGN STRICTURES OF THE ESOPHAGUS

Farzaneh Banki

Jeffrey A. Hagen

■ DEFINITION

Benign strictures of the esophagus are the result of scar formation and cicatricial contraction that occur after injury to the esophageal wall. The most common cause of this injury is gastroesophageal reflux disease (GERD), which results in ulceration of the squamous mucosa of the distal esophagus and formation of a peptic stricture. Other common causes of benign esophageal strictures include caustic ingestion; pill-induced injury; and stenoses after radiation therapy, laser or photodynamic therapy, or surgery. Because malignancy can present as an esophageal stricture, biopsy specimens always should be taken to exclude the possibility of esophageal cancer.

The most common presenting symptom in patients with a benign esophageal stricture is dysphagia. This usually becomes significant when the luminal diameter is less than 13 mm. The dysphagia typically begins with solid food, and it is usually predictable with respect to the types of food that cause difficulty. Over time, as the stenosis worsens, the dysphagia may progress to include semisolid and liquid foods. This is in contrast to patients with dysphagia due to an esophageal motility disorder who usually present with dysphagia for liquid and solid foods, which is more intermittent and less predictable.

■ PATHOPHYSIOLOGY

Peptic Esophageal Strictures

Peptic strictures account for nearly 80% of all esophageal strictures. These strictures always involve the squamocolumnar junction and are located in the distal esophagus, near the gastroesophageal junction, unless a long segment of Barrett's esophagus is present. In this case, the squamocolumnar junction is located more proximally, and the peptic stricture is found at a higher level. Most are less than 1 cm in length, but in rare cases peptic strictures may be 8 cm in length.

It has been estimated that peptic strictures occur in 7% to 23% of patients with untreated reflux esophagitis, usually as a complication of relatively advanced reflux disease. It has been shown that patients with peptic strictures have a higher degree of acid exposure than reflux patients without strictures, and there is an association between alkaline reflux and stricture formation. A defective sphincter also is present in most patients with an esophageal stricture. When a defective sphincter is present in combination with acid and alkaline reflux, a stricture may be present in 85%. Finally, hiatal hernias are common in patients with peptic strictures, with abnormal esophageal body function present in 64%. Other conditions that predispose to the development of peptic strictures in patients with reflux include chronic use of salicylates or nonsteroidal antiinflammatory drugs (NSAIDs), long-term nasogastric tube placement, and hypersecretion of acid or increased gastric volume in Zollinger-Ellison syndrome. Patients who have undergone treatment for achalasia and patients with scleroderma are at particular risk for peptic strictures due to the combined presence of impaired lower esophageal sphincter function and poor esophageal clearance.

Caustic Ingestion

Acid and alkali ingestion can cause severe injury to the esophagus, resulting in the formation of a nonpeptic stricture. Because they are odorless and tasteless, strong alkaline chemicals, such as those found in commercial drain cleaners, more commonly are ingested accidentally, especially by children. Because they are not particularly noxious, they often are ingested in relatively large quantities, resulting in an extensive chemical injury to the esophagus. Strong acid has a strong offensive odor and a bitter taste that make it more likely to be expelled rapidly if taken accidentally.

In contrast to peptic strictures, corrosive injuries are more likely to involve all layers of the esophagus, which may lead to perforation, mediastinitis, and tracheoesophageal fistula. Because of the diffuse distribution of the offending chemical, these strictures also tend to involve longer lengths of the esophagus and may occur at multiple levels.

Pill-Induced Strictures

Pill-induced injuries are an increasingly recognized cause of a benign esophageal stricture. Strongly acid medications, including NSAIDs, vitamins, and antibiotics, are implicated most often. They can occur as an isolated injury, particularly in the elderly or institutionalized patient, or they may be superimposed on strictures that result from other causes. A pill-induced stricture should be suspected in any patient with a benign esophageal stricture that occurs in the absence of significant reflux symptoms or when a patient has persistent signs of esophageal injury despite aggressive acid suppression therapy.

Postoperative Strictures

Postoperative stenoses account for less than 10% of all nonpeptic strictures. They most commonly occur at the site of an anastomosis, occurring in 44% of patients after a transhiatal esophagectomy with a cervical esophagogastrostomy. Risk factors that have been identified for the development of postoperative strictures include an anastomotic leak, the presence of cardiovascular disease, and the use of a circular stapled anastomotic technique. Radiation therapy also seems to impair healing and increase the likelihood of anastomotic stricture formation. A new technique for construction of the cervical esophagogastric anastomosis with a side-to-side stapled anastomosis seems to reduce greatly the frequency of anastomotic leaks and postoperative stricture formation.

■ MANAGEMENT OF BENIGN ESOPHAGEAL STRICTURES

Esophageal Dilation

The initial step in management of patients with an esophageal stricture, regardless of the cause, is dilation. Options include the blind passage of mercury-weighted, rubber, blunt-tipped (Hurst) or tapered (Maloney) bougies; wire-guided polyvinyl (Savary) bougies; and wire-guided, metal olives (Eder-Puestow). Dilation also can be accomplished at the time of endoscopy using inflatable balloons.

Maloney dilation is preferred by many as the initial step because it can be accomplished easily in the office using topical anesthetic supplemented with a short-acting sedative. The end point of dilation should be relief of dysphagia, which requires dilation to at least 42 Fr. In most cases, it is desirable to dilate to at least 50 Fr, however, preferably to 60 Fr to achieve long-term relief of dysphagia. If blind passage of the Maloney dilator is unsuccessful, wire-guided Savary dilation should be attempted. Although this also can be performed under topical anesthetic with supplemental sedation, it requires endoscopy for placement of the guidewire and fluoroscopy to monitor the dilation. For particularly difficult strictures, Eder-Puestow dilation under general anesthetic should be considered. Alternatively, these difficult-to-manage strictures may be dilated using a balloon passed through an endoscope.

The risk of perforation associated with esophageal dilation is 0.5% to 6% depending on the indication for dilation. The risk is highest in patients with a malignant obstruction and in patients with corrosive strictures, particularly early after the injury. In both of these situations, the entire thickness of

the esophageal wall may be involved, resulting in a higher risk of full-thickness injury during dilation. It has been suggested that multiple episodes of dilation be carried out to reduce the risk of perforation, using the "rule of threes." According to this principle, dilators are passed until resistance is encountered, with subsequent dilation limited to 3 French sizes above this point.

Elimination of Further Injury

After the stricture has been dilated successfully, the focus of therapy should be on eliminating any ongoing injury to the esophagus. In the case of peptic strictures, this involves elimination of further reflux. It also is important to recognize that acid exposure may aggravate all types of nonpeptic stricture. As a result, elimination of acid reflux is an important part of the management of all patients with an esophageal stricture.

Medical Antireflux Therapy

The most common treatment offered to control reflux is antisecretory therapy, usually with a proton-pump inhibitor. Although short-term success can be achieved in most patients with medical therapy combined with intermittent dilation, persistent reflux results in the need for repeat dilation in at least 30% within the first year. The high recurrence rate associated with medical therapy combined with the demonstrated superior outcome of antireflux surgery in patients with complicated GERD suggests that prolonged medical therapy should be reserved for patients who are not suitable candidates for antireflux surgery.

Surgical Antireflux Therapy

The potential for superior results after antireflux surgery are not surprising when one considers the association between peptic strictures and the hallmarks of severe GERD described previously. These same indicators of advanced GERD also generally are recognized as risk factors for medical treatment failure. Specific circumstances in which antireflux surgery should be strongly considered include patients in whom esophagitis fails to heal on medical therapy and individuals who remain symptomatic while on medical treatment. Patients who require increasing doses of acid suppression therapy to maintain symptom control should be considered for surgery. Because medical therapy affects only acid secretion, patients with documented duodenogastric reflux also should be considered for surgical therapy.

The choice of operation performed should follow the principles applied in the management of reflux disease in general. In the presence of preserved esophageal body function (amplitude of esophageal contraction >20 mm Hg and presence of peristaltic waves in >70% of wet swallows), a laparoscopic Nissen fundoplication is the procedure of choice. This procedure results in resolution of the stricture and relief of dysphagia in more than 87%. To minimize the risk of a persistent stricture, it must be determined whether or not dilation would control the stricture before performing an antireflux operation. If not, primary resection should be considered (see later). It also is important to recognize that the presence of an esophageal stricture has been described as a warning sign that the esophagus may be foreshortened, a complication that is present in 14% of patients who present for surgical treatment of GERD. If a short esophagus is suspected, a transthoracic approach is preferable because it allows a greater degree of esophageal mobilization. This mobilization can reduce the tension on the repair, which is the most common cause of failure after antireflux surgery. In our experience, a thoracotomy and complete mobilization allow construction of a tension-free Nissen repair in about 43% of patients suspected as having a short esophagus, with a Collis gastroplasty providing additional length in the remaining patients. It has been suggested that laparoscopy still can be performed in these patients, but the need for a gastroplasty and its attendant complications seems to be higher.

Esophageal Resection

Esophageal resection should be considered in patients with difficult-to-manage strictures. This includes patients in whom the stricture cannot be dilated to the point of relief of dysphagia and patients with strictures that recur shortly after dilation. Resection also should be considered in patients with strictures that persist after antireflux surgery and in patients in whom antireflux surgery fails. The reconstructive options include the use of a gastric tube and interposition of a segment of either jejunum or colon. In 1994, Akiyama et al described a vagal-sparing esophagectomy with colon interposition, which seems to result in better alimentary function. A vein stripper passed from the abdominal portion of the esophagus to the cervical incision is used to invert and remove the esophagus from the neck downward. The bed of the removed esophagus is dilated, and a colon interposition is performed. This procedure is ideal for patients with a benign disease requiring replacement because it preserves vagal innervation to the upper gastrointestinal tract, allowing preservation of gastric reservoir function.

■ SUMMARY

Effective management of a patient with an esophageal stricture requires knowledge of the potential causes and recognition of the importance of reflux control in preventing ongoing injury to the esophagus. If the stricture can be dilated successfully, control of reflux with either acid suppression therapy or antireflux surgery is usually successful in controlling the stricture, although long-term success seems to be more likely after surgery. Caution should be exercised in selecting the surgical approach, with particular attention required to exclude the presence of a short esophagus. Esophageal resection should be considered in patients with strictures that are refractory to dilation and when antireflux surgery fails.

SUGGESTED READING

Gastal OL, et al: Short esophagus: analysis of predictors and clinical implications, *Arch Surg* 134:633, 1999.

Hunter JG, et al: Laparoscopic fundoplication failures: patterns of failure and response to fundoplication revision, *Ann Surg* 230:595, 1999.

Orringer MB, et al: Transhiatal esophagectomy for benign and malignant disease, *J Thorac Cardiovasc Surg* 105:265, 1993.

Richter JE: Peptic strictures of the esophagus, *Gastroenterol Clin N Am* 28:875, 1999.

Spechler SJ: Comparison of medical and surgical therapy for complicated gastroesophageal reflux disease in veterans. The Department of Veterans Affairs Gastroesophageal Reflux Disease Study Group, *N Engl J Med* 326:786, 1992.

Watson TJ, et al: Esophageal replacement for end-stage benign esophageal disease, *J Thorac Cardiovasc Surg* 115:1241, 1998.

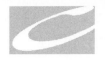

PHARYNGOESOPHAGEAL DYSFUNCTION AND CRICOPHARYNGEAL MYOTOMY

André Duranceau

Dysfunction at the pharyngoesophageal junction results in poor propulsion of food or liquid from the oral cavity into the cervical esophagus. This dysfunction is usually a manifestation of systemic disease, and the therapeutic approach, the indications, the timing of therapy, and the results of treatment are based on the etiologic diagnosis and the functional abnormalities present. The current standard approach in patients with oropharyngeal symptoms from pharyngoesophageal dysfunction includes the detection of the problem, its quantification, and an attempt at correction of these functional manifestations of dysphagia.

■ SYMPTOMS

Independent of the etiology of the dysphagia, three categories of symptoms result from misdirection of an alimentary bolus: pharyngonasal or pharyngooral regurgitations and laryngotracheal aspiration. Discomfort during meals and bronchopulmonary complications from aspiration are the main presenting patterns.

■ ETIOLOGIC CLASSIFICATION

Most patients presenting with oropharyngeal dysphagia symptoms resulting from pharyngoesophageal dysfunction can be classified into one of the following five categories.

Neurologic Disease
Symptoms in the patient with neurologic disease are the most difficult to assess and to treat. Cerebrovascular disease may result in difficulties of speech and expression. The dysarthric patient may show poor coordination of pharynx, larynx, and upper esophageal sphincter (UES) activity. The patient who has had a cerebrovascular accident often has difficulties in bolus formation and propulsion. Parkinson's disease

patients show hesitancy in bolus preparation and in initiating swallows. Patients with amyotrophic lateral sclerosis, with their loss of motor neurons and control mechanisms, show absence of voluntary deglutition, dysarthria, and repetitive aspiration.

Muscular Disease
Bilateral palpebral ptosis muscle weakness and repetitive efforts at swallowing suggest muscular disease. Hoarseness, dysphonia, and nasal speech, when accompanying oropharyngeal dysphagia, suggest dystrophic disease with poor control of laryngeal and uvulopharyngeal muscles.

Idiopathic Dysfunction of the Upper Esophageal Sphincter
When oropharyngeal dysphagia cannot be explained by neurologic or muscular disease, intrinsic dysfunction of the UES must be suspected. These patients are often tense individuals, although the underlying basis for a neuropsychogenic explanation of their condition is lacking. Dysphagia at the oropharyngeal level, frequent food incarceration, and bouts of aspiration are the most frequent symptoms. When a pharyngoesophageal diverticulum is present, fresh food regurgitation frequently accompanies the oropharyngeal symptom complex.

Iatrogenic Causes
Ablative or explorative surgery in the neck may cause poor function at the pharyngeal and UES level. Tracheostomy and thyroidectomy may result in limitations to normal laryngeal excursion. Irradiation causes dense ischemic fibrosis with strictures often difficult to dilate.

Functional Abnormalities of the Lower Esophagus
Reflux disease is known to present with referred oropharyngeal dysphagia symptoms in 9% to 15% of patients presenting with this condition. Idiopathic motor dysfunction and distal esophageal obstruction may present in the same way. Only a complete esophageal investigation allows the proper diagnosis to be made.

■ LABORATORY EVALUATION TO IDENTIFY THE UNDERLYING ETIOLOGY

Radiology
Radiologic assessment of the oropharyngeal dysphagia patient requires multiphasic, multipositional studies using fluoroscopic and video recording equipment. Due to the rapidity of events during the act of swallowing, dysfunction of the pharynx, larynx, and UES can be recorded accurately

only when using these techniques. They permit observation of the initiation of swallowing, the movements of the tongue and soft palate, the symmetry of pharyngeal contraction, the organization and activity of the larynx during its normal excursion, the aspiration of ingestate, and the activity of the UES at rest and during swallowing. Even minute abnormalities in the function of these muscle groups can be documented. Hypopharyngeal pooling and stasis and pooling in the piriform sinuses and in the valleculae suggest abnormal emptying.

Radionuclide Emptying Studies

Emptying assessment of the oropharynx is obtained easily during esophageal radionuclide transit evaluation. In all categories of oropharyngeal dysphagia patients, it provides quantification of emptying with a liquid, a semisolid, or a solid bolus. Objective documentation of results is allowed when using either medical or surgical treatment in these patients.

Endoscopy

Direct laryngoscopy and the use of the short rigid esophagoscope are preferred to obtain detailed evaluation of the larynx, pharynx, hypopharynx, and UES area. This technique rules out any endoluminal lesion. The flexible endoscope subsequently allows complete assessment of the distal esophagus. When a pharyngoesophageal diverticulum has been documented by radiographic studies, endoscopy is not considered a matter of urgency. Unless an underlying malignancy is suspected, endoscopy is considered dangerous. Its use can be delayed until correction of the oropharyngeal problem has been completed.

Motility Studies

Manometric evaluation of the esophagus and its sphincters is useful to quantify the distal esophageal function and the physiologic abnormalities present at the pharyngoesophageal junction. Physiologic evaluation of the UES needs to take into consideration two important factors: (1) the radial and axial asymmetry of the sphincter and (2) the upward and anterior excursion of the sphincter during swallowing. Because of this asymmetry, single-port recording catheters are considered less accurate to assess UES resting pressures. Multilumen recording catheters with port opening at the same level sum accurately the effects of the cricopharyngeus at rest. A circumferential pressure transducer probably provides the most accurate pressure values. The Dent sleeve catheter also has the advantage of recording sphincter pressures at any level along the sleeve membrane, even if sphincter movement occurs. Manometry performed concurrently with videofluoroscopy permits the integration of manometric data with fluoroscopic observations. In particular, impaired UES opening, impaired coordination and relaxation, and weak pharyngeal propulsion can be distinguished from increased outflow resistance as manifest by high intrabolus pressure. Methods of manometric recording, if performed as a stand-alone test, may provide accurate resting and closing pressures but they underestimate the true functional abnormalities present in patients with oropharyngeal dysphagia.

■ CRICOPHARYNGEAL MYOTOMY

Operations on the pharyngoesophageal junction aim at removing the obstructive effect of the functionally obstructive UES. The high-pressure zone, when significantly decreased or abolished, should decrease the resistance to bolus transit, although the dysfunction may persist.

The surgical approach to the pharyngoesophageal junction is the same, whether a diverticulum is present or not. We prefer a left-sided oblique incision along the anterior border of the sternocleidomastoid muscle for maximal exposure. The prethyroid muscles are divided along the axis of the incision. The plane for dissection is anterior and medial to the large vessels and lateral to the thyroid gland with successive division of the middle thyroid vein and inferior thyroid artery.

Extended Cricopharyngeal Myotomy

When performed for idiopathic oropharyngeal dysphagia or for oropharyngeal dysphagia secondary to neurologic muscular or iatrogenic reasons, a 6- to 7-cm myotomy is created across the pharyngoesophageal junction. The only well-identified reference point for location of the UES is the cricoid cartilage. It serves as a midpoint for the length of the myotomy. Two centimeters of cervical esophageal musculature initially is divided with progressive extension of the operation proximally. Two centimeters of the pharyngoesophageal junction is sectioned, and 2 cm of hypopharyngeal musculature subsequently is sectioned down to the mucosa. The posterior pharyngoesophageal junction is denuded of all muscle by dissecting a flap of muscularis from the mucosa with transverse section of the muscle at the proximal and distal ends of the myotomy. The muscle flap is resected for histologic analysis (Figure 1).

Cricopharyngeal Myotomy with Diverticulum Suspension or Resection

When a pharyngoesophageal diverticulum (Zenker's) is present, the only recognized treatment is surgical. The operation aims first at removing the restrictive UES. The diverticulum, seen as a complication of the sphincter dysfunction, either is suspended if less than 4 cm or is resected if larger. The diverticulum also is resected if there is any suspicion of a mucosal lesion within the diverticulum.

When the myotomy is completed, a nasogastric tube is introduced, and air is insufflated at the pharyngoesophageal junction to confirm the integrity of the mucosa. Nasogastric drainage is employed for 12 to 24 hours until normal peristalsis is perceived. After cricopharyngeal myotomy, nasogastric drainage prevents the need for blind insertion of a tube if gastric drainage problems become evident after the operation.

■ RESULTS OF OPERATIONS ON THE UPPER ESOPHAGEAL SPHINCTER

Neurologic Dysphagia

Patients with oropharyngeal dysphagia of exclusive neurologic origin show functional abnormalities of resting pressures in the UES and incoordination and relaxation defects.

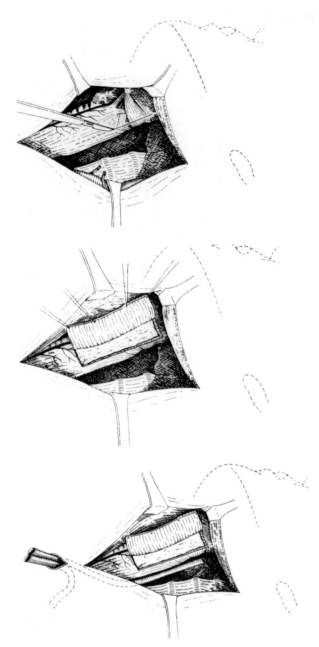

Figure 1
The cricopharyngeal myotomy is 6 to 7 cm in length. It extends 2 cm on the cervical esophagus and 2 cm across the pharyngoesophageal junction and includes 2 to 3 cm on the hypopharynx. The muscularis is dissected free from the mucosa, and with transverse division of the muscle at the proximal and distal ends of the myotomy, a muscle flap is lifted, and it usually is resected for histologic analysis.

UES hypertension has been reported by Ellis and Crozier, whereas Bonavina reported incoordination and poor relaxation of the sphincter during the pharyngeal contraction. In a preliminary observation, we recorded normal resting pressures but relaxation was incomplete for 7 of 20 patients with neurogenic dysphagia. Poor coordination of sphincter opening during pharyngeal contraction was observed in 80% of patients. Only neurologic oropharyngeal dysphagia patients have shown complete absence of relaxation or achalasia of the UES.

Cricopharyngeal myotomy is reported for more than 200 patients with dysphagia of exclusive neurologic origin. The operation aims at decreasing the resistance to pharyngoesophageal transit by removing or lessening the sphincter effects of the cricopharyngeus. The underlying motor abnormalities remain unchanged in our experience. Patients can be expected to improve (1) if they retain an intact voluntary deglutition, (2) if they show normal movements of the tongue, (3) if they present with normal phonation, and (4) if no dysarthria results from their central disease.

Results have been mixed and vary with the disease category. Overall, 50% of treated patients report excellent results. The remaining patients may show initial improvement with subsequent deterioration. Poor results are seen when the prognostic factors mentioned earlier cannot be met. Mortality after this operation for a neurologic condition may be 12% to 20%. Mortality results from persistent aspiration with subsequent pulmonary and cardiovascular complications.

Muscular Dysphagia

Weaker and longer contractions in the pharynx of patients with muscular dysphagia are not powerful enough to propulse the bolus past the cricopharyngeus area. The UES becomes a functional obstacle to food transit. Just as for neurologic patients, cricopharyngeal myotomy aims at abolishing the resistance at the pharyngoesophageal junction. These patients, although they have a powerless pharynx, still improve after operation in greater than 75% of cases. Patients retain adequate voluntary deglutition, and if they also retain appropriate muscular control of the larynx, comfortable swallowing is obtained after the myotomy with significant decrease in preoperative symptoms. Improvement in pharyngeal emptying usually is observed. Progression of the disease is the main factor controlling evolution after myotomy. The appearance of dysphonia and hoarseness suggests deterioration of muscular function with potentially increased aspiration episodes. In these patients, laryngeal exclusion or excision is necessary to stop the aspiration problems.

Idiopathic Dysfunction of the Upper Esophageal Sphincter

Dysfunction of the UES without any evidence of neurologic or muscular pathology to explain it is termed *idiopathic*. In these patients, no pharyngoesophageal diverticulum is present, and the same type of cricopharyngeal myotomy is used as for patients with neurologic or muscular dysphagia. More than 80 patients operated on for this condition have been reported, with seven eighths showing excellent improvement after operation.

The functional abnormalities present in the UES of patients when a pharyngoesophageal diverticulum is present have been assessed in a meticulous study by Cook and Jamieson. Using a sleeve sensor to assess the sphincter, they documented significantly higher intrabolus pressures in the hypopharynx during barium swallow studies. At the same time, they measured the maximal luminal area of the open sphincter. The computed surface of the sphincter showed significantly less surface than in controls. Documented histologic fibrosis and inflammation in the sphincter are responsible for a restrictive myopathy. The decreased sphincter compliance and the high hypopharyngeal intrabolus pressures eventually might lead to diverticulum formation through repeated efforts of the pharynx and hypopharynx. Myotomy with diverticular suspension or myotomy with resection of the diverticulum results in uniform excellent control of symptoms. Jamieson et al documented a normalization of intrapharyngeal pressures and disappearance of the UES opening abnormalities by these operations.

Iatrogenic and Distal Esophageal Dysfunction

Functional abnormalities of the UES are seen after extensive cervical operations, such as laryngectomy. After exclusion of any recurrent disease, cricopharyngeal myotomy may be helpful in relieving functional obstruction. When oropharyngeal symptoms are associated with the distal dysfunction of motor disorders or reflux disease, they usually are improved by appropriate treatment.

■ SUMMARY

Motor dysfunction of the pharyngoesophageal region can be classified by meticulous clinical, radiologic, and laboratory investigation. These abnormalities can be helped by cricopharyngeal myotomy in patients showing dysfunction but with intact voluntary swallowing.

SUGGESTED READING

Castell JA, et al: Manometric characteristics of the pharynx, upper esophageal sphincter, esophagus and lower esophageal sphincter in patients with oculopharyngeal muscular dystrophy, *Dysphagia* 10:22, 1995.

Duranceau A, Ferraro P: Pharyngeal and cricopharyngeal disorders. In Pearson FG, editor: *Esophageal surgery*, Philadelphia, Churchill Livingstone, 2002, p 477.

Pera M, et al: Sleeve recording of upper esophageal sphincter resting pressures during cricopharyngeal myotomy, *Ann Surg* 225:229, 1997.

Poirier NC, et al: Cricopharyngeal myotomy for neurogenic oropharyngeal dysphagia, *J Thorac Cardiovasc Surg* 113:233, 1997.

Sideris L, et al: The treatment of Zenker's diverticula: a review, *Semin Thorac Cardiovasc Surg* 11:337, 1999.

ACHALASIA

Steven R. DeMeester

Achalasia has an incidence of approximately 6 per 100,000 population and is the most common primary esophageal motility abnormality. It is characterized by failure of the esophagus to empty normally. Clinically this is manifested as dysphagia, typically for solids and liquids, and radiographically a barium swallow shows marked holdup of contrast material at the gastroesophageal junction, often creating the characteristic "bird's beak" deformity. The diagnosis is confirmed by esophageal motility testing that shows some or all of the following abnormalities: (1) a normal or hypertensive lower esophageal sphincter (LES) that fails to relax completely with swallowing; (2) simultaneous, low-amplitude contraction waves in the esophageal body; and (3) pressurization of the normally negative intrathoracic esophagus above gastric baseline. Primary achalasia must be differentiated from secondary achalasia (pseudoachalasia) caused by a malignancy near the gastroesophageal junction and Chagas' disease in patients with a history of travel to or living in rural areas of South America.

The cause of achalasia is unknown, but the disease produces irreversible destruction of the ganglion cells of Auerbach's plexus. Treatment is palliative and focuses on relief of the outflow obstruction produced by the nonrelaxing LES. Options include balloon dilation, surgical myotomy, *Botulinum* toxin injection, and in advanced disease esophagectomy. Medical therapy with nitrates or calcium channel blockers is largely ineffective and seldom used for long-term primary treatment.

■ TREATMENT

Botulinum Toxin Injection

Botulinum toxin (Botox) inhibits acetylcholine release from nerve endings, decreases cholinergic excitation at the LES, and lowers sphincter pressure when injected at this location. Approximately two thirds of patients note symptomatic improvement with *Botulinum* toxin injection, but in most patients the effects are temporary, and symptoms return within several months. Repeated injections are possible, but long-term treatment with *Botulinum* toxin probably is best suited to patients with significant medical comorbidities that prohibit more effective and durable treatment options.

Balloon Dilation

One of the earliest treatments for achalasia was dilation of the LES. Currently, dilation typically is performed using a 30- to 50-mm balloon fluoroscopically positioned across the LES. The objective is to stretch and rupture enough of the LES muscle to allow emptying of the esophagus, but not so much that gastroesophageal reflux or esophageal perforation occurs.

The likelihood and longevity of clinical improvement after pneumatic dilation have been correlated with the reduction in sphincter pressure. The best results (80% success at 2 years) occur in patients who have their sphincter pressure reduced to less than 10 mm Hg. Dilation also seems to be more successful in older individuals. Patients younger than 40, particularly patients younger than age 18, have been reported to have a poor response. Perforation rates vary based on the size of the dilating balloon, but most centers report an incidence of 5% to 10%. Frequently, repeated dilations are required for recurrent symptoms, in part depending on the aggressiveness of the initial dilation. In addition, increased gastroesophageal reflux has been shown to occur after successful balloon dilation for achalasia.

Surgical Myotomy

Surgical myotomy has been the gold standard treatment for achalasia for many years; however, enthusiasm for surgery has increased dramatically with the introduction of minimally invasive techniques. The traditional open procedure was a transthoracic Heller myotomy with or without an added partial fundoplication. The myotomy extends approximately 6 to 8 cm above the gastroesophageal junction, or until the thickened muscular layer has thinned out. On the gastric side of the gastroesophageal junction, there are two distinct approaches. One approach is to limit the myotomy to only several millimeters below the gastroesophageal junction to minimize the likelihood of inducing reflux and not add a fundoplication. The other approach is to carry the myotomy well down onto the stomach to ensure completeness, then add a partial fundoplication to minimize or protect against gastroesophageal reflux.

Currently, most patients are treated using a minimally invasive approach, either thoracoscopically or laparoscopically. A thoracoscopic myotomy is done identical to the open transthoracic myotomy with no added fundoplication. Intraoperative endoscopy facilitates identification of the gastroesophageal junction, and the myotomy is carried only 3 to 5 mm down on the stomach to minimize the incidence of postoperative gastroesophageal reflux. Experience in most centers has shown, however, that it is difficult to determine precisely the location of the gastroesophageal junction, and it is always a judgment as to where to end the myotomy distally to avoid either an incomplete or an excessive myotomy. Results after a thoracoscopic myotomy reflect the difficulty walking this fine line, with some reports suggesting that 27% of patients have persistent dysphagia secondary to an incomplete myotomy, whereas 60% of patients have evidence of increased esophageal acid exposure by 24-hour pH monitoring, suggesting that the myotomy was carried too far down onto the stomach.

In addition, compared with a laparoscopic approach, the thoracoscopic procedure seems to be associated with increased postoperative discomfort and greater difficulty addressing mucosal injuries intraoperatively. Consequently, most centers, including ours, prefer a laparoscopic approach, carry the myotomy well down onto the stomach (1.5 cm), and add a partial fundoplication to prevent reflux. I prefer to limit the dissection to the anterior aspect of the esophagus, perform the myotomy to the left of the anterior vagus nerve, and cover the myotomy site with an anterior Dor hemifundoplication. In the rare patient with achalasia and an associated hiatal hernia, I combine the myotomy with crural repair and a posterior Toupet hemifundoplication.

The incidence of complications, including the need for conversion to an open procedure, is extremely low after laparoscopic myotomy, and almost all patients are discharged home within 48 hours. Follow-up beyond 2 years has shown good to excellent results in greater than 90% of patients in most series. Similar to balloon dilation, excellent results correlate with reduction of sphincter pressure to less than or equal to 10 mm Hg. Previously, we tried intraoperative manometry to verify successful reduction of the sphincter pressure to less than 10 mm Hg, but found the measurements under general anesthesia to be difficult and unreliable.

Several centers have reported increased difficulty with a laparoscopic myotomy after *Botulinum* toxin injection or balloon dilation, both of which can produce scarring, making separation of the mucosa from the muscular layers difficult. Given the excellent visualization, safety, and results with a laparoscopic myotomy, it should be considered the preferred treatment for patients with achalasia. Although there have been no comparisons of laparoscopic myotomy and balloon dilation, a randomized, prospective trial comparing balloon dilation with open myotomy showed more consistent reduction of sphincter pressure and overall superior relief of symptoms with surgical myotomy. No significant difference in the incidence of gastroesophageal reflux was found between the two procedures. Patients with achalasia have such poor esophageal emptying that any improvement is noted immediately by the patient. Symptomatic success does not equate with true relief of outflow resistance, however. Consequently the best way to evaluate these patients is to compare esophageal emptying with a timed barium esophagogram before and after myotomy.

Esophagectomy for End-Stage Achalasia

A small percentage of patients with achalasia, whether previously treated or not, present with end-stage disease characterized by a dilated and sigmoid-shaped esophagus. Often symptoms in these patients include not only dysphagia, but also aspiration. In these patients, the results of myotomy are less reliable, and although the symptom of dysphagia may improve, the regurgitation and aspiration persist. In these patients, we recommend esophagectomy using a transabdominal vagal-sparing technique. With this procedure, the esophageal mucosa is stripped out, leaving the dilated muscular tube intact. After division of the cardia and a limited, highly selective vagotomy along the high lesser curve, the transverse colon based on the inferior mesenteric vessels is brought up posterior to the stomach and through the posterior mediastinum inside the esophageal muscular tube. Reconstruction consists of an end-to-end esophagocolostomy, side-to-side stapled cologastrostomy to the posterior fundus near the cardia, and end-to-end colocolostomy.

Early results show excellent function of the intact, innervated stomach with minimal regurgitation. Because these patients have an intact and functioning gastric reservoir, they eat extremely well. Preservation of the intact vagus nerves is problematic in patients with prior fundoplication or surgery at the hiatus, and in these patients transhiatal esophagectomy with gastric pull-up or colon interposition to the antrum after two thirds gastrectomy are the preferred options.

SUGGESTED READING

Csendes A, et al: Late results of a prospective randomised study comparing forceful dilatation and oesophagomyotomy in patients with achalasia, *Gut* 30:299, 1989.

Eckardt VF, et al: Predictors of outcome in patients with achalasia treated by pneumatic dilation, *Gastroenterology* 103:1732, 1992.

Kolbasnik J, et al: Long-term efficacy of Botulinum toxin in classical achalasia: a prospective study, *Am J Gastroenterol* 94:3434, 1999.

Patti MG, et al: Minimally invasive surgery for achalasia: an 8-year experience with 168 patients, *Ann Surg* 230:587, 1999.

Shoenut JP, et al: A prospective assessment of gastroesophageal reflux before and after treatment of achalasia patients: pneumatic dilation versus transthoracic limited myotomy, *Am J Gastroenterol* 92:1109, 1997.

DIFFUSE ESOPHAGEAL SPASM AND SCLERODERMA

John C. Ofenloch
Kamal A. Mansour

■ DIFFUSE ESOPHAGEAL SPASM

Diffuse esophageal spasm (DES) is an esophageal motility disorder characterized by simultaneous, repetitive, high-pressure muscular contractions within the esophagus. Increased esophageal wall tension and segmental contractions result in chest pain and dysphagia. Although the precise etiology is unclear, the esophageal musculature is markedly hypertrophic and is hypersensitive to stretching. Degeneration of the esophageal branches of the vagus nerve has been observed in patients with DES; however, this is not a consistent finding. In contrast to achalasia, the dysphagia associated with DES is typically less incapacitating, and some degree of peristalsis is retained.

Diagnosis

An esophageal neoplasm first should be excluded by contrast esophagogram in all patients with dysphagia. Classically a corkscrew appearance on esophagogram indicates severe DES. Esophageal emptying is delayed due to the high-pressure, segmental contractions. Subsequent esophageal manometry confirms repetitive, simultaneous contractions of abnormally high pressure. Lower esophageal sphincter (LES) function and pressure are normal in 70% of patients. Frequently, esophageal diverticula are identified in association with DES as a result of compartmentalized contractions and increased wall tension.

Medical Management

Medical treatment focuses on prevention of high-amplitude muscular contractions and attenuation of muscular hypersensitivity. Nitrates and calcium channel–blocking agents have been used successfully for treatment of this condition. Localized areas of muscular hypertrophy can be treated with pneumatic dilation or botulinum toxin injection. Both of these therapies have been used successfully. Most patients have diffuse involvement of the esophageal body and are not candidates for localized therapy. Medical management of patients with DES can be challenging because they frequently have a high degree of anxiety and seek medical attention aggressively.

Surgical Management

Indications for surgical intervention include failure of medical treatment to alleviate the pain associated with spasm or dysphagia. Patients with associated symptomatic esophageal diverticula or hiatal hernia also are candidates for surgical intervention. Surgical treatment should include a long esophagomyotomy performed through a left thoracotomy. The hypertrophied esophageal musculature is divided longitudinally to expose the esophageal mucosa. The divided muscle is dissected bluntly away from the myotomy to expose the mucosa over half the esophageal circumference. The myotomy extends from the level of the aortic arch to the LES. In patients with an abnormal LES, the myotomy should extend through the sphincter approximately 1 to 2 cm onto the cardia of the stomach. In these cases, the operation also should include a partial fundoplication to avoid the complication of postoperative gastroesophageal reflux. At our institution, we prefer a Belsey Mark IV partial fundoplication because this is accomplished easily from the left thoracotomy. A video-assisted thoracic surgery approach with esophageal myotomy is an acceptable alternative to a standard left thoracotomy, although we have found it more difficult when a fundoplication is required.

■ SCLERODERMA

Scleroderma is the most common collagen vascular disease affecting esophageal function, with 50% to 80% of patients eventually developing esophageal motor dysfunction. Scleroderma is characterized by progressive smooth muscle atrophy affecting the distal two thirds of the esophagus. The proximal one third of the esophagus comprises primarily striated muscle and is unaffected. Collagen deposition within the connective tissue matrix of the esophagus and subintimal arteriolar fibrosis lead to loss of peristalsis. Lower esophageal aperistalsis and poor or absent LES tone lead to symptoms of dysphagia and gastroesophageal reflux disease (GERD). Patients often develop esophagitis and esophageal strictures as a result of gastroesophageal reflux. Starnes et al reported a 9% to 12% incidence of Barrett's metaplasia in patients with scleroderma. We have encountered a significant incidence of Barrett's metaplasia in our own series.

Diagnosis

Esophageal involvement should be suspected in all patients with scleroderma, and a thorough evaluation should be performed, particularly in patients with symptoms of dysphagia or reflux. Initially an esophagogram should be obtained. Strictures can be identified clearly, and the classic lead pipe appearance of an atonic esophagus with reflux may be seen. Mass lesions of the esophagus can be excluded effectively from the differential diagnosis. Often this study shows reflux and the presence of an associated hiatal hernia. Esophagoscopy should be used to obtain biopsy specimens of suspicious lesions and to evaluate any changes consistent with Barrett's esophagus or dysplasia. In 1987, Katzka et al reported a 37% incidence of adenocarcinoma in three patients with scleroderma of the esophagus and Barrett's metaplasia. Manometry is essential in all patients with dysphagia and in patients with an aperistaltic distal esophagus as shown on esophagogram. Typically, patients with scleroderma show normal peristalsis within the proximal striated muscle of the esophagus and weak or absent peristalsis in the distal smooth muscle portion of the esophagus. Ineffective, low-amplitude contractions of the distal two thirds of the esophagus with diminished LES pressure are diagnostic of esophageal scleroderma. In patients with symptoms of reflux and a normal esophagogram or unremarkable esophagoscopy, 24-hour pH monitoring is a useful adjunct.

Medical Management

Control of systemic scleroderma typically is maintained with vasoactive medications and antiinflammatory agents. Antifibrotic agents may be used to reduce sclerosis. Patients with scleroderma and GERD without stricture or Barrett's esophagus should be treated aggressively with antireflux therapy. This therapy currently includes proton-pump inhibitors, such as omeprazole or esomeprazole magnesium. *Helicobacter pylori* eradication should be included when a biopsy specimen shows this organism. Patients with symptomatic strictures may be managed initially with bougie or pneumatic dilation to achieve symptom relief. Temporary relief can be obtained, but the risk of perforation must be assessed, especially in patients with poor nutritional status or patients taking steroids for treatment of the underlying systemic disease. Investigations of octreotide and intestinal motility may hold promise in improving distal esophageal motor function in patients with scleroderma.

Surgical Management

Surgery is reserved for the few patients who have reflux symptoms refractory to medical management and patients who develop strictures or Barrett's esophagus as a complication of GERD. The overall condition of the patient must be considered before surgical treatment, and the control of the systemic process must justify surgical treatment. Five-year survival from the time of diagnosis of scleroderma can approach 70%.

Antireflux operations, particularly the Collis gastroplasty combined with Belsey Mark IV repair, have been advocated for patients who have symptoms of GERD and have developed erosive esophagitis. Reconstruction of the esophagogastric junction in patients with scleroderma can be difficult due to the attenuated nature of the distal esophagus and the presence of esophageal shortening. Fundoplication without esophageal lengthening is a major reason for failure of the reconstruction. In 1976, Orringer et al reported successful resolution of symptoms after Collis-Belsey reconstruction of the esophagogastric junction. Manometric and pH monitoring confirmed these results 1 year postoperatively. Late recurrence of reflux symptoms was high, however, even after the authors changed to a Collis-Nissen repair. In addition, performance of a Nissen fundoplication in patients with poor esophageal motility can be complicated postoperatively by the gas-bloat syndrome and an inability to vomit.

Although resolution of reflux can be obtained with Collis-Belsey reconstruction of the esophagogastric junction, we have found that these results are not durable. Esophagitis or stricture formation recurs at an average of 4 years after antireflux procedures. Esophageal resection and colonic interposition should be considered as the initial treatment option for patients who are anticipated to have long-term survival. Motility disturbances and loss of the distal esophageal high-pressure zone compound the symptoms of reflux and dysphagia and are treated best with esophageal replacement. In addition, the incidence of adenocarcinoma in patients with Barrett's esophagus warrants aggressive therapy.

SUGGESTED READING

Feussner H, et al: The surgical management of motility disorders, *Dysphagia* 8:135, 1993.

Henderson RD, Pearson FG: Surgical management of esophageal scleroderma, *J Thorac Cardiovasc Surg* 66:686, 1973.

Katzka DA, et al: Barrett's metaplasia and adenocarcinoma of the esophagus in scleroderma, *Am J Med* 82:46, 1987.

Mansour KA: Update: surgery for scleroderma of the esophagus: a 12-year experience, *Ann Thorac Surg* 60:227, 1995.

Mansour KA, Malone CE: Surgery for scleroderma of the esophagus: a 12-year experience, *Ann Thorac Surg* 46:513, 1988.

Orringer MB: Surgical management of scleroderma reflux esophagitis, *Surg Clin North Am* 63:859, 1983.

Orringer MB, et al: Gastroesophageal reflux in esophageal scleroderma: diagnosis and implications, *Ann Thorac Surg* 22:120, 1976.

Orringer MB, et al: Combined Collis gastroplasty-fundoplication operations for scleroderma reflux esophagitis, *Surgery* 90:624, 1981.

Starnes UA, et al: Barrett's esophagus: a surgical entity, *Arch Surg* 119:563, 1984.

CONGENITAL AND ACQUIRED ESOPHAGEAL DIVERTICULA

Christopher T. Salerno

John D. Mitchell

Richard I. Whyte

Esophageal diverticula may arise from any location along the esophagus but classically are divided into three anatomic types: (1) pharyngoesophageal (Zenker's), (2) mid esophageal, and (3) epiphrenic. Other classification schemes refer to developmental origin (congenital or acquired), etiology (traction or pulsion), and structure (true or false). Most esophageal diverticula are acquired and occur in adults. Traction diverticula, which typically arise in the mid portion of the esophagus, result from an adjacent mediastinal inflammatory process that distracts the esophagus. Most esophageal diverticula encountered in the Western world are pulsion diverticula. These diverticula are the result of increased intraluminal pressure leading to mucosal and submucosal herniation through a weak point in the esophageal wall. Pulsion diverticula usually are associated with an esophageal motility disorder. Two types of pulsion diverticula commonly are recognized—pharyngoesophageal and epiphrenic diverticula. True diverticula are composed of all three layers of the esophageal wall, whereas false diverticula do not contain all three layers and typically consist of only the mucosa and submucosa.

■ CONGENITAL ESOPHAGEAL DIVERTICULA

Esophageal diverticula are extremely rare in infants and children. Diverticula that produce symptoms at a young age and on histologic examination contain all walls of the esophagus can be considered congenital diverticula. When a tracheoesophageal remnant is identified in the diverticulum, the lesion is identified more appropriately as a duplication rather than as a diverticulum. There are limited reports of true congenital diverticula in the literature, and most authors recommend diverticulectomy.

■ PHARYNGOESOPHAGEAL (ZENKER'S) DIVERTICULUM

Pharyngoesophageal (Zenker's) diverticula account for 60% to 65% of all esophageal diverticula. These diverticula originate in Killian's triangle, a weak point in the posterior esophagus, just proximal to the transverse fibers of the cricopharyngeal muscle and between the oblique fibers of the inferior pharyngeal constrictor muscle. Zenker's diverticulum is a pulsion diverticulum associated with incomplete, or discoordinate, upper esophageal sphincter relaxation. The resultant increased hypopharyngeal pressure produces a narrow-mouthed posterior diverticulum. The diverticulum progresses in size as saliva, food, and medications distend the sac.

Zenker's diverticula most commonly present in individuals in their 60s and have a twofold to threefold greater incidence in men than women. Symptoms depend on the stage of the disease. Early on, patients may complain of vague pharyngeal sensations, dysphagia, cough, and excess salivation. Later, more severe symptoms, such as severe (or frequent) dysphagia, regurgitation of food, halitosis, voice changes, aspiration, and odynophagia, may occur. One third of patients also complain of weight loss. Carcinoma arising in the diverticulum is rare (0.3% to 3%).

The diagnosis of a Zenker's diverticulum is made best by barium esophagogram, which shows a posterior midline protrusion just above the cricopharyngeus (Figure 1). Small diverticula may be transient. A posterior cricopharyngeal bar, or indentation, is a common radiographic finding and denotes a hypertrophic or nonrelaxing cricopharyngeus muscle. In evaluating patients with pharyngoesophageal diverticula, it is important to examine the remainder of the esophagus to exclude any additional esophageal pathology. Endoscopic assessment is controversial due to the risk of perforation. Esophageal manometry offers little in the evaluation of patients with pharyngoesophageal diverticula and is generally unnecessary.

Surgery is the only effective therapy for Zenker's diverticulum, and all patients should be considered surgical candidates. Respiratory or nutritional deficiencies, such as aspiration and weight loss, may be directly attributable to the diverticulum and should not be contraindications to surgery. Multiple different operative approaches have been proposed: diverticulum inversion, diverticulectomy, cricopharyngeal myotomy, diverticulectomy with myotomy, and myotomy with suspension of the diverticulum.

Diverticulum inversion should be avoided due to an unacceptably high rate of recurrence. Diverticulectomy alone is associated with a clinical recurrence rate of 20% and a radiographic recurrence rate approaching 85%. This is not surprising given the fact that diverticulectomy alone fails to deal with the underlying motor pathology.

Myotomy alone, which should correct the underlying physiologic abnormality, has been reported as 78% effective and may be considered for patients with small (<2 cm) diverticula. Diverticulectomy or suspension should be added if the diverticulum itself is large or dependent. Both procedures are performed via a left cervical incision and are associated with a low rate of recurrence and complications. Several reports suggest that avoiding opening the esophagus is associated with a lower rate of complications; however, these findings are not consistent, and it is likely that myotomy and diverticulectomy or diverticulum suspension are equivalent procedures.

The operation is performed using general anesthesia with endotracheal intubation. The patient is supine with the neck extended and the head turned to the right. An oblique incision is made at the anterior border of the sternocleidomastoid muscle. After the platysma is divided, the

Figure 1

Anteroposterior **(A)** and lateral **(B)** projections of a barium esophagogram of Zenker's diverticulum show a large midline barium-filled diverticulum.

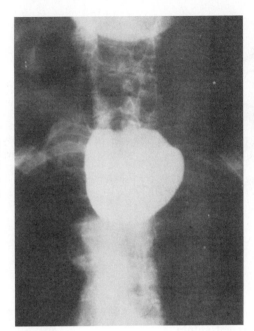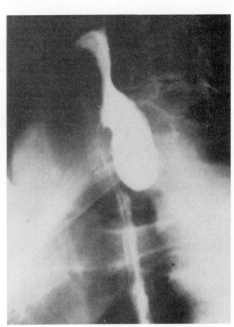

sternocleidomastoid muscle and the carotid sheath are retracted laterally. The thyroid gland and trachea are retracted medially; care is taken to avoid injury to the recurrent laryngeal nerve, which runs in the tracheoesophageal groove. The omohyoid muscle and inferior thyroid artery are divided. The diverticulum is identified, mobilized, and elevated. A myotomy is fashioned for a distance 4 to 6 cm caudally and 2 to 3 cm cranially, from the neck of the diverticulum (Figure 2). Passage of a bougie (36 Fr to 40 Fr) often helps to identify the correct submucosal plane and prevents narrowing of the esophagus if the diverticulum is excised. The divided muscle fibers of the esophagus and cricopharyngeus should be mobilized off the underlying submucosa and separated. Alternatively, some authors recommend resecting a segment of hypopharyngeal muscle.

The diverticulum may be either suspended or resected. If suspension is chosen, four to five fine silk sutures are used to tack the diverticulum to the posterior pharynx to allow for dependent drainage. Diverticulectomy may be performed using either a stapler or division and primary closure. Insufflating the esophagus while submerging the myotomy zone in saline can be useful to test mucosal integrity. A liquid diet is started on the first postoperative day, and the patient advances to a regular diet after discharge.

A large series of patients undergoing diverticulectomy at the Mayo Clinic showed a mortality of 1.2%, a leak rate of 1.7%, and a 3.1% incidence of unilateral vocal cord palsy. Almost all morbidity was seen in patients undergoing reoperative surgery. The success rate was 93% in follow-up ranging from 5 to 14 years.

Emphasis has been placed on endoscopic treatment of Zenker's diverticulum. In 1950, Dolhman described a procedure whereby a modified rigid esophagoscope and electrocautery were used to divide the wall between the true lumen and the diverticulum. With the development of endoscopic staplers, Collard et al proposed using a modified stapler to produce an esophagodiverticulostomy. The initial reports with a combined total of approximately 200 patients show excellent results. These early reports with limited follow-up show no increased risk of recurrence or mediastinal complications compared with standard surgical therapy.

■ MID ESOPHAGEAL DIVERTICULUM

By definition, mid esophageal diverticula occur in the middle one third of the esophagus. These "true" diverticula usually are found within 4 to 5 cm of the carina and constitute an estimated 10% to 17% of all esophageal diverticula. These diverticula often are wide-mouthed and more commonly occur on the right side. Classically, mid esophageal diverticula were classified as traction diverticula; however, more recent studies have shown that some mid esophageal diverticula are pulsion diverticula and are associated with an underlying esophageal motility disorder. Most mid esophageal diverticula are asymptomatic, although some patients may present with symptoms attributable to an underlying dysmotility syndrome. Occasionally, patients present with complications, including gastrointestinal bleeding, hemoptysis, pneumonia, or aspiration symptoms from an esophagobronchial or esophagovascular fistula.

The diagnosis of mid esophageal diverticula is made best by barium esophagogram. An effort should be made to identify any obvious underlying motility disorders during the radiographic evaluation, and preoperative manometry should be considered if the barium esophagogram is inconclusive. Endoscopy is helpful to assess complications of the diverticula. Computed tomography may be helpful in assessing the amount of mediastinal adenopathy, but other studies, such as magnetic resonance imaging or nuclear emptying studies, before surgery are not necessary.

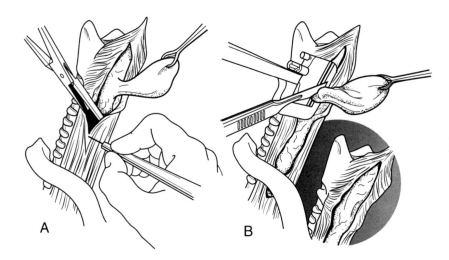

Figure 2
Repair of a cricopharyngeal diverticulum. Cricopharyngeal myotomy **(A)** and diverticulectomy **(B)**.

Most patients with mid esophageal diverticula do not require surgical intervention. In cases that present with a primary complication of the diverticulum, a right thoracotomy with excision of the inflammatory mass, primary closure of the fistula, and interposition of viable tissue should be performed. Mid esophageal diverticula associated with an esophageal motility disorder should be approached similarly. The diverticulum should be excised after passage of a bougie (46 Fr to 54 Fr). The diverticulum should be closed in two layers, and a contralateral myotomy should be performed.

■ EPIPHRENIC ESOPHAGEAL DIVERTICULUM

Epiphrenic diverticula arise in the distal 10 cm of the esophagus and are found more commonly projecting to the patient's right side. These diverticula are thought to be related to an underlying esophageal motility disorder and are considered to be pulsion diverticula. Most commonly present in individuals in their 50s, the clinical presentation is variable, with most patients presenting with symptoms related to the dysmotility syndrome, such as dysphagia, chest pain, or regurgitation. Rarely, patients may present with atrial fibrillation, hiccups, bleeding, or esophageal obstruction. Most patients with epiphrenic diverticula are asymptomatic, and there seems to be no relation between size of the diverticulum and symptoms.

All patients with suspected epiphrenic diverticula should undergo an esophagogram (Figure 3). This study establishes the diagnosis, rules out other pathology, and may show an associated motility disorder. Endoscopy has a limited role in the evaluation of these patients. Manometry should be attempted, although it may be difficult to perform because the catheter may pass into the diverticulum rather than through the true esophageal lumen. Surgery should be advised for symptomatic patients, whereas asymptomatic patients can be followed clinically.

The optimal operation for epiphrenic diverticula consists of diverticulectomy with esophagomyotomy. A common

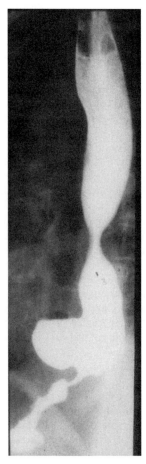

Figure 3
Barium esophagogram of a large epiphrenic diverticulum in a patient with known diffuse esophageal spasm.

approach involves a left thoracotomy through the seventh intercostal space. After the esophagus is mobilized and encircled with tapes, the diverticulum is mobilized. A diverticulectomy is performed over a 50 Fr bougie, and the esophagus may be closed with staples or sutures. The esophagomy-otomy should be performed opposite the diverticulectomy and should extend proximally above the diverticulum and distally onto the stomach. Because there is, by definition, an underlying motility disorder, the myotomy should be carried onto the stomach, and a nonobstructing fundoplication should be added to prevent significant postoperative reflux.

Controversy exists regarding the recommended length of the myotomy and the need for an antireflux procedure. Some authors have recommended a shorter myotomy, less mobilization of the hiatus and gastroesophageal junction, and no fundoplication. Most authors have advocated, however, a long myotomy—extending onto the stomach—arguing that a shorter myotomy results in continued functional obstruction with continued postoperative dysphagia at best and a dehisced esophageal suture line at worst. The longer myotomy and more extensive dissection around the hiatus predispose to reflux—hence the argument to add a nonobstructing partial fundoplication.

Laparoscopic diverticulectomy and myotomy have been described for diverticula in the distal 10 cm of the esophagus. The reported limited experience with this technique has been favorable with similar outcomes to those obtained with the open procedure. The surgical approach is similar to that used during laparoscopic fundoplication. The patient is placed in the lithotomy position, and the surgeon stands between the patient's legs. Five operating ports are placed after establishing a pneumoperitoneum. The peritoneum over the left and right crus is dissected, and the short gastric vessels are divided using a harmonic scalpel. The distal esophagus is encircled with a Penrose drain to facilitate downward traction of the gastroesophageal junction. The mediastinal dissection is performed in a blunt fashion. Dissection of the diverticula may be facilitated by the passage of a bougie or video endoscope. Using the endoscope, the esophagus can be inflated, deflated, or transilluminated to assist with the dissection. The diverticulum is amputated using an endoscopic stapler. The muscularis may be left open or closed with interrupted sutures. A myotomy is performed opposite the diverticula, and a partial (220 to 240 degrees) posterior fundoplication is fashioned. The patient can be started on a liquid diet on postoperative day 1 or 2 and can be advanced slowly.

■ INTRAMURAL ESOPHAGEAL DIVERTICULUM

Esophageal intramural diverticulosis is a rare condition usually identified on barium esophagogram. The intramural diverticula are dilated ducts of the esophageal submucosal glands, which are lined by squamous epithelium. The cause of these pseudodiverticula is unknown. Some authors have suggested an association with gastroesophageal reflux disease, diabetes mellitus, or esophageal candidiasis. Others have suggested that these are congenital lesions. Dysphagia is the primary symptom, and esophagectomy is the appropriate therapy.

■ SUMMARY

Esophageal diverticula most commonly are acquired pulsion diverticula. They may occur anywhere in the esophagus and are classified best by their anatomic location. The evaluation of almost all esophageal diverticula is similar—contrast esophagogram followed by manometry. Endoscopy plays a secondary role. There is no effective medical therapy for any esophageal diverticulum. Surgery should be offered to symptomatic patients. The procedure chosen should address the diverticulum and any underlying motility disorder.

SUGGESTED READING

Allen M: Treatment of epiphrenic diverticula, *Semin Thorac Cardiovasc Surg* 11:358, 1999.
Altorki N, et al: Thoracic esophageal diverticula: why is operation necessary? *J Thorac Cardiovasc Surg* 105:260, 1993.
Baker M, et al: Esophageal diverticula: patient assessment, *Semin Thorac Cardiovasc Surg* 11:326, 1999.
Eubanks T, Pelligrini C: Minimally invasive treatment of esophageal diverticula, *Semin Thorac Cardiovasc Surg* 11:363, 1999.
Rice T, Baker M: Midthoracic esophageal diverticula, *Semin Thorac Cardiovasc Surg* 11:352, 1999.
Rosati R, et al: Diverticulectomy, myotomy, and fundoplication through laparoscopy, *Ann Surg* 227:174, 1998.
Sidersis L, et al: The treatment of Zenker's diverticula: a review, *Semin Thorac Cardiovasc Surg* 11:337, 1999.

MEDICAL TREATMENT OF BARRETT'S ESOPHAGUS

William J. Ravich

Barrett's esophagus (BE) is a condition in which the squamous mucosa of the distal esophagus is replaced by columnar mucosa. BE is found in about 5% of gastroesophageal reflux disease (GERD) patients referred for endoscopy and 1% of patients undergoing endoscopy for any indication. The prevalence is higher in men than in women and in whites than in African Americans. A recognized complication of GERD, BE is of greatest clinical interest because of its role in the development of esophageal adenocarcinoma.

■ DIAGNOSIS

Diagnosis depends on endoscopy and endoscopy-directed biopsy. BE may appear as a circumferential band of columnar mucosa extending up into the esophagus, as tongue-like extensions of columnar mucosa protruding above an otherwise normal-appearing squamocolumnar junction, or as islands of columnar mucosa separated entirely from the squamocolumnar junction (Figure 1). Often, these findings are combined, with tongues or islands at the proximal margin of a length of circumferential columnar mucosa.

The characteristic histologic finding is incomplete intestinal metaplasia, a mixture of intestinal goblet cells and gastric mucin cells within the same microscopic fields. This histologic appearance commonly is referred to as *specialized columnar epithelium (SCE), specialized intestinal metaplasia,* or *distinctive-type Barrett's mucosa.* In addition to incomplete intestinal metaplasia, BE may contain areas of cardiac-type and fundic-type columnar mucosa.

Until about 1990, there was an additional widely accepted requirement for the diagnosis—that there be a minimum length of columnar-lined distal esophagus (most often stated as 3 cm). It is now recognized that shorter segments of SCE are relatively common, are associated with GERD, and carry an increased risk of malignant degeneration. Although no longer essential for the diagnosis of BE, a 3-cm length still commonly is used as the criterion separating long-segment BE from short-segment BE.

There is reason for concern that BE is currently underdiagnosed and overdiagnosed. Autopsy evidence suggests that most BE patients are not recognized before death. Reflux symptoms correlate poorly with severity of disease, and BE patients as a group are not more symptomatic than GERD patients without BE. Many patients never seek medical attention for reflux. Even among patients complaining of reflux symptoms, most probably never undergo endoscopy. The only way to improve the detection of BE would be to expand the criteria for endoscopy in GERD. It has been proposed that patients with long-standing GERD symptoms, especially patients older than age 50 years, are at particular risk for having BE and that this group should have a single endoscopy to look for BE.

In addition to underdiagnosis being a concern, there seems to be a lack of consensus and consistency in the criteria for diagnosis of BE, raising concern that some patients may be misdiagnosed with BE. A set of guidelines formulated by a committee of experts and accepted by the American College of Gastroenterology (ACG) requires the presence of incomplete intestinal metaplasia to make a diagnosis of BE. Although these guidelines have not been universally accepted, SCE is at risk for developing into adenocarcinoma.

A major problem involves the diagnosis of short-segment BE, which accounts for a substantial portion of the increased diagnosis of BE. Under normal circumstances, the junction of squamous and columnar mucosa clearly identifies the gastroesophageal junction. BE is precisely that condition,

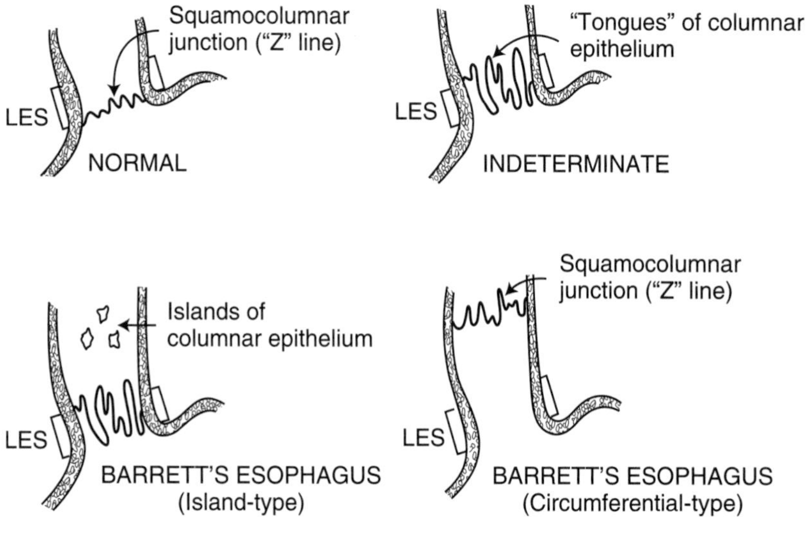

Figure 1

Variations in appearance of Barrett's esophagus. LES, lower esophageal sphincter. (*From Herlihy KJ, et al: Barrett's esophagus: clinical, endoscopic, histologic, manometric, and electrical potential difference characteristics,* Gastroenterology *86:436, 1984.*)

however, in which the squamocolumnar junction and gastroesophageal junction do not coincide. Many alternative endoscopic markers (the proximal margin of the gastric folds, the indentation produced by the lower esophageal sphincter, the change in luminal contour from saccular to tubular, and the loss of peristalsis) and histologic markers (cytokeratin staining characteristics) have been proposed, but the sensitivity and specificity of these markers are uncertain.

SCE sometimes is found in biopsy specimens obtained from a normal-looking squamocolumnar junction. Is the presence of SCE sufficient to make the diagnosis of BE? Biopsy specimens obtained from the gastric cardia have been reported to contain SCE in about 15% to 20% of individuals, show a different ethnic distribution than BE, and are not related to GERD. This information suggests that SCE is not specific to BE and casts into doubt the diagnosis of BE if there is any question about whether the biopsy specimens were taken from the esophagus.

I favor the proposal that a single endoscopy should be performed in patients with long-standing GERD that requires continuous drug therapy to maintain symptomatic control, especially in white men, who appear to be at particularly high risk for BE and Barrett's cancer. In the absence of erosive esophagitis or BE, the likelihood of developing BE in the future would seem to be remote, and the examination does not need to be repeated unless a change in the patient's clinical condition warrants.

The diagnosis of BE must be accepted with caution in the absence of SCE on histology, regardless of the apparent length of BE. In the presence of SCE, but with less than 3 cm of columnar looking epithelium, diagnostic certainty depends on the endoscopist's certainty that the tissue definitely was obtained from the distal esophagus and not the cardia. If there is any question, the diagnosis should be accepted as tentative only. Referral to a center with an established interest in BE might be appropriate for a second opinion. I do not consider specialized intestinal metaplasia at a normal-appearing gastroesophageal junction to represent BE.

■ REFLUX TREATMENT

Erosive esophagitis and continuing exposure to noxious gastric contents are prerequisites for the development of BE. The role of ongoing contact with gastric contents may explain why other forms of erosive esophagitis do not seem to cause BE and why patients with BE as a group have more severe acid reflux by continuous pH monitoring than patients with uncomplicated GERD or patients with reflux esophagitis without BE. When erosive disease is controlled effectively, BE does not increase in length.

Bile reflux has been proposed as a major factor in BE and Barrett's cancer. Bile seems to play a permissive role in reflux esophagitis, amplifying the damaging effect of refluxed acid. Studies suggest that proton-pump inhibitors (PPIs) not only diminish acid reflux, but also decrease bile reflux, possibly due to a general decrease in gastric secretions. Given the consensus that antireflux surgery does not seem to diminish the risk of Barrett's cancer, most gastroenterologists have been reluctant to accept the proposal that bile reflux is a major factor in malignant degeneration and that as a result antireflux

surgery should be considered the primary treatment for this condition.

Studies indicate that *Helicobacter pylori* gastritis may accelerate healing of reflux esophagitis and that eradication of *H. pylori* in GERD may exacerbate reflux disease. This purported protective influence of *H. pylori* in GERD has been disputed. Until this issue is resolved, it seems prudent to treat *H. pylori* gastritis for appropriate nonreflux indications, but not to attempt eradication as part of reflux management. Any exacerbation of reflux disease that does occur should respond to more intensive reflux therapy.

The treatment of reflux in BE is similar to that for severe reflux disease in general (Table 1) and usually includes behavioral changes and drug therapy. Behavioral changes include losing weight; eating smaller meals; avoiding lying down after eating; elevating the head of the bed; and avoiding foods, beverages, and drugs that overdistend the stomach, increase gastric acid secretion, decrease lower esophageal sphincter tone, or alter esophageal or gastric motility. (A full description of the dietary and lifestyle modifications lies beyond the scope of this chapter but can be found in any general review of the treatment of GERD.) Full compliance with all these measures can be disruptive and impractical. With PPI therapy, rigid adherence is not as crucial as it has been in the past. The greatest attention should be paid to the individual's actual behaviors that are most likely to be reflux provoking.

Because BE is associated with more severe reflux disease, PPIs usually are indicated. Occasional patients who are not on any treatment or already are taking H_2 receptor antagonists (H_2RAs) can be started or continued on these medications. In patients with active erosions, healing should be confirmed endoscopically. Drug therapy probably should be continued indefinitely. Attempting to fine-tune the intensity of therapy is probably misguided.

With current PPI drug therapy, truly refractory erosive disease is relatively rare. Compliance with medical therapy should be reviewed, and greater adherence to the commonly recommended dietary and lifestyle modifications should be instituted. A careful drug history should be taken looking for the use of drugs that cause pill-induced esophagitis (e.g., nonsteroidal antiinflammatory drugs, tetracycline, potassium, iron, bisphosphonates, quinidine, clindamycin).

Refractory erosive esophagitis usually can be controlled by increasing the intensity of acid suppression therapy. Choices include changing the specific PPI prescribed, increasing the dose of PPI therapy, or adding an evening dose of an H_2RA to a morning dose of PPI. Prokinetic agents have a modest incremental effect in reflux disease when added to either H_2RA or PPI therapy. With withdrawal of cisapride from the U.S. market because of life-threatening side effects and the often disturbing side effects seen with metoclopramide, prokinetic agents are being used less frequently than in the past. In countries where the prokinetic agent domperidone is available, it might be considered to supplement acid-suppressive agents.

Antireflux surgery should be considered for patients with refractory disease who find the necessary behavior modifications unacceptable or patients who are truly refractory to therapy. I consider severe esophageal paresis and marked gastroparesis to be relatively strong contraindications to surgery. It is crucial that the patient understand the risks of

Table 1 Medical Treatment of Gastroesophageal Reflux Disease Complicated by Barrett's Esophagus

CONDITION	THERAPEUTIC INVENTION
BE without erosions in patient who is not on reflux therapy	H_2RA therapy in standard doses
BE without erosions in patient who is on reflux therapy	Continue current reflux therapy
BE with erosions in patient who is not on reflux therapy	Look for and correct behavioral factors that might be exacerbating reflux
	Take careful drug history with attention to drugs that might impair UGI motility or cause drug-induced esophagitis
	Start PPI therapy in standard doses
BE with erosions in patient on standard-dose PPI therapy	Emphasize compliance with behavioral modifications and drug therapy
	Retake careful drug history with attention to drugs that might impair UGI motility or cause drug-induced esophagitis
	Increase intensity of acid suppression therapy
	Consider addition of prokinetic agent, especially in patients with documented gastroparesis
	Discuss and evaluate for possible antireflux surgery
BE with erosions in patient on intensive acid suppression therapy	Discuss and evaluate for possible antireflux surgery

BE, Barrett's esophagus; H_2RA, H_2 receptor antagonist; UGI, upper gastrointestinal; PPI, proton-pump inhibitor.

surgery, including the possibility of relapse, and the fact that surveillance of BE still will be required.

■ SURVEILLANCE

It is common practice to enter patients with BE into a surveillance program involving periodic endoscopies with biopsies of the BE. The risk of malignant transformation is reported to be about 10% in many retrospective studies. The prospective risk of developing cancer is difficult to determine, but an annual incidence of about 1% has been suggested. These statistics should be interpreted with some caution because of the possibility of reporting bias. Some studies have indicated that the number of patients found to have carcinomas during surveillance endoscopy is quite low, although when cancer is found as part of a surveillance program it is often at an early and surgically curable stage.

BE seems to pass through a series of stages of increasing cellular atypia, changes that resemble the cytologic changes of cancer. These microscopic changes, called *dysplasia*, can be detected with endoscopic biopsy. Most patients never develop dysplasia, but patients who do are at an increased risk of cancer. The more severe the dysplasia, the greater the risk of cancer. The detection of dysplasia is a secondary goal of surveillance endoscopy in BE.

Studies have shown substantial interobserver variation among trained gastrointestinal pathologists in the diagnosis of low-grade dysplasia (LGD) with the probability of progression increasing along with agreement in the pathologic interpretation of dysplasia. Confirmation of the diagnosis by a pathologist experienced in the use of the dysplasia grading system is advisable before any major and irreversible clinical decisions are made. Treatment of active esophagitis may be required before a final diagnosis or grade of dysplasia to avoid difficulty in distinguishing reactive changes from dysplasia. Although many surrogate markers have been proposed (aneuploidy, increased 4N fraction, overexpression of the *p53* tumor-expressor gene), none have gained wide acceptance as substitutes for the evaluation for dysplasia.

Because LGD and high-grade dysplasia (HGD) usually are not visible to the endoscope-assisted eye, a systematic approach to tissue sampling should be taken. Biopsy specimens should be obtained from the entire area of BE and not just from suspicious focal lesions. The more ardent practitioners of this systematic approach advocate the routine use of large-capacity ("jumbo") biopsy forceps to improve the quantity of tissue obtained. Alternatively the use of methylene blue, sprayed through the endoscope, has been proposed as a means of identifying areas of particular concern. The dye stains nondysplastic Barrett's mucosa more consistently than areas of dysplasia and cancer, permitting targeting of tissue sampling.

In recognition of the infrequency with which cancers are detected, recommendations have favored extending the intervals between surveillance endoscopies for nondysplastic BE. Patients with dysplasia on previous endoscopies are targeted for more frequent surveillance. The hope is that the number of endoscopies can be decreased without significantly diminishing the chance of cure should Barrett's cancer be detected.

I follow a modification version of the recommendations proposed by the ACG, expanded to account for a variety of scenarios not specifically covered in the ACG guidelines (Table 2). The length of Barrett's segment and dysplasia status affect the subsequent decisions. I obtain tissue samples, preferably using large particle biopsy forceps, from all obvious nodules, masses, and ulcers and systematically sample the entire length of flat Barrett's mucosa, generally

Table 2 Recommendations for Surveillance in Barrett's Esophagus

DYSPLASIA	RECOMMENDATIONS*
None	Determine adequacy of tissue sampling Repeat EGD in 1 and 2 yr with systematic tissue sampling to confirm absence of dysplasia If still no dysplasia, surveillance EGD at 2- to 3-yr intervals
SIM of normal-looking GE junction without dysplasia No dysplasia	Review endoscopic report to confirm location of biopsy specimens Avoid diagnosis of Barrett's esophagus Reassure patient No follow-up EGD unless required to confirm endoscopic description or for patient who is overwhelmed by anxiety
Low-grade	Repeat endoscopy in 6 and 12 mo, then every year If LGD absent on two consecutive endoscopies, increase intervals between surveillance EGD to that for no dysplasia If LGD persists, surveillance EGD at 12-mo intervals
High-grade	Confirm pathologic diagnosis If focal HGD only, repeat endoscopy and biopsies to confirm If HGD is reproducible or multifocal HGD, consider esophagectomy If patient is poor surgical candidate or refuses esophagectomy, follow with endoscopies every 3 mo

*Author's adaptation of American College of Gastroenterology Practice Guidelines (Sampliner R: The Practice Parameters Committee of the American College of Gastroenterology, *Am J Gastroenterol* 93:1028, 1998.)
EGD, esophagogastroduodenoscopy; SIM, specialized intestinal metaplasia; GE, gastroesophageal; LGD, low-grade dysplasia; HGD, high-grade dysplasia.

following what has been described as the Seattle protocol. I have not routinely incorporated the use of methylene blue staining, and I do not obtain surrogate markers, but I may consider their use in the future.

■ INTERVENTION

The risk of cancer in LGD is relatively modest. Simply modifying the surveillance program, with endoscopies at shorter intervals and perhaps more intensive tissue sampling, generally is suggested (see Table 2). Detection of invasive carcinoma should lead to the evaluation for possible esophagectomy. Most gastroenterologists favor esophageal resection, pointing to the high rate of coincident cancer reported in patients who undergo esophagectomy for endoscopically detected HGD and the high prospective risk of subsequently developing cancer. Others have followed patients with HGD without definite cancer and believe that although the risk of developing cancer is relatively high, patients who do not progress are spared unnecessary surgery, and curative surgery remains possible in patients who are found to have esophageal cancer on subsequent endoscopy.

Dysplasia of any grade in a nodule, polyp, or mass of any size, referred to as a *dysplasia-associated lesion or mass,* suggests that the lesion may contain undetected invasive carcinoma. Endoscopic ultrasound should be performed to stage the lesions for possible esophagectomy. For patients in whom the tumor appears to be limited to the mucosal layer, especially if elderly or poor operative risks, endoscopic mucosectomy has been suggested as an alternative approach. If the entire lesion is recovered and dysplasia is confined to the mucosal layer, the patient needs to be followed with frequent surveillance endoscopies.

Barrett's ablation has been proposed as an alternative to reflux treatment with periodic surveillance. The approach involves therapeutically induced ulceration of the involved mucosal surface, using one of a variety of techniques, along with aggressive acid suppression with PPIs. With repeated treatment sessions, total or near-total visual eradication can be achieved in a high proportion of patients. Complications include bleeding, perforation, and stricture formation.

Although the concept of Barrett's ablation has a certain appeal, experience with this approach is limited, and the long-term impact on outcome is unknown. Pseudoregression with reepithelialization of squamous mucosa over retained, and now hidden, islands of Barrett's mucosa has been described. There is concern that these islands may prove difficult to follow for malignant degeneration. It is unclear who should be considered for Barrett's ablation—patients with nondysplastic Barrett's mucosa, patients with LGD in hopes that ablation might result in regression of LGD, or patients with HGD without an obvious nodule or mass.

When cancer is found, the patient should be staged and evaluated for possible esophagectomy. Unless there is a strong contraindication, I encourage patients with HGD in flat Barrett's mucosa to consider esophagectomy, but I discuss the option of close follow-up with frequent surveillance endoscopies. Patients generally decide based on their willingness to accept the long-term risk of developing cancer and their anxiety that delay might affect the chances of cure. The mortality of esophagectomy in a good surgical candidate, particularly a patient younger than 70 years old, is extremely low, and the morbidity risk is reasonable. Clinically significant postoperative gastroparesis has occurred in a few patients postoperatively but can be extremely difficult to treat when it does occur. I consider Barrett's ablation and photodynamic therapy evolving interventions for BE complicated by cancer limited to the mucosal layer.

SUGGESTED READING

Drewitz DJ, et al: The incidence of adenocarcinoma in Barrett's esophagus: a prospective study of 170 patients followed 4.8 years, *Am J Gastroenterol* 92:212, 1997.

Levine DS, et al: An endoscopic biopsy protocol can differentiate high-grade dysplasia from early adenocarcinoma in Barrett's esophagus, *Gastroenterology* 105:40, 1993.

Peters JH, et al: Outcome of adenocarcinoma arising in Barrett's esophagus in endoscopically surveyed and nonsurveyed patients, *J Thorac Cardiovasc Surg* 108:813, 1994.

Sampliner RE, et al: Effective and safe endoscopic reversal of nondysplastic Barrett's esophagus with thermal electrocoagulation combined with high-dose acid inhibition: a multicenter study, *Gastrointest Endosc* 53:554, 2001.

Sampliner R: The Practice Parameters Committee of the American College of Gastroenterology: practice guidelines on the diagnosis, surveillance, and therapy of Barrett's esophagus, *Am J Gastroenterol* 93:1028, 1998.

SURGICAL THERAPY FOR BARRETT'S ESOPHAGUS

Dmitry Oleynikov
Carlos A. Pellegrini

Barrett's esophagus (BE) presents a unique challenge for a surgeon because it invariably arises as a result of chronic distal esophageal injury induced by reflux. The incidence of this disease is on the rise in the Western hemisphere. There are many theories that attempt to explain this phenomenon, but most agree that pathologic evidence of BE is a risk factor for malignancy. Investigators report an estimated 40-fold to 50-fold increase in incidence of adenocarcinoma over the general population if BE is diagnosed, and an even higher percentage of patients will progress to cancer if dysplasia is present at the time of diagnosis. Most patients come to medical attention after endoscopy for long-standing symptoms of gastroesophageal reflux. Prolonged exposure to gastric acid and bile is considered important in the pathogenesis of BE. Endoscopic surveillance is necessary to monitor Barrett's epithelium for progression to adenocarcinoma, and the interval between endoscopy varies with the pathologic findings at initial biopsy. There is a spectrum of therapeutic intervention when BE is discovered ranging from medical management to esophagectomy. This is an area of considerable controversy requiring the treating physician to tailor patient management depending on the clinical circumstances and pathologic findings.

◼ DIAGNOSIS

BE is a pathologic diagnosis based on the identification of specialized intestinal metaplasia at the gastroesophageal junction.

The presence of goblet cells that replace normal squamous columnar epithelium of the esophagus on microscopic examination is pathognomonic for BE. Because gross endoscopic inspection of the esophagus may be inaccurate, a biopsy specimen must be obtained when BE is suspected. BE may be seen in conjunction with esophagitis, and several areas should be sampled with biopsy technique to avoid sampling error. Traditionally, such intestinal metaplasia had to be present for a length of 3 cm when measured from the gastroesophageal junction for a patient to be diagnosed as having BE. BE less than 3 cm is defined as short segment disease, and contrary to previous thinking this distinction may be artificial. Evidence suggests that length in and of itself does not *stratify* risk for the development of malignancy. Any length of visible BE, if it contains intestinal metaplasia on histologic inspection, is diagnostic of BE. A long segment of BE may make surveillance difficult given the number of biopsy specimens that must be taken. Expertise in pathology is often necessary to confirm the diagnosis, especially if dysplasia is seen. This distinction is clinically important and can be divided further into low-grade or indeterminate-grade dysplasia and high-grade dysplasia. Pathologic grade of dysplasia is the best risk stratification technique currently in clinical use.

◼ TREATMENT

The presence or absence of dysplasia is the most important initial consideration when evaluating treatment options. BE without dysplasia may be managed by reducing or eliminating reflux either pharmacologically with proton-pump inhibitors or by performing antireflux surgery. Because chronic gastroesophageal reflux disease is implicated strongly in the development of BE, we pay special attention to patients' presenting symptoms. Fit, symptomatic patients who have BE should undergo a total fundoplication. To plan appropriately for the operation, several studies must be performed, including esophageal manometry, 24-hour pH studies, and barium upper gastrointestinal studies. By recreating a competent gastroesophageal valve, acid and bile reflux theoretically are eliminated. Because elimination is not achieved with proton-pump therapy, and medical therapy may render patients asymptomatic even when they are still refluxing, an operation is the best option. Medical therapy should be reserved for patients who are too frail to undergo surgery. We do not recommend endoscopic mucosal ablation of BE in patients without dysplasia. Asymptomatic patients also should be offered an antireflux procedure because there is mounting evidence that this may prevent patients from developing dysplasia and cancer by decreasing acid and alkaline exposure. Because regression of BE may not occur after antireflux surgery, patients need to undergo endoscopic survey every 2 to 3 years to search for progression of the disease to dysplasia or malignancy. This occurs infrequently if no dysplasia is present. The exact risk of developing malignancy is hard to determine but usually is quoted as 40 to 50 times that of the general population. A longitudinal study of patients with BE found that if the initial biopsy specimen showed absence of high-grade dysplasia, the risk of developing cancer over a 6-year (mean) follow-up was 0.7% per year. The risk rose to 23% per year if the patient's initial biopsy specimen showed high-grade dysplasia. In another study, the incidence of malignancy after 5 years of follow-up in patients initially diagnosed with low-grade dysplasia was 12%.

Patients who come to the clinic with a diagnosis of high-grade dysplasia are placed on double doses of proton-pump inhibitors for 2 months. At the end of 2 months, a repeat endoscopy is performed with special attention to any mucosal irregularity. Multiple biopsy specimens are obtained of all suspicious areas and every 1 cm of the BE segment. Endoscopic ultrasound is employed if a specific lesion is identified. In some cases, only BE without dysplasia is identified on the follow-up biopsy specimen. This finding simply means that the inflammation present before initiation of therapy led to an erroneous diagnosis. These patients must be followed at 3-month intervals once or twice to ensure that there is no high-grade dysplasia. If this proves to be the case (i.e., high-grade dysplasia has been ruled out), we offer antireflux surgery.

Postoperatively, we perform surveillance endoscopy and close follow-up.

When a patient is referred with a diagnosis of high-grade dysplasia and is proved eventually to have high-grade dysplasia, the situation is different. Using multiple biopsy specimens and endoscopic ultrasound, many of these patients are found to have an adenocarcinoma, and the patient is offered an esophagectomy after appropriate staging. For the subset of patients who persist with high-grade dysplasia, preoperative counseling is initiated. This discussion includes the risk of esophagectomy given the patients' age and their general state of health, length of BE, and their access to medical care. Younger patients who are able to undergo the operation are offered an esophagectomy. Older patients in poor health or patients with short segment disease who are willing to undergo close endoscopic follow-up may be watched. Endoscopic mucosal ablation is a promising alternative for this group of patients.

The rationale for proceeding directly to surgical intervention when the diagnosis of high-grade dysplasia is confirmed can be found in the pathologic findings after esophagectomy. Table 1 summarizes 15 studies that have looked at the rate of missed adenocarcinoma on final pathology in patients who were thought to have only high-grade dysplasia. Combining patients from all these studies, 43% of patients harbored adenocarcinoma at the time of resection. This finding can be contrasted with the relatively low operative mortality rates reported by these authors. As a result, early and aggressive resection may provide a safe alternative for patients who are at a particularly high risk of progression to malignancy.

■ SURGICAL TECHNIQUE

When a decision to proceed with esophagectomy is reached in patients with high-grade dysplasia, we perform a laparoscopically assisted transhiatal esophagectomy. Patients are placed in low lithotomy position, allowing the surgeon to

Table 1 Missed Adenocarcinoma and Operative Mortality in All Patients with High-Grade Dysplasia Only on Preoperative Esophagoscopy Who Underwent an Esophagectomy

REFERENCE	YEAR	NO. PATIENTS	n (%)	MORTALITY, n/%
Hamilton and Smith	1987	5	3 (60)	0
Altorki et al	1991	8	3 (38)	0
Pera et al	1992	18	9 (50)	0
Levine et al	1993	7	0 (0)	1/14
Rice et al	1993	16	6 (38)	1/6
Streitz et al	1993	9	2 (22)	0
Wright et al	1994	15	7 (47)	0
Peters et al	1994	9	5 (55)	0
Edwards et al	1996	11	8 (73)	0
Heitmiller et al	1996	30	13 (43)	1/3.3
Ferguson and Naunheim	1997	15	11 (73)	0
Cameron and Carpenter	1997	19	2 (10)	0
Falk et al	1999	12	4 (33)	0
Other		10	7 (70)	0
Total		184	80 (43)	3/2

Adapted from Pellegrini CA, Pohl D: *J Gastrointest Surg* 4:131, 2000.

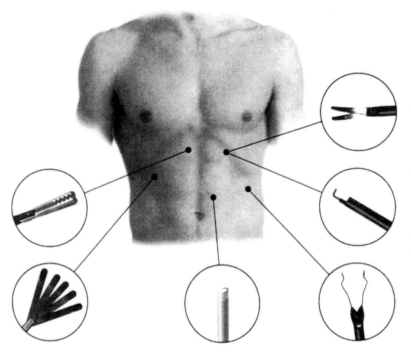

Figure 1
Trocar positioning and instrumentation. Camera port: 10-mm 30-degree scope. Right epigastric 5-mm port: atraumatic grasper. Left medial port: Endoshear and L-hook electrocautery-irrigation device. Right lateral port: fan liver retractor. Left lateral trocar: Endo-Babcock (United States Surgical Corporation, Tyco). (*From Kao CC, Pellegrini CA: In Cameron JL, editor:* Current surgical therapy, *ed 6, St. Louis, 1998, Mosby, p 1237.*)

operate between the patients' legs. Ports are placed in a location similar to that which would be used for an antireflux procedure (Figure 1). A careful gastric mobilization is performed by transection of short gastric vessels, mobilization of the esophagus from the hiatus, and careful dissection in the mediastinum for approximately 8 to 12 cm of the thoracic esophagus. The left gastric artery ligation and transection, mobilization of the duodenum with pyloromyotomy, and tubularization of the stomach are performed through a limited upper midline incision. The cervical esophagus is identified on the left side, and a stapled esophageal anastomosis is performed. It also is possible first to do a thorough thoracoscopic mobilization of the esophagus and follow with a laparoscopic mobilization of the gastric conduit. Several groups have reported good outcomes with this technique without excessive operative times, but most studies to date have failed to show a distinct advantage over the open approach. Another surgical option includes an en bloc esophagectomy, with abdominal and thoracic exposure. We reserve this procedure for patients who harbor transmural lesions, which seldom are encountered in patients with high-grade BE. Although we routinely use the stomach as a conduit, the colon and the small bowel remain viable options when an adequate gastric tube cannot be performed.

■ CONCLUSION

The management of BE continues to evolve as new insights in the pathogenesis are discovered. As a uniform standard of care is being debated, recommendations for diagnosis and management are also in flux. New molecular markers promise to stratify the risk of progression to malignancy with better accuracy. Novel medical and surgical techniques are being developed to target mucosa at risk, and a better understanding of the etiology may produce prevention strategies. Careful evaluation of BE can produce excellent outcomes for patients at risk.

SUGGESTED READING

DeMeester SR, DeMeester TR: Columnar mucosa and intestinal metaplasia of the esophagus: fifty years of controversy, *Ann Surg* 231:303, 2000.

Overholt BF, Panjehpour M: Photodynamic therapy in the management of Barrett's esophagus with dysplasia, *J Gastrointest Surg* 4:129, 2000.

Pellegrini CA: The role of minimal-access surgery in esophageal disease, *Curr Opin Gen Surg* 2:117, 1994.

Pellegrini CA, Pohl D: High-grade dysplasia in Barrett's esophagus: surveillance or operation? *J Gastrointest Surg* 4:131, 2000.

ESOPHAGEAL INFECTIONS

Manoel Ximenes Netto

Esophageal infections are a common cause of complications in immunosuppressed patients, including patients infected with human immunodeficiency virus (HIV) and less frequently patients with malignancies and transplants. In immunocompetent hosts, esophagitis is unusual, and the predisposing conditions include local or systemic factors, such as antibiotic treatment, the use of inhaled corticosteroids, potent antisecretory drugs (H_2 blockers), alcoholism, malnutrition, advanced age, diabetes mellitus, adrenal insufficiency, achalasia, and any other cause of long-standing esophageal obstruction. Patients usually present with painful swallowing (odynophagia), difficulty in swallowing (dysphagia), and retrosternal chest pain. When symptomatic, these opportunistic infections are associated with a poor outcome—hence the necessity of early diagnosis and treatment in individuals with acquired immunodeficiency syndrome (AIDS).

The causative agents in esophageal infections are various, and fungal, viral, bacterial, and parasitic organisms may be found. HIV-positive patients may be infected with several organisms, and 21% to 35% may present with esophageal symptoms that are sustained by the infecting microorganisms. Table 1 lists infecting agents in immunocompetent and immunocompromised individuals.

■ FUNGAL INFECTIONS IN HIV PATIENTS

Candidiasis is the most frequent infection in HIV patients, and *Candida albicans,* a normal inhabitant of the intestinal flora, is responsible for most infections in these patients. Other *Candida* species, such as *C. tropicalis, C. glabrata,* and *C. krusei,* are less numerous. The incidence of esophageal problems in HIV-infected patients when examined by the gastroenterologist showed the average following results in 207 cases: *Candida,* 60% (n = 119); cytomegalovirus (CMV),

15.3% (n = 40); herpes simplex virus (HSV), 11% (n = 22); Kaposi's sarcoma, 6% (n = 6); noninfectious ulcerations, 5.6% (n = 17); and no lesions 17.3% (n = 40). *Candida* esophagitis is present in 49% to 79% of the symptomatic population, but on the whole 25% have multiple fungal or viral infections.

The infecting mechanism has two steps. First, there is colonization with superficial adhesion and proliferation in the upper gastrointestinal tract. Second, there is epithelial infection, which requires a defect in the defense mechanism (cellular immunity). In clinical practice, the differentiation between the two (colonization and infection) is verified by means of the gross appearance of the exudate and the microscopic study of the biopsy specimens.

■ VIRAL INFECTIONS

Virus esophagitis is second in prevalence of infections in HIV-positive patients, although normal hosts also may be infected. HSV, varicella-zoster virus (VZV), and CMV are the most common infecting agents. Other less common viruses include Epstein-Barr virus (EBV), HIV, human papillomavirus (HPV), papovavirus, and poliovirus. The type of ulceration and the pathogenesis may vary among viruses: HSV and VZV cause epithelial necrosis, whereas in CMV infection the damage is on the submucosal tissue. HSV infection usually presents with the usual symptoms of all viral infections (painful swallowing, retrosternal pain, and heartburn), although other symptoms, such as nausea, vomiting, and hematemesis, may be the initial complaints. A presumptive diagnosis may be made when confronted with HSV infection of the mouth and nares. CMV differs from HSV in regard to transmission, which may be acquired from blood product transfusion and organ donation. It is usually part of a widespread infection involving the gastrointestinal system and solid viscera. The patient presents with anorexia, nausea, vomiting, and painful swallowing. Acute retrosternal pain is uncommon. VZV may cause severe damage to the esophagus in the immunocompromised patient. In rare instances, the esophagus may be involved in children carrying chickenpox and adults with herpes zoster.

EBV is unusual in immunocompetent and immunocompromised individuals. In patients with AIDS and esophageal symptoms, EBV was found by in situ hybridization at the

---

Table 1 Causative Organisms in Esophagitis

FUNGAL	VIRAL	BACTERIAL	PARASITIC
Candida albicans	Cytomegalovirus	Gram-positive coccobacilli	*Cryptosporidium*
Candida krusei	Herpes simplex virus	Gram-negative bacilli	*Pneumocystis carinii*
Candida glabrata	Epstein-Barr virus	*Actinomyces*	*Leishmania donovani*
Candida parapsilosis	Human immunodeficiency	*Mycobacterium avium-intracellulare*	*Trypanosoma cruzi*
Candida guilliermondii	virus	*Treponema pallidum* (syphilis)	(Chagas' disease)
Histoplasma capsulatum	Varicella-zoster virus	*Helicobacter pylori*	
Cryptococcus	Papillomavirus		
	Poliovirus		

esophageal ulcer base. HIV may be seen in giant ulcers, which may progress to fistulization into the mediastinum. Other viral infections, such as HSV, should be ruled out.

HPV, responsible for warts and condylomas in the genitalia of healthy individuals, occasionally may produce giant lesions in immunocompromised patients and, rarely, esophageal lesions. Papovavirus and poliovirus have been described in rare patients.

■ BACTERIAL ESOPHAGITIS

Infectious esophagitis due to bacteria is unusual in granulocytopenic patients and normal individuals. It may present as primary infection in patients with AIDS or as a secondary infection from adjacent organs, such as *Mycobacterium tuberculosis*. Gram-positive cocci and gram-negative bacilli normally present in the oropharynx may be the infecting agent in the esophagus, as ulceration distally. Bacterial esophagitis may be seen in 11% to 16% of autopsied material. High fever and bacteremia may be the only symptoms.

Tuberculosis, a rare condition in more recent years, has been on the rise secondary to the HIV epidemic. The usual presentation is secondary to pulmonary tuberculosis rather than primary, and it may be seen from the pharynx to the level of the carina. Symptoms include dysphagia, pain (retrosternal), and cough, with fistulization as a late event. *Mycobacterium avium-intracellulare, Treponema pallidum* (syphilis), *Corynebacterium diphtheriae* (diphtheria), *Clostridium tetani* (tetanus), and *Helicobacter pylori* occasionally may cause esophageal symptoms. *H. pylori*, a more recently described organism found in patients with gastritis and duodenal ulcers, has not been encountered in the normal esophagus.

■ IDIOPATHIC CHRONIC ULCERS

When all diagnostic studies fail to show other causes of an esophageal ulcer, the ulcerated lesion may be considered idiopathic. Even in these cases, HIV has been found by means of combinations of RNA in situ hybridization, immunohistochemistry, and antigen capture enzyme-linked immunosorbent assay of tissue homogenates. The suggestion is that these ulcerated lesions are due to a cytopathogenic effect of HIV infection.

■ PARASITIC INFECTION

Cryptosporidium and *Pneumocystis carinii* as opportunistic infections have been described in HIV-infected patients and found as nonspecific inflammations in the distal part of the esophagus. *Leishmania donovani,* a protozoan disorder found in epidemic areas of the Mediterranean basin, Asia, Africa, and South America, also has been described in HIV patients and involving other areas, such as the liver.

Chagas' disease, a trypanosomiasis caused by a protozoan, *Trypanosoma cruzi*, has been described throughout the Americas from Northern California to Southern Argentina and Chile. The human infection extends from the southern United States to the State of Chubut in Argentina. More than 100 vertebrate hosts have been naturally infected with the parasite. Trioatomines usually live in rural areas in easy contact with vertebrates, such as birds, reptiles, bats, and dogs. Even though only three authenticated cases have been described in the United States, the large number of Latin American immigrants contaminated with *T. cruzi* may be a source of contamination through blood transfusion and organ donation. In Latin America, 4.8 to 5.4 million people may be infected with Chagas' disease, and of these 10% to 12% have overt esophageal achalasia.

■ DIAGNOSIS AND TREATMENT

The clinical findings of esophagitis infection—due to fungus and virus—include odynophagia and heartburn, and in severe cases, melena and hematemesis may result. If left untreated, the disease may progress to necrosis with perforation and bleeding, and large tumor-like masses (fungus ball) may appear. When nausea, vomiting, abdominal pain, intestinal bleeding, cough, fever, and diarrhea also are present, other pathogenic organisms should be sought. Oral thrush is a frequent finding in esophageal infection, and when seen in the HIV-infected patient, the predictive value of candidiasis varies between 70% and 100%. Careful examination of the mouth and pharynx may give clues as to the type of infection. Oropharyngeal candidiasis may be an indication of esophageal disease. Of HIV-positive patients, 25% have concomitant diagnoses, including viruses. In most instances, there is no relationship between the cause of the esophageal infection and any particular type of symptoms.

The best and most accurate method to diagnose fungal esophagitis is by endoscopy with brushing and biopsy specimens. A grading scale has been described as follows: grade I, a few elevated plaques up to 2 mm without ulceration; grade II, many raised white plaques more than 2 mm, without ulceration; grade III, confluent, linear, and nodular elevated plaques with ulceration; and grade IV, the same findings of grade III plus narrowing of the lumen. The fear of contamination with the use of endoscopic techniques has been eliminated with standardization of disinfection procedures and protective measures used by the personnel.

Blind brush cytologic study is another method, with a sensitivity of 88% to 96% for *Candida* and a specificity of 85%. Cultures seldom are needed, unless unusual pathogens are suspected, such as *M. tuberculosis, Aspergillus,* or other bacilli. Viral cultures are more accurate than histology for the diagnosis of HSV and should be obtained to differentiate from fungus infection.

Imaging studies (barium swallow) have a limited value in the differential diagnosis of esophageal infection because the abnormalities are nonspecific. The classic findings on double-contrast studies are discrete longitudinal plaque lesions, making linear and irregular filling defects. In the unusual circumstance when the patient is thrombocytopenic, the esophagus is suspected of being perforated or strictured, or endoscopy is unavailable, contrast study should be done.

The medical armamentarium currently available to treat fungal infections includes (1) nonabsorbable topical medication, such as nystatin, clotrimazole, and oral amphotericin B; (2) oral medication, including fluconazole and itraconazole; and (3) parenteral drugs, such as amphotericin B, fluconazole, and flucytosine. The manner in which to treat these patients depends on the degree of immunocompetence. A topical agent such as clotrimazole when given as a 10-mg buccal troche five times a day for 1 week is effective in the immunocompetent patient and has a clear advantage compared with nystatin and oral amphotericin.

In AIDS patients, a more aggressive treatment schedule should be used. The drug of choice is fluconazole, 100 mg/day for 2 weeks. Clotrimazole, 100 mg vaginal tablets dissolved orally three times a day, may clear esophageal symptoms in almost 100% of patients. In granulocytopenic patients, the risk of dissemination is much higher, and these patients should be treated more aggressively with amphotericin B (0.5 mg/kg). The duration of treatment is modulated by the clinical response. In disseminated cases, the dosage is at least tripled for 6 to 12 weeks. For infections confined to the epithelial tissues, 0.3 mg/kg of amphotericin B for 1 week is sufficient. Intravenous amphotericin B is the treatment of choice in cases of *Aspergillus* infection.

Recurrence is common in HIV-infected patients. Prophylaxis is recommended with fluconazole (150 mg/day orally). In intensive care unit patients, amphotericin B is effective as a preventive measure.

The diagnosis of HSV can be suspected on clinical grounds alone in a patient who presents with sudden onset of herpetic lesions on the nasolabial area with esophageal symptoms. The endoscopic findings include rounded 1- to 2-cm vesicles forming ulcers with discrete and raised edges. By esophagogram, the lesion resembles a "volcano." In this instance, the course of the disease may resolve spontaneously in a short time. Immunologic stains from centrifugated material are more sensitive than the usual histologic pattern. In difficult cases, monoclonal antibodies to HSV antigen or in situ hybridization may result in improved diagnostic yield. The treatment of esophagitis due to HSV is acyclovir, 250 mg/m^2 orally every 8 hours for 7 to 10 days. In cases of an acyclovir-resistant strain, foscarnet is the drug of choice. Another medication that may replace acyclovir is its analogue famciclovir, which has better gastrointestinal absorption and may be used for treatment and prophylaxis. Nonresponsive patients may have serious complications, such as extensive necrosis, hemorrhage, stricture, tracheoesophageal fistula, and dissemination of the disease. If detected early (within 1 hour of the first sign), high-dose acyclovir may shorten the duration of symptoms by 36%.

CMV is present in most adults worldwide, and healthy people may harbor a latent infection in many tissues of the body. It may be part of a systemic disease with slow onset when compared with HSV or *Candida* infections. Nausea, vomiting, fever, abdominal pain, and weight loss are the initial symptoms and reflect the diffuse process. The diagnosis is based on the tissue specimens obtained at endoscopy and from the base of the ulcer, not the edges, because this is the site where the subepithelial and endothelial cells are found. Tissue specimens also should be sent for other culture to rule out concurrent fungal, viral, or bacterial agents.

Acyclovir and foscarnet are the drugs of choice in the treatment for CMV infection. Both agents are potent inhibitors of herpesvirus replication by inhibiting viral DNA polymerase. Acyclovir is administered as the drug of choice, with a standard dose of 5 mg/kg every 12 hours for 14 days. Response is slow and recurrence common, and maintenance therapy should be given for several weeks, sometimes indefinitely, especially in cases of concomitant opportunistic infection if zidovudine is used. In cases of gancyclovir-resistant CMV strains, foscarnet, 90 to 120 mg/kg intravenously every 12 hours for 2 to 3 weeks, should be administered with close surveillance of adverse effects.

VZV, a DNA virus that causes chickenpox and herpes zoster, is an unusual cause of esophagitis but may produce severe esophagitis in the immunocompromised patient. The symptoms of varicella encephalitis, pneumonia, and hepatitis are more common in cases of fulminating infection. The diagnosis is made easily when the dermatologic lesion is seen, which consists of erythematous macules that vesiculate over 12 to 24 hours. The pustules begin to dry, and crusting occurs by 10 to 12 days. The dermatomes most frequently involved are from the third thoracic to the second lumbar segments and the first division of the trigeminal nerve (ophthalmic). The lesions seen at endoscopy should be sent for routine histology, cytology, and viral cultures. Immunohistochemical staining using monoclonal antibodies to VZV antigens should help differentiate from HSV infection. The treatment of choice for VZV infection is acyclovir, its analogue famciclovir, or foscarnet as an alternative therapy in cases of resistant organism.

EBV infection is the cause of almost all typical infectious mononucleosis syndromes, characterized by malaise, fever, pharyngitis, lymphadenopathy, and IgM heterophil antibody production. In the immunocompetent person, odynophagia and hematemesis due to esophageal ulceration may complicate a case of mononucleosis. The histologic findings in the esophageal lesions are similar to those found in oral hairy leukoplakia in HIV-positive patients. Acyclovir is the therapy of choice in these cases of esophageal lesions; because relapse is common, long-term therapy is advised.

HIV may account for esophageal ulcerations with no visible or identifiable pathogenic organisms. The ulcerative lesions may be accompanied by fever, chills, and rash; later in the clinical course, complications such as giant ulcer, fistula, hemorrhage, and perforation can occur. These lesions may fail to respond to conventional therapy (antiviral or antifungal drugs) but respond to systemic corticosteroid, which should be continued for more than 30 days. Occasionally, thalidomide can be used in such cases due to its immunomodulatory effects.

HPV, a double-stranded DNA virus, occasionally may be seen as a cause of esophageal infection but usually is asymptomatic. In a healthy person, warts and condylomas form in the squamous epithelial layer. In the esophagus, the lesion appears like white plaques, nodules, or large lesions. Treatment may not be necessary, but large exuberant lesions may have to be removed endoscopically, with the diagnosis established by immunohistochemical stains. Other treatments, such as interferon-alfa and chemotherapeutic agents (bleomycin, etoposide), have been tried with varying results.

Three strains of poliovirus exist and are classified in the genus *Enterovirus*. A late postpolio dysphagia has been described as a consequence of direct involvement of the brain stem reticular formation leading to abnormal control of the swallowing mechanism.

Bacterial esophagitis is a rare finding in immunocompromised and immunocompetent patients. The symptoms, similar to other esophageal infections, include painful swallowing and retrosternal pain. At endoscopy, plaques, pseudomembranes, and small ulcerations are identified. Gram stains and cultures may show the flora usually seen in the upper respiratory tract (bacilli, *Staphylococcus aureus, Staphylococcus epidermidis, Streptococcus viridans*). The treatment should include a β-lactam antibiotic in combination with an aminoglycoside, adjusted to the clinical response and cultures.

M. tuberculosis when involving the esophagus almost in all cases is due to adjacent mediastinal infection and rarely to primary esophageal involvement. Symptoms are those due to the mycobacterial infection (i.e., cough, weight loss, chest pain, and low-grade fever); in advanced cases, bleeding, perforation, and esophageal respiratory fistula may result. Endoscopy is mandatory for the diagnosis, and specimens are sent for routine bacteriologic and acid-fast stain. Treatment of esophageal tuberculosis is standard and not different from other locations of this disease. Surgery seldom is required to correct the fistulous tract between the esophagus and the respiratory tract. *Mycobacterium avium* complex infection has been reported commonly in patients with advanced AIDS, but esophageal infection is seen rarely. The treatment is usually with a multidrug regimen including isoniazid, rifampin, ethambutol, cycloserine, ethionamide, and amikacin. Ansamycin (150 to 300 mg/day orally) and clofazimine (100 to 200 mg/day orally) are still in the experimental phase and may offer some promise.

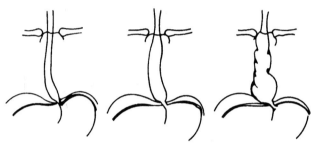

Figure 1
Radiographic classification of Chagas' achalasia. Stage I with a transverse diameter of 3 cm or less *(left)*. Stage II with a transverse diameter between 3 and 7 cm *(middle)*. Stage III beyond 7 cm *(right)*.

Table 2 Medical and Surgical Treatment Options for Chagas' Achalasia

MEDICAL TREATMENT
Pharmacologic (acute phase)
   Nifurtimox, benzimidazole
Nonsurgical
   Bougienage
   Dilation
   Botulinum toxin
SURGICAL TREATMENT
Cardiomyotomy
   With antireflux valve (180, 270, or 360 degrees)
   Without antireflux valve
Cardioplasty
   With endoluminal valve (Thal)
   With extraluminal valve
Excision of gastroesophageal junction and replacement
   Jejunum
   Ileocecal valve
Cardiomyotomy and graft
   Round ligament
   Diaphragm
Triple operation
   Esophagogastric anastomosis, hemigastrectomy, and
      Roux-en-Y
Esophagectomy
   Transpleural, transhiatal, and endoesophageal pull-through

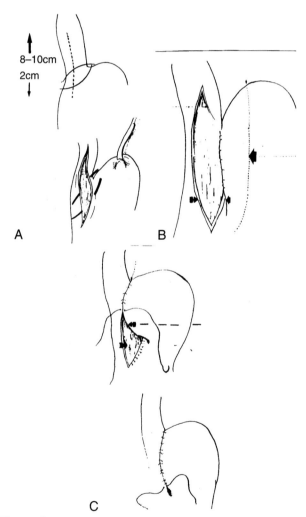

Figure 2
Technique of esophagomyotomy and 180-degree anterior fundoplication. **A,** Myotomy 8 to 10 cm above the esophageal gastric junction and 2 cm below. **B,** Suturing of the gastric fundus on the left gastric border. **C,** Completion of the plication on the right edge of the myotomy.

The treatment for idiopathic (aphthous) esophageal ulcerations is not well defined. Thalidomide has been used in a few patients; however, neurotoxicity prevents its use on a large scale. Corticosteroid is the treatment of choice with the average dose of 40 mg for a 1-month course, tapering to 10 mg/week. Syphilis, diphtheria, tetanus, nocardiosis, and actinomycosis occasionally may cause esophagitis in immunocompetent individuals. In a patient with tertiary syphilis and esophageal stricture, the syphilitic etiology should be considered. In diphtheria, the esophagus becomes secondarily infected when the patient presents with the characteristic membranes of the oropharynx, nose, and throat. In rare cases of tetanus infection, dysphagia may be present due to the toxin *Clostridium tetani* acting on the central nervous system. Anecdotal cases of nocardiosis and actinomycosis have been reported in the era of the AIDS epidemic, with doxycycline and penicillin G being the drugs of choice. *H. pylori* may be found in the esophagus of patients with gastric *H. pylori* infection, but does not cause esophagitis.

Chagas' disease of the esophagus usually is seen 7 to 10 years after the primary infection and in the young and active population. Three stages may be observed: acute, intermediate asymptomatic, and symptomatic. In the initial stage, the diagnosis is made by direct examination of a tiny blood sample in which the parasite is identified. In the chronic phase, indirect methods (xenodiagnosis, blood culture) have a sensitivity of 20% to 50%. The serologic tests (complement fixation, indirect immunofluorescence, direct agglutination, and enzyme-linked immunosorbent assay) have a sensitivity of greater than 95%. In the chronic symptomatic phase, the diagnosis is made on clinical grounds; symptoms include dysphagia, hiccups, salivation with hypertrophy of the salivary gland, cough, constipation, and weight loss. Additional studies include barium swallow, scintigraphy, endoscopy, manometry, and laboratory tests. The three stages of Chagas' achalasia may be differentiated based on radiographic studies (Figure 1).

The medical and surgical treatment options for Chagas' achalasia are outlined in Table 2. In the acute phase, nifurtimox (a nitrofuran derivative) or benzimidazole (a nitroimidazole) may be used. The first drug is given in a dose of 10 mg/kg/day in adults and 15 mg/kg/day in children for 2 or 3 months; the dose for the second medication is 5 to 10 mg/kg/day for the same amount of time.

Bougienage by the patient or physician seldom is used currently. Dilation in large series has accomplished good results in 69%, 18% required subsequent dilation, and 12% had esophagomyotomy.

Surgical therapy applies to achalasia and idiopathic Chagas' disease. If surgery is considered, it should be kept simple, safe, and effective with a morbidity and mortality near 0%. The simplest procedure for achalasia is esophagomyotomy as described by Heller in 1914. Czendes compared dilation and esophagomyotomy in 81 patients and found that 85% of patients operated had good results, whereas only 56% had

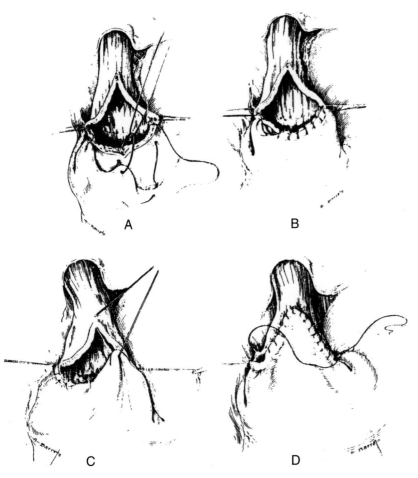

Figure 3
Technique used in advanced cases of achalasia. **A,** After opening the esophageal gastric junction 8 to 10 cm above and 2 to 4 cm below, an endoluminal valve is constructed with the anterior gastric wall. The first row of stitches is placed 2 cm at the edges and 4 cm in the middle. **B,** Additional sutures complete the endoluminal valve. **C** and **D,** The onlay patch with gastric fundus is sutured to the esophageal opening like an inverted V. (*Courtesy of H. Barreto, MD.*)

the same results after dilation. A depiction of this technique and an antireflux anterior fundal plication are shown in Figure 2. In a collected series of 1363 patients with this procedure, 93% obtained good to excellent results. In advanced stages of achalasia, simple myotomy with or without an antireflux valve is inappropriate. More sophisticated operations have been used for achalasia stage III or IV. Cardioplasty with an endoluminal valve as described by Thal to treat distal esophageal stenosis has been used by many surgeons throughout South America in advanced megaesophagus on an elective and emergency basis. In major series by Brazilian authors comprising 755 patients, mortality was 0.32%, morbidity was 4.72%, and good to excellent results were obtained in 91%. This technique is depicted in Figure 3.

Esophageal resection for this benign disease has major complications. In a collected review of 301 cases of esophagectomy for achalasia (idiopathic and Chagas' disease), a mortality rate of 4% and complication rate of 24% were found. The new technology of minimally invasive videoscopic surgery has been applied to achalasia, and several reports have shown good results with this approach. Several complications have been described, such as subcutaneous emphysema, atelectasias, pneumothorax, delayed gastric emptying, and esophageal perforation. Injection of the esophagogastric junction with botulinum toxin A, a potent inhibitor of acetylcholine release from nerve endings, has been used as an alternative conservative option for patients with Chagas' disease associated with achalasia, with relief of symptoms in 14 of 19 patients, as described by D'Onofrio et al in 2000. Long-term results are awaited, however.

SUGGESTED READING

Czendes A: Late results of a prospective randomized study comparing forceful dilatation and esophagomyotomy in patients with achalasia, *Gut* 30:299, 1989.

D'Onofrio V, et al: Long-term follow-up of achalasia patients treated with botulinum toxin, *Dis Esophagus* 13:101, 2000.

Gaissert HA, et al: Surgical management of necrotizing candida esophagitis, *Ann Thorac Surg* 85:296, 1999.

Ximenes M III: Esophageal resection for recurrent achalasia, *Ann Thorac Surg* 62:322, 1996.

Ximenes M III: Chagas's disease of the esophagus. In Shields TW, et al, editors: *General thoracic surgery*, ed 5, Philadelphia, 2000, Lippincott Williams & Wilkins, p 1807.

Ximenes M III, et al: Primary surgical treatment of Chagas' megaesophagus: results in 450 cases, *HFA Pub Tec Cient* 2:247, 1987.

ESOPHAGEAL DUPLICATION CYSTS

Malcolm V. Brock

Esophageal duplication cysts are a subset of congenital abnormalities of the foregut. Duplications can occur anywhere in the alimentary tract, with ileal duplications being the most common and gastric duplications the least. Esophageal duplication cysts account for 10% to 15% of all foregut duplication cysts.

In the thorax, esophageal duplication cysts are part of a larger differential diagnosis, accounting for only 5% to 10% of all mediastinal cysts. Bronchogenic cysts represent 50% to 60% of mediastinal cysts.

■ DEFINITION OF ESOPHAGEAL DUPLICATION CYST

Esophageal duplication cysts are defined by histologic features rather than by location. Difficulty in distinguishing esophageal duplication cysts from bronchogenic cysts, owing to their close embryonic relationship, has caused much confusion. An esophageal duplication cyst is a cystic remnant of the embryonic foregut that is lined with gastrointestinal epithelium and covered by two well-developed smooth muscle layers (usually complete with a myenteric plexus) that has no cartilage. The important point histologically is that the alimentary epithelium can be composed of squamous, columnar, cuboid, pseudostratified, or ciliated cells. The presence of cilia in the epithelium does not indicate that the cyst is respiratory in origin. The 18- to 32-week embryo and even some newborns have esophageal linings that contain areas of ciliated and nonciliated epithelium.

Of duplication cysts, 50% to 60% contain ectopic gastric mucosa (especially in children), and some may have pancreatic tissue. Esophageal duplication cysts are usually spherical or tubular structures, fairly adherent to the esophagus. Communication with the esophageal lumen is uncommon. If there is luminal communication, it is seen most often with the 20% of duplication cysts that have longer tubular structures. Cyst contents vary but usually contain mucoid fluid. Duplication cysts usually are unilocular and occur at any level of the esophagus.

■ PRESENTATION

Clinical presentation is highly variable and often depends on the age of the patient. One quarter of cases present in childhood, usually in infants younger than 2 years of age, and involve the upper third of the esophagus. In children, duplication cysts tend to produce tracheal and esophageal compression with associated respiratory or obstructive esophageal symptoms. Of patients with esophageal duplication cysts, 12% have associated congenital anomalies, usually related to the neural system or the gastrointestinal tract. Adults with esophageal duplication cysts are usually asymptomatic, and many present incidentally. If left untreated, however, most become symptomatic, especially if there is acute enlargement of the cyst due to bleeding, infection, or retention of secretions from the cyst lining. Dysphagia is the most common symptom of presentation but occurs only if there is significant compression of the esophageal lumen by the cyst. The risk of symptomatic compression varies not by the volume of the cyst, but by its topography. Duplication cysts located in the upper mediastinum tend to produce more compression symptoms on the esophagus than cysts located in the middle and inferior mediastinum. Other common symptoms include anorexia, regurgitation, weight loss, chest pain (which can simulate anginal pain), gastrointestinal bleeding, vomiting, arrhythmias, dyspnea, wheezing, coughing, and recurrent pneumonitis. Duplication cysts can cause life-threatening complications, including bleeding, ulceration, and cyst rupture with subsequent mediastinitis.

■ ETIOLOGY AND NATURAL HISTORY

The genesis for duplication cysts is unknown, but one commonly accepted theory is that these anomalies result from an error during recanalization of the embryonic gastrointestinal tract. Another theory proposes that they develop during early embryogenesis when the primitive solid esophagus forms vacuoles that coalesce into a patent lumen. A persistent isolated vacuole may enlarge into an intramural or paraesophageal cyst. The natural history is variable. Bleeding from an esophageal duplication is associated with a cyst lined with gastric mucosa. Malignant degeneration, even metastatic disease from a primary arising in an esophageal duplication cyst, has been reported but is extremely rare.

■ DIAGNOSIS

Duplication cysts are the second most common cause of benign esophageal masses in adults after leiomyoma. The major diagnostic consideration is to differentiate an esophageal duplication cyst from other mediastinal masses, especially bronchogenic cysts. Table 1 lists other lesions that should be considered in the differential diagnosis of esophageal duplication cysts. Table 2 summarizes the distinctive features of esophageal duplication cysts compared with other cysts of the mediastinum. Most esophageal duplication cysts are found in the distal right aspect of the esophagus, specifically in the right posterior-inferior mediastinum. Bleeding from an esophageal duplication cyst may elude endoscopic evaluation but can be elucidated with a technetium 99m pertechnetate scan (Meckel scan). These scans usually can localize bleeding at a rate of 0.1 to 0.3 ml/min or 500 ml/day.

Intermittent bleeding can be detected 5 days after scanning because red blood cells remain labeled for this time in the circulation.

Barium studies show a smooth intramural mass often extending into the esophageal lumen. Typically, no erosions of the mucosa are seen. The difficulty with a barium esophagogram is that it is incapable of distinguishing a fluid-filled cyst from a solid mass, making the differentiation between a leiomyoma and an esophageal duplication cyst difficult. Computed tomography (CT) scan is useful to confirm the location and size of the extrinsic mass. On CT, duplication cysts are round, homogeneous masses with smooth margins located in the posterior mediastinum. They do not enhance with intravenous contrast material and do not invade adjacent structures. A clue on the CT scan in differentiating an esophageal duplication cyst from other esophageal masses is its low density. The typical CT density of an esophageal duplication cyst approximates the CT attenuation of water (0 to 20 Hounsfield units), but cysts of higher attenuation (80 to 90 Hounsfield units) can occur. If CT alone is used as the diagnostic imaging modality, cysts with higher attenuation units can be misinterpreted as leiomyomas.

Esophagoscopy should be performed after radiographic examination to ensure that the mucosa overlying the mass is normal. Biopsies of the mucosa are not advised because the biopsy forceps rarely reach the lesion and may leave a mucosal membrane laceration, producing an infection that complicates surgical removal. Endoscopic ultrasound (EUS) has emerged as one of the most important tools to diagnose esophageal duplication cysts and is a useful adjunct after obtaining a thoracic CT scan. EUS not only defines the relationship of the cyst to the esophagus (as an intramural or extramural lesion), but also distinguishes between cystic and solid lesions. We employ an Olympus GF EUM-20 radially scanning echoendoscope (Olympus America Inc, Melville, NY) scanning at 7.5 and 12 MHz. Typically the EUS appearance is that of a cystic thin-walled structure. The cyst itself may be filled with debris or with an air-fluid level. Endoscopically guided needle aspiration and transcutaneous needle aspiration can be used to characterize the cyst's contents.

Table 1 Differential Diagnosis of Esophageal Duplication Cyst
Primary and metastatic malignancies
Lymphatic cyst
Teratoma
Lymphoma
Thymoma
Thyroid
Neurogenic tumor
Leiomyoma
Sarcoma
Granular cell tumor
Lipoma
Neurofibroma
Fibrovascular tumor
Dermoid tumor
Myoblastoma

Table 2 Features Differentiating Mediastinal Cysts

DISTINGUISHING FEATURES	ESOPHAGEAL DUPLICATION CYST	BRONCHOGENIC CYST	NEUROENTERIC CYST	PERICARDIAL CYST
Histology	Squamous, columnar, cuboid, pseudostratified, or ciliated epithelium Presence of two layers of smooth muscle No cartilage present	Respiratory epithelium (ciliated, pseudostratified, columnar), cartilaginous plates, bronchial glands, smooth muscle in the walls	Squamous or enteric epithelium	Unilocular cystic lesions with a thin connective tissue wall and clear fluid
Radiology	Right posterior inferior mediastinum	Right posterior middle mediastinum	Posterior mediastinum usually superior to the carina	Spherical or teardrop mass abutting the heart, diaphragm, and anterior chest wall
Associated anomalies	Associated with alimentary tract anomalies	None	50% associated with vertebral anomalies	None

We typically do not aspirate these cysts because the risk of introducing infection into the cyst outweighs the added diagnostic information from tissue pathology.

In addition to EUS, magnetic resonance imaging (MRI) can be used as the imaging modality of choice for esophageal duplication cysts, even if a CT scan obtained gives a plausible diagnosis. MRI has a high signal intensity of T2-weighted images (because of the watery contents of the cyst) and is a sensitive method for detecting fluid-filled soft tissue masses. Additionally, MRI allows multiplanar imaging, such as coronal and sagittal views.

■ SURGICAL TREATMENT

The gold standard that properly diagnoses an esophageal duplication cyst is surgical excision and appropriate pathologic examination. All symptomatic patients require resection. This is especially true if the onset of the symptoms is recent because this may be an indication of malignancy. In the past, many advocated resection in virtually all patients regardless of symptoms. With advances in diagnostic modalities, in particular EUS, asymptomatic patients at high risk for surgery (e.g., the elderly) are being followed with "watchful waiting." Given the benign nature of the lesion, conservative management is a reasonable option if there is a definitive diagnosis of an esophageal duplication cyst in a high-risk patient. If the patient is a good surgical candidate, however, complete cyst removal is encouraged to avoid the risks of cyst enlargement, compression on surrounding structures, ulceration with resultant hemorrhage, infection, rupture, and possible malignancy.

Surgical treatment is usually by enucleation of the cystic mass. Video-assisted thoracic surgery seems ideally suited to resect esophageal duplication cysts because these lesions are often benign, asymptomatic, and easily dissected surgically and can be extracted through a trocar incision. Alternatively a "limited" or "utility" thoracotomy can be made through which the dissection is carried out and the light source inserted via the proposed chest tube site. These minimally invasive approaches allow a relatively faster postoperative recovery time for the patient than a full posterolateral thoracotomy.

SUGGESTED READING

Cioffi U, et al: Presentation and surgical management of bronchogenic and esophageal duplication cysts in adults, *Chest* 113:1492, 1998.

Geller A, et al: Diagnosis of foregut duplication cysts by endoscopic ultrasonography, *Gastroenterology* 109:838, 1995.

Hocking M, Young DG: Duplications of the alimentary tract, *Br J Surg* 68:92, 1981.

Salo JA, Ala-Kulju KV: Congenital esophageal cysts in adults, *Ann Thorac Surg* 44:135, 1987.

Van Dam J, et al: Endoscopic ultrasonography and endoscopically guided needle aspiration for the diagnosis of upper gastrointestinal tract foregut cysts, *Am J Gastroenterol* 87:762, 1992.

Whitaker JA, et al: Esophageal duplication cyst, *Am J Gastroenterol* 73:329, 1980.

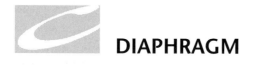

DIAPHRAGM

MORGAGNI AND BOCHDALEK HERNIAS IN THE ADULT

Juan A. Cordero, Jr.
Darroch W. O. Moores

Most diaphragmatic hernias present in the neonatal period or childhood. The adult presentation of congenital diaphragmatic hernias is exceedingly rare, and few thoracic surgeons have significant experience in their treatment. These hernias can occur through the posterolateral foramen of Bochdalek, the anterior foramen of Morgagni, or the esophageal hiatus. The presentation of congenital diaphragmatic hernias in adults is varied and relates to the size and location of the defect.

■ EMBRYOLOGY AND ANATOMY

Morgagni and Bochdalek hernias are defects that result from failure of fusion of the embryologic elements of the diaphragm. The diaphragm develops from four structures: transverse septum, pleuroperitoneal membranes, esophagus and its mesentery, and ingrowth of muscular components from the lateral body wall. The foramen of Morgagni arises from failure of the transverse septum to fuse to the sternum. The resulting triangular space is located between the xiphisternum and the costal margin fibers that insert on the central tendon. Most defects (>90%) are right-sided because the pericardium protects the left side, but left-sided and bilateral defects do occur. Morgagni hernias are direct hernias that usually contain a true peritoneal sac. These hernias tend to be large, and they usually contain large bowel or omentum within their sac. A few rare cases of small bowel and stomach herniation have been reported in association with these hernias.

The foramen of Bochdalek represents a posterolateral defect in the diaphragm and results from failure of the pleuroperitoneal membranes to develop. These defects more commonly occur on the left side (>90%) but can occur on the right side, where the liver often covers the defect and prevents detection. The posterolateral location of the defect commonly allows for herniation of the stomach, spleen, and colon.

■ PRESENTATION AND DIAGNOSIS

Foramen of Morgagni hernias in adults are often asymptomatic and are diagnosed incidentally on radiographic examinations. Usually a mass is seen in the right pericardiophrenic space on a computed tomography (CT) scan obtained for unrelated symptoms. Symptomatic patients most commonly present with gastrointestinal manifestations that include crampy abdominal pain or constipation from partial large bowel obstruction. Although complete large bowel obstruction is a rare presentation, the last patient we operated on with a Morgagni hernia presented in this fashion. In this patient, a barium enema study obtained to evaluate large bowel dilation revealed an incarcerated Morgagni hernia. Cardiorespiratory symptoms are less common and include nonspecific chest pain, palpitations, and dyspnea. Although chest radiographs can suggest a Morgagni hernia, the diagnosis usually is made with a CT scan. The usual CT finding is a retrosternal mass representing herniated omentum. An air-filled viscus also may be seen if colon herniation has occurred. A barium enema study can be used to delineate any colonic involvement.

In contrast to Morgagni hernias, the adult presentation of foramen of Bochdalek hernias frequently is associated with severe symptoms and episodes of intermittent obstruction. The posterolateral location of the defect on the left usually leads to the herniation of stomach or colon with resultant obstruction. The most common symptoms associated with Bochdalek hernias are episodes of intermittent obstruction as the involved viscera herniate and subsequently spontaneously reduce. Other rare presentations include progressive respiratory symptoms, such as dyspnea or wheezing; bowel herniation from pregnancy; gastric, colonic, or splenic volvulus; and even sudden death from gastric ulcer perforation. The diagnosis of a Bochdalek hernia can be made by seeing a mass on posteroanterior and lateral chest radiographs; this can be confused with a neoplastic process. The gastrointestinal symptoms usually result in a CT scan that is diagnostic, however.

■ SURGICAL THERAPY

All diaphragmatic hernias should be repaired because of the potential for complete obstruction and strangulation. Signs of incarceration or strangulation should prompt emergency surgical intervention. Rare patients with prohibitive operative risk and asymptomatic hernias may be observed closely.

Morgagni hernias should be approached transabdominally via a midline or subcostal incision. The transabdominal approach allows for simple reduction of the hernia, assessment of bowel viability, and the ability to inspect the contralateral side. After reducing the hernia contents, the sac is identified and resected, exposing the extent of the defect. The defects are usually large and are closed by approximating the diaphragm up to the posterior part of the sternum and rectus sheath using nonabsorbable interrupted suture material. Adequate repair may necessitate placement of sutures around the ribs anteriorly or into the periosteum of the sternum. In our experience, we have not had to use prosthetic material or drain the pleural space.

Foramen of Bochdalek hernias may be approached via a transabdominal or transthoracic approach. There are strong proponents of both approaches. We approach these hernias in a similar fashion to paraesophageal hernias and are strong advocates of a transabdominal approach. The transabdominal approach has several advantages, including complete access to the abdominal cavity for inspection of the involved viscera and the contralateral side and simple reduction of the hernia contents by gentle traction. We have not encountered any intrathoracic adhesions in any of these patients.

We approach these patients through an upper midline incision. The contents of the hernia are reduced, and the extent of the hernia sac is evaluated. The hernia sac is excised, and the defect is closed primarily with heavy nonabsorbable suture material. These defects are usually small, and prosthetic patch closure rarely is needed, although it frequently is used in children. Tube thoracostomy drainage of the affected hemithorax completes the procedure. In our experience, repair of adult congenital diaphragmatic hernias is associated with low morbidity and mortality in the elective setting. Only the rare asymptomatic patient with prohibitive operative risk should be denied surgical therapy.

Minimally invasive techniques using laparoscopic or video-assisted thoracic surgical techniques have been reported in the repair of diaphragmatic hernias. As with the open technique, a transabdominal approach seems favored because of the ability to inspect the entire abdomen. Although these minimally invasive options seem to be more attractive, they should be used only in the elective setting. The early results with these techniques are promising; however, long-term follow-up is needed. Regardless of the surgical approach, morbidity and mortality are low, and results are excellent. Mortality can be 15% if surgical intervention is required on an emergent basis, however.

SUGGESTED READING

Karanikas ID, et al: Complications of congenital posterolateral diaphragmatic hernia in adults, *J Cardiovasc Surg* 35:555, 1994.

Naunheim KS: Adult presentation of unusual diaphragmatic hernias, *Chest Surg Clin N Am* 8:359, 1998.

EVENTRATION OF THE DIAPHRAGM

Benedict D. T. Daly

Eventration is a condition characterized by extreme elevation of the diaphragm. Most commonly, it involves a hemidiaphragm, but it may involve only a portion of the diaphragm or may be bilateral. There are two types of eventration. In the congenital type, a thin fibroelastic membrane characterized by a lack of cross-striated muscle or highly degenerated muscle separates the thorax and abdomen. The acquired type is associated with phrenic nerve paralysis. The diaphragm is flaccid, and with time atrophy and interstitial fibrosis become prominent.

Eventration results in paradoxical motion of the affected diaphragm with respiration. Although ventilation on the paralyzed side is maintained by the transmission of cyclic pressure changes across the mediastinum, significant reductions in the forced vital capacity (FVC), total lung capacity (TLC), and forced expiratory volume in 1 second (FEV_1) occur. Physiologic dead space is increased, and there is a reduction in Po_2. In infants and small children, weakness of the intercostal muscles, a more horizontal orientation of the ribs, and a mobile mediastinum accentuate these abnormalities. Recumbence adversely affects these patients. Congenital eventration of the diaphragm may be associated with ipsilateral pulmonary hypoplasia and may be difficult to distinguish from diaphragmatic hernia and sac.

Most adults are asymptomatic, but some exhibit dyspnea or orthopnea. Symptoms in infants and young children may be respiratory or gastrointestinal. Respiratory symptoms vary from tachypnea, retraction, or cyanosis on feeding to frank respiratory insufficiency. Gastrointestinal symptoms include inability to gain weight, vomiting, epigastric pain, or frank intestinal obstruction often associated with organoaxial or mesenteroaxial gastric volvulus.

The diagnosis is suspected by chest radiography that shows elevation of the diaphragm and is confirmed by fluoroscopy, ultrasonography, or phrenic nerve conduction studies. Fluoroscopy used to be the most common method of showing paradoxical motion of the paralyzed hemidiaphragm during sudden inspiration off the ventilator or with the classic sniff test. Ultrasonography has become the most popular method of making the diagnosis, however, because it can be performed at the bedside and be repeated easily. Computed tomography and magnetic resonance imaging of the chest sometimes are useful for showing unusual abnormalities of the diaphragm or other associated abnormalities, but these modalities generally do not have a role in patient management. Eventration usually manifests itself at three times: shortly after birth, after a palliative or corrective congenital heart procedure, or later in life from a known or unknown cause. Special considerations apply to each of these.

Eventration in the newborn is rare, usually associated with severe respiratory distress, and may be secondary to congenital eventration or phrenic nerve injury at birth. Congenital eventration is often partial, whereas the acquired form is usually complete. The latter often is associated with Erb's palsy. It is often difficult to distinguish between the two types, and most cases are managed as phrenic nerve injury. Phrenic nerve recovery rarely is seen after 1 month, and there is little justification in delaying surgical treatment beyond that time. Returning the diaphragm to a position of full inspiration prevents paradox and helps maintain the position of the mediastinum and the stability of the chest wall. This usually is accomplished by plication with or without a prosthesis. Plication does not prevent the later recovery of diaphragmatic function, and early plication may help prevent some of the pathologic changes that are seen in the lungs of these patients. Most patients can be weaned from the respirator within a few days of plication unless there are more severe underlying associated abnormalities. Persistent dyspnea and relapsing bronchitis and bronchopneumonia are indications for plication in patients not requiring immediate ventilatory support.

In large series of patients, the incidence of phrenic nerve injury after congenital heart procedures generally varies from 1.5% to 3%. It occurs more commonly in patients who have had previous operations and in younger patients. The procedure most commonly associated with phrenic nerve injury is the creation or takedown of a systemic-to-pulmonary artery shunt, particularly the Blalock-Taussig shunt. Procedures on the branch pulmonary arteries also are associated with a relatively high incidence of phrenic nerve injury. Injury should be suspected in any patient in whom there are unexplained difficulties in weaning from the respirator. There are no concrete rules regarding the timing of surgical intervention. Most authors recommend waiting 2 to 3 weeks to allow for recovery. More than half of patients are weaned successfully without surgery, although a return of normal diaphragmatic function is observed in only half. Plication rarely is required in children older than 18 months of age. If it is known that the nerve was severed, however, operation should not be delayed because plication leads to early extubation, usually within 2 to 4 days. Although diaphragmatic plication does not preclude diaphragmatic recovery, some recommend earlier plication in all patients because it reduces morbidity and hospital stay.

Nonmalignant diaphragmatic paralysis is rare, and many causes have been described. Operative trauma may occur during procedures in the mediastinum or neck, whereas paralysis has been reported after cardiac operations secondary to clamping or cold injury. Paralysis of the right hemidiaphragm has been reported after liver transplantation.

It also has occurred in association with viral or bacterial infection, chronic neurologic disease, disease of the cervical vertebrae, aortic aneurysms, or trauma involving sudden deceleration or blast injury. In many cases, the cause is idiopathic. A 20% to 30% reduction in vital capacity and TLC frequently returns toward normal after 6 months. A few patients experience dyspnea and orthopnea that interfere with their daily activities. In these patients, plication should be considered but with rare exception only after sufficient time has elapsed to preclude regeneration. This is generally 1 year.

Plication also has benefited an occasional patient with postsurgical diaphragmatic paralysis and significant underlying lung disease who cannot be weaned from a ventilator. Plication may benefit the patient with a paralyzed diaphragm after pneumonectomy because it improves function in the intact diaphragm. Plication results in significant improvements in FVC, FEV_1, TLC, and functional reserve capacity. Residual volumes do not change. The Po_2 and diffusing capacity of lung for carbon monoxide also improve significantly. These changes occur in association with an increase in maximal transdiaphragmatic pressure, maximal voluntary ventilation, and ventilatory muscle recruitment. More importantly, the objective improvement in mechanics and oxygen exchange that is seen after plication seems to be durable.

Plication can be accomplished by a variety of similar operations. Commonly the lateral and posterior portions of the diaphragm are plicated with interrupted horizontal mattress sutures reinforced with polytetrafluoroethylene (Teflon) pledgets (Figure 1). These nonabsorbable sutures are placed circumferentially in a radial fashion beginning near the outer margin of the diaphragm, avoiding the branches of the phrenic nerve and placed approximately 0.5 cm apart in the infant and 1 cm in the adult. In the adult, the sutures are carried into the central tendon. In infants and small children, the central tendon is not sutured to avoid any compromise to nerve or arterial blood supply. Enough diaphragm has to be included in each pleat to make the diaphragm taut. Another technique that has been used is to incise the diaphragm and imbricate one side over the other with two layers of interrupted sutures. In cases of congenital eventration, some surgeons have preferred to stretch the diaphragm out and reattach it to the costal margin. When plication fails to bring the diaphragm into the position of near full inspiration, a prosthetic material may be required. Although we prefer to use an eighth interspace thoracic incision, others prefer to use the seventh or even the sixth interspace. Plication also may be accomplished thoracoscopically using sutures or a mechanical stapling device, gathering the leaf of the affected diaphragm in successive pleats until it is taut. The operation sometimes is performed through the abdomen, especially if intraabdominal abnormalities must be dealt with at the same time.

Long-term complications after plication are rare. The most common reported complication is gastroesophageal reflux. Experimental studies suggest that an increased transdiaphragmatic inspiratory pressure gradient and a decreased lower esophageal sphincter pressure contribute to reflux. Recurrence of eventration or rupture has required reoperation in a few patients.

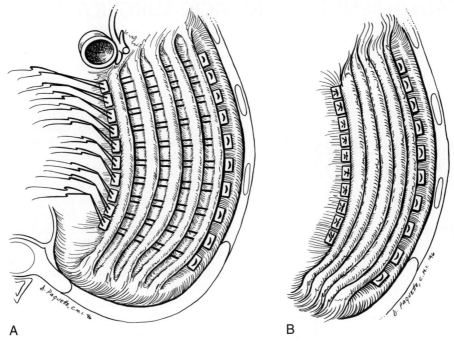

A   B

Figure 1
Plication of the right diaphragm in an adult. **A,** Sutures buttressed with polytetrafluoroethylene (Teflon) pledgets extend anteriorly to the level of the vena cava. **B,** Plicated diaphragm. (*From Daly BDT, Feins NR: In Kaiser LR, et al, editors:* Mastery of cardiothoracic surgery, *Philadelphia, 1988, Lippincott-Raven.*)

SUGGESTED READING

Ciccolella DE, et al: Improved diaphragmatic function after surgical plication for unilateral diaphragmatic paralysis, *Am Rev Respir Dis* 146:797, 1992.

DeLeeuw M, et al: Impact of diaphragmatic paralysis after cardiothoracic surgery in children, *J Thorac Cardiovasc Surg* 118:510, 1999.

Deslauriers J: Eventration of the diaphragm, *Chest Surg Clin N Am* 8:315, 1998.

De Vries TS, et al: Surgical treatment of diaphragmatic eventration caused by phrenic nerve injury in the newborn, *J Pediatr Surg* 33:602, 1988.

Graham DR, et al: Diaphragmatic plication for unilateral diaphragmatic paralysis: a 10-year experience, *Ann Thorac Surg* 49:248, 1990.

Langer JC, et al: Plication of the diaphragm for infants and young children with phrenic nerve palsy, *J Pediatr Surg* 23:749, 1988.

Tonz M, et al: Clinical implications of phrenic nerve injury after pediatric cardiac surgery, *J Pediatr Surg* 31:1265, 1996.

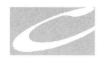

GENERAL PRINCIPLES OF VIDEO-ASSISTED THORACIC SURGERY

Anthony P. C. Yim

For a century since the first lung resection was reported in 1891 by Tuffier, posterolateral thoracotomy (and occasionally median sternotomy and clam-shell incision for bilateral pulmonary procedures) has been the preferred mode of surgical access. Although these incisions provide excellent surgical exposure, they also are among the most painful incisions ever to be encountered by patients—not only because of the lengths of the incisions and division of muscles, but also primarily because ribs (or sternum) have to be separated to gain access into the chest. In contrast to other incisions, this pain does not last for weeks, but often persists for decades.

Although it has been realized for some time that the trauma of access is often worse than that of the procedure itself, the use of smaller incisions alone to access the chest (i.e., without video assistance), such as the French incision, never gained wide popularity in the surgical community. Conventional wisdom relates minimal access to limited surgical exposure, and complicated intrathoracic procedures performed under suboptimal surgical exposure are generally not considered safe. Any attempt to spread the ribs to compensate for the smaller skin incision would defeat the purpose of minimal access surgery. This situation was changed by the advent of videoendoscopic surgery. Fueled by the success of laparoscopic cholecystectomy in the 1980s, video-assisted thoracic surgery (VATS) plays a part in a revolution that now affects all surgical disciplines. The thoracoscope-camera unit with its own light source provides a well-illuminated, magnified operative view with high resolution for details, which surpasses that provided by the conventional headlight and magnifying loops. The hemithorax is arguably the best body cavity for minimal access surgery. Bound by the rigid rib cage, when the lung is collapsed (using single-lung ventilation), there is plenty of room to work. Carbon dioxide is unnecessary, and valved ports and dedicated endoscopic instruments are not mandatory.

VATS as it is practiced today exists as a spectrum ranging from a purely endoscopic technique with port access at one end to the other end in which a minithoracotomy is used for later specimen retrieval, and the surgeon operates primarily by looking at the video monitor but also occasionally through the minithoracotomy wound. VATS implies that no rib spreading is required throughout the entire procedure. For surgeons who routinely use the rib spreader and operate by primarily looking through the minithoracotomy, we suggested the term *minithoracotomy with video assistance* and consider that a completely different technique.

It is important to be able to be flexible in the application of a new technology. Video assistance has a role to play even in open surgery. Video assistance, or simply making use of the illumination it brings, can help with a difficult adhesiolysis in the lung apex or base, or when median sternotomy is used for bilateral lung surgery, resection of a posteriorly located nodule could be difficult, and video assistance can help easily in these situations. This is not VATS; one can call this *thoracotomy/median sternotomy with video assistance*, but regardless of the names given, the possibility of combining a new technology with an existing, established surgical technique to improve outcome should not be ignored. Video assistance also could serve as an intermediate step for some practicing surgeons trying to acquire a new skill.

■ INDICATIONS, PATIENT SELECTIONS, AND CONTRAINDICATIONS

VATS represents a new approach, not a new procedure. Common indications for VATS are summarized in Table 1. With increased experience and refinement of technique, the list almost certainly can be lengthened in the future.

Table 1 Some Common Indications for Video-Assisted Thoracic Surgery

PLEURAL DISEASES
Diagnosis of indeterminate pleural effusions and masses
Drainage of empyema (fibrinopurulent phase) and hemothorax
SPONTANEOUS PNEUMOTHORAX
Bleb resection
Bullectomy and pleurodesis
MEDIASTINAL DISEASES
Biopsy of mediastinal masses and lymph nodes
Thymectomy
Excision of clinically benign cysts or masses
Pericardial window
Thoracodorsal sympathectomy
Esophageal mobilization
Spinal surgery
PARENCHYMAL DISEASES
Major lung resections
Nonanatomic resections

The use of VATS as a diagnostic modality or treatment of benign conditions has long been accepted into mainstream thoracic surgery, so much so that it is now increasingly difficult for surgeons to justify not using VATS as the surgical approach of choice for several conditions. For pleural diseases, VATS not only offers an excellent means for diagnosis, but also an ideal approach to treat breakdown of loculations, to guide placement of chest drains, and possibly to treat with talc insufflation. Conversion to a thoracotomy should not be viewed as a technical failure, but a sign of good judgment. We generally do not recommend VATS resection for established mediastinal malignancy. When there is a sign of tissue plane invasion intraoperatively, the safest approach currently is to proceed with an open dissection.

The indications for VATS major resections remain the same as for conventional resection but are more controversial. For primary lung cancer, preresectional staging (including mediastinoscopy) is a crucial step in cancer management and should be strictly adhered to. There are few absolute contraindications that are specifically applicable to VATS major resections; they are listed in Table 2. Apart from the inability to tolerate single-lung ventilation, all of them are anatomic considerations. We do not recommend VATS for tumors larger than 4 cm, not primarily because of technical difficulties, but because ribs have to be spread excessively to retrieve the specimen, and this tends to negate any benefit of minimal access surgery. True pleural symphysis that leads to abandonment of the VATS approach is uncommon in our experience. When the correct plane in the pleural space is entered and a space is created, endoscopic adhesiolysis can proceed quickly and safely. We have reported our experience on redo VATS surgery, and we no longer consider prior surgery an absolute contraindication to VATS resection.

■ OPERATIVE TECHNIQUE

Compared with conventional surgery, VATS demands a new set of manual skill and eye-hand coordination. For someone who is experienced with open surgery, however, the learning curve is usually steep. Similar to any technical procedure, attention to fine details is crucial to ensure a successful, reproducible outcome.

Anesthesia

The procedure should be carried out under general anesthesia with selective single-lung ventilation. This usually can be accomplished using a double-lumen endobronchial tube (usually left-sided intubation unless a left pneumonectomy is anticipated). We prefer this rather than the commercially available endotracheal tube with a built-in bronchial blocker because the latter technique makes it more difficult to collapse the lung, especially in patients who have emphysema. There is currently no endobronchial tube commercially available for young children, and in those situations, we use a single-lumen endotracheal tube and position its tip in the appropriate main stem bronchus.

Patient Positioning

The patient is turned into a full lateral decubitus position. We advocate flexing the operating table to open up the intercostal spaces for insertion of the thoracoscope and instruments. When a utility minithoracotomy is required for the procedure, this flexion naturally opens up the wound to render rib spreading unnecessary. If there is any doubt, the position of the endobronchial tube should be confirmed or reconfirmed at this time using a fine-bore flexible bronchoscope before the patient is prepared and draped as for thoracotomy.

Instruments

We prefer a 10-mm thoracoscope and a three-chip camera system for complex procedures such as major resection. We use two television monitors so that the surgeon and the assistants can view simultaneously without having to turn their heads. We use a 0-degree lens for most procedures, including resections of the lower lobes and middle lobe, and a 30-degree lens for the upper lobes. The correct choice of lens for each operation cannot be overemphasized. It is crucial that the assistant is reminded at all times to avoid torquing the thoracoscope; because of the leverage, even slight torquing could result in significant pressure on the intercostal nerve and postoperative neuralgia.

We generally do not use ports except for the thoracoscope and for introducing mechanical staplers. This is done not only to save money on the ports, but also because the presence of a trocar port makes it difficult to use conventional thoracic instruments. We prefer these (e.g., sponge holding forceps and Metzenbaum scissors) rather than dedicated endoscopic instruments because they are light, easy to use, familiar to all surgeons, universally available, and cheap.

For some technically simple procedures that do not require extensive dissection and retrieval of large specimens (e.g., thoracodorsal sympathectomy), we have been using 2-mm "needlescopic" instruments (MiniSite; US Surgical, Norwalk, CT) with excellent results. In contrast to conventional VATS, in which the initial port was created by finger-clamp technique, a 2-mm port (with the blunt introducer) was placed percutaneously (and blindly) into the chest after a tiny stab incision was made in the dermis. The lung should be collapsed before the introduction of a 2-mm port, which

---

Table 2 Contraindications for Video-Assisted Thoracic Surgery Major Resections

ABSOLUTE CONTRAINDICATIONS
Inability to tolerate single-lung ventilation
Large tumor (>4 cm maximal diameter)
Pleural symphysis
Established N2 disease
T3 tumor (main stem bronchial involvement)
Planned sleeve resection

RELATIVE CONTRAINDICATIONS
Hilar lymphadenopathy
Previous surgery (VATS or thoracotomy)
Completely fused fissures
Prior irradiation to the hilum
T3 tumor (chest wall involvement)

From Yim APC: In Pearson FG, et al, editors: *Thoracic surgery*, ed 2, Philadelphia, 2002, WB Saunders.

then is advanced slowly until a characteristic "pop" is felt, which signifies the pleural cavity has been entered. With the use of these miniaturized instruments, postoperative pain is minimized further, and no suturing of wounds is required. Scars generally are not detectable after a few weeks postoperatively.

Intercostal Strategy and Instrument Maneuvering

The surgeon normally stands behind the patient except for major pulmonary resections or when the pathology is located in the posterior lung or mediastinum. We generally explore by placing the thoracoscope in the seventh or eighth intercostal space over the mid to anterior axillary line depending on the patient's body build and the location of the pathology. From this position, a panoramic view of the hemithorax can be obtained. The basic principle here is to align the thoracoscope, the pathology, and the television monitor so that the surgeon can look straight ahead when he or she operates; this provides the best ergonomic position for instrument placement.

The instruments should not be placed too close to the thoracoscope or to each other to avoid "fencing" during manipulation. As mentioned earlier, one fundamental difference between laparoscopy and VATS is that carbon dioxide insufflation is not required in the latter. This not only means that valved ports and dedicated endoscopic instruments are largely unnecessary, but also that digital palpation is permissible and should be encouraged. By bringing the lung toward the palpating finger placed through different port sites, a large portion of the lung surface can be palpated. This is important because small nodules (<0.5 cm) that are not subpleurally located almost certainly would go undetected by thoracoscopic examination alone.

Experienced VATS surgeons all have learned to feel with the tips of their instruments. One important reason why we advocate using conventional tools is because they are familiar to the surgeons and shorten the time needed to acquire this technique. The inherent decrease in tactile information due to the lack of manual palpation during VATS is compensated by the enhancement of visual information—the monitors provide a magnified view of the operative field with high resolution for details. Subtle displacement of a structure during dissection (which is usually not noticeable in open surgery) provides important clues to an experienced VATS surgeon.

Paradoxical motion is generated when the camera and instruments are facing each other. This sometimes is unavoidable when there is a wide operating field. We have found that by turning the camera 180 degrees, a normal spatial relationship is restored for the operator. This simple maneuver allows the surgeon to use the camera and existing ports to his or her best advantage.

Retrieval of Specimen

We routinely use a specimen bag (for small specimens <3 cm) or a wound protector (for larger specimens) during retrieval to avoid contamination or tumor cell implantation. In major pulmonary resection, if the primary tumor is less than 4 cm, we generally have not found a mechanical rib spreader to be necessary (even for removal of the entire lung), although some manual rib retraction may be needed at the time of retrieval.

Complications

Major complications from VATS are relatively uncommon. Persistent air leak is the most common complication after VATS and can be minimized by careful patient selection, meticulous dissection, and use of endoscopic suturing. Tumor implantation after VATS resection for cancer has been reported. This implantation could be avoided by gentle handling of tissue, routine use of a wound protector, and copious irrigation of the hemithorax before closure. One of the most dreaded complications for surgeons is massive bleeding from pulmonary vessels. Mechanical failure of the vascular staplers resulting in massive bleeding has been reported, but these are anecdotal cases, and the staplers available now are generally reliable.

■ SUMMARY

VATS is an established, alternative approach to conventional open surgery in the management of a variety of intrathoracic conditions. Because VATS is merely a new approach and not a new procedure, the surgical indications and objectives remain unchanged. Postoperative pain is significantly less after VATS. Other documented advantages over conventional surgery include better preservation of pulmonary function in the early postoperative period, earlier return to full activities, and better quality of life. Older and sicker patients who otherwise would be poor-risk candidates for a thoracotomy approach can be recruited for surgery. The long-term results of VATS have been shown to be at least as good, if not superior to, its open counterparts. VATS demands a new set of manual skills and should be an integral part of thoracic surgical training.

SUGGESTED READING

Yim APC: Minimizing chest wall trauma in video assisted thoracic surgery, *J Thorac Cardiovasc Surg* 109:1255, 1995.

Yim APC, et al: Counteracting paradoxical motion in videoendoscopic surgery, *Ann Thorac Surg* 66:965, 1998.

Yim APC: Video assisted pulmonary resections. In Pearson FG, et al, editors: *Thoracic surgery,* ed 2, Philadelphia, 2002, WB Saunders.

Yim APC, et al, editors: *Minimal access cardiothoracic surgery,* Philadelphia, 2000, WB Saunders.

VIDEO-ASSISTED THORACIC SURGERY FOR MEDIASTINAL DISEASES

Michael J. Mack

Michal Savcenko

With the introduction of new video imaging techniques in the early 1990s, diagnostic thoracoscopy evolved into video-assisted thoracic surgery (VATS) with broader diagnostic applications and a limited therapeutic role. Although still in evolution, the indications for a thoracoscopic approach in mediastinal disease include the diagnosis of mediastinal masses, removal of small noninvasive masses from the anterior or posterior mediastinum, excision of symptomatic mediastinal cysts, staging of lung cancer, sympathectomy, and possibly thymectomy with or without thymoma (Table 1). VATS management of pericardial effusive and esophageal diseases is discussed in another chapter. We first discuss our general approach to VATS procedures followed by specific modifications for each indication.

■ GENERAL TECHNIQUE

Our VATS approach to mediastinal disease uses the same principles as other VATS procedures with some modifications.

Anesthesia and Monitoring
General endotracheal anesthesia is employed with a double-lumen endotracheal tube to allow single-lung ventilation and collapse of the ipsilateral lung. Because we use single-lung anesthesia, arterial pressure and oxygen saturation monitoring and end-tidal carbon dioxide concentration are routine.

Position and Incision
Although in most intrathoracic procedures we position the patient in the lateral decubitus position, we keep the patient supine for most mediastinal procedures; the exception is posterior mediastinal masses and lung cancer staging, when we use the decubitus position. With the patient in the supine position, we place a pillow or a roll underneath the ipsilateral posterior hemithorax to allow a 10- to 15-degree elevation. The operating table is slanted away from the surgeon and from the center to ensure maximal excursion of the intercostal spaces and lowering of the patient's pelvis away from the chest. All of these positioning manipulations are helpful to prevent limitation of excursion of the camera or instruments. The table also is placed in a reverse Trendelenburg position, and the patient's arm is tucked at the side posterior to the operative field. These maneuvers allow the lung to drop away from the mediastinum with little—if any—retraction necessary for exposure.

The basic VATS principle of placing three scope and instrument incisions in an inverted triangle is followed with the scope at the apex and the two instruments superior and lateral to the scope. Instruments should be positioned as far away from the scope as possible so that "sword fighting" does not occur.

Instruments and Technique
With improvement in camera and scope quality, most mediastinal procedures can be performed with 5-mm scope, instrument, and trocars. We employ carbon dioxide (CO_2) insufflation for most mediastinal procedures in contradistinction to most lung procedures. CO_2 insufflation has the advantage of displacing the lung to the periphery of the operative field and opening up the mediastinum for better exposure during the resection and minimizing any bleeding that occurs. CO_2 insufflation is safe up to 8 to 10 cm H_2O. Sealed laparoscopic trocars are used rather than the traditional open thoracic trocars. In the procedures in which a large amount of tissue is going to be removed, a 10-mm trocar is used instead of the usual 5 mm. We find that a 5- or 10-mm, 30-degree angled scope is most versatile for visualization.

Most procedures in the mediastinum can be performed with a minimum of complex instruments. An endoscopic grasper and a hook cautery are sufficient to perform most dissections. If bleeding is anticipated, a suction irrigation device can be used. For extensive dissection or if collapse of the lung is a problem, a fan retractor can be placed through a fourth port. If an extensive amount of electrocautery is used with smoke building up in the thoracic cavity, CO_2 can be insufflated with a separate port open to keep a constant "breeze" through the thoracic cavity to clear the smoke. An alternative is the use of the harmonic scalpel for resection of mediastinal tissue without smoke. If there is any question of malignancy or if a large amount of tissue is to be removed from the thoracic cavity, an endoscopic bag is placed through an anterior trocar site for extraction through the chest wall.

Table 1   Role of Video-Assisted Thoracic Surgery in Mediastinal Disease

PREFERRED APPROACH	ACCEPTABLE APPROACH	POSSIBLE BUT NOT PROVEN
Sympathectomy	Staging of lung cancer	Thymectomy
Benign anterior mediastinal masses	Posterior neurogenic tumors	
Mediastinal cysts		

Postoperative Care

Extubation is immediate in the operating room. Ketorolac is used liberally for postoperative pain. Most procedures in the mediastinum can be performed as an outpatient or at the most, in the case of thymectomy, an overnight hospital stay.

■ ANTERIOR MEDIASTINAL MASSES

Indications

The differential diagnosis of most anterior mediastinal masses is thymoma, lymphoma, and germ cell tumors. VATS offers a superior access for the diagnosis of masses of the anterior mediastinum, largely supplanting the second interspace mediastinotomy (Chamberlain procedure). The advantages include superior visualization of the mass, information about involvement of surrounding structures, and multiple access sites for biopsy. The avoidance of an anterior chest incision also allows prompt initiation of postoperative radiation therapy.

Technique

Anterior masses are approached with incisions placed posterior to the mid axillary line. Masses should be approached from the side to which they are more prominent. If the mass is in the middle, the right side is preferred because of easy visibility of the superior vena cava and innominate vein and more room for maneuverability in the hemithorax because of the absence of the pericardium and heart. Smaller well-encapsulated or cystic anterior mediastinal masses, believed to be noninvasive, can be resected completely by the VATS approach. If invasion is suspected or detected intraoperatively, conversion to an open thoracotomy is appropriate. This situation usually can be anticipated preoperatively, however, and conversion is seldom necessary.

Results

The largest reported experience is that of Roviaro et al, who reported 133 VATS procedures for primary mediastinal disease. The procedure was diagnostic in 50 and therapeutic in 83. Conversion to thoracotomy was required in five cases, owing to size of the mass, extensive adhesions, or tumor infiltration of surrounding structures.

■ POSTERIOR MEDIASTINAL MASSES

Indications

Posterior mediastinal masses account for 30% of all mediastinal pathology requiring intervention, with most posterior masses being neurogenic in origin. In adults, only 2% to 4% are malignant. The presence of a tumor is an indication for resection, although asymptomatic patients with a small tumor and no intraspinal extension can be managed expectantly. Preoperative computed tomography or magnetic resonance imaging should be obtained to rule out an intraspinal component. For the most part, VATS is reserved for lesions without intraspinal extension.

Technique

The patient is placed in the lateral decubitus position to approach the posterior mediastinum. The approach is from anterior to the mid axillary line, and a 30-degree scope is preferred. The parietal pleura is incised around the tumor, and the dissection, using a hook cautery and grasper for retraction, is usually not difficult. The main focus of the operation is to control the neurovascular pedicle with adjacent intercostal and vertebral vessels. Endoscopic hemoclips should be used when the vascular supply is identified. Complete resection should be achieved with placement of the tumor in an endoscopic bag for removal through an anterior trocar site.

Results

Because these tumors are relatively unusual, only small series exist in the literature. Our own experience is removal of 15 neurogenic tumors in 10 years with no significant problems encountered.

■ MEDIASTINAL CYSTS

Indications

Most masses in the middle mediastinum are cystic and benign in origin, and most mediastinal cysts are contained in the middle mediastinum. The most frequently encountered cysts include bronchogenic, pericardial, esophageal duplication, and neurenteric cysts. Resection is indicated for simple cysts if symptomatic or if malignancy is suspected on the basis of septation or accompanying mass. Successful management of cysts with aspiration only has been reported; however, there is a high recurrence rate associated with this approach.

Technique

The VATS technique for excision of a simple cyst is relatively straightforward. Dissection planes are usually easiest to identify if the dissection is initiated with the cyst wall intact. As much of the dissection should be completed without rupture of the cyst as possible. When the dissection is completed, or if the cyst is inadvertently ruptured, cyst fluid should be aspirated before removal. If in the rare instance a safe plane of dissection between the cyst and the adjacent vital structure cannot be developed easily, leaving a small portion of the cyst wall attached to that structure is acceptable, with the cyst lining being obliterated with electrocautery.

Results

No significant series of mediastinal cysts exist in the literature, with most reports limited to case reports or single-digit series. Our own experience is relatively small but with no problems occurring with simple excision.

■ STAGING OF LUNG CANCER

Indications

Mediastinal lymphadenopathy typically is staged before lung resection for cancer. Surgical mediastinoscopy remains the gold standard approach for lymph nodes in the superior middle mediastinum. For staging of left-sided lesions, however, VATS has replaced the Chamberlain procedure as our primary method of staging. The additional advantage of the VATS approach is that it also stages the pleural cavity for pleural metastasis, further decreasing the rate of needless exploratory thoracotomies. VATS allows staging of lymph nodes in the aortopulmonary window (level 5), preaortic (level 6), subcarinal (level 7), paraesophageal (level 8), inferior pulmonary ligament (level 9), tracheobronchial (level 10), and hilar lymph nodes (level 11).

Operative Technique

The patient is placed in the usual decubitus position for planned pulmonary resection for cancer. The inverted triangle is used for trocar placement, and if a VATS lobectomy is planned, the anterior incision is placed at the site of the accessory thoracotomy. On entering the chest cavity, the pleural space is explored to rule out pleural metastasis. The mediastinal pleura is opened to examine the lymph node stations. A panoramic view of the lateral hemithorax is possible. In the left hemithorax, good visualization can be obtained of the preaortic level 5 and subaortic level 6 spaces. The posterior mediastinum, near the distal left main stem bronchus (level 7), also can be examined easily. In the right hemithorax, paratracheal lymph nodes to the level of the azygos vein levels 4 and 2 can be identified and sampled adequately. From either hemithorax, it is possible to biopsy the subcarinal lymph (level 7), paraesophageal lymph nodes (level 8), and inferior pulmonary ligament (level 9). Based on the results of the staging, the procedure either is continued or, in the case of positive N2 staging, the procedure is completed with plans for adjuvant therapy.

Results

The largest published series of staging for lung cancer is that of Roviaro et al, in which they showed a reduction in the rate of exploratory thoracotomy to 2.9%. Further published series of lymph node sampling in lung cancer by Naruke et al showed the accuracy of this approach for staging.

■ SYMPATHECTOMY

Indications

Sympathectomy for hyperhidrosis has become one of the most common indications for the VATS approach. Although there is significant experience with the use of sympathectomy for reflex sympathetic dystrophy, the existence of a minimally invasive approach for the treatment of palmar hyperhidrosis has popularized the procedure. Although sympathectomy has been known to be effective for most of the 20th century, the morbidity of the open approaches limited its application. At present, multiple series of thoracoscopic sympathectomy for hyperhidrosis of more than 1000 patients exist in the United States and in Asia.

Technique

We perform a bilateral approach at a single setting. The procedure can be done in a spontaneously breathing patient under local anesthesia and sedation or with general endotracheal anesthesia. We prefer to employ a double-lumen tube and collapse of the lung. With the patient in the supine position, the table is rotated away from the operative side, and three 5-mm incisions are made in the inframammary fold. This leads to a superior cosmetic result in women, who frequently have this disease. A 5-mm, 30-degree scope is inserted through the middle incision, and CO_2 insufflation is used to retract the lung. The ribs are counted carefully, and the sympathetic trunk is identified over the head of the second rib. We use electrocautery to excise the T2 ganglion only. When the ganglion is excised, hemostasis is obtained, and a rubber catheter is placed into the chest cavity while the lung is reinflated. After the chest is deaired under water seal, the catheter is removed, and no chest tubes are used postoperatively. The contralateral side is approached, and the procedure is performed in a similar manner. Bilateral procedures seldom take longer than 30 minutes, and the procedure routinely can be done as an outpatient.

Results

The results of sympathectomy for hyperhidrosis are excellent, with many series reporting virtually a 100% success rate for palmar hyperhidrosis. The procedure also has proved beneficial for axillary hyperhidrosis, facial blushing, and scalp sweating and occasionally benefits plantar hyperhidrosis. Rare cases of Horner's syndrome have been reported, being more common when stellate ganglion is ablated for pain syndromes. The main complication is compensatory hyperhidrosis, with some degree occurring in approximately 65% of patients. Common areas of compensatory hyperhidrosis include the inframammary area, the lower back, and the inner aspect of the thighs. Limiting excision to below the T2 ganglion seems to diminish the compensatory hyperhidrosis.

■ THYMECTOMY

Indications

Thymectomy usually is performed for management of myasthenia gravis and occasionally for thymoma. Benign, circumscribed, and well-encapsulated thymomas can be removed by a VATS approach with extraction via an endoscopic bag. If invasion is suspected, the VATS approach should not be employed. Although we have significant experience with VATS in myasthenia gravis, the experience is limited to few centers beyond our own. One of the basic tenets of myasthenia surgery is that a complete thymectomy with excision of all thymic tissue, including ectopic foci, is necessary to maximize the chance of remission. Concern exists on the part of some surgeons of the ability to resect completely all thymus tissue by a VATS approach.

We have found the VATS approach preferable because a less invasive, superior cosmetic approach is more accepted by young, predominately female myasthenic patients. No significant perioperative management for the myasthenia is required.

Technique

The thymus gland can be accessed through either the left or the right thoracic cavity. We usually choose the right

VATS approach because of wider access to the mediastinum without the pericardium and heart limiting the view and easier identification of the superior vena cava and innominate vein for landmarks. The patient's right side is elevated to allow placement of instrumentation in the mid to posterior axillary line. Four incisions are used because a fan retractor is necessary in the latter stages of dissection to distract the extensive amount of dissected tissue. CO_2 insufflation is used, and it is especially helpful to open up and expose the cervical area for resection. Dissection is begun anterior to the phrenic nerve and continued in the retrosternal area. All anterior mediastinal tissue is excised, including the fat at the pericardiophrenic angle. Thymic veins are identified at the junction with the innominate vein and doubly clipped with endoscopic hemoclips. By downward traction with a fan retractor, the superior poles into the cervical area can be identified. Dissection can be tedious in the cervical area, but the superior poles can be identified reliably and excised completely. Identification of the contralateral phrenic nerve can be difficult, and we use blunt dissection to sweep all mediastinal tissue off of the contralateral pleura. Because of this, some surgeons perform bilateral thoracoscopy to simplify the dissection process. When exenteration of all anterior mediastinal tissue is performed, the specimen is put in an endoscopic bag because it simplifies extraction out of the chest cavity. If a rent in the contralateral pleura exists, it is of no consequence. At the completion of the procedure, the chest cavity is deaired, and unless inadvertent lung injury has occurred no chest tube is placed. Extubation is in the operating room, care in the intensive care unit is not necessary, and discharge is routinely on the first postoperative day.

Results

We have performed thymectomy in 36 patients for myasthenia gravis. Although it is difficult to compare series due to the heterogeneity of the disease and the undulating nature of the disease course, we believe that our results are comparable to the open approaches. Although our complete remission is lower than other published series, our overall remission rate is the same. The new classification of the Myasthenia Gravis Foundation should allow better comparison of the results of different series.

■ CONCLUSION

VATS is a valid alternative for mediastinal disease in which a relatively simple operative procedure contrasts with the morbidity of the classic thoracotomy and sternotomy approaches. In many centers, VATS now is considered the procedure of choice for excision of anterior and posterior mediastinal masses and mediastinal cysts and for the staging of lung cancer. Because of the existence of VATS, the volume of sympathectomy procedures has increased dramatically over the last 5 years. The role of VATS in the management of myasthenia gravis is controversial, and we suspect will remain so for the foreseeable future.

SUGGESTED READING

Demmy TL, et al: Mutlicenter VATS experience with mediastinal tumors, *Ann Thorac Surg* 66:187, 1998.

Gossot D, et al: Early complications of thoracic endoscopic sympathectomy: a prospective study of 940 procedures, *Ann Thorac Surg* 71:1116, 2001.

Mack MJ: Video-assisted thoracoscopy thymectomy for myasthenia gravis, *Chest* 11:389, 2001.

Naruke T, et al: Lymph node sampling in lung cancer: how should it be done? *Eur J Cardiothorac Surg* 16:S17, 1999.

Roviaro GC, et al: Videothoracoscopic approach to mediastinal pathology, *Chest* 17:1179, 2000.

VIDEO-ASSISTED THORACIC SURGERY AND ESOPHAGEAL DISEASE

Ziv Gamliel
Mark J. Krasna

There has been a rapid and steady increase in the number of video-assisted thoracic surgery (VATS) procedures being performed worldwide. Using thoracoscopic instruments, access to the entire left and right hemithoraces and the mediastinum can be obtained. Large, painful, muscle-dividing, rib-spreading incisions no longer are required to provide access to thoracic structures. Most reported cases involve the use of VATS for pulmonary, pleural, mediastinal, and pericardial disease. The use of VATS for functional disorders of the esophagus and for benign and malignant esophageal lesions is becoming more widespread as experience with thoracoscopic instrumentation increases.

■ BENIGN STRUCTURAL LESIONS

The usefulness of VATS techniques in esophageal surgery has been shown most clearly in the surgical management of benign lesions. The surgical approach to benign lesions classically has involved making a big incision to perform a small operation requiring limited dissection. The rapidly increasing number of published case reports of thoracoscopic esophageal operations suggests that such generous access to the surgical field is not always necessary.

The list of benign structural lesions of the esophagus that have been approached thoracoscopically is steadily growing. These VATS operations have included excision of benign lesions, such as leiomyomas and esophageal duplication cysts, and repair of structural lesions, such as fistulas, diverticula, and perforations. VATS repair of a paraesophageal hernia also has been reported. The increasing variety of available endoscopic staplers and clip appliers and endoscopic retracting, dissecting, and suturing instruments has contributed to the increasing use of thoracoscopy to manage benign structural lesions of the esophagus.

VATS enucleation of leiomyoma often can be accomplished easily. Placement of a nasogastric tube or flexible esophagoscope before starting the procedure can be helpful. With the patient in the left lateral decubitus position, ports are established in the seventh interspace in the posterior axillary line, in the fifth interspace in the anterolateral line, and in the sixth interspace in the posterolateral line. The operating thoracoscope is placed via the inferior port. The lung is retracted anteriorly via the anterior port. Via the posterior port and via the operating thoracoscope, the mediastinal pleura

overlying the leiomyoma is opened with endoscopic scissors. Enucleation of the leiomyoma can be accomplished sharply with endoscopic scissors and bluntly with an endoscopic Kittner dissector. A heavy silk retraction suture can be passed through the leiomyoma via the anterior port site to facilitate the enucleation. Hemostasis is achieved with electrocautery and endoscopic clips, avoiding injury to the mucosal layer. The specimen is delivered via the anterior port site using an endoscopic retrieval bag.

The decision to approach benign structural lesions of the esophagus thoracoscopically should be governed by several factors. The familiarity of the surgeon with the surgical anatomy of the esophagus and open techniques of esophageal surgery is crucial. Less technically demanding procedures, such as enucleation of leiomyomata, should be attempted before advancing to more challenging procedures, such as excision of diverticula or repair of perforations. The size and location of the lesion sometimes may influence the ease with which VATS can be performed. Port placement may be high or low, from the left or right, and should be dictated by the specific location of the lesion. The same management principles governing open surgical techniques must be applied in VATS approaches. The ability to convert immediately to an open incision approach is essential.

Benign Functional Disorders

VATS for benign esophageal disease is not limited to structural lesions. Various functional disorders of the esophagus can be managed thoracoscopically. These VATS procedures include truncal vagotomy, esophageal myotomy, Collis gastroplasty, and fundoplication. The indications for these thoracoscopic procedures are the same as those for the standard open procedures. Using endoscopic instrumentation, these procedures should be performed using the same intraoperative management principles as their respective standard open procedures.

VATS truncal vagotomy can be accomplished from either the left or the right side. Its chief advantage is in the reoperative setting, where it obviates the need for dissection through scar tissue formed after previous surgery on the intraabdominal esophagus. In such a situation, the thoracoscopic approach allows a less invasive, shorter, and safer operation. An operating thoracoscope with a working channel is recommended. Typically, three ports are used. The mediastinal pleura is incised, and a short length of distal esophagus is mobilized circumferentially. The left and right vagus nerves are identified and dissected off the esophageal wall. A short segment of each vagus nerve is excised after the proximal and distal ends are clipped. The circumference of the esophagus is inspected carefully for additional vagal branches. No gastric drainage procedure is performed initially, but balloon dilation of the pylorus can be used in case of prolonged gastric atony.

To avoid thoracotomy for extramucosal esophagomyotomy, pneumatic balloon dilation has been used in the treatment of achalasia. Several series of VATS myotomy have been published with good results reported. A flexible esophagoscope can be positioned in the esophagus to insufflate and transilluminate. With the patient in the right lateral decubitus position, superior and inferior ports are established at the left sixth and ninth interspaces in the posterior axillary line. An anterior port is established in the fifth interspace in the anterior axillary line, and a posterior port is established in the eighth interspace in the posterolateral line. Using an operating thoracoscope with a working channel, the inferior pulmonary ligament is divided with endoscopic scissors aided by electrocautery. Next, with the monitor at the foot of the table, the diaphragm is retracted downward via the inferior port, and the lateral wall of the esophagus is held taut via the anterior and posterior ports. This allows the myotomy to be performed via the superior port using endoscopic scissors aided by electrocautery. The esophagus is not encircled. An endoscopic Kittner dissector can be used to dissect bluntly the circular esophageal muscle over 50% of the esophageal circumference. Mucosal perforation can be ruled out by insufflation via the esophagoscope and repaired by endoscopic suturing.

The widespread performance of laparoscopic Nissen fundoplication has created concerns about its indiscriminate use in cases of esophageal shortening to avoid a thoracotomy. There have been increasing numbers of reports of VATS stapled, uncut Collis gastroplasty. This procedure has been performed in association with thoracoscopic fundoplication. At this time, there are few follow-up data available on thoracoscopic fundoplication. As the popularity of laparoscopic Nissen fundoplication soars, the ability to offer a thoracoscopic alternative in cases of esophageal shortening will become increasingly important. For now, much more study of long-term results is warranted.

■ STAGING OF ESOPHAGEAL CANCER

The modern treatment of esophageal cancer is based on disease stage. The presence of lymph node metastases may dictate the use of preoperative neoadjuvant chemotherapy or radiotherapy. The location of lymph node metastases may influence neoadjuvant radiation fields. Accurate preresection staging of esophageal cancer has remained a challenging problem. Nonsurgical staging tools, such as computed tomography, magnetic resonance imaging, and endoscopic ultrasound (EUS), have contributed greatly to the accuracy of presurgical staging. Nonetheless, these techniques have inherent limitations that lower their accuracy.

Imaging modalities such as computed tomography, magnetic resonance imaging, and EUS often fail to determine clearly whether an esophageal cancer is locally invading surrounding structures. Size criteria alone are inaccurate in evaluating for lymph node metastases, making such imaging modalities unhelpful in this regard. EUS occasionally has been useful in detecting invasion of local structures but is not able to assess accurately invasion of the membranous wall of the airway due to technical limitations. Although EUS-guided fine needle aspiration of suspicious lymph nodes has been performed with increasing success, the number of specimens that can be obtained usually is limited. Lymph nodes may be beyond the reach of an endoscopic needle. Because of the possibility of specimen contamination by passage of the needle through the primary tumor, peritumoral nodes cannot be sampled accurately by EUS.

VATS staging of esophageal cancer is especially useful in distinguishing between T3 and T4 tumors and in assessing for lymph node metastases. This technique usually involves a right thoracoscopy, allowing close inspection or even partial mobilization of the primary tumor to rule out local invasion of adjacent structures. Right thoracoscopy allows sampling of peritracheal, periesophageal, subcarinal, and inferior pulmonary ligament nodes. Occasionally, unsuspected metastatic disease can be detected in the lung parenchyma or on the pleural surfaces. When aortic invasion or aortopulmonary window lymph node involvement must be ruled out, a left thoracoscopy is performed.

Staging thoracoscopy is performed with a nasogastric tube in place and with the patient tilted slightly forward in the lateral decubitus position. The number of ports may vary from one to five, but the procedure typically involves three port sites. On the right side, the chest usually is entered bluntly at first in the eighth intercostal space in the mid axillary line. Under thoracoscopic guidance, two additional sharp trocars are placed in the fifth intercostal space in the anterior axillary line and in the sixth intercostal space in the posterior axillary line.

The anterior port is used for lung retraction. The other two ports are used for endoscopic scissors or cautery dissection and suction and retraction of the pleura. The use of an operating thoracoscope with a working channel is highly recommended. Before partially mobilized lymph nodes are excised completely, an endoscopic clip applier is used for ligation of the vascular pedicle. To facilitate thorough sampling of the lower paratracheal lymph nodes on the right, the azygos arch can be divided with a vascular endoscopic stapler. To allow sampling of the inferior pulmonary ligament node, the ligament is divided with electrocautery with the patient in steep Trendelenburg position. If necessary, the primary tumor can be mobilized to assess local invasion.

After the completion of thoracoscopic staging, a single straight chest tube is introduced via the inferior port site and passed posterosuperiorly toward the apex of the chest cavity. When the chest tube drainage permits, the chest tube is removed. Depending on what other procedures have been performed concomitantly (e.g., laparoscopic staging, jejunostomy, Mediport insertion), the patient usually is discharged later on the day of VATS staging or the following morning. Complications of VATS staging are rare.

The accuracy of computed tomography in assessing regional lymph node status is less than 70%. EUS may overstage the depth of tumor invasion in 6% to 11% of cases. The diagnostic accuracy of thoracoscopic lymph node staging is approximately 95%. The accuracy of VATS assessment of local invasion (T3 versus T4 stage) approaches 100%. Coupled with its accuracy and low morbidity, the ability of thoracoscopy to sample lymph nodes that are remote from the esophagus and suspected lung/pleural metastases makes it a useful staging tool.

■ RESECTION OF ESOPHAGEAL CANCER

When performed for malignant disease, esophageal resection classically has involved exposure in the chest. Right thoracotomy used in the Lewis-Tanner and McKeown approaches has been associated with postoperative pain, dysfunction, and other morbidity. Esophagectomy without thoracotomy has been performed successfully via the transhiatal approach but limits the ability to obtain a radial resection margin and precludes methodical lymphadenectomy. As a result of an increased incidence of intraoperative bleeding and injuries to the membranous wall of the airway, several series have failed to document a significant reduction in pulmonary complications using this approach.

With the intent of reducing postoperative pain, dysfunction, and morbidity from thoracotomy without resorting to blind, blunt transhiatal esophagectomy, VATS mobilization of the intrathoracic esophagus has been performed with increasing frequency. This technique affords excellent visualization, allowing meticulous dissection and lymphadenectomy, and can be performed safely by surgeons with a thorough knowledge of the surgical anatomy of the esophagus and extensive experience with VATS techniques. If there is any doubt about the possibility of local tumor invasion (T4 stage), VATS mobilization should be abandoned in favor of open thoracotomy.

VATS mobilization of the esophagus most commonly has been used in conjunction with open cervical esophagogastric anastomosis. Intrathoracic esophagogastric anastomosis also has been performed thoracoscopically using a double-stapling technique. Results have been mixed, with at least one series reporting no reduction in the anticipated rate of postoperative complications, including atelectasis, anastomotic leaks, pleural effusions, pneumonia, and stricture. Seeding of port sites with tumor also has been reported. Until more experience is gained with this technique and until further refinements in instrumentation are made, thoracoscopic esophagogastric anastomosis cannot be regarded as the preferred approach.

■ SUMMARY

It rapidly is becoming apparent that almost any thoracic esophageal operation can be performed thoracoscopically. In the case of some procedures, VATS already is preferred over open thoracotomy. In the case of other esophageal operations, it remains to be seen whether thoracoscopy offers any overall advantage. Continual refinement of thoracoscopic instruments and techniques will help minimize the disadvantages of this sometimes tedious and difficult approach. While gaining further experience with thoracoscopy for esophageal disease, it is important to adhere to the same surgical management principles that guide open surgical approaches and to evaluate long-term results.

SUGGESTED READING

Gamliel Z, Krasna MJ: The role of video-assisted thoracic surgery in esophageal disease, *Chest Surg Clin N Am* 8:853, 1998.

Krasna MJ, et al, CALGB Thoracic Surgeons: CALGB9380: a prospective trial of the feasibility of thoracoscopy/laparoscopy in staging esophageal cancer, *Ann Thorac Surg* 71:1073, 2001.

Luketich JD, et al: Minimally invasive esophagectomy, *Ann Thorac Surg* 70:906, 2000.

Wiechmann RJ, et al: Video-assisted surgical management of achalasia of the esophagus, *J Thorac Cardiovasc Surg* 118:916, 1999.

VIDEO-ASSISTED THORACIC SURGERY FOR PLEURAL DISEASE

Joseph I. Miller, Jr.
Russel S. Ronson

Since the first documented thoracoscopy by Jacobaeus in 1910, diseases of the pleura and pleural space have been the most frequent indication for its diagnostic and therapeutic use. With the introduction of video assistance in the 1980s and improved instrumentation, video-assisted thoracic surgery (VATS) has become an important part of the diagnostic and therapeutic armamentarium of a thoracic surgeon's practice. Although video technology and instrumentation have changed dramatically since the 1980s, the indications for thoracoscopy in pleural disease have changed minimally. VATS procedures for the diagnosis of unknown pleural effusion, lysis of pleural pulmonary adhesions, installation of pleurodesis agents, and biopsy and excision of pleural base masses have been performed in Europe and the United States. The evident change is the ease with which these procedures can be performed with greater sensitivity and diagnostic accuracy, coupled with a broader range of therapeutic maneuvers that can be done safely and definitively.

■ INDICATIONS

The indications for VATS in pleural disease are listed in Table 1. Thoracoscopy to identify the cause of undiagnosed

Table 1 Indications for Video-Assisted Thoracic Surgery in Pleural Disease

Determine cause of undiagnosed pleural effusion
Drainage, débridement, and decortication of early empyema
Chemical and mechanical pleurodesis for benign and malignant effusions
Evacuation of traumatic and postoperative hemothorax
Biopsy of pleural-based lesions
Excision of primary lesions of the pleura

pleural effusions is a routine practice and is the most common indication for VATS in most hospital centers.

VATS not only allows for drainage and adequate sampling of fluids for laboratory evaluation, but also biopsy of pleural and parenchymal nodules, should they exist. The diagnostic accuracy of biopsy with direct visualization surpasses any of the closed techniques, while allowing for additional treatment planning of the physician and patient without the morbidity of a thoracotomy. Débridement of early empyemas and loculated effusions, evaluations of postoperative traumatic hemithoraces, and pleurodesis for persistent or life-threatening hemithoraces also are recognized indications for initial thoracoscopic intervention.

The success of VATS has led to the expansion of its use to the pediatric and elderly populations. Thoracoscopic drainage of empyemas in children is frequently the only treatment necessary and allows avoidance of a thoracotomy and its subsequent morbidity. The indications for VATS in the elderly and pediatric populations still are controversial, however, in some areas, and the limited data on these subsets of the patient population make conclusions about efficacy and cost-effectiveness difficult. Following are descriptions of some of the specific indications.

Undiagnosed Pleural Effusion

The major indication for VATS is the undiagnosed cause of a pleural effusion. Approximately 30% of pleural effusions have inconclusive diagnoses after thoracentesis, owing to negative and inadequate evaluation of pleural cytology.

The inadequacy of a needle thoracentesis also is highlighted by the yield of only approximately 20% sensitivity in the effusion of patients with mesothelioma. With the use of thoracoscopy, the diagnostic yield approaches 100%. Harris et al reported a series 124 patients with undiagnosed pleural effusions; the diagnostic sensitivity of thoracoscopy for malignancy in undiagnosed effusions was 95%, specificity was 100%, and negative predicted value was 94%. In this cohort of patients, many had two to three negative needle thoracenteses before thoracoscopic examination. Reports documenting malignancy as the origin for previously undiagnosed pleural effusions range from 46% to 91%. The Video Assisted Thoracic Surgery Study Group (VATSSG) reported the largest series of VATS treatment to date. Of the 1820 thoracoscopic cases reported from 40 institutions since 1992, 274 had previously undiagnosed cause of their pleural effusions; 36.9% were benign, and 63.1% were malignant.

VATS also allows the adequate sampling of effusion fluid for specific pathologic examination after definitive diagnosis has been made. Cell markers for patients with suspected lymphoma and hormonal receptor analysis for patients determined to have metastatic breast cancer have been used for further therapeutic decision making after VATS at our institution. With the advent of molecular markers, molecular staging is becoming more commonplace in lung carcinoma. It is likely that VATS will be used to sample malignant pleural tissue to determine marker behavior and to determine a more effective therapeutic oncologic drug regimen.

The diagnosis of benign pleural effusion is often more difficult and less successful than with malignant processes. Benign diseases found at thoracoscopy include empyema, pulmonary tuberculosis, bile pleuritis, sarcoidosis, and nonspecific inflammatory disease.

Empyema

Empyema is the most common benign pleural collection diagnosed and treated with VATS. Empyema is an age-old problem first described by Hippocrates, which has plagued thoracic surgeons since the beginning of the 20th century. Although the incidence has decreased markedly since the introduction of antibiotics, empyemas have not disappeared from the spectrum of diseases treated by thoracic surgeons. Less than 1% of antibiotic-treated bacterial pneumonia results in empyema, but 5% of patients develop a parapneumonic effusion associated with their parenchymal disease. Of these parapneumonic effusions, 20% develop into empyemas. The spectrum of empyema thoracis ranges from thin free-flowing intrapleural fluid (phase 1), to a fibrinopurulent exudate with thin loculations and the beginnings of an organized inflammatory reaction (phase 2), to a well-organized, loculated, thick purulent fluid that forms a peel or rind to the pleural surfaces (phase 3). The acuteness of the fluid accumulation combined with the viscosity of the fluid and the state of loculation make it easy for VATS to be performed in the early course (phases 1 and 2) of developing organized empyema with complete evacuation of all fluid and early débridement of the pleural space. Late organized fluid collections frequently require open decortication with drainage.

Initial therapy with VATS does not preclude later thoracotomy needed for better exposure, difficult dissection, and disruption of dense loculations. Incisions placed in the line of a future potential thoracotomy do not affect a later procedure cosmetically or technically; however, delays in diagnosis make thoracoscopy significantly more technically difficult, with increased prolonged illness, increased complications, and an inability to treat the advanced process with VATS alone. We do not recommend VATS for the third phase of empyema, in which fluid is highly organized and a thick rind is formed on the pleural surfaces.

Success rates of empyema treated with VATS treatment modalities vary widely. Outcomes of empyema treatment with VATS are summarized in Table 2. In a prospective randomized trial of VATS compared with tube thoracostomy and instillation of streptokinase done in 1997 by Wait et al, VATS resulted in significantly shorter hospital stays, shorter intensive care unit stays, and fewer days requiring a chest tube. In addition, the success rate of complete resolution of

Table 2 Thoracoscopic Treatment of Empyema

AUTHOR	PATIENTS (N)	SUCCESS WITHOUT FURTHER TREATMENT (%)
Wait et al (1997)	11	100
Karmy-Jones et al (1997)	13	92
Mack et al (1992)	4	75
Ridley (1991)	30	60

Modified from Ronson RS, Miller JI: Video-assisted thoracoscopy for pleural disease, *Chest Surg Clin N Am* 8:919, 1998.

Table 3 Talc Regimen for Pleurodesis

COMPONENT	AMOUNT
Talc	5 g
Saline	50 ml
1% Lidocaine (Xylocaine)	5 ml

pleural disease was 100% with VATS compared with 44% with tube thoracostomy and streptokinase alone.

The extent of disease, organization of the empyema, and time course of the infection must determine individualized therapy for each patient, rather than uniformly using a specific treatment for all patients presenting with empyema thoracis. Strategic planning and integrated use of all therapies available is needed to optimize patient outcome.

Hemothorax

Hemothoraces are being treated with VATS with increasing frequency because of the high success rates and limited morbidity and mortality. Evacuation of a retained hemothorax with VATS after coronary artery bypass surgery has become commonplace for thoracic surgeons. The increased use of off-pump coronary artery bypass surgery and the rush to get patients out of the hospital have led to the development of an increasing number of postpericardiotomy syndromes with a collection of fluid in the pleural space, particularly on the right, frequently representing blood or an exudative effusion. Techniques to address these problems are discussed later.

Pleurodesis

Pleurodesis, both chemical and mechanical, has become a mainstay of treatment of malignant pleural effusions, persistent pneumothorax, and empyemas. Mechanical abrasion has been done using Kittner sponges, cautery scratch pads, endoscopic lasers, and endoscopic cautery. The most effective means of accomplishing thoracoscopic pleurodesis has been with the instillation of chemical talc to produce an inflammatory pleuritis, resulting in obliteration of the pleural space by parietal and visceral pleural symphysis. Agents used for chemical pleurodesis include talc, doxycycline, fibrin glue, kaolin derivatives, and silver nitrate. The advantage of using VATS for pleurodesis is the ability to perform adhesiolysis and chemical instillation and distribution with a single intervention that has minimal morbidity.

Talc pleurodesis is the standard with which all chemical pleurodesis is compared. Hartman et al performed talc insufflation in 51 patients with malignant effusions using local anesthesia and video assistance in the endoscopy suite. At 30- and 90-day follow-up, 97% and 95% of patients had complete resolution of effusion. This was compared with success rates of 33% and 47% in a similar group treated only with tube thoracostomy and insufflation of bleomycin

or tetracycline. Average hospital stay in the VATS group was 4 days, and no significant complications ensued. Other authors have reported success rates using VATS-assisted pleurodesis for malignant and benign effusions of 87% to 99% with limited morbidity, including patients with significant metastatic disease. The advantages of talc are its ease in instillation, effective distribution with good visualization, and high success rate. The regimen used for talc instillation at our institution is presented in Table 3. Operative cost, general anesthesia, and poor healing of severely debilitated patients must be taken into account before scheduling VATS in patients with limited life spans. Alternative techiques through closed chest tube thoracostomy and talc instillation can be carried out in these debilitated individuals.

Pleural Masses

Video techniques have enabled definitive diagnosis and treatment of large and more complex benign, malignant, and metastatic pleural lesions. The diagnosis of pleural-based mass lesions with closed needle biopsy is often difficult, and repeated attempts at diagnosis with blind punctures and radiographically directed catheters are becoming more infrequent with the increased use and high success of VATS. Inadequate tissue sampling and difficulty differentiating between mesothelioma and metastatic lesions make closed biopsy techniques difficult in many cases. Sensitivities for correct diagnosis of pleural mass using VATS-directed biopsy range from 80% to 100%. Pleural processes in the absence of an effusion mandate VATS as the diagnostic technique of choice to avoid injury of the parenchymal tissues adjacent to the parietal pleura that can occur with closed techniques.

Although benign lesions of the pleura are seen infrequently, they may be diagnosed and treated using thoracoscopy without the need for open thoracotomy. Solitary fibrous nodules and benign mesothelioma often are excised easily under direct vision using VATS. The primary advantage of thoracoscopy for benign pleural disease is the ability to rule out a concomitant or undiagnosed malignant process.

Malignant mesothelioma is the primary pleural malignancy most often seen by thoracic surgeons. Traditionally, this highly lethal disease has been treated with supportive measures and palliative interventional therapy. The role of VATS in the management of mesothelioma is still being debated, but some of the initial reports indicate that it may be useful in select patients. Cytology in mesothelioma is frequently nondiagnostic, making needle thoracocentesis a poor diagnostic technique. For these reasons, thoracoscopy is strongly advocated for all patients with the preliminary diagnosis of malignant mesothelioma.

The sensitivity of thoracoscopic diagnosis for malignant mesothelioma is high, with rates of 95% being reported, comparable to open techniques. The role of VATS treatment for malignant mesothelioma, other than diagnosis, is yet to be defined.

Elderly

The studies using VATS for diagnosis and treatment of pleural disease in the elderly are limited. In 1996, Jaklitsch et al reported an excellent review of 296 patients older than age 65 who underwent thoracoscopic evaluation of thoracic disease. Of these patients, 25% had pleural pathology as their indication for intervention. The low mortality in their cohort is in contrast to previous reports of increasing mortality with thoracotomy. The threshold for diagnostic and therapeutic intervention with VATS should be less with the elderly population, given the potential increased benefit without compromise of treatment success.

Pediatric

The hallmark of thoracoscopic treatment of pleural disease in children is for empyema. Débridement and decortication in children usually is fraught with less difficulty than in adults. Milanez de campo et al reported a success rate of 88.2% for complete treatment of empyema in children younger than age 18 without the need for further intervention. In our own institution, this is the treatment of choice for all pediatric empyema, and it is rare that an open thoracotomy in a pediatric patient is required for the treatment of pleural empyema.

■ TECHNIQUE

Operative techniques for VATS are varied, ranging from local to general anesthesia, one-lung versus two-lung ventilation, single versus multiple ports of entry, 0- to 90-degree endoscopes, and even operative or endoscopic suites for performing the procedure. Simple diagnostic thoracoscopy using a mediastinoscope can be done today if only a pleural effusion is present. The patient is placed in an anterolateral position using single-lumen ventilation. A 0.5-inch incision is made in the fifth or sixth intercostal space in the anterior axillary line. Fluid is removed for culture, cytology, and chemical studies; digital palpation is performed; and the endoscope is introduced. Simple pleural biopsy and examination of all pleural surfaces are carried out. This technique is cost-effective and avoids the set-up fee for VATS and double-lumen anesthesia. A single chest tube is brought out through the port site. Although considered old-fashioned, this technique can be used effectively. We performed this technique until 1990, when VATS became available. It is still used in selected cases.

When VATS is performed, the patient is placed in the lateral decubitus position with the pathologic side superiorly. Appropriate padding is placed so that there is no undue pressure placed on the elbow, arms, torso, or legs.

Anesthetic technique consists of double-lumen endotracheal intubation, arterial line, continuous pulse oximetry, and, if necessary, central venous pressure monitoring. Anesthesia is introduced, and the ipsilateral lung is deflated.

The number of ports needed for procedures treating pleural-based disease depends on the extent and nature of the preoperative goal. The Stortz operating thoracoscope (W. Stortz, Zurich, Switzerland) gives excellent visualization and allows disruption of the pleural space, loculated fluid pockets, and biopsy of pleural masses. One can use a 0-degree scope, a 30-degree scope, or a 45-degree scope. Either a 10- or 5-mm scope can be used depending on which size is available. The initial incision for a single-port placement is in the anterior axillary line in the fifth or sixth intercostal space. The scope is directed slightly posteriorly to allow for investigation of the entire cavity. Adhesions from the visceral to the parietal pleura may need to be divided on entrance into the thoracic space. This should be done slowly and with caution to avoid bleeding, which makes visualization more difficult as the scope is introduced. When the pleural space is entered, complete visualization of all surface and structures is available. The surgeon should examine visceral and parietal pleura, diaphragm, and pericardium. Pleura and lung biopsy specimens are obtained easily as indicated.

Multiple ports provide for more complex exposures to be done, allowing assistants access to help retract, cauterize, or stabilize tissue. The second port generally is placed in the mid axillary line, again in the fifth intercostal space. On completion of the procedure, a single chest tube is brought out through the port site.

■ SUMMARY

The techniques available for any one particular procedure are as numerous as the number of surgeons performing that procedure. Mechanical abrasion for pleurodesis can be done with sponges, cotton-tip applicators, electrocautery, and endoscopic lasers. Disruption of fluid loculations by blunt-tip suction devices, digital manipulation, ring forceps, or Metzenbaum scissors is another example of the diversity of methods used to achieve the same results. Regardless of the technique, the important factor is complete and adequate visualization of all structures and maintenance of the same operative principles and standards set for the same procedure as if it were done using conventional open techniques. VATS has become the standard for diagnosing pleural disease when conventional modalities fail.

SUGGESTED READINGS

Harris RJ, et al: The diagnostic and therapeutic utility of thoracoscopy: a review, *Chest* 108:828, 1995.

Hazelrigg SR, et al: Video Assisted Thoracic Surgery Study Group data, *Ann Thorac Surg* 56:1039, 1993.

Jaklitsch MT, et al: Video-assisted thoracic surgery in the elderly: a review of 307 cases, *Chest* 110:751, 1996.

Kaiser LR: Video-assisted thoracic surgery: current state of the art, *Ann Surg* 220:720, 1994.

Ronson RS, Miller JI: Video-assisted thoracoscopy for pleural disease, *Chest Surg Clin N Am* 8:919, 1998.

Wait MA, et al: A randomized trial of empyema therapy, *Chest* 111:1548, 1997.

Yim APC, et al: Thoracoscopic management of malignant pleural effusions, *Chest* 109:1234, 1996.

COMPLICATIONS OF VIDEO-ASSISTED THORACIC SURGERY

Walter E. McGregor
Rodney J. Landreneau

Video-assisted thoracic surgery (VATS) is the evolutionary development of thoracoscopy, which first was performed by the Swedish internist Jacobaeus in 1913. He introduced a primitive cystoscope into the thorax to lyse pleural adhesions and enhance the collapse therapy for pulmonary tuberculosis popular in that period. The development of effective antimicrobial therapy for tuberculosis in the 1940s led to declining use of this minimally invasive thoracic procedure. Interest in the use of thoracoscopy as a diagnostic approach to pleural pathology persisted, particularly among European physicians.

Improvements in fiberoptics, video optics, and endoscopic instrumentation in the 1980s led to the development of successful videoscopic surgical techniques for a wide variety of intraabdominal and orthopedic problems previously managed through open surgical approaches. Thoracic surgeons were relatively late to join the surgeons engaged in these minimally invasive videoscopic surgical approaches. Today many thoracic surgeons have come to use VATS, however, selectively for a variety of thoracic surgical problems. As the experience with VATS approaches has matured since the 1990s, it has become important to be aware of the complications related to these approaches. Most of these complications are a direct result of faulty surgical judgment or inadequate technical experience with VATS.

This chapter reviews results and general concepts related to VATS, summarizes possible adverse consequences associated with VATS, and identifies measures that can be taken to reduce their occurrence. The VATS approach has been explored as an alternative to open thoracotomy for the management of a wide variety of thoracic surgical problems. The results of critical analysis have shown that VATS is versatile and safe when used by experienced surgeons. The reported surgical mortality is low (0.07% to 2.0%). Postoperative deaths are almost uniformly related to the virulence of the thoracic disease process being approached by VATS (i.e., malignant pleural and pericardial effusions, empyema with associated pneumonia, or interstitial lung disease with pulmonary hypertension and progressive hypoxia). Nonfatal intraoperative and postoperative complication rates also are low (3.6% to 10.9%) (Table 1). Complication rates tend to decline as the surgeon develops skills with videoscopic surgery.

A few key videoscopic surgical skills must be mastered to optimize the results with VATS. The surgeon must overcome the dissociation between the visual field (video monitor) and his or her reliance on direct palpation and manipulation of the target intrathoracic pathology. The two-dimensional limitations of videoscopic visibility of the thorax also must be recognized and overcome. Understanding the importance of strategic intercostal access necessary to conduct the proposed VATS intervention is crucial for a timely and safe procedure. To achieve appropriate intercostal access, several basic principles should be applied. First, the initial intercostal access site should be placed at a distance from the lesion to achieve a panoramic view and provide full visibility of hand instrumentation that is introduced lateral to the target pathology. Second, instrument crowding should be avoided, which otherwise may result in "fencing" during instrument manipulation. Third, mirror imaging should be avoided by positioning instruments and thoracoscope within the same 180-degree arc. That is, the lesion should be approached in the same general direction with instruments and camera. Fourth, instruments should be moved serially, rather than synchronously, to avoid operative chaos and should be manipulated only when seen directly through the thoracoscope. Familiarity with the limitations and the utility of endosurgical instrumentation is important. Refinement of endosurgical technical skills and mature surgical judgment are necessary to choose VATS appropriately over open thoracic approaches.

We now specifically review the complications that can be seen with the VATS approach to a variety of intrathoracic problems (see Table 1). We also discuss some technical maneuvers aimed at overcoming these problems and offer some insight into clinical decision making that can aid in avoiding adverse consequences of VATS.

■ PULMONARY PARENCHYMAL INJURY AND PERSISTENT BRONCHOPLEURAL FISTULA

By definition, VATS is used to address intrathoracic conditions requiring surgical diagnosis or treatment. The most commonly addressed problems by the VATS approach are those of the lung and pleura. Several circumstances inherent to the underlying thoracic pathology place the pulmonary parenchyma at risk for injury. Careful review of the patient's preoperative radiographic studies are critical before the VATS intervention. Computed tomography (CT) may show significant pleural thickening or pleural adhesions, which must be avoided during intercostal access to avoid inadvertent pulmonary parenchymal injury. This is of particular concern when VATS is used to manage complex/loculated pleural fluid collections. To avoid this, initial port placement should be directly into an area of pleural fluid.

The nature of the target pathology identified by CT scan must be scrutinized closely before committing to the VATS approach. Large areas of dense consolidation present within a background of interstitial lung disease are best avoided as sites of VATS lung biopsy. The use of VATS for excision biopsy of indeterminate deep-seated pulmonary lesions and pulmonary lesions greater than 3 cm in diameter also should be avoided. The presence of endobronchial extension of the target pathology also precludes the use of VATS wedge approaches to accomplish excisional biopsy of the lung. Attempting VATS wedge resection in this setting is likely to

Table 1 Complications in 5280 Thoracoscopies

COMPLICATION	INCIDENCE (%)
Persistent air leak	1.76
Hemorrhage	0.44
Pneumonia	0.25
Atelectasis	0.19
Infection	0.17
Lung parenchyma tear	0.13
Horner's syndrome	0.13
Chest wall pain	0.07
Emphysema	0.05
Bronchopleural fistula	0.04
Pulmonary edema	0.04
Esophageal mucosal laceration	0.04
Recurrent nerve injury	0.04
Arrhythmia	0.04
Respiratory failure	0.04
Chylothorax	0.02
Port implantation metastasis	0.02
Cerebral ischemia	0.02
Total	3.6

From Inderbitzi RGC, Grillet MP: Risks and hazards of videothoracoscopic surgery: a collective review, *Eur J Cardiothorac Surg* 10:483, 1996.

result in fracture of the pulmonary parenchyma because the jaws of the endostapler device are opposed on the thick or indurated tissues. The margins of resection are likely to be compromised and the physiologic integrity of the remaining lobar tissue impaired when deep wedge resections are directed toward such large or centrally located lesions.

Pulmonary parenchymal injury also can result from inadequate isolation and collapse of the ipsilateral lung with double-lumen intubation or bronchus blocking techniques. We believe it mandatory for the thoracic surgeon to confirm bronchoscopically proper positioning of the endotracheal tube before and after lateral positioning of the patient. This endoscopic inspection can reduce the possibility of inadequate pulmonary parenchymal collapse and reduce the inadvertent puncture of the lung during the establishment of intercostal access for the VATS procedure. Inadequate collapse of the lung also can lead to difficulty in identifying the pulmonary pathology. Lung injury can result as endosurgical instruments are used in the limited intrathoracic space. The use of the endostapling device also is made more difficult when it is insinuated across partially expanded lung tissue. Skewering of the lung parenchyma can result as the stapling device is advanced on the pulmonary tissue.

Faulty or "rough" surgical technique also can lead to pulmonary parenchymal injury. The surgeon must manipulate the lung tissue gently and precisely separate foci of visceral to parietal pleura adhesion. Proper application of the endostapler device is crucial to avoid parenchymal injury. Overzealous purchase of pulmonary parenchyma during endostapler application can result in staple line dehiscence. Repeated application and closure of the stapler across the pulmonary parenchyma to improve resection margins also can result in fracture of the fragile intraparenchymal pulmonary vessels, leading to intraparenchymal hematoma. Distortion of anatomic detail can result, which can compromise

the accuracy of subsequent stapler application during the course of VATS wedge resection. Physiologic impairment of the pulmonary lobe from which the wedge resection is being taken also can occur as a result of the intraparenchymal hemorrhage.

The manipulation and resection of emphysematous pulmonary tissue must be done with great care and precision. These flimsy pulmonary tissues are prone to injury when pulmonary adhesions are separated and during the conduct of pulmonary wedge resection. Staple line separation and leakage are seen commonly with reexpansion of the lung on completion of the lung resection procedure. This was a problem despite all efforts of care after "lung reduction" surgical procedures until the introduction of bovine pericardial reinforcement of the resection staple line. It also seems that polytetrafluoroethylene strip (Gore-Tex Inc, Flagstaff, AZ) buttressing of the suture line can reduce effectively the occurrence of prolonged air leak after resection of emphysematous lung tissues. Application of a polymerized polyethylene glycol–based gel, FocalSeal (Genzyme, Tucker, GA, and Focal, Inc, Lexington, MA), over the staple line through an intercostal access site also can assist in sealing microscopic areas of air leak.

Inability to identify an anatomic source of bullous disease for spontaneous pneumothorax at the time of VATS exploration is associated with an unacceptable rate of prolonged postoperative air leak and recurrent pneumothorax after discharge from the hospital. This can occur in 20% of patients operated on for spontaneous pneumothorax. Careful inspection of the apex of the upper lobe, the upper aspect of the superior segment of the lower lobe, and all pleural edges of the lung must be done. The primary site of pleural disruption and secondary loci of bullous disease that may lead to subsequent pneumothorax problems all should be addressed with wedge resection at the time of VATS exploration. When these direct inspection methods fail to identify the source of the pneumothorax, we attempt to observe bubbling from suspicious areas of the lung surface, while partially reexpanding the lung under a small amount of saline. If these measures fail to identify a discrete site of air leak, we recommend the performance of a subtotal apical pleurectomy to facilitate pleurodesis in this area of greatest anatomic likelihood of a small/microscopic visceral pleural disruption. Pleurectomy must be undertaken cautiously at the apex of the chest near the area of the first rib to avoid irritation/injury to the stellate ganglion. This injury may result in the development of a postoperative Horner's syndrome of variable duration.

■ WOUND HEMATOMA AND INTRATHORACIC HEMORRHAGE

Intercostal access site hematoma can occur from a variety of causes. The sites of intercostal access generally should be made closely above the lower rib of the chosen intercostal space to avoid injury to the intercostal vascular pedicle. Intercostal arterial injury also can result in the development of intrathoracic, subpleural, and chest wall hematomas.

Injury to the vascular pedicle of the major chest wall musculature also can occur with the establishment of intercostal access. Intercostal access through the thick belly of the pectoralis major, serratus anterior, and latissimus dorsi musculature should be avoided. Intercostal access through these muscles may be necessary sometimes. Under these circumstances, small intercostal access ports are used to protect entry into the chest rather than introducing instrumentation repeatedly through unprotected intercostal sites. This can reduce trauma to the larger chest wall musculature.

Excessive bleeding also can occur from the lung surface during or after pulmonary decortication. This parenchymal surface bleeding is often less dramatic and resolves with lung reexpansion and adequate drainage of the pleural space. Any coagulopathy that may be present also must be corrected.

Significant and dangerous bleeding from the major pulmonary vasculature can occur during the course of VATS interventions. VATS lobectomy and VATS biopsy of pathologic mediastinal adenopathy are procedures in which particular caution must be applied to avoid vascular injury. The pulmonary vasculature injury should be controlled initially with tamponade. The lung itself can be compressed against the site of injury until a sponge stick is introduced through an appropriate intercostal access to compress the site of vascular injury directly. The surgeon must decide if conversion to open surgery to repair the injury is required.

Vascular injury during VATS thymectomy and VATS resection of posterior mediastinal tumors may occur. Injury to the innominate vein or its tributaries has been the most commonly discussed vascular injury with thymic resection. Subclavian arterial injury can occur during the dissection required to remove posterior neurogenic tumors that commonly are located in the apex of the chest. As described for pulmonary vascular injuries, tamponade of the injury with a sponge stick should be the first maneuver for control of bleeding. Conversion to thoracotomy may be required to repair the problem.

An additional source of bleeding can occur due to injury of intercostal vessels at the sites of intercostal access used for the VATS procedure. Care should be taken to accomplish intercostal access over the top of the lower rib of the interspace chosen for access. Protected trocar access also should be used to reduce the likelihood of intercostal vascular injury that may occur when repeated reentry into the chest with hand instruments is required. Inspection for bleeding at the sites of intercostal access is recommended at the termination of the procedure.

Significant intrathoracic and intraabdominal bleeding also can occur as a result of transdiaphragmatic hepatic or splenic injury when intercostal access is attempted at too low of an intercostal space. This bleeding is seen most commonly when pleural disease processes are approached thoracoscopically. The diaphragm may be elevated due to associated ipsilateral pulmonary collapse or pleural scarification. Careful attention to the CT scans of the chest can assist in establishing the initial intercostal access within the center of the pleural fluid collection at the appropriate interspace.

■ NERVE INJURY

The most common nerve injury seen after VATS is to the intercostal nerves at the sites of intercostal access used for the procedure. Mild-to-moderate paresthesias occurring over the dermatomal innervation of the intercostal nerves injured are the most common acute postoperative symptoms seen. These paresthesias usually resolve over several weeks. They usually manifest as burning and heaviness over the breast and upper abdomen. Injury of intercostal nerves at sites of low intercostal access for VATS also can lead to ipsilateral rectus muscle and abdominal oblique muscular dysfunction. This dysfunction may manifest as a sensation of upper abdominal bloating, particularly after meals or when straining this musculature. This acute intercostal nerve dysfunction seems to occur less frequently than after open thoracotomy. Mild chronic postoperative chest wall discomfort after VATS seems to be similar to that seen after open thoracotomy. This discomfort may be experienced in 28% of patients. Chronic, disabling intercostal neuralgia after VATS can be seen in nearly 1% of patients beyond 1 year of surgery. This rate of significant chronic postoperative pain is similar to that seen after open thoracotomy. Acute and chronic pain after VATS may be prevented by avoiding excessive torque of the thoracoscope and endosurgical instruments against the ribs at the intercostal access site. This torque can result in local rib bruising or fracture or intercostal nerve injury with neuroma formation. Strategic intercostal access for the endosurgical instruments can eliminate the need to lever the thoracoscope against the chest wall to gain visibility.

We also recommend the use of anterolateral locations for intercostal access whenever possible so as to minimize the occurrence of injury at the intercostal access site. This recommendation is based on the greater breadth of the intercostal spaces at a lateral and anterior location. Posteriorly the interspaces are more narrow, and the thoracic musculature is more prominent. These anatomic considerations explain the increased risk of direct and torque injury to the neurovascular bundle and the rib periosteum posteriorly. The use of small-diameter thoracoscopes and hand instrumentation also may reduce such complications. The selective use of angled thoracoscopic optics and flexible or curved endosurgical hand instrumentation may reduce the risk of intercostal nerve injury. Management of patients with chronic pain can be difficult and often is best achieved through consultation with an anesthesiologist interested in chronic chest wall pain issues.

Injury to mediastinal nervous structures is second in order of occurrence with VATS interventions. The recurrent laryngeal branch of the left vagus nerve and the phrenic nerve are especially susceptible to injury during VATS biopsy of aortopulmonary window lymph nodes. The thoracic surgeon must be certain of the anatomic relationships as viewed through the thoracoscope and be sure to visualize the vagus and phrenic nerves before dissecting and obtaining the biopsy specimen of mediastinal pathology in this location (Figure 1). Similar risk of injury to these nerves can occur when adenopathy in the right periazygous mediastinal area is approached. Phrenic nerve injury can occur during pericardial window for the diagnosis/treatment of idiopathic or known malignant pericardial effusions. This injury is more common with left-sided VATS approaches to the pericardium because of the reduced working space available. This is particularly the case when a large pericardial effusion

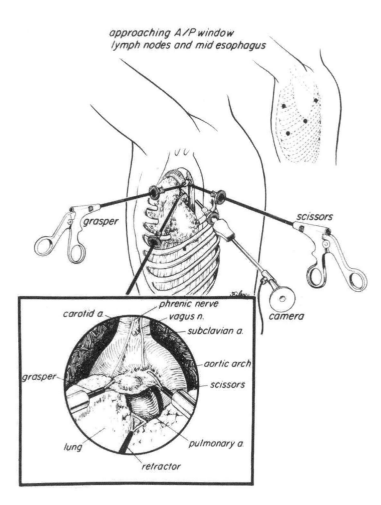

Figure 1
Contents of the aorticopulmonary window visualized during video-assisted thoracic surgery (VATS) exploration of adenopathy in this location. Significant vascular and neural injury can occur if care is not taken during the VATS procedure. (*From Landreneau RJ, et al: Thoracoscopic mediastinal lymph node sampling: useful for mediastinal lymph node stations inaccessible by cervical mediastinoscopy,* J Thorac Cardiovasc Surg *106:554, 1993.*)

is present. We commonly use a right-sided approach to pericardial pathology, unless associated left-sided pathology also is present, which requires thoracic surgical management. As mentioned earlier, stellate ganglion injury can occur during the course of pleurectomy. Injury to this ganglion is also at risk during thoracodorsal sympathectomy performed for the management of a variety of sympathetic syndromes (i.e., hyperhidrosis, causalgia, and Raynaud's phenomenon). As for the prevention of other complications associated with VATS, a full understanding of the surgical anatomy is crucial.

Most sympathectomy procedures involve ablation or isolation of the sympathetic ganglion chain from the level of the second ganglia distally for various lengths. Discrimination between the stellate ganglion and the second thoracodorsal ganglia is important. The stellate ganglion is located beneath the pleural vale at the level of the first rib. This pleura should be incised to identify this nervous structure, which is in close proximity to the subclavian vessels. Management of nerve injuries consists of watchful surveillance. Traction and minor electrocautery injury to the stellate ganglia usually improves or resolves over 3 to 6 months; however, transection or ablation of the ganglia is often a permanent problem of variable degrees.

Finally, brachial plexus injury can occur during VATS approaches to sympathectomy and during attempts at resection of upper thoracic posterior mediastinal neurogenic tumors. These injuries may be associated with important subclavian vascular injuries mentioned earlier. Careful inspection of preoperative chest CT is important to assess the proximity of posterior neurogenic tumors to the axillary neurovascular structures. In some circumstances, primary thoracotomy or early conversion to thoracotomy is the most prudent course in the management of these conditions.

■ MAJOR LYMPHATIC INJURY

Lymphatic disruption is a rare event but occurs during right-sided or left-sided VATS approaches. Right-sided procedures, such as mediastinal tumor resection, esophageal mobilization, or mechanical pleurodesis, can result in injury to the main thoracic duct. Left-sided procedures, such as aortopulmonary node biopsy and thoracodorsal sympathectomy, disrupt important lymphatic channels. Chylous leak can be prevented by the use of endosurgical vascular clips to control lymphatic tissues transected during dissection in these fields.

When performing mechanical pleurodesis or pleurectomy, abrading the mediastinum should be avoided to spare not only lymphatic disruption, but also mediastinal nerve injury. If a lymphatic leak is suspected at the time of surgery, localization of the lymphatic injury can be facilitated by instilling cream through a nasogastric tube, which increases the output of chyle through the lymphatic disruption. The site of lymphatic injury can be localized and appropriately ligated.

The chylous fistula may not be appreciated until the postoperative period. Conservative management with a low-fat diet or primary reliance on hyperalimentation can be used for the short-term. Patients with high-output drainage continuing beyond 1 week of conservative management should be reexplored with VATS or thoracotomy to ligate directly the site of lymphatic disruption as described earlier.

■ TRACHEOBRONCHIAL INJURY

Injury to the tracheobronchial tree is an uncommon problem seen with VATS. Disruption of the bronchial closure due to faulty staple closure can be seen with VATS lobectomy. Leakage from the staple line cannot be accepted, and assurance of its integrity is crucial before completion of the intervention.

VATS procedures directed toward the management of bronchogenic cysts also have been complicated by tracheobronchial disruption. This risk seems to be similar to that seen with open approaches to bronchogenic cyst resection. These cysts can be tightly adherent to airways, and the cyst may not separate easily from the posterior membranous airway. To prevent tracheobronchial injury, the posterolateral wall of the cyst adherent to the membranous airway usually is left behind. After this marsupialization technique, electrocautery or argon beam coagulation of the remaining lining mucosa is performed to prevent recurrence of the cyst.

Finally, tracheobronchial injury may occur during VATS mediastinal dissection of the esophagus for staging of esophageal carcinoma or during esophageal resection for benign or malignant disease. The risk of membranous tracheobronchial injury is increased in the setting of significant subcarinal or periesophageal lymphadenopathy. Induction radiotherapy to the mediastinum before esophageal cancer resection also increases the risk of membranous tracheal injury during the necessary mediastinal dissection of the esophagus.

■ ESOPHAGEAL INJURY

Few intrathoracic complications have the potential impact on the patient's outcome comparable to that seen with an esophageal injury. Mediastinal and pleural sepsis resulting from esophageal perforation may be associated with tremendous postoperative morbidity and a mortality approaching 50%.

Esophageal pathologic conditions for which the VATS approach has been used include resection of esophageal leiomyomata and enteric cysts, esophagomyotomy for the management of esophageal achalasia, and direct dissection of the intrathoracic esophagus during esophagectomy.

Esophageal injury has occurred during thoracodorsal sympathectomy when the surgeon has become disoriented to the apical thoracic anatomy as viewed through the thoracoscope. VATS approaches to transthoracic vagotomy as part of the management of upper abdominal splanchnic pain syndromes or for the treatment of incomplete vagotomy also can be complicated by esophageal injury.

Surgical experience is the most important consideration in avoiding esophageal injury when working with the various pathologic conditions. Only a few surgeons today have developed proficiency with these esophageal problems using VATS or laparoscopic approaches.

The use of the fiberoptic esophagoscope not only can assist the surgeon in assessing the adequacy of the esophageal surgery, but also can facilitate the identification of esophageal mucosal injury during the operation. Immediate repair of the esophageal injury is of primary importance. Although VATS repair can be done, there should be no hesitation to convert to open thoracotomy to repair the esophageal injury if any concern exists regarding the integrity of the esophageal repair.

■ CARDIAC INJURY

Cardiac injury is a rare occurrence with VATS interventions. The most important risk for the development of this injury is the presence of significant cardiomegaly. Careful attention to proper intercostal access for left-sided VATS approaches is important when approaching these patients. When performing a VATS pericardial window or resection, caution should be taken to avoid direct injury to the heart. The pericardium must be elevated with the aid of a skin hook to allow for safe penetration through the sac with an endo-scissors. Thick-walled pericardial processes with minimal effusions or intrapericardial adhesions can increase the risk of possible cardiac injury. Careful study of the preoperative CT scan and echocardiogram are important to identify these processes associated with minimal pericardial fluid. Injury can occur to the epicardial fat, atrial appendage, or ventricular myocardium (Figure 2).

A distended pericardium causes crowding of instrumentation within the left chest. Because of the risk of cardiac injury, we usually approach pericardial drainage or biopsy procedures through the right chest as greater visibility of the pericardial process and increased mobility of instrumentation is available. Left-sided approaches are chosen only when important pleural or pulmonary parenchymal processes also are present within the left chest. When a left-sided approach is chosen, we also ask the cardiologist involved to attempt temporary catheter drainage of the pericardial sac before the VATS intervention. This latter maneuver can increase greatly the room available within the left hemithorax to accomplish the VATS procedure.

■ COMPROMISE OF SURGICAL ONCOLOGY PRINCIPLES

Concerns regarding the adequacy of VATS for the therapeutic treatment of intrathoracic malignancy continue among

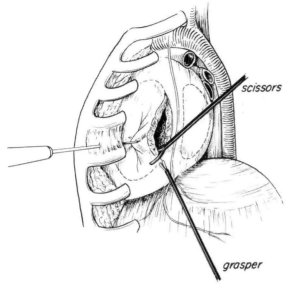

Figure 2
Left-sided video-assisted thoracic surgery interventions used to manage pericardial effusive processes. Myocardial injury and injury to the phrenic nerve must be guarded against. (*From Mack MJ, et al: Video thoracoscopic management of benign and malignant pericardial effusions,* Chest 103:390S, 1993.)

many physicians. The key issues of concern regarding the VATS approach are addressed with an emphasis on avoidance of these adverse possibilities.

Compromise of Surgical Margins of Resection

Wedge resection is the most commonly performed VATS resection of the lung. VATS may be used to accomplish excisional biopsy of indeterminate pulmonary nodules or as compromised primary resectional therapy of lung cancers in patients with significant cardiopulmonary impairment who cannot withstand anatomic lobectomy. It is vital in both of these clinical circumstances that a clear resection margin be obtained. Spillage of tumor within the pleural space with its potentially devastating consequences can be anticipated if the tumor is fractured and the visceral pleura is violated. The thoracic surgeon should assess carefully the location of the nodule within the pulmonary parenchyma with digital palpation through an intercostal access site. We also recommend introduction of grasping tools of sufficient working length through an intercostal access site to test compression of the pulmonary parenchyma along the proposed length of endostapler application for the wedge resection. This maneuver can assist in estimating the thickness of the tissue being transected with the endostapler to obtain adequate surgical margins. If the thickness of the purchase is too great or if the margin is inadequate, the surgeon should consider some other approach to resection of the target lung pathology. This may require initial intraoperative True-Cut needle biopsy, followed by anatomic resection or conversion to a limited lateral thoracotomy so

that standard stapling devices can be used for the deeper wedge resection.

The rate of local recurrence after sublobar resection when used as definitive therapy is known to be two to three times that after anatomic resection of small (T1) lung cancers. This local recurrence rate may be acceptable when sublobar "compromise" resections are thought to be necessary. Adjunctive intraoperative radiobrachytherapy may reduce the possibility of local recurrence, but inordinately high local recurrence rates remain the rule if resection margins are inadequate.

Inability to Identify and Resect All Malignant Disease

This concern primarily relates to the use of VATS techniques for the therapeutic management of pulmonary metastases. It is appreciated that all foci of metastatic disease must be cleared to provide any therapeutic benefit from pulmonary metastasectomy. Opponents to the use of VATS for therapeutic metastasectomy believe that potentially curative resection may be compromised due to the inability to palpate manually the entire lung during the course of metastasectomy. Accordingly, sites of metastasis may be missed when the VATS approach is used.

Proponents of the use of VATS for therapeutic metastasectomy point out that today's CT techniques can identify sites suspicious for metastasis with equal efficiency to manual palpation. If the sites of disease are amenable to VATS resection (i.e., small and located in the periphery of the lung), the use of VATS may be a reasonable approach to resection. They also argue that prognosis with metastasectomy is related primarily to the biology of the metastatic process. These conclusions are strengthened by the results of the international review of survival after therapeutic metastasectomy. In that retrospective analysis, the primary determinants of survival after metastasectomy were the presence of a limited disease burden (one site of metastasis) and a long disease-free interval from primary tumor resection to the development of pulmonary metastases.

This controversy is likely to continue until proper randomized studies addressing this issue are conducted. One can conclude, however, that the VATS approach should be considered only when the disease burden is limited, and small metastatic lesions are located in the periphery of the lung.

Inadequate Intraoperative Staging of the Malignancy

Another concern with VATS approaches to pulmonary resection is the possibility of inadequate nodal staging of the pulmonary hilum and mediastinum for metastatic spread. This is a risk when an inadequate effort to sample the proper nodal stations is undertaken. This understaging reduces the likelihood that patients will be considered for novel adjuvant therapies for lung cancer. This understaging also adulterates the results of primary surgical therapy for early stage lung cancer by including patients with occult, more advanced stage disease within the cohort of patients who truly have early disease. Complete nodal staging is possible with VATS techniques. We advocate this staging be a part of all VATS lung resections for primary bronchogenic carcinoma.

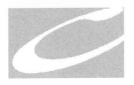

CARDIOVASCULAR SURGERY

EVALUATING PATIENTS BEFORE CORONARY ARTERY BYPASS SURGERY

Thomas A. Traill

There is substantial literature about preoperative evaluation of cardiac patients before noncardiac surgery. It can be summarized simply by the rule that management of coronary artery disease in such a patient is generally the same as the management when the patient is not about to have an operation. Therefore, operative candidates who have not been worked up at another time should be risk-stratified, then evaluated and treated according to the noninvasive assessment of risk; stable patients, previously evaluated, do not need another round of testing, even those with severe disease. Much less has been written about assessing patients with coronary heart disease before advising surgical revascularization. However, as every heart surgeon knows, judicious referral of patients likely to benefit from an operation is preferred over an approach that bases the decision to operate only on the cardiologic situation at hand without reference to whether the patient will survive intact and enjoy a useful result of the procedure.

■ INITIAL ASSESSMENT

Against the severity and potential threat posed by a patient's coronary artery disease must be weighed the risk presented by heart function, the extent of noncardiac vascular disease, preexisting neurologic disease that may be aggravated by cardiopulmonary bypass, lung function, kidney function, and overall physical condition. Issues familiar to the surgeon that may affect the conduct of surgery and subsequent healing are steroid treatment, previous chest or breast surgery, and prior irradiation. Except to the extent that it influences wound healing, diabetes need not be considered as a separate risk factor because the risks it presents stem from secondary vascular, renal, and neurologic effects. Postoperative management of diabetes is not difficult and does not significantly add to the problems in the intensive care unit.

The same might be said of age; age after all only increases the likelihood that individual organ systems may have their own particular kinds of dysfunction. However, it must also be recognized that advanced age necessarily limits the time available to enjoy the results of a successful operation. When recommending an operation to an elderly patient, thought should be given to the likely duration of convalescence, the time, for example, that it may take to recover the preoperative weight and strength, and to deduct this period from the increased life span that one is promising as the result of a successful procedure. "Quality of life" is a much-used but ill-defined expression. One of its constituents must be independence, and if the duration and difficulty of convalescence are likely to jeopardize a person's ability to live independently, this must be taken into consideration. "Successful" surgery that entails moving from one's own home to assisted living may not be seen as a boon by the patient.

■ CORONARY ARTERY DISEASE

It goes without saying that patients evaluated for coronary bypass have coronary artery disease, but this can take many forms. In the patient perceived as being potentially at high risk, it is important to be confident that the benefit of surgery is plain. Since the days of the Coronary Artery Surgery Study (CASS), it has been known that with the exception of left main coronary stenosis, it has been difficult to develop angiographic criteria that allow identification of patients for whom coronary bypass offers special advantage. The urge to improve on the picture displayed in a coronary arteriogram must be tempered by the findings on clinical and noninvasive assessment, particularly when the treatment is to be surgical rather than by percutaneous angioplasty. A decision to recommend coronary bypass therefore entails analyzing, first, whether the patient needs revascularization; second, whether bypass is preferable to angioplasty and stenting, and, third, whether there is excessive risk, based on the factors discussed in the following paragraphs.

This chapter is not the place for an extended discussion of the first two of these issues. In brief, a recommendation that revascularization is appropriate depends on an assessment that a patient has medically intractable symptoms, has an unstable clinical picture, or is at high risk without a coronary procedure. High risk is signaled clinically, by crescendo or progressive symptoms, by the results of stress testing that demonstrates early, global, or hypotensive ischemia or by the fact that there has already occurred extensive ischemic left ventricular injury. The choice between bypass and angioplasty (often made without a surgical consultation, because the cardiologist inevitably has the first look at the angiographic films) depends on technical issues—whether a stent can safely be placed—and on how much revascularization needs to be done. In patients with multivessel disease, this same decision is also influenced by extent of involvement of the left anterior descending coronary artery. It is generally inappropriate to open the chest for bypass if the left anterior descending artery does not need a procedure. By the same token, repeated angioplasty of the left anterior descending is a poor substitute for internal mammary bypass, an elegant and extremely effective procedure that carries minimal risk and morbidity. Clinical trial data from, for example, the Bypass Angioplasty Revascularization Investigation (BARI), have been taken by some to imply that diabetes should influence the choice of whether to perform angioplasty or bypass for multivessel disease. It seems likely, however, that the reason a difference has emerged in the diabetic patient subpopulation in such trials is that these patients have a higher event rate, hence more likelihood of revealing a difference that attained statistical significance. In nondiabetic patients also, coronary bypass is probably preferable to multivessel stenting, but with a difference too small to meet a statistical threshold in trials involving only limited numbers of patients.

■ CARDIAC FUNCTION

Ejection fraction is a poor guide to a patient's operability. Indeed some of the greatest benefit from coronary bypass occurs in patients with impaired left ventricular function, but it should not be assumed that the benefit lies in clinically useful improvement in left ventricular function. For that reason it is important to decide whether the indication for operation is to relieve ischemia or to improve function. The former may be very successful. The latter has a tendency to be disappointing. Although the concept of hibernating myocardium has been much written about and reproduced in short-term animal models, there is a dearth of clinical studies attesting to improvement in overall cardiac performance after successful revascularization. In this respect, hibernation is very different from stunning, which may easily be observed in patients recovering from acute coronary syndromes. With the exception of those operated on for large left ventricular aneurysms, coronary bypass patients taking medication for left ventricular failure before surgery need just as much after surgery.

Nowhere is ejection fraction less of a concern than in patients with aortic stenosis. When the aortic valve is heavily calcified, either on fluoroscopy or echocardiography, and the physical signs imply aortic stenosis to be severe, even the most unpromising left ventricle may be dramatically improved. A recent patient at the author's institution, a priest, provided such a striking example of this that his case was referred to the Vatican as having been a miraculous cure.

In contrast, patients with mitral regurgitation may have a misleadingly high ejection fraction of the partly unloaded left ventricle. It is important to be confident that, regardless of left ventricular function, the volume of mitral reflux is sufficiently high to make surgical valve replacement or repair hemodynamically worthwhile.

■ PULMONARY HYPERTENSION

In adult practice, and Eisenmenger syndrome aside, pulmonary hypertension is seldom in itself a reason to advise against cardiac surgery. High pulmonary artery pressure is generally an issue in patients referred for aortic or mitral valve disease, in whom intraoperative right ventricular failure is unusual, and often successfully managed with nitric oxide and other pulmonary vasodilators. However, pulmonary hypertension does predict a longer stay on the ventilator postoperatively. Why this should be so is not obvious, and it seems most likely that in older patients with valvular problems, pulmonary vascular disease tends to coexist with injury to the lung parenchyma in the form of fibrosis or bronchiectasis. Whatever the reason, the fact that pulmonary hypertensive patients may spend an extra day or few days in the intensive care unit before they can be mobilized should be taken into account when, as is often the case in chronic valvular disease, the patient is already not strong.

■ CAROTID DISEASE

Because stroke has always been the most feared of the perioperative complications of cardiac surgery, considerable energy has been devoted to minimizing its incidence. Currently, the rate of perioperative stroke is reported as between 1% and 5%, and that has probably increased in the past 20 years, presumably because patients are older. There is probably a comparable percentage incidence of overall cognitive impairment, not caused by cerebral infarction. Of strokes, the majority are caused by embolism, and it seems plain enough that most such emboli are from the ascending aorta, with relatively few from the cardiac lumen and valves, and a few from the carotids. The remaining strokes are caused by low cerebral pressure during cardiopulmonary bypass, from extracranial disease (which might therefore be preventable), and from intracranial atherosclerosis.

Preventing adverse neurologic outcomes therefore requires identifying patients at greatest risk. Preoperative carotid endarterectomy has gained a place, because it is easily accomplished and nowadays carries minimal risk even in the patient with fairly extensive coronary disease. I only recommend against it in the occasional patient with a very unstable coronary picture. Whether it makes a lot of difference is open to question. Because bruits are a poor guide to finding significant narrowings, a practice of preoperative carotid surgery can be effective only if all patients above a certain age or with certain other risk factors are screened. Even if we decide to correct all carotid narrowings, this will not influence the rate of embolism from the aorta, and it will save only a small number of patients from low-pressure watershed infarctions. However, the data from studies of carotid endarterectomy do imply that in operating on patients with lesions of more than 70%, patients with bilateral disease, and those with previous transient ischemic attacks, the long-term incidence of stroke is reduced. When carotid surgery is indicated on general grounds, doing it before coronary bypass makes sense. The so-called combined procedure, in which two teams operate consecutively in the same room, is best reserved for patients with very threatening carotid disease who have unstable angina or severe left main coronary artery disease. There is more detailed discussion on this topic in the chapter "Combined Carotid and Coronary Disease".

DEMENTIA AND STROKE

Dementia is worsened by cardiopulmonary bypass more often than not. For reasons not clear, this is particularly true in the context of alcoholism. The implications are two-fold. First, worse dementia will prejudice the result of surgery, by slowing convalescence, potentially requiring sedation and neuroleptic agents in the postoperative period, prolonging the period of bed rest, and increasing the chance of respiratory complications. Second, the survival benefit of surgery becomes much less valuable in someone whose cognitive function has been reduced, or in whom recovery from surgery entails the end of independent living. There is no absolute score from the Mini-Mental Status Examination that provides a cutoff for declaring a patient inoperable. In my practice, some forgetfulness would not preclude surgery in a patient who otherwise needs it, especially if the patient reported it. However, a history of mistaking the time of day, getting lost, or being confused would strongly militate against surgery.

Previous stroke is generally less of a problem, provided the vascular supply to the head is currently stable. Generally it seems best to wait 2 or 3 months after a stroke before placing a patient on cardiopulmonary bypass. This is an accepted rule of thumb, not really based on specific experience so much as an impression of the time it takes for neurologic function to plateau after stroke and for the healing within the brain to be complete. In patients with remote cerebral infarction, there is seldom substantial neurologic change after cardiopulmonary bypass.

Patients with significant parkinsonism require considerable care and effort on the part of the nursing staff during their recovery, and they may require a more extended period of rehabilitation than other patients. However, heart surgery does not by itself aggravate Parkinson's disease, and these patients generally have good coughs, so that the disease presents less of a contraindication to operation than might be thought on first meeting the patient. Some patients with Parkinson's disease have abnormal peripheral circulatory regulation, seen at its most extreme in the Shy-Drager syndrome (central orthostatic hypotension), and still others seem to have abnormalities of cardiac reflexes affecting heart rate. These may require particularly careful attention to fluid balance postoperatively and intelligent use of perioperative temporary epicardial pacing.

AORTIC DISEASE

Finding aortic calcification on first entering the mediastinum is a discouraging beginning to a cardiac surgical procedure. Such palpable or even visible calcification carries a risk of stroke even if it proves possible to perform coronary revascularization off bypass and with ingenious avoidance of conventional aortocoronary saphenous vein grafts, or even combined with ascending aortic replacement. Accordingly, when a patient's overall operability is in question, perhaps on account of age or some disability, preoperative radiology of the aorta may be helpful. When ascending aortic calcification is identified on a plain radiograph, once a sure sign of syphilis but today no longer, the surgeon will certainly find extensive, even eggshell calcification of the ascending aorta. Lesser degrees of calcification may be identified by computed tomography (CT) scanning. Such disease, although not automatically precluding successful operation, might well prove to be a deciding factor in a borderline patient, and we may expect to see CT scanning used increasingly along with carotid screening as part of the preoperative evaluation in the elective patient.

PERIPHERAL VASCULAR DISEASE

Many patients referred for coronary revascularization have a history of claudication and may have undergone surgery for peripheral vascular disease. Others may have known or occult abdominal aortic aneurysm. They are at particular risk for several reasons: leg ischemia may develop postoperatively; problems may develop with healing the leg; leg ischemia may develop after use of the balloon pump; and other issues may be involved such as aortic dissection, atheroembolism, and mesenteric ischemia. Generally there is not a great deal to be done in this setting other than to proceed with cardiac surgery, because the unstable cardiac picture is likely to take precedence over vascular surgery that might otherwise reduce risk. The exception is the patient who has an ischemic toe or foot with rest pain or infection. Here, in a patient who is already at high risk, it may be better to temporize with coronary angioplasty, then take care of the foot by revascularization or amputation rather than to attempt coronary bypass surgery first, after which losing the foot would be only the best of several bad outcomes.

Atheroembolism after cardiac catheterization or heart surgery carries a bad prognosis for kidney function and implies extensive aortic disease. In patients with persistent "trashing," it may be best to refrain from using antithrombotic agents, because these may interfere with clotting over the denuded atheroma and delay healing of the soft, cholesterol-bleeding plaque.

■ LUNG FUNCTION

The parameters that are conventionally measured to assess lung function before heart surgery are forced expiratory volume in 1 second (FEV_1), forced vital capacity, diffusing capacity, and arterial blood gases. Severe airways obstruction (FEV_1 <800 ml or 30% of expected) carries significant surgical risk, with an expectation of difficulty weaning from the ventilator and the possibility of tracheostomy. Similarly, preoperative hypercarbia (pCO_2 > 50 mm Hg) carries a very high concern for postoperative problems with CO_2 retention and a prolonged intensive care unit stay. The intangibles that may enter into making a final decision in this area are the volume of sputum and secretions in the patient with chronic bronchitis, the conformation of the chest, and the patient's energy level and drive. The patient with severe emphysema who is slim, with a straight back and a low CO_2 level—the so-called pink puffer—stands a much better chance of early weaning than the blue bloater—the obese, kyphotic patient with increased P_{CO_2} even before surgery. Kyphosis is an important factor to consider even in the absence of restrictive or obstructive spirometry values, because the sternotomy may compromise cough and the ability to clear secretions.

■ KIDNEY FUNCTION

Impaired kidney function in patients undergoing cardiac surgery is less feared than it used to be. Due to contemporary perfusion methods, cardiac catheterization and angiography nowadays cause more renal injury than does cardiac surgery. Accordingly, in patients with renal dysfunction, it is usually the cardiologist who decides whether a patient with suspected coronary artery disease is at sufficient risk to require angiography rather than the surgeon who advises against bypass. In patients with contrast-induced nephropathy who need urgent coronary revascularization, delaying surgery for a few days until serum creatinine normalizes seems to be preferable to a double insult to the kidney in only a few days.

Patients with end-stage renal disease on dialysis are easier to manage than are those with severe chronic renal insufficiency in whom angiography and bypass may supply the *coup de grace*.

Thus in the patient with known chronic ischemic heart disease and deteriorating kidney function, it may be best to wait until he or she begins dialysis before considering coronary revascularization.

■ CONCLUSION

Most of the issues discussed in this chapter, if taken individually, can be worked around, some obviously more easily than others. At my institution, judgment on occasion calls on "the Traill eyeball test," an assessment of a patient's overall vigor, which will influence their ability to battle their way off the ventilator and out of bed postoperatively despite being debilitated by their heart disease and perhaps by an extended intensive care unit stay. Here, muscle mass, posture, and motivation are the key. Often the most useful clue comes from finding out how the patient was before their heart disease caused symptoms. A patient who 3 months earlier was able and keen to perform physical tasks or to travel stands a much better chance of surviving to enjoy the result of their surgery than does one who has been accustomed for some years to a passive, sedentary lifestyle. Patients often know the answer, even as their physicians grope for tests to document the details. An elderly or infirm patient who demurs from surgery is usually right; someone keen to go ahead—"I can't live like this, doctor"—should generally be offered the chance.

SUGGESTED READING

Cohn SL, Goldman L: Preoperative risk evaluation and perioperative management of patients with coronary artery disease, *Med Clin North Am* 87:111, 2003.

Handbook of preoperative assessment and management, Philadelphia, 2000, Lippincott Williams and Wilkins.

Krupski WC, et al: Preoperative cardiac risk management, *Cardiovasc Surg* 10:415, 2002.

Merli GJ, et al, editors: *Medical management of the surgical patient*, Philadelphia, 1998, WB Saunders.

McKhann GM, et al: Predictors of stroke in coronary bypass patients. *Ann Thorac Surg* 63:516, 1997.

CARDIAC ANESTHESIA

Daniel Nyhan
K. Gage Parr

Although cardiac anesthesia is one of the older anesthesia subspecialties, it continues to evolve and grow as a result of better understanding of basic pathophysiology and the application of new techniques in patient management. The now widespread practice of intraoperative transesophageal echocardiography (TEE), new surgical techniques, and an increasingly senescent population with greater comorbidities has resulted in an increasing need for subspecialty-trained cardiac anesthesiologists. The fundamentals of cardiac anesthesia, such as principles of anesthetic technique, indications for and types of monitoring used, management of the various underlying cardiac conditions, pharmacologic principles, and the interplay with specific disease states, TEE, "fast tracking," and other areas are first outlined in broad terms. These areas each form the basis of textbooks in and of themselves, and many excellent sources are available. Thereafter, we highlight specific areas, including some novel and/or controversial issues in the management of this patient population. The seminal features of disorders of coagulation, off-pump coronary artery bypass grafting (CABG), robotic surgery, and neurologic complications after cardiac surgery are discussed in the context of implications for intraoperative management.

■ ANESTHESIA FOR CARDIAC SURGERY

Successful intraoperative management of cardiac surgery patients requires a thorough understanding of underlying cardiac disease and relevant comorbid issues, the details of the specific surgical procedures, and potential contribution to overall morbidity (both cardiac and noncardiac morbidity, such as neurologic, renal, pulmonary, etc). These anesthesia principles also require knowledge of airway management and pharmacology (pharmacokinetics and pharmacodynamics) of the multiple agents administered during surgery. In the context of patient care, these core issues are best outlined by discussing (1) the preoperative assessment, (2) intraoperative monitoring, and (3) induction and maintenance of anesthesia in the setting of commonly encountered cardiac lesions.

Preoperative Assessment
The preoperative evaluation must include examination and assessment of the patient's airway, including determination of the presence or absence of airway issues during any previous operations. These include oral excursion, temporomandibular distances, dentition, and extent of neck flexion and extension. The Mallampati gradation refers to the ability or inability to visualize the uvula and faucial pillars. There are several medical conditions that should alert the physician to the possibility of a difficult airway (Table 1). Two such conditions that occur more commonly in cardiac patients include obesity and ankylosing spondylitis (associated with aortic regurgitation).

The preoperative cardiac evaluation involves a review of the patient's history, physical findings, and diagnostic imaging and hemodynamic data. An assessment of the functional status (exercise, daily activities, temporal changes therein, anginal symptoms, etc.) of the patient cannot be overemphasized. A discord between the latter and the diagnostic data should be a red flag. For example, a poor or deteriorating functional status in the setting of incomplete or equivocal diagnostic data (coronary angiography without ventriculography, aortic or mitral systolic bruit without hemodynamic measurements, or measurements determined under different clinical conditions) may alter not only intraoperative monitoring (TEE, pulmonary artery [PA] catheter) but also the surgical procedure. The diagnostic data should be evaluated to determine (1) the major anatomic lesion or lesions (coronary arteriographic assessment of coronary anatomy, echocardiographic evaluation of valve structure) and (2) the functional status of the heart (radionucleotide imaging, ventriculography, echocardiography, hemodynamic data, and oxygen saturation).

The evaluation of comorbid issues (cerebrovascular disease, peripheral vascular disease, impaired renal function, and compromised pulmonary reserve) is a critical component of the preoperative evaluation in that the findings may modify not only the anesthesia but also the surgical management with the objective of improving outcome. Again, the history (e.g., symptoms of transient ischemic attack), patient examination (e.g., carotid bruit), and a basic battery of laboratory tests (liver and renal function tests, coagulation tests, blood counts, electrolytes, chest radiography, electrocardiography, urinalysis) and, if appropriate, carotid duplex studies and pulmonary function tests are used to accomplish this objective.

Cardiac patients are placed on multiple medications with a view to optimizing primary and secondary preventive strategies. These and any allergies should be noted. Some specific medications may alter management (timing of discontinuation of aspirin and oral anticoagulants), use of glycoprotein IIb/IIIa inhibitors and the specific inhibitor used, heparin (potential for FFP administration to augment antithrombin III activity), angiotensin-converting enzyme (ACE) inhibitors (potential for problematic hypotension and acidosis, especially postbypass), prior cardiac surgery with potential aprotinin use (risk of sensitization and anaphylaxis). Some medications should be continued because they represent essential treatments for what are ongoing conditions (e.g., β-blockers, Ca^{2+} antagonists, antiarrhythmic agents, etc.). Indeed, there is some evidence to suggest that aspirin falls into this category in that outcomes are improved in patients with acute coronary syndromes after CABG if aspirin is continued. Other medications (e.g., amiodarone, digitalis) have especially long half-lives such that their continuation or discontinuation preoperatively has little impact on tissue levels.

The preoperative evaluation would be incomplete without emphasizing the important role of patient education in allaying inevitable preoperative anxiety. A relatively brief period invested in developing rapport with patients can yield rich dividends.

Table 1 Selected Pathologic States that Influence Airway Management

PATHOLOGIC STATE	DIFFICULTY
Infectious epiglottis	Laryngoscopy may worsen obstruction
Abscess (submandibular, retropharyngeal, Ludwig's angina)	Distortion of airway renders mask ventilation or intubation extremely difficult
Croup, bronchitis, pneumonia (current or recent)	Airway irritability with tendency for cough, laryngospasm, bronchospasm
Papillomatosis	Airway obstruction
Tetanus	Trismus renders oral intubation impossible
Traumatic foreign body	Airway obstruction
Cervical spine injury	Neck manipulation may traumatize spinal cord
Basilar skull fracture	Nasal intubation attempts may result in intracranial tube placement
Maxillary/mandibular injury	Airway obstruction, difficult mask ventilation and intubation; cricothyroidotomy may be necessary with combined injuries
Laryngeal fracture	Airway obstruction may worsen during instrumentation
	Endotracheal tube may be misplaced outside larynx and may worsen the injury
Laryngeal edema (postintubation)	Irritable airway, narrowed laryngeal inlet
Soft tissue, neck injury (edema, bleeding, emphysema)	Anatomic distortion of airway
	Airway obstruction
Neoplastic upper airway tumors (pharynx, larynx)	Inspiratory obstruction with spontaneous ventilation
Lower airway tumors (trachea, bronchi, mediastinum)	Airway obstruction may not be relieved by tracheal intubation
	Lower airway distorted
Radiation therapy	Fibrosis may distort airway or make manipulations difficult
Inflammatory rheumatoid arthritis	Mandibular hypoplasia, temporomandibular joint arthritis, immobile cervical spine, laryngeal rotation, cricoarytenoid arthritis all make intubation difficult and hazardous
Ankylosing spondylitis	Fusion of cervical spine may render direct laryngoscopy impossible
Temporomandibular joint syndrome True ankylosis "False" ankylosis (burn, trauma, radiation, temporal craniotomy)	Severe impairment of mouth opening
Scleroderma	Tight skin and temporomandibular joint involvement make mouth opening difficult
Sarcoidosis	Airway obstruction (lymphoid tissue)
Angioedema	Obstructive swelling renders ventilation and intubation difficult
Endocrine/metabolic acromegaly	Large tongue, bony overgrowths
Diabetes mellitus	May have reduced mobility of atlanto-occipital joint
Hypothyroidism	Large tongue, abnormal soft tissue (myxedema) make ventilation and intubation difficult
Thyromegaly	Goiter may produce extrinsic airway compression or deviation
Obesity	Upper airway obstruction with loss of consciousness
	Tissue mass makes successful mask ventilation unlikely

From Stone DJ, Gal TJ: Airway management. In Miller RD, editor: *Anesthesia,* Philadelphia, 1998, Churchill Livingstone, Table 39-3.

Intraoperative Monitoring

As with any surgery, cardiac surgery patients' basic physiologic parameters are monitored using pulse oximetry, electrocardiography, blood pressure (cuff), temperature, and ventilation/oxygenation (FIO_2, gas flows, respiratory rate, ventilatory pressures and volumes). Neuromuscular blockade is assessed using a neuromuscular monitor. All patients have arterial and central lines placed. Arterial lines are placed preinduction unless circumstances dictate otherwise. Central venous access usually involves placement of a large-bore cannula ("volume line"), as well as monitoring/drug infusion line(s), and can be placed either before or after induction, depending on patient circumstances and physician preference. In the presence of adequate peripheral venous access, most practitioners secure central venous access postinduction. The use of PA catheters and TEE in cardiac patients is variable.

There are clear indications for using these monitoring techniques (elevated pulmonary vascular pressures/resistance, valve disease, aortic disease, etc). However, many patients do not have hard indications for using either PA catheters or TEE. In these circumstances, the practice is variable, ranging from the routine placement of either PA catheters or TEE to either or neither. Pacing and defibrillating capabilities should always be readily available.

Induction and Maintenance of Anesthesia

Induction is one of most critical times in the management of cardiac patients. The safe conduct of induction requires a detailed/thorough understanding of the agents used and their cardiovascular depressant effects in the setting of the specific cardiac pathology in that patient. The choice of agents should be determined by these principles. In general, one specific agent from each of four categories is used for induction and maintenance, as follows.

1. Intravenous opioids (e.g., fentanyl, sufentanil, etc) (the dose determined by patient response, the type and dose of other agents used, and the time frame to extubation).

2. Major tranquilizers (e.g., benzodiazepines, etomidate, propofol).

3. Volatile anesthetic agents (e.g., isoflurane, enflurane, etc). Note that the issue of precipitating coronary steal (in patients with steal prone coronary anatomy) with isoflurane administration has probably not held up to rigorous scientific scrutiny.

4. Muscle relaxants (e.g., succinylcholine, pancuronium, vecuronium, etc). The dose chosen should be determined by airway considerations and have minimal cardiovascular depressant effects. However, some muscle relaxants are deliberately chosen because of their cardiovascular modulating effect and their ability to counteract the effects of other agents (e.g., the vagolysis induced by pancuronium counteracts the vagotonic effects of fentanyl).

The specific anesthetic technique can be modified depending on the time frame to extubation (fast-tracking), although extubation is often also determined by other issues, such as bleeding, hemodynamic stability, and so on.

The management of patients (incorporating the administration of pharmacologic agents including anesthetics) with coronary artery disease should be predicated on optimizing the determinants of myocardial oxygen supply and demand by the prudent use of appropriate anesthetic agents and doses and of cardiovascular modulating drugs. Note that some agents can decrease myocardial oxygen supply but improve myocardial supply/demand ratios because of their differential effects on the latter. Intravascular volume and slow sinus rhythm must be maintained in patients with aortic stenosis and left ventricular hypertrophy to avoid hemodynamic decompensation. This is even more important if there is coexisting coronary artery disease (especially left main or left main equivalent disease). Patients with mitral stenosis, especially if associated with elevated pulmonary vascular pressures and atrial fibrillation (frequently the situation by the time surgery is indicated), are equally challenging. Pulmonary vascular assessment and the maintenance of intravascular volume, myocardial contractility, and systemic vascular resistance are essential if these patients are to be managed successfully. Hemodynamic parameters are more amenable to manipulation in regurgitant lesions. However, optimizing heart rate in patients with aortic regurgitation (cardiac output is maximized at heart rates of 80 to 100 bpm) is critical. Optimizing contractility and afterload can be achieved with appropriate infusions (catecholamines, nitrosovasodilators). Patients with mitral regurgitation should be managed with a view to optimizing forward flow. These latter patients are frequently more problematic after mitral valve replacement/repair in that the surgical procedure may unmask underlying poor left ventricular function. Finally, other specific lesions require specific management consideration, such as avoiding hypertension in patients with aortic dissections, ability to readily volume resuscitate, and deliver inotropes in pericardial tamponade.

Regional Anesthesia and Cardiac Surgery

Regional anesthesia techniques can be used in both adult and pediatric cardiac surgery. Neuroaxial blocks (spinal, epidural, paravertebral, and caudal) are most commonly used. The purported salutary effects of regional anesthetic techniques include (1) effective attenuation of the stress response to surgery, (2) optimizing coronary blood flow and ventricular function, (3) improving parameters of pulmonary function postoperatively, and (4) facilitating extubation postoperatively.

These techniques undoubtedly effectively obtund the stress response, but there is no evidence that they are more effective than general anesthesia in suppressing the stress response. Moreover, although neuroaxial techniques may provide more effective analgesia and shorter extubation times, these have not been shown to translate into shorter hospital stays for these patients. Neuroaxial techniques are not more widely used because of the risks of developing hematomas in anticoagulated patients. These techniques are effective and some clinical trials suggest safety, but the definitive clinical trials required to determine if regional adjuncts confer unique advantages that would outweigh the rare but disastrous neurologic complications have not been conducted.

■ SPECIFIC CONSIDERATIONS

Coagulation and Anticoagulation in Cardiac Surgery

Despite recent trends toward performing CABG without CPB (OPCAB), in the majority of cardiac operations, CPB is still used. Even with adequate anticoagulation with heparin, CPB results in coagulation abnormalities that predispose the patient to postoperative bleeding and the need for transfusion of blood and blood products. This proclivity is increasingly exacerbated by preoperative medications, including aspirin, glycoprotein IIb/IIIa inhibitors, fibrinolytics, etc. Although a complete discussion of this area is beyond the scope of this chapter, we emphasize the seminal issues.

Heparin, the anticoagulant of choice for CPB, potentiates the effects of antithrombin III. It can be reversed by protamine, which binds heparin and creates an inactive complex. Although large doses of heparin (e.g., 300 IU/kg) given for cardiac surgery are adequate to prevent clot formation during CPB, significant activation of and changes in the coagulation and fibrinolytic systems still occur. Thrombin is generated during CPB even in the setting of adequate heparin. In this setting, thrombin generation may be induced by mechanisms that are both coagulation pathway-dependent and -independent (e.g., the kallikrein pathway). The resultant factor consumption and secondary fibrinolysis can result in significant bleeding after CPB, even if the heparin has been adequately reversed with protamine.

CPB-induced abnormalities in coagulation include changes in platelet number and function, alterations in concentration and function of coagulation factors, and the aforementioned increases in fibrinolytic activity and activation of inflammatory pathways. The hemodilution that occurs with the onset of CPB causes a decrease in platelet count. The platelet count is also depleted as a result of platelet adhesion to the CPB tubing and as a result of platelet consumption during hemostasis. Despite this, platelet counts less than 100,000/µl are uncommon during CPB and counts usually return to normal within a few days of surgery. Platelets are also activated by contact with the CPB tubing, causing platelet degranulation and dysfunction. Heparin-bonded CPB circuits have been developed with the hope of preventing platelet activation and platelet adherence to CPB circuits. However, the benefits of using these circuits remains uncertain.

Hemodilution also decreases the concentration of coagulation factors during CPB. However, levels of factors II, VII, VIII, IX, X, and XIII are usually adequate for homeostasis. Normovolemic hemodilution before CPB has been used in an attempt to minimize the decrease in coagulation factor concentration and the decrement in platelet and red blood cell counts that occur with CPB. Vasopressors may be required to maintain optimal hemodynamics before CPB. Blood is reinfused after the termination of CPB and reversal of heparin. In theory, the patient should have a higher hematocrit and platelet count and higher concentrations of coagulation factors and a decreased risk of transfusion with its attendant risks. Studies addressing the efficacy of normovolemic hemodilution in cardiac surgery patients have not demonstrated benefit, however. This may be in part related to small study numbers and inadequate study power. Moreover, it is generally the healthier patients who can tolerate normovolemic hemodilution; this group has a low incidence of transfusion even without normovolemic hemodilution.

Antifibrinolytics are now commonly used to minimize fibrinolysis during CPB. There are two major classes of antifibrinolytic agents currently in use—lysine analogues (ε-aminocaproic acid and tranexamic acid) and serine protease inhibitors (e.g., aprotinin)—with the latter having mechanisms of action that extend beyond that of inhibition of fibrinolysis. Lysine analogues have been demonstrated to be effective in reducing chest tube drainage and transfusion requirements after CPB. Aprotinin (a serine protease inhibitor) has been shown to decrease post-CPB chest tube drainage and transfusion and to reduce the inflammatory response associated with CPB. Importantly, only the "high-dose regimen" of aprotinin has been shown to confer these benefits. A meta-analysis comparison of lysine analogues and aprotinin and their efficacy in reducing chest tube output and transfusion requirements in cardiac surgery failed to demonstrate a statistical difference between these two regimens. Notwithstanding the inherent deficiencies in meta-analysis (e.g., potential differences in the patient population groups in the analysis), analysis of subgraphs suggested the possible superiority of aprotinin in certain circumstances.

Aprotinin is expensive and is most effective at the higher recommended dose. In contrast, lysine analogues are inexpensive. Aprotinin can induce antibody formation and the risk of anaphylaxis on subsequent exposure. This is not a feature of lysine analogues. For these reasons, many centers reserve aprotinin for "high-risk" cases. Patients at high risk of developing intracoronary thrombosis (e.g., patients with unstable angina) should not receive antifibrinolytics or have aprotinin therapy initiated until the patient is fully anticoagulated with heparin.

Unfractionated heparin can cause thrombocytopenia (Table 2) via a number of mechanisms that result in very different clinical syndromes that have specific implications for perioperative management and reanticoagulation with heparin for CPB. The most common occurrence (>20% of patients on therapeutic intravenous heparin) is the development of non–antibody-mediated heparin-associated thrombocytopenia that is usually of modest severity, reverses on stopping heparin, and does not preclude heparin use for CPB. Heparin-induced thrombocytopenia (HIT) is much less frequent (occurs in 2% to 4% of patients receiving therapeutic heparin). HIT is antibody mediated and results from heparin-induced IgG antibody formation against platelet factor 4. A small percentage (0.4%) of patients on heparin who develop an IgG antibody response develop a more serious clinical syndrome, HIT associated with intravascular thrombosis. The underlying mechanisms that distinguish these two groups are currently unknown. These two patient groups (HIT with and without intravascular thrombosis) pose a dilemma for the clinician when cardiac surgery and CPB are required. However, is seems that HIT does not recur in patients with serologically confirmed HIT after the disappearance of heparin-induced antibodies. In contrast to platelet antibody formation following quinidine or sulfonamide exposure, which can persist for years, antibodies induced by heparin therapy decline rapidly with a median time to seroconversion to a negative antibody test of 50 days. Patients with the less common thrombotic form of HIT (HIT, type II) are more problematic, but emerging studies offer the potential for managing these patients during CPB with a combination of unfractionated heparin and glycoprotein IIb/IIIa inhibitors.

Preexisting inherited coagulation defects (thrombocytopenia, hepatic dysfunction, hemophilia, or other coagulation factor defects such as von Willebrand's factor deficiency) can contribute to severe coagulopathies after CPB. This can also occur with some acquired coagulation defects. For example, preoperative administration of platelet inhibitors may exacerbate the platelet dysfunction that occurs in response to CPB. Although aspirin does not seem to result in significant

Table 2 Heparin and Thrombocytopenia		
	TYPE I (HEPARIN-ASSOCIATED THROMBOCYTOPENIA)	**TYPE II (HEPARIN-INDUCED THROMBOCYTOPENIA)**
Incidence (%)	10-33	3
Etiology	Non–immune mediated: platelet margination, aggregation, and sequestration	Immune mediated: IgG antibodies to heparin platelet complexes
Platelet count	>100,000	<100,000
Resolution	Occurs in 1-5 days, often even if patient is on heparin	Occurs in 5 days, with discontinuation of heparin
Thrombosis	No	Yes, can occur (in a small percentage) (See text)

post-CPB bleeding, administration of glycoprotein IIb/IIIa inhibitors may result in severe post-CPB bleeding. With the exception of abciximab, the half-life of currently used glycoprotein IIb/IIIa inhibitors (tirofiban and eptifibatide) is relatively short (≈2 hours). Deferring surgery until the effect of these agents has diminished should allow return of platelet function and reduce postoperative bleeding.

Preoperative warfarin and heparin therapies have been studied to determine their effect on post-CPB bleeding. Warfarin administration has not been shown to increase post-CPB bleeding. In fact, it may have a protective effect by reducing thrombin generated during CPB. The presence of preoperative intravenous heparin also has not been shown to increase postoperative bleeding. Reversal of heparin with protamine after CPB negates its effects. Most practitioners discontinue heparin infusion 1 to 2 hours before the start of surgery to prevent bleeding with central venous and arterial line placement and to attenuate surgical bleeding (especially from the sternum) before CPB. Patients with unstable angina may require heparin therapy up to the time of surgery.

In contrast to unfractionated heparin, preoperative administration of low-molecular-weight heparin (LMWH) may result in significant post-CPB bleeding. These drugs are not reversed by protamine, and the activity levels are not reliably measured by the activated partial thromboplastin time (aPTT) or the activated clotting time (ACT). Half-lives of these drugs vary significantly. Therefore, if one wishes to delay surgery until the effect of the drug has worn off, it is important to know which LMWH was administered and its half-life. Fibrinolytics, such as streptokinase, can also cause severe postoperative bleeding. Unfortunately, the only treatment for this problem is transfusion of large amounts of coagulation factors.

Heparin/protamine titration curves have been developed to prevent underdosing or overdosing of protamine and to prevent heparin rebound. Systems such as the heparin management system not only measure ACT but are also able to determine the quantity of heparin in the blood by titrating IT to known quantities of protamine. This allows protamine doses to be based on the actual concentration of heparin in the blood, not weight or total heparin dose. OPCAB procedures attempt to avoid the coagulopathy associated with CPB by avoiding CPB altogether.

Several intraoperative factors are associated with an increased incidence of bleeding. These include the type of surgery (combined valve/coronary procedures and repeat surgeries), an especially long duration of CPB, deep hypothermic circulatory arrest, older patient age, lower body temperature on admission to the intensive care unit, and abnormal coagulation parameters after CPB.

Finally, therapies aimed at reducing the need for blood products after CPB have been implemented. If time allows, anemic patients may benefit from treatment with erythropoietin before surgery. By increasing the preoperative hemoglobin concentration, the effects of hemodilution may be decreased and the requirements for transfusion attenuated.

Blood Substitutes

Artificial blood and red blood cell substitutes are subjects of ongoing research and offer the potential to provide an alternative to blood transfusion. There are three types of compounds currently under investigation: (1) perfluorocarbons (which can carry more oxygen than human plasma), (2) free hemoglobins (human, bovine, and recombinant), and (3) liposome-encapsulated hemoglobin. None of these compounds have been approved for human use, although some have reached the level of phase III clinical trials. All have potential problems. Perfluorocarbons carry oxygen in proportion to the inspired oxygen concentration; therefore, they are of more benefit if the PO_2 can be increased. Although perfluorocarbons do not pose an infectious risk, the emulsions that carry the perfluorocarbons may cause cytokine release. Free hemoglobins have the advantage that these molecules are designed to load and unload oxygen. They are also very stable and can be stored for a long period of time. In addition, they can be sterilized and viruses can be inactivated, although the ability to inactivate prions is unknown. However, problems do exist with these hemoglobins. They are rapidly cleared from the body and therefore have a limited half-life. There is the potential that these molecules can be modulated to limit clearance. Free hemoglobin causes vasoconstriction, perhaps in part related to its affinity to bind nitric oxide. Although these molecules do not carry an infectious risk, they can be immunogenic. Liposomal hemoglobin has many of the advantages of free hemoglobin. Additionally, liposomal hemoglobin is not rapidly cleared from the circulation and does not cause the hypertension commonly associated with free hemoglobin. However, producing uniform liposomes is difficult; therefore, this area of research is still in the early stages of development.

Disorders of coagulation in the setting of CPB represent an area of intense, ongoing investigation. Interventions directed at decreasing blood loss and minimizing transfusions often have a sound theoretical basis but frequently fail to confer a benefit in practice. This likely reflects the multifaceted complex mechanisms that are involved but not yet completely understood.

Neurologic Complications in Cardiac Surgery

Neurologic sequelae after cardiac surgical procedures are among the most devastating complications associated with contemporary cardiac surgery. These neurologic complications are especially frustrating, as they frequently occur in patients in whom the primary cardiac surgical objective has been achieved. Despite an apparent increase in our understanding of the underlying mechanisms from innumerable studies in this area, the frequency of these devastating complications has not materially decreased. This likely reflects the multifactorial etiology; the changing patient population, which is increasingly older with more advanced cardiac and noncardiac disease (especially vascular disease); and the lack of effective interventions.

Perioperative neurologic complications can be classified into (1) focal deficits, (2) postoperative delirium, (3) short-term neurocognitive deficits, and (4) long-term neurocognitive deficits. Focal neurologic deficits occur in 1.5% to 5.2% of patients, especially in those with significant cardiovascular risk factors (increased age, hypertension, diabetes, carotid bruits, and history of a cerebrovascular event). Although the majority of these focal lesions develop intraoperatively, up to one third of all perioperative focal deficits appear in the early postoperative period. The precise mechanisms underlying this latter subgroup is no better understood than its intra-operative counterpart. It is likely that multiple factors are involved, including microembolic phenomena and hypoperfusion, perhaps in part resulting from the desire for aggressive blood pressure control to promote homeostasis. Hemodynamic manipulation and blood pressure control are often difficult, especially in patients with long-standing hypertension (shifted autoregulatory curve) and/or latent underlying cerebral vascular disease. The medical, economic and social costs of perioperative focal and nonfocal neurologic complications are well recognized.

Postoperative delirium is reported to occur in 10% to 30% of patients undergoing cardiac surgery. However, it is well recognized that this specific complication also occurs in patients undergoing noncardiac surgery. Changes in the metabolic, endocrine, and pharmacologic (including psychoactive drugs and, by definition, all anesthetic agents) milieu are important contributors, as is a history of stroke.

Short-term cognitive changes are well recognized after cardiac surgery, and these changes may persist in the long term (up to 5 years). Although many studies have been done in this area, the results are often not consistent. For example, short-term neurocognitive changes have been reported with a frequency as low as 33% and as high as 83%. In one study, long-term (5 years) complications were reported in 42% of patients, but intermediate-term (6 weeks and 6 months) deficits in this same patient population were less prevalent (36% and 24%, respectively). This observation might be explained by the progression of underlying cerebral vascular disease in this patient population, due to advancing age. The authors, however, thought that cognitive deficits at the time of hospital discharge were an independent and significant predictor of long-term cognitive decline. This suggests a different underlying etiology.

Why do counterintuitive and inconsistent results emerge from these neurocognitive studies? These types of studies are notoriously difficult to conduct, and there are several methodologic issues that beset this field. For detailed information, the interested reader is strongly urged to refer to Slade's review of this area. Neurocognitive data can be analyzed using either individual patient data or data for the group as a whole. When evaluating early postoperative neurocognitive deficits, both methods yield the same results. However, when these methods are applied to longer-term data (>2 months) different results and conclusions emerge. Individual data analysis clearly demonstrate that longer-term deficits occur, whereas group data analysis demonstrates either no change or an improvement. Even more problematic is the issue of repeat testing (the phenomenon whereby a subject's performance on a repeated test is influenced by having previously taken the same test). This could obviously lead to an apparent improvement on repeat testing compared with that which would be observed otherwise. Fatigue and the circumstances that may exist postoperatively (especially early postoperatively) would have the opposite effect, especially if the neurocognitive assessment was complex.

Methods that have been used to compensate for the confounding variable of repeat testing include parallel testing (a different test or set of tests is used to assess the same function or set of neurocognitive functions) and the incorporation of control groups into study designs. The specific control group or groups used are critically important. Ideally, an operative control group undergoing noncardiac surgery should unmask the confounding variables of perioperative stress (metabolic changes, neuroendocrine changes, anesthetic effects, etc). A second nonoperative control group should also be included. Common nonoperative controls used in neurobehavioral studies include spouses (which does not control for gender) and friends (which can control for age, gender, and level of education). Finally, the definition of a change in neurocognitive performance is highly variable across studies. The consensus statement on neurocognitive testing in cardiac research studies has attempted to address this and other methodologic issues. An approach that uses a reliable change index and incorporates a control group has the greatest sensitivity and is the method of choice for determining individual neurocognitive changes. The conclusions of studies in this area should always be interpreted in light of the above issues.

Perioperative Management and Neurological Complications

The neurologic sequelae associated with cardiac surgery have multiple etiologies. These can be grouped into three broad categories: embolic phenomena (both microemboli and macroemboli), hypoperfusion, and the inflammatory response to CPB. Clearly, there are important interactions between these mechanisms. For example, the neurologic consequences of a microembolic event are likely to differ in a patient with cerebral vascular disease and long exposure to CPB from those in a patient without cerebral vascular disease for whom the duration of CPB was short. There are innumerable intraoperative variables that can influence the incidence of neurologic complications. It is exceedingly difficult in the clinical setting to definitively identify one or more variables that are causally related to neurologic events. For example, manipulation of pressure and flow patterns on CPB has not been shown to modulate neurologic outcome. However, other variables have been correlated with adverse neurologic outcomes. Microemboli (generated from atheromatous debris, platelets, air, products of red blood cell hemolysis, glove powder, etc) detected by transcranial Doppler (TCD) of the middle cerebral artery are associated with adverse neurologic outcome.

Several subtle but important intraoperative management issues also influence the frequency of microembolic events. Frequency of manipulation of the aorta, frequency of injection into the CPB circuit, use of cardiotomy suction to retrieve blood from the surgical field, and cerebral blood flow (CBF) all correlate with adverse neurologic outcomes. The desire to limit aortic manipulation drives many intraoperative decisions, including potential use of epiaortic mapping, use of pedicle grafts, and use of alternative sites for proximal anastomosis. Minimizing the amount of blood loss on CPB through the use of antifibrinolytics and/or aprotinin can decrease damage from the use of cardiotomy suction. Higher CBF is associated with an increased incidence of TCD-detected microembolic phenomena. CBF itself is modulated by temperature and by the type of acid-base management used. Higher CBF is observed when pH-stat is used to manage blood gases and higher P_{CO_2} levels are maintained. The converse is observed with an alpha-stat approach to blood gas management. Valve surgery is also associated with a higher incidence of embolic events, perhaps due to embolized valve debris or entrapment of air in open cardiac chambers.

The belief that both microembolic and macroembolic events and the injurious effects of CPB are important in mediating neurologic injury has motivated the development of OPCAB techniques. Approximately 20% of all coronary surgeries in the United States are performed as OPCAB procedures. Neurologic complications also occur after OPCAB but may be significantly decreased. The studies designed to compare OPCAB and conventional CAB have either had a small number of patients and/or were subject to the criticism that the two patient populations were dissimilar. Nevertheless, the preponderance of emerging evidence suggests that OPCAB may decrease the incidence of neurologic complications. As experience with this technique improves (improved hemodynamic management) and newer technologies are used (automated proximal anastomotic devices that eliminate the need for aortic manipulation), a clearer picture should emerge.

■ NEW TECHNIQUES IN CARDIAC SURGERY AND THEIR EFFECTS ON ANESTHETIC CARE OF THE PATIENT

Off-Cardiopulmonary Bypass Coronary Artery Bypass Grafting

OPCAB has become increasingly popular. The purported benefits of this approach include: decreased cerebral microemboli and stroke rates due to reduced aortic manipulation, decreased bleeding and blood product utilization due to the avoidance of CPB, decreased time to extubation, decreased length of stay, and decreased overall cost. OPCAB cases challenge the anesthesiologist who must manage with profound hemodynamic fluctuations, ischemia, and changes in myocardial function that result from manipulation of the heart.

Decreases in preload resulting in decreased cardiac output are frequent problems during OPCAB. The placement of pericardial sling sutures in the posterior pericardium can cause constriction of the inferior vena cava and/or pulmonary veins, thus limiting venous return to the right and/or left side of the heart. This decrease is exacerbated when the heart is lifted out of the pericardium so that conduit anastomoses can be performed on the posterior surface. To overcome these effects, the patient is usually placed in steep Trendelenburg and crystalloid or colloid is administered to augment preload. Monitoring pulmonary vascular and central venous pressures helps to optimize loading conditions of the heart. Experience and judgment are required to interpret vascular pressure measurements in this setting because aberrant heart position, ischemia, and atrioventricular valvular regurgitation may alter pressure readings and confound interpretation of the data. TEE allows direct visualization of the heart to determine adequacy of preload. It may also detect new onset valvular regurgitation or diastolic dysfunction. However, the placement of pericardial sutures, lifting the heart out of the pericardium, and sponges placed behind the heart all obscure the images of the heart on TEE. Generally, all available data should be used to determine adequacy of preload during OPCAB.

Ischemic changes and new regional wall motion abnormalities (RWMAs), as well as global cardiac dysfunction, are not uncommon during OPCAB procedures. Ischemia can result from the temporary occlusion of a coronary artery for the purpose of completing a distal anastomosis. New-onset ischemia may be seen on the electrocardiogram in the distribution of the occluded coronary artery. Transient and minor ST-segment and axis changes are usually seen after the heart is positioned or the coronary is occluded. These changes may be minor and not progressive, but if associated with RWMAs, they are indicative of significant ischemia. TEE manifestations of ischemia include the development of new RWMAs, new-onset valvular regurgitation due to papillary muscle ischemia, and diastolic dysfunction. Ischemia may also manifest as an increase in pulmonary artery pressures (dysfunction, mitral valve regurgitation). Ischemia should be managed in the standard way by optimizing the determinants of myocardial oxygen supply and demand. Blood flow to an ischemic region can be increased by the use of shunts, opening the occluded coronary artery or via a new graft. Ischemia can also result in heart block, necessitating pacing. If the myocardium becomes profoundly ischemic, refractoriness to pacing may ensue. Importantly, failure to pace may be physiologically based and not a mechanical problem with lead placement.

Robotic Cardiac Surgery

Robotic assisted surgery is likely to gain increasing acceptance. It has the potential to allow precise movements in small spaces, increasing the potential for port-access surgery. There is also the potential for remote or telesurgery. The current generation of robots used for cardiac surgery consists of three main components.

1. The robot, with three arms: one holds a stereoscopic camera and the other two hold specially designed instruments
2. Control unit contains a stereoscopic viewer that allows the surgeon to view the field in three dimensions; two control handles, which allow manipulation of the instruments; and pedals, which allow the surgeon to switch control between the instruments and the camera
3. A central processing unit (CPU) tower

Anesthesia for these procedures is similar to that of other port-access cardiac surgery cases. Double-lumen endotracheal tubes, external defibrillator pads, TEE, and lateral positions may all be necessary. The robot component of the system is large, and once the arms are locked to the trocars, the operating table cannot be moved. The challenges for the anesthesiologist include coordinating their care with that of others in the operating room and maintaining the ability to resuscitate the patient in the circumstances dictated by the patient's position and use of the robot.

SUGGESTED READING

Koster A, et al: Anticoagulation during cardiopulmonary bypass in patients with heparin-induced thrombocytopenia type II and renal impairment using heparin and the platelet glycoprotein IIb-IIIa antagonist tirofiban, *Anesthesiology* 94:245, 2001.

McKhann GM, et al: Predictors of stroke risk in coronary artery bypass patients, *Ann Thorac Surg* 63:516, 1997.

Murkin JM, et al: Statement of consensus on assessment of neuro-behavioral outcomes after cardiac surgery, *Ann Thorac Surg* 59:1289, 1995.

Newman MF, et al: Longitudinal assessment of neurocognitive function after coronary-artery bypass surgery, *N Engl J Med* 344:395, 2001.

Slade P, et al: The use of neurocognitive tests in evaluating the outcome of cardiac surgery: some methodologic considerations, *J Cardiothorac Vasc Anesth* 15:4, 2001.

Stone DJ, Gal TJ: Airway management. In Miller RD, editor: *Anesthesia,* Philadelphia, 2000, Churchill Livingstone, p 1414.

Warkentin TE, Kellton JG: Temporal aspects of heparin-induced thrombocytopenia, *N Engl J Med* 344:1286, 2001.

ADULT CARDIOPULMONARY BYPASS

Terry Gourlay

Ken Taylor

The safe application of cardiopulmonary bypass (CPB) depends largely on attention to detail with regard to the configuration and management of the CPB system. The use of protocols specific to both the routine clinical scenario and the abnormal or accidental is also an essential part of this approach. Management strategies for patients who present with atypical conditions must be determined before surgery if these patients are to benefit from the flexibility of modern perfusion technology and management techniques; hence, an informed team approach to the delivery of clinical CPB is integral to safety.

■ PATIENT EVALUATION

It is imperative that the perfusion technique used is selected in light of full awareness of patient history. The patient's cardiovascular and operative history may have an impact on the perfusion protocol and cannulation technique. For example, patients presenting with a history of systemic arterial hypertension, diabetes, cerebrovascular, or renal disease may require a specific protocol designed to be protective of these patients. Such protocols may involve modifications to the perfusion circuitry or the use of specific pharmacologic agents in the priming solution, such as the addition of mannitol to the prime, higher blood flow index, or the use of hemoconcentrators. Overall, a team approach and awareness of case history, together with well-developed protocols and technology, aid in the delivery of a quality perfusion and in the prevention of potentially major complications.

■ THE HEART-LUNG MACHINE STRUCTURE AND MANAGEMENT

Circuit Component

The perfusion apparatus we use is designed to permit the highest possible level of flexibility while maintaining safe and effective delivery of CPB. In common with modern practice, and to ensure continuity of supply, we select our perfusion products from more than one manufacturer. Our basic system comprises:

Sorin/Dideco Avant 903, or Jostra Safe Maxi blood oxygenators
Pall AV6 40 micron Arterial line blood filter
Jostra or Sorin custom tubing pack
Medtronic Myotherm Blood cardioplegia delivery system
Stockert SIII Modular heart/lung machine
Stockert 3T Heater/Cooler for systemic and cardioplegia temperature control

These perfusion system components represent, in our view, a simple, safe, and effective CPB delivery solution. The arterial line filter is vented to the venous reservoir, and line pressure is measured premembrane using an isolated pressure gauge. An air bubble detector, positioned at the outlet of the arterial pump, and a level sensor positioned on the venous/cardiotomy reservoir provide early warning of any potentially injurious embolic event. The suction, vent, cardioplegia, and arterial flow delivery are provided by separate roller pump heads. To prevent the entrainment of air and the separation of blood-carrying connectors, all connectors, on both the positive and negative pressure aspects of the circuit, are solvent bonded. Also, all connectors on the arterial/high-pressure side of the circuit have nylon ties applied for extra safety and security.

Cannulae

For routine valve and coronary artery bypass surgery, we use a Sarns 28 Fr 6672 right-angled aortic cannula positioned through a stab incision in the ascending aorta below the innominate artery, secured with two concentric purse-string sutures. Correct placement of the cannula is confirmed by vigorous pulsing of blood within the cannula and smooth and unrestricted deflection of the line pressure gauge indicator arm before initiating bypass. This is further confirmed by close monitoring of the line pressure in the early stages of the initiation of bypass, ensuring that line pressure remains within acceptable normal limits. Excessively high line pressure at this stage may indicate improper placement of the cannula. In the event that the aorta is not appropriate for cannulation, for example, due to excessive atherosclerosis or dissection, we will cannulate the femoral artery.

We use a dual-stage single cannula for the venous cannulation (Sarns 46 to 34 Fr Two-Stage). This cannula is positioned through the right atrial appendage with the tip positioned in the inferior vena cava. When the single, two-stage cannula is inappropriate, for example, when working within the chambers of the right heart, we use two 8-mm whistle tip caval cannulae positioned via the right atrium into the superior and inferior vena cavae.

Priming Solution

When the prebypass hemoglobin is 14 or above, we use the following priming solution for routine elective procedures.

> 1700 ml Hartmann's solution
> 5000 IU heparin
> 25 ml of 8.4% sodium bicarbonate solution
> Total priming volume = 1730 ml

In patients who present with a prebypass hemoglobin of less than 14 we use the following.

> 1200 ml Hartmann's solution
> 500 ml Gelofusine (a gelatin-based solution)
> 5000 IU heparin
> 25 ml of 8.4% sodium bicarbonate solution
> Total priming volume = 1730 ml

When the prebypass hemoglobin is excessively low (<11), we may substitute a unit of blood for an equivalent volume of Hartmann's solution.

Cardioplegia Solution

We routinely use blood cardioplegia, which is delivered using the Medtronic Myotherm system. This system delivers to the patient a 4:1 mixture of blood taken from the oxygenator outlet and cardioplegic solution taken from a separate delivery bag, with flow being controlled via a single roller pump. The blood cardioplegia is delivered to the patient through a Sorin R502-15 cardioplegia needle in the ascending aorta. The cardioplegic solution routinely used is as follows.

> Initial dose: Cardioplegia solution A—50 ml St. Thomas' solution in 500 ml Hartmann's solution

> Follow-up doses: Cardioplegia solution B—25 ml St. Thomas' in 500 ml Hartmann's solution

An initial dose of 800 to 1000 ml of the cardioplegia solution is delivered at 4°C, and this is followed by additional doses at no greater than 30-minute intervals, or earlier where surgery permits.

■ CARDIOPULMONARY BYPASS TECHNIQUE

Temperature

During routine CPB, nasopharyngeal, rectal, and arterial and venous blood temperatures are monitored. We use only moderate cooling, to a core temperature of 32°C, for routine cases of less than 1 hour, with cooling initiated at the onset of CPB. For longer procedures, the patient may be cooled to a core temperature of 30°C to 32°C using a blood–water temperature difference of no more than 12 degrees during both the cooling and rewarming phases.

Blood Flow

We routinely use a cardiac index of 2.4 L/m² throughout the period of CPB. On the rare occasion when significant hypothermia is used, this index can be reduced to 1.8 L/m². Regardless of the cardiac index, mean blood pressure is maintained at a minimum of 50 mm Hg, with blood flow adjustment being the primary source of control. In older patients or those with cerebrovascular disease, a higher mean arterial pressure may be used (>60 mm Hg), again by increasing blood flow when possible, rather than resorting to pharmacologic means.

We routinely use pulsatile blood flow during total CPB, primarily because of its effect in preventing the vasoconstrictive response to nonpulsatile flow. We use nonpulsatile flow during the periods of initiation of bypass and when the heart is actively ejecting at the end of CPB. Pulsatile pump–driven counterpulsation may be used during the termination of routine bypass or in those patients requiring more prolonged periods of mechanical assist before terminating perfusion. Roller pump–generated counterpulsation may be triggered and timed in a similar manner to that for controlling a balloon pump, either from arterial pressure or ECG. Most modern pulsatile roller pump systems have a facility for controlling the timing of the pulse generated by the pump head, and this can be a very effective support mechanism while balloon support is being prepared for longer-term support.

Blood Gas Control

Because we use a temperature drift technique, cooling occasionally to below 32°C, we use an alpha-stat blood gas regimen. A gas blender is used in delivering the ventilating gas.

Heparin Management

An initial dose of 3,000 IU/kg of heparin is administered to the patient by the anesthetist to achieve systemic anticoagulation. The activated clotting time (ACT) is measured before initiation of bypass to ensure that it is in excess of 500 seconds. These measurements are repeated every 30 minutes during the CPB procedure, and additional heparin is administered when necessary to maintain an ACT in excess of 500 seconds, or 750 seconds in the presence of aprotinin.

Aprotinin

We use aprotinin as our major hemostatic strategy in those patients considered to be at increased risk of bleeding (reoperations, coagulopathies, septic patients, Jehovah's witnesses, etc). In the majority of cases, we use the standard Hammersmith high-dose regimen.

- Test dose to check for allergic reactions
- Loading dose—2×10^6 KIU after anesthetic induction
- Pump prime dose—2×10^6 KIU in the CPB circuit prime
- Maintenance dose—0.5×10^6 KIU during CPB period

We are currently extending our use of aprotinin in view of our recent discovery of its specific antiinflammatory effect.

Blood Pressure Management

During bypass, the patient may experience periods of hypotension and hypertension. During the early phase of the procedure, hypotension is commonly encountered, but this is generally transient and associated with the changing viscosity resulting from hemodilution by the priming solution. This condition rarely requires intervention but may be effectively treated with the administration of blood if it persists. Hypertension is a far more common condition during bypass and may be dealt with using many vasodilatory strategies, including the administration of sodium nitroprusside, or putting the patient deeper under anesthesia.

Line Pressure

The arterial line pressure gauge is one of the most critical elements of the perfusion system, giving essential information regarding the condition of the arterial side of the circuit, including the oxygenators, filter, arterial line itself, and the cannula and aorta. Under normal conditions and at normal flow levels ($2.4 L/m^2$), we routinely see line pressures of 180 to 230 mm Hg. Any substantial increase in line pressure above these levels may indicate a blockage in the membrane oxygenator or arterial filter, or a kink in the arterial line, and must be acted on immediately.

Filtration

Common to most perfusion systems, our system incorporates a number of filters—some built into the venous and cardiotomy aspects of the reservoir—positioned to remove inappropriate materials from the input side of the perfusion system, particularly in the form of surgical debris. We also routinely use an arterial line filter, positioned between the membrane oxygenator outlet and the patient end of the arterial line. This filter's main purpose is to remove particulate microemboli and air emboli from the output side of the system. These filters, particularly the arterial line filter, are essential components of the perfusion system. The arterial line filter currently used in our system is the Pall AV6 40 micron filter, a configuration that our laboratory studies have shown to offer significant protection to patients from circuit generated gaseous and particulate emboli, while offering little resistance to blood flow. We consider the arterial line filter to be the last, and most important, safety device in the perfusion circuit.

Leukocyte-depleting filters, a recent development in filter technology, were designed to perform the traditional functions of the arterial line filter with the added benefit of removing activated neutrophils associated with reperfusion injury. These new filters have been undergoing assessment in our unit for some time. We have used these filters (Pall LG6) over the past few years with some measured benefit, particularly with regard to reduction in blood transfusion requirements and duration of ventilatory support in the postoperative phase.

These filters have been promising, and we continue to evaluate them, with particular emphasis on their effect on moderating the neutrophil-mediated aspect of the systemic inflammatory response syndrome.

Cerebral Protection

Patients with a history of stroke, carotid bruit, or cerebrovascular disease are given our cerebroprotective perfusion protocol. In these patients, we add 200 ml of 20% mannitol to the priming solution and perfuse at a flow index of $2.8 L/m^2$, or at a level that maintains a mean arterial blood pressure at least 60 mm Hg. Additionally, these patients may receive intravenous thiopentone.

Renal Failure

Patients who present with a serum creatine greater than 200 are transfused with Hartmann's solution at a rate of

Table 1 Complications Associated With Cardiopulmonary Bypass

SYSTEM	COMPLICATION
Nervous	Cerebral
	Stroke
	Seizure
	Behavior alteration
	Brachial plexopathy
Cardiac	Myocardial injury
	Arrhythmia (supraventricular, ventricular)
	Coronary artery spasm
	Pericardial tamponade
Hematologic	Surgical bleeding
	Medical bleeding
	Inadequate heparin reversal
	Platelet defects
	Hyperfibrinolysis
	Isolated clotting deficiencies
	Disseminated intravascular coagulation
	Inherited coagulopathies and dyscrasias
	Cold agglutinins
Vascular	Aortic bleeding and dissection (cannula insertion)
	Arterial emboli
	Leg ischemia (femoral cannulation)
Pulmonary	Atelectasis
	Edema
	Pleural effusion
	Pneumothorax
	Pneumonia
	Anaphylaxis (protamine, albumin)
	Adult respiratory distress syndrome
	Interstitial hemorrhage (Swan-Ganz catheter)
Gastrointestinal	Gastritis
	Peptic ulcer
	Mesenteric ischemia and infarction
	Acute pancreatitis
	Cholecystitis
	Colonic perforation/diverticulitis
	Liver failure
	Splenic rupture
Immune	Postpericardiotomy syndrome
Renal	Acute tubular necrosis
	Chronic renal failure

30 to 50 ml/hr for a period of 8 to 12 hours preoperatively up to a maximum volume of 50% of patient's body mass. In addition, these patients receive intraoperative dopamine infusion (3 to 4.5 μg/kg/min). Patients with marginal renal function, but with serum creatinine of less than 200, receive the renal dopamine regimen only.

Diabetes
In diabetic patients, blood glucose levels are checked every 30 minutes. Insulin is administered via the venous reservoir if the blood glucose level falls below 250 mg%.

Hematocrit
Although monitored regularly (every 15 to 30 minutes) during the CPB procedure, it is rare that the level of hematocrit gives cause for concern. With diminishing hemodilution associated with a smaller priming load, hematocrit rarely falls below 25% to 27% in our practice. In the event that the hematocrit is lower than 20% to 22% and volume administration is required, blood would be our first choice additive. However, this is an increasingly rare occurrence.

Termination of Bypass
Moderate, rather than profound, cooling of the patient results in a less complicated CPB termination phase. We rewarm to a nasopharyngeal temperature of 37°C, with a venous blood temperature not exceeding 37.5°C. An aortic needle is routinely used for venting purposes, and proper function of this is ensured before starting the termination procedure. Once a stable cardiac rhythm has been achieved, the heart is filled to the predetermined filling pressure, and the arterial pump output is slowly reduced to zero output, with a proportionate reduction in venous return. Once off bypass, blood spilling into the chest cavity from the aortic vent is slowly returned via the aortic cannula, until both the vent and the cannula are removed.

■ COMPLICATIONS

Routine uncomplicated cases have a minimal risk of complications, ranging from 1% to 2%. As the technique of CPB has evolved over the decades, so too have the safety and prevention of problems associated with the technique and physiologic undesirable affects of CPB. A partial list of the more common complications associated with CPB is outlined in Table 1.

SUGGESTED READING

Hornick P, Taylor K: Pulsatile and nonpulsatile perfusion: the continuing controversy, *J Cardiothorac Vasc Anesth* 11:310, 1997.

Hsu LC: Heparin-coated cardiopulmonary bypass circuits: current status, *Perfusion* 16:417, 2001.

Potger KC, et al: Coronary artery bypass grafting: an off-pump versus on-pump review, *J Extracorp Technol* 34:260, 2002.

Utley JR: Pathophysiology of cardiopulmonary bypass: current issues, *J Card Surg* 5:177, 1990.

Wan S, et al: Inflammatory response to cardiopulmonary bypass: mechanisms involved and possible therapeutic strategies, *Chest* 112:676, 1997.

MYOCARDIAL PROTECTION

Vinod H. Thourani
Robert A. Guyton

The increasing use of percutaneous transluminal coronary angioplasty, atherectomy, and stent placement (with or without radiation) has resulted in surgical referral of older patients with more severe coronary artery disease, diminished ventricular function, and more prevalent concomitant systemic disease, decreasing the margins of safety for cardiac surgical procedures. Integral to the initiation and successful performance of routine or complex cardiac surgical procedures are sophisticated techniques of myocardial protection.

The goals of myocardial protection during cardiac surgery are to facilitate the operation by providing a quiet, bloodless field; enhancing the precision of the operation; and avoiding iatrogenic injury from cardiopulmonary bypass and surgically imposed ischemia. In addition, myocardial protective strategies are geared to prevent reperfusion injury on resolution of the coronary occlusion and the release of the aortic cross-clamp. Currently, myocardial protection may be achieved by (1) either crystalloid or blood cardioplegia delivered antegrade into the aortic root proximal to the aortic cross-clamp, alone or combined with retrograde (coronary sinus) delivery; (2) continuous retrograde blood cardioplegia delivered under normothermic or hypothermic core conditions; (3) continuous ventricular fibrillation under moderate hypothermia without aortic cross-clamping; (4) no cardioplegic solution administration during off-pump coronary artery bypass (OPCAB); or (5) perfusion-assisted direct coronary artery bypass (PADCAB).

Well-orchestrated and methodical protection of the heart throughout the surgical procedure is essential. Although coronary artery bypass graft (CABG) surgery remains the cornerstone of the practicing cardiac surgeon, valve surgery dominates the practice of some surgeons. The resurgence of OPCAB surgery has led cardiac surgeons to reevaluate myocardial protection for these patients. This chapter outlines the current strategy and practice of myocardial protection for cardiac surgical procedures with emphasis on CABG and OPCAB procedures.

■ FACTORS CONTRIBUTING TO MYOCARDIAL PROTECTION

Preoperative Preparation

Optimal myocardial protection requires that a calm, well-medicated, well-hydrated, and well-nourished patient be brought to the operating room. Patients who are to undergo operation late in the day should receive intravenous fluids or medications during the several-hour period before surgery. β-Blockers and calcium channel blockers can be given by mouth on the morning of surgery.

Anesthetic induction should proceed smoothly with minimal physiologic derangement; tachycardia, hypertension, hypotension, elevated cardiac filling pressures, and myocardial ischemia must be avoided. This can be accomplished in simple cases with minimal monitoring, but in more complex cases a Swan-Ganz catheter is necessary. In cardiac reoperations or when preparation of the conduit for coronary bypass may be prolonged, careful anesthetic technique is important when the interval between anesthetic induction and the onset of cardiopulmonary bypass may be prolonged. Emergency situations, such as an acute myocardial infarction, may force the anesthesiologist to make speed a major priority, altering usual techniques.

The performance of cardiopulmonary bypass offers a unique opportunity for the surgeon to manipulate the metabolic state of the heart before ischemic or cardioplegic arrest. Oxygen consumption of the heart during ischemic arrest or even during hypothermic cardioplegic arrest is related directly to oxygen consumption of the heart before ischemic arrest. Some blood cardioplegic techniques (particularly warm blood cardioplegic techniques) allow metabolic restoration of the heart at the beginning of the cross-clamp period. This is not the case with cold crystalloid cardioplegia. For this reason, a hypertrophied or hyperdynamic heart may benefit from β-blocker administration at the initiation of cardiopulmonary bypass to decrease metabolic stimulation of the heart. If the heart is metabolically stressed (e.g., a heart that has deteriorated because of acute mitral insufficiency), the heart should be rested on cardiopulmonary bypass for a few minutes in an empty beating state before aortic cross-clamping. Ischemic or chemical preconditioning of the heart before the initiation of cardiopulmonary arrest has been successful in experimental situations, but so far it has not been proved consistently efficacious in human clinical trials as a myocardial protectant.

Cannulation Techniques

Cannulation of the ascending aorta for arterial return from the pump is a standard technique. In coronary reoperations, cannulation should be accomplished sufficiently distal to the proximal anastomoses that the aortic cross-clamp can be placed without obstruction of the vein grafts. Venous cannulation remains highly variable from surgeon to surgeon. A two-stage single cannula introduced into the atrium with holes positioned in the inferior vena cava and right atrium allows adequate venous drainage for most procedures. This cannula has a distinct *disadvantage* in that warming of the heart, particularly the right atrium and right ventricle, occurs because of warm venous blood flowing through these chambers. Double venous cannulation with separate snared cannulae in the inferior vena cava and superior vena cava is the most secure method to isolate the heart and prevent warming.

Hypothermia

Hypothermia, introduced by Bigelow et al and Shumway and Lower, has become a cornerstone of myocardial protection. Hypothermia reduces metabolic rate, oxygen demand, and energy depletion during ischemia (Figure 1). Hypothermia for cardiac surgery may be accomplished by systemic cooling, local irrigation, or perfusion hypothermia. Perfusion hypothermia (administered with cardioplegia) is the most efficient way to cool the myocardium, but coronary pathology may lead to wide variation in myocardial temperature from region to region. These variations can be minimized by systemic cooling and local irrigation. Systemic cooling is simple to accomplish and does not unduly prolong the operation if rewarming is initiated in a timely manner. Local irrigation of the pericardium with a cold, balanced electrolyte slush can be an important adjunct to myocardial hypothermia but may be difficult when distal anastomoses are performed on the lateral or inferior walls of

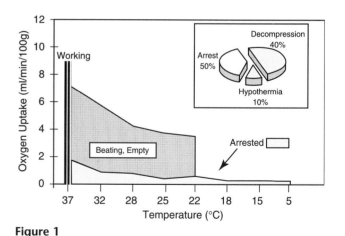

Figure 1

Myocardial oxygen uptake (reflecting oxygen demand) versus temperature. Compared with the oxygen uptake of a normally beating working heart, nullifying cardiac work with total vented bypass reduces oxygen uptake by 30% to 60%, whereas arresting the heart reduces the oxygen demands a further 50% (total reduction 90%). Hypothermia further reduces oxygen demands significantly between 37°C and 22°C. (*From Vinten-Johansen J, et al: Surgical myocardial protection. In Gravlee GP, et al, editors:* Cardiopulmonary bypass: principles and practice, *ed 2, Philadelphia, Lippincott Williams & Wilkins, 2000, p 232.*)

the heart. The exposed anterior surface of the heart may not cool with this technique. Care should be taken not to expose the phrenic nerves to the ice slush.

Avoidance of Ventricular Distention

Ventricular distention while the heart is perfused with blood before aortic cross-clamp impairs endocardial blood flow and should be avoided. Ventricular distention is less damaging if it occurs during the period of cardioplegic arrest. Left ventricular distention during the arrest invariably is accompanied, however, by elevated pressure in the aortic root, washout of cardioplegic solution, rapid warming of the heart, and sometimes initiation of contraction with consequent ischemic damage. Ventricular distention is particularly likely to occur when the vigor of the cardiac contraction is diminished by systemic cooling, when the aortic valve is incompetent, when the aortic cross-clamp initially is removed and reperfusion hyperemia leads to a flood of coronary sinus efflux, or when ventricular fibrillation occurs before or immediately after the aortic cross-clamp interval. As depicted in Figure 1, oxygen consumption is reduced substantially by decompressing the left ventricle compared with a beating heart working to support the systemic circulation. This reduction in oxygen demand is achieved by reducing pressure and volume work of the heart. If distention occurs, it should be relieved promptly by active or passive techniques.

For mild ventricular distention before or just after the aortic cross-clamping, manual massage of the heart may be adequate. If ventricular distention persists, the heart may be vented passively by elevating the operating table to increase venous return to the pump, amputating the tip of the left atrial appendage, or making an incision in the pulmonary artery to allow efflux of blood. The heart may be actively vented by placing a suction catheter into the left atrium, pulmonary artery, or left ventricle (via the right superior pulmonary vein or the apex of the left ventricle). During the cross-clamp interval, the heart may be vented actively by placing the suction catheter in the ascending aorta (or using the cardioplegia infusion cannula for this purpose) or passively by punching proximal anastomosis holes in the ascending aorta or allowing the cardioplegia infusion cannula to drain into the pericardium. Many surgeons avoid active cardiac venting during coronary operations because entrained air may be difficult to remove, particularly after one has performed three or four proximal anastomoses.

Cardioplegia Administration

Introduced in 1955 by Melrose et al and popularized by Gay and Ebert in 1973, cardioplegia plays an important role in myocardial protection strategies. Acting as a selective myocardial perfusion agent, cardioplegic solutions can alter or inhibit ischemic injury by virtue of hypothermia and asystole. In addition, cardioplegia can be used to avoid reperfusion injury through alteration of its delivery and composition using various adjunctive agents and pharmacologic therapies. In its simplest formulation, cardioplegia leads to decreased ischemic injury primarily by reducing oxygen demand to less than 10% of the working heart by initiating rapid hypothermia and by cardiac asystole. Cardioplegia avoids reperfusion injury by targeting detrimental pathophysiologic

mechanisms and mediators (e.g., leukocytes, cytokines). In our practice at Emory University, crystalloid and blood cardioplegia techniques are used.

The composition of crystalloid cardioplegia should be an analogue of the extracellular fluid. The optimal potassium concentration for initial arrest seems to be approximately 20 to 25 mEq/liter. The optimal pH of the crystalloid cardioplegic solution seems to be approximately 7.8 (measured at 37°C). The calcium level of the cardioplegic solution should be low, but probably not 0. Glucose seems to be useful in providing energy supply during the anaerobic intervals. At Emory University, Plasma-Lyte A intravenous solution is supplemented with 25 mEq of potassium chloride, 20 mEq of sodium bicarbonate, and 3 ml of 50% dextrose in water (final concentrations in mEq/liter: sodium 160, potassium 30, magnesium 3, chloride 98, acetate 27, gluconate 23, and bicarbonate 20; dextrose 1500 mg/liter).

An adequate quantity of cardioplegic solution should be delivered to the most vulnerable region of the myocardium to achieve electrical quiescence and a myocardial temperature of 15°C or less. Because cardioplegic delivery may be distinctly heterogeneous (secondary to the aberrations in critical coronary stenoses), some regions of the heart may be exposed to 10 times as much cardioplegic solution as other regions. Not only is delivery of the cardioplegic solution heterogeneous, but also the pressure to which various regions of the coronary vasculature are exposed is heterogeneous, depending on proximal coronary stenoses. For instance, in a patient with left main disease, it may be necessary to use high aortic root pressures to achieve cardioplegic infusion. Aortic infusion pressures of 150 mm Hg may be used without damage to unprotected coronary beds and may be necessary to force solution past critical stenoses.

Generally, in the average-size heart, infusion of 1 liter of 4°C crystalloid cardioplegic solution decreases septal myocardial temperature to approximately 12°C, if infusion pressure is maintained between 60 and 80 mm Hg. Repeat infusion is needed every 15 to 20 minutes to maintain this regional hypothermia. Studies have shown that cardioplegic infusion temperatures of 2°C can be used safely for myocardial cooling.

Popularized by Salerno and Buckberg, administration of blood cardioplegia has become an integral component of myocardial protection for patients undergoing CABG or valvular surgery. Experimental and clinical investigations have shown that administration of blood cardioplegia affords the benefit of enhanced oxygen-carrying capacity, active resuscitation, avoidance of reperfusion damage, limitation of hemodilution, provision of oncotic pressure, buffering, rheologic effects, and endogenous oxygen free radical scavengers. Blood cardioplegia may be administered antegrade or retrograde, intermittent or continuous, and tepid or cold. Although blood cardioplegia initially was used for patients considered high risk due to ischemic or hibernating myocardium, poor left ventricular function, or concomitant CABG and valve procedures, it has become the standard myocardial protection used by cardiac surgeons at Emory University.

Retrograde cardioplegic infusion via the coronary sinus also has been used for difficult situations involving valve surgery, an incompetent aortic valve, ischemic myocardium, or severe proximal coronary obstruction. This technique also may lead to heterogeneous delivery of cardioplegia, and administration is usually concomitant with antegrade cardioplegia infusion. The ventricular septum and right ventricular free wall are particularly susceptible to inadequate protection with retrograde cardioplegic infusion.

Reperfusion Techniques

Myocardial protection does not end with removal of the aortic cross-clamp. Changes in myocardial function, metabolism, and ultrastructure continue during reperfusion. Conditions should be optimized during this time to prevent "reperfusion injury," which may ensue after aortic cross-clamp removal.

During reperfusion, the same caveats apply as before the cross-clamping: avoid tachycardia, hypotension or hypertension, and ventricular distention or fibrillation. If asystole is maintained during reperfusion, the heart must be vented, either actively or passively, to avoid ventricular distention. Reperfusate modification with Krebs cycle intermediates, such as glutamine or aspartate, and with adenosine triphosphate precursors may be useful. Other reperfusion modifications include warming the cardioplegic solution and infusion of the solution into the aorta at a rate of 70 to 100 ml/min. The aortic cross-clamp may be partially removed, allowing blood to flow into the ascending aorta and mix with the cardioplegic solution; this leads to infusion of a variable mixture of blood and cardioplegic solution into the coronary circulation for 3 to 5 minutes before the cross-clamp is removed completely. This infusion maintains cardiac arrest during the first few minutes of warm blood reperfusion.

Myocardial recovery after removal of the aortic cross-clamp is gradual, and a period of myocardial rest with a decompressed, beating heart and a good aortic perfusion pressure for 20 to 30 minutes allows the best opportunity for myocardial recovery and a good functional result.

Overall Scheme for Cardiopulmonary Bypass

The optimal system of myocardial protection cannot be prescribed in any protocol or even set of protocols; it must be tailored to suit the individual patient. Many of the schemes outlined previously are complicated and require prolongation of the operation. Each surgeon should have a standard system of myocardial protection and many alternative options to accommodate the individual patient. In this modern era of sophisticated and sometimes complicated technologic advancement, it is important to remember that the shortest and gentlest operation gives the patient the best chance for a smooth postoperative convalescence.

Cardiopulmonary bypass equipment includes a roller pump, membrane oxygenator, and open reservoir system. Blood and crystalloid cardioplegia are used in our institution, with indications for each determined by the presence or absence of myocardial ischemia and surgeon preference. Generally, for on-pump, low-risk patients (not including patients with acute ischemia, redo CABG surgery, or concomitant valve procedures), coronary artery bypass consists of systemic cooling to 30°C; local irrigation of the pericardium; aortic cross-clamping when the cardiac temperature has

reached approximately 32°C; antegrade infusion of a cold (2°C to 4°C), oxygenated crystalloid cardioplegic solution in sufficient volume (1 liter) at 70 mm Hg into the aortic root to lower the temperature of the myocardium to 15°C; infusion of cardioplegic solution (approximately 200 ml) down each vein graft as each distal anastomosis is completed; rewarming as the last distal anastomoses are completed; and removal of the aortic cross-clamp and reperfusion while the proximal anastomoses are performed. In all patients undergoing cardiac surgery, the following drugs are administered intravenously just before removal of the aortic cross-clamp: 37.5 g of mannitol, 2 mg/kg of lidocaine, 50 mg of esmolol and 2 g of magnesium sulfate. Ventricular distention is avoided by passive cardiac decompression. This standardized system has many possibilities for enhancement in special situations: Cardioplegic solutions can be reinfused at intervals into the aortic root or into the coronary sinus; systemic temperature can be lowered to 22°C, 20°C, or 18°C; local irrigation can be applied continuously or intermittently; the aortic cross-clamp can be left in place while distal and proximal anastomoses are completed; active rather than passive venting of the cardiac chambers may be accomplished; or reperfusion may be modified by administration of cardioplegia just before removal of the aortic cross-clamp or by partial removal of the aortic cross-clamp while cardioplegia is infused slowly in the aortic root, maintaining asystole while the heart is reperfused.

Our standard system for on-pump moderate-risk to high-risk patients (including patients with acute myocardial ischemia, hibernating myocardium, poor left ventricular function, redo CABG surgery, or associated valve procedures) consists of antegrade hypothermic blood cardioplegia supplemented with near-continuous retrograde cardioplegia. Some surgeons within our group have changed their practice to include blood cardioplegia for all patients undergoing on-pump cardiac surgery. We use systemic cooling to 28°C to 30°C, local cold irrigation of the pericardium, and aortic cross-clamping when the cardiac temperature has reached approximately 28°C to 32°C. Our antegrade and retrograde blood cardioplegia protocol uses four parts blood to one part Plasma-Lyte A solution. Antegrade infusion of a cold (8°C to 10°C) oxygenated blood cardioplegia (500 ml) with high potassium (105 mEq/liter Plasma-Lyte A solution) is administered at 400 to 500 ml/min in the aortic root after aortic cross-clamping. After this, retrograde cold (8°C to 10°C) blood cardioplegia (5 liters) with low potassium (35 mEq/liter Plasma-Lyte A solution) is administered with a maximum retrograde pressure of 38 to 40 mm Hg. After the 5-liter retrograde infusion, cold (8°C to 10°C) blood cardioplegia (near-continuous rate) with low potassium (20 mEq/liter Plasma-Lyte A solution) is administered retrograde throughout the quiescent state of the heart. Antegrade infusion of blood cardioplegia is performed every 15 to 20 minutes into the aortic root. In addition, blood cardioplegic solution (approximately 100 to 200 ml) is infused down each vein graft as each distal anastomosis is completed. Rewarming is initiated as the last distal anastomoses are completed, and removal of the aortic cross-clamp and reperfusion are initiated while the proximal anastomoses are performed.

■ OPERATIVE SCENARIOS FOR MYOCARDIAL PROTECTION

Coronary Artery Disease
Severe Obstruction of Proximal Coronary Arteries

Severe triple-vessel disease or left main disease requires that hypotension judiciously be avoided before aortic cross-clamping. If the initiation of cardiopulmonary bypass leads to hypotension, the aorta should be cross-clamped at once and cardioplegic infusion implemented. The use of α-agonists to elevate aortic pressure is not without hazard, as subendocardial ischemia in collateralized regions has been shown. Ventricular distention and ventricular fibrillation are particularly hazardous with severe triple-vessel or left main coronary disease.

As the cardioplegia infusion is begun, the resistance of the coronary arteries can be gauged by the pressure in the ascending aorta. If the pressure is particularly high or if the cardioplegic infusion has to be reduced to a particularly low rate, one should assume that the patient has severe triple-vessel or left main coronary disease, and one should not rely on the native circulation for reperfusion of the heart. In this instance, the distal and proximal anastomoses should be completed during a single cross-clamp period to allow adequate reperfusion of the heart when the cross-clamp is removed. Extensive local irrigation should be accomplished. If the cross-clamp interval is to be longer than approximately 45 to 50 minutes, the systemic temperature may be lowered to 22°C to augment myocardial protection further. The portion of the myocardium most vulnerable (by the preoperative angiogram or measurement of regional myocardial temperatures) should be grafted first and cardioplegic solution infused into this area down the grafted saphenous vein, if applicable. The use of retrograde and antegrade infusions of cardioplegic solution may be helpful.

Acute Myocardial Infarction

In the present era, patients require surgical intervention for acute myocardial ischemia primarily because of angioplasty or stent failure. In these instances, the overwhelming priority is rapid revascularization of the infarcting myocardium. The chest is opened expeditiously, and the patient is placed on cardiopulmonary bypass while vein grafts are harvested from the leg. We have found oxygenated crystalloid cardioplegia to be inferior to blood cardioplegia for reperfusion of acutely ischemic myocardium. Internal mammary arteries are not ordinarily used in this situation because one seeks to infuse cardioplegic solution into the infarcting muscle as rapidly as possible. This generally can be accomplished within 45 minutes of the patient's arrival to the operating room. Proximal anastomoses are constructed with the aortic cross-clamp in place. The heart is decompressed passively, and reperfusion is modified by infusion of cardioplegia as the aortic cross-clamp is partially removed.

Another situation in which the surgeon confronts acute ischemia is the occurrence of ischemia after induction of anesthesia. In this instance, it may not be possible to identify which portion of the heart is ischemic because the manifestation of ischemia may be global ventricular dysfunction rather than localized electrocardiographic changes. If available, intraoperative transesophageal echocardiography may identify specific dyskinetic myocardial segments. Rapid initiation of cardiopulmonary bypass, aortic cross-clamping, cardioplegic infusion, ventricular decompression, and subsequently cardioplegia delivery via vein grafts must be accomplished quickly.

Coronary Disease with Poor Left Ventricular Function

Patients with chronic congestive heart failure, low ejection fraction, or recent myocardial infarction with a large area of akinetic or dyskinetic myocardium must receive special care to avoid further myocardial damage during revascularization. Cardiopulmonary bypass can be initiated slowly and aortic pressure maintained (with an α-agonist infusion if necessary). The ventricle is decompressed passively, and tachycardia is treated with β-blockade. The decompressed heart is allowed to rest for a few minutes with a good aortic perfusion pressure before aortic cross-clamping and cardioplegia infusion. Proximal and distal anastomoses are accomplished during a single cross-clamp interval. The aortic cross-clamp is removed, and the heart is allowed to rest, decompressed via the amputated left atrial appendage for 10 to 20 minutes before weaning from cardiopulmonary bypass.

Coronary Artery Reoperations

Coronary artery reoperations pose challenging surgical problems. The aortic cross-clamp must be placed sufficiently high to allow infusion of cardioplegic solution down patent vein grafts. If there is atherosclerotic buildup in vein grafts, manipulation of the heart is minimized until cardioplegic arrest has been accomplished. Side-biting aortic clamps are avoided; only the aortic cross-clamp is placed on the ascending aorta, following which proximal and distal anastomoses are accomplished during a single period of cross-clamping. Infusion of cardioplegic solution into several vein grafts simultaneously may be facilitated by the use of multiple-port cardioplegic infusion cannulae. Some surgeons in our institution advocate dissection of the femoral vessels before opening the chest to facilitate femoral bypass if problems arise during the dissection of the heart from the sternum.

Coronary artery reoperations for acute myocardial ischemia present a special problem. This is one instance in which preoperative placement of an intraaortic balloon pump preoperatively is particularly useful. The intraaortic balloon pump allows improved coronary perfusion while the chest is opened and dissection of the heart is accomplished.

Coronary artery reoperations with patent internal mammary artery grafts present an even greater challenge. If the internal mammary artery graft supplies a coronary artery that is partially perfused from the aortic root, cardioplegic infusion may be accomplished via the aortic root while the internal mammary artery is occluded with a soft clamp or snare. Alternatively the operation may be accomplished by cooling the patient to 20°C, venting the heart actively with a left ventricular vent, maintaining aortic root pressure at 80 mm Hg, and operating on a fibrillating, cold, well-perfused heart with local isolation of coronary artery segments. Another alternative is occlusion of the internal mammary artery graft with a soft bulldog clamp, clamping of the aortic root, and antegrade and retrograde infusion of cardioplegic solution to protect the region supplied by the internal mammary artery.

Off-Pump Coronary Artery Bypass

Concern for myocardial protection during multivessel OPCAB stems from the knowledge that the brief periods of ischemia necessary to visualize the target vessels during the distal anastomoses produce myocardial injury that not only may affect the individual target areas, but also cause cumulative global dysfunction. Strategies to protect the myocardium from ischemia and reperfusion injuries may improve outcomes of OPCAB procedures.

Ischemic preconditioning enjoyed brief popularity as a cardioprotective strategy during OPCAB. The theoretical benefit of brief occlusion and reperfusion preceding the longer occlusion necessary to construct a coronary anastomosis was supported by abundant laboratory evidence showing improved myocardial protection in that region of the heart. In humans, ischemic preconditioning has not been shown universally to attenuate myocardial contractile dysfunction or "stunning." Although ischemic preconditioning seemed appropriate and acceptable for single-vessel bypass via small thoracotomy (minimally invasive direct coronary artery bypass), as the number of bypass grafts performed during OPCAB increased, the enthusiasm of surgical practitioners to perform repeated episodes of ischemic preconditioning for each coronary artery has diminished. Although presently a few OPCAB surgeons perform surgical ischemic preconditioning, future development of chemical preconditioning is more attractive.

As OPCAB is increasingly applied to complex multivessel cases, several practical considerations regarding myocardial protection should be mentioned. Perhaps the simplest and most important is graft sequence during multivessel OPCAB. As a general rule, it is important to graft the *collateralized* vessels first and reperfuse them by performing proximal anastomoses or releasing clamps on the internal mammary artery pedicles, then graft the *collateralizing* vessels. By this approach, vital coronary flow provided by collateralizing vessels is not interrupted before restoration of flow to the collateralized vessels via the newly constructed coronary grafts. The preferred sequence at our institution is as follows:

1. Graft completely occluded, collateralized vessels first. There is little decrement in myocardial perfusion during construction of this distal anastomosis. When this graft has been constructed and reperfused, the collateralizing vessel may be occluded and grafted more safely.
2. Be flexible with the timing of the left internal mammary artery–left anterior descending artery (LIMA-LAD) anastomosis. It should be done first when the LAD is collateralized and in most cases of tight left main stenosis. LIMA-LAD grafting should be performed last, however, if the LAD is the least diseased, collateralizing vessel. To occlude the lightly diseased, collateralizing LAD first is to limit critically total myocardial blood flow during construction of the LAD-LIMA anastomosis because the collateralized vessels are effectively occluded simultaneously.

3. Be flexible with the timing of proximal anastomoses. Aortosaphenous or aortoradial anastomoses may be done first or early in the case after the distal anastomosis of critical collateralized targets. The collateralized vessels are reperfused via the grafts before the collateralizing coronary artery is occluded and grafted. This limits global ischemia and dysfunction. In most routine cases, however, the proximal aortosaphenous anastomoses may be constructed after all distal anastomoses have been completed, allowing graft length to be estimated most easily.
4. Be aware that occlusion of the large right coronary artery may result in heart block. Epicardial pacing should be immediately available and a selection of appropriately sized intracoronary or aortocoronary shunts. Reperfusion of an adjacent or collateralizing coronary graft either by completion of the proximal anastomosis or via perfusion-assisted techniques (see later) before occlusion of the right coronary artery may reduce the likelihood of untoward events.
5. Hearts with ischemic mitral regurgitation may be stabilized by early grafting and reperfusion of the culprit vessels causing papillary muscle dysfunction.
6. Above all, customize the graft sequence for each individual case, considering coronary anatomy, pattern of collateralization, myocardial contractility, atherosclerosis of the ascending aorta, conduit availability, and graft geometry.

In specific cases of OPCAB (particularly anastomoses of the lateral and inferior wall coronary vessels), manipulation of the heart may lead to deterioration of hemodynamics. In these cases, PADCAB provides a disconnect between coronary perfusion pressure and systemic arterial pressure and may interrupt this deterioration of hemodynamics. During PADCAB, distal anastomoses are constructed as usual in OPCAB, and grafts are connected immediately to the outflow of a small pump circuit. Inflow to the circuit is provided by placement of a small cardioplegia-type catheter in the ascending aorta or femoral artery. A servo-controlled pump (Quest Medical, Allen, TX) system is the principal component of this circuit and allows exact control of coronary perfusion pressure and temperature. Chemical additives may be administered in the outflow circuit at precisely controlled concentrations. Consequently, distal anastomoses may be constructed with venous or radial arterial grafts and perfused at a predetermined pressure, regardless of systemic arterial pressure. Flows can be measured precisely to confirm graft patency. Grafted, collateralized coronary arteries may be used to drive coronary perfusion retrograde through the collaterals to the collateralizing native coronary artery during grafting of that target. Perfusion via collaterals of adjacent myocardial regions also may contribute to improved myocardial protection. The addition of nitroglycerin, adenosine, or other coronary vasodilators may improve further regional and collateral myocardial perfusion.

In OPCAB, the cardioprotective armamentarium against ischemic injury includes ischemic or chemical preconditioning, coronary shunting, PADCAB, and possible preload and afterload reduction using axial pumps.

Valve Disease
Aortic Regurgitation

Aortic regurgitation is a threat to myocardial protection in many ways. A low aortic diastolic pressure may lead to subendocardial ischemia before or during cardiopulmonary bypass just before aortic cross-clamping. Ventricular distention easily occurs and may result in early ventricular fibrillation. Cardioplegic solutions cannot be readily infused into the aortic root. Associated ventricular hypertrophy further stresses the system of myocardial protection. In this setting, great care is taken to avoid ventricular distention as cardiopulmonary bypass is initiated. β-Blockade is used to protect the myocardium during subsequent ischemic arrest and to allow the heart to continue beating as it is cooled down slowly to 25°C or 23°C. Copious local irrigation is used for myocardial cooling. The aorta is opened immediately after ventricular fibrillation occurs, and cardioplegia is infused into each coronary ostium. Retrograde cardioplegia also may be used via the coronary sinus. The preoperative angiogram is reviewed to determine the length of the left main coronary artery, taking care that the cardioplegic solution is not infused selectively into either the circumflex artery or LAD. Cardioplegic solution is reinfused into each ostium as the valve operation is accomplished. Concomitant CABG is accomplished before valve placement to allow infusion of cardioplegic solution via a multiple-port cardioplegic infusion cannula into all vulnerable regions of the myocardium simultaneously. The heart is reperfused carefully and rested because one must presume that with aortic regurgitation myocardial protection in some regions of the heart has been compromised.

Aortic Stenosis

Aortic stenosis, particularly in the elderly, often is accompanied by at least mild aortic regurgitation so that many of the aforementioned problems apply. Hypertrophy of the ventricle creates a particular vulnerability to subendocardial ischemia. Systemic cooling and local irrigation (particularly intracavitary irrigation with a cold solution after the valve is excised) improve myocardial protection.

Mitral Valve Disease

Options for myocardial protection during mitral valve operations include (1) avoidance of aortic cross-clamping, operating on a beating empty heart; (2) antegrade infusion of cardioplegic solution into the aortic root; and (3) retrograde infusion of cardioplegic solution via the coronary sinus.

The first option, avoidance of aortic cross-clamping, does not provide optimal exposure of the mitral valve and increases the risk of introducing air into the ascending aorta as the operation is completed. The second option, antegrade infusion of cardioplegic solution, raises a particular hazard if a second infusion of cardioplegic solution must be accomplished: The right coronary artery in this case is particularly vulnerable to introduction of air as a second dose of cardioplegia is delivered into the air-filled ascending aorta. Special care must be taken to avoid coronary air embolism. Retrograde cardioplegia is attractive, but concerns exist about adequate protection of the septum and right ventricle, particularly if pulmonary hypertension is present and right ventricular function must be preserved early after operation.

■ SUMMARY

In contrast to in the experimental laboratory, the human heart is not diseased in a consistently reproducible fashion. As a result, the strategy for myocardial protection must be modified by the cardiac surgeon not only according to the pathology of the patient, but also the talent and experience of the surgeon. Many effective techniques are available; surgeons must combine them intelligently for each patient. Future strategies for myocardial protection may incorporate systemic or local cardiac infusion of therapeutic agents that will have broad-spectrum effects using multiple windows and multiple targets in multiple organs and will address the multiple organ effects of ischemia that occur with on-pump or off-pump cardiac surgery.

SUGGESTED READING

Brown WM, Jones EL: First operation for myocardial revascularization. In Edmunds LH, editor: *Cardiac surgery in the adult,* New York, 1997, McGraw-Hill, p 535.

Buckberg GD, Marelli D: Myocardial protection. In Kaiser LR, et al, editors: *Mastery of cardiothoracic surgery,* Philadelphia, 1998, Lippincott-Raven, p 287.

Puskas JD, et al: Myocardial protection for off-pump coronary artery bypass surgery, *Semin Thorac Cardiovasc Surg* 13:82, 2001.

Vinten-Johansen J, et al: Surgical myocardial protection. In Gravlee GP, et al, editors: *Cardiopulmonary bypass: principles and practice,* ed 2, Philadelphia, Lippincott Williams & Wilkins, 2000, p 215.

Vinten-Johansen J, Thourani VH: Myocardial protection: an overview, *J Extra-Corporeal Tech* 32:38, 2000.

BLOOD CONSERVATION STRATEGIES IN CARDIAC SURGERY

Jerrold H. Levy

Cardiopulmonary bypass (CPB) is associated with defective hemostasis, which results in bleeding and the requirement for allogenic blood product transfusions in many patients undergoing cardiac surgery and/or coronary artery bypass graft surgery (CABG). Conservation of blood has become a priority during surgery because of the shortages of donor blood, the risks associated with the use of allogeneic blood products, and the costs of these products. Further, transfusions expose patients to a variety of potential cellular and humoral antigens, pose risks of disease transmission and immunomodulation, and may alone represent proinflammatory stimuli in the perioperative period. Multiple approaches are important when considering strategies to limit blood transfusions. Strategies to reduce bleeding and transfusion requirements include recognizing risk factors, developing transfusion practices, conserving red blood cells (RBCs), using new alternatives to RBCs, altering inflammatory responses, and also potentially improving anticoagulation/reversal. Pharmacologic approaches to reduce bleeding and transfusion requirements in cardiac surgical patients are based on either preventing or reversing the defects associated with the CPB-induced coagulopathy, and represent one of the mainstay approaches in cardiac surgery. Pharmacologic strategies to reduce the need for allogeneic blood requirements will be reviewed.

■ RISK FACTORS

Certain risk factors are important when evaluating patients for bleeding potential. The patient who comes to surgery anemic or with a low preoperative RBC mass based on low weight (i.e., children) poses important risk factors for the need of transfused RBCs. Also, associated diseases and preoperative pharmacologic strategies are important because hemostasis is involved with platelet and coagulation factor interaction; also, the preexisting use of antiplatelet agents, especially IIb/IIIa receptor antagonists and clopidogrel (Plavix), is important to consider. Current studies suggest more patients with atherosclerotic vascular disease will be receiving antiplatelet strategies. Further, preexisting liver disease is important to consider because these patients have complex multifactorial coagulopathies. Also, although widely thought that warfarin preexposed the patient to bleeding, more recent data suggest this may not be true. Finally, redo cardiac surgical procedures requiring repeat sternotomy, multiple valve replacements, and other procedures providing long CPB times may also pose potential risk factors for bleeding.

■ DEVELOPING TRANSFUSION PRACTICES

Coagulation factor administration in patients with excessive post-CPB bleeding is generally empirical related to turnaround times of laboratory tests and empirical factor administration. Transfusion-based therapy with excessive bleeding should be based on objective reasons to give factors; unfortunately, there are few validated tests to assess platelet function. Point-of-care coagulation monitoring using thromboelastography resulted in fewer transfusions in the postoperative period. If hemostatic tests are relatively normal and the patient is actively bleeding, reexploration should be considered. The use of thromboelastography and/or an algorithm to guide transfusion therapy in cardiac surgery, especially after complex surgery, should be considered.

■ RED CELL CONSERVATION AND SUBSTITUTES

Because the preexisting red blood mass is important, conserving RBCs is equally important. The use of RBC-saver techniques for high-risk patients is important to consider especially by reprocessing shed blood. Whether in low-risk patients this is effective or not remains to be seen. The use of autologous normovolemic hemodilution is an interesting concept that allows the removal of both red cells and coagulation factors before bleeding. This is also done at the time of surgery and often cannot be performed in a hemodynamically unstable patient. The role of erythropoietin is also interesting, but erythropoietin requires several weeks of therapy to be effective and requires the need to replete iron as well, and so should be considered in a Jehovah's witness or other patient who can be operated on electively.

Artificial blood products and hemoglobin-based oxygen-carrying solutions are currently under development. Blood substitutes are solutions that can be used in resuscitation emergencies or during surgery when rapid intravascular volume expansion is needed in view of acquired red cell losses. The main types of products in development are primarily based on cell-free hemoglobin solutions called hemoglobin-based oxygen-carrying solutions or perfluorocarbon emulsions. None of the agents are currently approved for clinical use in the United States, but they are in different stages of clinical development. Free hemoglobin solutions are subject to more rapid degradation when packaged outside of the RBC membrane. Further, the iron moiety of free hemoglobin readily diffuses in the plasma space and effectively scavenges nitric oxide from pulmonary and systemic vascular endothelia, altering both pulmonary and systemic vascular tone. One mechanism for the reduced need for blood products may be due to the administration of iron and stimulation of erythropoiesis.

■ DESMOPRESSIN

Desmopressin acetate (1-deamino-8-D-arginine vasopressin [DDAVP]) is a synthetic analogue of vasopressin with decreased vasopressor activity. Desmopressin therapy causes a 2- to 20-fold increase in plasma levels of factor VIII and stimulates vascular endothelium to release the larger multimers of von Willebrand factor. Desmopressin also releases tissue plasminogen activator (tPA) and prostacyclin from vascular endothelium. Although definitive studies are lacking supporting its routine use, patients who might benefit from its use include those with mild to moderate forms of hemophilia or von Willebrand disease undergoing surgery and uremic platelet dysfunction. Despite initial enthusiasm for desmopressin, only recently have data suggested that it may be useful to treat platelet dysfunction after cardiac surgery based on specific testing. DDAVP should be considered in the cardiac surgical patient with renal failure or evidence of platelet dysfunction.

■ LYSINE ANALOGUES

Epsilon-aminocaproic acid (EACA, Amicar) and its analogue, tranexamic acid (TA), are derivatives of the amino acid lysine and have been reported in clinical studies of cardiac surgical patients. Both of these drugs inhibit the proteolytic activity of plasmin and the conversion of plasminogen by plasminogen activators. Plasmin cleaves fibrinogen and a series of other proteins involved in coagulation. TA is 6 to 10 times more potent than epsilon-aminocaproic acid. Most of the early studies using antifibrinolytic agents showed decreased mediastinal drainage in patients treated with EACA. However, many of these studies lacked controls, were retrospective, and were not blinded. In the literature, there have been a small number of thrombotic complications in patients receiving lysine analogues, but the studies were not designed to prospectively capture many of these complications. Although the designs of these studies have not been routinely prospective, the incidence of these complications in routine CABG is low and a small number of patients have been studied. Prospective studies evaluating safety issues including the risk of perioperative myocardial infarction, graft patency, and renal dysfunction still need to be studied. TA is approved for use in the United States to prevent bleeding in patients with hereditary angioedema who are undergoing teeth extraction. Most studies report lysine analogues in first-time CABG where the risk of bleeding is low, and not in complex cases. One of the major driving factors in the use of EACA is that it is inexpensive.

■ APROTININ

Aprotinin is a serine protease inhibitor isolated from bovine lung that produces antifibrinolytic effects, inhibits contact activation, reduces platelet dysfunction, and attenuates the inflammatory response to CPB. It is used to reduce blood loss and transfusion requirements in patients with a risk of hemorrhage. Data from clinical trials indicate that aprotinin is generally well tolerated, and the adverse events seen are those expected in patients undergoing open-heart surgery and/or CABG with CPB. Hypersensitivity reactions (i.e., anaphylaxis) occur in less than 0.6% of patients receiving aprotinin for the first time and seem to be greatest within 6 months of reexposure. The results of original reports indicating that aprotinin therapy may increase myocardial infarction (MI) or mortality rates have not been supported

by more recent studies specifically designed to investigate this outcome. There are little comparative tolerability data between aprotinin and the lysine analogues aminocaproic acid and TA. Aprotinin is often used in patients at high risk of hemorrhage, in those for whom transfusion is unavailable, or in patients who refuse allogeneic transfusions.

Multiple studies support the efficacy of aprotinin and include approximately 45 studies involving 7000 patients. In 1992, Cosgrove reported 171 redo CABG patients who received either high-dose aprotinin (Hammersmith dose), low-dose aprotinin (half–Hammersmith dose), or placebo. They found that low-dose aprotinin was as effective as high-dose aprotinin in decreasing blood loss and blood transfusion requirements. Despite the efficacy of reducing both the need for allogeneic blood and chest tube drainage, retrospective analysis of the data suggested a higher risk for MI and graft closure that was not statistically significant. Despite the question about adequacy of anticoagulation, the study created safety concerns that were addressed in two additional prospective studies reported by Levy in redo CABG patients and by Alderman in primary CABG patients. In patients undergoing repeat (CABG) surgery, donor RBC transfusions in the high- and low-dose aprotinin groups was reduced compared with the placebo groups. More important, there was also a significant difference in total blood product exposures among treatment groups (high-dose aprotinin, 2.2 ± 0.4 U; low-dose aprotinin, 3.4 ± 0.9 U; pump prime only, 5.1 ± 0.9 U; placebo, 10.3 ± 1.4 U). There were no differences among treatment groups for the incidence of perioperative MI. Both high- and low-dose aprotinin significantly reduce the requirement for allogeneic blood transfusion in repeat CABG patients without increasing the risk for perioperative MI. There also was a statistically significant reduction in strokes in the aprotinin-treated patients.

To assess the effects of aprotinin on graft patency and MI in patients undergoing primary coronary surgery with CPB, 870 patients were randomized to receive intraoperative aprotinin (n = 436) or placebo (n = 434). Graft angiography was obtained a mean of 10.8 days after the operation. Among 703 patients with assessable saphenous vein grafts, occlusions occurred in 15.4% of aprotinin-treated patients and 10.9% of patients receiving placebo. After adjusting risk factors associated with vein graft occlusion, the aprotinin-placebo risk ratio decreased from 1.7 to 1.05. These factors included female gender, lack of prior aspirin therapy, and small and poor distal vessel quality (1.5 mm). At U.S. sites, saphenous vein occlusions occurred in 9.4% of the aprotinin group and 9.5% of the placebo group. At Danish and Israeli sites, where patients had more adverse characteristics, occlusions occurred in 23.0% of aprotinin- and 12.4% of placebo-treated patients. Aprotinin did not affect the occurrence of MI (aprotinin, 2.9%; placebo, 3.8%) or mortality (aprotinin, 1.4%; placebo, 1.6%). In this study, the probability of early vein graft occlusion was increased by aprotinin, but this outcome was promoted by multiple risk factors for graft occlusion.

■ STUDIES IN CHILDREN

Aprotinin consistently reduces blood loss and transfusion requirements in adults during and after cardiac surgical procedures, but its effectiveness in children is debated. Miller evaluated the hemostatic and economic effects of aprotinin in children undergoing reoperative cardiac procedures with CPB. Control, low-dose aprotinin, and high-dose aprotinin groups were established with 15 children per group. Platelet counts, fibrinogen levels, and thromboelastographic values at baseline and after protamine sulfate administration; number of blood product transfusions; and 6- and 24-hour chest tube drainage were used to evaluate the effects of aprotinin on postbypass coagulopathies. Time needed for skin closure after protamine administration and lengths of stay in the intensive care unit and the hospital were recorded prospectively to determine the economic impact of aprotinin. Coagulation tests performed after protamine administration rarely demonstrated fibrinolysis but did show significant decreases in platelet and fibrinogen levels and function. The thromboelastographic variable indicated a preservation of platelet function by aprotinin. Decreased blood product transfusions, shortened skin closure times, and shortened durations of intensive care unit and hospital stays were found in the aprotinin groups, most significantly in the high-dose group, with a subsequent average reduction of nearly $3000 in patient charges. In children undergoing reoperative cardiac surgical procedures, aprotinin is effective in attenuating postbypass.

■ DEEP HYPOTHERMIC CIRCULATORY ARREST

Early experience with aprotinin in deep hypothermic circulatory arrest (DHCA) raised concerns about hazards associated with its use. Based on what little is known about possible mechanistic interactions among hypothermia, stasis, and aprotinin, there is no evidence that aprotinin becomes unusually hazardous in DHCA. Excessive mortality and complication rates have been reported only in clinical series in which the adequacy of heparinization is questionable. Benefits associated with the use of aprotinin in DHCA have been inconsistently demonstrated. The only prospective, randomized series showed significant reduction in blood loss and transfusion requirements. Use of aprotinin in DHCA should be based on the same consideration applied in other cardiothoracic procedures.

■ COMPARISON STUDIES AND META-ANALYSES

There are little data to compare the efficacy and safety of pharmacologic agents available for reducing allogeneic blood administration in cardiac surgical patients. Levi reported a meta-analysis of all randomized, controlled trials of the three most frequently used pharmacologic strategies to decrease perioperative blood loss (aprotinin, lysine analogues [aminocaproic acid and TA], and desmopressin). Studies were included if they reported at least one clinically relevant outcome (mortality, emergent reoperation, proportion of patients receiving a transfusion, or perioperative MI) in addition to perioperative blood loss. In addition, a separate meta-analysis was done for studies concerning complicated cardiac surgery. A total of 72 trials (8409 patients) met the inclusion criteria. Treatment with aprotinin decreased mortality almost two-fold (odds ratio, 0.55) compared with placebo. Treatment with aprotinin and with lysine analogues decreased the frequency of surgical reexploration (0.37 and 0.44, respectively). These two treatments also significantly decreased the proportion of patients receiving any allogeneic blood transfusion. By contrast, the use of desmopressin resulted in a small decrease in perioperative blood loss but was not associated with a beneficial effect on other clinical outcomes. Aprotinin and lysine analogues did not increase the risk of perioperative MI; however, desmopressin was associated with a 2.4-fold increase in the risk of this complication. Studies in patients undergoing complicated cardiac surgery showed similar results.

■ SUMMARY

Blood conservation for cardiac surgery requires multiple strategies for reducing bleeding and the need for donor blood products. Of all of the strategies, aprotinin has been demonstrated to be highly effective in reducing bleeding and transfusion requirements in high-risk patients undergoing repeat median sternotomy or in high-risk patients. Results from multicenter studies of aprotinin show there is no greater risk of early graft thrombosis, MI, or renal failure in aprotinin-treated patients. Antiinflammatory strategies on the horizon may further add to our pharmacologic armamentarium for cardiac surgery and CPB.

SUGGESTED READING

Alderman EL, et al: International Multi-center Aprotinin Graft Patency Experience (IMAGE), *J Thorac Cardiovasc Surg* 116:716, 1998.

Levi M, et al: Pharmacological strategies to decrease excessive blood loss in cardiac surgery: a meta-analysis of clinically relevant endpoints, *Lancet* 354:1940, 1999.

Levy JH, et al: A multicenter, placebo-controlled, double-blind trial of aprotinin for repeat coronary artery bypass grafting, *Circulation* 92:2236, 1995.

Miller BE, et al: Hematologic and economic impact on aprotinin in reoperative pediatric cardiac surgery, *Ann Thorac Surg* 66:535, 1998.

Mojcik C, Levy JH: Systemic inflammatory response syndrome and anti-inflammatory strategies, *Ann Thorac Surg* 71:745, 2001.

BleedingWeb.com

INOTROPIC SUPPORT

Susan Garwood
Roberta L. Hines

Inotropic agents are traditionally regarded as pharmacologic adjuncts that are clinically used to attain the goals of improved cardiac output and perfusion pressure. Typically, therefore, inotropes are based on adrenergic and/or dopaminergic receptor activity, increasing left ventricular contractility, and vasomotor tone. However, the ideal agent should be expected to achieve these goals with a minimal change in myocardial oxygen consumption; the enhanced cardiac output and perfusion pressures should not occur at the expense of an increase in heart rate that is commonly seen with adrenergic and dopaminergic agents. Most drugs that interact with adrenergic and dopaminergic receptors are nonspecific, particularly at higher doses, and do effect changes in heart rate and rhythm. Although these effects may be desirable in certain clinical scenarios, clinicians are moving away from uptitrating the dose of a single agent to the target blood pressure or cardiac output and are now more likely to use two or more agents that have more specific actions or add a drug that will balance the undesirable effects of the primary inotrope. In that way, for example, an increased heart rate may be avoided with a lower dose of epinephrine while increasing afterload with a pure vasopressor.

If the definition of an inotrope given here is reviewed, then a number of noncatecholamine agents should be considered, including some that do not affect myocardial contractility but rather alter loading conditions of the left and right ventricles to reduce myocardial oxygen consumption and stroke work, thereby enhancing cardiac output and peripheral perfusion.

■ CATECHOLAMINE INOTROPES

The inotropic and vascular effects of directly acting catecholamines are achieved by activation of receptors that have been classified as adrenergic (alpha-1 and -2, beta-1 and -2) and dopaminergic (DA-1 and -2). Indirectly acting catecholamines such as ephedrine stimulate neurotransmitter release from sympathetic nerve terminals but may act directly as the dose increases.

Epinephrine
Standard teaching dictates that epinephrine administered at lower doses stimulates beta-1 and -2 receptor activity, resulting in an increased contractility and velocity of conduction, peripheral vasodilation, and relaxation of the bronchioles, whereas higher doses increase heart rate and activate alpha receptors, increasing peripheral vascular resistance and initiating the undesirable side effects of tachyarrhythmias,

increased myocardial oxygen consumption, and ischemia. However, the specific effects of a given dose in a particular patient are not entirely predictable. A number of patient-related factors affect the response, the most variable of which is the downregulation of beta receptors. Patients with chronically elevated catecholamine levels experience a reduction in the number and density of beta receptors along with a reduction in the binding affinity for epinephrine. This decline in the sensitivity of the receptor leads to a subnormal response to a given dose of the inotrope.

Acute beta receptor downregulation has also been observed during and after cardiopulmonary bypass, thoracic and abdominal surgeries, and after reversible myocardial ischemia. There is an abrupt decline in receptor affinity along with a proliferation of lymphocyte beta-adrenergic receptors resulting in an attenuation of the cardiovascular response to the inotrope.

Further factors that affect the response to epinephrine are prior administration of β blockers, the availability of the calcium ions that are required for the contractile response, and intracellular factors, including hypoxia, acidosis, or adenosine triphosphate (ATP) depletion. Hypoperfusion states (such as cardiopulmonary bypass), sepsis, or hypovolemia leads to increased intracellular lactate levels, decreased ATP levels, and/or intracellular hypoxia. Such changes in the intracellular milieu allow the myocyte K^+_{ATP} channels to open with resulting hyperpolarization of the membrane, inhibition of the voltage-gated calcium channels, and apparent resistance to the catecholamine inotrope. It is therefore essential to maintain rigorous control over adequate oxygenation and respiratory and metabolic acidosis, when considering the use of epinephrine or other catecholamine inotropes. These may not be the agents of choice when trying to separate the patient from bypass after exceedingly long bypass runs or for circulatory support in septic patients or those with respiratory distress syndrome.

Other concerns with the use of epinephrine focus on tachycardia, vasoconstriction, and myocardial ischemia, secondary to the tachycardia, increased myocardial O_2 consumption, and possibly increased platelet aggregation. However, after cardiac surgery, for a similar hemodynamic improvement, epinephrine at 0.01 to 0.03 µg/kg/min elicits less tachycardia than dobutamine at 2.5 to 5.0 µg/kg/min. Factors to measure and manage appropriately during epinephrine administration are hypokalemia and hyperglycemia.

Dopamine
As with epinephrine, traditional teaching suggests that the effects of dopamine are dose dependent, escalating from predominantly dopaminergic effects through beta-adrenergic and finally achieving alpha-adrenergic effects. Thus, the lower doses of dopamine (<3 µg/kg/min) have been termed "renal dose" dopamine and are used extensively in the expectation of preserving or enhancing renal performance. However, the supposed dose-dependent effects of dopamine are not specific and vary enormously from patient to patient. There is clearly a receptor regulation effect, noticeable particularly in chronic illness, and it has been demonstrated in healthy volunteers that a specific micrograms per kilogram per minute dose results in quite marked differences in individual serum dopamine concentrations.

Furthermore, a number of commonly used drugs exhibit dopaminergic and antidopaminergic effects that compound the interindividual variability.

Although it has been demonstrated in human volunteers that low-dose dopamine increases renal artery blood and enhances glomerular filtration rate, producing marked natriuresis and diuresis, these effects are often not confirmed in clinical trials. It has now been conclusively demonstrated by meta-analyses of large numbers of clinical trials that dopamine does not confer any renal protective effects—that is to say that the preemptive use of dopamine does not prevent the onset of renal dysfunction in the perioperative period or intensive care setting. Several reasons have been offered for this lack of effect: (1) the onset of renal failure is not a terribly common event in cardiac surgery, and clinical studies would require several hundreds of patients to detect an improvement in renal outcome—clinical trials to date have therefore been grossly underpowered; and (2) although dopamine may increase overall renal blood flow, it also promotes the intrarenal redistribution of blood flow with a preferential flow away from the relatively hypoxic medulla to the cortex. This may be particularly inappropriate during cardiopulmonary bypass when renal blood flow, renal autoregulation, and regional renal blood flow are already severely compromised by hypothermia and loss of pulsatile flow. Also, (3) animal and in vitro experiments reveal that although DA-1 receptor stimulation causes renal vasodilation, unopposed DA-2 stimulation produces renal vasoconstriction. Animal experiments of renal failure rely on renal ischemia with intense renal vasoconstriction, so that administration of dopamine induces renal vasodilation, there being no further effect of the vasoconstrictor DA-2 activity. Clinical scenarios are unlikely to produce such intense renal vasoconstriction as the experimental models; therefore, the administration of dopamine may produce some or further vasoconstriction by stimulation of the DA-2 receptor.

With respect to the cardiovascular system, dopamine increases inotropy, chronotropy, dromotropy, and lusitropy. Dopamine is useful when a combination of inotropic support and vasoconstriction is required, as in sepsis. It is also particularly useful in cardiogenic shock, allowing for a brisk diuresis and a relief of acute pulmonary edema. For similar hemodynamic indices, mean systemic and filling pressures are significantly higher with dopamine compared with dobutamine. However, it has been demonstrated that, after cardiac surgery, dopamine causes more tachycardia than epinephrine at doses that produce comparable improvement in contractile function. Dopamine has a number of other undesirable features, including arrhythmias, interference with the function of the anterior pituitary axis, potentiation of lipolysis, and aggravation of ischemic injury. It is also extremely venoirritant and should only be administered via a central venous cannula. Extravasation may cause marked tissue damage.

Dobutamine

Dobutamine produces dose-dependent increases in cardiac output and reductions in diastolic filling pressures. Increased venous return, due to "reduced venous capacitance," contributes to the increased cardiac output. Based on chronic heart failure studies, dobutamine has been recommended as an agent to increase cardiac output without increasing heart rate. However, in the setting of chronic failure, there often is significant beta receptor downregulation so that the effect on heart rate is lost. Because heart rate is a major determinant of myocardial oxygen consumption, the favorable effects of dobutamine are negated if tachycardia is produced (this is the basis for dobutamine stress-echocardiography). For a given increase in cardiac output, dobutamine causes more tachycardia than epinephrine after cardiac surgery. In fact, a recent study of graded dobutamine infusion at up to 40 μg/kg/min immediately after cardiopulmonary bypass suggested that dobutamine improves left ventricular performance predominantly by increasing heart rate. However, in paced cardiac surgery patients, dobutamine increases myocardial oxygen uptake and coronary blood flow compared with dopamine, which increases oxygen use without increasing oxygen supply. Dobutamine also increases systemic vascular resistance after cardiopulmonary bypass, presumably by a predominance of alpha receptor stimulation during this period of low vascular tone and possible acute beta receptor downregulation. Dobutamine may therefore not be the inotrope of choice in this setting because of the possibility of a significant increase in myocardial oxygen consumption for relatively modest improvement in cardiac output.

Norepinephrine

Norepinephrine is experiencing renewed popularity for management of cardiovascular dysfunction. Alpha-adrenergic agonists benefit certain patients with circulatory failure refractory to inotropic and fluid therapy, allowing restoration of mean arterial pressure.

Isoproterenol

Isoproterenol has a potent chronotropic action; current applications therefore include treatment of bradycardia (especially after orthotopic heart transplantation) and atrioventricular heart block. It reduces refractoriness to conduction and increases automaticity. The tachycardia seen with isoproterenol is a result of both direct effects of the drug on the sinoatrial and atrioventricular nodes and reflex response to peripheral vasodilation. As such, it is routinely used following cardiac transplantation for increasing automaticity and inotropy.

Isoproterenol also has a place in the management of right ventricular dysfunction associated with pulmonary hypertension. Although isoproterenol is an excellent pulmonary vasodilator, decreased perfusion pressure secondary to a reduced diastolic period and a low vascular resistance may in fact lead to inadequate perfusion of the right coronary artery and confound right ventricular failure.

Dopexamine

Dopexamine is a new synthetic catecholamine that is not currently available in the United States but is used extensively in Europe and Australasia. It is structurally related to dopamine and dobutamine and has affinity for beta-2-adrenergic receptors (60 times that for dopamine) and dopaminergic (DA-1) receptors (about one third of the activity of dopamine), minimal DA-2 activity, and no alpha activity. It also inhibits neuronal catecholamine uptake, enhancing the positive inotropic action. As would be predicted from this receptor profile, the hemodynamic effects result in increased inotropy, chronotropy, and vasodilatory effects at the peripheral, pulmonary, renal, and splanchnic beds. Clinical studies demonstrate that dopexamine's effects are most pronounced when used as a continuous infusion of 1 to 4 μg/kg/min.

In healthy volunteers, incremental infusions of dopexamine 1.0 to 4.0 μg/kg/min resulted in proportional increases in plasma dopexamine concentrations. On termination of the infusions, plasma concentrations decreased monoexponentially with a half-life of 7 minutes. Clearance was rapid. The elimination half-life is prolonged to approximately 11 minutes in patients with a low cardiac output. The plasma clearance in postsurgical patients is also prolonged over that of healthy volunteers but not to such an extent that it would be expected to cause clinical problems in this patient population. Like most catecholamines, there is no transfer across the blood-brain barrier. Dopexamine is extensively metabolized to pharmacologically inactive products. Excretion of unchanged drug and metabolites is via urine and stool.

In volunteer studies, dopexamine given in incremental doses of up to 8 μg/kg/min increased cardiac output in a dose-dependent manner. Heart rate was increased particularly at the higher doses, to a greater extent than that seen with the same dose of dopamine, and is thought to be baroreceptor reflex mediated. In low cardiac output syndrome after cardiopulmonary bypass, dopexamine increases cardiac output, heart rate, and stroke volume, accompanied by a reduction in systemic and pulmonary vascular resistance. However, post–cardiopulmonary bypass tachycardia is a consistent observation in clinical trials of dopexamine, and the increase in cardiac output has frequently been attributed to this rather than an increased contractility. In head-to-head comparisons with dobutamine in post–cardiac surgery low output syndromes, there were no discernible differences between the two treatment groups, with the observed increases in cardiac output resulting from similar increases in both heart rate and contractility.

There is some controversy as to whether dopexamine has specific renal effects separate from its beta-2 effects. Clearly, dopexamine improves cardiac function. The question is whether the increase in renal performance can be attributed to factors other than the increase in cardiac output. The relative effects between dopamine, dobutamine, and dopexamine with respect to renal function are given in Table 1.

Although the literature has not been favorable for direct renal effect for dopexamine, there may be special circumstances in which dopexamine proves to be a renoprotective agent. A series of animal studies suggests that dopexamine may prevent ischemia-reperfusion–induced organ damage. The phenomenon of reperfusion injury has been attributed to several complex processes that include the production of oxygen free radicals. In a rat model of oxygen free radical toxicity, pretreatment with the natural scavengers significantly promoted the survival rate. Prior administration of dopexamine was as effective in providing protection against lethal toxicity but simultaneous administration of a selective beta-2-adrenergic receptor antagonist significantly prevented the beneficial effect of dopexamine. In contrast, simultaneous pretreatment with both a DA-1 antagonist and a beta-1 antagonist did not modify the beneficial effects of dopexamine. Infusions of dobutamine, prenalterol, or fenoldopam failed to prevent mortality. Dopexamine was also tested in a canine hemorrhagic shock model where an intense ischemic state is produced by hemorrhage and then perfusion restored by reinfusion of the shed blood. In the control dogs, despite recovery of the circulation, renal hemodynamics and renal function were severely impaired. In the animals pretreated with dopexamine, both renal hemodynamics and renal function were restored to baseline. The data suggest that tubular function was protected by DA-1 receptor activation, whereas improvements in renal blood flow appeared to be due to activation of both vascular DA-1 and beta-2 receptors. Renal failure after cardiopulmonary bypass has often been claimed to be a reperfusion injury. All of the studies on dopexamine and cardiac surgery used dopexamine after cardiopulmonary bypass, that is, after the ischemic insult. In animal studies, dopexamine was given before the ischemic injury. Perhaps if dopexamine were used in a more preemptive manner, beneficial renal effects, separate from the effects on cardiac output, may be seen.

Other features of DA-1 stimulation have brought dopexamine into recent focus. In septic shock models, dopexamine has increased splanchnic blood flow and results in an improved oxygen uptake and delivery, which has afforded some protection against endotoxemia. Furthermore, dopexamine appears to have an antiinflammatory role with a ramping down of complement and other inflammatory cascades during and after cardiopulmonary bypass.

Phosphodiesterase Inhibitors

Phosphodiesterase inhibitors increase cyclic adenosine monophosphate (cAMP) levels in myocytes, enhancing calcium entry with a resultant positive inotropic action. The increase in contractility is also accompanied by an improved

Table 1 Comparative Renal Effects of Dopamine, Dopexamine, and Dobutamine						
	DOSE (μg/kg/min)	**ERFP**	**GFR**	**C_{Li}**	**RVR**	**RENAL FRACTION**
Dopamine	3	23% Increase	No change	35% Increase	Reduced	No change
Dopexamine	1	10% Increase	7% Increase	30% Increase	No change	No change
Dobutamine	5	No change	No change	No change	Increased	Decreased

ERFP, effective renal plasma flow; GFR, glomerular filtration rate; C_{Li}, lithium clearance; RVR, renal vascular resistance.

myocardial diastolic relaxation (which does not occur with catecholamine inotropes), decreased left ventricular wall tension, increased left ventricular end-diastolic area, and augmented coronary and internal mammary artery perfusion. The increased arteriolar smooth muscle cAMP also produces pulmonary vasodilation, making these phosphodiesterase inhibitors agents of choice in low output syndrome associated with pulmonary hypertension and in right heart failure. Nevertheless, arteriolar vasodilation also affects the systemic vasculature so that low peripheral vascular resistance and a reduction in mean arterial and perfusion pressures may actually accompany the increased inotropy and cardiac output. Compared with catecholamine inotropes, phosphodiesterase inhibitors have a greater direct vasodilatory effect with subsequent lower filling pressures and mean arterial pressures when used in doses that give similar increases in cardiac output. In this case the perfect solution is to add a pure vasopressor such as low-dose vasopressin that is not active at the pulmonary bed. Clinically, the increased inotropy and cardiac output after the administration of a phosphodiesterase inhibitor is not accompanied by a tachycardia, other than a reflex tachycardia that may accompany the lowered mean arterial pressure secondary to the low systemic vascular resistance. The efficacy of phosphodiesterase inhibitors has been demonstrated in large clinical trials of cardiopulmonary bypass and intensive care therapy. Significant increases in stroke volume and cardiac index are consistently noted with improved oxygen delivery and clinically relevant reductions in filling pressures.

Phosphodiesterase inhibitors are not classified as catecholamines as they are nonadrenergic and do not require beta receptor stimulation for activity. A synergistic inotropic effect is therefore obtained if used together with a catecholamine inotrope. Furthermore, phosphodiesterase inhibitors are not affected by concomitant or prior use of β blockers and lose none of their potency in beta receptor downregulation. Similarly, there is no loss of inotropic support if a cardioselective β blocker is added for rate control in a patient. During the rewarming phase of cardiopulmonary bypass, a loading dose of 50 μg/kg of milrinone followed by a continuous infusion of 0.50 μg/kg/min results in a significant increase in cardiac output and oxygen delivery. Using this protocol, the elimination half-life is approximately 50 minutes.

Because of the potent effect of pulmonary vasodilation, milrinone is used in acute and chronic congestive heart failure and is routinely used as a long-term at-home therapy to optimize patients on the cardiac transplant list, particularly in those refractory to other inotropes who may otherwise require intraaortic balloon counterpulsation.

However, the use of milrinone in acute exacerbations of chronic congestive heart failure has recently come into question. In a recent study of almost 1000 patients, milrinone versus placebo was added to standard treatment and infused for 48 hours in patients with exacerbation of chronic left-sided failure. Milrinone was associated with a higher rate of early treatment failure, more hypotension, and new atrial arrhythmias, plus a nonsignificant higher number of deaths in hospital. The editorial accompanying the article suggested that the use of milrinone for circulatory support in other conditions should therefore now be questioned.

B-Type Natriuretic Peptide

Human B-type natriuretic peptide (hBNP, originally called brain natriuretic peptide) is a 32-sequence amino acid, endogenously produced in the ventricular myocardium in response to elevated end-diastolic pressure and volume. Unlike other neurohormonal pathways that are affected by the failing left ventricle, natriuretic peptides appear to improve loading conditions by their diuretic, natriuretic, and vasodilator properties. hBNP also inhibits the renin-angiotensin axis and the endothelin pathway.

As the drug nesiritide, it is manufactured from *Escherichia coli* using recombinant DNA. hBNP binds to the guanylate cyclase receptor of vascular smooth muscle and endothelial cells, leading to an increase in intracellular guanosine cyclic monophosphate (GMP) and therefore smooth muscle relaxation. In preclinical trials, nesiritide relaxed arterial and venous tissue that had been previously been exposed to vasoconstrictors and did not affect cardiac indices of myocardial contractility or electrophysiology. In large prospective, randomized, controlled human studies, nesiritide produced dose-dependent reductions in pulmonary capillary occlusion pressure and systemic arterial pressure in patients with acute or chronic congestive heart failure, with a more pronounced effect on hemodynamic parameters and some modest improvement of symptoms than either placebo or the standard of care, nitroglycerin. Nevertheless, despite the improved cardiovascular parameters and self-reporting of symptoms, none of the trials of nesiritide to date have demonstrated improvement in short- or long-term outcome in either acute or chronic failure.

With respect to the perioperative period, the use of nesiritide has been primarily limited to patients in severe congestive heart failure on long-term infusions as a bridge to transplantation. Although symptoms of failure are clearly improved during this period, it must be remembered that with long-tem infusion, nesiritide has a prolonged half-life and hypotension can be persistent long after the drug has been discontinued, with implications for the bypass and postbypass periods.

Arginine Vasopressin (Vasopressin)

Arginine vasopressin is an endogenous peptide synthesized exclusively in the hypothalamus and released from the posterior pituitary. Vasopressin release is stimulated by changes in vascular volume and vascular time and is bound to two distinct types of receptors: vasomotor (V_1) and renal (V_2).

In normotensive volunteers, endogenous vasopressin levels are found to be in the range of 5 to 15 pg/ml. The administration of exogenous vasopressin produces very little effect with respect to blood pressure response under these normal basal conditions. However, if hypotension is induced, the physiologic response in these healthy individuals is to increase endogenous levels of vasopressin to greater than 60 pg/ml with a resulting normalization of blood pressure. In contrast, in shocklike states (sepsis, post–cardiopulmonary low output state, hemorrhage), endogenous vasopressin levels are found to be inappropriately low (<20 pg/ml); the normal physiologic response of an increased vasopressin secretion from the posterior pituitary is severely blunted. However, under these circumstances, a bolus or infusion of vasopressin rapidly achieves a significant increase in systemic vascular resistance and mean arterial blood pressure.

Vasopressin has been shown to be effective in patients refractory to other inotropes and vasopressor. The reason vasopressin can remain active in these situations while other catecholamines and vasopressor do not is explained by the observation that vasopressin blocks the hyperpolarization of the cell membrane in response to K^+_{ATP} channel activation (secondary to hypoxia, acidosis or ATP depletion), allowing the voltage-gated calcium channels to open.

In addition to the blocking of the K^+_{ATP} channels, vasopressin increases vascular tone via three other mechanisms. Binding of the V_1 receptor results in (1) an inositol triphosphate–mediated release of calcium from intracellular stores, (2) a decreased accumulation of the second messenger cGMP in vascular smooth muscle that inhibits nitric oxide–mediated vasodilation, and (3) blunts the rise in cAMP attenuating the vasodilation.

A review of a large number of post–cardiopulmonary bypass shock patients who required left ventricular device insertion revealed that unlike other vasopressors, the administration of vasopressin is not accompanied by an elevation in pulmonary artery pressures or problems with right heart failure. Furthermore, there may be some advantage to using vasopressin in patients who have existing or are at risk for renal dysfunction. Vasopressin V_1 receptors are present only on the efferent arteriole; therefore, filtration fraction is increased, possibly promoting a maintenance of glomerular filtration. In contrast, catecholamine receptors are present at both the afferent and efferent arterioles; renal blood flow and filtration fraction may be compromised. Theoretically, vasopressin might be expected to cause vasospasm of the coronary arteries or grafted arterial conduits. However, no ischemic changes were noted in the large series of post–cardiopulmonary bypass shock patients mentioned earlier.

In practical terms, a bolus of 1 to 2 U of vasopressin produces a brisk and significant increase in systemic vascular resistance and mean arterial blood pressure. An infusion rate of 2 to 5 U/hr appears to be the optimal range, with a plateau effect at greater than 8 U/hr. At these higher doses, peripheral vasoconstriction becomes intense with poor perfusion and digital/limb ischemia. Clinically, it is preferable to use a lower dose of vasopressin together with a modest dose of an inotrope and to use the vasopressin to wean the patient off of the higher doses of inotropes or catecholamine vasopressors. Vasopressin is now included in the advanced cardiac life support protocol; in this scenario a bolus of 40 U of vasopressin is administered.

Fenoldopam

Fenoldopam is a selective DA-1 agonist and therefore a potent vasodilator at both the renal and systemic vascular beds. Fenoldopam has a rapid onset and offset of a few minutes, both of which are independent of dose; its clearance is not affected by end-stage liver or kidney disease. Fenoldopam has no inotropic activity and does not cross the blood-brain barrier. Unlike other vasodilators, it causes a dose-related increase in cardiac output without tachycardia, reduced preload, or hypotension in patients with heart failure. It increases renal plasma flow and stimulates diuresis and natriuresis via a direct tubular effect in patients with congestive heart failure and renal impairment. DA-1 receptor activity also increases myocardial blood flow. Fenoldopam is presently available and effective for the management of perioperative hypertension in the dosage range of 0.01 to 0.8 µg/kg/min. Fenoldopam has a significantly shorter median time to hemodynamic response compared with nifedipine (10 minutes as opposed to 40 minutes) and is free of the toxicity and rebound effects that are associated with sodium nitroprusside.

Most of the earlier studies on fenoldopam concentrated on the secondary renal effects of the drug while acting as a hypotensive agent; thus, it has been shown that there is a dose-related increase in renal blood flow that plateaus at an infusion rate of 0.5 µg/kg/min. This increase in renal blood flow is accompanied by a dose-related increase in urine flow, fractional excretion of sodium, filtration fraction, and a concomitant decrease in renal vascular resistance. The natriuretic effect may be blunted by activation of the renin-angiotensin-aldosterone system. Nevertheless, fenoldopam augments renal blood flow in mildly to moderately hypertensive patients, during the period of blood pressure reduction.

Because it is speculated that perioperative renal insults are usually secondary to a period of relative ischemia, renal blood flow augmentation during blood pressure reduction would prove to be a very attractive property of an adjunct drug. At times when hypotensive therapy is required to facilitate surgery and reduce blood loss, for example, during spinal surgery, neurosurgery, or joint replacement, renal blood flow would at least be preserved, if not increased. In a head-to-head comparison with sodium nitroprusside, fenoldopam, but not sodium nitroprusside, improved renal function at all levels of baseline renal function while lowering blood pressure. There is no question that fenoldopam is a potent renal vasodilator. It has been used in the clinical context of intense renal vasoconstriction during cyclosporine administration in organ transplantation surgery with the results that the nephrotoxicity of cyclosporine is clearly ameliorated.

■ COMBINED THERAPY

The combination of catecholamines is controversial. Rather than being synergistic, there appears to be a "pseudoantagonism" with clinical interactions between drugs with affinity for the same receptor being complex and unpredictable. In contrast, phosphodiesterase inhibitors are synergistic when added to a catecholamine mediating increased cellular cAMP concentrations through mechanisms independent of the beta receptor. After cardiopulmonary bypass, a combination of epinephrine and phosphodiesterase inhibitors is additive, augmenting ventricular performance. Even small doses of phosphodiesterase inhibitors added to catecholamines can markedly increase cardiac index without having a significant effect on arterial pressure in medical or surgical cardiac patients, and clinicians often give a "half-loading dose" of milrinone before separation from bypass with an epinephrine infusion.

The combined use of norepinephrine, amrinone, and nitroglycerin in the management of severe low cardiac output has been reported. The advantages of using an inotrope and a vasodilator in combination include lower filling pressures, less metabolic demand, and fewer side effects. The choice of which combination to use must be based on the underlying disease, preoperative drug therapy, and response to the individual inotropes and vasodilators.

SUGGESTED READING

Garwood S: Perioperative renal issues: dopexamine and fenoldopam—new agents to augment renal performance, *Semin Anesthesiol* 14:308, 1998.

Morales DLS, et al: Therapy for vasodilator shock: arginine vasopressin, *Semin Anesth Perioper Med Pain* 19:98, 2000.

Poole-Wilson PA: Treatment of acute heart failure: out with the old, in with the new (editorial), *JAMA* 287:1578, 2002.

CARDIAC PACING IN ADULTS

Jeffrey Brinker

The evolution of the cardiac pacemaker has been an amazing medical success story and serves as a paradigm for many implantable medical devices. The efforts of physicians, surgeons, engineers, and entrepreneurs have combined to produce highly reliable and multifunctional systems that address an ever-increasing spectrum of cardiac disabilities. Recent estimates of pacemaker implants in the United States (about 153,000 primary and 38,000 replacements per year) represent an increase of 22% from 1990 to 2000 in the number of patients having such a device. In its simplest form, the pacing system consists of a generator (housing the electronics and power supply) and lead(s) that connect the latter to the heart. At one time the implantation procedure was the greatest hurdle in cardiac pacemaking and required a surgeon's expertise; however, with miniaturization of devices and techniques facilitating central venous access, appropriate choice, programming, and monitoring of the increasingly sophisticated devices have become greater concerns in most situations. Although the practice of permanent pacing now includes surgeons, cardiologists, and teams of both, it has gradually shifted from the operating room to the catheterization/electrophysiology laboratory where the specialist in rhythm disorders has assumed an increasingly dominant role. Still, there are many circumstances in which a surgeon is needed and it is important that he or she has a working knowledge of how these devices work, implantation techniques, and the management of complications.

■ HISTORICAL ASPECTS*

The history of artificial cardiac pacing systems can be traced to attempts by two ingenious individuals to develop a

*A number of historical reviews of pacing have been published. The original references used in this section were taken from Siddons H, Sowton E: *Cardiac pacemakers*, Springfield, IL, 1967, Charles C Thomas, p 4–7.

device capable of resuscitating an asystolic heart. Both were aware of the occasional success of intracardiac injections of various pharmacologic "cocktails" and recognized that stimulation of the heart just by the penetration of a needle could result in a ventricular contraction. They were also aware of physiologic experiments demonstrating the ability of electrical stimuli to cause muscle contraction. Mark Lidwill, an Australian anesthesiologist, presented a paper in 1929 describing a portable device that used a unipolar transthoracic needle to deliver stimuli at rates between 80 and 120 per minute. This proved successful in at least one stillborn infant. Hyman, aware of Lidwill's work, developed a self-contained device in which electricity could be generated by a hand crank. This was delivered to the heart by a transthoracic bipolar needle. In a series of carefully devised animal experiments, he demonstrated the use of the device to support cardiac rhythm over a wide set of circumstances in 1932. Unfortunately, neither the lay public nor organized medicine was ready for electrical attempts to resuscitate the dead and pacemaker therapy lay dormant until midcentury. Bigelow and Callaghan explored the use of electrical stimulation to support the cardiac rhythm during hypothermic heart surgery in 1951. In 1952, Zoll demonstrated the ability to treat Stokes-Adams attacks with transcutaneous electrical stimulation (a methodology still in use for emergent situations).

As cardiac surgery evolved, the need for a reliable pacing system led to the development of a small transistorized device that could be worn by the patient and stimulate the heart via wires placed on the heart by the surgeon. In 1958 the first fully implantable "permanent" pacemaker was implanted by Senning in a patient with refractory Stokes-Adams attacks. This device was powered by rechargeable cells and was connected to the heart by epicardial wires. Furman demonstrated the ability to stimulate the heart via an endocardial catheter in 1958, and within 5 years permanent transvenous pacing systems were being used routinely. The concept of P synchronous pacing was introduced in 1963 by Nathan, and, with the improvement of atrial pacing leads, physiologic pacing was fully realized by the early 1980s with the "fully automatic" (DDD) pacemaker. Sensor-driven pacemakers capable of increasing the heart rate in relation to a perceived increase in metabolic demand (e.g., motion, minute ventilation, etc.) became available in single-chamber devices shortly thereafter.

By 1990 dual-chamber sensor-driven pacemakers became available, and they now account for about 63% of all implants.

Essential to the evolution of the modern pacemaker has been the development of noninvasive means to communicate with and alter the function of the device. Thus, the modern-day generator can be programmed to well over a million different combinations of parameters. It can track and store information about its functioning and the patient's intrinsic cardiac activity, and it can convey this information to the physician in a matter of seconds by placing a programming "head" on the skin above the device.

Preimplant Assessment

The first step in the implant process should be careful consideration of the need for a permanent device. Perceived abuses in the past have focused attention on clearly establishing the indication for pacing. It is good practice to characterize the specific indication for a given patient in accordance with published guidelines. Documentation of symptoms and demonstrative electrocardiographic strips are important. Some indications remain controversial such as dual-site atrial pacing for the limitation of atrial fibrillation, whereas others are new and not fully defined (pacing for obstructive and congestive cardiomyopathies). In these situations, it may be advisable to have a consultant's endorsement of the proposed therapy.

The type of pacing system to be implanted is related to the indication for pacing as well as patient-specific factors such as age, size, overall physical condition, life expectancy, and underlying cardiac and central venous pathology. A good history, physical evaluation, and review of pertinent laboratory and radiographic data are essential. Table 1 lists some of these concerns. Based on these factors, the implanting physician must make decisions between the alternatives outlined in Table 2. This process provides the data set necessary for the physician to plan the procedure, secure appropriate logistical support (hardware, personnel, etc.), and obtain informed consent from the patient and his or her family.

The informed consent should realistically present the potential risks and benefits as well as alternatives to the planned procedure. Because the decision to implant a pacemaker usually (but not always) confers a lifelong commitment to this form of therapy, the importance of continued follow-up and the eventual need for generator replacement should be specified. Short- and long- term risks should be relevant to the specific individual as opposed to representing the idealized "typical" patient.

Pacing Mode

The multiprogrammability of modern pacemakers provides great flexibility in patient management. Specific devices vary in size, battery capacity, and, most important, functionality. Pacing mode is characterized by a five-position code (Table 3), of which only the first three positions are commonly used because multiprogrammability and telemetry are now universal and antitachycardia capability is rare in devices without defibrillation capability. Rate adaptation (also termed "rate responsive") is distinguished by using the letter "R" in the fourth position of the code. A pacemaker is defined by its maximal capability; thus, a DDDR generator is capable of dual-chamber rate adaptive pacing. It may, however, be programmed to function in a "lesser" mode (e.g., VVI, AAI, DVI, DDIR, etc.) as the clinical situation demands.

Table 1 Factors Influencing Implant Procedure
GENERAL CONDITION
Age, life expectancy, size
Pacing indication
Ancillary rhythm disturbance (e.g., atrial fibrillation)
VENOUS SYSTEM
Documented or suspected thrombosis or stenosis
Presence of preexisting lines (e.g., temporary pacer, Hickman catheter, etc.)
Presence of a dialysis shunt
Congenital anomaly
CARDIAC PATHOLOGY
Tricuspid valve disease (regurgitation, stenosis, valve replacement)
Congenital cardiac disease (e.g., single ventricle, corrected transposition)
Right ventricular enlargement
OTHER FACTORS
Prior mastectomy
Infection/dermatitis
Prior radiation therapy
Paresis
Cosmetic concerns
Hobbies (sports, hunting, etc.)

Table 2 Implantation Alternatives
GENERATOR
Capabilities (single/dual/triple site, sensor(s), programmability, diagnostics, etc)
Size
Battery longevity
Cost
Manufacturer
LEAD(S)
Uni/bipolar
Active/passive fixation
Steroid eluting
Diameter/length
Polarization and impedance properties
Special characteristics or shapes
ACCESS
Cephalic, subclavian, axillary, internal/external jugular, femoral
Via direct venotomy or Seldinger's technique
Epicardial or endocardial via atrial access
GENERATOR PLACEMENT
Pectoral (right/left, subcutaneous/submuscular, retromammary)
Abdominal
SPECIAL CONSIDERATION FOR PACING SITE
Coronary venous system for left ventricular pacing
RV apex, outflow, septum
Right atrial appendage, septum, lateral wall, low right atrial

Physiologic Pacing

The traditional use of a pacemaker has been to ensure an adequate "lowest" heart rate in a patient who exhibits symptomatic bradycardia. This can be accomplished by the implantation of a VVI device, which is relatively inexpensive and simplest to implant, program, and monitor. This mode of pacing, however, has been likened to slow ventricular

Table 3 Pacing Modes

FIRST POSITION: CHAMBER PACED
(A)trium
(V)entricle
(D)ual
(S)ingle—implies device is limited to single chamber
    function: A or V
(O) no pacing
SECOND POSITION: CHAMBER SENSED
(A)trium
(V)entricle
(D)ual
(S)ingle—implies device is limited to single chamber
    function: A or V
(O) no sensing
THIRD POSITION: RESPONSE TO SENSED EVENT
(I)nhibit pacer output
(T)rigger pacer output
(D)ual—both inhibit and trigger pacer outputs
(O) No response
FOURTH POSITION: RATE MODULATION
(R)ate adaptive
FIFTH POSITION: MULTISITE PACING
(A)trial multisite pacing
(V)entricular multisite
(D)ual chamber multisite

Examples: DDD dual chamber pacing and sensing with atrial tracking.

VVIR ventricular pacing and sensing with rate adaption.

DDDOV dual chamber pacing without rate adaption but with multisite ventricular pacing (e.g., biventricular).

From Berstein AD, et al: The revised NASPE/BPEG generic code for antibradycardia, adaptive-rate, and multisite pacing, *PACE* 25:260, 2000.

tachycardia and imparts a hemodynamic burden by sacrificing the benefits of a coordinated atrioventricular (AV) contraction sequence as well as the ability to adjust heart rate in response to metabolic demands. In some patients, retrograde electrical activation of the atria by ventricular pacing causes simultaneous contraction of atria and ventricles. This may result in a clinical condition termed "pacemaker syndrome" in which there is symptomatic hypotension and elevation of venous pressures during pacing. Although there are still situations in which a VVI pacemaker may be used (e.g., rare episodes of bradycardia in which only a "safety net" backup device is needed), modern pacing should attempt to mimic normal cardiac physiology as closely as possible. Ideally, this involves initiation of cardiac electrical activity by a normal sinus node, the rate of which is appropriately influenced by neural and humeral factors that relate to the body's instantaneous demand for cardiac output, and maintenance of an appropriate AV contraction sequence. In traditional use, the term "physiologic pacing" was applied to any dual chamber pacing systems, but it is now realized that "physiologic" is a relative term. Depending on the nature of the underlying disease, "physiologic" pacing might be accomplished by the use of an AAIR, a VDD, a DDD, a DDDR, or, in the case of chronic atrial fibrillation, a VVIR pacing system. As noted, a DDDR device can be programmed down to almost any other mode, but a simple single chamber (SSI) generator can sense and pace in only one chamber. Thus, a patient with sick sinus syndrome and intact AV conduction will do very well with an SSIR pacer functioning in the AAIR mode but should he or she develop AV block, this device would be useless. Careful evaluation of the patient's AV conduction and chronotropic competence is an essential part element of the preimplant evaluation.

Stimulation from the right ventricular apex results in an abnormal activation of the ventricles as evidenced by the appearance of a left bundle-branch block (LBBB) pattern in the electrocardiogram (ECG). This results in some degradation of ventricular function compared with the normal ventricular activation pattern. This, however, is usually of only minor consequence. Attempts to pace from the septal area or right ventricular outflow tract have been associated with claims of improved hemodynamics coupled with a more narrowed paced QRS pattern. In patients with congestive dilated cardiomyopathy and wide-complex LBBB, biventricular or left ventricular pacing has been used to provide a more coordinated interventricular activation and contraction. Early results suggest that this form of therapy, even in patients with no underlying bradyarrhythmia, can improve overall heart function. Thus, a truly "physiologic" pacing system would now optimize interventricular as well as AV contraction sequence.

There are some situations in which a pacemaker is used to produce a nonphysiologic activation pattern to address a preexisting pathophysiologic state. The most striking example of this is the deliberate preactivation of the right ventricle in patients with hypertrophic obstructive cardiomyopathy. This has resulted in a reduction of left ventricular outflow gradient in the majority of patients, presumably by causing a perturbation in left ventricular contraction pattern. To be effective the ventricle must be continuously paced and the optimal pacing site is said to be the right ventricular apex. The ultimate role of this form of therapy in patients with medically refractory hypertrophic obstructive cardiomyopathy remains to be determined.

Pacing Leads

Although modern pacemakers are technically complex and have a limited life span determined by their power source, these devices are extremely reliable. They have advanced diagnostics that allow for replacement before end of battery life and are relatively easy to remove and replace. The pacing lead, on the other hand, is subject to unpredictable failure that may arise because of a defect in material or construction and/or the interaction of the lead and body (e.g., compressive forces on the lead body, tissue reaction at the electrode/myocardial interface, or microdislodgment/macrodislodgment). The vast majority of pacing systems use endocardial leads because of their less invasive placement, maintenance of acceptable electrical characteristics, and superior long-term integrity compared with epicardial leads. Removal of a chronically implanted endocardial lead, however, is difficult and carries with it the risk of serious adverse events, including death. Epicardial leads are now usually restricted to situations in which venous access to the heart is precluded, there is a risk of embolization of clot from the lead to the systemic circulation (e.g., single ventricle), there is a prosthetic tricuspid valve, or in very small pediatric patients. In some of these cases, the surgeon may choose to implant endocardial leads transatrially by limited thoracotomy. Most endocardial lead systems used currently are bipolar in configuration and have either a passive (fins or tines) or active (fixed or extendable helix) means of securing close contact of the electrodes with the endocardium. The choice of fixation is usually one of physician preference because both have advantages and disadvantages (Table 4). There are some specialty leads that are required by particular pacing systems (e.g., single-lead VDD systems), but in general, the advent of an industry wide standard (IS-1) connecting configuration has allowed the mixing of leads and generators from all manufacturers. Some patients, however, may have lead systems that precede IS-1, requiring the use of special adapters to match current pacemaker generators. Thus, the importance of confirming the specific hardware in a patient who presents for generator replacement.

There has been considerable controversy surrounding the type of insulation used in lead construction. In general, this relates to the propensity of some polyurethane insulation (primarily P80A) to degrade, resulting in inner and outer insulation defects and lead failure. Although no insulation is perfect, polyurethane is uniquely subject to environmental stress cracking (ESC) and metal ion oxidation (MIO). Silicone rubber insulation and polyurethane 55D are considered to have reasonable reliability.

Implantation Logistics

Permanent pacemakers may be implanted in an operating room or a catheterization laboratory with similar success and complication rates. Procedures performed in the catheterization laboratory have been shown to be less costly. Personnel, in addition to the operator, include a nurse or anesthesiologist to administer conscious sedation and a technologist to assist with fluoroscopic imaging. Often a representative of a pacemaker company is present to provide specific information about the device to be used as well as to assist with operation of the pacing system analyzer and device programming. An adequate imaging system is necessary; it must be able to be rotated so that anteroposterior and oblique projections are possible and the resolution must be good enough to distinguish objects such as guidewires and the extension of an active fixation helix. A magnification mode is desirable, as is the ability to record and archive images. Digitally equipped devices

may provide additional features such as "road mapping," which may facilitate venous access and catheter manipulation. Pulsed fluoroscopy can significantly reduce radiation to patient and staff. The procedure table should be flat and fully radiolucent. Ideally, it should be capable of assuming the Trendelenburg and reverse Trendelenburg positions.

Monitoring of the ECG, blood pressure, and pulse oximetry is mandatory. The ECG should be continually observed, and a multilead display or capability is desirable. Special electrode pads that can monitor the cardiogram, deliver direct current defibrillatory shock, and provide for emergency transcutaneous pacing, if necessary, offer advantages. Automated noninvasive blood pressure monitoring is adequate in most cases. Pulse oximetry may provide the first evidence of over sedation or large air embolism.

Surgical instruments required for pacemaker implantation may vary with the specifics of the case, but a basic tray with preidentified "add-ons" is usually adequate. Suction, electrocautery, and cables for connection of leads to a pacing system analyzer (PSA) are essential. The PSA acts as an external pacemaker generator and can provide information such as lead impedance, capture threshold, and sensing characteristics as well as act as a temporary pacemaker.

Special guidewires, sheaths, stylets, etc. should be available as separate add-ons. Intravascular contrast may be necessary as well. Appropriate drugs, intravenous infusion devices, and resuscitation equipment must be readily available. A pericardiocentesis set should be in the room. Relatively rapid access to an echocardiographic device is necessary.

■ PREOPERATIVE PREPARATIONS

Routine preoperative testing includes a 12-lead ECG, complete blood and platelet counts, prothrombin and partial thromboplastin times, routine electrolytes, blood urea nitrogen, and creatinine. Posteroanterior and lateral chest films may be helpful but are not usually considered necessary. Patients receiving anticoagulation therapy present a difficult problem. The options for those receiving an oral agent include cessation of therapy 4 to 5 days before implantation; conversion to intravenous heparin either in hospital or through a home care agency (discontinued 6 to 8 hours before the procedure); and conversion to a fractionated (low-molecular-weight) heparin (e.g., enoxaparin), which is discontinued 12 hours before the procedure. The choice is

Table 4 Endocardial Lead Fixation	
ACTIVE	**PASSIVE**
Can be placed at almost any site	Placement in trabeculated area
Easier removal of chronic implant	More difficult to remove
Good for difficult anatomy (amputated atrial appendage, tricuspid regurgitation, RVH)	Higher incidence of dislodgment in these situations
Higher capture threshold*	Lower thresholds
Increased incidence of "microperforation"	Perforation rare
Helical mechanism may malfunction if repetitive attempts are made to find optimal fixation site	Repositioning easier

*Use of steroid eluting leads lowers chronic thresholds for both active and passive leads such that the difference between the two is small.

dependent on the indication for anticoagulation and patient preference. Restarting heparin before 24 hours postimplantation carries with it a significant risk of pocket hematoma. This problem may be approached by restarting Coumadin at the maintenance dose on the day of the procedure and low-molecular-weight heparin about 12 to 18 hours after implantation. The latter is continued on an outpatient basis until the INR is therapeutic.

The patient is kept on nothing-by-mouth status usually overnight; however, this is shortened to at least 6 to 8 hours before implantation by some operators. An intravenous line is placed in the upper extremity ipsilateral to the proposed site of implantation. This is used for hydration, drug administration, and, if necessary, the injection of contrast to outline the venous anatomy.

Although antibiotic prophylaxis is controversial, there is the suggestion that such therapy reduces the incidence of infection, and we routinely give a systemic antibiotic with "staph-cidal" activity immediately before the procedure and for 24 hours thereafter. If there is a concern about a higher risk of infection (e.g., prolonged procedure, questionable breach of sterility, preexisting dermatitis), especially in a diabetic patient, this course is extended. Oral sedation with diazepam and diphenhydramine given before the procedure is augmented as necessary during the procedure with midazolam and fentanyl, which achieves a level of conscious sedation adequate for the procedure.

■ IMPLANTATION PROCEDURE

The vast majority of permanent pacemaker implants use endocardial leads that may be placed into subclavian, axillary, cephalic, internal or external jugular, or iliofemoral veins. The pacemaker generator is placed in proximity to the venous access site in a subcutaneous or submuscular pocket. The decision with regard to implant site is made after consideration of the parameters listed in Table 1. The "routine" implant uses the subclavian technique, and discussion of the implantation will be restricted to this approach.

The patient is scrubbed from the anterior angle of the jaw to the nipple line bilaterally. This area is then prepped and draped. The inferior border of the clavicle and the deltopectoral groove provide important landmarks. Operators vary in technique, but we commonly make a 5-cm incision parallel to and about 2 cm below the inferior margin of the clavicle. For percutaneous venous access this incision begins at the deltopectoral groove; however, if a cephalic venotomy is anticipated, this is extended about 1 cm laterally. The incision is carried to the prepectoral fascia. The pocket for the generator can be made subcutaneously or under the muscle. In most cases the former is satisfactory, but care should be taken to ensure that it is subcutaneous and not subcuticular.

Venous Access
The standard technique for percutaneous subclavian venous access using the Seldinger technique uses an 18-gauge needle attached to a 10-ml syringe containing a few milliliters of anesthetic. The needle is placed, bevel down, through the incision and towards the clavicle at the junction of its medial

and middle thirds. Upon touching the clavicle, the needle is directed underneath it and toward the sternal notch. Once under the clavicle, the needle should not be redirected because of the danger of lacerating underlying structures. Small injections of anesthetic may be used if patient discomfort is experienced. Negative pressure is applied as the needle is advanced under the clavicle so that entrance into the vein is immediately recognized. If the vein is not entered, the entire needle is withdrawn, flushed, and reinserted with slightly different angulation. If venous entry is not obtained after three attempts, consideration should be given to the performance of a venogram to confirm venous patency and road-map its course for the next attempt. This is accomplished by injection of 20 to 40 ml of a low osmolal contrast agent followed by a saline or dextrose and water push to hasten the bolus of contrast into the central circulation. Using fluoroscopic guidance, the exploring needle can be advanced directly into the contrast-filled vein. Entrance into the vein is accompanied by aspiration of dark nonpulsatile blood into the syringe. The syringe is removed while the needle is held carefully in place with a finger over the hub to avoid air embolism. A J-shaped guidewire is advanced through the needle and into the right atrium, and then into the inferior vena cava, which confirms venous entry. A guidewire coursing over the right heart border could still be within a dilated tortuous ascending aorta, and failure to recognize this can result in significant complication.

Once venous entry is confirmed, a large peel-away sheath/dilator set can be advanced over the wire into the superior vena cava. The sheath size should be the smallest capable of accommodating both the desired lead and the guidewire. The dilator is removed and the guidewire retained within the sheath. A pacemaker lead is advanced through the sheath and into the right atrium, at which time the sheath is removed and the retained guidewire used for the insertion of a second sheath for the advancement of the second pacing lead. The second sheath is then removed, but the guidewire is left so that it could be used again should there be a problem with one of the leads. During these maneuvers, one should take care to prevent air from being sucked through the sheath into the right heart and then into the lungs. The use of sheaths with hemostatic valves has been helpful in this regard.

Although this traditional method of gaining subclavian venous access is popular and highly successful, recent evidence suggests that leads placed by this method may be entrapped by the subclavius muscle and the costoclavicular ligament. Forces exerted by these structures on the lead may contribute to insulation degradation and lead failure. Because of this, attention has been directed at a more lateral approach into the axillary vein. The cephalic vein can be found by surgical exploration of the groove between the deltoid and pectoralis muscles. Prior to the availability of peel-away sheaths, cephalic venotomy was the most common approach for introducing pacemaker leads. An appeal of the direct venotomy is the elimination of the risk of a blind needle stick (see later). It is possible to place two leads into even a very small vein by using a guidewire followed by sheaths in the same fashion as described earlier for the percutaneous technique. Often the cephalic vein is sacrificed by this technique.

The success of the cephalic approach varies with the skill and experience of the operator but may be as low as 75%.

This is because the vessel may be too small, exists as a plexus of tiny vessels rather than a larger single vessel, lies very deeply, or takes a circuitous route. Techniques for the percutaneous access of the lateral subclavian or axillary vein have been described using radiographic landmarks or contrast venography. These methodologies combine the ease of the traditional subclavian approach with the avoidance of the compressive structures achieved by the cephalic cutdown.

Alternative venous access sites include the jugular and femoral veins. Permanent implant via the femoral route may be elected in the situation of superior vena caval occlusion; however, experience with this methodology is small and epicardial pacing may be a better choice in most cases.

Persistent Left Superior Vena Cava
Lead insertion may be complicated by the persistence of a left superior vena cava draining into the coronary sinus. This situation is usually unrecognized before implantation and can occur in almost 0.5% of patients undergoing this procedure. In many cases the procedure can be carried out by appropriately shaping stylets to direct the leads to their sites in the atrial appendage and ventricular apex. Active fixation leads have been recommended. In some cases, it may be difficult or impossible to obtain good lead positioning from the left side, and this must be abandoned. Venography should be performed showing a patent right superior vena cava entering the atrium before attempting a right-sided implant because rarely the right vena cava is absent. Epicardial or femoral access remains an option in such cases.

Ventricular Lead Placement
Once both leads have been introduced into the right atrium or inferior vena cava, the ventricular lead is usually placed first. This is most often done by shaping a stylet into a "dog's leg" curve and directly advancing the lead through the tricuspid valve into the ventricular apex. Alternatively, the stylet may be withdrawn and the lead looped in the atrium, rotated anteriorly, and slightly withdrawn to flop across the tricuspid valve into the ventricle. A straight stylet is then introduced and the lead guided to the apex. Entry into the ventricle usually is signaled by ventricular ectopy. If such is not the case, one should be suspicious of entry into the coronary venous system through the coronary sinus. In some cases, advancing a lead into the pulmonary artery using a large-curved stylet, withdrawing the stylet, and slowly retracting the lead will ensure entry into the ventricle. A stable position in the right ventricular apex is signaled by absence of ectopy and little movement of the lead tip with cardiac motion when the stylet is withdrawn. The electrical characteristics are then tested.

If an active fixation lead is used, preliminary electrical testing is done before extrusion of the helix. Acceptable values are noted in Table 5. One should check that electrical parameters are stable, indicating a reliable position, and that a reasonable "heel" of lead remains in the right atrium with deep inspiration so that excessive tension is not applied to the lead when the patient assumes an upright posture.

Atrial Lead Placement
The atrial lead is positioned after the ventricular lead. In positioning of the atrial lead, care must be taken not to dislodge the ventricular lead. Some atrial leads are preformed into a J shape, but most leads used in the atrium are shorter versions of those used in the ventricle. An active fixation device is more commonly used in the atrium. The J shape is obtained by the advancement of a precurved stylet. The lead is "shaped" in the body of the right atrium and rotated toward the tricuspid valve. It is then withdrawn such that the tip enters the atrial appendage. This is manifest by the tip catching on the appendage as the lead is withdrawn. Slight advancement at this time allows the lead to assume the characteristic J shape. The tip of lead takes on the characteristic to-and-fro movement of the appendage. When position appears satisfactory by fluoroscopy, the electrical parameters are tested (before helix extension in active fixation leads). Acceptable values for these measurements are noted in Table 5. If satisfactory positioning is not obtained in the appendage, the use of an active fixation lead provides an opportunity to explore other areas of the atrium. The stability of placement is checked by having the patient take a deep inspiration. The electrical values should remain satisfactory and the J should not open up to more than an L shape.

Left Ventricular Pacing
Demonstration of improved cardiac function accompanying ventricular "resynchronization" in patients with heart failure accompanied by significant intraventricular conduction delay has focused considerable attention on methods of pacing the left ventricle. Although there remains some debate as to the relative benefits of biventricular versus left ventricular pacing, it is clear that a key element is stimulation of the left ventricle. Endocardial pacing has been performed in this chamber, but rarely so because of the threat of systemic embolization of clot forming on the leads. Traditional epicardial pacing carries with it all the disadvantages that this technique has for routine pacing (i.e., morbidity of an invasive procedure and relatively high rate of lead failure) and is used infrequently. Fortunately, the left ventricle pacing can be accomplished by a lead placed in the coronary

Table 5 Optimal Parameters for Permanent Endocardial Lead Placement		
	ATRIUM	**VENTRICLE**
Capture threshold	<1.5 V	<1.0 V
Sensed P/R amplitude	>1.5 mV	>4.0 mV
Slew rate	>0.2 V/sec	>0.5 V/sec
Impedance*	400 to 1000 ohms	400 to 1000 ohms
	10-V output†	Absence of diaphragmatic pacing for both leads

*High impedance leads exceed usual values.
†Both leads should be free of diaphragmatic pacing when temporarily programmed to 10V output.

venous system. These are introduced by a sheath placed in the coronary sinus from which the leads are advanced into tributaries from the left ventricular free wall. The best hemodynamic results are obtained with leads placed over the lateral wall of the heart in a marginal vein. A variety of specialized lead systems are currently available, including some low-profile devices that are placed over a guidewire. Early iterations of these leads were associated with high rates of failure due to dislodgment or rise in capture threshold; current devices, however, perform considerably better. Successful placement of left ventricular and biventricular systems is more time consuming than routine dual-chamber pacing and requires a knowledge of the coronary venous system as well as basic catheterization skills.

■ COMPLICATIONS OF PACING

Complications associated with permanent cardiac pacemaking may result from the implant process itself, may be due to a defect in the system, or may be the consequence of an interaction between the hardware and the body. Table 6 lists some of the more frequent complications in each respective category. In one study, "early" and "late" complications each occurred in about 7% of patients. The majority of complications were evident within 3 months of implant. Pacemaker infection occurred in 1.8% and erosion in 0.9%. Eleven percent of all patients required an invasive procedure to address a complication. The PASE study enrolled patients over 65 years of age to receive dual-chamber devices. Complications occurred in 6.1% of the patients, of whom 70% required repeat surgery. Pneumothorax and lead dislodgment each occurred in about 2%, whereas cardiac perforation was encountered in 1%.

Table 6 Complications Associated With Pacemaking

IMPLANTATION
Sedation (oversedation, adverse or paradoxical reaction to drug)
Venous access
   Seldinger's technique: pneumothorax, hemothorax,
      arteriovenous fistula, chylocele, hemoptysis, injury
      to nerve
   Sheath insertion: perforation of heart or great vessel,
      air embolism
Lead placement: brady/tachyarrhythmia, perforation of heart
   or vein, disruption of tricuspid valve, damage to lead,
   misplacement into left heart
Generator placement: subcuticular placement, pocket hematoma,
   improper connection to lead(s)
SYSTEM FAILURE
Degradation of insulation
Conductor fracture
Generator fault: e.g., short circuit
HARDWARE AND THE BODY
Microdislodgment/exit block
Infection
Thromboembolism
Erosion of hardware
Twiddler's syndrome (patient manipulates generator/lead)

Implant-Associated Complications

Blind needle puncture of the subclavian vein is by its very nature associated with the possibility of puncture or laceration of a number of structures, including lung, subclavian artery, thoracic duct, and nerves. The risk of this is higher in the very aged and in patients with anatomic distortions, whereas it is obviated when access is achieved by direct cephalic venotomy. Pneumothorax is the most common significant complication of the subclavian Seldinger's approach. It may be recognized only by the postprocedure chest films or signaled by cough, dyspnea, pleuritic pain, or severe respiratory distress. When small (<10%), it can be managed conservatively; however, a large pneumothorax is treated with a chest tube as are significant hemothoraces. Inadvertent needle entry into the subclavian artery usually is without sequelae; however, laceration of the artery may be associated with significant bleeding. On occasion, the artery is mistaken for the vein, and a large-bore sheath and even pacing leads are introduced. If this is recognized, the sheath should be left in situ and consideration given to surgery or an endovascular repair. The latter may be accomplished by a balloon tamponade of the artery or insertion of a stent/graft. Rarely, a pacing wire is passed from the subclavian artery through the aortic valve and into the left ventricle without recognition. This may later be accompanied by systemic thromboembolic phenomena.

Passage of a large-bore sheath and delivery of pacing leads may also cause complication. The most common complication accompanying this part of the implant process is air embolism through the sheath. This may be manifest by fluoroscopic detection of air coursing through the heart and pulmonary artery, chest discomfort, shortness of breath, hypotension, and a drop in arterial oxygen saturation. Treatment is usually just supportive and includes oxygen supplementation, inotropic cardiovascular support, and, on occasion, attempts at catheter aspiration. Positioning the patient to trap the air for catheter aspiration is not often helpful. The natural history of this complication is breakup and resorption of the air with resolution of symptoms over a relatively short time. Prevention of this complication includes increasing the central venous pressure during sheath and lead insertion by increasing fluids, elevation of the legs, and having the patient elevate intrathoracic pressure by humming. Avoidance of deep inspiration and use of hemostatic sheaths are helpful. Other complications accompanying sheath insertion include obstruction or injury to an internal mammary artery graft or perforation of a central vein if the sheath dilator system is forcibly advanced without proper guidewire protection.

Placement of pacing leads may be accompanied by bradyarrhythmia or tachyarrhythmia, damage to the tricuspid valve, cardiac perforation, and inadvertent passage into the left ventricle through a patent foramen ovale or atrial septal defect. Perforation appears to be more common in elderly women. It may be accompanied by pericardial effusion and tamponade manifest acutely by hypotension or subacutely as an inflammatory reaction to a small amount of blood introduced by a sealed perforation. On occasion, the pacing lead may be seen by echocardiocardiography to be in the pericardial space; however, in most cases the lead has already been repositioned because of poor pacing and sensing characteristics.

Delayed perforations have also occurred. Treatment of tamponade is usually achieved by pericardiocentesis and catheter drainage over a 12- to 24-hour period. Rarely, there is a need for surgical repair of the perforation site signaled by brisk bleeding requiring volume resuscitation, continued significant pericardial drainage, or inability to effectively drain an effusion. It goes without saying that anticoagulant, thrombolytic, and antiplatelet therapy may adversely influence the course of patients with perforation.

Inadvertent placement of a lead in the left heart may not be obvious during placement if only the anteroposterior fluoroscopic view is monitored. It will be noted if a steep left anterior oblique view and/or a lateral postprocedure chest radiograph is obtained. A right bundle-branch block pattern to the paced ventricular complex suggests a left ventricular position. The major risk of left-sided pacing is systemic embolization of clot forming on the lead. Percutaneous extraction should be performed if this condition is recognized early after implant. In the chronic situation, it may be reasonable to leave the system in place and treat with anticoagulation.

Implantation of the pulse generator may be complicated by incorrectly connecting the leads, malplacement in a subcuticular position, or by the introduction of bacteria (usually local flora) during the process. Pacing leads may be connected to the wrong channel of the generator or the connection might be too loose such that electrical potentials are generated by repetitive contact between the connecting pin of the lead and set screw of the device. Such will cause abnormalities of pacing function, including oversensing. Mismatch between the generator mass and the pocket may lead to migration of the generator or pressure necrosis of overlying skin. A pocket hematoma may occur early after implantation due to lack of adequate hemostasis before closure; a subacute hematoma may occur upon the reinstitution of anticoagulation. Large and tense hematomas that threaten the integrity of the pocket should be explored and drained. It is usually considered ill advised to try to drain them by needle aspiration. Smaller hematomas can be treated conservatively.

Infection

Infection may be limited to a superficial incisional site, involve the pacemaker pocket itself, or be associated with the intravascular course of the pacing leads. Superficial skin infections usually respond to medical treatment. Infections of the pacemaker pocket may be considered to be of three sorts: a purulent process presenting with swelling pain, and erythema; a frank erosion of the skin in which part of the pacing hardware is exposed; and a localized cellulitis not infrequently at a point at which the generator is causing pressure of the overlying skin. In the first case, the causative bacteria is most often *Staphylococcus aureus,* and clinical presentation is acute, occurring within the first few weeks of implantation. In the latter, more indolent situations, a less-virulent organism (e.g., *S. epidermidis*) is involved, and presentation may be months or years after implantation. Most experts favor removal of all pacing hardware in all of these situations, although there have been cases in which the pacing leads have been salvaged by extensive pocket débridement and antibiotic therapy. In patients who present with a "preerosion" (i.e., a localized discoloration over a pressure

point) replacement of the generator under the pectoralis muscle has been successful. The major risk factor for pocket infection is reoperation.

Otherwise unexplained sepsis (especially *S. aureus*) in a patient with an endocardial lead(s) should arouse suspicion of the latter as a source. Transesophageal echocardiography has been extremely helpful in identifying vegetations on leads and should be used if transthoracic ultrasound is negative. Even in the absence of echocardiographic confirmation of vegetation, recurrent sepsis with the same organism shortly after a course of antibiotics in the absence of an alternative source suggests a lead-associated etiology. Involvement of the leads generally mandates complete removal of all pacing hardware because it is virtually impossible to eradicate infection even with very prolonged courses of antibiotics.

Thromboembolism

Detectable thrombus formation is very common in the subclavian vein after lead insertion. In most situations this is asymptomatic, but occasionally acute thrombosis extending into the axillary vein is associated with considerable pain and swelling of the upper extremity. In such cases, conservative therapy, a course of thrombolytic therapy, and/or anticoagulation have all been used with reasonable success. The dangers of venous thrombosis include pulmonary embolism, extension of thrombus retrograde and antegrade to obstruct the cerebral venous sinuses and the superior vena cava, and the inability to access the central venous system from an ipsilateral vein. There is no evidence that prophylactic anticoagulation is either safe or effective in preventing thrombosis. Intuitively, the number of leads or total obstructive mass might be thought an important factor in the development of venous thrombosis, but this has not been proved. Although rare, the superior vena cava syndrome presents a difficult problem, and the role of thrombus versus a fibrous constriction remains enigmatic. Endovascular treatment is often successful but is associated with a fairly high recurrence rate. When there is concomitant obstruction of the more distal venous system, surgical reconstruction may be necessary.

Lead Failure

Failure of a lead to pace or sense appropriately may be due to macrodisplacement or microdisplacement, exit block due to a fibrous reaction at the site of electrode–myocardial interface, fracture of a conductor wire, or insulation failure. Early lead failure is most often due to displacement, and it requires repositioning. Late lead failure due to exit block is becoming less frequent with the introduction of electrodes of superior design and the inclusion of steroid eluting technology. A moderately high rise in threshold in a chronic lead can often be compensated for by programming a higher energy output from the generator. Conductor fracture is infrequent and is usually due to some physical stress to the lead either during insertion or from stress and strain exerted on the lead within the body. Insulation failure is far more frequent and may involve either the outer insulation or the inner insulation (that which separates the coaxial conductor wires in a bipolar pacing lead). A major risk for insulation failure is entrapment by the subclavius muscle and/or the subclavicular ligaments. Certain forms of polyurethane insulation appear more susceptible to insulation degradation.

Insulation failure is associated with a low telemetered impedance, whereas conductor fracture is manifest by a very high impedance. In either case these findings may be intermittent. The inner insulation defect may result in absence of pacing due to potentials generated by contact of the two conductors simulating cardiac activity. Lead replacement is necessary when either insulation or conductor failure occur. A unique lead problem has occurred in a number of preformed atrial J leads manufactured by Telectronics. A small strip of curved metal wire used to create the J shape of the distal lead was found susceptible to fracture under the stress and strain of cardiac activity. The fractured wire fragment could wear through the insulation and lacerate the myocardium and other mediastinal structures potentially causing effusion, tamponade, and death. Because this J retention wire is not electrically active, its fracture does not affect the electrical integrity of the lead. Risk of significant complication of wire fracture is almost exclusively limited to the Accufix family of atrial J leads.

Although these leads have been withdrawn from the market since 1994, a significant number of patients still have them in place. Treatment alternatives include elective lead extraction, fluoroscopic monitoring, selective extraction of leads showing fracture and protrusion of the wire fragment, and snare catheter selective extraction of the wire fragment. The risks of spontaneous wire injury and elective extraction have recently been summarized and suggest the former to be less than the latter, indicating a conservative approach for most patients.

Recalls

The increasingly complex nature of implantable pacemakers and defibrillators renders them susceptible to potential malfunction. Over a 10-year period (1990 to 2000), advisories affecting 408,500 pacemakers were issued. Pacemaker and lead advisories usually do not require replacement of the device, although in select pacer-dependent patients such may be the case. More often reprogramming or more frequent monitoring is implemented. Still, the cost of managing device advisories and recalls is quite high, especially for the Medicare system, which absorbs much of this burden. Although the replacement of a generator requires only minor surgery and offers little risk, the extraction of chronically implanted leads is often a difficult process that can result in significant morbidity and mortality.

Lead Extraction

Endocardial leads begin to form fibrous attachments to the great veins and cardiac chambers soon after implantation. The degree of lead ensheathment increases over time such that it becomes increasingly difficult to remove a lead by simple traction after 3 to 6 months. A variety of tools have been developed to aid in the extraction of chronically implanted leads. These include interlocking stylets to maintain lead integrity while traction is applied, telescoping sheaths that are designed to peel the lead away from adhesions, and devices to catch and extract the lead from a femoral or jugular access. These tools provide a way for lead removal by the process of countertraction. Although this process has a high success rate, there is about a 2% risk of major complication and about a 0.4% risk of death. The recent introduction of laser and electrodissection sheaths has facilitated the procedure but has not reduced the risk of complication. Because of the risk of complication, alternatives to lead extraction should be carefully considered. The early characterization of indications for lead extraction as "mandatory," "necessary," and "discretionary" have been revised into the class I (conditions for which there is general agreement that leads should be removed), class II (conditions for which leads are often removed but there is some divergence of opinion with respect to the risk/benefit ratio of removal), and class III (conditions in which there is general agreement that lead removal is unnecessary) (Table 7).

Leads in patients with infection are often easier to remove, whereas more difficulty is encountered when less-experienced physicians attempt extraction and when the implant has been of longer duration. Complications appear related to less-experienced physicians, female patients, and when multiple leads require extraction. The majority of complications associated with lead extraction involve the perforation of the heart or a central vein. Because of this, procedures should be performed with the same type of backup afforded the elective coronary angioplasty.

Most extractions are accomplished in the electrophysiology or catheterization laboratory where excellent imaging and logistical support for intravascular catheterization are available. We have found that conscious sedation is adequate. A small-bore arterial line is placed in the left femoral artery while a larger sheath is placed in the right femoral vein in case a femoral retrieval system is necessary. On occasion, a temporary pacing system (usually active fixation) is placed before extraction via the right internal jugular vein. We usually attempt manual traction with a stylet in place before using a device. Care is taken to apply only gentle traction manually so as not to damage the lead such that an extraction sheath might not be used. If this is not successful, a laser or an electrodissection sheath may be used or, alternatively, a snare device might be introduced from the femoral vein.

There may be many reasons for hypotension to occur during the course of extraction. This, however, should mandate an echocardiogram as well as fluid therapy. Laceration of a great vein is not detected by echocardiography, and a level of suspicion should be maintained for this diagnosis should hypotension be present with a negative echocardiogram.

Care should be given when reimplantation of a pacing system is undertaken soon after extraction. Perforation may be more likely in veins that have been intervened upon. Extraction via a sheath introduced through the original access site provides a means of entrance to the central circulation for the immediate reimplantation of leads in those cases where there is no infection. A variety of techniques have been proposed to wedge a guidewire into the lead such that it can be withdrawn into the circulation when the lead is extracted from a femoral or jugular access. Patients with systemic infection should probably not receive a new system until several days of antibiotics have been given postexplantation. Reimplantation should be performed at an alternative site when the system has been infected.

The extraction of chronically implanted leads can be very difficult and is associated with a higher rate of major

Table 7 Indications for Lead Extraction

CLASS I (GENERAL AGREEMENT THAT LEADS SHOULD BE REMOVED)
Sepsis
Life-threatening arrhythmias due to lead
Retained lead or fragment posing immediate physical threat to patient
Clinically significant thromboembolic events related to lead or lead fragment
Lead interfering with the operation of another implantable device
Occlusion of all useable veins with the need to implant a new transvenous device
CLASS II (CONDITIONS IN WHICH THERE IS A DIVERGENCE OF OPINION WITH RESPECT TO BENEFIT VERSUS RISK OF REMOVAL)
Localized pocket infection, erosion, or chronic draining sinus that does not involve the transvenous portion of the lead system
An occult infection for which no source can be found and for which the pacing system is suspected
Chronic pain at the pocket or lead insertion site that causes significant discomfort for the patient not manageable by alternative techniques
A lead that due to its design or mode of failure may cause threat to patient but this is not immediate or imminent
A system that interferes with the treatment of a malignancy
Traumatic injury to the entry site of the lead for which the lead may interfere with reconstruction of the site
Leads preventing access to the venous circulation for newly required implantable device(s)
Nonfunctional leads in a young patient
CLASS III (RISK OF REMOVAL HIGHER THAN BENEFIT)
Any situation where the risk of removal is higher than the benefit achieved
A single nonfunctional lead in an older patient
A normally functioning lead that may be reused at the time of pulse generator replacement assuming the lead has a reliable performance history

Love CJ, et al: Recommendations for the extraction of chronically implanted transvenous pacing and defibrillator leads: indications, facilites, training, *Pacing Clin Electrophysiol* 23(4 Pt 1):544, 2000.

complication than most other activities performed in the electrophysiology laboratory. The procedure should only be performed by those who have had experience in these procedures at a site with excellent logistical support. Guidelines for the performance of extraction have been suggested.

SUGGESTED READING

Bernstein AD, Parsonnet V: Survey of cardiac pacing and implanted defibrillator practice patterns in the United States in 1997, *Pacing Clin Electrophysiol* 24:842-855, 2001.

Calkins H, et al: Prospective randomized comparison of the safety and effectiveness of placement of endocardial pacemaker and defibrillator leads using the extrathoracic subclavian vein guided by contrast venography versus the cephalic approach, *Pacing Clin Electrophysiol* 24:456-464, 2001.

Cazeau S, et al: Effects of multisite biventricular pacing in patients with heart failure and intraventricular conduction delay, *N Engl J Med* 344:873-880, 2001.

Gregoratos G, et al: ACC/AHA guidelines for implantation of cardiac pacemakers and antiarrhythmia devices: a report of the American College of Cardiology/American Heart Association Task Force on Practice Guidelines (Committee on Pacemaker Implantation), *J Am Coll Cardiol* 31:1175-1209, 1998.

Linde C, et al: Long-term benefits of biventricular pacing in congestive heart failure: results from the multisite stimulation in cardiomyopathy (MUSTIC) study, *J Am Coll Cardiol* 40:111-118, 2002.

Maisel WH, et al: Recalls and safety alerts involving pacemakers and implantable cardioverter-defibrillator generators, *JAMA* 286:793-799, 2000.

Spittell PC, Hayes DL: Venous complications after insertion of a transvenous pacemaker, *Mayo Clin Proc* 67:258-265, 1992.

Westerman GR, et al: Transthoracic transatrial endocardial lead placement for permanent pacing, *Ann Thorac Surg* 43:445, 1987.

INTRAOPERATIVE TRANSESOPHAGEAL ECHOCARDIOGRAPHY

João A. Lima

Since its introduction in the early 1980s, transesophageal echocardiography (TEE) has become an integral part of intraoperative monitoring in cardiac surgery. Intraoperative TEE is a safe, relatively noninvasive tool that can dramatically affect surgical management. A recent review of the use of intraoperative TEE at the Mayo Clinic showed 14% of patients had previously undetected cardiac defects necessitating changes in surgical management. Other studies have shown that intraoperative TEE findings can change the operative plan in up to 19% of cases involving cardiac valve surgery. Current applications include preoperative visualization of previously undetected cardiac defects; appraisal of ventricular size, function, and wall motion abnormalities; assessment of preoperative valvular structure and function; and visualization of aortic atheromatous disease. Postoperative applications include evaluation of adequacy of surgical repair, detection of intracardiac air, and management of hemodynamics.

Typically, the cardiac anesthesiologist or cardiologist inserts the TEE probe and interprets the study in the operating room. Absolute contraindications to TEE insertion include esophageal stricture, tumor, or recent surgical resection. Relative contraindications are esophageal varices, esophagitis, and coagulopathy. The incidence of esophageal perforation during TEE is less than 1 in 10,000.

■ MITRAL VALVE REPAIR/REPLACEMENT

Mitral valve repair has become the preferred treatment for severe mitral regurgitation (MR). Valve repair versus replacement provides the advantages of lower short- and long-term morbidity and mortality. Mitral valve repair also better preserves left ventricular anatomy and function and frees the patient from postoperative anticoagulation.

The use of intraoperative TEE can provide key information to the cardiac surgeon regarding the underlying anatomy and pathophysiology of the mitral valve. Feasibility of repair depends on the location, extent, and mechanism of the MR. After general examination of the atria, ventricles, and other valves, a careful and systematic evaluation of the mitral valve apparatus is required.

Severity of MR as measured by TEE is typically determined with color flow Doppler. Mitral valve jets that reach the posterior wall of the left atrium or have a width greater than 6.5 mm are highly predictive of severe MR. The true severity of MR is often underestimated in patients with eccentrically directed jets because of decreased color flow representation.

The presence of rapid heart rate or decreased left ventricular function can also cause underestimation of MR. Severity of intraoperative MR as measured by color flow imaging is often less than that seen in the ambulatory setting because of decreased cardiac output or arterial blood pressure during general anesthesia. Normalization of blood pressure with phenylephrine can significantly increase MR grade, stressing the importance of recreating normal hemodynamics during color Doppler grading. The use of pulsed wave Doppler to interrogate pulmonary vein blood flow also has utility in grading MR severity. Reversal of pulmonary vein blood flow during systole is a sensitive and specific indicator of severe MR. Severe left atrial enlargement (>5.5 cm) also suggests the existence of severe MR.

Careful measurement of the mitral valve annulus provides information regarding the need for mitral annuloplasty. MR caused by annular dilation is usually seen as a centrally directed color flow jet resulting from failure of leaflet coaptation. Further description of the mitral valve apparatus should also include presence or absence of calcification, which is important in determining feasibility of mitral repair.

Examination of mitral leaflet structure and mobility provides important information regarding the mechanism and etiology of MR. The presence of fixed, thickened, severely calcified leaflets implies rheumatic etiology and may present a contraindication to repair. Redundant, myxomatous valve leaflets as seen in mitral valve prolapse are highly amenable to surgical repair, particularly if alterations are predominantly in the posterior leaflet. Eccentricity of color flow Doppler jets during TEE can localize a specific mitral valve leaflet requiring repair. Prolapsed or flail leaflets result in flow jets directed away from the affected leaflet, whereas fixed leaflets show color flow directed toward the site of pathology. The correlation of valvular pathology and location ascertained during surgery with alterations detected by preoperative TEE is very accurate (>90%). Precise localization of mitral valve pathology can aid in planning surgical technique. For example, anterior leaflet prolapse often requires complicated and time-consuming chordal reconstruction.

Intraoperative TEE is also important in postrepair assessment. TEE has been found to be more effective than direct palpation of the left atrium or filling the arrested ventricle in detecting residual MR after repair. A close examination of the mitral valve should be performed after separation from cardiopulmonary bypass when the hemodynamic state is stable.

Mild residual MR after repair is frequently present, and follow-up of these patients suggests that long-term morbidity and mortality are not different from that for patients without residual MR. Moderate-severe residual MR requires reinstitution of cardiopulmonary bypass and reexploration. Patients with moderate residual MR after repair present a clinical dilemma, as these patients often have poorer long-term results compared with patients with mild residual regurgitation. Reinstitution of cardiopulmonary bypass, however, is also associated with certain risks. Decisions regarding moderate MR after repair should use TEE findings to determine the potential feasibility of valve repeat repair or replacement, while taking into consideration the patient's current hemodynamic state, age, and underlying medical conditions.

In addition to assessment of residual MR, TEE in the immediate postrepair state should also focus on detection of systolic anterior motion (SAM) of the anterior mitral valve leaflet. This rare complication (1% to 2%) can cause dynamic left ventricular outflow obstruction. Postrepair SAM presents more commonly with inflexible annuloplasty rings and is thought to be due to the posterior portion of the annuloplasty ring pushing the anterior leaflet too far forward.

Patients undergoing annuloplasty as part of a mitral valve repair should have assessment of annular area with TEE in the immediate postrepair period. The short-axis view of the mitral valve can use planimetry to directly measure valve area. Similarly, use of continuous-wave Doppler to measure pressure half-time and calculate mitral valve area with the continuity equation can reveal whether a significant mitral stenosis exists.

■ AORTIC, TRICUSPID, AND PROSTHETIC VALVE SURGERY

Intraoperative TEE is also useful in evaluating the aortic valve. Significant aortic regurgitation may require the use of retrograde cardioplegia for myocardial protection. Intraoperative measurement of the left ventricular outflow tract aids in selection of aortic homograft size in aortic valve replacement. Postbypass examination of the "freehand" aortic homograft and root with TEE typically reveals a "cylinder within a cylinder" resulting from the homograft around the patient's native ascending aorta. Flow between the homograft layer and aortic root suggests failure of either proximal or distal suture lines. Distortion of the aortic homograft may also be secondary to hematoma or bleeding into this space between the graft and aortic root wall.

Tricuspid valve regurgitation (TR) is often detected during intraoperative TEE for left sided valvular disease. Up to 25% of patients receiving mitral or aortic surgery require concurrent tricuspid valve repair. TEE can often suggest the etiology of TR: thickened, immobile leaflets imply rheumatic, carcinoid, or drug-induced disease. In many patients with TR secondary to left-sided pathology, TR will diminish after aortic or mitral repair or replacement. Severe TR in the setting of a dilated tricuspid annulus or right ventricle may require separate repair. As with the mitral valve, assessment of TR should take place under normal hemodynamic conditions, as variables such as volume status and pulmonary artery pressure can dramatically affect TR.

TEE is an excellent tool for evaluating function of prosthetic valves after valve replacement surgery. Proper evaluation of prosthetic valves with echocardiography requires knowledge of the structure and flow characteristics specific to each prosthesis. Primary surgical issues in the immediate postcardiopulmonary bypass period include proper mechanical function and detection of perivalvular leaks. For example, intraoperative TEE can easily determine whether both leaflets of a St. Jude aortic valve are opening properly and whether there is perivalvular regurgitation. Small leaks in the immediate postbypass period after replacement typically diminish over time after correction of coagulopathy and tissue healing. Larger leaks may require a second look, and TEE can help direct the cardiac surgeon to the site of the problem. All prosthetic devices normally have some intrinsic regurgitation. Color flow jets are usually less than 2.5 cm long with mitral valves and have characteristic patterns. For example, the St. Jude mitral valve typically has one central regurgitation jet and two peripherally located centrally directed regurgitation jets, whereas the Medtronic mitral prosthesis has one large centrally located jet.

■ OBSTRUCTIVE HYPERTROPHIC CARDIOMYOPATHY

Obstructive hypertrophic cardiomyopathy is a progressive disease with high mortality. Surgical intervention typically consists of myectomy after development of clinical symptoms. Intraoperative TEE is invaluable in guiding surgical therapy. Pinpointing the site of septal contact by the anterior mitral leaflet during SAM allows precise localization of myectomy. Distance from this point of septal contact to the aortic annulus should be measured so that apical extension of the myectomy is adequate to relieve outflow obstruction. Septal thickness can also be determined, providing information to the cardiac surgeon regarding safe depth of the myectomy. Although aortic outflow tract gradients are often difficult to accurately measure with TEE, an attempt to measure premyectomy gradient should be made. Finally, examination of the mitral valve should be performed to determine whether MR is secondary to SAM or due to coincident mitral disease requiring separate repair.

Postmyectomy evaluation should include interrogation of the left ventricular outflow tract with continuous wave Doppler for evidence of residual obstruction. Attempts at inducing obstruction with pharmacologic agents such as isoproterenol are used at some centers. Close examination of the ventricular septum with color flow Doppler may reveal a ventricular septal defect from overzealous septal resection. Mild residual SAM often exists in the immediate postbypass period and usually improves in subsequent examinations. MR should be markedly improved. Lingering MR may be due to either inadequate myectomy with continuing SAM or coexisting mitral pathology.

■ DETECTING AORTIC ATHEROMATOUS DISEASE

Intraoperative TEE can be useful to detect atheromatous disease of the aorta. Studies have suggested an association between the degree of atheromatous disease of the aortic arch and risk of systemic embolization and stroke. Elderly patients with atheromatous disease of the aorta may have significantly higher rates of postoperative neurologic change after cardiopulmonary bypass. It is hypothesized that aortic atheromas embolize during aortic cross-clamping and cannulation. Direct palpation by the surgeon has been shown to be an insensitive method to detect aortic atheromatous disease and can miss over 80% of significant disease. While palpation of the aortic arch may detect calcific aortic disease, TEE is clearly superior in displaying soft, "cheesy" atheromatous disease and intimal thickening. Intimal thickening (>5 mm by TEE) predicts higher risk of postoperative neurologic complications after cardiac surgery.

Modification of surgical technique in the presence of severe atheromatous disease has been proposed, but the impact of these changes on neurologic outcome has not been well validated. This may be due to the inability of TEE to image the aortic arch because of the air–tissue interface of the overlying lung and right main bronchus. Intraoperative epiaortic B-mode scanning in combination with TEE may better detect aortic atherosclerotic disease and reduce perioperative neurologic complications.

LEFT VENTRICULAR FUNCTION AND WALL MOTION ANALYSIS

Intraoperative TEE can provide useful information to the cardiac anesthesiologist and cardiac surgeon regarding patient hemodynamics. The midpapillary short-axis view of the left ventricle (LV) can serve as an important window for cardiac monitoring. Estimates of LV preload and filling have been found to be as accurate as radionucleotide studies. TEE better evaluates preload in the patient with poor LV function or valvular disease than pulmonary artery catheter measurements. Abnormal LV compliance in this patient population nullifies assumptions in the use of the Swan-Ganz catheter to estimate LV volumes by pulmonary capillary wedge pressures. LV end-diastolic areas less than 5.5 cm^2 or LV cavity obliteration are TEE signs that are highly indicative of decreased preload.

The LV fractional area change, as determined from the short-axis view, allows qualitative estimation of LV contractility. Through estimates of LV function, TEE can guide use of inotropic support during weaning from cardiopulmonary bypass. Contractility estimates based on short-axis views of LV fractional shortening are preload and afterload dependent and require caution in interpretation.

Diastolic dysfunction is easily measured by TEE using pulsed-wave Doppler interrogation of mitral inflow to determine the ratio of early diastolic LV filling to atrial diastolic LV filling. This ratio is normally greater than 1.0. Impaired early diastolic filling results in a ratio less than 1.0 and implies poor myocardial relaxation, characteristic of diastolic dysfunction. These patients require higher filling pressures to maintain preload and may require lusitropic agents to facilitate separation from bypass.

TEE for intraoperative monitoring of LV regional wall motion abnormalities has also been advocated. Abnormal inward motion and thickening of the myocardium starts within seconds of ischemia in the affected region. These changes begin as mild hypokinesis and progress to dyskinesis as ischemia progresses. Wall motion abnormalities precede changes on ECG or in pulmonary capillary wedge pressure by several minutes. Detection of early changes may allow more rapid and effective treatment of intraoperative ischemia. Wall motion abnormalities may be an early signal of bypass graft spasm or obstruction. Precise anatomic localization of the ischemia is facilitated by the TEE short-axis view. Long-axis views are useful to detect apical ischemia. However, several factors limit TEE as a monitor for ischemia in the cardiac patient. The TEE probe is typically placed after anesthetic induction and removed prior to leaving the operating room, thus missing the periods at highest risk for perioperative ischemia. Furthermore, detection of abnormalities requires frequent TEE examinations, possibly distracting the anesthesiologist from other aspects of patient care. Finally, not all wall motion abnormalities are due to ischemia. Ventricular pacing and bundle branch conduction blocks can produce discordant septal motion, which can be misinterpreted as ischemia.

FUTURE DIRECTIONS

Intraoperative TEE has progressed from providing simple estimates of LV function to providing detailed information about cardiac valvular abnormalities. Future directions include refinement of techniques for determining intravascular pressure and flow, automated endocardial border detection for continuous feedback of myocardial performance, and three-dimensional reconstructive techniques for precise cardiac modeling.

SUGGESTED READING

Click RL, et al: Intraoperative transesophageal echocardiography: 5 year prospective review of impact on surgical management, *Mayo Clin Proc* 75:241, 2000.

Heitmiller ES, et al: Transesophageal echocardiography. In Blitt CD, Hines RL, editors: *Monitoring in anesthesia and critical care medicine*, New York, 1995, Churchill-Livingstone, p 261.

Zaroff JG, Picard MH: Transesophageal echocardiographic evaluation of the mitral and tricuspid valves, *Cardiol Clin* 18:731, 2000.

CONCOMITANT CARDIAC AND THORACIC OPERATIONS

John R. Doty
Stephen C. Yang

A small percentage of patients referred for thoracic surgery have disease in more than one thoracic organ system. The most common situation is when a solitary pulmonary nodule is found incidentally on a preoperative chest x-ray. Alternatively, significant coronary disease is revealed during preoperative cardiac clearance in patients with known pulmonary or esophageal disease. Occasionally the surgeon identifies a mediastinal or lung mass at the time of cardiac surgery and must decide intraoperatively whether to perform a biopsy, resection, or further workup of this lesion. The surgeon also must weigh in the risks and operative approaches if a second staged procedure is performed.

Surgical approaches for combined procedures on the heart, lung, esophagus, and other structures in the thorax can be tailored to the specific disease processes if careful attention is given to diagnosis and staging before surgery. Median sternotomy is the preferred approach for most cardiac operations and provides adequate exposure for biopsy and resection of all mediastinal masses. This incision also provides adequate but suboptimal exposure for pulmonary resections of the upper and middle lobes. Lower lobectomy is difficult to perform through a median sternotomy, however, particularly on the left because of difficulty gaining control of the pulmonary veins that lie posterior to the heart. Thoracotomy is the preferred approach for most pulmonary operations and provides adequate exposure for some cardiac procedures, particularly mitral valve surgery through a right thoracotomy or lateral wall coronary bypass through a left thoracotomy.

■ SOLITARY PULMONARY NODULE DURING CARDIAC EVALUATION

As the age of patients referred for cardiac surgery continues to rise, and the use of computed tomography (CT) scans to diagnose coronary disease becomes popular, an incidental solitary pulmonary nodule may be found and need to be addressed. Careful history should be elicited on tobacco use, asbestos exposure, tuberculosis, family history of lung cancer, and exposure to fungal sources. A previous chest surgical procedure would require adequate exposure to lyse pleural adhesions. Chest CT should be performed to evaluate the mediastinum for nodal involvement. Positron emission tomography scans may help in determining malignant potential and if there is involvement elsewhere. If imaging studies suggest cancer, an attempt should be made to obtain a tissue diagnosis before cardiac surgery. Bronchoscopy with brushings or transbronchial biopsy of paratracheal nodes

can be done with minimal risk if the patient's cardiac disease is stable but is usually of low yield. Percutaneous biopsy of a solitary pulmonary nodule is not advised because pneumothorax or hemothorax would not be well tolerated by a patient with cardiac disease. Mediastinal lymphadenopathy can be evaluated with node biopsy at the time of cardiac surgery because the patient will require treatment of the cardiac disease to tolerate chemotherapy or radiation should this represent advanced cancer. Pulmonary function tests should be documented before surgery.

Most patients who are found to have concomitant cardiac and other intrathoracic disease should be treated in a staged fashion, with the first operation performed on the organ system with the most life-threatening disease. Typically, myocardial revascularization is required followed by pulmonary or esophageal resection after recovery from cardiac surgery. Care should be taken during the sternotomy to avoid entry into the pleural space where the next operation is planned to prevent formation of adhesions. Prior sternotomy is not a contraindication for mediastinoscopy because the latter is performed in a different plane. Similarly, esophageal resection via the transhiatal, three-incision, or thoracoabdominal incision approach is through previously unoperated fields. Thoracotomy is well tolerated after median sternotomy and does not require reentry into the previous operative field. While mobilizing structures off of the mediastinum during the subsequent thoracotomy, however, the internal mammary conduit (if used, particularly on the left) should be identified carefully and left undisturbed.

■ UNSUSPECTED PULMONARY OR MEDIASTINAL MASS

Occasionally the surgeon is faced with a lung or mediastinal mass at sternotomy without adequate preoperative diagnosis or staging, such as during emergent coronary artery bypass graft (CABG) procedures. Definitive surgery for these masses should not be performed at the time of cardiac surgery because the extent of disease is unknown and unwisely may prolong an urgent or emergent operation. Often these patients have been transferred directly from the cardiac catheterization suite and are coagulopathic and hemodynamically compromised. Biopsy of these masses is acceptable and can be performed with sharp incision or large-bore hollow needle core biopsy techniques. Excessive biopsy should be avoided because uncontrollable bleeding can result due to anticoagulation for cardiopulmonary bypass (CPB).

■ CONCOMITANT OPERATIONS

Several authors have reported small series of patients undergoing concomitant operations for cardiac and other intrathoracic disease. Most commonly, these are patients with coronary artery disease and a lung mass, and the typical concomitant operation is CABG surgery and pulmonary resection through a median sternotomy. If tissue diagnosis of the lung mass has been unyielding before surgery, a wedge resection should be performed if the mass is peripheral before the initiation of CPB with frozen section diagnosis.

If the results come back malignant, completion lobectomy should be performed during rewarming while the lungs are collapsed.

Posterior and inferior lung masses are difficult to resect through a median sternotomy, and therein lays the disadvantage in doing these simultaneous procedures. These operations probably should be limited to upper or middle lobe resections. Assessment of the mediastinal lymph nodes also would be difficult, if not impossible, especially if nodal dissection is one's preference. These patients are at higher risk for bleeding (staple lines, lung and mediastinal dissected tissue) and pulmonary complications in the postoperative period. The surgeon should consider CABG surgery without CPB (off-pump CABG surgery) in appropriate patients because this allows for a smaller total dose of heparin. Double-lumen endotracheal intubation is required to perform lung resection in these patients.

Concomitant pulmonary resection and cardiac surgery should be considered if the patient has cardiac disease that can be approached easily through a thoracotomy, such as atrial septal defect, mitral valve disease, or repair of a descending thoracic aortic aneurysm. These combined procedures can obviate the need for a second operation if appropriately selected and can be particularly useful in the reoperative cardiac patient in whom reentry through a previous sternotomy can be avoided. A slightly larger thoracotomy is employed to provide adequate exposure for cannulation.

A second group of patients with concomitant disease are those with end-stage chronic obstructive pulmonary disease and cardiac disease who are candidates for lung volume reduction surgery (LVRS). Median sternotomy is an ideal approach for these patients, offering not only traditional exposure for CABG surgery, but also excellent exposure for bilateral upper lobe lung volume reduction. Valve repair or replacements in combination with LVRS should be avoided. Similarly, off-pump CABG surgery should be encouraged. Median sternotomy is well tolerated by these patients and is preferable to bilateral thoracotomies. Patients with severe end-stage lung disease who are not candidates for LVRS could be considered for combined lung transplantation and CABG surgery.

Anterior-superior mediastinal masses can be resected easily at the time of cardiac surgery through a median sternotomy and do not require preoperative tissue diagnosis, unless imaging studies suggest advanced disease outside the mediastinum. Resection of the thymus and anterior fat pad enhances exposure for the cardiac procedure and should be performed before the initiation of CPB. Combined esophagectomy and CABG surgery has been reported only twice in the literature and is indicated only in the most unusual of circumstances.

■ INDICATIONS FOR COMBINED INTRATHORACIC OPERATIONS

Most patients presenting with concomitant disease within the thorax are treated most appropriately and conservatively with staged procedures because the cardiac disease typically requires more immediate intervention, whereas the pulmonary or mediastinal disease can be evaluated thoroughly

Table 1 Suggested Indications for Concomitant Cardiac and Thoracic Operations

DIAGNOSIS	OPERATION
Coronary artery disease and stage I lung cancer in upper lobe	Median sternotomy, coronary artery bypass graft, lobectomy
Coronary artery disease and end-stage chronic obstructive pulmonary disease	Median sternotomy, coronary artery bypass graft, bilateral upper lobe lung volume reduction
Coronary or valvular disease and mediastinal mass	Median sternotomy, cardiac operation, resection of mediastinal mass
Coronary or valvular disease and unexpected mediastinal or pulmonary mass	Cardiac operation, biopsy of mass
Right lung mass and mitral valve disease	Right thoracotomy, pulmonary resection, cardiac operation

and treated in a subsequent operation. Although there has been concern that CPB can affect adversely the immune system and subsequent response to malignancy, there are currently no published data to support or refute this concept. If patients are appropriately selected, concomitant procedures can be performed safely without adversely affecting mortality, morbidity, or long-term outcomes. Operative mortality ranged from 0% to 7%, and perioperative morbidity rates ranged from 37% to 50% for small series of patients undergoing concomitant cardiac and pulmonary operations reported in the literature. A significant percentage of these deaths were due to pulmonary complications, such as intrapulmonary hemorrhage, acute respiratory distress syndrome, or aspiration.

Long-term outcomes have not been evaluated fully for patients undergoing concomitant procedures, and published data are contradictory. Five-year survival rates for patients with lung cancer in these series ranged from 35% to 88% and depended on the tumor stage. A significant difference in survival for stage I lung cancer patients was found by investigators at the Mayo Clinic. Stage I patients in their series undergoing cardiac surgery followed by pulmonary resection had a 100% 5-year survival compared with a 36% 5-year survival in stage I patients undergoing a combined procedure.

Our current indications for combined intrathoracic operations are listed in Table 1. All patients should undergo appropriate preoperative staging with thoracic CT and a diligent attempt at tissue diagnosis.

SUGGESTED READING

Canver CC, et al: Pulmonary resection combined with cardiac operations, *Ann Thorac Surg* 50:796, 1990.

Mariani MA, et al: Combined off-pump coronary surgery and right lung resections through midline sternotomy, *Ann Thorac Surg* 71:1343, 2001.

Miller DL, et al: Combined operation for lung cancer and cardiac disease, *Ann Thorac Surg* 58:989, 1994.

Rao V, et al: Results of combined pulmonary resection and cardiac operation, *Ann Thorac Surg* 62:342, 1996.

Schmid RA, et al: Lung volume reduction surgery combined with cardiac interventions, *Eur J Cardiothorac Surg* 15:585, 1999.

TREATMENT OF STERNAL WOUND INFECTIONS

Michael F. Chiaramonte
E. Gene Deune
Craig A. Vander Kolk

Patients undergoing prolonged cardiac procedures that require a sternotomy incision are often critically ill and are prone to infectious complications. Obesity and diabetes mellitus also are well-known risk factors for infection. The incidence of superficial wound infections is 4% to 6.2%. Incision and drainage followed by local wound care is usually all that is required. The incidence of deep suppurative mediastinitis is less than 2%. Early and aggressive management that includes débridement of infected tissue and bone followed by closure using a muscle flap is essential to achieve a successful outcome.

■ DIAGNOSIS

The combination of fever, leukocytosis, drainage, and sternal instability suggests acute suppurative mediastinitis. Occasionally, computed tomography is necessary to exclude an undrained collection. If mediastinal infection is suggested clinically, however, surgical exploration should be undertaken.

If the diagnosis is definite or highly suspicious, blood and wound cultures should be obtained. A broad-spectrum antibiotic effective against gram-positive and gram-negative organisms is given. *Staphylococcus epidermidis* is the most common organism. Vancomycin is required if sensitivities show the organism to have methicillin resistance.

■ TREATMENT

Débridement

Operative exploration is performed, especially if the patient is septic. The patient's entire chest and abdomen are prepared and draped. The sternal wound is opened and débrided of necrotic tissue. The sternum is separated carefully from the ventricle, and infected bone is débrided using a rongeur until healthy, bleeding bone is identified. Care is taken to protect vein grafts and the internal mammary arteries (IMAs). If cartilage becomes exposed, it should be removed entirely or débrided within the perichondrium. Bone and wound swabbings are sent for culture. The sternum is irrigated with warm saline with or without antibiotics. Although some authors have recommended delaying the muscle flap based on the degree of contamination and possible need for further débridement, we almost uniformly perform a muscle flap at the initial débridement with good results.

Reconstruction: Muscle Flaps

The pectoralis major muscle is the most common muscle used for reconstruction of sternal wounds. The pectoralis major muscle has a dual blood supply from the thoracoacromial and the IMA. Most sternal defects require a pectoralis major muscle advancement flap on the side where the IMA was used and a pectoralis major muscle turnover flap on the contralateral side. Rarely the rectus abdominis muscle is used as a turnover flap to provide coverage of the inferior aspect of the sternum.

When the wound has been débrided of all nonviable tissue and bone, the muscle flaps are elevated. We always start with a left pectoralis major muscle advancement flap, based on the thoracoacromial vascular pedicle, followed 95% of the time with a right pectoralis major turnover flap because the right IMA commonly is spared. The pectoralis major muscle advancement flap is harvested by first elevating the skin and subcutaneous tissue from the pectoralis major muscle. The humeral insertion is divided. Placing the arms at the patient's side and using a lighted retractor are helpful. The pectoralis major muscle is elevated starting at the sternal origin until reaching the loose areolar plane beneath the muscle. The thoracoacromial vessels can be visualized on the undersurface of the pectoralis major muscle and palpated. Extreme care should be taken when cautery is used near the vessels. The clavicular attachments are divided carefully. The pectoralis major muscle is advanced into the sternal defect and sutured to the soft tissue on the contralateral side.

If more muscle is required, a right pectoralis major turnover flap is harvested. The skin and subcutaneous tissue are separated from the pectoralis major muscle leaving the fascia intact. The dissection extends to the insertion on the humerus. The humeral attachment is divided using the cautery; rarely a counterincision over the insertion is required.

The pectoralis major muscle is divided from its clavicular attachment until the thoracoacromial vessels are identified. The location coincides with the crossing of the cephalic vein as it enters the subclavian vein. The vessels are ligated with large Surgiclips and divided. The pectoralis major muscle easily separates from the underlying pectoralis minor muscle in a loose areolar plane. The pectoralis major is held vertically and split in the direction of the muscle fibers so that one half may be directed superiorly and the other inferiorly. If the muscle is substantial, a turnover flap occasionally can be used as the sole muscle flap to fill the defect. The muscle is inset using 3-0 polyglactin 910 (Vicryl) suture so that the defect between the sternal borders is obliterated. A 3/16 round Jackson Pratt drain is placed deep and superficially to the flaps. Two 3/16 round Jackson drains are placed in the donor site created by harvesting the pectoralis major muscle and secured with a 3-0 nylon suture. The wound is irrigated with saline and closed with interrupted deep and dermal 3-0 polyglactin 910 suture. The skin is closed with staples.

Defects involving the lower third of the sternum may not be covered adequately with a pectoralis major muscle flap and may require a rectus abdominis muscle turnover flap. This muscle is based on the superior epigastric artery and should be harvested from the side where the IMA was not used. There also are intercostal arteries, however, that support the rectus abdominis muscle if the IMA has been used on the side from which the rectus abdominis is to be harvested. The sternal incision is extended inferiorly and centered over the rectus abdominis muscle. The fascia is incised and elevated off the surface of the muscle. The insertion of the rectus abdominis muscle on the pubic symphysis is divided, and inferior epigastric arteries are identified and suture ligated. The muscle is elevated in the loose areolar plane that exists on the posterior surface. Care must be taken to identify and preserve the superior epigastric arteries as they exit from the costal margin approximately 3 cm laterally to the midline. The muscle is turned over and inserted into the sternal defect. The fascia is closed with a running 0 Ti-Cron suture; Scarpa's fascia and the dermis are closed with 3-0 interrupted polyglactin 910 suture. The skin is closed with a running 4-0 polyglactin 910 subcutaneous suture. A 3/16 round Jackson Pratt drain is placed in the subcutaneous space and secured with a 3-0 nylon suture. Infrequently a split-thickness skin graft is placed over the muscle flaps when there is inadequate chest skin for coverage.

■ STERILE STERNAL DEHISCENCE

Occasionally, patients develop sterile sternal nonunion after sternotomy. The most common approach to this problem has been no treatment at all. Patients are told to accept and tolerate the clicking and the discomfort from the motion and subluxation of the sternal edges. A few patients have severe pain, however, and are unable to resume their preoperative occupation and activity. Some of these patients are taken back to the operating room for removal of sternal wires or for rewiring. Rewiring has been less than optimal because of the transverse sternal fractures from the wires eroding through the bone.

A few centers have employed rigid internal fixation for sternal nonunion in infected and noninfected sternal dehiscence. The guiding principle is that rigid fixation with plates and screws achieves far better stability than wires. Many techniques have been proposed for the internal fixation. An increasingly popular technique described by Chase has been the use of parallel plates on both sides of the sternotomy. Currently, one plate manufacturer is developing dedicated implantable sternal plates for use in infected and noninfected sternal nonunion reconstructions, but these plates are not yet available for clinical use.

■ CONCLUSION

A spectrum of muscle flap procedures is available for coverage of sternal defects. The selection of muscle flap is dictated by the size of the defect and the vessels used for cardiac revascularization. Early and aggressive débridement combined with muscle flap placement lessens the morbidity and mortality associated with mediastinitis.

SUGGESTED READING

Chase WC, et al: Internal fixation of the sternum in median sternotomy dehiscence, *Plast Reconstr Surg* 103:1667, 1999,

Georgiade GS, Rehnke R: Mediastinitis. In Georgiade GS, et al, editors: *Georgiade plastic, maxillofacial and reconstructive surgery*, ed 3, Baltimore, 1997, Williams & Wilkins, p 829.

Nelms B: Infections. In Pearson FG, editor: *Thoracic surgery*, New York, 1995, Churchill Livingstone, p 1367.

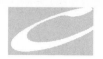
CARDIAC TUMORS

Cornelius M. Dyke
Eric R. Skipper

■ INCIDENCE AND DISTRIBUTION

Primary cardiac tumors are rare, although a busy surgeon sees several in his or her practice lifetime. The incidence of primary tumors of the heart in autopsy series ranges from 0.002% to 0.3%. Three quarters of these tumors are benign, and myxomas constitute approximately 50% of all benign tumors. Myxomas are found predominantly in adults between age 30 and 60 and are slightly more common in women. Nonmyxomatous benign tumors arise from many different cell lines (Table 1), whereas malignant tumors are predominantly sarcomas (angiosarcomas, rhabdomyosarcomas, fibrosarcomas). Primary pericardial tumors are predominantly mesotheliomas. In children, rhabdomyomas are the most common type of intracardiac tumor, whereas myxomas are rare.

Metastatic tumors of the heart are much more common than primary tumors, occurring in approximately 1% of patients with metastatic disease. Metastatic endocardial lesions are rare; pericardial or epicardial lesions predominate. Lung, breast, melanoma, lymphoma, and leukemia metastasize most frequently to the heart. Lesions that infiltrate the myocardium or are associated with bloody effusions are more likely to be malignant. These findings may be evident on cardiac magnetic resonance imaging (MRI) or computed tomography (CT).

■ PRESENTATION

Tumors of the heart typically present in one of four ways: (1) found incidentally; (2) after embolization and/or stroke; (3) with obstruction of blood flow; or (4) with vague constitutional symptoms such as fatigue, myalgias, or fevers. Tumors of the heart may present with symptoms of either right-sided or left-sided heart failure depending on the anatomic location of the tumor and the chamber obstruction. Tumor embolization occurs suddenly and may affect any arterial branch. Presentation may be catastrophic and debilitating when brain embolization and infarction occurs. The propensity of myxomas to embolize is evidenced by the fact that tumor fragments from peripheral embolic sites may be found in 60% of patients with left atrial myxomas.

Occasionally, diagnosis may be made on biopsy and pathologic examination of embolic tissue.

The systemic symptoms of atrial myxomas are vague, nonspecific, and thought to be due to a proinflammatory state induced by the tumor. Patients may complain of lethargy, fatigue, and fever, which are thought to result from proinflammatory mediators, particularly interleukin-6 (IL-6). Myxomas constitutively produce and secrete IL-6, and patients with myxomas may have markedly elevated levels. Whether IL-6 influences tumor recurrence or may be used as a marker for recurrence is unclear.

Symptoms of heart failure may occur when intracardiac tumors enlarge and obstruct blood flow. Symptoms of mitral stenosis or mitral regurgitation occur with mitral annular obstruction by the tumor mass or leaflet destruction from tumor involvement or trauma. Pulmonary hypertension may complicate valve involvement. Uncommonly, right-sided atrial myxomas may obstruct venous return and cause liver engorgement, ascites, and peripheral edema.

Many patients are asymptomatic and diagnosed during evaluation of unrelated medical problems. Incidental findings on chest x-ray, chest CT, echocardiogram, or cardiac catheterization may lead to the diagnosis of a cardiac tumor. Occasionally an intracardiac mass may be identified during cardiac surgery for an unrelated problem.

■ DIAGNOSIS

Nonneoplastic intracardiac masses, such as thrombus or infectious vegetations, usually can be excluded on the basis of the history and physical examination. Carney's syndrome, a hereditary disorder of cardiac myxomas, skin pigmentation, and endocrine abnormalities, may be suspected after careful physical examination. Pigmentation in patients with Carney's syndrome is spotty and may occur on the trunk or face and frequently involves the vermilion border of the lips (distinguishing them from common freckles). Pituitary adenoma or Cushing's syndrome has been reported in association

Table 1 Benign Nonmyxomatous Tumors of the Heart (Descending Order of Frequency)
Rhabdomyomas
Fibromas
Papillary fibroelastomas
Hemangiomas
Lipomas
Hamartomas
Teratomas
Pheochromocytomas

with cardiac tumors and is a component of the syndrome. Preoperative identification of Carney's syndrome is important for patient counseling because myxomas in Carney's syndrome are frequently multicentric and prone to recurrence (or missed at initial resection). Intraoperative transesophageal echocardiography (TEE) with a thorough search of all cardiac chambers at the time of operation is mandatory in patients with Carney's syndrome.

The initial test for patients suspected of having a cardiac tumor is transthoracic echocardiography (Figure 1). The differential diagnosis of an intracardiac mass includes thrombus, cardiac tumor, and bacterial or fungal vegetation. The diagnosis may be narrowed considerably based on the location of the mass and other clinical circumstances. Echocardiography can identify the size of the mass, whether it is solitary or multifocal, and the anatomic location and relationship to other intracardiac structures, particularly the mitral valve. Other intracardiac masses, such as thrombus or bacterial vegetations, usually can be differentiated based on echocardiographic characteristics. Although echocardiography remains the gold standard for intracardiac imaging, limitations include significant operator dependence, inability to visualize adjacent thoracic structures such

as the pericardium, and less precise differentiation of soft tissue characteristics.

Tumors that have an atypical appearance on echocardiography deserve special consideration. Careful attention to the history and physical examination can help differentiate primary tumors from metastatic lesions. Ultrafast chest CT and MRI are excellent cardiac imaging modalities and frequently useful for atypical or potentially malignant lesions. MRI is excellent for soft tissue contrast and identification of vascular structures (without contrast material), although patients with indwelling devices, such as pacemakers or defibrillators, are not candidates for study. Newer CT techniques allow for multiplanar imaging and three-dimensional reconstructions, but intravenous contrast material is required. MRI and CT are extremely useful imaging techniques in nonmyxomatous cardiac tumors. Frequently, MRI can help differentiate cell type based on T1-weighted and T2-weighted images (e.g., lipoma versus fibroma), excluding the need for preoperative biopsy. Cardiac lesions that infiltrate from the pericardium are likely metastatic. Tumor infiltration of the myocardium or endocardium can be identified with either MRI or CT (rather than echocardiography) and is a sign of primary cardiac malignancy. Transvenous biopsy

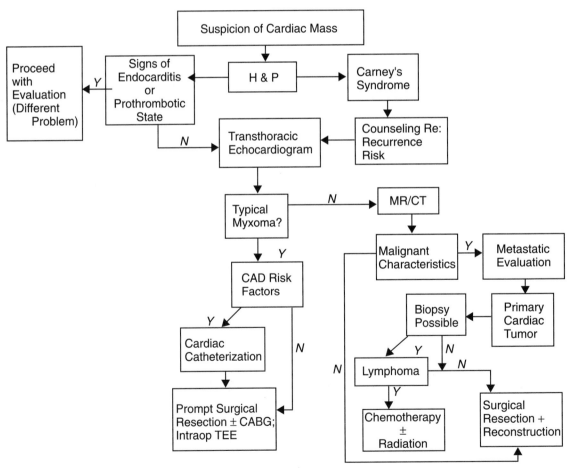

Figure 1
Treatment algorithm for patients with a cardiac mass. H&P, history and physical examination; MR/CT, magnetic resonance/computed tomography; CAD, coronary artery disease; CABG, coronary artery bypass graft; TEE, transesophageal echocardiography.

may be warranted when anatomically feasible, and in cases of lymphoma, surgery can be obviated by a tissue diagnosis preoperatively. Other signs of malignancy detected on contrast-enhanced CT or MRI include vascularity of the tumor and the presence of hemopericardium. When a large pericardial effusion is present, fluid sampling and cytologic examination can be diagnostic. Subxiphoid pericardiotomy, drainage of fluid, and pericardial biopsy may identify pericardial implants from metastatic disease.

Patients with an intracardiac mass and classic echocardiographic features of a myxoma should be prepared for the operating room and do not require multiple imaging studies. Surgical resection of a typical myxoma should not be delayed because the consequences of embolization in the interim between diagnosis and treatment can be catastrophic. Appropriate counseling and informed consent should be followed by surgical resection within 24 hours. In patients with risk factors for coronary artery disease, preoperative cardiac catheterization should be performed to determine need for concomitant coronary artery bypass graft surgery. Ventriculography is not necessary and carries a risk of dislodgment of tumor fragments and embolization. Patients with Carney's syndrome should undergo TEE, either preoperatively or intraoperatively, to evaluate thoroughly all cardiac chambers for multicentric lesions.

■ INDICATION FOR SURGERY

All patients with a cardiac mass having typical myxomatous characteristics should be considered for surgery because a curative resection is likely. Patients with atypical cardiac tumors also should be considered for resection because tumor growth and impingement or obstruction of blood flow may occur. Patients with potentially malignant lesions merit attempts at surgical resection because alternative therapy is usually ineffective. Malignant tumors may progress rapidly from localized, resectable lesions to become diffuse infiltrative and unresectable lesions within weeks. This aggressive growth precludes cardiac transplantation for most patients. There is little room for observation of intracardiac tumors except in children. Rhabdomyoma is the most common intracardiac mass in infants and children; 80% of these tumors regress spontaneously, so observation is indicated. Surgical resection in children occasionally is necessary due to obstructive symptoms.

■ TREATMENT

Standard cardiac anesthetic techniques are used. For patients with right atrial myxomas, Swan-Ganz catheterization is not necessary and risks tumor embolization. We consider TEE to be a routine component of intraoperative monitoring and recommend its use in all patients undergoing resection of cardiac tumor, unless specific contraindications apply. Median sternotomy is the preferred incision because it allows easy access to all cardiac chambers and is well tolerated. Full sternotomy is used; although partial sternal incisions are possible, we have found no significant advantage to this approach. Cardiopulmonary bypass is mandatory, and aortic cannulation is routine. Bicaval venous cannulation is used; direct cannulation of the superior vena cava improves exposure of the atrium. Right atriotomy is the incision most commonly used for resection of right and left atrial myxomas. Although a simultaneous left atriotomy incision can be used to facilitate location of a left atrial myxoma (the biatrial approach), precise TEE usually obviates the need for a left atriotomy. For the typical myxoma arising from the atrial septum, full-thickness resection of the septum and attached stalk from the right side allows deliverance of the tumor mass into the right atrium. Patching of the septum is performed routinely; we prefer autologous pericardium. Ventricular tumors are approached best through the tricuspid or mitral valves. Occasionally, transaortic resection is necessary. Full-thickness resection of ventricular myxomas is not necessary and carries undue risk. Only a small thickness of endocardium need be resected along with the mass.

The principle of complete resection applies to all cardiac tumors. Reconstruction of the right atrial free wall is frequently necessary with large, nonmyxomatous atrial tumors. Bovine pericardium makes an excellent passive right atrial conduit. Malignant tumors diagnosed preoperatively should be considered for complete resection when possible; cardiectomy and transplantation are possible, although logistically difficult and best performed at high-volume transplant centers.

Care of the patient after resection of an atrial myxoma is routine. General principles of cardiac surgical postoperative care, such as early extubation, early ambulation, and aggressive rehabilitation, apply. Patching of the atrial septum does not mandate anticoagulation with warfarin; aspirin therapy is sufficient. More extensive reconstructions of the heart may warrant short-term anticoagulation at the discretion of the surgeon.

■ PATHOLOGY

The typical myxoma has a gelatinous, smooth, "bunch-of-grapes" appearance with a short stalk arising from the endocardium, with varying sizes. More infrequently, myxomas may be hard, smooth, and sessile. Pedunculated tumors may be extremely friable; given their gross appearance and the aggressive motion of the cardiac cycle, it is remarkable that embolization does not occur more frequently. Histologically, myxomas are lined by a layer of endothelium cells and filled with a mucoid matrix. Mitotic figures are rare.

Malignant primary cardiac tumors are nearly all sarcomas, and nearly all types have been reported. Many are undifferentiated and defy classification by cell type. Tumors of the pericardium are usually metastatic, although primary mesotheliomas can occur. Benign cardiac tumors generally have a less friable gross appearance and can grow large depending on type, especially lipomas. Histologic type can be variable. A list of benign, nonmyxomatous cardiac tumors in descending order of frequency is given in Table 1.

■ RESULTS

The operative risk for resection of atrial myxoma is low. Perioperative mortality in a series of 100 patients over 40 years from the Mayo Clinic was 1%. Five-year survival free of recurrence of myxoma was 94% in this series. The 20-year Kaplan-Meier survival estimate was no different in patients after myxoma resection than in the general population. Recurrent myxomas are associated most frequently with Carney's syndrome. When recurrence occurs, reresection is indicated. Complete resection of nonmyxomatous benign cardiac masses would be expected to yield results comparable to myxomas, but large series do not exist. Life expectancy in patients with a malignant primary cardiac tumor is poor. Complete resection of sarcomas is difficult, and life expectancy is usually less than 1 year when complete resection is not possible. It is only slightly longer in patients after a complete resection.

Chemotherapy and radiation therapy are rarely effective, although case reports of longer survival exist.

SUGGESTED READING

Araoz PA, et al: CT and MR imaging of benign primary cardiac neoplasms with echocardiographic correlation, *Radiographics* 20:1303, 2000.

Becker AE: Primary heart tumors in the pediatric age group: a review of salient pathologic features relevant for clinicians, *Pediatr Cardiol* 21:317, 2000.

Schaaf HV, Mullany CJ: Surgery for cardiac myxomas, *Semin Thorac Cardiovasc Surg* 12:77, 2000.

Silverman NA: Primary cardiac tumors, *Ann Surg* 191:127, 1980.

TRAUMA TO THE HEART AND GREAT VESSELS

Anees J. Razzouk
Randall S. Fortuna

The two main mechanisms of injury to the heart and great vessels are blunt and penetrating trauma. The spectrum of injury varies from asymptomatic cardiac contusion to sudden death from rupture of the heart or thoracic aorta. Severe injuries most commonly are related to high-speed motor vehicle accidents and civilian violence. Modern advances in trauma care, including prehospital management and rapid transport, have allowed victims with serious injuries to survive long enough to reach the hospital. The trauma surgeon is presented with the challenge of providing rapid evaluation and prompt surgical intervention. Timely use of echocardiography (transthoracic or transesophageal), spiral computed tomography (CT), or angiography is essential for rapid diagnosis of complex injuries. With expeditious management, significant survival rates can be achieved even in patients who arrive at the emergency department in extremis and appear unstable or lifeless.

■ BLUNT INJURIES

Myocardial Contusion

Myocardial contusion is the most common injury in salvageable patients after blunt chest trauma. Although this clinical entity remains ill defined, it may result in cardiac

arrhythmia, valvular rupture, thromboembolism, congestive heart failure, late ventricular aneurysm, and chronic constrictive pericarditis. Tachyarrhythmias and conduction disturbances are the most common clinical manifestations of cardiac contusion; an initial electrocardiogram (ECG) is a useful diagnostic tool. CPK-MB and troponin levels are measured when concomitant myocardial infarction is suspected. Radionuclide scanning is not useful in the evaluation of patients with blunt chest trauma. Echocardiography is used as an adjunct in patients with persistent ECG abnormalities or unexplained hypotension to exclude functional and structural abnormalities of the heart. Because of its location immediately posterior to the sternum, the right ventricle is the most frequently injured chamber.

The prognosis of patients with cardiac contusion is generally excellent. Careful cardiac monitoring is essential for all patients. Arrhythmias are usually transient, a few require treatment, and most resolve before discharge without long-term therapy. Significant cardiac impairment with frank pump failure or instability should be treated aggressively with invasive hemodynamic monitoring, volume resuscitation, inotropic support, and, rarely, intraaortic balloon pump counterpulsation. With proper precautions, patients with myocardial contusion can undergo emergency surgery for associated injuries safely.

Coronary Artery Injuries

Coronary artery injuries from blunt chest trauma are rare. In descending order of frequency, left anterior descending artery, right coronary artery, and circumflex coronary artery injuries have been described. Laceration or rupture of a coronary artery can cause cardiac tamponade. Myocardial infarction in the setting of blunt trauma may result from acute coronary dissection, thrombosis, or aneurysm formation and warrants urgent coronary angiography. Early treatment of these injuries can limit the resultant infarct size and usually is associated with a low mortality. Asymptomatic, stable patients and patients with distal coronary artery thrombosis may be managed conservatively. Appropriate lesions may be treated with angioplasty and coronary artery stenting. Patients with ongoing ischemia or bleeding require direct intervention. Ligation of a distal or a secondary coronary artery commonly results in a small infarct but is well tolerated. Repair of a proximal injury to a large vessel usually requires urgent coronary artery bypass graft surgery, which often can be done without cardiopulmonary bypass. Use of a heparin-bonded circuit can obviate the need for full systemic heparinization when cardiopulmonary bypass is unavoidable. Access to the proximal left anterior descending and left main coronary arteries is improved by transecting the proximal main pulmonary artery using cardiopulmonary bypass.

Ventricular Aneurysms

Ventricular aneurysms, most commonly of the anterolateral wall of the left ventricle, are the result of myocardial damage with necrosis and scarring. Findings of recurrent arrhythmia, heart failure, and systemic emboli may develop weeks to years after the initial injury. Although the broad-based neck and paradoxical wall motion are seen easily by echocardiography, angiography is necessary to rule out associated coronary lesions. Elective surgical endoaneurysmorrhaphy improves left ventricular function and curtails potentially life-threatening complications. Long-term results are excellent.

Ventricular Septal Rupture

Ventricular septal rupture should be suspected in any patient with cardiac failure or a new systolic murmur after blunt chest trauma. Rupture of the septum may occur acutely after injury due to compression of the full heart during a vulnerable period or days later when a contused or aneurysmal septum subsequently perforates. The defect is identified easily by echocardiography. Right and left heart catheterization and coronary angiography allow precise calculation of the shunt and rule out associated coronary artery injury. Small defects with minimal shunting (pulmonary-to-systemic flow ratio <1.5) close spontaneously and are managed medically. Patients with severe congestive heart failure require early surgical closure to reduce the high mortality of this lesion. A prosthetic patch is usually necessary, and exposure of the defect may require a ventriculotomy through contused myocardium. If the patient can tolerate the shunt with medical therapy, however, repair can be delayed for 2 to 3 months to allow fibrosis of the defect edges, reducing the operative risk. Traumatic atrial septal defects are extremely rare.

Valvular Injuries

Valvular injuries due to blunt trauma are rare and most commonly involve the aortic valve, followed by the tricuspid and mitral valves. Patients with a small tear in an aortic cusp, most commonly noncoronary, may be asymptomatic for a week or more and can await elective repair. Rupture of one or more cusps causing acute aortic insufficiency is poorly tolerated, however. Findings of hemodynamic decompensation, arrhythmia, dyspnea, heart failure, or respiratory failure indicate the need for immediate surgical intervention. When primary repair of the damaged aortic valve is not possible, valve replacement becomes necessary and carries a low operative mortality. Damage to the mitral or tricuspid valve usually results in some degree of insufficiency caused by papillary muscle rupture, chordae tendineae disruption, or leaflet tear. The onset of symptoms may be immediate or delayed days to years after injury. Acute severe mitral valve regurgitation precipitates cardiac and respiratory decompensation with left-sided heart failure and pulmonary edema. Urgent management includes early surgical repair of chordal and leaflet rupture and possible annuloplasty, or in the case of papillary muscle rupture, valve replacement may be necessary. Although many patients tolerate traumatic isolated tricuspid regurgitation for many years, elective valvuloplasty is recommended to prevent progressive right ventricular dysfunction. Rupture of a papillary muscle is least favorable for repair and may require valve replacement.

Free Cardiac Rupture

Free cardiac rupture may occur at the time of blunt injury or a few days after myocardial contusion or infarction. The clinical presentation is dramatic; patients usually develop cardiac tamponade if the pericardium is intact or exsanguinate with massive hemothorax if the pericardium is injured. Sites of blunt cardiac rupture in survivors are the right atrium, left atrium, right ventricle, and left ventricle in descending order of frequency. When echocardiography is not available, pericardiocentesis may aid diagnosis of hemopericardium and provide temporary hemodynamic improvement. The key to survival is aggressive resuscitation in the emergency department and rapid transport to the operating room. The incision of choice is median sternotomy, which provides good exposure of all four cardiac chambers. If the patient shows hemodynamic deterioration and cannot be stabilized, left anterior thoracotomy through the fourth or fifth intercostal space is performed in the emergency department to open the pericardium, relieve tamponade, and control bleeding. For large injuries, a Foley catheter may be inserted through the rupture and inflated to control hemorrhage. Atrial injuries are controlled with vascular clamps and oversewn. Ventricular ruptures are controlled with digital compression and repaired primarily using pledgeted nonabsorbable mattress sutures. Cardiopulmonary bypass may be necessary for repair of complex wounds located in difficult areas, such as the atrioventricular groove.

Rupture of the Thoracic Aorta

Rupture of the thoracic aorta after blunt trauma causes immediate death in 80% to 90% of cases. In survivors, only the adventitia and mediastinal surrounding tissue precariously contain the acute pseudoaneurysm formed at the site of disruption. Successful outcome in these patients, who usually have multiple injuries, requires early recognition and prompt treatment. A strongly suggestive history (i.e., sudden deceleration in a motor vehicle accident or motor vehicle/pedestrian crash) or an abnormal chest radiograph (i.e., widening of the paraspinal line, contralateral deviation of an endotracheal or nasogastric tube, obscuring of aortic contour, presence of apical pleural capping, or depression of left main stem bronchus) warrants further diagnostic screening. High-quality spiral CT allows for rapid scanning of the entire chest and abdomen. Absence of mediastinal hemorrhage or direct signs of aortic injury by CT exclude the diagnosis of aortic disruption. Transesophageal echocardiography is useful in detecting aortic tears at the isthmus but is not reliable in evaluating injuries of the distal ascending aorta and proximal arch and arch vessels. Associated injuries, such as cervical spine or maxillofacial fractures, may render transesophageal echocardiography difficult to perform safely. In patients with stable hemodynamics, aortography (standard or intraarterial digital subtraction) has been the study of choice for definitive identification of injuries of the thoracic aorta and its branches.

Most aortic tears (90% to 95%) are located at the junction of the isthmus and the proximal descending aorta. Surgical repair is performed via left posterolateral thoracotomy through the fourth intercostal space. Double-lumen endotracheal intubation or the use of a bronchial blocker allows deflation of the left lung to improve surgical exposure. Rapid volume infusion for resuscitation or use of β-blockers can prevent fluctuation in blood pressure. Proximal control of the aortic arch between the left carotid artery and the left subclavian artery can be achieved via a transpericardial incision anterior to the phrenic nerve or an extrapericardial approach. Dissection of the distal aorta is minimized, and all uninterrupted intercostal arteries are preserved. Primary, direct repair of the torn aorta has several advantages over use of a prosthetic tube or patch and is the preferred method of repair in children. In complex injuries (i.e., spiral transection, or distal dissection with flap), an interposition tube graft expedites reconstruction of the disrupted aorta. Controversy continues regarding the optimal method of spinal cord protection during repair of aortic injury. The clamp and sew technique is simple; does not require extra incisions; and avoids complications associated with cannulation, bypass, and heparinization. When the repair cannot be completed in less than 30 minutes of aortic cross-clamping, however, the use of bypass to perfuse the distal aorta may reduce spinal cord ischemia. Distal circulatory support can be passive using a shunt (from ascending aorta or left ventricle to descending aorta or femoral artery) or active using a femoral artery–femoral vein bypass, left heart bypass (e.g., left atrial to femoral artery), or total cardiopulmonary bypass. The use of a heparin-coated circuit or heparin-free centrifugal pump can reduce the bleeding complications associated with systemic heparinization of trauma victims. The incidence of paraplegia (5% to 7%) and mortality rates of 15% to 20% are independent of the technique of repair.

Injuries of the ascending aorta are approached via median sternotomy and may require cardiopulmonary bypass. Profound hypothermic circulatory arrest or low flow may be necessary to repair rare complex injuries of the aortic arch. Early surgical repair has been the standard treatment for any aortic injury. Patients with severe associated injuries, particularly to the brain, lungs, or heart, may benefit from delayed repair, however. Meanwhile, close hemodynamic and radiographic monitoring and aggressive antihypertensive therapy (β-blockers and vasodilators) can minimize the risk of rupture. Endovascular stent grafts have been used successfully to defer repair of subacute or chronic aortic pseudoaneurysms. Occlusion of the left subclavian artery, arm ischemia, and compression of the left main bronchus by the thrombosed pseudoaneurysms may complicate use of these stent grafts. It is likely that future technical developments will make endoluminal grafting an effective and less invasive treatment for acute aortic tears from blunt trauma.

Injuries to the Brachiocephalic and Left Carotid Artery

Injuries to the brachiocephalic and left carotid artery are approached via a limited upper sternotomy (Figure 1A and B). Repair may consist of patch angioplasty or oversewing of the aorta at the site of tear and constructing a bypass graft from the ascending aorta to the avulsed vessel (Figure 1C). Injury of the proximal left subclavian artery is best approached via a left thoracotomy.

■ PENETRATING CARDIAC TRAUMA

The clinical presentation of penetrating cardiac injuries ranges from deceptive hemodynamic stability to acute circulatory collapse and cardiac arrest. Of patients with penetrating cardiac wounds, 80% die at the scene of injury or in transit. Prompt transport to a trauma center without delay from attempting field resuscitation increases survival in patients with penetrating heart injury. High-velocity missile injuries produce massive tissue destruction and hemorrhage with little chance for survival. Stab wounds to the ventricles can often seal, allowing patients to arrive alive at the hospital. The right ventricle most commonly is injured, followed by the left ventricle and right atrium. Injury to the heart is suspected in any patient who sustains penetrating trauma in an area inferior to the clavicles, superior to the costal margins, and medial to the midclavicular lines.

Cardiac Penetration

Cardiac penetration may lead to severe hemorrhage when the pericardial sac is open or may cause cardiac tamponade. Pericardial tamponade offers a protective effect by limiting extrapericardial bleeding and is a critical independent factor in patient survival. The classic Beck's triad of tamponade (distended neck veins, muffled heart sounds, and hypotension) and pulsus paradoxus are present in less than 10% of cases. Echocardiography is the diagnostic test of choice in stable patients to detect pericardial effusion before clinical signs of impending collapse. Patients with stable vital signs and hypotensive patients who respond to resuscitative measures should be transported to the operating room for definitive repair. Median sternotomy is the incision of choice for exploring penetrating injuries of the heart and mediastinum. An additional anterior thoracotomy or "hook" incision is helpful for repair of coexisting thoracic trauma. The left anterolateral thoracotomy incision is used most often in the emergency department for resuscitating patients in extremis. This incision can be extended across the sternum as bilateral anterolateral thoracotomies if the patient's injuries involve the right hemithorax. Both internal mammary arteries are sacrificed and must be ligated at the completion of the procedure.

Immediate intubation, aggressive fluid resuscitation, and early emergency department left anterolateral thoracotomy

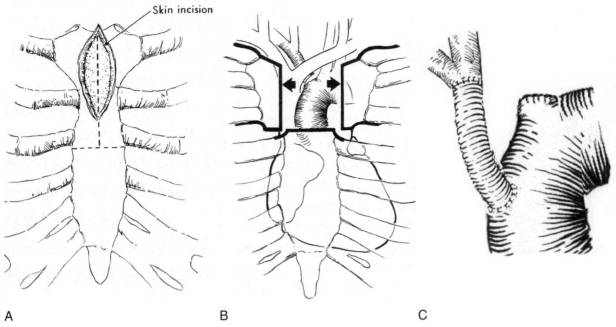

Figure 1
A, Limited skin incision and inverted T upper sternotomy. **B,** Exposure of ascending aorta, brachiocephalic artery, and left common carotid artery through a limited upper sternotomy. **C,** Repair of brachiocephalic artery transection with bypass graft from the ascending aorta. *(Adapted from Sakopoulos AG, et al:* J Vas Surg *31:200, 2000.)*

are indicated for penetrating heart wounds with agonal state or recent cardiac arrest, deterioration or cardiac arrest after initial stabilization, or uncontrolled hemorrhage from a thoracostomy tube. In the case of exsanguinating hemorrhage, clamping the descending aorta preserves cerebral and coronary blood flow. Tamponade is relieved by opening the pericardial sac through a longitudinal incision anterior to the phrenic nerve. Patients with tamponade from an anterior penetrating stab wound of the heart, a short prehospital time, and vital signs on admission have the highest survival (80%) after emergency department thoracotomy. The use of a skin stapler to occlude temporarily lacerations in the cardiac muscle provides effective control of hemorrhage and allows expedient transfer to the operating room for definitive cardiorrhaphy.

Hemodynamically stable patients suspected by echocardiography of having a cardiac injury should undergo subxiphoid pericardial window in the operating room. When the exploration is dry, pericardial lavage to liberate any clotted blood within the sac can improve the specificity of this procedure. If a cardiac injury is confirmed, the vertical incision is extended as a median sternotomy for cardiorrhaphy.

Ventricular Wounds
Ventricular wounds are repaired by digitally occluding the laceration while placing horizontal mattress sutures over polytetrafluoroethylene (Teflon) or pericardial pledgets. Lacerations in proximity to the coronary arteries require placement of the mattress sutures beneath the vessels.

Coronary Artery Lacerations to Major Vessels
Coronary artery lacerations to major vessels may be repaired primarily or bypassed using a vein graft, with or without cardiopulmonary bypass. Smaller coronary branches that are lacerated are managed by ligation.

Atrial and Vena Cava Injuries
Atrial and vena cava injuries are repaired with running, nonabsorbable suture. Initial control of bleeding is achieved using a vascular clamp, bullhorn, or Foley balloon. A short period of total inflow occlusion of the heart (1 to 3 minutes) may help the repair of complex injuries on the superior or inferior atriocaval junction.

Ventricular Septal Defects
Ventricular septal defects usually are detected late after penetrating cardiac trauma. Small defects close spontaneously. Delayed symptoms of congestive heart failure are associated with a pulmonary-to-systemic shunt ratio of greater than 2:1, and these defects should be closed surgically. Repairs are done similar to repairs for congenital defects.

Foreign Bodies
Foreign bodies in the pericardial cavity or the myocardium should be removed to avoid pericarditis, delayed tamponade, or conduction defects. Missiles in the cardiac chambers are localized by transesophageal echocardiography and removed to avoid embolization.

Iatrogenic Cardiac Injuries

Iatrogenic cardiac injuries may occur during cardiac catheterization. Urgent surgical intervention is indicated in traumatic coronary artery injuries complicating balloon, laser, and atherectomy angioplasties and transmyocardial perforation associated with radiofrequency ablation. Survival exceeds 97% despite the 5% incidence of perioperative infarction.

SUGGESTED READING

Asensio JA, et al: Penetrating cardiac injuries, *Surg Clin North Am* 76:685, 1996.

Feliciano DV, Rozycki GS: Advances in the diagnosis and treatment of thoracic trauma, *Surg Clin North Am* 79:1417, 1999.

Razzouk AJ, et al: Repair of traumatic aortic rupture, *Arch Surg* 135:913, 2000.

Wall MJ, et al: Acute management of complex cardiac injuries, *J Trauma* 42:905, 1997.

SURGICAL MANAGEMENT OF PERICARDIAL DISEASE

Patrick DeValeria

Steven J. Lester

The pericardium can be affected by a variety of disease processes. The three conditions that most frequently require surgical intervention are constrictive pericarditis, cardiac tamponade, and recurrent effusive disease. In recent years, advances in invasive hemodynamic measurements, echocardiography, computed tomography, and magnetic resonance imaging have led to improvements in the diagnosis of these disease states, have demonstrated the physiology of tamponade and constriction, and have aided in the often difficult differentiation between pericardial constriction and myocardial restriction.

■ ETIOLOGY

The spectrum of pericardial disease is changing. Tuberculous pericarditis, once common, is now a rare disease. Iatrogenic pericardial disease resulting from cardiac surgery and interventional cardiovascular procedures is becoming a common cause of symptomatic pericardial disease. As more cancer patients are diagnosed and treated, more malignant and radiation-induced pericardial disease is being seen. Many patients with pericardial disease still have an idiopathic disease presumed to be infectious, but the majority are likely due to an autoimmune or autoreactive process.

■ CLINICAL PRESENTATION AND DIAGNOSTIC MODALITIES

Constrictive Pericarditis

Any condition that causes pericardial inflammation can result in constrictive pericarditis. Regardless of etiology, the final common pathway is adherence of the visceral and parietal pericardial layers, reducing pericardial compliance and impairing diastolic filling. As with cardiac tamponade, the basic physiologic abnormality is the inability of the cardiac chambers to fill sufficiently during diastole. In constriction, early diastolic filling is normal with subsequent abrupt cessation of filling when the maximum volume of the pericardium is reached. In cardiac tamponade, ventricular filling is impaired throughout diastole.

The two basic physiologic principles in constrictive pericarditis are ventricular interdependence and dissociation of intrathoracic and intracardiac pressures. In the appropriate clinical setting, the diagnosis of constriction is based on the physical examination and investigations that can detail constrictive physiology.

Physical Examination

Distended neck veins are essentially always present in constriction. In constriction, filling occurs in early diastole and the elevated pressures result in a rapid y descent as opposed to the absent or delayed y descent seen in tamponade. In constriction, Kussmaul's sign (absence of an inspiratory drop in the mean venous pressure) is seen. An early diastolic sound ("pericardial knock") may be heard on auscultation as ventricular filling is abruptly halted.

Cardiac Catheterization

Traditionally, the diagnosis of constrictive pericarditis in the heart catheterization laboratory has been based on the following findings:

1. A dip-and-plateau diastolic pressure tracing ("square-root sign") with elevated and equalized end-diastolic pressures in all four cardiac chambers

2. Left ventricular end-diastolic pressure/right ventricular end-diastolic pressure less than 5 mmHg
3. Pulmonary artery systolic pressure less than 50 mmHg
4. Right ventricular diastolic pressure divided by the right ventricular systolic pressure greater than one third

These hemodynamic criteria are characteristic but not pathognomonic of constriction; they can be seen in restrictive diseases that alter diastolic filling. Therefore, it is important to obtain additional hemodynamic data that will highlight the basic physiology of constriction, ventricular interdependence, and dissociation between intrathoracic and intracardiac pressures, such as the following.

1. Simultaneous right and left ventricular pressure tracings to highlight ventricular interdependence (Figure 1). During inspiration, right ventricular pressure will increase while left ventricular pressure will decrease in apposition to the concordant respirophasic changes in right and left ventricular pressures seen in normal circumstances. In addition, during inspiration right ventricular filling will be more complete.
2. Simultaneous pulmonary capillary wedge pressure (PCWP) and left ventricular pressure tracings to highlight the dissociation between intrathoracic and intracardiac pressures (Figure 2). During inspiration, the drop in intrathoracic pressure is not transmitted to the cardiac chambers, resulting in a reduction in the pressure gradient seen between the PCWP and the left ventricle.

Echocardiography

Two-dimensional and Doppler echocardiography provide the cornerstone for the diagnosis of constrictive pericarditis. The tomographic images provided by the echocardiogram may reveal a thickened and calcified pericardium, a dilated inferior vena cava, and the characteristic septal bounce resulting from ventricular interdependence. However, it is the unique respirophasic changes in ventricular filling and venous flow detailed in the Doppler examination that are most helpful. These include:

1. Respiratory variation in the early mitral filling (E wave) velocity. Due to the dissociation between intrathoracic and intracardiac pressures, during inspiration there will be a drop in the E wave velocity. It has been suggested that one should see a greater than 25% respirophasic variation in the E wave velocity. However, the magnitude of the respirophasic change in the E wave velocity lacks the sensitivity needed to be the sole criterion used to definitively exclude constrictive pericarditis. A more important screen for the diagnosis of constrictive pericarditis is a restrictive mitral filling pattern (Figure 3). If a restrictive filling pattern is noted, additional Doppler data, as outlined later, are mandated.
2. Increased diastolic flow reversal velocity in the hepatic vein with expiration. Although there are respirophasic changes in the flow reversal velocities in restrictive heart disease, in difference to constriction, these occur during inspiration (Figure 4). *I find a dilated IVC with*

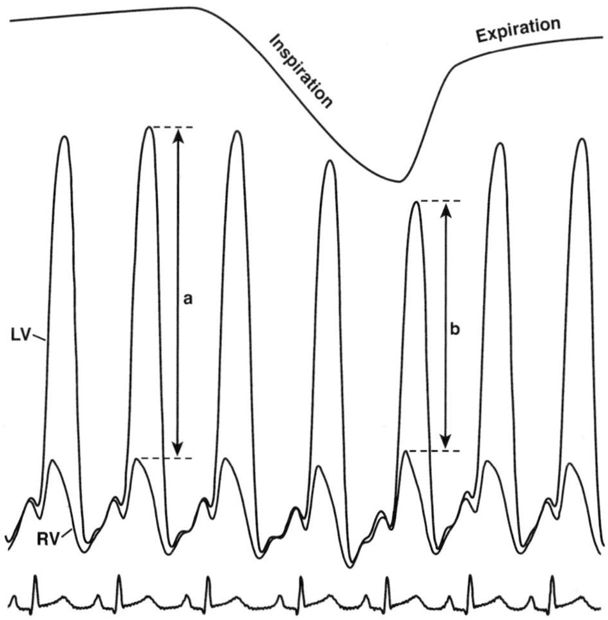

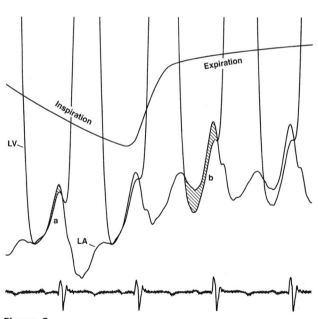

Figure 1
Simultaneous left (LV) and right (RV) ventricular pressure tracings highlighting ventricular interdependence. During inspiration RV filling is increased, increasing RV pressure at the expense of LV filling where LV pressure is reduced (a>b).

Figure 2
Simultaneous left ventricular (LV) and left atrial (LA) pressure tracings highlighting the dissociation between intrathoracic and intraventricular pressures. During inspiration there is little separation in the LV and LA diastolic pressures in difference to the separation seen during expiration (b>a).

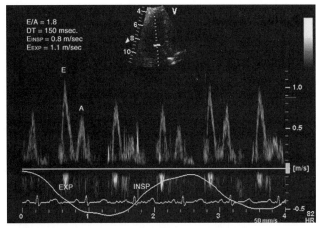

Figure 3
Pulsed-wave Doppler recording of the mitral inflow from a patient with constrictive pericarditis. A restrictive filling pattern, E/A ratio > 1.5 and a deceleration time (DT) < 160 ms, is noted along with an accentuated change in the E-wave velocity between inspiratory (INSP) and expiratory (EXP) phases of respiration.

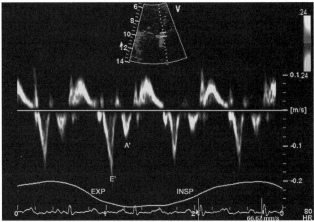

Figure 5
Doppler tissue imaging recording of the mitral annular velocities from a patient with constrictive pericarditis. Note that although the early filling component (E') varies with respiration, the velocity remains > 10 cm/sec. A', annular motion following atrial contraction; EXP, expiration; INSP, inspiration.

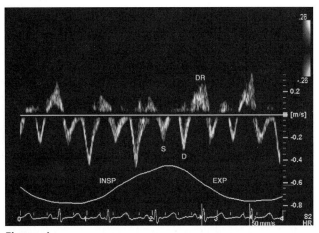

Figure 4
Pulsed-wave Doppler recording of hepatic vein flow velocities from a patient with constrictive pericarditis. Note the reduced diastolic forward flow (D) and the accentuated diastolic flow reversal (DR) during the expiratory (EXP) phase of respiration. S, systolic forward flow velocity; INSP, inspiratory phase of respiration.

the characteristic respirophasic changes in the hepatic venous flow velocities most faithful in confirming the diagnosis of constrictive pericarditis.
3. Mitral annular velocity during the early contribution to filling (E') greater than 10 cm/sec (Figure 5). Because restrictive heart diseases directly affect the myocardium, the relaxation properties of the left ventricle are impaired, in difference to constriction; hence in restrictive heart diseases the mitral annular velocities will be reduced.

4. Respirophasic change in the superior vena caval (SVC) flow velocities less than 20 cm/sec. Enhanced respiratory effort can cause respirophasic changes in Doppler flow velocities. The SVC Doppler data help to exclude this.

Computed Tomography and Magnetic Resonance Imaging

These two imaging modalities may be useful to confirm the diagnosis of constrictive pericarditis by further detailing the thickness of the pericardium. However, constrictive physiology *may* be present even if pericardial thickness is normal. The diagnosis of constriction should *never* be excluded simply on anatomic criteria alone.

Cardiac Tamponade

Cardiac tamponade is impairment of ventricular filling due to increased intrapericardial pressure. The elevated intrapericardial pressure results from increased pericardial contents, such as effusions, pus, gas, or blood. Unless recognized and promptly treated, cardiac tamponade can be fatal.

The diagnosis of tamponade should be considered in any patient with hypotension and elevated neck veins. Cardiac tamponade is a *clinical* diagnosis; investigations such as echocardiography confirm the presence of pericardial contents and evaluate their hemodynamic significance.

Physical Examination

A clinically significant elevation in intrapericardial pressure will usually result in increased resting heart rate (>90 bpm). The neck veins will be distended with the characteristic reduced or delayed y descent (see Constrictive Pericarditis, above). Kussmaul's sign (see Constrictive Pericarditis, above) is absent in tamponade and, if noted, signifies a component of constriction. A careful evaluation of the blood pressure may show pulsus paradoxus, defined as a drop in systolic arterial pressure greater than 10 mm Hg during inspiration. Although characteristic of tamponade, pulsus paradoxus is not specific for this condition. It may be seen in conditions where there is a reduction in inspiratory forward stroke volume, such as massive pulmonary emboli, pulmonary hypertension, right ventricular infarction, acute hypotension, and obstructive lung disease. In addition, when there is focal cardiac compression (usually localized postsurgical thrombus), extreme hypotension, severe aortic regurgitation, or an atrial septal defect, pulsus paradoxus may be absent despite the presence of a hemodynamically significant elevation in intrapericardial pressures.

Echocardiography

An echocardiogram should be obtained in all patients in whom the history and physical examination suggest tamponade. The initial approach is to identify the contents, most often fluid, in the pericardial space. M-mode, two-dimensional, and Doppler evaluations are then used to determine the hemodynamic significance of the pericardial contents.

M-Mode and Two-Dimensional Echocardiographic Findings

1. Dilated inferior vena cava (IVC) with an inappropriate respiratory response (<50% reduction in IVC size with inspiration). If the IVC is not dilated, the diagnosis of cardiac tamponade should be questioned. However, patients who are mechanically ventilated with positive end-expiratory pressures have a dilated IVC; hence this finding is of little clinical value in these patients.
2. Diastolic inversion or collapse of right ventricle and right atrial free wall. The heart rate in patients with tamponade is elevated. Because of its increased temporal resolution, M-mode echocardiography best facilitates appreciation of the diastolic collapse of the cardiac chambers. In patients with pulmonary hypertension or those who have had cardiac surgery or trauma, diastolic collapse of the right ventricle may be absent because of pericardial adhesions or loculated effusions. Loculated, usually postsurgical effusions adjacent to the left ventricle can cause isolated left ventricular diastolic collapse.
3. Abnormal motion of the interventricular septum.

Doppler Echocardiographic Findings

These include accentuated reciprocal respirophasic changes in the ventricular filling velocities and stroke volumes. During inspiration, the transmitral E wave velocity will decrease and the transtricuspid E wave velocity will increase. These Doppler findings are sensitive to the increase in intrapericardial pressure and generally occur prior to the anatomic abnormalities (see earlier). If the respirophasic changes in ventricular filling velocities do not resolve after pericardiocentesis, a component of constriction is likely present.

■ SURGICAL INDICATIONS

We consider all patients with a well-documented diagnosis of pericardial constriction to be surgical candidates provided there are no significant medical contraindications. Primary surgical therapy is used in cases of symptomatic effusions that are either inaccessible or loculated (primarily the posterolateral regions of the pericardium), recurrent effusions, and frequently for symptomatic effusions after coronary artery bypass graft surgery.

A careful preoperative evaluation is essential when radiation-induced constrictive pericarditis is a possibility, as these patients often do poorly with surgical intervention and have an early mortality approaching 25% to 35%. Radiotherapy has late effects on all cardiac tissue and causes mediastinal fibrosis, interstitial pulmonary disease, and impaired wound healing. These factors contribute to poor outcome in this subgroup of patients. Evaluation must also address concomitant coronary artery or valvular heart disease.

■ SURGICAL APPROACHES

Pericardiocentesis

Pericardiocentesis should be the first modality for effusive diseases, and is generally performed under echocardiographic guidance. Transthoracic echocardiography is used to identify the largest accumulation of fluid and the target for the pericardiocentesis needle. The two-dimensional ultrasound image will provide an estimate of the distance the needle must travel to reach the pericardial space. Our practice is to use a long angiocath (intravenous line). Confirmation that the angiocath is in the pericardial space is obtained by use of agitated saline contrast injections and echocardiographic imaging. A wire is then placed through the angiocath. The angiocath is removed, and a 6 Fr sheath with a dilator is inserted over the wire. The wire and dilator are then removed, and the position of the sheath is confirmed with the use of agitated saline and echocardiographic imaging. A pigtail catheter is inserted through the sheath. The sheath is pulled back, and the pigtail catheter is secured in place. The side port of the sheath is then cut off, and the sheath is secured to the catheter with tape. The authors prefer this method, which incorporates the insertion of the sheath as it facilitates the insertion of the pigtail catheter. To avoid the potential of collapsing the drainage catheter, it is our practice to drain most of the effusion by hand through a syringe before attaching to a Hemovac-style drainage system.

Subxiphoid Pericardial Window

A subxiphoid pericardial window may be used to drain recurrent or loculated effusions that compromise hemodynamics. A significant amount of tissue can be removed for culture and pathologic assessment as well. Only a limited amount of the pericardium is accessible, so it is not an effective therapy for constriction. The subxiphoid approach is less effective than complete pericardiectomy in preventing recurrent effusions. However, the recurrence rate is still less than 10%.

The subxiphoid approach can be performed under local anesthesia if there is significant concern over hemodynamic collapse with the use of general anesthesia. A 4- to 8-cm vertical incision is created in the midline over the xiphoid and upper abdomen. The dissection is carried down through the soft tissues, with mobilization of the xiphoid and division of the linea alba. The xiphoid may be removed if necessary to aid exposure. A retractor is used to lift the xiphoid and inferior sternum, and the soft tissue and diaphragmatic fibers dissected inferiorly to identify the pericardium. The pericardium may be grasped with forceps, tissue clamp, or a suture passed through it for retraction and then opened to release the tension of the effusion. Care must be taken to not damage the myocardium during this initial incision. A 4- to 6-cm patch of pericardium may be excised and sent for pathologic assessment and culture. Fluid is also collected for culture and cytology. A finger or suction catheter is used to break up fluid loculations inferiorly and laterally. A right-angled chest tube is placed beneath the cardiac apex and brought out through a separate stab incision lateral to the midline. The linea alba is closed with interrupted, nonabsorbable sutures, and the soft tissues are reapproximated. We typically leave the drainage tubes in place for a minimum of 36 hours or until the drainage is less than 100 ml for a 24-hour period. It is important to completely evacuate the effusion. Intraoperative transesophageal echocardiography (TEE) can be helpful in determining that adequate drainage has been accomplished.

Median Sternotomy

The authors prefer the median sternotomy approach in cases of complete pericardiectomy for constriction and recurrent effusion. This provides excellent exposure of the atria, ventricles, and cavae and gives easy access for cardiopulmonary bypass if required for instability or bleeding. Manipulation of the heart is required to free the lateral aspect of the left ventricle, but this can be minimized by placing the table in steep Trendelenburg position and rotating the patient to the right when freeing the lateral left ventricle.

The operative procedure uses standard cardiovascular monitoring techniques, including use of TEE. Once sternotomy is completed, great care should be taken to identify and mobilize the innominate vein and release the adhesions between the inner table of the sternum and surrounding tissues to prevent bleeding when the retractor is spread. While we attempt to perform complete pericardiectomy off cardiopulmonary bypass in every case, cardiopulmonary bypass should be available for all patients. The dissection is typically begun at the diaphragmatic surface of the pericardium, where small fluid collections are often located, and extended over the left ventricle first. A plane of dissection must be identified between the parietal pericardium and epicardium to prevent epicardial bleeding. If no free space can be identified, a knife blade is used to incise the thickened pericardium, until the bulging myocardium protrudes into the incision. As a flap is created, it can be used as a retraction handle to develop the dissection plane. It is important to free the left ventricle first to prevent acute right ventricular failure. This is believed to be caused by releasing the right side of the heart, allowing for increased right ventricular filling in the face of persistent high right ventricular afterload created by persistent constriction of left ventricular filling.

The pericardium is removed, leaving approximately a 1-cm margin of pericardium anterior to the left phrenic nerve. The diaphragmatic pericardium is removed to free the inferior aspect of the left ventricle and apex of the heart. The dissection plane is then carried over the right ventricle,

again leaving a margin of pericardium around the phrenic nerve. Identification of the phrenic nerves can be difficult in some cases. Opening the pleural spaces may aid in determining the course of the nerves. The plane of dissection ultimately is carried out over the cavae and atria, if they are involved in the constrictive process. Islands of pericardium can be left behind and is preferable to causing cardiac injury. Calcified plates and plaques should be resected and often a Freer elevator and rongeurs are required for the task. Calcification embedded into the myocardium should be left alone.

In some cases, a constricting layer of visceral pericardium or epicardium may be encountered. This must either be resected or scored with a knife until the myocardium bulges through the constrictive layer. Once the procedure is completed, any associated pleural effusions should be drained and the chest closed over mediastinal drains in standard fashion.

Left Anterior Thoracotomy

Some surgical groups prefer left anterior thoracotomy to perform complete pericardiectomy for recurrent effusion or constrictive pericarditis. Although initially described for draining pericardial effusions, a limited pericardiectomy via thoracotomy approach has no benefit over subxiphoid pericardiectomy and is less well tolerated by debilitated patients. There is no evidence to suggest that the surgically created "pleuropericardial window" remains patent. In constrictive disease states, a left anterior thoracotomy affords good access to the left ventricle but limits exposure to the lateral right ventricle and right atrium.

The patient is positioned with the left chest angled to 45 angles and the left femoral region prepared into the field to allow access for femoral-femoral cardiopulmonary bypass, if necessary. The incision is made over the fifth interspace from the lateral aspect of the sternum to the posterior axillary line. The mammary artery frequently must be divided. A retractor is placed, and the parietal pleura and intercostal muscles further divided to improve exposure. The lung is mobilized superiorly and a linear incision made in the pericardium, anterior to the phrenic nerve. This is carried out from the pulmonary artery to the diaphragm. The proper plane between the parietal pericardium and epicardium must be identified and maintained to prevent epicardial tears. Resection can be carried out anterior and posterior to the left phrenic nerve, preserving a strip of pericardium in which the nerve and companion vessels course to the diaphragm. The resection is carried out over the right ventricle as far as possible. Technical details regarding the dissection are the same as described with the median sternotomy approach.

Thoracoscopic Pericardial Window

Some authors have advocated a video-assisted thoracic surgery (VATS) approach for management of pericardial effusions. This allows for removal of a larger section of the pericardium than the subxiphoid approach but requires use of a double-lumen endotracheal tube. The VATS approach also allows for drainage of any associated pleural effusion. This can be performed from either side of the chest, but the left is preferable. Three access ports are commonly used, one in the region of the anterior axillary line at the sixth interspace and two more in the posterior axillary line at the fifth and eighth interspaces. Not only is a free pleural space required for the technique, but a free pericardial space is necessary to prevent possible cardiac injury. Any evidence of pericardial thickening or fusion should cause the surgeon to reconsider use of VATS techniques.

Once the ports are in place the inferior pulmonary ligament should be mobilized with cautery and the phrenic nerve identified. The bulging pericardium is grasped and incised with endoscopic scissors. A 3-by-3-cm window can be created both above and below the phrenic nerve. Care must be taken to leave a margin of pericardium around the phrenic nerve. Closure over a chest tube is by standard techniques.

The indications for VATS drainage of pericardial effusions are still under debate. There is no indication for VATS pericardiectomy in constrictive pericarditis.

■ RESULTS

Pericardiectomy can be a challenging and tedious operation. Myocardial injury, phrenic nerve damage, acute right ventricular failure, and incomplete decortication of the ventricles are potential complications. Cardiac deconditioning with myocardial atrophy, acute right ventricular overload, and direct myocardial injury may contribute to immediate postoperative low-output syndrome. Early recognition of this state with institution of appropriate inotropic or mechanical support can stabilize the patient and allow time for myocardial recovery. Milrinone, with its properties of both inotropic augmentation and reduction in pulmonary vascular resistance, can be particularly beneficial in cases of acute right ventricular distention.

Pericardiectomy is usually well tolerated by patients; the 30-day operative mortality is between 5% and 8% in most series. Incomplete pericardiectomy has been shown to correlate with worse operative survival. Long-term survival varies depending on the patient population. Actuarial survival at 5 and 10 years is approximately 70% and 50%, respectively. Patients with a history of malignancy, prior radiation exposure, advanced New York Heart Association (NYHA) symptoms, and advanced age all have a poorer survival after pericardiectomy. Patients with a history of radiation exposure have not demonstrated a substantial benefit from pericardiectomy. Several studies have shown that this subpopulation of patients has a markedly increased early and late mortality and a 1-year survival of 50% or less. This poor outcome has been attributed to radiation-induced myocardial damage, difficulty in obtaining a complete resection, and associated pulmonary fibrosis from the radiation.

Patients without a history of radiation exposure demonstrate a significant improvement in NYHA functional class. Several retrospective studies have shown that nearly 90% of patients improve in functional class, and approximately 80% remain free of congestive heart failure symptoms at 5 years.

SUGGESTED READING

Boonyaratavej S, et al: Comparison of mitral inflow and superior vena cava Doppler velocities in chronic obstructive pulmonary disease and constrictive pericarditis, *J Am Coll Cardiol* 32:2043, 1998.

DeValeria PA, et al: Current indications, risks and outcome after pericardiectomy, *Ann Thorac Surg* 52:219, 1991.

Hatle LK, et al: Differentiation of constrictive pericarditis and restrictive cardiomyopathy by Doppler echocardiograph, *Circulation* 79:357, 1989.

Hurrell DG, et al: Value of dynamic respiratory changes in left and right ventricular pressures for the diagnosis of constrictive pericarditis, *Circulation* 93:2007, 1996.

Ling LH, et al: Constrictive pericarditis in the modern era: evolving clinical spectrum and impact on outcome after pericardiectomy, *Circulation* 100:1380, 1999.

VIDEO-ASSISTED THORACIC SURGERY AND PERICARDIAL EFFUSIVE DISEASES

Malcolm M. DeCamp, Jr.

Patients with effusive diseases of the pericardium present a challenge and a dilemma for the surgeon. Most patients have significant comorbidities or an advanced underlying malignancy confounding clinical decision making. The dilemma is the acute life-threatening hemodynamics of tamponade juxtaposed with the often dismal prognosis relative to their associated diseases. The challenge is to palliate effectively the acute cardiovascular compromise with minimal morbidity. Historically, surgical intervention required either formal thoracotomy or a subxiphoid approach; the former was associated with substantial incisional morbidity, and the latter was complicated by a higher risk of recurrence. The advent of video-assisted thoracic surgery (VATS) allows for the superior exposure offered by thoracotomy coupled with the patient comfort issues associated with port-access surgery.

■ PRESENTATION AND EVALUATION

More than half of patients requiring intervention for asymptomatic pericardial effusion have a history of malignancy. Other predisposing factors include uremia, viral infection, collagen vascular disease with associated serositis, drug-induced, radiotherapy-induced, post–myocardial infarction syndrome, and postcardiotomy syndrome. Symptoms are frequent and range from dramatic, such as syncope, dyspnea, palpitations, or acute chest pain, to more subtle complaints, including fatigue, dull aches, or chest heaviness. Most patients manifest Beck's triad of hypotension, tachycardia, and muffled heart tones. Evidence of cervical and abdominal venous hypertension, such as distended neck veins and hepatomegaly, and a pulsus paradoxus is common.

Standard chest radiographs support the clinical suspicion of pericardial effusion but are not diagnostic. Cardiomegaly is a consistent finding. One third of patients have a coexistent pleural effusion, an important observation when planning surgical intervention. Echocardiography is the diagnostic study of choice to confirm a pericardial effusion. Whether transthoracic or transesophageal, echocardiography can define the anatomy (size, location, and character) and the physiologic implications of the fluid. Echocardiographic signs of tamponade include diastolic collapse of the right atrium and right ventricle, dilation of the inferior vena cava, and reversal of the flow across the mitral valve. These are all signs indicative of inadequate diastolic filling, leading to decreased stroke volume and rate-dependent cardiac output. Echocardiography has largely supplanted right heart catheterization in the diagnosis of tamponade. The classic catheterization findings of equilibration of diastolic pressures across the right and left cardiac structures (right atrium, right ventricle, pulmonary artery, left atrium, and left ventricle [pulmonary capillary wedge pressure]) are definitive. When preload is severely limited, patients manifest signs and symptoms of cardiogenic shock with cool extremities, oliguria, and altered mental status. With this extreme presentation, an acute intervention, such as pericardiocentesis, is necessary to facilitate diagnosis and allow safer but more definitive therapy at a later date.

■ INDICATIONS

Definitive pericardial drainage is necessary therapy for patients with symptomatic recurrent, loculated, or malignant effusions. Malignant pericardial effusions are almost certain to recur after pericardiocentesis. The choice of definitive drainage technique should be based on an assessment of the prognosis of patients. Patients who have viable oncologic treatment options (i.e., many breast cancer patients) are reasonable candidates for a pericardial window. Viable treatment options include creation of a window into the pleural space, the peritoneum, or the preperitoneal space. Usurping the large absorptive surface of the pleura or peritoneum is a more appealing approach physiologically, and these techniques have better long-term success rates compared with the subxiphoid approach. Specific clinical indications favoring VATS include posterior loculated pericardial collections, such as seen after cardiac surgery, coexistent pleural or pulmonary/parenchymal disease. VATS allows the surgeon to address the pleural or parenchymal pathology and the pericardial process with a single surgical approach.

■ TECHNIQUE

Any pericardial resection for effusive disease requires appropriate treatment of tamponade physiology before the induction of general anesthesia. These patients have a fixed stroke volume and rate-dependent cardiac output with high levels of circulating endogenous catecholamines. The induction of general anesthesia is sympatholytic and can precipitate cardiovascular collapse. Recognition of these physiologic principles underscores the need for cooperation between surgeons, cardiologists, and anesthesiologists. With effective teamwork, there is rarely the need for an emergent pericardial window.

VATS pericardial resection requires selective lung ventilation. I prefer a double-lumen endotracheal tube, although bronchial blockers can be employed. The existence of associated pleural/pulmonary pathology takes precedence in defining which side to approach. When there are no associated findings, a left VATS approach provides access to a larger pericardial surface to allow creation of a larger window (Figure 1). Posterior pericardial loculations mandate a left-sided approach. A left VATS approach is done best via the 90-degree, full right lateral decubitus position, whereas a right VATS approach with its limited right-facing pericardium needs only 30- to 45-degree anterolateral positioning.

Single-lung ventilation is established during preparing and draping to allow ample time for atelectasis in the operative field. The initial camera port incision is in the sixth intercostal space in the mid axillary line, acknowledging the fact that the distended pericardium (especially on the left) may be displaced well laterally. Digital followed by camera inspection allows confirmation of a free pleural space.

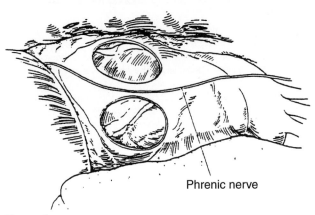

Figure 1
Left-sided approach with two windows created anterior and posterior to the phrenic nerve. The posterior defect is between the nerve and the pulmonary veins. *(From Jaklitsch MT, et al: In Loughlin KR, Brooks DC, editors:* Principles of endosurgery, *Cambridge, MA, 1996, Blackwell Science, p 230.)*

Pleural effusions should be drained on entering the chest to allow the lung to fall posteriorly, enhancing exposure. A three-port technique is most common, with the second and third operative ports placed under videoscopic guidance in the fourth and seventh intercostal spaces in or anterior to the anterior axillary line.

The key structure requiring identification before proceeding with creation of a window is the phrenic nerve pedicle. There is a variable amount of fat associated with this structure. On the left and often on the right there is a relatively bare area of exposed fibrous pericardium anterior to the phrenic nerve pedicle. With cephalad retraction of the lung on the left side, a similar free exposed area of fibrous pericardium can be visualized posterior to the phrenic pedicle. The more anterior aspects of the pericardium seen through the right or the left chest may be invested in thymic and pericardial fat. There is variable vascularity to this fat, which mandates its elevation or resection if the target area of pericardium to be resected involves this anterior space.

Initiating the creation of a window can be challenging because the tensely distended fibrous pericardium is often difficult to grasp. Preoperative drainage simplifies this. A nerve hook, Kocher clamp, or other similar jawed instrument is useful to elevate a portion of the pericardium, which is incised with scissors or endo-shears. Aspiration of a small aliquot (approximately 10 ml) may facilitate initial drainage by creating a small amount of laxity in the fibrous pericardium. The ideal window should be 4 to 8 cm × 4 to 8 cm in size (Figure 2). On the left, it is also possible to create a similar window posterior to the phrenic pedicle (see Figure 1).

Figure 2
Right-sided pericardiectomy with a large window anterior to the lung hilum and the phrenic nerve. Creating the window is simplified with the D-loop forceps retracting. Electrocautery is used to create the window facilitated by the use of D-loop forceps to resect the portion of pericardium to be excised. *(From Jaklitsch MT, et al: In Loughlin KR, Brooks DC, editors:* Principles of endosurgery, *Cambridge, MA, 1996, Blackwell Science, p 230.)*

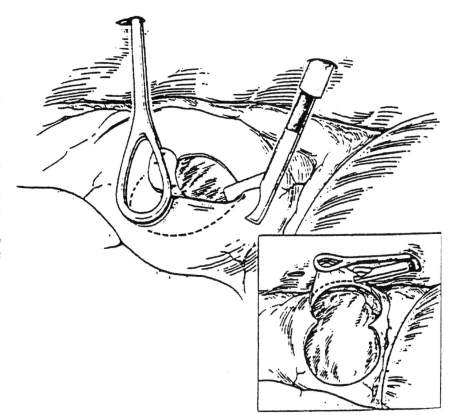

Associated pericardial fat should be included with the pericardial resection to allow the visceral pleura when the lung is inflated to come in direct contact with the heart. Attention to hemostasis in these areas is crucial because the expanded pericardium is often hyperemic. When coexistent malignant pleural disease is suspected or confirmed, talc insufflation into the ipsilateral pleural space has proved effective and has not led to cardiac constriction or irritability. Pleural drains are placed to ensure good dependent drainage of the posterobasal hemithorax. With the creation of an adequate window, placement of intraoperative pericardial drains is not necessary.

■ RESULTS

Durable control of pericardial effusive disease after VATS window creation can be expected in 95% of cases. This is superior to the 80% to 85% efficacy associated with subxiphoid windows and is comparable to the results reported using thoracotomy. Mortality is related most often to the underlying disease and underscores the need to evaluate the patient globally before proceeding to surgery. Only patients with reasonable physiologic reserve, an otherwise preserved quality of life, reliable therapeutic options for their malignancy, or benign disease are likely to benefit from VATS therapy. Patients with excessive comorbidities or a poor oncologic prognosis (expected survival <90 days) would be better served with alternative attempts at palliation using catheter-based or subxiphoid approaches.

SUGGESTED READING

DeCamp MM Jr, et al: Malignant effusive disease of the pleura and pericardium, *Chest* 112:2915, 1997.

DeCamp MM Jr, et al: The safety and versatility of video-thoracoscopy: a prospective analysis of 895 consecutive cases, *J Am Coll Surg* 181:113, 1995.

Flores RM, et al: Video-assisted thoracic surgery pericardial resection for effusive disease, *Chest Surg Clin N Am* 8:835, 1998.

Geissbuhler K, et al: Video-assisted thoracoscopic pericardial fenestration for loculated or recurrent effusions, *Eur J Cardiothorac Surg* 14:403, 1998.

Hazelrigg SR, et al: Thoracoscopic pericardiectomy for effusive pericardial disease, *Ann Thorac Surg* 56:792, 1993.

PULMONARY THROMBOENDARTERECTOMY

Michael M. Madani
Stuart W. Jamieson

Pulmonary thromboendarterectomy is the definitive surgical treatment of pulmonary hypertension from chronic pulmonary thromboembolic disease. It is estimated that every year in the United States approximately 2 million people have deep vein thrombosis, about one third of whom develop acute symptomatic pulmonary embolism. With an incidence of about 630,000 cases annually, symptomatic pulmonary embolism is about half as common as myocardial infarction and three times more common than cerebrovascular accidents. Many patients with symptomatic and asymptomatic pulmonary embolism progress to develop chronic pulmonary hypertension. Although it is impossible to determine accurately the incidence of pulmonary hypertension caused by chronic pulmonary embolism, it is estimated that there are at least 100,000 cases annually in the United States alone.

The pathophysiology of the disease relates to the inability of the body to lyse and resolve the embolic material, with an additional factor being the secondary vasculopathy that sometimes follows. It is likely that most cases result from one acute embolic episode, but the condition also can result from recurrent smaller embolic material from chronic indwelling lines, catheters, and leads. Why some people are unable to resolve their emboli is uncertain, but many factors play a role, including large volumes of emboli; chronic repetitive emboli; and congenital or acquired coagulation disorders, such as inherited deficiencies of antithrombin III, protein C, and protein S and the presence of lupus anticoagulant.

When the clot is lodged and secondary fibrosis and vasculopathy have developed, pulmonary hypertension ensues. This progresses to right ventricular hypertrophy and failure, arrhythmias, severe systemic venous congestion, and death.

Patients with chronic pulmonary hypertension do not have a particular clinical presentation, and in most cases their symptoms are nonspecific. They usually present with progressive exertional dyspnea, which is out of proportion to the clinical findings. They also may present with atypical chest pain, palpitations, hemoptysis, and a chronic productive cough. Some may have a clear history of acute pulmonary emboli in the past, whereas others may present with recurrent episodes of thrombophlebitis. Many patients give no history of deep vein thrombosis or pulmonary embolism. The physical findings in these patients relate to signs of right heart failure as a result of severe pulmonary hypertension. These signs may include cyanosis and chronic venous stasis with or without skin discoloration.

The diagnosis is based mostly on the clinical suspicion by the physician. Although a variety of diagnostic tests are available and are used routinely, pulmonary angiography remains the gold standard. Generally, right heart catheterization is performed in the same setting. When the diagnosis is established, patients undergo a comprehensive cardiopulmonary workup to assess candidacy for pulmonary thromboendarterectomy.

■ MEDICAL MANAGEMENT

The curative treatment for pulmonary hypertension from chronic pulmonary embolism is surgical removal of the obstruction; medical therapy plays only a supportive and palliative role. The mainstay of medical management is long-term anticoagulation. This therapy not only helps prevent future embolic episodes, but also limits propagation of thrombus already present within the pulmonary vasculature. Anticoagulation therapy does not help resolve the existing obstructive material, which is fibrotic in nature.

Additional drugs, such as diuretics, vasodilators, and inotropes, are used to treat right ventricular failure. Furosemide is the most common diuretic agent used for patients with signs of volume overload and right heart failure, usually with only transient improvement. Vasodilators can improve pulmonary hypertension, but the effects are generally minimal and short-lived because the obstruction is mechanical in nature and secondary to thromboembolic material. All classes of vasodilators, such as β-blockers, α-blockers, calcium channel blockers, nitrates, angiotensin-converting enzyme inhibitors, and nitric oxide, have been used with only varying degrees of success. Other medical agents used to improve right ventricular failure are inotropes, such as phosphodiesterase inhibitors (e.g., amrinone) and cardiac glycosides (e.g., digoxin). Phosphodiesterase inhibitors have vasodilatory and inotropic effects and are used in patients with severe heart failure on an inpatient or outpatient basis.

■ SURGICAL MANAGEMENT

Chronic embolic pulmonary hypertension is caused by pulmonary artery obstruction by the fibrotic residua of unresolved clot. As such, the only effective curative treatment is surgical removal of the obstruction. When performed by an experienced surgeon, pulmonary thromboendarterectomy has a low morbidity and mortality and produces excellent results. The only other curative alternative is lung transplantation, which we strongly believe is inappropriate. Considering the long waiting period for a donor, the mortality during the waiting period, lifetime antirejection medications with their associated problems, and the lower morbidity and mortality associated with pulmonary thromboendarterectomy, transplantation should not be offered as the primary treatment.

There are four treatment goals for thromboendarterectomy: (1) a hemodynamic goal of alleviating right ventricular failure, (2) a respiratory goal of improving oxygenation by removing ventilation-perfusion mismatch, (3) a prophylactic goal of preventing progression of right ventricular failure and preventing retrograde extension of the obstruction, and (4) a preventive goal of avoiding the secondary vasculopathy that continues in the remainder of the pulmonary circulation. Contraindications to pulmonary thromboendarterectomy include the absence of thromboembolic disease (e.g., patients with primary pulmonary hypertension) and irreversible underlying pulmonary disease. There is no degree of right heart failure that we consider irreversible.

When an appropriate candidate has completed the full diagnostic workup, an inferior vena cava filter is placed before surgery. In combination with lifetime anticoagulation therapy, this filter prevents further thromboembolic episodes.

Pulmonary thromboendarterectomy has evolved to its current stage over many years of experience, but certain principles form the basis of the operation as it currently is practiced. A median sternotomy is always used because thromboembolic disease is almost invariably a bilateral process (otherwise the degree of pulmonary hypertension would not be significant). Median sternotomy allows easy access to both pulmonary arteries. Cardiopulmonary bypass is used, not only to provide cardiovascular stability, but also to allow cooling of the patient for periods of circulatory arrest. Circulatory arrest is essential for effective and complete pulmonary endarterectomy, which cannot be performed without a bloodless field. Lastly, recognition of the correct endarterectomy plane is one of the most important principles of this operation; a successful outcome is not possible without recognition of this plane or without a complete endarterectomy all the way to the feathered tail in each one of the branches.

The conduct of the operation is as follows. When the patient is anesthetized, prepared, and draped as for other open-heart operations, a median sternotomy is made, and the pericardium is attached to the wound edges. The patient is anticoagulated with 400 U/kg of beef-lung heparin sodium to achieve an activated clotting time greater than 400 seconds. Cardiopulmonary bypass is provided through one aortic cannula and two venous cannulae. These patients generally have a large right heart and tricuspid regurgitation. They may become hemodynamically unstable with manipulation of the heart, and care must be taken in handling the heart during cannulation and initiation of cardiopulmonary bypass.

When on bypass, the heart is emptied, and a pulmonary artery vent is placed in the main pulmonary artery. This marks the origin of the pulmonary arteriotomy on the left side. The patient's temperature is lowered on bypass to 18°C to 20°C. When the heart fibrillates, an additional vent is placed through the right upper pulmonary vein. Cooling takes about 45 minutes, during which time dissections of the pulmonary artery, aorta, and superior and inferior vena cavae are completed.

When the core temperature reaches 20°C, an aortic cross-clamp is applied, and cold crystalloid cardioplegia is administered into the aortic root as a single dose. A cooling jacket around the heart provides additional myocardial protection. The entire procedure is performed using a single cross-clamp period and no additional cardioplegia. The superior vena cava and aorta are separated using a modified cerebellar retractor, and the right pulmonary artery is incised between the fully mobilized superior vena cava and the aorta, allowing a direct view into the pulmonary artery.

With the surgeon on the left side of the patient, thrombi within the vessel are removed. It is important to recognize that any thrombotic material, fresh or old, in the main pulmonary arteries is incidental. Most patients have a normal-appearing main pulmonary artery and no evidence of thrombus. Thromboembolectomy without complete endarterectomy is ineffective.

At some point, good, clear visualization is impaired by backbleeding from large collateral vessels. The patient then is placed on full circulatory arrest to provide a completely bloodless field. Using a microtome knife, the correct endarterectomy plane is identified over the posterior wall of pulmonary artery, and the endarterectomy is carried out down each of the branches. Using traction and a fine, blunt-tip suction-dissector device specially designed for this procedure, each one of the branches in the pulmonary tree is endarterectomized to a feathered tail. With experience, this generally is performed in less than 20 minutes, at which point the circulation is resumed, and the pulmonary arteriotomy is closed.

The surgeon moves to the right of the patient and prepares for endarterectomy of the left pulmonary artery. During this time, the patient remains on cardiopulmonary bypass at 18°C to 20°C until the left pulmonary arteriotomy is performed and further dissection is impaired by backbleeding. The circulation is arrested again, and a complete left-sided endarterectomy is performed similar to the right side. We have found that 20 minutes of circulatory arrest time for each side is adequate; only rarely does the surgeon require more time to complete the endarterectomy. In these unusual circumstances, 25 to 30 minutes of circulatory arrest time has been well tolerated, but longer times increase the risks of a neurologic event. Should more than 25 to 30 minutes be needed, circulation is restarted for 10 minutes before another arrest period is initiated.

The patient is rewarmed to normal body temperature, and the right atrium is explored for intraatrial shunts (seen in approximately 25% of patients). The patient is weaned from cardiopulmonary bypass. Depending on body habitus of the patient, warming may take 45 to 120 minutes. When off cardiopulmonary bypass, standard wound closure is performed. We perform a pericardial window into the left chest before closure. This is because of a high incidence of delayed pericardial effusions postoperatively, probably due to the bilateral hilar dissections.

■ POSTOPERATIVE RESULTS AND CONCLUSIONS

Most of the complications associated with this operation are not different from other open-heart operations. These include arrhythmia, postoperative bleeding, pericardial effusion, infection, and fluid overload. Pulmonary reperfusion injury or the reperfusion response, which occurs in about 10% of patients, is directly related to this procedure. This is a self-limited process and in most cases resolves within 72 hours. It probably stems from extensive denuded endothelium and the prolonged obstruction of the pulmonary vessels.

We have performed 1600 cases of pulmonary endarterectomy at University of California San Diego (UCSD). We now offer this procedure to high-risk patients with anticipation of a good clinical outcome and low mortality and morbidity. In the last 1000 cases performed at UCSD over 10 years, the mortality has been 5.5% to 6%, and overall morbidity was 10%. The most common complication is the reperfusion response. Occasionally a patient may continue to have persistent pulmonary hypertension late postoperatively. This is usually due to a preoperative diagnostic error, leading to operation in a patient with pulmonary hypertension unrelated to thromboembolic disease. These patients tend to be quite ill postoperatively, and most of our mortality occurs in these patients.

Chronic thromboembolic pulmonary hypertension remains an underdiagnosed entity in the United States and around the world. These patients are debilitated in their daily lives and if untreated carry a poor prognosis. Medical management is limited and at best palliative. Surgical removal of the thromboembolic obstruction by full endarterectomy is the best curative option and carries a low and currently acceptable mortality and morbidity. The success of the operation and good clinical outcome depend on correct clinical diagnosis, comprehensive preoperative workup, experienced surgical and anesthesia teams, and excellent postoperative nursing care.

SUGGESTED READING

Benotti JR, et al: The clinical profile of unresolved pulmonary embolism, *Chest* 84:669, 1983.

Holister LE, Cull VL: The syndrome of chronic thromboembolism of the major pulmonary arteries, *Am J Med* 21:312, 1956.

Jamieson SW, Kapelanski DP: Pulmonary endarterectomy, *Curr Probl Surg* 37:165, 2000.

Madani MM, Jamieson SW: Chronic thromboembolic pulmonary hypertension, *Curr Treat Options Cardiovasc Med* 2:141, 2000.

SURGICAL TREATMENT OF ATRIAL FIBRILLATION

A. Marc Gillinov
Patrick M. McCarthy

In recent years, there has been a resurgence of interest in the surgical treatment of atrial fibrillation (AF). This is attributable to several factors, including high prevalence of AF in the cardiac surgical population, improved understanding of the anatomic basis of AF, and development of new, simple surgical techniques for AF ablation.

Traditional surgical treatment of AF is the Cox-Maze III procedure. Relatively underused, the Cox-Maze III procedure cures AF in more than 90% of patients and virtually eliminates the risk of stroke. Recent understanding of the importance of the pulmonary veins and left atrium in the pathogenesis of AF has resulted in the development of new surgical approaches. New operations to ablate AF use alternate energy sources (cryothermy, microwave, radiofrequency, and laser) and simplified left atrial lesion sets that include pulmonary vein isolation. These operations cure AF in 70% to 80% of patients.

■ SURGICAL PROCEDURES AND THEIR RESULTS

The Cox-Maze III Procedure

The Cox-Maze III procedure is the gold standard for surgical treatment of AF. Cox and colleagues designed the procedure based on experimental and clinical evidence concerning the pathophysiology of AF. To improve results and simplify the operation, they modified the procedure twice, culminating in the Cox-Maze III.

In the Cox-Maze III operation, incisions and cryolesions are strategically placed to interrupt the macroreentrant circuits that characterize AF (Figure 1). Right and left atrial incisions interrupt the most common reentrant circuits and direct the sinus impulse from the sinoatrial node to the atrioventricular node along a specified route. Multiple "blind alleys" off the main conduction pathway (the Maze analogy) allow electrical activation of the entire atrial myocardium.

In the left atrium, the Cox-Maze III includes encircling and isolating the pulmonary veins and excising the left atrial appendage. These features are maintained in most operations designed by others to ablate AF. The right atrial lesions of the Cox-Maze III serve primarily to prevent postoperative atrial flutter. Many of the newer operations for AF do not include right atrial lesions. In experienced hands, the Cox-Maze III procedure requires about 1 hour on cardiopulmonary bypass.

The Cox-Maze III is extraordinarily effective, eliminating AF in 90% or more of patients. While perioperative AF is common, affecting 30% to 40% of patients, this is easily treated with standard antiarrhythmic drug therapy. By 3 to 6 months, cardiac healing is complete and atrial refractory periods have returned to normal. At that time, if pharmacologic therapy has been instituted, it is withdrawn, and more than 90% of patients maintain sinus rhythm. Left and right atrial contractility are demonstrated in more than 80% of patients after the Cox-Maze III procedure. Pacemaker implantation is required postoperatively in 5% to 10% of patients; these individuals usually have underlying sick sinus syndrome, and are maintained with atrioventricular pacing.

Although the Maze procedure is a relatively complex operation, it carriers very low risk. From January 1991 through January 2002, 309 patients had the Maze procedure performed at The Cleveland Clinic Foundation. Overall operative mortality was 1.9%. Operative mortality was zero for patients with lone AF, 2.1% for patients having the Maze with mitral valve repair, and 4.2% for patients having the Maze with mitral valve replacement. Maze success, designed as freedom from AF more than 6 months after surgery, was 97.7% for lone AF, 95.8% for Maze with mitral valve repair, and 95.5% for Maze with mitral valve replacement.

Cryothermy

Cryoablation is a well-established modality in arrhythmia surgery and an important component of the Cox-Maze III procedure. Application of a cryoprobe to atrial tissue for 2 minutes at −60°C produces a transmural lesion that can be confirmed visually. Tissue architecture is preserved, leaving

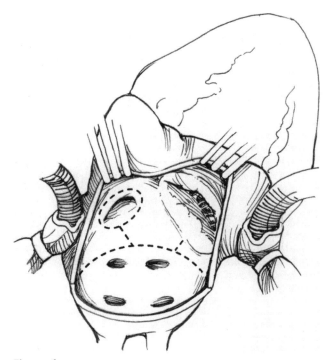

Figure 1
Left atrial incisions of the Cox-Maze III procedure. The pulmonary veins are encircled by a single incision. There are connecting incisions to the left atrial appendage, which is excised, and to the mitral annulus. (From Gillinov AM, et al: Ann Thorac Surg 74:2210, 2002.)

a smooth endocardial surface. Endocardial cryolesions can be created using reusable rigid probes or disposable flexible probes. In addition, cryolesions may be created from the epicardial or endocardial surface. Application of cryothermy to replace incisions of the Cox-Maze III procedure reduces operative time. Experience with cryoablation on the beating heart is limited.

Left atrial cryoablation that includes pulmonary vein isolation cures AF in 70% to 80% of patients. These results were achieved in patients with mitral valve disease. Superior results might be expected in patients without structural heart disease. When all of the incisions of the Cox-Maze III are replaced by cryolesions, AF is ablated in more than 90% of patients.

Microwave

Microwave creates lines of conduction block by thermal damage and subsequent scar formation. Microwave heating results in a deep lesion without producing char on the endocardial surface. This feature may reduce the risk of thromboembolism. At present, 2-cm, 4-cm, and 10-cm catheters are available for microwave ablation of AF.

Microwave energy may be applied from the endocardial or epicardial surface of the heart. With either approach, pulmonary vein isolation is easily accomplished (Figure 2). In addition, there is experience with off-pump, epicardial pulmonary vein isolation. The 10-cm microwave probe is designed to enable thoracoscopic, off-pump pulmonary vein isolation, a procedure that is under development. This 1-hour procedure, which includes pulmonary vein ablation and excision of the left atrial appendage under direct vision, requires a 1- to 2-day hospitalization.

Perioperative AF after microwave ablation is common, occurring in approximately two-thirds of patients. Although 30% to 40% of patients leave the hospital in AF, many return to sinus rhythm over the ensuing 3 months. Thus discharge in AF is not necessarily an indication of procedure failure. Late results document 80% cure of AF.

Radiofrequency

Several different radiofrequency catheter systems are available for surgical application. These include flexible probes, rigid probes, pencil-like probes with a cooled tip, and a probe that is configured as a bipolar clamp. Bipolar radiofrequency ablation is particularly rapid and allows assessment of lesion transmurality, which is important to procedural success. Radiofrequency probes may be placed on either the epicardial or the endocardial surface of the heart. As with microwave, epicardial radiofrequency energy can be utilized to perform beating heart, or "off-pump," ablation.

Creation of left atrial lesions, including pulmonary vein ablation, generally requires 10 to 20 minutes (Figure 2). Although specific lesion sets created with radiofrequency energy vary, results are similar; AF is ablated in 70% to 80% of patients. As with microwave ablation, most treated patients have organic heart disease and undergo a mitral valve procedure in addition to ablation of AF. For such patients, results with radiofrequency fall just short of those reported with the Cox-Maze III procedure. Success is similar regardless of whether right atrial lesions are included.

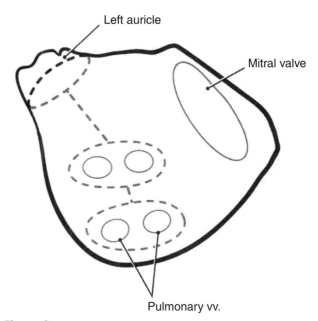

Figure 2

Typical left atrial lesion set produced with radiofrequency or microwave ablation. Each set of pulmonary veins (VV) is isolated separately. There are connecting lesions between the left and right pulmonary veins and from the left pulmonary veins to the left atrial appendage. The importance of an additional lesion to the mitral annulus is controversial. *(Adapted from Kress DC, et al: Validation of a left atrial lesion pattern for intraoperative ablation of atrial fibrillation,* Ann Thorac Surg *73:1160, 2002; reproduced with permission from The Society of Thoracic Surgeons.)*

■ CHOICE OF OPERATION

The Cox-Maze III Procedure

The traditional "cut-and-sew" Cox-Maze III procedure is remarkably effective at curing AF. Because of perceived complexity associated with this operation, it is relatively underused.

The Cox-Maze III procedure is used in patients with lone AF and in those with structural heart disease. For patients with lone AF, the Cox-Maze III procedure should be considered in good-risk patients with (1) previous thromboembolism or (2) left atrial thrombus and contraindications to anticoagulation or (3) highly symptomatic AF and failed medical or catheter-based intervention. In patients with AF who require cardiac surgery for other reasons, the Cox-Maze III procedure should be used as an adjunct to valve surgery, coronary artery bypass grafting, or myectomy in good-risk patients.

Pulmonary Vein Isolation and Left Atrial Connecting Lesions and Appendage Excision

Using alternate energy sources, pulmonary vein isolation with left atrial connecting lesions can be accomplished in less than 30 minutes. Such procedures ablate AF in 70% to 80% of patients. These operations, with left atrial appendage excision are recommended for AF patients requiring complex cardiac surgery, elderly patients, and those with extensive comorbidities that increase operative risk. Any of the alternate energy sources can be used to isolate the pulmonary veins. Surgeons may choose to incorporate connecting lesions between the left and right pulmonary veins or from the left pulmonary veins to the mitral annulus; the importance of these connecting lesion is unproved. The left atrial appendage is easily removed; excision is preferable to oversewing the orifice as an incompletely oversewn appendage may serve as a nidus for clot formation. Failure to add right atrial lesions leaves patients vulnerable to atrial flutter. However, atrial flutter develops in fewer than 10% of patients after pulmonary vein isolation; when it does occur, it is effectively treated by percutaneous, catheter-based techniques.

■ CONCLUSION

Surgical treatment of AF is highly effective and carries very low risk. Improved understanding of the pathogenesis of AF and technological advances have resulted in a variety of new surgical procedures that can be performed rapidly and safely.

Minimally invasive, thoracoscopic pulmonary vein isolation is now possible. Given these options, nearly all cardiac surgery patients with preexisting AF should have concomitant AF ablation. In addition, selected patients with lone AF should be offered surgical cure.

SUGGESTED READING

Gillinov AM, et al: Atrial fibrillation: current surgical options and their assessment, *Ann Thorac Surg* 2002.

Cox JL, Ad N: New surgical and catheter-based modifications of the Maze procedure, *Semin Thorac Cardiovasc Surg* 12:68, 2000.

Cox JL, et al: Current status of the Maze procedure for the treatment of atrial fibrillation, *Semin Thorac Cardiovasc Surg* 12:15, 2000.

Cox JL, et al: Impact of the Maze procedure on the stroke rate in patients with atrial fibrillation, *J Thorac Cardiovasc Surg* 108:833, 1999.

Haissaguerre M, et al: Spontaneous initiation of atrial fibrillation by ectopic beats originating in the pulmonary veins, *N Engl J Med* 339:659, 1998.

Kress DC, et al: Validation of a left atrial lesion pattern for intraoperative ablation of atrial fibrillation, *Ann Thorac Surg* 73:1160, 2002.

McCarthy PM, et al: The Cox-Maze procedure: the Cleveland Clinic experience, *Semin Thorac Cardiovasc Surg* 12:25, 2000.

CARDIAC TRANSPLANTATION

David D. Yuh
John V. Conte

Cardiac transplantation is an established, effective therapy for patients with end-stage heart failure, resulting in marked improvements in long-term survival and quality of life. This chapter outlines the important perioperative and operative considerations in cardiac transplantation.

PREOPERATIVE CONSIDERATIONS

Recipient Selection Criteria

Significant advances in the medical management of recipients before and after transplantation have led to modifications of traditional recipient selection criteria, including upper age limits, concomitant disease, and level of disability. The criteria outlined in this section have been adopted by most transplant centers in the United States.

Indications

Generally accepted indications for cardiac transplant evaluation are listed in Table 1. Generally, patients with severe cardiac disability despite maximal medical therapy, but who are otherwise healthy, are considered for cardiac transplantation. Most potential cardiac transplant recipients have end-stage, inoperable coronary artery disease (CAD) (one third of patients) or idiopathic cardiomyopathy and often require multiple hospitalizations. Other diagnoses include defined cardiomyopathy (e.g., viral, postpartum, familial), congenital anomalies, and valvular disease. More than half of patients fall into the cardiomyopathy category. Disabling symptoms typically include symptoms associated with congestive heart failure (e.g., dyspnea, orthopnea, generalized edema, weakness), although recurrent symptomatic ventricular arrhythmias and severe ischemic symptoms (i.e., unstable angina) often are observed. Transplant candidates generally fall into New York Heart Association (NYHA) functional classes III and IV.

Although the NYHA functional classification is used widely in the assessment of transplant candidates, a more accurate and objective measure of functional capacity is provided by peak oxygen consumption during treadmill exercise testing. Peak oxygen consumption is a function of peak cardiac output and peripheral oxygen extraction, correlates well with functional class, and is an independent predictor of prognosis in heart failure patients. Patients with severely reduced peak oxygen consumption (<15 ml/kg/min; approximately 50% of normal) have a 1-year mortality greater than 50% and benefit significantly from transplantation, both in survival and in functional capacity.

Contraindications

There are several well-established contraindications to cardiac transplantation, based on significant risks of recurrent cardiac dysfunction, severe symptomatic limitations, and limited rehabilitation potential or survival after transplantation (Table 2). Some of these conditions are relative or temporary contraindications; exceptions can be made on a selective basis, or corrective measures may be taken.

Severe, fixed pulmonary hypertension (pulmonary vascular resistance >5 Wood units) is a significant independent risk factor for early mortality after orthotopic cardiac transplantation, due to a heightened incidence of acute posttransplant right ventricular failure. In some cases, pulmonary vascular resistance can be lowered to acceptable levels with supplemental oxygen, vasodilators, or inotropes. Patients with severe, fixed pulmonary hypertension should be considered for combined heart-lung transplantation.

Evaluation and Management of Patients Awaiting Cardiac Transplantation
Candidate Evaluation and Listing

Screening and diagnostic tests used in the formal evaluations of potential heart transplant candidates at most centers are listed in Table 3. Patients deemed suitable for cardiac transplantation are categorized and listed on the basis of clinical status, time on the waiting list, body size, and ABO blood group. Clinical status is composed of two broad status

Table 1 Indications for Adult Cardiac Transplantation
Severe cardiac disability despite maximal medical therapy
History of recurrent hospitalizations for congestive heart failure
New York Heart Association functional class III or IV
Peak metabolic oxygen consumption <15 ml/kg/min
Symptomatic cardiac ischemia refractory to conventional treatment
Unstable angina not amenable to coronary artery bypass graft surgery or percutaneous transluminal coronary angioplasty with left ventricular ejection fraction <30%
Recurrent symptomatic ventricular arrhythmias
Exclusion of all surgical alternatives to cardiac transplantation
Revascularization for significant reversible ischemia
Valve replacement for critical aortic valve disease
Valve replacement or repair for severe mitral regurgitation

Table 2 Contraindications to Adult Cardiac Transplantation

ABSOLUTE CONTRAINDICATIONS
Advanced age (>70 years)
Significant, irreversible pulmonary, hepatic, or renal dysfunction
  Severe obstructive or restrictive lung disease
    (e.g., FEV_1 <1.5 liters, D_{LCO} <50% predicted)
  Severe hepatic failure
  Severe renal insufficiency (e.g., creatinine clearance
    <40 ml/min, albuminuria >500 mg/24 hr)
Severe pulmonary hypertension (e.g., pulmonary vascular
  resistance >5 Wood units)
Unresolved, recent malignancy
Significant systemic disease
  Diabetes mellitus with significant end-organ dysfunction
  Severe peripheral or cerebral vascular disease
Psychiatric illness or history of medical noncompliance
POTENTIALLY REVERSIBLE CONTRAINDICATIONS
Active infection
Active peptic ulcer disease
Diverticulitis
Symptomatic cholelithiasis
Current tobacco, alcohol, or drug use
Cachexia
Morbid obesity (>150% predicted ideal body weight)

FEV_1, forced expiratory volume in 1 second; D_{LCO}, carbon monoxide diffusion in the lung.

Table 3 Commonly Used Tests in the Evaluation of Potential Heart Transplant Candidates

SUITABILITY FOR TRANSPLANTATION (PHASE I)
Required Laboratory Tests
Complete blood count with differential, platelet, and
  reticulocyte count
Blood type and antibody screen (ABO, Rh)
Prothrombin and activated partial thromboplastin time
Bleeding time
Immunology panel (FANA, rheumatoid factor)
Electrolytes, Mg^{2+}
General survey panel
CK with isoenzymes
Serum protein electrophoresis
Urinalysis
Viral serologies
  Compromised host panel (cytomegalovirus, adenovirus,
    varicella-zoster, herpes simplex, Epstein-Barr virus)
  Hepatitis A and B antibodies, surface antigen, hepatitis C
  Cytomegalovirus—quantitative antibodies and IgM
  Human immunodeficiency virus
Studies Obtained as Indicated
Echocardiography with bubble study
MUGA for right and left ventricular ejection fraction
Cardiac catheterization
Thoracic CT scan
Quantitative ventilation-perfusion scans
Carotid duplex
Mammogram
Colonoscopy
Sputum for Gram stain; AFB smear; KOH; and routine
  bacterial, mycobacterial, and fungal cultures
REQUIRED FOR LISTING (PHASE II)
HLA and DR typing
Transplant antibody
Quantitative immunoglobulins
Histoplasma, Coccidioides, and *Toxoplasma* titers
Purified protein derivative
Pulmonary function tests with arterial blood gases
12-hour urine collection for creatinine clearance and total protein
Urine viral culture

FANA, fluorescent antinuclear antibody; MUGA, multiple gated acquisition (blood pool scan); CT, computed tomography; AFB, acid-fast bacillus; KOH, potassium hydroxide.

classifications developed by the United Network for Organ Sharing. Status IA patients require an intensive care unit (ICU) setting with invasive hemodynamic monitoring (i.e., Swan-Ganz catheter) and need parenteral inotropes or mechanical device support (e.g., intraaortic balloon pump [IABP], ventricular assist device [VAD], ventilator) to maintain adequate cardiopulmonary function. Status IB patients comprise inpatients or outpatients who require low-to-moderate levels of parenteral inotropes without Swan-Ganz catheterization or who are on VAD support for more than 30 days. Status II includes all other waiting patients. Listed patients are monitored by the transplant cardiologist or surgeon at varying intervals based on the patient's condition with selected tests, particularly peak oxygen consumption and hemodynamic measurements. Although most listed patients continue to deteriorate over time, a significant number stabilize or improve with medical therapy, prompting inactivation or removal from the list.

Medical Management

Medical management of listed patients is directed toward (1) relieving debilitating symptoms from end-stage congestive heart failure and (2) preserving organ function and optimizing the patient's condition for transplantation. Clinically stable transplant candidates with end-stage heart failure usually are treated with a combination of digoxin, diuretics, and afterload-reducing agents on an outpatient basis. Oral anticoagulants are used selectively by some transplant programs to reduce the risk of pulmonary and systemic emboli, which may occur asymptomatically in 60% of patients with idiopathic cardiomyopathy. Patients with recurrent sustained episodes of ventricular arrhythmias are treated with antiarrhythmics or implantation of an automatic cardioverter defibrillator or pacemaker cardioverter defibrillator. Parenteral vasodilators (i.e., nitroprusside, nitroglycerin) and inotropes (i.e., dopamine, dobutamine, milrinone) are used when oral medications prove inadequate.

Mechanical Support

Heart failure and clinical deterioration refractory to parenteral support necessitates mechanical support in the form of IABP counterpulsation or VAD placement. IABP counterpulsation improves coronary perfusion and reduces afterload and mitral regurgitation. Extended IABP use is associated with vascular complications. IABP should be used to provide moderate, short-term support in acute circulatory failure with end-organ dysfunction or ischemic dysrhythmias.

VADs are implanted mechanical pumps designed to assume a significant portion of the systolic workload from the left ventricle (LVAD), right ventricle (RVAD), or both ventricles (BiVAD) and are intended for intermediate-term to long-term circulatory support for patients in severe ventricular failure. Mechanical support generally is considered when the cardiac index is less than 2.0 liters/min/m^2, the ventricular filling pressures are greater than 20 mm Hg, the urinary output is less than 20 ml/hr (adults), and the systemic vascular resistance is greater than 2100 dynes·sec·cm^5 despite maximal parenteral inotropic and vasodilator therapy. The three most widely used ventricular assist systems include the Novacor LVAD (Novacor Medical Division, Baxter Healthcare, Oakland, CA), the Thoratec VAD (Thoratec Corp, Pleasanton, CA), and the HeartMate IP LVAD (Thoratec Corp, Pleasanton, CA). All three systems have been used successfully to reduce the mortality of end-stage cardiac patients awaiting transplantation. Complications observed in LVAD-supported patients include hemorrhage (40%), infection (20% to 75%), and right ventricular failure (10% to 30%).

Donor Selection and Management
Donor Criteria
Cardiac donors must have sustained irreversible brain death, usually as a result of blunt or penetrating head trauma or cerebrovascular accidents. Suggested criteria for cardiac donors and guidelines for recipient matching developed by the American Heart Association in 1992 are listed in Table 4. Normal cardiac function and the absence of a significant cardiac history and significant coronary atherosclerosis must be established. Donors less than 50 years old are preferred, but donors 55 years old and older are considered at most centers with a more detailed evaluation, including coronary angiography to rule out significant CAD.

Absolute contraindications for donation include severe coronary or structural disease, prolonged cardiac arrest, prior myocardial infarction, a carbon monoxide/hemoglobin level

greater than 20%, arterial oxygen saturation less than 80%, malignancy (sometimes excluding primary brain and skin cancers), and positive human immunodeficiency virus status. Relative contraindications include thoracic trauma, sepsis, prolonged severe hypotension (i.e., mean arterial pressure <60 mmHg for >6 hours), noncritical coronary artery stenosis, hepatitis B surface antigen or hepatitis C antibodies, multiple resuscitations, severe left ventricular hypertrophy, and a prolonged high inotropic requirement (e.g., dopamine >20 µg/kg/min for 24 hours). It is important to rule out reversible metabolic or physiologic causes of impaired cardiac function, rhythm disturbances, and electrocardiogram anomalies (e.g., brain herniation, hypothermia, hypokalemia).

Despite these guidelines, the donor organ shortage and critical clinical situations have prompted the use of cardiac grafts from "high-risk" donors with satisfactory short-term results. These include grafts that are potentially compromised by advanced age, high-dose inotropic support, donor-to-recipient undersizing, potential infection, echocardiographic abnormalities, or prolonged ischemic transport time.

Donor Management
The primary goal of managing the cardiac donor is the maintenance of hemodynamic stability. Patients with acute brain injury are often hemodynamically unstable, owing to neurogenic shock/pulmonary edema, excessive fluid losses, and bradycardia. Continuous hemodynamic monitoring, aggressive fluid resuscitation, vasopressors, and inotropes usually are required. Judicious fluid management prevents intraoperative hemodynamic instability and minimizes the need for inotropes and vasopressors, both of which increase myocardial wall stress. Intravascular volume should be given to maintain the central venous pressure between 5 and 12 mm Hg. Diabetes insipidus is common in organ donors and requires the use of intravenous vasopressin (0.8 to 1.0 U/hr) to reduce excessive diuresis. To maintain adequate perfusion pressures, dopamine and β-agonists commonly are used. Blood transfusions are used sparingly to maintain the hemoglobin concentration at 10 g/dl to facilitate adequate myocardial oxygen delivery. Hypothermia should be avoided because it predisposes to ventricular arrhythmias and metabolic acidosis.

Donor-Recipient Matching
Donor-recipient matching parameters include ABO compatibility and body size. ABO compatibilities are strictly observed because isolated episodes of hyperacute rejection have been observed in cardiac transplants performed across this barrier. Size matching and graft ischemic time are particularly important for recipients with an elevated pulmonary vascular resistance. Grafts from donors weighing less than 70% to 80% of the recipient or donors with ischemic times greater than 3 hours are used cautiously for recipients with pulmonary hypertension.

When an appropriate donor-recipient pairing is made, the recipient is screened for preformed antibodies against a standardized panel of random donors. A percent reactive antibody level greater than 5% prompts a prospective specific crossmatch between the donor and recipient.

Table 4 Suggested Criteria for Cardiac Donors and Guidelines for Recipient Matching

Age <40 years (may be extended)

Negative serologies for human immunodeficiency virus and hepatitis B

No active severe infection

No malignancy with possibility of metastases (i.e., most extracranial malignancies disqualify person as donor)

No evidence of significant cardiac disease or trauma

Low probability of coronary artery disease (coronary angiograms may be required)

Normal or acceptable ventricular function after intravascular volume normalization; dopamine <10 µg/kg/min

Blood type (ABO) compatibility with recipient

Donor body weight usually between 80% and 120% of recipient's body weight

If required, negative prospective cytotoxic T-cell crossmatch (retrospective crossmatch usually is performed)

Allograft ischemic time <4-5 hr

■ OPERATIVE TECHNIQUES

Donor Cardiac Procurement

After median sternotomy, a retractor is placed, and the pericardium is opened and suspended (Figure 1A). The heart is inspected and palpated for contusions, perforations, thrills, and coronary atherosclerosis. If the heart is deemed satisfactory, its final acceptance is communicated immediately to the recipient team. The aorta and pulmonary artery are dissected superiorly to the level of the arch and bifurcation to ensure adequate length for implantation. The superior vena cava is mobilized superiorly to the origin of the azygos vein and encircled with two ligatures, taking special care to preserve the sinoatrial node. An adequate length of the inferior vena cava is dissected free from its pericardial reflection and is surrounded with an umbilical tape. The aorta is encircled with an umbilical tape, and a 14-gauge cardioplegia perfusion cannula is inserted into its ascending segment. Intravenous heparin is administered at a dose of 300 U/kg and allowed to circulate for 3 to 5 minutes.

Extraction of the heart begins with ligation and division of the superior vena cava. The inferior vena cava is clamped and partially divided just above the diaphragm, and the heart is allowed to beat several times until it is empty. The ascending aorta is clamped distal to the perfusion cannula at the level of the innominate artery, and a hyperkalemic cardioplegic solution at 10°C is infused rapidly into the aortic root at a pressure of 150 mm Hg, arresting the heart in diastole. The left inferior pulmonary vein is partially divided to avoid left ventricular distention, and cold saline (4°C) is poured onto the heart and into the pericardial well. When the heart is fully arrested, cooled, and perfused with cardioplegia, it is elevated from the pericardial well, and each of the pulmonary veins is divided at their pericardial reflections. The pulmonary artery and aorta are divided at the level of the bifurcation and innominate artery. The explanted heart is placed into two sterile plastic bags with a cold saline interface, then placed within an airtight container filled with ice-cold saline and transported in a standard ice-filled cooler.

Standard Orthotopic Cardiac Transplantation

After intravascular monitoring and access lines are placed and anesthesia is induced, the supine patient's chest and groin areas are prepared and draped. Central venous access via the left internal jugular vein is usually obtained, sparing the right side for future endomyocardial biopsies. After a median

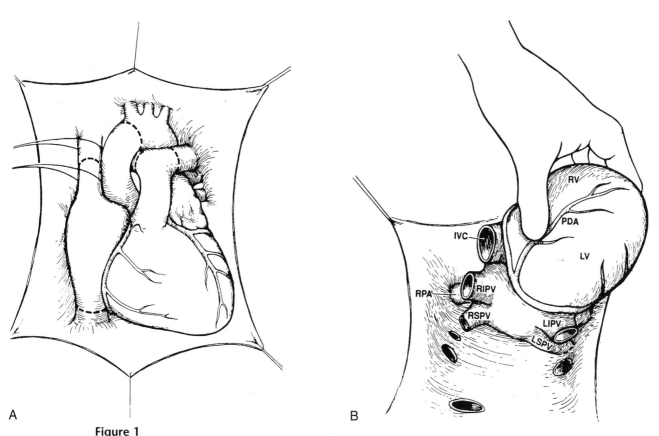

A   B

Figure 1
Donor cardiac procurement. **A,** Anticipated lines of transection of the venae cavae, aorta, and pulmonary arteries. **B,** Donor heart excision starting with transection of the inferior vena cava (IVC) and pulmonary veins (PV) and proceeding superiorly before transecting the pulmonary arteries and aorta. R, right; L, left; I, inferior; S, superior; RPA, right pulmonary artery; RV, right ventricle; LV, left ventricle; PDA, posterior descending artery. *(From Smith JA, et al: The Stanford manual of cardiopulmonary transplantation, Armonk, NY, 1996, Futura Publishing.)*

sternotomy is performed, the pericardium is opened and suspended followed by routine cannulation of the aorta and both venae cavae (Figure 2A). The arterial cannula is inserted in the most distal aspect of the ascending aorta just below the innominate artery. The venous cannulae are placed in the superior and inferior venae cavae and snared with umbilical tapes. Some surgeons opt to place a vent in the right superior pulmonary vein to prevent graft left ventricular distention. After institution of cardiopulmonary bypass with moderate hypothermia (28°C to 30°C) and snugging of caval snares, the ascending aorta is cross-clamped, and the aorta and pulmonary artery are divided at the level of the sinotubular junctions. The left atrium is divided at the atrioventricular groove, and the venae cavae are divided close to their atrial junctions.

After the donor heart is placed in a bowl of cold saline, the aorta and pulmonary artery are separated from each other. The left atrium is opened by connecting the pulmonary vein orifices, fashioning the donor atrial cuff. The atrial septum is inspected, and if a patent foramen ovale is present, it is closed. Under continuous application of topical cold saline into the pericardial well, implantation begins with the direct anastomosis of the donor and recipient left atrial cuffs with a continuous 3-0 polypropylene (Prolene) suture. On completion of this anastomosis, a cold bubble-free saline infusion line is placed into the left atrium through the atrial appendage for continuous endocardial cooling and evacuation of air from the left heart. Inferior and superior vena caval anastomoses are performed in end-to-end fashion with continuous 4-0 polypropylene sutures. Systemic rewarming is initiated at this time (Figure 2B).

The pulmonary artery and aortic anastomoses are completed in an end-to-end fashion using continuous 4-0 polypropylene sutures. At this time, the caval snares are released, the head of the bed is lowered, and endocardial cooling is halted, permitting blood into the heart and lungs and displacing any air trapped in the left-sided chambers through an aortic needle vent. Lidocaine is infused into the bypass circuit, the aortic cross-clamp is removed, and deairing procedures are continued to vent any residual air from the

heart. The left atrial line is removed, and the hole is oversewn. Although spontaneous defibrillation usually occurs at this time, electrical defibrillation may be required. While still under cardiopulmonary bypass, all suture lines are inspected for hemostasis before bypass is weaned. The superior vena caval cannula is repositioned into the right atrium, and the inferior vena caval cannula is removed just before discontinuation of bypass. An epinephrine infusion (10 to 50 ng/kg/min) is titrated to achieve a heart rate of 90 to 110 beats/min to maximize chronotropically and inotropically cardiac output and to lower pulmonary vascular resistance. Temporary ventricular and atrial pacing wires are placed. The pericardium is left open, and mediastinal chest tubes are placed. Pleural space violations or effusions are treated with chest tubes. The sternum and overlying fascia and skin are closed in the usual fashion.

Heterotopic Cardiac Transplantation

Originally described by Demikhov, heterotopic transplants account for about 2.5% of current cardiac transplants. The operative technique bypasses the left heart and involves anastomoses between the left atria, aorta, pulmonary arteries, and donor superior vena cava to recipient right atrium. The major indication for this operation is the presence of fixed, severe pulmonary hypertension whereby the native right heart continues to work against the elevated pulmonary vascular resistance while the graft bypasses the left heart. Other indications include cases in which the graft is a temporary support in the setting of reversible cardiac failure.

■ POSTOPERATIVE MANAGEMENT OF CARDIAC TRANSPLANT RECIPIENTS

Early Postoperative Period

The acute postoperative management of cardiac transplant recipients resembles that of most common open-heart operations. On completion of the operation, the intubated transplant recipient is transported from the operating room to

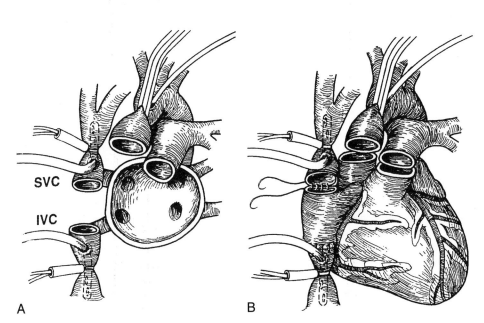

Figure 2
A and **B**, Standard orthotopic cardiac transplantation. SVC, superior vena cava; IVC, inferior vena cava. *(From Smith JA, et al: The Stanford manual of cardiopulmonary transplantation, Armonk, NY, 1996, Futura Publishing.)*

the ICU where cardiac rhythm and hemodynamics are monitored. Swan-Ganz pulmonary artery balloon catheters usually are reserved for recipients with significant pulmonary hypertension. Strict isolation, previously enforced to reduce the incidence of infection in these immunocompromised patients, is not required; hand washing and facemasks generally are considered adequate. Precautions are taken, however, to minimize patient contact with objects or persons harboring active infectious agents.

The primary objective in the immediate postoperative period is to maintain adequate perfusion of the recipient, while minimizing cardiac work. Approximately 10% to 20% of transplant recipients experience some degree of transient sinus node dysfunction in the immediate postoperative period, often manifest as sinus bradycardia that usually resolves within 1 week. Because cardiac output is primarily rate dependent after transplantation, the heart rate should be maintained between 90 and 110 beats/min during the first few postoperative days, using temporary pacing or β-agonists as needed. Persistent sinus node dysfunction and bradycardia is rare (<5%) but may require a permanent transvenous pacemaker. The systolic blood pressure should be maintained between 90 and 110 mm Hg, using afterload reduction in the form of nitroglycerin or nitroprusside if necessary. Low-dose dopamine (3 to 5 μg/kg/min) frequently is used to augment renal blood flow and urine output. The adequacy of cardiac output is indicated by warm extremities and a urine output greater than 0.5 ml/kg/hr without diuretics. Cardiac function generally normalizes within 3 to 4 days, after which parenteral inotropes and vasodilators can be tapered.

Several factors may contribute to some form of depressed global myocardial performance in the acute postoperative setting. The myocardium is potentially subject to prolonged ischemia, inadequate preservation, or catecholamine depletion before implantation. Right heart failure is common in the early postoperative period and often is caused principally by pulmonary hypertension. Inotropes with pulmonary vasodilatory effects (e.g., milrinone) and nitric oxide, a selective pulmonary vasodilator, have been effective in treating early right heart failure. Rarely a temporary RVAD may be necessary.

Optimizing pulmonary function is crucial, and standard ventilator management is applied in the immediate postoperative period. Ventilatory weaning is initiated after the patient is deemed stable, awake, and alert and is performed through successive decrements in intermittent mandatory ventilation rate, followed by a trial of continuous positive airway pressure. When acceptable ventilatory mechanics and arterial blood gases are achieved, the patient is extubated, usually within 24 hours. Postextubation pulmonary care consists of supplemental oxygen for several days, aggressive pulmonary toilet, and serial chest radiographs.

Expedient removal of indwelling lines reduces the incidence of line-related infections. Pleural and mediastinal thoracostomy tubes are removed when drainage has decreased to less than 25 ml/hr, and pacing wires are removed after 7 to 10 days if pacing is not required. After several days, barring significant complications, the patient is transferred from the ICU to a cardiac surgery ward for the remainder of the hospitalization, when patient instruction, immunosuppressant adjustment, an initial endomyocardial biopsy, and rehabilitation occur.

Graft Physiology

The grafted heart presents several unique physiologic characteristics. During procurement, the heart graft is denervated and is isolated from normal autonomic regulatory mechanisms. The resting heart rate is generally higher due to the absence of vagal tone, and sinus arrhythmia and carotid reflex bradycardia are absent. The denervated heart graft develops an increased sensitivity to catecholamines, which is important in maintaining an adequate cardiac response to exercise and stress. During exercise, the cardiac transplant recipient experiences a steady but delayed increase in heart rate, primarily owing to a rise in circulating catecholamines. This initial rise in heart rate subsequently is accompanied by an immediate increase in filling pressures resulting from augmented venous return. Resultant increases in stroke volume and cardiac output are sufficient to sustain the increase in activity. Graft coronary circulation maintains its capacity to dilate and increase blood flow in response to increased myocardial oxygen demand.

Immunosuppression

Currently, conventional immunosuppression in cardiac transplant recipients consists of the triple-drug combination of cyclosporine or FK506, azathioprine or mycophenolate mofetil (CellCept), and glucocorticoids. Initially, high doses of these drugs are given, with eventual tapering for long-term administration. Cyclosporine potently inhibits T-lymphocyte activation, presumably by blocking the release of interleukin-2 from helper T cells. Cyclosporine is titrated to maintain a trough serum concentration between 150 and 250 ng/ml in the first few weeks after transplantation and between 50 and 150 ng/ml thereafter. Azathioprine, a cytotoxic agent and bone marrow suppressant, is dosed to maintain the white blood cell count greater than 5000/mm^3. Glucocorticoids exhibit potent immunosuppressive effects by inhibiting leukocyte elaboration of inflammatory mediators (e.g., lymphokines, colony-stimulating factors). A methylprednisolone bolus (500 mg intravenously) is given intraoperatively after coming off cardiopulmonary bypass and during the first 24 hours postoperatively (125 mg intravenously every 8 hours). Prednisone is dosed at 1.0 mg/kg/day during the first posttransplant week and, in the absence of acute rejection, tapered thereafter to a maintenance dose of 0.2 mg/kg/day.

Prophylactic induction therapy with OKT3 monoclonal antibodies is an adjunct to standard triple-drug regimen. Directed against the T-cell (CD3) receptor, OKT3 antibodies rapidly remove circulating T lymphocytes without affecting erythrocytes, granulocytes, or platelets. OKT3 induction therapy, given over the first 10 postoperative days, has delayed the time to first rejection and has reduced early rejection rates. Other induction agents include antithymocyte globulin and interleukin-2 blockers (daclizumab [Zenapax]).

Judicious doses of these drugs are usually well tolerated but are associated with side effects. Cyclosporine commonly is associated with nephrotoxicity, hypertension, hepatotoxicity, hirsutism, and an increased incidence of lymphoma. The primary toxicity of azathioprine is generalized bone marrow depression manifested as leukopenia, anemia, and thrombocytopenia. Steroids are associated with a myriad of side effects, including the appearance of cushingoid features, hypertension, diabetes, osteoporosis, and peptic ulcer disease. Initial doses of OKT3 may cause significant hypotension, bronchospasm, or fever, presumably due to T cell–mediated release of lymphokines. Patients receiving OKT3 are monitored closely and premedicated with acetaminophen, antihistamines, and corticosteroids. Most of these adverse effects are manageable or reversible with dosage reduction.

Postoperative Complications

Accelerated graft CAD, infection, and rejection are the foremost postoperative complications observed in cardiac transplant recipients. At the Johns Hopkins Hospital, these conditions accounted for 25%, 24%, and 15% of all deaths from 1983 to 2000.

Acute Rejection

Acute graft rejection is a major cause of death after cardiac transplantation. The incidence of acute graft rejection is highest during the first 3 months after transplantation. At the Johns Hopkins Hospital, 64% of cardiac transplant recipients experience acute rejection during this period. After this initial 3-month period, the incidence of acute rejection averages about 0.6 episode per patient-year.

Surveillance endomyocardial biopsies permit rejection to be diagnosed before significant graft injury and dysfunction occurs. The procedure, performed under local anesthesia, involves the percutaneous introduction of a Caves-Schultz bioptome into the right ventricle via the right internal jugular vein, under fluoroscopic guidance. Multiple biopsy specimens are taken from the interventricular septum per session, taking care not to injure the tricuspid valve apparatus. Safe, simple, and relatively well-tolerated, endomyocardial biopsies of the cardiac allograft start 7 to 10 days after transplantation and are repeated periodically at progressively longer intervals.

Acute rejection is characterized histologically by lymphocytic infiltration and myocytic necrosis. The classic Stanford classification developed by Billingham in 1979 was the first grading system widely used to characterize rejection severity. Since then, many grading systems have evolved from different transplant groups, culminating in uniform criteria developed by the International Society for Heart and Lung Transplantation in 1990 (Table 5).

The timing and severity of rejection episodes determine therapy. Severe or moderate rejection episodes occurring in the early posttransplant period are treated with pulsed steroid dosing (methylprednisolone, 1000 mg/day for 3 days). Subsequent severe or moderate rejection episodes detected on routine surveillance biopsy are treated with steroid pulsing or by merely increasing the oral prednisone dosage to 100 to 200 mg/day for 3 consecutive days, followed by a taper back to baseline dosages over 2 weeks. Mild rejection usually is not treated with augmented immunosuppression unless it is persistent.

Acute rejection refractory to steroid therapy is treated with antilymphocyte preparations in the form of antithymocyte globulin and OKT3 monoclonal antibodies, adding CellCept or substituting FK506 for cyclosporine. Second-line therapies used in difficult, persistent cases of rejection include methotrexate and total lymphoid irradiation. Endomyocardial biopsies are repeated 10 to 14 days after antirejection therapy to assess resolution of the rejection episode.

Chronic Rejection

Accelerated graft CAD or atherosclerosis is a major limiting factor for long-term survival in cardiac transplant recipients. Significant graft CAD resulting in diminished coronary blood flow may lead to arrhythmias, myocardial infarction, sudden death, or impaired left ventricular function with congestive graft failure. Typical angina from myocardial ischemia usually is not noted in the denervated graft. In a retrospective analysis of cardiac transplants performed at the Johns Hopkins Hospital from 1983 through 2000, the actuarial freedom from graft

---

Table 5 Histologic Grading Systems for Acute Cardiac Rejection

GRADE	HISTOLOGIC CHARACTERISTICS
Stanford Classification	
Mild rejection	Interstitial and endocardial edema
	Scanty perivascular and endocardial lymphocytic infiltrate
	Pyroninophilia of endocardial and endothelial cells
Moderate rejection	Interstitial, perivascular, and endocardial lymphocytic infiltrate
	Early focal myocytolysis
Severe rejection	Interstitial hemorrhage
	Infiltrate of lymphocytes and polymorphonuclear leukocytes
	Vascular and myocyte necrosis
Resolving rejection	Active fibrosis
	Residual small lymphocytes, plasma cells, and hemosiderin deposits
International Grading System	
0	No rejection
1A	Focal (perivascular or interstitial) infiltrate without necrosis
1B	Diffuse but sparse infiltrate without necrosis
2	One focus with aggressive infiltration and/or focal myocyte damage
3A	Multifocal aggressive infiltrates and/or myocyte damage
3B	Diffuse inflammatory process with necrosis
4	Diffuse aggressive polymorphous with or without infiltrate, edema, hemorrhage, or vasculitis
	Necrosis

CAD at 1, 5, and 10 years was 95%, 54%, and 30%. Clinically observed risk factors for developing this condition have included advanced donor/recipient age, human leukocyte antigen incompatibility, hypertriglyceridemia (serum concentration >280 mg/dl), frequent acute rejection episodes, and recipient cytomegalovirus (CMV) infection.

Multiple causes for graft CAD have been proposed, but they all invoke chronic, immunologically mediated damage to the coronary vascular endothelium. Transplant atherosclerosis is a diffuse vascular narrowing extending symmetrically into distal branches and is characterized histologically by concentric intimal proliferation with smooth muscle hyperplasia. Coronary arteriography is performed periodically to identify recipients with accelerated CAD. Because graft CAD manifests as diffuse coronary intimal thickening, intracoronary ultrasound has been advanced as a more sensitive means to detect graft atherosclerosis due to its ability to assess vascular wall morphology in addition to luminal diameter.

Coronary angioplasty, stenting, and coronary artery bypass graft surgery have been used to treat discrete proximal lesions in some cases of graft CAD; however, the only definitive therapy for diffuse disease is retransplantation. Effective prevention of graft CAD relies on developments in improved immunosuppression, recipient tolerance induction, improved CMV prophylaxis, and inhibition of vascular intimal proliferation.

Infection

Infection is the leading cause of morbidity and mortality after cardiac transplantation. The risk of infection and infection-related death peaks early during the first few months after transplantation and rapidly declines to a low persistent rate thereafter. In a retrospective analysis of cardiac transplants performed at the Johns Hopkins Hospital from 1983 through 2000, the actuarial freedom from infection-related death at 3 months, 1 year, and 5 years was 94%, 88%, and 75%.

Postoperative infections can be classified broadly into infections that occur early and late after transplantation. Early infections occurring during the first month after transplantation are commonly bacterial (especially gram-negative bacilli) and manifest as pneumonia, mediastinitis, catheter sepsis, and urinary tract and skin infections. Treatment of these infections generally involves identification of the infective agent (e.g., cultures, antibiotic sensitivities), source control (e.g., catheter removal, débridement), and appropriate antibiotic regimens. In the late posttransplant period, opportunistic viral, fungal, and protozoan pathogens are more prevalent. The lungs, central nervous system, gastrointestinal tract, and skin are the usual sites of invasion.

CMV infection is recognized widely as the most common and important viral infection in transplant patients, with an incidence of 73% to 100% in cardiac transplant recipients. It presents either as a primary infection or as reactivation of a latent infection, most commonly 1 to 4 months after transplantation. By definition, primary infection results when a previously seronegative recipient is infected via contact with tissue or blood from a seropositive individual. The donor organ itself is thought to be the most common vector of primary CMV infections. Reactivation infection occurs when a recipient who is seropositive before transplant develops clinical CMV infection under immunosuppression.

Seropositive recipients also are subject to infection by new strains of CMV. Clinically, CMV infection has protean manifestations, including leukopenia with fever, pneumonia, gastroenteritis, hepatitis, and retinitis. CMV pneumonitis is the most lethal of these, with a 13% mortality, whereas retinitis is the most refractory to treatment, requiring indefinite treatment. CMV has been identified as a trigger for accelerated graft CAD and as an inhibitor of cell-mediated immunity. Most cases of CMV infection respond to ganciclovir and hyperimmune globulin. Both of these agents are used prophylactically, especially in seronegative patients receiving a graft from a seropositive donor.

Fungal infections are less common than bacterial or viral infections. Early recognition is important because these infections are generally more refractory to therapy and are more lethal. Therapy consists of antifungal agents, including amphotericin B, fluconazole, and flucytosine.

Long-term antibiotic prophylaxis typically includes nystatin mouthwash for thrush, sulfamethoxazole-trimethoprim for opportunistic bacterial and *Pneumocystis carinii* infections, and antivirals such as acyclovir or ganciclovir.

Neoplasm

Transplant recipients are at significantly greater risk for developing malignancy, undoubtedly due to long-term immunosuppression. Tumors to which recipients are predisposed include skin cancer, B-cell lymphoproliferative disorders, carcinoma in situ of the cervix, carcinoma of the vulva and anus, and Kaposi's sarcoma. The incidence of B-cell lymphoproliferative disorders in transplant patients is many times greater than seen in the normal age-matched population. Thought to be caused by unchecked Epstein-Barr virus infection in the setting of T-cell suppression, B-cell lymphoproliferative disorders generally are treated with a reduction in immunosuppression and administration of an antiviral agent, such as acyclovir or ganciclovir. Neoplasms of the breast, lung, prostate, and colon are not increased in these patients.

Retransplantation

The primary indications for cardiac retransplantation are graft failure due to accelerated graft atherosclerosis or recurrent acute rejection. Patients in need of retransplantation generally are held to the same standard criteria as initial candidates. Survival rates after retransplantation are diminished significantly compared with those achieved in primary transplant patients. At the Johns Hopkins Hospital, 1-year survival was 88% after cardiac retransplantation.

■ RESULTS OF CARDIAC TRANSPLANTATION

According to the Registry of the International Society for Heart Transplantation (ISHLT), 57,220 heart transplants were performed at more than 300 transplant centers worldwide between 1982 and 2000. A review of 325 heart transplants performed at the Johns Hopkins Hospital between 1983 and 2000 placed 1-, 5-, and 10-year actuarial survival estimates at 83%, 66%, and 49%. ISHLT data show that 96% of surviving recipients achieve and sustain NYHA class I functional status after 4 years.

SUGGESTED READING

Baumgartner W, et al: *Heart and heart-lung transplantation*, Philadelphia, 2001, WB Saunders.

Fleischer KJ, Baumgartner WA: Heart transplantation. In Edmunds LH, editor: *Cardiac surgery in the adult*, New York, 1997, McGraw-Hill, p.1409.

Kormos R, et al: Transplant candidate's clinical status rather than right ventricular function defines need for univentricular versus biventricular support, *J Thorac Cardiovasc Surg* 111:773, 1996.

Lower R, Shumway N: Studies on the orthotopic homotransplantation of the canine heart, *Surg Forum* 11:18, 1960.

HEART-LUNG TRANSPLANTATION

Douglas N. Miniati
Robert C. Robbins

Since the first successful human heart-lung transplantation in 1981, many advances have been made in the arena of thoracic transplantation. One of the major changes has been a decline in the use of heart-lung transplantation in cases of suppurative lung diseases and primary pulmonary hypertension, which have attained similar survival rates when treated with double-lung transplantation. As a consequence, the total number of heart-lung transplantations performed per year has decreased. Nevertheless, heart-lung transplantation continues to be the primary mode of treatment for patients with congenital heart disease and Eisenmenger's physiology and other particular subgroups of patients with primary pulmonary pathology. Some of these groups include patients with severe right ventricular dysfunction accompanying diagnoses such as primary pulmonary hypertension, cystic fibrosis, emphysema, idiopathic pulmonary fibrosis, and α_1-antitrypsin deficiency. Other patients who may benefit from heart-lung transplantation include patients with the aforementioned pulmonary diseases plus end-stage coronary artery disease or left ventricular failure. For all of these patients, heart-lung transplantation offers palliation and improvement in quality of life.

■ RECIPIENT AND DONOR SELECTION

Currently the most common indications for heart-lung transplantation are congenital heart disease and primary pulmonary hypertension, together accounting for approximately 60% of all indications. Congenital heart diseases that may lead to Eisenmenger's syndrome and the need for transplantation include atrial and ventricular septal defects, patent ductus arteriosus, and truncus arteriosus. Other congenital indications include univentricular heart with pulmonary atresia and aortic atresia–hypoplastic left heart syndrome. Pulmonary disease processes with concordant severe myocardial dysfunction also are indications for heart-lung transplantation (see earlier). The decision to list these patients for heart-lung transplantation as opposed to bilateral-lung transplantation rests mainly on the degree of ventricular failure (e.g., at our institution, patients with primary pulmonary hypertension are listed for heart-lung transplantation if the right ventricular ejection fraction is <20%). Advantages to using heart-lung transplantation in these patients include a potentially shorter waiting period, a simpler operative procedure, and fewer postoperative airway complications. Disadvantages include subjecting the patient to the risks associated with a denervated heart and the development of graft coronary artery disease and an inefficient allocation of donor organs if a domino-donor heart transplantation is not possible.

The key to determining which patients may benefit most from heart-lung transplantation is identifying patients with progressive cardiopulmonary dysfunction who still have the ability to tolerate the operation, postoperative rehabilitation, and immunosuppressive protocols employed. Candidates for transplantation generally should be less than 50 years old with a life expectancy of 12 to 18 months (the life expectancy for patients with Eisenmenger's physiology may be longer, 3 to 5 years, because of right ventricular compensation). As is the case for other forms of transplantation, the benefits of expert medical and other surgical therapy must be exhausted. Contraindications may include age older than 50 years, significant systemic disease (e.g., peripheral vascular disease, cerebrovascular disease, portal hypertension), active infection, irreversible liver or kidney dysfunction, active or recent malignancy, preoperative corticosteroid use, wide deviation from ideal body weight, peptic ulcer disease, current cigarette smoking or drug or alcohol abuse, psychiatric illness/noncompliance, severe osteoporosis, and mechanical ventilation for greater than 1 week. Diabetes mellitus is no longer a contraindication in and of itself but may be a contraindication if it is poorly controlled. In addition, previous thoracic surgery (with the potential development of dense adhesions and bleeding complications) must be considered a relative contraindication on a case-by-case basis.

Donor selection, evaluation, and management must be performed meticulously to achieve optimal graft function. In general, donors younger than 40 years of age are preferred, but many centers use donors 50 years old, provided that a complete evaluation, including coronary angiography, is performed. The donor's arterial P_{O_2} should be greater than 100 mm Hg on 30% oxygen and greater than 400 mm Hg on 100% oxygen. In addition, the peak airway inspiratory pressure should be less than 30 cm H_2O, and a bronchoscopy should be performed to prove that there are no purulent secretions or signs of aspiration. Other routine screening tests include a chest x-ray, 12-lead electrocardiogram, arterial blood gases, echocardiogram, and serologic studies. Absolute contraindications for using a donor's heart and lungs include severe coronary artery disease or structural heart disease, a prolonged circulatory arrest, previous history of myocardial infarction, carbon monoxide hemoglobin level of greater than 20%, arterial oxygen saturation less than 100%, active malignancy, significant smoking history, and positive human immunodeficiency virus status. Relative contraindications include thoracic trauma, sepsis, mean arterial blood pressure less than 60 mm Hg for more than 6 hours, noncritical coronary artery disease, positive hepatitis serologies, multiple resuscitations, severe left ventricular hypertrophy, and prolonged requirement for high inotrope levels. Before explantation, the donor is given a dose of broad-spectrum antibiotics for infection prophylaxis and intravenous steroids to attenuate the systemic inflammatory response associated with brain death.

Other important points of donor management are centered on preventing or minimizing the neurogenic pulmonary edema that may occur in brain-dead patients. Bolus fluids should be avoided, and the central venous pressure should be maintained at 5 to 8 cm H_2O. To maintain an appropriate blood pressure, vasopressors, such as dopamine or phenylephrine, may be required. From a respiratory standpoint, a positive end-expiratory pressure of 3 to 5 cm H_2O should be maintained to prevent atelectasis, and the fraction of inspired oxygen should not exceed 40%. Appropriately selected donors should be managed such that hemodynamic stability and pulmonary function are preserved as well as possible.

■ DONOR-RECIPIENT MATCHING

Donors are matched to recipients first by ABO blood type, then by body size and, in particular, by thoracic cavity dimensions. Although weight, height, and chest circumference all are considered, height seems to correlate best with an appropriate size match. Generally, there should be a height difference of no more than 4 inches, although in some select cases a difference of 6 to 8 inches may be allowable. The chest x-ray may be helpful in matching vertical and transverse thoracic cavity dimensions, although computer-generated images often lack the quality necessary to make these assessments. Ideal donor organs are usually slightly larger than those of the recipient and may depend on the recipient's underlying disease.

■ DONOR ORGAN PROCUREMENT

The donor operation is performed via median sternotomy. During the donor procurement, intravenous prostaglandin E_1 (PGE_1) is used for pulmonary arterial dilation, starting approximately 15 minutes before aortic cross-clamping. The dosage typically starts at 20 ng/kg/min, increasing to a target PGE_1 infusion rate of 100 ng/kg/min in 10-ng/kg/min increments, maintaining an arterial blood pressure of at least 55 mm Hg. When the chest is opened, the pleural spaces are entered and the lungs are inspected. After briefly deflating the lungs, the pulmonary ligaments are divided, and ventilation is resumed. The thymic remnant is excised, and the pericardium is incised vertically and laterally. After dissecting the great vessels, umbilical tapes are placed around the ascending aorta, the venae cavae, and the trachea, as high as possible between the aorta and the superior vena cava (Figure 1A-D). The pericardium is excised as far posteriorly as each pulmonary hilum, and the azygos vein is ligated and divided.

The cardioplegia cannula is placed into the mid ascending aorta just proximal to the site for the aortic cross-clamp, and the pulmonary preservation solution is delivered via an 18 Fr aortic cannula placed into the proximal main pulmonary artery, just distal to the pulmonic valve (Figure 1E). The donor is heparinized, the venae cavae are ligated, the heart is allowed to empty, and the aortic cross-clamp is applied. Although cold crystalloid cardioplegia (10 ml/kg) is infused to arrest the heart, the inferior vena cava and left atrial appendage are incised to avoid right and left ventricular distention. Pulmonary preservation solution, consisting of cold modified Euro-Collins solution with 8 mEq/liter magnesium sulfate and 65 ml/liter of 50% dextrose (15 ml/kg/min for 4 minutes), is infused into the pulmonary artery simultaneously. In addition, 4°C saline or physiologic irrigating solution (PhysioSol; Abbott Laboratories, North Chicago, IL) is poured over the heart and lungs for topical cooling, and ventilation is maintained with half-normal tidal volumes of room air.

After the infusion of the preservation solutions and pouring of topical cold solution, fluid is aspirated from the thoracic cavity, and the lungs are deflated. The venae cavae are completely divided, and the aorta is divided at the cross-clamp. The heart-lung bloc is dissected free from the esophagus from the diaphragm superiorly, avoiding injury to the trachea, lung, or great vessels. A full normal tidal volume is delivered to the lungs, and the trachea is stapled at least four rings above the carina with a TA-55 stapler. The trachea is divided above the staple line, and the heart-lung bloc is removed, wrapped in sterile lap pads, immersed in 4°C saline, and packaged for transportation. Improvements in preservation protocols, including the use of PGE_1, free radical scavengers, leukocyte depletion, and colloid-based perfusates, have allowed for procurement 1000 miles from the transplant center and cold ischemia times of 6 hours.

■ RECIPIENT OPERATIVE TECHNIQUE

The first part of the recipient operation focuses on the safe removal of the native organs, avoiding injury to nerves and minimizing bleeding. Routinely, median sternotomy is performed, but if dense adhesions are expected (e.g., patients with previous thoracotomies or cystic fibrosis), a bilateral "clamshell" thoracotomy may provide better exposure. The use of aprotinin and an argon beam coagulator for control

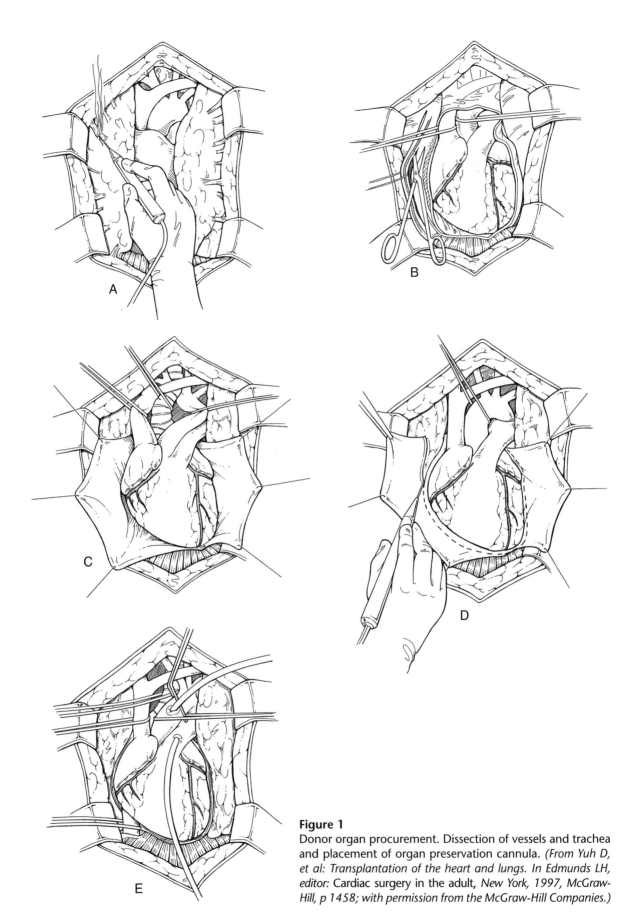

Figure 1
Donor organ procurement. Dissection of vessels and trachea and placement of organ preservation cannula. *(From Yuh D, et al: Transplantation of the heart and lungs. In Edmunds LH, editor:* Cardiac surgery in the adult, *New York, 1997, McGraw-Hill, p 1458; with permission from the McGraw-Hill Companies.)*

of chest wall bleeding from pleural and posterior mediastinal adhesions have been important adjunctive measures to decrease postoperative bleeding. After the chest is opened, the pleurae are opened from the diaphragm up to the great vessels, and any pleural adhesions are lysed. Next the anterior portion of the pericardium is excised, and a 3-cm pedicle is fashioned on each side to contain and protect the phrenic nerve and pericardiophrenic vessels (Figure 2B). The patient is fully heparinized, then cannulation for cardiopulmonary bypass is performed, with the aortic cannula near the base of the innominate artery and the venae cavae cannulated individually. Routine cardiopulmonary bypass is instituted with systemic cooling to 28°C. An aortic cross-clamp is applied, and the heart is excised. The aorta is divided just above the aortic valve, the pulmonary artery at the bifurcation, and the right and left atria at the mid atrial level. If a bicaval anastomosis is to be performed, the cavae are divided individually. Care must be taken to leave a small amount of right atrial tissue at the inferior vena cava–right atrial junction to facilitate this anastomosis to the donor heart (Figure 2C).

The superior vena cava should be divided at the superior vena cava–right atrial junction proximal to the azygos vein. The remaining right and left atrial tissues are excised. Next, attention is directed toward removal of the lungs. The left atrial remnant is divided such that the left superior and inferior pulmonary veins can be rotated laterally and dissected free. The left pulmonary ligaments are divided, and the lung is rotated medially to gain access to the posterior left pulmonary hilum. In dissecting the hilum, great care must be taken not to damage the vagus nerve. The left main pulmonary artery is divided, followed by the left main stem bronchus, which is stapled with a TA-30 stapler before division. The left lung is removed, and the same technique of hilar dissection is performed to remove the right lung (Figure 2DE).

The last step in preparing the thorax for insertion of the heart-lung bloc entails removal of the pulmonary arterial and main stem bronchial remnants. When the native pulmonary artery is removed, a portion near the ligamentum arteriosum is left behind to avoid damage to the left recurrent laryngeal nerve. Next, the stapled main stem bronchi are grasped with clamps to assist dissection superiorly to the level of the trachea. Care is taken to dissect the membranous portion of the trachea away from the esophagus. Meticulous attention must be paid to achieving hemostasis during this dissection, especially in patients with congenital heart disease who may have large bronchial collaterals because this represents the most important part of the operation. Metal clips are usually sufficient to ligate these branches, and a perfusion pressure of 60 mm Hg at this time is helpful in unmasking potential postoperative bleeding points. Excessive bleeding can produce not only hemodynamic instability, but also damage to the transplanted lungs. This damage can occur because of increased capillary permeability secondary to ischemia and reperfusion and subsequent need to transfuse large volumes of blood and blood products. The dissection is carried out to the level of the carina, where the trachea is divided.

The heart-lung graft is prepared by irrigating the tracheobronchial tree with normal saline and suctioning, then trimming the trachea to leave one or two rings above the carina. The bloc is lowered into the chest (Figure 2F), manipulating the right lung under the right phrenic pericardial pedicle, followed by the left lung under the left pericardial pedicle. Next the tracheal anastomosis is performed using a running 3-0 polypropylene suture. This anastomosis can be facilitated by inferior traction on stay sutures placed at the junction of the membranous and cartilaginous portions of the recipient's open trachea. When the anastomosis is complete, ventilation with half-normal tidal volumes of room air and topical cooling are instituted. In addition, another cooling line is placed into the left atrial appendage to enhance endomyocardial cooling and to deair the left side of the heart. The posterior pericardium is closed over the tracheal anastomosis to provide separation from the aortic anastomosis should a small tracheal leak occur.

If a bicaval technique is used, the recipient and donor inferior venae cavae are anastomosed, followed by the superior vena cava and aortic anastomoses, all with a running 4-0 polypropylene suture. If the atrial cuff technique is used, the donor right atrium is incised from the inferior vena cava to the base of the right atrial appendage, taking care to avoid the sinoatrial node, and the anastomosis is performed using a running 3-0 polypropylene suture, followed by the aortic anastomosis. During the right atrial or caval anastomosis, rewarming to 37°C is begun. After the aorta and pulmonary artery are deaired, the aortic cross-clamp, caval tapes, and left atrial catheter are removed, and the left atrial stump is oversewn. The pulmonary preservation solution infusion site is repaired, the heart is resuscitated, and cardiopulmonary bypass is weaned. Techniques that have been employed in an attempt to reduce allograft reperfusion injury include the use of a heparin-bonded cardiopulmonary bypass circuit, leukocyte filtering of the perfusion blood just before the removal of the aortic cross-clamp, and the use of modified ultrafiltration after separation from cardiopulmonary bypass. After all cannulae are removed, heparinization is reversed with protamine sulfate, and methylprednisolone is administered (500 mg intravenously).

The chest is closed in routine fashion, and ventilation with a positive end-expiratory pressure of 3 to 5 and 40% inspired fraction of oxygen is continued. On graft reperfusion, intravenous dopamine, epinephrine, or phenylephrine is used to maintain a heart rate of 100 to 110 beats/min and a mean arterial blood pressure of 60 mm Hg, and nitroglycerin or inhaled nitric oxide is used to decrease pulmonary vascular resistance. Before transport to the intensive care unit, the tracheal anastomosis is checked via bronchoscopy, and the airways are suctioned.

■ EARLY POSTOPERATIVE CARE

Much of the postoperative care of heart-lung transplant recipients is similar to that of other open-heart surgery patients. Inotropes, vasopressors, and vasodilators are used to achieve optimal hemodynamics, while ventilator support is employed to maintain adequate gas exchange. These supports are weaned as tolerated, usually within the first few postoperative days. A small percentage of patients have early lung graft dysfunction due to pulmonary edema or alveolar damage associated with ischemia and reperfusion. With improvements in graft preservation, the incidence of this phenomenon, which

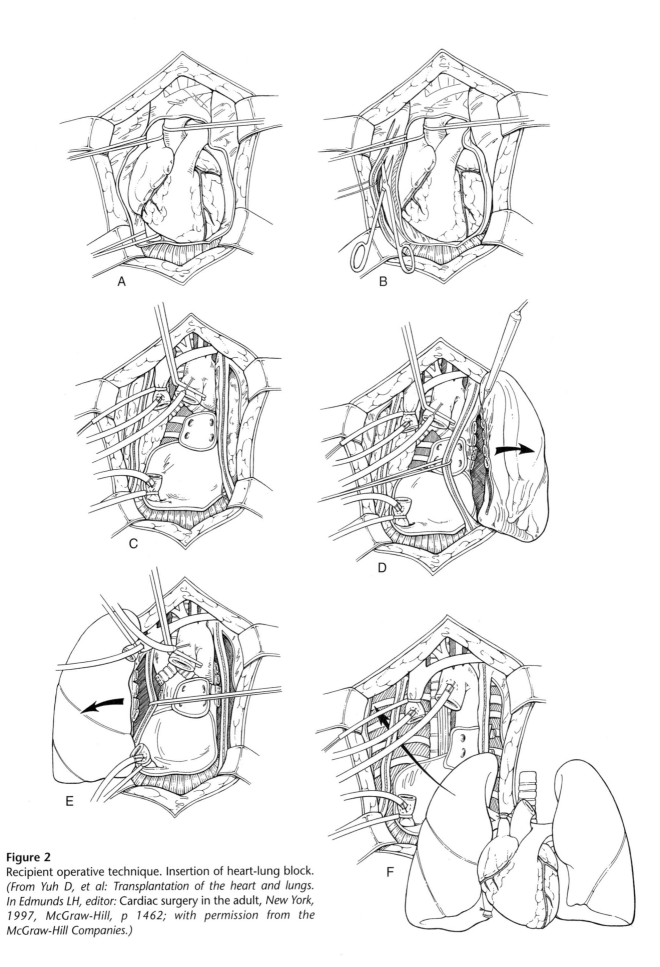

Figure 2
Recipient operative technique. Insertion of heart-lung block.
*(From Yuh D, et al: Transplantation of the heart and lungs.
In Edmunds LH, editor:* Cardiac surgery in the adult, *New York,
1997, McGraw-Hill, p 1462; with permission from the
McGraw-Hill Companies.)*

previously has been called the *reimplantation response*, is expected to diminish. In severe cases that are unresponsive to appropriate fluid balance maintenance and mechanical ventilator maneuvers, inhaled nitric oxide or extracorporeal membrane oxygenation may be required.

■ IMMUNOSUPPRESSION

Most patients receive a standard triple-drug immunosuppressive maintenance protocol consisting of cyclosporine, azathioprine, and prednisone. Typically, after the intraoperative dose of methylprednisolone (500 mg), three additional doses of 125 mg are administered intravenously at 8-hour intervals; all steroids then are withheld for 2 weeks to permit healing of the tracheal anastomosis. Oral prednisone is given after this healing period, starting at 0.6 mg/kg/day and tapered to 0.1 to 0.2 mg/kg/day over the next few weeks. Cyclosporine is initiated as soon as normal renal function is confirmed, with a target serum drug level of 150 to 250 ng/ml for the first few weeks, then tapered down to 100 to 150 ng/ml. Azathioprine is given as a loading dose of 4 mg/kg preoperatively, then maintained at 2 mg/kg/day, but adjusted to keep the white blood cell count greater than 5000 cells/mm³. In addition to the aforementioned regimen, induction therapy is performed using rabbit antithymocyte globulin (RATG) on postoperative days 1, 2, 3, 5, and 7 or OKT3 on days 1 through 14 if there is an adverse reaction to RATG therapy.

New immunosuppressive medications are being developed constantly in an effort to find substances with increased efficacy but lower toxicity. In particular, tacrolimus and mycophenolate mofetil have shown promise in heart transplant patients and currently are undergoing trails in the treatment of heart-lung transplant patients. Other agents on the horizon include sirolimus (rapamycin) and IL-2 receptor monoclonal antibodies, which may permit the avoidance of RATG induction therapy.

■ ACUTE REJECTION

Surveillance and diagnosis of heart-lung transplant acute rejection have changed since this procedure first was performed. Several centers have verified that cardiac allograft rejection and lung allograft rejection often occur asynchronously and that cardiac rejection seldom occurs in the absence of pulmonary rejection. For these reasons, surveillance and initial diagnosis of acute rejection in heart-lung recipients depend on fiberoptic bronchoscopy with transbronchial parenchymal lung biopsy and bronchoalveolar lavage, which is the current gold standard. This surveillance, along with routine arterial blood gases and pulmonary function tests, is performed at 1, 2, 3, 4, 8, and 12 weeks posttransplantation, then every 3 months for the first 2 years. This is a controversial area, however, and some centers choose to follow spirometry and clinical indicators to guide selective pulmonary biopsies. Endocardial biopsies are performed only if there is a high clinical index of suspicion for isolated cardiac rejection, if there is a decrease in myocardial function by echocardiogram, or if a patient is unable to undergo transbronchial biopsy. Other indicators of rejection include impaired respiratory

function and the development of characteristic bilateral infiltrates on chest x-ray, although these radiologic findings may be absent in the first postoperative month.

Treatment of acute rejection generally consists of an augmentation of steroids, using intravenous methylprednisolone (1000 mg/day for 3 days) for early or severe rejection and oral prednisone (100 mg/day for 3 days) for later or mild rejection, followed by a steroid taper. Refractory cases may be treated with antithymocyte antibodies such as OKT3 or RATG or, if these are unsuccessful, total lymphoid irradiation. As additional immunosuppressive agents and strategies evolve, the treatment of acute heart-lung allograft rejection likely will employ these new methods. As in the case of early graft failure, inhaled nitric oxide and extracorporeal membrane oxygenation may be useful adjuncts to immunosuppressive therapy for acute rejection.

■ LONG-TERM MANAGEMENT AND OUTCOMES

During the first posttransplantation year, infection is the most common cause of death. After the first year, infection and obliterative bronchiolitis (OB) contribute nearly equally as the main causes of death, with graft coronary artery disease also playing a significant role. Because infections are the leading cause of morbidity and mortality in heart-lung recipients, a high index of clinical suspicion must be maintained. In the early postoperative period, bacterial pathogens predominate, whereas opportunistic viral and fungal pathogens are more often the culprits in late cases of infection. Cytomegalovirus, in particular, causes a significant amount of morbidity, prompting treatment of any donor-recipient cytomegalovirus serology mismatch with intravenous ganciclovir and hyperimmune globulin for 6 to 8 weeks. Infection prophylaxis may vary from center to center but typically consists of nystatin mouthwash, oral trimethoprim-sulfamethoxazole, aerosolized amphotericin B, and acyclovir.

The development of OB can decrease significantly a patient's long-term survival, causing death from respiratory insufficiency or via a superimposed respiratory infection. According to Reichenspurner's review of the Stanford data, the incidence of OB is approximately 18%, 49%, 56%, and 71% at 1, 2, 3, and 5 years after heart-lung transplantation. Risk factors for the development of OB include multiple episodes of acute rejection and the occurrence of cytomegalovirus pneumonitis. Diagnosis of this condition can be made with the aid of pulmonary function tests and transbronchial biopsy; treatment consists of augmentation of immunosuppression.

Neoplasms resulting from immunosuppression affect heart-lung transplant recipients as they do all other transplant patients. Skin cancer; non-Hodgkin's lymphomas; Kaposi's sarcoma; and cervical, vulval, uterine, and perineal tumors usually arise around 5 years posttransplantation. Treatment consists of decreasing immunosuppression and instituting chemotherapy or various immunologically based therapies.

According to the 2000 ISHLT Registry report, the 1-year survival after heart-lung transplantation is 63%, decreasing to 23% at 12 years posttransplantation. Survival beyond the first year, during which acute rejection and infection claim the most lives, confers a survival half-life of approximately 9 years.

Risk factors for 1-year mortality include pretransplantation ventilator dependence, repeat transplantation, transplantation occurring between 1988 and 1991, and recipient male gender. At the 5-year point, pretransplantation ventilator dependence and transplantation occurring between 1988 and 1991 further increase the mortality risk, along with recipient age, which increases mortality in a linear fashion, whereas the indications of cystic fibrosis and α_1-antitrypsin deficiency significantly decrease mortality risk.

At Stanford, approximately 175 heart-lung transplantations have been performed. The 1-, 5-, and 10-year survival values are 71%, 48%, and 33%. The major causes of death are infection (30%), OB (21%), graft coronary artery disease (8.6%), and hemorrhage (6.7%). Early and late survival after heart-lung transplantation continues to improve with experience, and aggressive rehabilitation programs have been successful in returning patients to a normal lifestyle with moderate levels of physical activity. Heart-lung transplantation continues to provide palliation to patients who are not candidates for bilateral lung transplantation with cardiac repair. As recipient selection, donor evaluation, and organ preservation improve, the most promising organs will be transplanted into those who will benefit most from this procedure. Additional innovations in immunosuppression and in the detection and treatment of infection most likely will result in less morbidity, decreased incidence of OB, and improved survival.

SUGGESTED READING

Barlow CW, et al: Heart-lung versus double-lung transplantation for suppurative lung disease, *J Thorac Cardiovasc Surg* 119:466, 2000.

Kown MH, Robbins RC: Controversies surrounding the current status of heart-lung transplantation, *Semin Resp Crit Care Med* 20:439, 1999.

Reichenspurner H, et al: Stanford experience with obliterative bronchiolitis after lung and heart-lung transplantation, *Ann Thorac Surg* 62:1467, 1996.

Sarris GE, et al: Long-term results of combined heart-lung transplantation: the Stanford experience, *J Heart Lung Transplant* 13:940, 1994.

Whyte RI, et al: Heart-lung transplantation for primary pulmonary hypertension, *Ann Thorac Surg* 67:937, 1999.

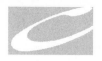

MECHANICAL CIRCULATORY SUPPORT

INTRAAORTIC BALLOON PUMP

Hans H. Scheld
Christof Schmid

In the 1990s, usefulness of the intraaortic balloon pump (IABP) to support the failing left ventricle became increasingly evident. The IABP provides a simple and economical method to improve oxygen supply to the myocardium and reduce its oxygen consumption with a low rate of adverse events. In some institutions, IABPs are implanted in 1 out of 10 cardiac patients, usually prophylactically for high-risk conventional surgery. In contrast, right ventricular support with the IABP has not seen widespread use because pulmonary vasodilators are an excellent nonsurgical alternative.

■ PHYSIOLOGIC PRINCIPLES

The IABP provides diastolic counterpulsation, by which it assists the heart in series with the cardiac cycle. Its effect is variable and depends on the preexisting cardiovascular condition. During systole, collapse of the IABP balloon leads to afterload reduction and a decrease in left ventricular wall tension and myocardial oxygen demand. In diastole, balloon inflation increases coronary flow, which in the failing heart may increase 100%. Increases in the coronary blood flow and in the coronary blood flow velocity result in important changes in distribution of blood flow, which explain the beneficial effects in patients with myocardial ischemia (Figure 1).

Initiation of the IABP first increases cardiac output. Left ventricular filling pressure and wedge pressure decrease, whereas stroke index increases. Pulmonary venous congestion is reduced, relieving pulmonary artery hypertension and right ventricular failure. Mean blood pressure and heart rate show no consistent response, but systolic pressure usually is decreased, and diastolic pressure is increased. Systemic vascular resistance decreases as a consequence of the baroreceptor reflex, as does tension time index, an estimate of myocardial oxygen demand.

■ INDICATION

Heart failure is a common indication for IABP and includes a wide spectrum of underlying cardiac diseases and clinical settings. In general, cardiac index less than 2.0 liter/min/m²

indicates imminent or present low cardiac output state. Because the IABP is a simple-to-use tool and associated with a low complication rate, it is usually the first invasive countermeasure against heart failure if medical treatment is insufficient. Frequently, it is used liberally on clinical grounds only, without measurement of the cardiac index. An important caveat is that patients must have a certain minimal degree of ventricular pump function because the IABP alone is not sufficient to provide cardiovascular perfusion without ventricular ejection.

The most common indication is acute myocardial ischemia. When patients deteriorate early or later after myocardial infarction and require increasing inotropic and vasopressor support, insertion of an IABP effectively improves coronary perfusion and reduces afterload of the weakened left ventricle. Insertion of an IABP should be considered whenever dopamine is insufficient to maintain cardiac pump function and addition of epinephrine is being considered. If emergent cardiac catheterization shows significant coronary stenoses, insertion of the IABP should be performed in the catheterization laboratory so that proper placement of the balloon can be confirmed by fluoroscopy. The aim is to stabilize the patient and reduce catecholamine support.

In the case of a ventricular septal defect or mitral regurgitation after acute myocardial infarction, patients may benefit dramatically from diastolic counterpulsation because left ventricular afterload reduction decreases the left-to-right shunt and left atrial pressure. The IABP may allow these patients to recover and undergo surgery electively.

Diastolic counterpulsation also has been proved effective when elevated levels of serum creatinine kinase and troponin I indicate periprocedural myocardial ischemia after percutaneous transluminal coronary angioplasty (PTCA) or surgical coronary revascularization (coronary artery bypass graft surgery). As in the setting of acute myocardial infarction, patients benefit from improved coronary perfusion and less myocardial work. Patients are supported for several days until the enzyme release has subsided, and the need for catecholamine support has passed.

Further causes of acute heart failure amenable to IABP support include decompensation due to various cardiomyopathies; dilated cardiomyopathy and end-stage ischemic cardiomyopathy are the most common, followed by acute myocarditis. If hemodynamic recovery and weaning from the device are not possible, mechanical support can be continued with a "bridge-to-transplant" intention.

In addition to emergency indications, elective insertion of an IABP before surgery has gained widespread acceptance and is favored by many cardiothoracic surgeons operating on patients with severely impaired ventricular pump function. Preoperative IABP reduces postoperative oxygen demand and the need for catecholamines, decreasing the length of intensive care unit (ICU) stay. Mortality does not seem to be affected.

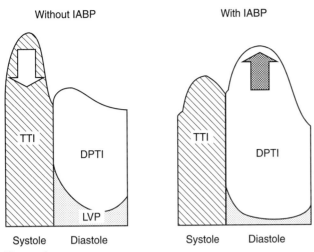

Figure 1
The intraaortic balloon pump (IABP) diminishes the tension time index (TTI) and increases the diastolic pressure time index (DPTI). LVP, left ventricular pressure.

Similarly, cardiologists performing high-risk PTCA (e.g., for stenosis of the left main coronary artery and severely compromised left ventricular function) rely on periprocedural mechanical support, either on an IABP or extracorporeal membrane oxygenation.

Another indication for IABP implantation is to provide pulsatile flow in patients supported by a continuous-flow mechanical assist device. It is not clear whether continuous nonpulsatile flow is harmful or has hemodynamic and metabolic consequences. Although axial flow pumps have shown intriguing results as long-term assist devices, in the immediate postoperative period patients may benefit from pulsatile flow provided by IABP. Other rare indications include septic shock, drug-induced cardiac failure, and myocardial contusion.

Contraindications are mainly relative and occasionally absolute. An IABP catheter cannot be advanced if the femoral artery is occluded. When severe occlusive arterial disease of the lower extremities is present, further obliteration of the femoral artery lumen may critically affect perfusion of the leg. A cold pulseless leg and compartment syndrome may develop, mandating immediate removal of the IABP to repair the vessel. Other absolute contraindications include acute aortic dissection and severe aortic valvular insufficiency. An IABP should not be placed in patients with irreversible myocardial failure except as a bridge-to-bridge or bridge-to-transplant or in patients with terminal illnesses.

A kink of the iliac artery or descending aorta is rarely a contraindication, but abdominal aortic aneurysms are controversial. Some surgeons argue the advantages, whereas others fear thromboembolism and rupture. Prosthetic replacement of the femoral artery is usually not considered a contraindication, but it is more hazardous.

◼ SURGICAL IMPLANT TECHNIQUE

Routine IABP placement consists of insertion of the balloon catheter into a femoral artery using Seldinger's technique in a widely prepared sterile field. The common femoral artery is palpated and punctured with an 18-gauge cannula in a 45-degree cephalad direction. A long flexible J-shaped guidewire is inserted through the cannula up the descending thoracic aorta. Use of the guidewire is especially important when there is known or suspected kinking of the iliac artery or descending thoracic aorta. The cannula is removed, and access to the vessel is successively widened with dilators. An introducer sheath with a hemostasis valve to prevent backbleeding is inserted over the guidewire. With the guidewire and introducer sheath in place, the IABP with its balloon collapsed is threaded carefully over the guidewire. The length of insertion can be estimated by laying the IABP onto the patient's surface from the inguinal insertion site to the distal end of the aortic arch, approximately the sternomanubrial junction.

When the IABP is in place, the guidewire can be removed and the lines for balloon inflation and pressure measurement connected. If the tip of the IABP catheter floats freely in the aortic lumen at a proper position, a good arterial blood pressure signal can be obtained. If the IABP catheter has been advanced too far, the blood pressure signal is damped; pulling the IABP catheter back restores a good pressure signal and ensures a good position.

In some centers, it is general policy not to use an introducer sheath. There may be an advantage to this, at least in patients with severe occlusive arterial disease. If the patient has a noncalcified femoral vessel, an IABP catheter can be inserted without a sheath even in obese patients. Appropriate dilation of the puncture channel is important because inserting the IABP catheter by force may damage the balloon. A problem that can arise lies in repositioning of the catheter if it has not been inserted far enough. In most systems, the external part of catheter is protected by a sterile cellophane bag, which is fixed to the introducer sheath. If no sheath is used, the external part of the catheter cannot be kept sterile. Sheathless insertion is attractive when an IABP is inserted during surgery and its proper position can be confirmed immediately by transesophageal echocardiography. It is less optimal in the ICU, where a chest radiograph is needed to confirm position. Small body size is another scenario for sheathless insertion and use of smaller balloons. Secure fixation of the catheter to the skin of the thigh is necessary to avoid displacement of the catheter. In patients previously operated on for infrarenal aortic aneurysm with a Y-prosthesis and bifemoral anastomoses, puncture of the Dacron prosthesis also can be done, but dilation is more difficult due to the resistance of the graft.

Sometimes percutaneous cannulation of the femoral artery is not possible. In these cases, a surgical cutdown is required. A longitudinal incision starting just below the inguinal ligament or a transverse incision 1 to 2 cm below the inguinal ligament is possible. When the femoral artery is exposed, one may decide whether to puncture the vessel (large caliber) or to anastomose a 6-mm vascular graft end-to-side (small caliber). In the former situation, a purse-string suture is placed around the puncture site and brought out through the incision so that the suture can be tied after removal of the IABP catheter. This may obviate reopening of the wound. If a vascular graft (usually a Dacron tube) is sewn to the femoral artery, the flow through that vessel is only minimally compromised. The IABP catheter is inserted through the Dacron tube and tied at its end with one or two hemostatic sutures. Removal requires a second operation with occlusion and oversewing of the Dacron tube just distal to the anastomosis.

Infrequently an IABP cannot be inserted via the femoral artery and must be placed directly into the thoracic aorta instead. As with the femoral access, there are two possibilities for insertion into the ascending aorta or proximal aortic arch. If the aortic wall is not fragile, two polytetrafluoroethylene (Teflon) felt–reinforced purse-string sutures with tourniquets may secure hemostasis after puncture and insertion of the IABP catheter. The proper length of insertion must be estimated before placement and should be confirmed by transesophageal echocardiography. If purse-string sutures fail to control bleeding, a 6-mm vascular graft (e.g., Dacron) can be anastomosed end-to-side to the aorta. To avoid redo sternotomy for removal of the IABP catheter, a long Dacron graft can be used and brought up to the subcutaneous tissue in the subxiphoid region. For later removal of the IABP catheter, only a few centimeters of the skin incision need to be reopened. The hemostatic sutures at the end of the Dacron graft can be cut, the IABP removed, and the graft oversewn and positioned below the fascia. Other approaches to IABP insertion include the iliac artery, subclavian artery, and axillary artery, although these are used rarely.

■ BALLOON MANAGEMENT

After careful deairing, the arterial pressure line of the IABP catheter is connected to a transducer, and the trace is inspected on the monitor. An important consideration for optimal timing of counterpulsation is that the shape of the arterial pressure wave may depend on the arterial access (i.e., the arterial pressure trace in the thoracic aorta is different from the radial or femoral artery). The trigger for inflation and deflation must be chosen because arterial blood pressure, electrocardiogram (ECG), or an intrinsic pump rate may be used. Usually the arterial pressure waveform is preferred because it is exact, readily available, and not disturbed by electrocautery during surgery. The ECG trigger demands fixation of additional ECG skin pads but can be used if problems arise with pressure monitoring. When the pneumatic drive line is connected to the IABP controller, counterpulsation is initiated, preferably in a 1:2 beat ratio. This allows comparison with the patient's own ventricular beats and facilitates optional timing of balloon inflation and deflation. Ideally, inflation should start after closure of the aortic valve, which can be identified in the pressure waveform as the dicrotic notch. Earlier inflation increases afterload resistance, whereas delayed inflation is inefficient counterpulsation. Deflation should occur immediately before the arterial upstroke. Some prefer to start counterpulsation with only 50% augmentation and increase it stepwise to the maximum.

■ COMPLICATIONS

Complications can occur at any step of the insertion procedure. The incidence is influenced by several parameters, such as condition of the patient (worse in cardiogenic shock), site of insertion (higher after aortic insertion), gender (higher in females), duration of pumping, and expertise of the team.

Puncture of the femoral artery can damage the vessel and lead to an inguinal hematoma. If the guidewire is not introduced properly, dissection or perforation of the vessel may occur. The same can happen with insertion of the sheath when there is kinking or calcification of the vessel. Vascular traumatic injuries usually occur in the iliac artery vessels or lower abdominal aorta (about 1% of patients), whereas lacerations of supraaortic vessels are uncommon. When abdominal aortic aneurysms are present with intraluminal thrombus, thromboembolism can develop as a dangerous consequence. Intrinsic problems of the IABP catheter, including balloon rupture or leak (0.2% to 0.7% of patients), can occur especially in the presence of aortic calcification. Because helium dissolves easily in the blood, this is not dangerous. It is easily recognized, however, when there is no longer adequate diastolic augmentation, and the pneumatic drive line is filled with blood. With the sheath in place, it is not difficult to exchange the catheter, but it is also possible without a sheath. In either situation, it is advisable to reinsert a guidewire to the level of the thoracic aorta. Paraplegia is another dreaded complication, which occurs in about 0.01% of cases.

One of the most important and frequent problems is inadequate perfusion of the extremity distal to the IABP insertion site, which occurs in 5% to 30% of patients. Mild differences in skin temperature between the two extremities are usually not important but may indicate a potential problem. When pulses vanish, the IABP catheter must be removed urgently because leg ischemia and compartment syndrome are imminent. Lower leg ischemia also may develop after nonsurgical removal of the catheter. Overaggressive manual pressure on the vessel for hemostasis (if no purse-string suture is present) may lead to thrombotic occlusion, mandating immediate surgical embolectomy.

If the diastolic IABP waveform is small and low amplitude, the balloon itself may be too small. Because an oversized balloon can be only partially filled, one should favor larger balloon sizes if there is doubt.

■ SPECIAL CONSIDERATIONS

Use of the IABP in children is possible because small balloons are available (minimum 5 cc). IABP is used rarely in infants, however, probably due to the lack of experience and fear of complications. In small infants, it is advised to use an aortic access and leave the chest open for the duration of IABP support, whereas in older children, femoral cutdown should be used.

Mobilization of a patient during mechanical support is often problematic. In the adult, rigid introducer sheaths may lead to laceration or perforation of iliac vessels, which occurs rarely. The sheathless systems allow the patient to be mobilized to a chair. Similarly, transport of the patient from one institution to another is no longer a problem. Modern consoles are equipped with on-board batteries that permit operation for several hours.

■ SUMMARY

IAPBs have gained widespread use because they are effective, simple to use, and inexpensive. The main indications are treatment of unstable angina and low cardiac output related to myocardial ischemia in acute myocardial infarction, in PTCA, and after surgical revascularization procedures. More recently, it has been shown that patients with severely impaired left ventricular function benefit from preoperative IABP placement, resulting in less need for catecholamine support and shorter ICU stay after surgery. Insertion of the IABP can be accomplished percutaneously in almost all situations. Complications are few when the IABP is inserted properly and removed as soon as possible.

SUGGESTED READING

Akomea-Agyin C, et al: Intraaortic balloon pumping in children, *Ann Thorac Surg* 67:1415, 1999.

Christenson JT, et al: Optimal timing of preoperative intraaortic balloon pump support in high-risk coronary patients, *Ann Thorac Surg* 68:934, 1999.

Dietl CA, et al: Efficacy and cost-effectiveness of preoperative IABP in patients with ejection fraction of 0.25 or less, *Ann Thorac Surg* 62:401, 1996.

Schmid C, et al: Prophylactic use of the intra-aortic balloon pump in patients with impaired left ventricular function, *Scand Cardiovasc J* 33:194, 1999.

Torchiana DF, et al: Intraaortic balloon pumping for cardiac support: trends in practice and outcome, 1968-1995, *J Thorac Cardiovasc Surg* 113:758, 1997.

MECHANICAL CIRCULATORY ASSISTANCE

Vivek Rao
Mehmet C. Oz

Congestive heart failure remains the only cardiovascular diagnosis that is increasing in prevalence. In the United States, more than 5 million people experience heart failure, and almost 600,000 new patients are diagnosed each year. In 2000, there were 2243 heart transplants performed in the United States. Most patients who have heart failure unresponsive to maximal medical therapy require an alternate form of therapy. This chapter reviews surgical considerations in patients with acute or chronic heart failure and the potential role of mechanical circulatory assistance.

A wide variety of circulatory support devices currently are available in North America. Major advances in device technology have allowed physicians to broaden the range of salvageable patients to include patients with acute myocardial infarction and postcardiotomy shock. The concept of bridge-to-bridge support is important for nontransplant centers that do not have the resources to provide long-term mechanical support. Early hemodynamic stabilization with user-friendly temporary devices can have a significant impact on clinical outcomes after insertion of an implantable long-term system.

■ INDICATIONS

The criteria for left ventricular assist device (LVAD) insertion depend on the type of support required. For patients in whom myocardial recovery is expected (bridge to recovery), the indications for LVAD support are far less rigid than for patients in whom a bridge to transplantation is required. In general, hemodynamic criteria suggesting the need for mechanical support include a pulmonary capillary wedge pressure greater than 20 mm Hg, systolic blood pressure less than 80 mm Hg, a cardiac index of less than 2 liters/min/m^2 in the setting of maximal inotropic or intraaortic balloon pump support. We consider maximal inotropic support to include a minimum of two intravenous agents, such as the phosphodiesterase inhibitor milrinone at a concentration greater than 0.5 µg/kg/min and dobutamine at a concentration greater than 5 µg/kg/min. In the chronic heart failure patient, device insertion should be considered when a low-output state persists despite maximal medical therapy or end-organ failure is imminent (mixed venous saturation <60%). A rising serum creatinine value in association with oliguria is a frequent indication to proceed with LVAD insertion in an otherwise hemodynamically stable patient.

Bridge to Recovery

The Abiomed (Abiomed Corp, Danvers, MA) and Thoratec (Thoratec Corp, Pleasanton, CA) devices are approved by the U.S. Food and Drug Administration (FDA) and used widely to support patients in whom myocardial recovery is expected. Common indications include postcardiotomy syndromes, viral cardiomyopathies, anterior wall myocardial infarctions (with revascularization), and posttransplant reperfusion injury.

Both systems can be configured for univentricular or biventricular support. The Abiomed requires systemic heparinization but has the advantage of requiring minimal setup and adjustment to initiate and maintain support. Anticoagulation of the Thoratec device consists of warfarin (Coumadin) therapy to maintain an international normalized ratio (INR) of 3 to 3.5. Although the Abiomed system is significantly less expensive than the Thoratec pump, the latter has the advantage of providing long-term support should the heart not recover. One advantage of the Abiomed system, when used as a right ventricular assist device (RVAD), is the capability to provide continuous venovenous hemodialysis as renal replacement therapy without the need for additional vascular access.

In transplant-eligible patients who receive an Abiomed, conversion to an implantable long-term device is considered after 7 to 10 days of temporary support if no recovery is detected. Although a return to the operating room for a device change has added risk and cost, these may be offset by the improved patient outcome and outpatient capability of the implantable devices.

There has been an interest in long-term support for recovery. Contradictory results and the inability to predict which patients can be weaned successfully from long-term support have suppressed the initial enthusiasm surrounding myocardial recovery. Newer adjuvant technologies, such as cell transplantation and therapeutic angiogenesis, may allow more patients to be weaned successfully from long-term mechanical assist and delay or avoid the need for transplantation.

Bridge to Transplantation

Transplant-eligible patients are referred often for mechanical assist support. These patients present with either acute hemodynamic deterioration or chronic deterioration and impending end-organ failure despite maximal medical therapy. In addition, some patients are candidates for high-risk alternatives to transplantation, such as myocardial revascularization, aneurysmorrhaphy, or valvular repair/replacement. These procedures may pose prohibitive risk to the patient in the absence of LVAD backup. Lastly, patients in whom myocardial recovery was expected but did not occur often are referred for conversion to a long-term implantable device.

Several risk factors have been identified as independent predictors of survival after LVAD insertion, including preoperative oliguria, respiratory failure requiring mechanical ventilation, right heart failure, liver failure, and previous cardiac surgery. A 10-point screening score has been developed to predict mortality in LVAD recipients based on these criteria (Table 1). Patients presenting with screening scores greater than 5 face a 50% operative mortality compared with less than 15% in patients with scores less than 5.

■ SURGICAL CONSIDERATIONS

The surgical implant techniques for the more common ventricular assist devices (VADs) are discussed here. Common to all devices are management strategies to deal with preexisting coronary and valvular disease. Decisions must be made with respect to the eventual outcome of the patient and whether the device is meant to be a bridge to bridge, bridge to recovery, or bridge to transplant.

The management of coronary artery disease depends on the indication for LVAD support. In patients with severe left ventricular dysfunction who are undergoing high-risk revascularization with LVAD backup, the sites of the aortic proximal anastomoses need to be considered carefully. We recommend construction of the proximal anastomoses on the lesser curvature of the aorta, leaving enough room on the anterolateral aspect of the aorta to accommodate the LVAD outflow graft if necessary.

In patients presenting for primary LVAD support as a bridge to transplantation, the treatment of underlying coronary artery disease is entirely different. We usually do not perform bypasses on left-sided lesions, regardless of the severity, because angina after LVAD insertion is extremely rare. Significant (>70%) stenoses of the right coronary artery are bypassed routinely, however, to improve right ventricular perfusion. Although the short-term and medium-term patency of saphenous vein grafts is unknown in the presence of LVAD support, we believe that revascularization of the right coronary artery territory affords right ventricular protection in the critical early postoperative period. In patients presenting with postcardiotomy shock, we advocate repositioning of the right coronary artery graft to either the anterior aorta or the outflow graft itself.

Valvular Disease in LVAD Candidates

Despite the small number of patients who require management of valvular disease at the time of LVAD insertion, our results suggest that these patients can be supported successfully with mechanical circulatory assistance. On the basis of our clinical experience with the management of these patients, we have formulated guidelines for the intraoperative treatment of native or prosthetic valve disease (Figure 1).

Aortic Valve

During LVAD support, an untreated incompetent aortic valve results in a circulatory loop where blood is returned directly to the device via the insufficient valve. LVAD rates and flows are artificially elevated, and inadequate systemic perfusion occurs. The diagnosis of moderate aortic insufficiency can be difficult in the preoperative setting. We advocate the routine use of intraoperative transesophageal echocardiography for the assessment of all valvular structures and to assess for possible intracardiac shunts. Aortic competence can be assessed during cardiopulmonary bypass (CPB), when transvalvular gradients more closely resemble

Table 1 Risk Factor Summation Score

VARIABLE	SAMPLE SIZE	RELATIVE RISK	*p* VALUE	WEIGHTING
Ventilated	66	5.3	<.0001	4
Postcardiotomy shock	57	3.5	<.0001	2
Pre-LVAD	26	3.4	<.0001	2
CVP >16 mm Hg	83	2.1	.04	1
PT >16 sec	72	2.1	.02	1

LVAD, left ventricular assist device; CVP, central venous pressure; PT, prothrombin time.

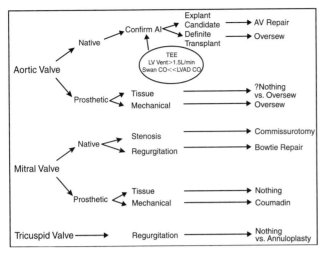

Figure 1
Algorithm for the management of valvular disease during left ventricular assist device (LVAD) support. AI, aortic insufficiency; AV, aortic valve; TEE, transesophageal echocardiography; LV, left ventricle; CO, cardiac output.

those of an LVAD-supported patient. Additional diagnostic information can be obtained by quantifying the amount of left ventricular vent return. For the average patient with a flow rate of 5 liters/min on CPB, a vent return of 1.5 liters/min implies significant aortic insufficiency and would prompt us to consider surgical correction.

In patients requiring long-term LVAD support as a bridge to transplant, our preferred strategy is to oversew an incompetent aortic valve. In patients who have the potential for myocardial recovery and subsequent LVAD explant, the valve is repaired by resuspending the prolapsing cusp or by suturing it to the adjacent normal cusp, creating a bicuspid valve. Our current strategy for patients with a mechanical aortic prosthesis is to prevent thromboembolism by using a Dacron graft to occlude the outflow of the valve. All surgical interventions on the aortic valve can be performed easily through the aortotomy created for the LVAD outflow graft after aortic cross-clamping and cardioplegia arrest. For patients with bioprosthetic aortic valves, we have elected not to occlude the valve. Reports of bioprosthetic valve thrombosis suggest, however, that even tissue valves should be oversewn.

Isolated aortic stenosis is not critical to the LVAD recipient because systemic blood flow is not dependent on antegrade flow through the aortic valve. In the patient undergoing aortic valve replacement with LVAD backup, consideration should be given, however, to the use of a tissue valve to prevent thromboembolism during device support.

Mitral Valve
Because native cardiac contraction and LVAD ejection are not synchronous, left ventricular ejection during device systole results in blood flow against the mitral valve (due to a closed aortic valve). Depending on the unloading characteristics of the device in situ, a significant volume of blood may be ejected through an incompetent mitral valve and result in pulmonary edema. We advocate repair of severe mitral insufficiency at

the time of LVAD insertion. We have found that the "bow-tie" repair described by Alfieri is accomplished easily via the apical left ventriculotomy at the time of device implant. This repair satisfactorily diminishes the severity of mitral regurgitation and may allow for weaning and device explantation in selected patients.

Severe mitral stenosis restricts blood flow to the left ventricle and consequently to the device. A low-output syndrome develops due to impaired LVAD flow and can lead to right heart failure secondary to increased pulmonary vascular resistance. Simple mitral commissurotomy can be performed via the apical ventriculotomy and should be performed carefully to avoid converting mitral stenosis into severe mitral regurgitation. In patients considered for LVAD backup during surgery for mitral pathology in the setting of poor ventricular function, a bioprosthesis should be considered to reduce the risk of valve thrombosis. Although normal flows across a mechanical mitral valve can allow for the presence of a mechanical prosthesis, the avoidance of postoperative anticoagulation is desirable.

Tricuspid Valve
Isolated tricuspid stenosis is a rare entity and has not presented in any patient in our experience. The treatment of tricuspid stenosis is similar to that of mitral stenosis, with the goal of reducing right atrial pressure and improving forward flow through the pulmonary circulation. Tricuspid insufficiency is extremely common secondary to either right ventricular failure or, more commonly, elevated pulmonary vascular resistance secondary to left ventricular failure. In the immediate postoperative period, LVAD flows are limited by output across the pulmonary vascular bed. LVAD patients require high-volume loading conditions and frequently require blood product transfusion. Both of these factors exacerbate right heart failure and predispose to tricuspid insufficiency. Early in our experience, we treated even moderate tricuspid insufficiency with an annuloplasty ring. We found, however, that tricuspid repair did little to improve right ventricular performance. We no longer advocate prophylactic tricuspid repair, unless the insufficiency is severe and ascites is present. We have found that as left ventricular failure resolves with ongoing device support, right-sided failure improves and tricuspid regurgitation abates. The early use of nitric oxide also has led to improved right ventricular hemodynamics.

Implant Techniques
Each of the devices described subsequently is easier to implant with the establishment of CPB, with the possible exception of the ABIOMED BVS system. We prefer to use standard ascending aortic cannulation and single two-stage right atrial venous return. Infrequently in patients with previous surgery and severe pulmonary hypertension, we employ femoral cannulation for the establishment of CPB. We prefer to keep patients normothermic during the implantation period and attempt to perform all cannulations on a beating heart to preserve right ventricular perfusion.

ABIOMED BVS 5000
The ABIOMED BVS 5000 is a dual-chamber temporary external pulsatile VAD composed of smooth-surfaced

polyurethane bladders and trileaflet valves (to ensure unidirectional flow) that may be used either for isolated left or right ventricular assistance or for combined biventricular assistance. Inflow from either the right or the left atrium can be established using specially designed atrial cannulae. We favor left and right ventricular cannulation, however, because of improved inflow capabilities. Two concentric purse-string sutures, buttressed with polytetrafluoroethylene (Teflon) or pericardial pledgets, are placed at the proposed cannulation site, and the catheters potentially can be inserted without the support of CPB. The outflow to either the pulmonary artery (often via the right ventricular outflow tract) or the aorta is established using an arterial cannula with a Hemashield (Meadox Medical, Wayne, NJ) (10 mm) or coated woven Dacron (12 mm) graft. The cannulae exit the skin in a subcostal position to permit closure of the chest while on BVS support. We prefer to tunnel the LVAD under the right costal margin and the RVAD under the left costal margin. The device adjusts itself to maintain a stroke volume of approximately 80 ml and a cardiac output of 4 to 5 liters/min.

The potential need for a longer-term device should be considered when implanting the Abiomed device. Cannulae should be positioned laterally to avoid interference with the midline pocket necessary for an implantable device. The site for the aortic anastomosis should be chosen carefully to allow for the 10- or 12-mm outflow graft to be replaced by the larger 19-mm grafts of the implantable devices.

Thoratec Extracorporeal VAD

The Thoratec VAD pump is composed of a rigid plastic case containing an elastomeric blood pumping sac derived from a proprietary polyurethane multipolymer (Thoralon). The pump can be used for left, right, or biventricular support. The blood sac is compressed by air from a pneumatic drive console to achieve ejection. Mechanical Bjork-Shiley valves, mounted in the inflow and outflow ports of the blood pump, control the direction of blood flow. The pump has a stroke volume of approximately 65 ml and is capable of an output of 6.5 liters/min at a pump rate of 100 beats/min. Two separate inflow cannulae are available for either atrial or apical insertion. The arterial outflow cannula consists of a 30-cm polyester graft suitable for anastomosis to either the aorta or the pulmonary artery.

We prefer to use the left ventricular apex for LVAD inflow and a right ventricular site for RVAD inflow. The left ventricular apex is exposed with the aid of a deep pericardial retraction suture placed just above the left inferior pulmonary vein. The apex is cored to a diameter of approximately 14 mm. A semirigid Ferguson vent is placed into the left ventricle to aid visualization. The inflow tract is inspected, and any thrombus or obstructing muscle tissue is removed. The mitral valve also is inspected, and any reparative procedures can be performed at this time via the apical ventriculotomy. Interrupted mattress sutures of 2-0 Tevdek pledgetted with Teflon are placed in a circumferential fashion around the inflow site. Full-thickness bites are taken through left ventricular muscle and, in the setting of acutely infarcting or edematous myocardium, can be reinforced with a strip of glutaraldehyde-preserved bovine pericardium. These sutures are passed through the felt sewing cuff of the blunt-tip ventricular cannula. The inflow cannula is inserted into the apex,

and the sutures are secured. The beveled end is situated such that the longer lip of the cannula lies flat against the ventricular septum. The LVAD inflow cannula is tunneled to exit the chest in a subcostal position so that the LVAD pump lies on the left upper abdominal quadrant.

If biventricular support is required, we proceed with insertion of the RVAD inflow cannula in a similar fashion. Pledgetted 2-0 Tevdek sutures are passed full thickness in a circumferential mattressed fashion around the proposed cannulation site, then passed through the felt sewing cuff of the blunt-tip ventricular cannula. A cruciate incision is made in the acute margin of the right ventricle, and the cannula is inserted and secured as described previously. The RVAD inflow cannula is tunneled to exit the right chest to position the pump on the right upper abdominal quadrant. For the RVAD outflow cannula, the arterial graft is trimmed to the appropriate length, then anastomosed to the main pulmonary artery using continuous 4-0 polypropylene (Prolene) suture. We have modified this standard technique to avoid an anastomosis to a friable pulmonary artery or to avoid CPB altogether. Two purse-string sutures are placed on the anterior aspect of the right ventricular outflow tract using 3-0 polypropylene sutures pledgetted with glutaraldehyde-preserved bovine pericardium. The Thoratec angled right atrial inflow cannula is immersed in hot water and fashioned into a straight outflow cannula. A cruciate incision is made in the right ventricular outflow tract, maintaining hemostasis with digital pressure. The outflow cannula is inserted and advanced just proximal to the pulmonary artery bifurcation. Then the purse-string sutures are tightened and secured. The outflow cannula is tunneled to exit the chest lateral to the RVAD inflow cannula.

Lastly, the LVAD outflow arterial cannula is anastomosed to the greater curvature of the ascending aorta. A partial occluding clamp is placed on the aorta, and a linear aortotomy is created. The superior and inferior aspects of the aortotomy are revised with a 5-mm punch, and the outflow graft is secured with a running 4-0 polypropylene suture buttressed with a Teflon felt strip. Then the LVAD outflow cannula is tunneled to exit the left chest medial to the LVAD inflow cannula.

All four cannulae are trimmed and attached to the pump housing after adequate deairing. Hand pumping of the LVAD device is started during the initial attempt to wean from CPB. After CPB is discontinued, the device is set to "volume" mode, and the RVAD device is initiated. Initial biventricular VAD flows are usually in the 4.5 to 5 liters/min range. Ejection pressures are adjusted to maintain a 100 mm Hg gradient above the systolic arterial or pulmonary pressure. Vacuum is set initially to −25 mm Hg until the sternum and chest are closed, at which time VAD filling can be augmented by increasing the suction to −50 mm Hg. Postoperatively, anticoagulation is started after chest tube losses are less than 50 ml/hr. The initial target for heparinization is to maintain an activated coagulation time of approximately 160 seconds. After extubation, warfarin therapy is initiated to maintain an INR of 3 to 3.5.

HEARTMATE Vented Electrical LVAD and NOVACOR N100 LVAS

The Novacor LVAS (WorldHeart Corp, Ottawa, Ontario, Canada) and the HeartMate LVAD (Thoratec Corp, Woburn, MA) are implantable long-term, left-sided devices.

The techniques of implantation are similar. The HeartMate is a single pusher-plate device with a maximum stroke volume of 85 ml. It is implanted through a median sternotomy with an inflow cannula inserted into the ventricular apex and an outflow graft anastomosed to the ascending aorta (Figure 2). The pumping chamber can be placed in the abdomen in a preperitoneal position, although some centers insert the device intraperitoneally. The sternotomy is performed before dissecting the preperitoneal pocket to improve the exposure of the diaphragm and to provide access to the heart in the event that these hemodynamically unstable patients decompensate.

The linea alba is divided above the umbilicus, and using a knife or low-power electrocautery, the preperitoneal fat is dissected from the undersurface of the rectus sheath. We avoid entering the peritoneum for several reasons. First, we have had significant morbidity from intraabdominal adhesions and device pressure on the stomach. Second, removal of a properitoneal device is made simpler because no bowel is adherent to the drivelines and valve housings. Third, if significant postoperative bleeding occurs, management of the patient is complicated by the heat loss from the intestines and blood loss into the peritoneal cavity. If the peritoneum is entered during the dissection, the larger holes are closed with absorbable sutures to prevent herniation of intestinal contents. Small holes often are left to facilitate drainage of this space into the peritoneum. If the desired plane is difficult to develop, the rectus sheath can be entered and the posterior rectus sheath left as a patch on the peritoneum. Some surgeons routinely stay in this plane and place the device anterior to the posterior rectus sheath. The dissection is carried laterally and inferiorly, dividing the transversalis fascia as needed, to allow room for the device. Superiorly the dissection is carried to the undersurface of the diaphragm until the apex of the heart can be palpated. The multiple small blood vessels in this plane should be divided with electrocautery before systemic heparinization. The properitoneal space to the right of the linea alba also is opened for approximately 2 to 3 inches to facilitate closure of the linea alba at the completion of the case and to allow room for the device outflow valve and graft conduit. The muscular attachment of the right diaphragm to the medial edge of the sternum also must be divided to allow room for the graft.

The device is inserted into the created pocket, and the site for the driveline is selected, attempting to create as long a tunnel as possible to which the Dacron coating of the driveline can adhere. We usually bring the driveline out in the right upper quadrant to facilitate fixation of the Dacron to the skin near the immobile costal margin. After making a skin incision smaller than the diameter of the driveline, the tunneling device is inserted and angled inferiorly below the umbilicus and into the preperitoneal space. This technique avoids trauma to the driveline and provides the longest tunnel possible in the hope of reducing the infection rate. Rubber finger cots are left on the device inflow and outflow to prevent the entrance of foreign material into the pumping chamber.

After establishing CPB, the apex of the heart is elevated with the use of a posterior pericardial suture. A Foley catheter is inserted through the vent site and a coring knife cuts down to the Foley catheter to remove a circular section of the left ventricular apex. Residual muscle or scar that may impinge on the cannula site is resected. A thorough search for thrombus also should be accomplished and does not require aortic cross-clamping, unless significant aortic insufficiency is present. Full-thickness horizontal mattress pledgetted 2-0 Tevdek sutures are placed around the sewing cuff, remembering that more ventricle must be gathered at the perimeter of the sewing circle than at its center.

When the apical cuff is secure, a cruciate incision in the diaphragm opposite the ventricular apex is made, and the TCI device inflow cannula is brought into the chest. Alternatively a linear incision is made down to the desired point in the diaphragm to facilitate tension-free connection of the device to the heart. The inflow cannula is inserted through the silicone apical cuff until the entire sintered titanium surface is within the cuff. Inflow complications are uncommon, owing to the short length of the inflow cannula; however, special modifications of the described technique sometimes are required in patients with acute infarctions, left ventricular aneurysms, or a calcified left ventricular apex. The Dacron tie of the inflow cuff is secured, and additional reinforcements (umbilical tape or heavy sutures) are applied to prevent air entrainment.

Next the outflow Dacron graft is cut to the appropriate length, usually 13 cm, keeping in mind that too long a graft kinks as the chest is closed. Postoperatively the device migrates

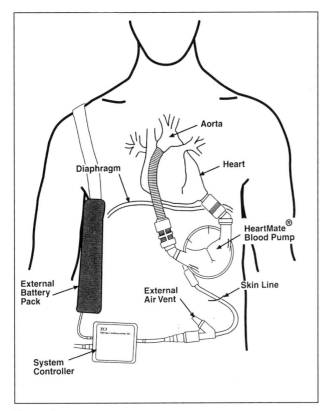

Figure 2
Preperitoneal placement of the HeartMate (Thoratec Corp, Woburn, MA) left ventricular assist device.

inferiorly and displaces the outflow graft; ample length to allow graft stretch should be allowed. A partial occluding clamp is placed on the right lateral aspect of the ascending aorta, and a longitudinal aortotomy is performed. The periaortic adventitia is left in place and helps provide hemostasis. Two 5-mm punch holes are made in either end of the linear incision, and the tissue between the punch holes is excised, leaving an elliptical hole. The distal end of the Dacron graft is sewn end-to-side to the aorta using continuous 4-0 polypropylene sutures. Even relatively small bleeding sites can be problematic postoperatively, so this anastomosis must be inspected meticulously.

We follow several steps to reduce the chance of air embolism. After placing the patient in steep Trendelenburg position, the patient is loaded with volume and ventilated while the LVAD is filled with blood. Next, the hand pump is used to eject blood through a vent hole in the partially occluded outflow graft. The field is flooded with fluid, and the CPB flow is reduced to minimize the chance of the device sucking air. Finally, we search for residual air with transesophageal echocardiography.

When deaired, the required inotropic support is instituted as the patient is weaned from CPB and the LVAD is fully activated. The graft is positioned to prevent kinking and to reduce the chance of injury at the time of reoperation.

CardioWest Total Artificial Heart

The CardioWest (CardioWest Technologies, Inc, Tucson, AZ) is currently the only total artificial heart approved for use in the United States under an FDA investigational device exemption (Figure 3). This device is pneumatically driven

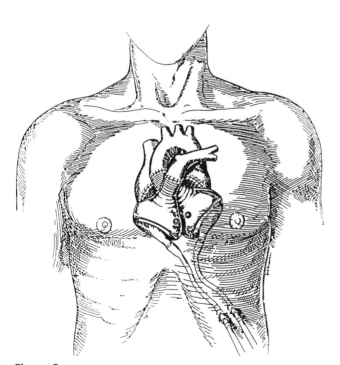

Figure 3
The CardioWest (CardioWest Technologies, Inc, Tucson, AZ) total artificial heart.

and implanted in the orthotopic position. The pump consists of a rigid pump housing that contains dual spherical polyurethane chambers. A four-layer polyurethane diaphragm ejects a maximal volume of 70 ml, and together the pump generates flows of 6 to 8 liters/min. Inflow and outflow conduits are constructed of Dacron and contain Medtronic-Hall mechanical valves. The dual ventricular chambers are anastomosed to native atrial cuffs, and the outflows are anastomosed to the great vessels. Dual pneumatic drivelines exit transcutaneously to an adjacent control system, which monitors pump pressures and performance. Antiplatelet and systemic anticoagulation are needed.

■ AXIAL FLOW PUMPS

Axial flow pumps represent the next generation of assist devices. They can provide full cardiac support in a much smaller pump with fewer moving parts and less blood-contacting surfaces than pusher-plate devices. In addition to their small size, their design is notable for nonpulsatile flow. Several studies have shown metabolic and neurohumoral changes in organ perfusion with uniform versus pulsatile flow. Clinical and long-term animal studies have failed, however, to show significant differences in morbidity and mortality with axial flow pumps. The most promising devices are the HeartMate II, DeBakey VAD, and Jarvik 2000. These devices weigh between 53 and 176 g and can generate flows in excess of 10 liters/min.

The Jarvik 2000, HeartMate II, and DeBakey axial flow pumps all have similar features as just mentioned. Their small size allows implantation into smaller patients than most pulsatile pumps. Although there is controversy over long-term nonpulsatile flow, most patients maintain some native cardiac function and continue to have pulsatile blood flow.

In the event of a device failure, there are few options or backup mechanisms in place other than replacement. Additionally, owing to the lack of valves, device malfunction can result in the equivalent of wide-open aortic insufficiency. The DeBakey and HeartMate II pumps already have been implanted successfully in a few patients in Europe. These pumps use the standard median sternotomy, apical cannulation, and ascending aortic outflow anastomosis similar to the HeartMate I and Novacor N100 LVADs. The Jarvik 2000 is implanted through a left thoracotomy in the sixth intercostal space. The pump itself is situated in an intraventricular position via an apical cannulation site. The 16-mm outflow graft is sewn to the descending thoracic aorta with the aid of a partial occluding clamp. CPB is achieved with femoral arterial and venous cannulation.

■ CLINICAL OUTCOMES

The operative mortality associated with LVAD support is approximately 20% with an additional 5% mortality at the time of LVAD explant and heart transplantation. Hospital discharge after transplantation is approximately 75%. The predominant causes of death include persistent multiorgan failure despite mechanical support and overwhelming sepsis. Right heart failure is common, occurring in almost 50% of patients receiving isolated left-sided support, but the need for right-sided mechanical assistance is less than 20%. Similarly the posttransplant survival to hospital discharge in total artificial heart recipients approaches 80%.

Postoperative neurologic complications occur in a few patients but are reported to be higher with the Novacor LVAS. After prolonged mechanical support, inflow valve regurgitation develops in the HeartMate LVAD, which manifests by increased flow rates (>8 liters/min) that are not comparable to thermodilution cardiac outputs. In addition, with valve incompetence, the device fails to decompress the left ventricle adequately and can lead to pulmonary edema.

The current-generation VADs were designed to function as bridge-to-transplant or bridge-to-recovery devices. They have relatively high rates of device-related infection and stroke. In addition, they remain expensive relative to the cost of transplantation and may not provide equivalent quality of life. The current-generation devices may not be ideal for "destination" therapy as an alternative to transplantation.

The next generation will comprise smaller, more durable, and completely implantable devices that ultimately may serve as destination therapy. In addition, these devices feature longer battery life and decreased rates of infection due to the lack of percutaneous lines. The potential patient population that ultimately may benefit from prolonged mechanical circulatory support will dwarf the current population of heart transplant recipients.

SUGGESTED READING

Farrar DJ, Hill JD: Univentricular and biventricular Thoratec VAD support as a bridge to transplantation, *Ann Thorac Surg* 55:276, 1993.

Hunt SA, Frazier OH: Mechanical circulatory support and cardiac transplantation, *Circulation* 97:2079, 1998.

Oz MC, et al: Screening scale predicts patients successfully receiving long-term implantable left ventricular assist devices, *Circulation* 92(Suppl II):II-169, 1995.

Oz MC, et al: Preperitoneal placement of ventricular assist devices: An illustrated stepwise approach, *J Card Surg* 10:288, 1995.

Rao V, et al: Surgical management of valvular disease in patients requiring left ventricular assist device support, *Ann Thorac Surg* 71:1448, 2001.

Smedira NG, Blackstone EH: Postcardiotomy mechanical support: risk factors and outcomes, *Ann Thorac Surg* 71:S60, 2001.

EXTRACORPOREAL LIFE SUPPORT IN THE ADULT

Kenneth J. Woodside
Scott K. Alpard
Joseph B. Zwischenberger

Extracorporeal life support (ECLS), including extracorporeal membrane oxygenation (ECMO), extracorporeal carbon dioxide removal ($ECCO_2R$), and arteriovenous carbon dioxide removal ($AVCO_2R$), has undergone a revolution over the past 30 years, allowing such techniques to leave the animal laboratory and significantly improve clinical outcomes in critically ill patients. These techniques, developed from engineering principles of cardiopulmonary bypass (CPB) for heart surgery, provide temporary replacement or augmentation of ventilation, oxygenation, and cardiac function. ECMO circuits use a modified heart-lung bypass machine, usually with a distensible venous blood drainage reservoir, a servoregulated roller pump, a membrane for gas exchange, and a countercurrent heat exchanger for thermoregulation (Figure 1). Continuous heparin anticoagulation prevents circuit thrombosis and thromboembolism. Although most initial work has been done in neonatal and pediatric populations, recent advances in adult ECLS have extended the application of these techniques to populations traditionally thought to have worse outcomes. The Extracorporeal Life Support Organization (ELSO) has maintained the voluntary Neonatal, Pediatric, and Adult ECMO Registry since 1989 and provided improved outcomes data for all populations since that time.

The first attempts at ECLS were in the 1960s, although it was not until the mid-1970s that Bartlett reported the first successful use of ECMO for newborn respiratory failure. Early trials established the therapeutic effectiveness of ECMO in infants whose predicted mortality was greater than 80%. Since then, ECMO has become the standard of care for unresponsive severe respiratory failure in neonates, with an overall survival rate of 77%. Older pediatric populations with respiratory failure have slightly inferior survival rates, with ECMO registry data demonstrating an overall survival of 63%, whereas children requiring cardiac support have an overall survival rate of 54%. Pediatric patients are thought to have a somewhat worse outcome from the effects of progressive mechanical ventilation with high fraction of inspired oxygen (FIO_2) and pressures, secondary organ damage and other comorbidities, and the longer duration of ECMO usually needed in this population. Small trials and case reports have described the expanded use of ECMO in patients with conditions previously thought to be contraindications, including major burns, malignancy, and disseminated infection.

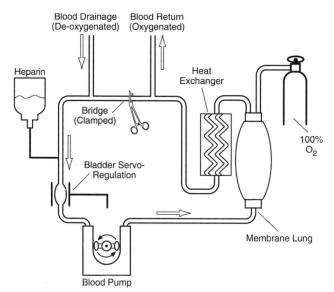

Figure 1
A typical ECMO circuit.

ADULT RESPIRATORY DISTRESS SYNDROME AND EXTRACORPOREAL LIFE SUPPORT IN ADULTS

Traditional ventilatory management of adult respiratory distress syndrome (ARDS) is associated with barotrauma from high inspiratory pressures, volutrauma from overdistention of alveoli, and toxicity due to high oxygen concentrations. These lung injuries lead to progressive deterioration in lung compliance, functional residual capacity, and gas exchange, with impairment of cardiac function by associated high positive pressures. Recent advances in pulmonary management suggest that lower airway pressures will lessen barotrauma and volutrauma. In particular, the ARDS Network Trial demonstrated improved survival with lower tidal volumes (6 ml/kg). However, low tidal volume ventilation can cause alveolar hypoventilation and hypercapnic acidosis and may require higher levels of peak end-expiratory pressure (PEEP) and FIO_2 to maintain adequate oxygenation. These factors may contribute to oxidant-induced lung injury. Use of ECMO can remove excess carbon dioxide and improve oxygenation, while avoiding the volutrauma and barotrauma associated with normal mechanical ventilation.

Despite numerous advances in critical care, ARDS still carries a mortality rate of 40% to 50%, which has stimulated an interest in expanding ECLS to adult populations. Hill reported the first successful use of adult ECMO in 1972. After a number of small, moderately successful studies, a national study of adult ECMO sponsored by the National Heart, Lung, and Blood Institute was performed in the late 1970s. However, the study was halted after 90 patients, because of greater than 90% mortality in both the control and treatment groups. In the mid-1980s, renewed interest in adult ECMO led to the development of the criteria now used by most adult ECMO centers: acute reversible respiratory or cardiac failure unresponsive to optimal ventilator and pharmacologic management, a potentially reversible underlying disease process, a predicted mortality greater than 80%, and expected recovery within a relatively short period of ECLS (several days to <1 month).

The specific inclusion criteria for adult ECMO are controversial and depend on the experience and capabilities of the ECMO center. The etiology of acute respiratory failure must be taken into account, although both primary and secondary ARDS can be supported by ECMO. Largely reversible processes, such as bronchospasm from severe reactive airway disease or severe hypothermia, can be supported or corrected by ECMO. Patients with factors once thought to be contraindications to ECMO, such as sepsis, bacteremia, or even trauma, can receive extracorporeal support. Other reversible processes amenable to ECMO include fat emboli syndrome, near-drowning, and thoracic trauma. Irreversible processes, such as pulmonary fibrosis, should exclude patients from consideration for extracorporeal support. A PaO_2-to-FIO_2 (P/F) ratio of less than 100 or transpulmonary shunts (Q_p/Q_s ratio) greater than 30% is often seen as an indication for ECMO. Until larger ECMO trials are complete, specific indications and criteria remain institution dependent.

There are several different ECLS techniques: ECMO, CPB, $ECCO_2R$, $AVCO_2R$, and the nascent artificial lung (Table 1). The optimal method of ECLS depends on the disease pathophysiology and the experience of the ECMO center. Patients requiring cardiac support need venoarterial (VA) ECMO, whereas those only requiring respiratory support receive venovenous (VV) ECMO (Table 2) or one of the carbon dioxide removal circuits ($ECCO_2R$ or $AVCO_2R$). VA ECMO is generally reserved for patients with cardiovascular instability and those with inadequate cardiac output. Once ECMO is initiated, ventilator settings are rapidly decreased, and low-rate sustained inflations above alveolar opening pressures applied to prevent total lung collapse. As this technique has significant risk for arterial thromboemboli, reduced pulmonary blood flow, impaired left ventricular function from volume overload, and circulatory dependence on the extracorporeal circuit, the other extracorporeal techniques are preferred when applicable. Patients initiated on a VA circuit may be converted to VV bypass if cardiac function improves.

Most adult patients with unresponsive severe respiratory failure require VV ECMO or $ECCO_2R$. VV ECMO is used when oxygenation and ventilation need to be supported, but cardiac output is adequate to maintain intracorporeal circulation. This technique uses higher flow rates (5 L/min) and parallel oxygenators for increased membrane surface area. During VV ECMO, right ventricular output is normal, or even somewhat higher than before ECMO, as cardiac output increases after severe hypoxia has been corrected. $ECCO_2R$ supports carbon dioxide removal by using low flow (about 1 L/min, or approximately 20% to 30% of cardiac output) partial VV bypass and low-frequency positive pressure ventilation (15 to 20 cm H_2O) by the natural lungs. Oxygenation and ventilation are dissociated; oxygenation occurs in the lungs, and carbon dioxide is cleared via the extracorporeal circuit. Overall survival rates in adults with these techniques range from 45% to 65%.

Like $ECCO_2R$, $AVCO_2R$ uncouples oxygenation and ventilation, with oxygen diffusion occurring across the native lungs and carbon dioxide removal occurring across the

Table 1 Comparison of Extracorporeal Membrane Oxygenation (ECMO), Cardiopulmonary Bypass (CPB), Low-Flow Positive Pressure Ventilation With Extracorporeal Carbon Dioxide Removal (LFPPV-ECCO$_2$R), Arteriovenous Carbon Dioxide Removal (AVCO$_2$R), and Artificial Lung

	ECMO	CPB	ECCO$_2$R	AVCO$_2$R	ARTIFICIAL LUNG
Setting	Respiratory and/or cardiac failure	Cardiac surgery	Respiratory failure	Respiratory failure (investigational)	Respiratory failure (experimental)
Location	Extrathoracic	Intrathoracic	Extrathoracic	Extrathoracic	Extrathoracic
Type of support	VA (cardiac) VV (respiratory)	VA (total bypass)	VV (respiratory) (CO$_2$)	AV (respiratory) (CO$_2$)	PA-PA or PA-LA
Cannulation	VA: neck VV: neck and groin 2 Cannulas (surgical or percutaneous) 1 Cannula (VVDL)	Direct cardiac 2 Cannulas (surgical)	Neck and groin 2 Cannulas (surgical or percutaneous) 1 Cannula (VVDL)	Groin 2 Cannulas (percutaneous)	Transthoracic to major vessels
Blood flow	High (70% to 80% CO)	Total (100% CO)	Medium (30% CO)	Low (10% to 15% CO)	Total (100%)
Ventilatory support	Pressure-controlled ± high PEEP 10 to 12 breaths/min	None (anesthesia)	High PEEP 2 to 4 breaths/min High F$_{IO_2}$	Pressure and/or volume controlled (algorithm driven)	None necessary
Blood reservoir	Small (50 ml)	Yes (>1 L)	Small (50 ml)	No	No
Arterial filter	No	Yes	No	No	No
Blood pump	Roller or centrifugal	Roller or centrifugal	Roller or centrifugal	None	None
Heparinization	ACT 200 to 260	ACT >400	ACT 200 to 260	ACT 200 to 260	ACT 200 to 260
Average length of extracorporeal support	Days to weeks	Hours	Days to weeks	Days to weeks	Days
Complications	Bleeding Organ failure	Intraoperative	Bleeding	Bleeding	Bleeding
Causes of death	Support terminated: PAP >75% systemic Irreversible lung disease Cardiac dysrhythmias	Intraoperative Air embolism	Multiorgan failure Septic shock Hemorrhagic	Respiratory failure	Right heart failure

From Alpard SK, Zwischenberger JA: Extracorporeal membrane oxygenation for severe respiratory failure, *Chest Surg Clin North Am* 12:355, 2002.

Table 2 Comparison of Venoarterial and Venovenous Extracorporeal Membrane Oxygenation (ECMO)

	VENOARTERIAL ECMO	VENOVENOUS ECMO
Cannulation sites	Internal jugular vein, right atrium, or femoral vein plus right common carotid, axillary, or femoral artery or aorta (directly)	Internal jugular vein alone (double-lumen or single-lumen tidal flow) Jugular-femoral Femorofemoral Saphenosaphenous Right atrium (directly)
Organ support	Gas exchange and cardiac output	Gas exchange only
Systemic perfusion	Circuit flow and cardiac output	Cardiac output only
Pulse contour	Reduced pulsatility	Normal pulsatility
CVP	Unreliable	Accurate guide to volume status
PA pressure	Unreliable	Reliable
Effect of R → L shunt	Mixed venous into perfusate blood	None
Effect of L → R shunt (PDA)	Pulmonary hyperperfusion may shunt	No effect on flow Require increased flow usual PDA physiology
Blood flow for full gas exchange	80 to 100 ml/kg/hr	100 to 120 ml/kg/hr
Circuit $S\text{v}O_2$	Reliable	Unreliable
Circuit recirculation	None	15% to 30%
Arterial PO_2	60 to 50 mm Hg	45 to 80 mm Hg
Arterial oxygen saturation	≥95%	80% to 95%
Indicators of O_2 insufficiency	Mixed venous saturation or PO_2 Calculated oxygen consumption	Cerebral venous saturation Da-VO_2 across the membrane Patient PaO_2 Premembrane saturation trend Combinations of all of the above
Carbon dioxide removal	Sweep gas flow and membrane lung size dependent	Sweep gas flow and membrane lung size dependent
Oxygenator	0.4 or 0.6	0.6 or 0.8
Ventilator settings	Minimal	Minimal-moderate (dependent on patient size)
Decrease initial vent settings	Rapidly	Slowly

From Alpard SK, Zwischenberger JA: Extracorporeal membrane oxygenation for severe respiratory failure, *Chest Surg Clin North Am* 12:355, 2002.
PDA, patent ductus arteriosus.

membrane gas exchanger. By using a low-resistance gas exchanger in a simple percutaneous arteriovenous shunt, near-total extracorporeal removal of carbon dioxide can be achieved with approximately 1 L/min of flow, allowing lower respiratory rates, tidal volumes, and peak airway pressures. In contrast to the other techniques, however, $AVCO_2R$ eliminates the roller pump and many of the other components of a typical ECMO circuit, resulting in significantly less exposure to foreign materials and priming fluids. Initial safety trials suggest that peak inspiratory pressures are less than 30 cm H_2O, with less complement activation and less leukocyte and platelet consumption. Severe progressive ARDS with P/F ratios less than 100 and profound hypoxia can exceed the capacity of $AVCO_2R$ to adequately correct the pathophysiology despite adequate carbon dioxide removal. Trials are currently under way to determine the effect of percutaneous extracorporeal $AVCO_2R$ with low tidal volume (6 ml/kg) mechanical ventilation on mortality and ventilator-free days in adults with ARDS (P/F ratio <200) and in children with severe acute respiratory failure from burn injury with or without smoke inhalation injury.

■ INITIATION AND MANAGEMENT TECHNIQUES

If cardiac support is required for hemodynamic instability or for transportation of a patient on ECLS, VA ECMO is initiated. Access is usually obtained in the neck and/or groin (Table 2). For patients without hemodynamic instability, VV ECMO is usually the technique of choice, with adult flow rates usually between 80 and 100 ml/kg/min. We normally use the right internal jugular vein for drainage and the right femoral vein for reinfusion (Figure 2). Other centers report

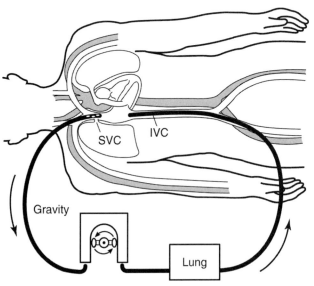

Figure 2
Venovenous bypass circuit using the superior vena cava (SVC) as the outflow tract and the femoral vein as the inflow tract.
(From Bartlett RH: Extracorporeal life support for cardiopulmonary failure, Curr Probl Surg *27:621, 1990.)*

improved flow rates and pulmonary artery mixed venous oxygen saturations with femoroatrial flow schemes. Venovenous double-lumen (VVDL) catheters are also available, allowing for single-site access. Survival results with VVDL ECMO are thought to be equivalent to VA ECMO. As these patients often have a number of comorbid conditions, access is dependent on the exact clinical situation and experience of the ECMO center.

After ECMO is initiated, ventilator settings are substantially reduced to minimize barotrauma and volutrauma. Typical settings include a peak inspiratory pressure of 15 to 20 cm H_2O and a respiratory rate of 10 breaths/min. PEEP levels are variable but typically 12 to 15 cm H_2O and mean airway pressure is 13 to 16 cm H_2O. In addition, oxygen toxicity is minimized by reducing inspired oxygen concentration to 30%. As many of these values are based on neonatal large animal studies, the optimal pressures vary according to individual ECMO center experience. As blood flow levels are high, titrated pharmacologic paralysis is maintained throughout ECMO therapy and an ECMO nurse remains at the bedside at all times.

Ventilatory techniques can be customized to the pathophysiology of the patient. For example, patients with large alveolar air leaks or even bronchopleural fistulas can be treated with selective ventilation of the opposite lung, selective occlusion of the ipsilateral bronchus, or cessation of mechanical ventilation, as breathing is not required for gas exchange. After 48 hours without an air leak, continuous static airway pressure (20 to 30 cm H_2O) is applied for lung conditioning and alveolar recruitment.

ECMO can be used for a number of primary and secondary obstructive processes, including reactive airway disease and severe airway plugging by blood clots or mucus. Flexible bronchoscopy with or without lavage can be used to clear clots or retrieve foreign materials. ECMO support is maintained until the obstruction is removed or the disease process adequately resolves; ECLS is continued until extracorporeal respiratory support is no longer required or therapy is deemed futile.

ECMO has been used postoperatively after congenital heart surgery or heart transplantation. If possible, there should be a brief period between operation and initiation of ECMO to allow hemostasis. In addition, ECMO has been used for lung transplant patients as preoperative support for severe pulmonary sufficiency, as postoperative support in the event of primary graft failure or severe ischemia-reperfusion injury, and as respiratory support for graft dysfunction during acute rejection episodes.

A number of surgical procedures have been performed on patients on ECMO (Table 3). Although the details and level of success of these operations are left to the individual reports, extreme diligence for maintaining hemostasis is mandatory for all of these procedures, as patients remain anticoagulated while connected to the ECMO circuit. Skin incisions are made with the cutting mode of electrocautery, and electrocautery and hemostatic glues are used liberally. ECMO has demonstrated particular promise for complex tracheal reconstructions for the maintenance of oxygenation. ECMO can provide intraoperative gas exchange and eliminate the need for an endotracheal tube. Postoperatively, ECMO can support respiratory function and allow fragile

Table 3 Operations Performed on Neonates, Children, or Adults while on Extracorporeal Life Support

PERFORMED WHILE ON ECLS
Tracheostomy
Video-assisted thoracoscopic bullectomy
Open lung biopsy
Hemothorax evacuation
Intracranial hematoma evacuation
Cardiac catheterization
Gastrointestinal reconstruction
Abscess drainage
Diagnostic peritoneal lavage
Laceration repair
Open reduction and internal fixation of fractures
Skin homografting (without débridement)
FACILITATED BY ECLS FOR INTRAOPERATIVE CARDIORESPIRATORY SUPPORT
Complex tracheal reconstructions for congenital tracheal stenosis
Tracheobronchial stent placement for tracheobronchial stenosis from a metastatic tumor mass
Laryngotracheoesophageal cleft repair
Pneumonectomy
Lung transplant
Heart transplant

ECLS, extracorporeal life support.

reconstructions time to heal without the burden of positive pressure ventilation.

COMPLICATIONS

Critically ill patients are complication prone, and ECMO patients are even more so. However, there are a few complications unique to ECMO patients. Hemorrhage and embolic complications require exact titration of anticoagulation for prevention. Although rare, vascular damage during cannulation can occur and can be fatal if control of the vessel is lost and it retracts into the chest or if aortic dissection occurs. Surprisingly, sepsis is uncommon; only 5% of ECMO patients develop positive blood cultures. Mediastinitis can be particularly morbid in patients with transthoracic cannulae or recent cardiac surgery.

ECMO circuits alter platelet function and survival. Thrombocytopenia develops as platelets aggregate in the circuit; sequester in the lung, liver, and spleen; and are damaged by the roller pump. Platelet counts should be maintained above 50,000, with platelet transfusion as needed. With the combined effects of anticoagulation and thrombocytopenia, care must be taken to monitor for the development of hemothorax, hemopericardium with pericardial tamponade, intracranial bleeding, or other such complications. Hemothorax and pneumothorax often require urgent tube thoracostomy placement to effect rapid drainage. An echocardiogram may be required to diagnose a pericardial effusion or hematoma. Tension hemopneumothorax and pericardial tamponade often present with the triad of increased P_{AO_2}, decreased peripheral perfusion with decreased pulse pressure and S_{VO_2}, and decreased ECMO flow with progressive hemodynamic deterioration. This triad indicates that emergent intervention is required. In addition, postoperative patients and trauma patients must be monitored for region-specific bleeding.

WEANING AND DECANNULATION

As native lung function improves, flow rates are decreased until the native lung is supporting the majority of gas exchange. The patient is then subjected to ventilator trials, with the circuit excluded. If gas exchange and hemodynamic parameters remain adequate, decannulation occurs. Patients requiring cardiac support undergo a similar trial but also have ECMO flow reduced to 10% to 20% of supportive flow. If filling pressures remain low and ventilator contractility is adequate, with or without inotropes, the patient may be decannulated. If percutaneous catheters were used, they are removed and local pressure is applied for at least 1 hour. If operative placement of the cannulae was required, operative removal and hemostatic control are necessary. Femoral vessels usually require repair. Repair of neck vessels is controversial, because immediate embolism or late stenosis can result. Many centers prefer ligation of the vessels, because the vessel was already obstructed by the cannula. If not already present, a tracheostomy should be placed for ventilator weaning and patient comfort.

CONCLUSIONS

ECLS can favorably affect survival in adults with expected survival rates of less than 20%. With such critically ill patients, extreme vigilance is required as almost every physiologic function is at least partially regulated during ECMO. In addition to the issues described in this chapter, numerous other issues must be addressed during the care of the patient. Specific circuit components must be integrated. Fluid and electrolyte status, as well as nutrition, are essential. Renal and endocrine function must be monitored and maintained. Daily neurologic checks while free of pharmacologic paralysis must occur. Protocols must be in place for the numerous minor and major complications that these patients experience. This approach requires an integrated multispecialty ECMO team of surgeons, intensivists, nurses, respiratory therapists, and other allied health professionals for effective ECLS and potentially improved patient survival.

SUGGESTED READING

Bartlett RH, et al: Extracorporeal life support: the University of Michigan experience, *JAMA* 283:904, 2000.

Conrad SA, Bidani A: Management of the acute respiratory distress syndrome, *Chest Surg Clin North Am* 12:325, 2002.

Duncan BW, editor: *Mechanical support for cardiac and respiratory failure in pediatric patients,* New York, 2001, Marcel Dekker.

Zwischenberger JB, et al: Percutaneous extracorporeal CO_2 removal for severe respiratory failure, *Ann Thorac Surg* 68:181, 1999.

Zwischenberger JB, et al, editors: *ECMO: extracorporeal cardiopulmonary support in critical care,* ed 2, Ann Arbor, MI, 2000, Extracorporeal Life Support Organization (ELSO).

AORTIC DISSECTION

Paul C. Y. Tang

John A. Elefteriades

Aortic dissection is the most common lethal condition affecting the human aorta and has an incidence of approximately 5 to 10 patients per 1 million population per year. Dissection is most common in men 50 to 70 years old. Dissection is defined as the entry of blood into the layers of the aortic wall through an intimal tear, with propagation of the split through the false lumen. There is a dissection flap that separates the true lumen from the false lumen. Reentry of blood into the true lumen can occur through an additional intimal tear downstream. Retrograde propagation of dissection can occur, leading to an ascending dissection from an intimal tear originating in the descending aorta.

Dissection is associated with multiple pathologic conditions, including hypertension (approximately 80% of patients), Marfan syndrome, bicuspid aortic valve, coarctation, trauma, and pregnancy. A bicuspid aortic valve is the most common congenital cardiac anomaly, with an incidence of 1% to 2% in the general population and associated with a 5% risk of aortic dissection overall. Bicuspid aortic valves cause more dissections than Marfan syndrome, which has an incidence of only 0.01% of the population but a 40% risk of dissection.

It now is established that genetics plays a large part in the development of aortic dissection and aneurysm. A positive family history is highly predictive for the development of these conditions. Iatrogenic causes of dissection include cannula insertion during surgery (e.g., cardiopulmonary bypass), catheter manipulation, and balloon angioplasty of a coarctation. Early recognition of these complications is essential, and prompt corrective procedures are required.

Complications from dissection are potentially lethal, especially complications involving the ascending aorta (Figure 1). Potentially lethal complications can be categorized into four groups: (1) intrapericardial rupture leading to cardiac tamponade, (2) acute aortic insufficiency, (3) aortic dilation with rupture into the pleural space, and (4) occlusion of branch vessels from dissection propagation. Occlusion of the coronary arteries causing myocardial ischemia and extracranial cerebral vessels leading to stroke are particularly lethal.

The Stanford classification for aortic dissections currently is used:

Type A—dissections involving the ascending aorta
Type B—dissections involving only the descending aorta

This classification correlates well with the natural history and therapeutic implications (see later) and is simpler and more practical than the older DeBakey classification:

Type I—arising from ascending aorta and extending to descending aorta
Type II—arising from and limited to ascending aorta
Type III—arising from and limited to descending aorta

Patients with acute dissection usually present with a pain that is "tearing" in quality. The pain typically is substernal in an ascending dissection and interscapular in the back if the descending aorta is affected. The pain can propagate as the dissection progresses, extending into the lower back and flanks. We consider persistent or renewed pain unresponsive to medical management worrisome for impending rupture. Symptoms such as syncope, shortness of breath, and limb pain also can occur. Paraplegia from spinal cord ischemia is an occasional presenting symptom. On examination, hypertension is usually present. It is important to look for physical signs of complications, such as the murmur of aortic insufficiency, unequal or absent pulses, signs of limb ischemia, or signs of cardiac tamponade from intrapericardial rupture.

■ DIAGNOSIS

Early diagnosis of thoracic aortic dissection first and foremost depends on clinical suspicion in a patient presenting with a consistent clinical picture and suggestive initial investigations. The initial workup may reveal a widened mediastinum on chest x-ray and evidence of myocardial ischemia on an electrocardiogram.

For definitive diagnosis and assessment for complications, transesophageal echocardiography (TEE) is an excellent initial investigation. TEE can identify the intimal flap, show intraluminal thrombus, and assess flow within true and false lumens. TEE also can evaluate complications, such as fluid collections in the periaortic, pleural, and pericardial spaces indicative of rupture; pericardial tamponade; aortic insufficiency from aortic root distortion; and disruption of the coronary ostia. TEE yields all the information necessary to decide on the need for surgical intervention. TEE differentiates between ascending and descending dissection. Advantages include the ability to be performed within a short time, avoidance of intravenous contrast material, and wide availability. A large multicenter European study found an impressive 99% sensitivity and 98% specificity for TEE in the diagnosis of aortic dissection.

Computed tomography (CT) and magnetic resonance imaging (MRI) are alternatives for investigating suspected aortic dissection. CT and MRI can be used as an adjunct to TEE for investigation of the carotid arteries, abdominal

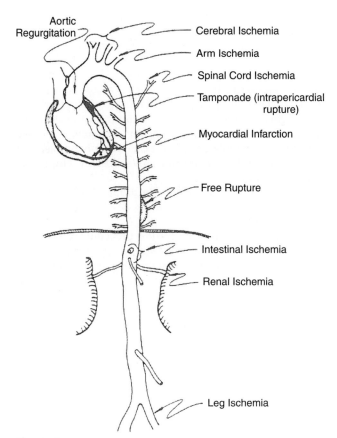

Aortic Regurgitation
Cerebral Ischemia
Arm Ischemia
Spinal Cord Ischemia
Tamponade (intrapericardial rupture)
Myocardial Infarction
Free Rupture
Intestinal Ischemia
Renal Ischemia
Leg Ischemia

Figure 1
Schematic illustration of potential complications of aortic dissection.

aorta, and renal arteries or alone if TEE is not available. These investigations are less operator dependent but require more time in the context of a potentially unstable patient. CT also is associated with the risks of contrast exposure. MRI may not be readily available on an emergency basis, and the MRI environment may be inappropriate for critically ill or unstable patients.

We no longer perform angiography routinely for investigation of aortic dissection because angiography may be unrevealing (no entrance for contrast media due to thrombosis of the false lumen), and it may miss the dissection if a tangential view of the intimal flap is not obtained. Large intimal tears may lead to misleadingly similar opacification of the true and false lumens. In addition, angiography is invasive and accompanied by the risks of contrast exposure.

■ MANAGEMENT

Initial Management—Antiimpulse Therapy

Wheat et al suggested that the impulse of blood from cardiac contraction acting on the aortic wall, not just hypertension, has an important role in continuing the propagation of aortic dissection. Impulse is a function of the blood acceleration, which in turn is related to the rate of ventricular fiber shortening. Wheat et al reasoned that drugs that decrease

myocardial contractility and blood pressure are necessary for success of medical therapy in slowing dissection. This view was supported in subsequent studies and now is generally accepted.

Antiimpulse therapy is used in all patients presenting with aortic dissection. We use an intravenous β-blocking agent (if contraindicated, a calcium channel antagonist is an alternative), and an afterload-reducing agent. The target is to reduce heart rate to less than 60 beats/min and systolic blood pressure to less than 100 mm Hg. These target ranges may be modified if there is oliguria or other signs of organ ischemia. After intravenous therapy for 48 hours, the regimen can be switched to oral therapy. This antiimpulse therapy is appropriate initial therapy for type A and type B dissection.

Acute Ascending Aortic Dissections (Type A)

There is a 1% to 2% per hour mortality rate in ascending dissection. The need for urgent and immediate operation in this scenario is well established and constitutes the standard of care. Patients surviving after 48 hours from the onset of symptoms due to delayed presentation or diagnosis may represent a separate prognostic group, however, who have "weathered the eye of the storm." For these delayed transfer cases, we do not perform urgent nocturnal surgery, but rather prefer semiurgent surgery during daytime hours. Severe comorbidities or advanced age may make operation for acute type A dissection inappropriate. These patients are treated with antiimpulse therapy and occasionally survive long-term.

Choice of a specific operation for acute type A dissection is controversial. Acute ascending aortic dissection is a lethal disease; that we consider the highest priority for immediate surgery to be achieving patient survival. Because composite graft replacement of the ascending aorta and aortic valve with coronary artery reimplantation is a dangerous procedure in acute type A dissection, composite grafting should be avoided whenever possible. Coronary button mobilization and anastomosis in the acutely dissected aorta is associated with a high risk of complications. In most cases, a supracoronary tube graft replacement of the ascending aorta is sufficient for acute type A dissection.

In patients with a connective tissue disorder, such as Marfan syndrome or annuloaortic ectasia (in which the annulus itself is significantly enlarged), composite graft replacement with coronary button implantation is appropriate. The proximal anastomosis can be constructed onto the strong aortic annulus to yield a secure proximal anastomosis. Sewing to a thin friable proximal aortic wall in a patient with connective tissue disease is technically difficult and often lethal. Subsequent dilation of the residual aortic segment can occur with the risk of late rupture.

The distal anastomosis should be carried out using an open technique under deep hypothermic arrest. A nonopen anastomosis leads to a cramped, distorted region at the posterior tip of the clamp and is a frequent site of bleeding. With clamp application, the anastomosis often is forced considerably more proximally, resulting in less complete resection of the ascending aorta. Only the ascending aorta normally is replaced in operations for acute type A aortic dissection; this essentially prevents the lethal complications, including coronary dissection, intrapericardial bleeding, and severe aortic insufficiency. The distal descending and abdominal aorta remain dissected and require treatment and follow-up similar to a type B dissection. Replacement of the ascending aorta usually restores perfusion to all vascular beds previously shut off by the dissection.

Concomitant aortic valve replacement is indicated only if insufficiency is severe (≥3+). The status of the aortic valve can be assessed with intraoperative TEE before cardiopulmonary bypass. Most cases require no valve intervention at all or can be handled by resuspending the aortic valve. Aortic insufficiency often improves with simple graft replacement of the ascending aorta because the leaflets are brought into closer coaptation, and root distortion is corrected.

A beveled, hemiarch replacement can be part of the open distal technique of tube grafting if necessary. A low rate of subsequent arch aneurysm formation occurs with this technique. With intimal tears originating in the aortic arch, it is still not clear whether the arch should be excised. Including the arch in the replacement may have long-term benefits, but a full arch replacement in the setting of acute aortic dissection is a challenging procedure. A tube graft suffices if the surgeon believes that full arch replacement is too formidable given the circumstances.

In acute dissection, the two aortic layers should be reapposed to obliterate the false lumen. This reapposition may be facilitated by use of surgical adhesives. In chronic dissections, the two layers must not be reapproximated, however, because major branch vessels of the aortic arch may be chronically dependent on flow through the false lumen. Relatively new valve-sparing operations for root replacement have been applied to acute type A dissections. It is still too early to judge their merit in this condition, however.

Although the surgical management of ascending aortic dissections is a challenging clinical problem, these operations can be performed with relatively low morbidity and mortality. In a review of our most recent data, postoperative mortality rate was 14% (8 of 57 patients) for acute type A dissection.

Acute Descending Aortic Dissection (Type B)

It generally is agreed that the management of uncomplicated acute descending aortic dissections is largely medical. This involves the use of antiimpulse therapy to decrease heart rate and peripheral constriction. The patient is monitored closely for development of complications, including rupture, dissection, extension, and organ ischemia.

We studied 100 consecutive, acute type B dissections treated at our center. Two thirds of these patients did well with only medical, antiimpulse therapy. Ten percent died during the acute hospitalization. About 20% required surgical intervention for various complications.

A surgical approach is required when complications develop, such as organ ischemia and impending or realized rupture. Direct graft replacement of the proximal descending aorta has been the standard treatment but is associated with significant morbidity and mortality.

Published series show overall mortality rates of 26% to 65%, with 35% of patients dying from bleeding in contiguous or distant aortic segments. The acutely dissected descending aorta is difficult to work with surgically. A daunting paraplegia rate of 30% to 36% was observed with direct graft replacement of the descending aorta for acute type B aortic dissection. Also, direct aortic replacement does not always correct organ ischemia.

In a Stanford series in which replacement of the thoracic aorta was performed, 8% required an additional operation to correct a persistent peripheral vascular deficit.

In view of these complication rates from direct aortic replacement, we have elected to follow a "complication-specific" approach. In our experience, the use of different surgical techniques directed at specific complications has yielded encouraging results. In some instances, this approach has allowed us to avoid certain complications associated with direct graft replacement of the aorta. Our approach has centered around three possible scenarios in complicated acute descending aortic dissection: (1) organ ischemia; (2) threatened rupture, continuing propagation of the dissection, or rapid enlargement of the descending aorta; and (3) realized rupture.

We have found the fenestration procedure particularly useful for patients presenting with organ ischemia. This procedure was first described by Guerin et al in 1935 and modeled after the phenomenon of "reentry" seen in spontaneous survivors of aortic dissection. The reentry of blood back into the true lumen allows the release of pressure inside the false lumen and decreases branch ostial obstruction, with improved flow through the true lumen. From our studies, reestablishment of flow to these arterial branches occurs above and below the site of fenestration.

In an early series of 14 patients who underwent the fenestration procedure, 12 had lower limb ischemia, 2 had renal ischemia, and 2 patients with lower limb ischemia also had spinal cord ischemia and paraplegia. Reperfusion was achieved in 13 (93%) of these patients, including restoration of renal and spinal cord perfusion. In these patients, we had no mortality in the operating room and documented a long-term actuarial survival rate of 77% and 52% at 1, 5, and 5 years. Compared with direct graft replacement of the aorta, fenestration does not require thoracotomy and avoids the issues of proximal hypertension, distal ischemia, and cord protection during high aortic clamping. Catheter techniques for fenestration are being developed.

The fenestration procedure is performed with the left flank elevated and an incision made at the level of the umbilicus extending from the midline to the posterior axillary line. The abdominal aorta is approached retroperitoneally and encircled just below the renal arteries proximally and above the iliac bifurcation distally. After heparin is administered, the aorta is cross-clamped proximally and distally. The aorta is divided transversely in the midportion of the isolated segment. In the proximal section, the intimal flap is excised as high as possible up to the clamp level. In the distal segment, the intima and adventitia are reapproximated with a continuous over-and-over suture (4-0 polypropylene). The proximal adventitial and distal reconstituted aortic segments are anastomosed with a continuous suture.

We have found the fenestration procedure to be a relatively simple and effective operation that is targeted specifically at organ ischemia in these critically ill patients. Some significant limitations pertain, however, to the application of the fenestration procedure. Only dissections that reach the infrarenal aorta can be managed with this technique. Fenestration is useful only in the acute setting because after 24 to 48 hours thrombosis of the false lumen often occurs, creating a fixed obstruction near the branch ostia that is less responsive to decompression of the false lumen. The rare patient needing late treatment may require direct grafting of the obstructed blood vessel.

In most cases of threatened rupture, rapid dissection propagation, or enlargement of the aorta, direct graft replacement of the aorta is recommended. An alternative surgical option that is occasionally helpful is the thromboexclusion procedure developed by Carpentier. Thromboexclusion involves permanent iatrogenic occlusion of the descending aorta distal to the left subclavian artery and an end-to-side anastomosis of a large-bore graft extending from the ascending aorta to the abdominal aorta. This leads to the creation of a blind pouch distal to the site of occlusion and gradual thrombosis of the entire descending aorta. Thrombosis extends only down to areas of high flow—the vicinity of the T8-L2 intercostal vessels, which maintain perfusion to the spinal cord. Postoperative angiography and TEE in these patients have confirmed the rapid occurrence of thrombosis within a few days and continued patency of these low intercostal vessels. We apply this procedure rarely when we believe that direct aortic replacement is contraindicated. This technique may have an advantage in lowering the incidence of paraplegia because the gradual thrombosis of the descending aorta allows time for collateral circulation to develop.

In realized rupture, there is no alternative to direct aortic replacement, with the priority being control of catastrophic bleeding. Because extensive replacement of the descending aorta is associated with a high rate of morbidity and mortality, we practice a limited resection of the bleeding site whenever possible. This site commonly is located in the proximal descending aorta, just distal to the left subclavian artery.

Following are technical tips we find useful for graft replacement of the aorta in aortic dissection:

1. Left atrial-to-femoral artery bypass is most useful for operations on the descending aorta. Either the superior or the inferior pulmonary vein is used for atrial access.
2. Deep hypothermic circulatory arrest is most useful for operations on the acutely dissected ascending aorta.
3. A "sandwich" technique with polytetrafluoroethylene (Teflon) felt strips inside the intima and outside the adventitia is used to reinforce the acutely dissected aorta.
4. The posterior suture line should be reinforced with interrupted, pledgetted sutures, which virtually eliminates anastomotic bleeding problems. This site is difficult to access if bleeding occurs after completion of the anastomosis.
5. For procedures involving the aortic arch, the left innominate vein can be divided safely to improve exposure.
6. If the ascending aorta is flaccid during perfusion via the femoral artery for surgery on an ascending dissection, cannulation of the false lumen is likely to have occurred. The surgeon needs to establish ascending perfusion immediately to restore flow.
7. The false lumen in chronic dissection should never be obliterated because branch vessels may derive their perfusion from flow through the false lumen.
8. Spinal cord ischemia with resulting paraplegia is a serious sequela after replacement of the descending aorta.

Various approaches for this problem are used. Limited aortic resection can spare the intercostal arteries. A sharply beveled anastomosis may be used to replace a long segment of the anterior aorta, while leaving the posterior aortic wall intact. Formal implantation of the intercostal arteries also can be performed by a side-by-side, graft-to-aorta anastomosis using the inclusion technique, but we prefer our "cobrahead" graft technique (Figure 2) for addressing the problem of spinal cord ischemia. A 10- to 12-mm, collagen-impregnated graft is anastomosed to the intercostal zone of the aorta with an end-to-side technique. This is the first graft performed before any other anastomosis, with immediate reperfusion of the spinal cord from a side arm off the arterial circuit within minutes. As soon as the main aortic graft is completed, the cobrahead graft is brought behind the main graft and quickly anastomosed to the front of the main graft with minimal ischemic time. This technique has been effective in preventing paraplegia. The main advantages of the cobrahead technique are that all anastomoses are easily accessible for control of bleeding and cord reperfusion is immediate.

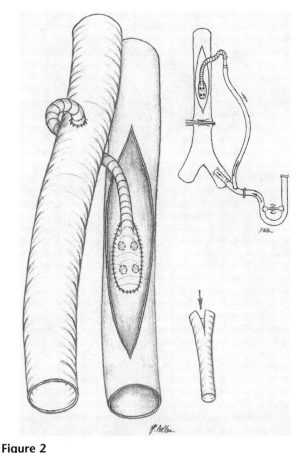

Figure 2
The cobrahead graft for intercostal artery implantation during descending aortic replacement. Spatulation of the graft and connection to an arterial perfusion circuit promptly restores spinal cord blood flow as shown in inserts.

Chronic (Descending) Aortic Dissection

Many descending aortic dissection patients (and an occasional nonoperated ascending dissection patient) survive to reach chronic states. In chronic descending dissections, we recommend regular monitoring with CT or MRI to monitor disease progression, such as aortic dilation or propagation of the dissection. Criteria for intervention are similar to those for aortic aneurysms. From our previous studies, a marked increase in complication rate occurs when descending aortic aneurysms exceed 7 cm in diameter. A similar increase is seen with ascending aneurysms exceeding 6 cm. We recommend surgery for descending and ascending thoracic aortic aneurysms at 6.5 cm and 5.5 cm before the extreme danger zone is reached. For Marfan syndrome patients, we recommend intervention at an earlier stage of 6 cm for descending and 5 cm for ascending aneurysms.

Identification of branch vessels can be difficult in chronic dissection. The dissected lumen in the abdominal aorta must be widely exposed to permit identification and reimplantation of all visceral arteries. When less than the total aorta is replaced, the intimal layer must be resected from the distal aortic cuff and subsequent anastomosis to the distal adventitial layer to prevent organ ischemia.

■ CONCLUSION

The challenge of managing aortic dissections and their associated aneurysms continues to test clinical and surgical skills. True today, as it was 100 years ago when said by Osler: "There is no disease more conductive to clinical humility than aneurysm of the aorta."

SUGGESTED READING

Anagnostopoulos CE: *Acute aortic dissections,* Baltimore, 1976, University Park Press.

Coady MA, et al: What is the appropriate size criterion for resection of thoracic aortic aneurysms? *J Thorac Cardiovasc Surg* 113:476, 1997.

Coady MA, et al: Familial patterns of thoracic aortic aneurysms, *Arch Surg* 134:361, 1999.

Elefteriades JA, et al: Management of descending aortic dissection, *Ann Thorac Surg* 67:2002, 1999.

ASCENDING AORTIC ANEURYSM

Thomas G. Gleason

Derek R. Brinster

Joseph E. Bavaria

The indications for repair of ascending aortic aneurysms are now more apparent than ever before. The operative and hospital mortality risks of ascending aortic and/or aortic root replacement have been reduced to acceptably low levels. This reduction in operative risk has generated a gradual trend toward repairing the diseased ascending aorta earlier for prophylaxis rather than waiting for an aortic catastrophe. The spectrum of options for aortic root reconstruction ranges from repair of native tissues to the use of autografts, homografts, xenografts, or full prosthetic composite grafts. Each technique has its share of proponents often attendant with good results, but each falls short of the perfect valve conduit, that is, the normal human aortic root.

The etiologies of ascending aortic diseases are protean and poorly understood. Generally, ascending aortic disease relates to genetic abnormalities as in the Marfan syndrome, atherosclerosis with calcification of the aortic wall, degeneration of the aortic wall, or some combination. In the last decade our increased understanding of the Marfan syndrome and its genetic basis of defective fibrillin metabolism underscore our ignorance of the vast complexity of molecular issues inherent to aortic disease. Although it is clear that the majority of patients with ascending aortic aneurysms have medial degeneration with loss of elastin in the media, it is not clear why or what causes the degenerative process to occur. Regardless, the physical law of Laplace is at play in all of these patients: as aortic diameter increases and aortic wall thickness decreases (e.g., degenerative aneurysms), the rate of aortic dissection or rupture increases. This is the basis for identifying and treating aneurysms before they dissect or rupture.

Normal aortic root and ascending aortic dimensions are predictable based on age and body size. Accrual of large amounts of echocardiographic and cross-sectional imaging data from normal individuals has allowed the development of regression formulas and nomograms to assist in defining abnormal aortic dilation. For example, an individual 18 to 40 years old will have an average aortic diameter at the sinus level equal to $0.97 + (1.12 \times$ body surface area $[m^2])$ (cm). The upper limit of normal is 2.1 cm/m² for the sinus segment in most adults. By definition, the aorta is pathologically dilated if its diameter exceeds the norm for a given age and body surface area. It is defined as an aneurysm if its diameter is 50% greater than the norm.

Aside from the presentation of an ascending aortic catastrophe (i.e., acute dissection, rupture, or intramural hematoma), most ascending aortic aneurysms are diagnosed incidentally at the time of an echocardiogram, catheterization, or cross-sectional imaging study for cardiac valvular disease, coronary arterial disease, or other thoracic disease. Rarely, patients will present with symptoms of chest discomfort, prompting one of these studies to reveal an aneurysm. People with the Marfan syndrome or with a strong family history of premature aortic rupture, dissection, or sudden death should undergo imaging via echocardiogram and/or cross-sectional imaging to rule out aortic aneurysm regardless of symptoms.

Once an ascending aortic aneurysm is identified, it is important to clarify several issues. First, an echocardiogram should be performed to evaluate the aortic valve for insufficiency, to assess the aortic root and sinus segment diameter, and to identify evidence of aortic dissection. Cross-sectional imaging with either computed tomography or magnetic resonance angiography is optimal to determine the extent and dimensions of the aneurysm. Patients over age 45, patients with bicuspid aortic valve, or patients in whom there is a history of hyperlipidemia or premature coronary artery disease should undergo cardiac catheterization. The result will direct concomitant revascularization at the time of aneurysm repair. Bicuspid aortic valve is often associated with aberrant proximal coronary arterial anatomy, notably a displaced right coronary os or a right, retroaortic circumflex artery. These findings have obvious implications during aortic root replacement.

■ SURGICAL INDICATIONS

There are two absolute indications for replacement of the ascending aorta: acute ascending aortic dissection (Stanford type A or DeBakey type I or II) and spontaneous or traumatic aortic rupture. Management of aortic dissection is discussed at length in the previous chapter, but it is our practice to repair all type A dissections in a standard fashion similar to our technique for aneurysm repair. Spontaneous aortic rupture typically occurs with ascending aneurysms over 6.0 cm in diameter that have dissected. The incidence of traumatic rupture of the ascending aorta is unknown, but survival to medical care with traumatic ascending disruption is exceedingly rare. There are a few reported cases of successful salvage of patients with this injury. Rather, the majority of traumatic aortic disruptions that do survive to medical care occur at the level of the distal isthmus, and these injuries are regularly repaired successfully. They are discussed in a subsequent chapter.

Acute intramural hematomas of the ascending aorta probably represent a variant of acute dissection, although they are less clearly understood. In a reasonable operative candidate we manage intramural hematomas in the same fashion as type A dissection because of the fear of impending extension of the dissection or rupture. Elderly patients or patients with multiple comorbidities may be appropriately treated with aggressive antihypertensive medications including β blockade for reduction of aortic wall stress (i.e., $\Delta p/\Delta t$) while following the hematoma with serial imaging studies. Medical therapy in this cohort will generate an expected short-term survival rate of 40%.

Bacterial or fungal endocarditis with destruction of the aortic root is also an indication for root and proximal ascending aortic replacement. Root replacement for endocarditis is discussed later in this textbook.

The focus of the remaining discussion is on the relative indications for repair of the ascending aorta. These include degenerative aneurysms, annuloaortic ectasia, aortic dilatation associated with the Marfan syndrome, chronic aortic dissection, calcified (i.e., porcelain) aorta, aneurysm with bicuspid aortic valve, and perhaps bicuspid aortic valve alone. Surgery on the ascending aorta for these indications is both elective and prophylactic. Aortic replacement serves to prevent aortic rupture, dissection, progression of aortic valvular insufficiency, and embolization of atheromata or to facilitate coronary revascularization in a patient with a calcified aorta.

The most common indication for elective ascending aortic replacement is for a degenerative aneurysm. In these cases there is age-related fragmentation and loss of elastin in the media that weakens the aortic wall. These patients often have associated aortic insufficiency despite the appearance of normal valve leaflets. Dilation of the sinotubular junction compromises the support structure for normal leaflet coaptation. Replacement of the ascending aorta and reestablishing a normal-sized sinotubular ridge is often all that is required for restoration of aortic valvular competency. Dilation of the aortic annulus or sinus segments generally mandates either full aortic root replacement or valve-sparing replacement.

Chronic ascending aortic dissections should be managed like aneurysms with the caveat that these aortas are likely to dilate and disrupt at a faster rate than degenerative aneurysms because the media in these aortas has already been disrupted. They are held together simply by the adventitia. Therefore, the threshold for repair should be lowered in these cases.

Ascending aortic replacement is also prudent in the patient with high-grade aortic calcification who requires coronary revascularization. This type of replacement should proceed with caution and the careful guidance of an intraoperative transesophageal echocardiogram. If it becomes apparent that the coronary ostia and their surrounding aortic tissue are heavily calcified, this can be a contraindication to aortic root replacement. Moreover, an appropriate site for proximal aortic transection at the sinotubular junction that is relatively free of calcification must be identified to facilitate a safe proximal aortic anastomosis.

There is evolving evidence of an association between congenital bicuspid aortic valve and aneurysmal dilation of the ascending aorta. In cases when both coexist and there is associated aortic insufficiency, we recommend full root and ascending aortic replacement. Occasionally, these bicuspid valves can be repaired facilitating a valve-sparing root replacement. There is current controversy as to whether patients with an insufficient bicuspid valve but a normal or near-normal ascending aortic diameter should undergo root and/or ascending aortic replacement, or simply aortic valve repair or replacement. Circumstantial evidence suggests that there is an underlying inherent defect or abnormality of the material properties of the aortic wall in these patients that predispose it to subsequent dilation, dissection, or rupture because so many patients with bicuspid aortic valve develop ascending aneurysms.

■ TIMING OF SURGERY

The timing of elective replacement of the ascending aorta should be determined on a given patient based on age, comorbid condition, size of the aneurysm, pathology of the aneurysm (e.g., Marfan syndrome), and degree of concomitant aortic valvular pathology. Griepp's experience of over 500 cases in the 1990s demonstrated that the hospital mortality of ascending aortic replacement is 4 times higher among patients older than 60 compared to those younger than 60. Patients with severe chronic obstructive pulmonary disease or patients with renal failure also have a higher mortality rate after thoracic aortic surgery. Importantly, Elefteriades' group has recently reported the natural history of thoracic aortic aneurysms in 570 patients (219 with ascending aneurysms) who were followed prospectively. This allowed for the prediction of rupture, dissection, or death based on size of aneurysm. Aneurysms over 6.0 cm had a yearly rupture rate of 3.7%, dissection rate of 3.9%, and mortality rate of 11.8%. The average yearly rate of rupture, dissection, or death was 15.6% for aneurysms over 6.0 cm (Figure 1). The risk of rupture for aneurysms over 6.0 cm is 27 times worse than for those less than 4.0 cm and is 11 times worse for those 5.0 to 5.9 cm. The survival estimates over 5 years when comparing elective surgical repair, emergent repair, and medical therapy are striking. Elective surgery in patients with thoracic aneurysms restores their 5-year survival curve to that of a normal population (85%), whereas emergent surgery for rupture or dissection reduces it to 37%. These data clearly justify elective surgical intervention in these patients.

Griepp and colleagues point out that use of aortic indices or ratios (i.e., measured diameter/predicted diameter) based on the formulas or nomograms for a given age group and body size probably provides a more accurate means of establishing guidelines for intervention in a given patient. We agree with this approach and use a paradigm that takes into account aortic pathology as depicted in Table 1. The intervention point is an aortic index of 1.5. We have lowered the threshold for elective surgery in patients with the Marfan syndrome, concomitant bicuspid aortic valve, and chronic dissection to 4.3 to 4.9 cm (index 1.3 to 1.4) unless a patient's comorbidities preclude a low operative mortality risk.

■ SURGICAL TECHNIQUE

We recommend and use a standardized approach to all ascending aortic and aortic root replacements. Time permitting, patients are evaluated and prepared for cardiac surgery in a typical fashion. Intraoperative monitoring should include transesophageal echocardiography and both pulmonary and systemic arterial catheters. Use of antifibrinolytic therapy with either aprotinin or epsilon-aminocaproic acid is recommended. Intravenous lidocaine, magnesium, methylprednisolone, and mannitol are delivered in all cases with a planned period of hypothermic circulatory arrest (HCA) for their theoretical neuroprotective attributes. When HCA is planned, patients are monitored with continuous electroencephalography (EEG).

Acute dissection or aortic rupture prompts peripheral arterial cannulation. We prefer direct femoral arterial cannulation for emergent cases because of ease of access and its long-term success. However, when severe peripheral vascular disease is present, the right axillary artery is cannulated via attachment of an end-to-side 8-mm Dacron graft.

The distal ascending aorta itself is cannulated in cases of elective ascending aortic and/or root replacement. Exact site of aortic cannulation requires a thoughtful approach. Several factors should be taken into account including: degree of atheromata, integrity of the aortic wall, extent of calcification, and operative plan for the distal aortic anastomotic site. Our preference is to perform open distal aortic anastomoses in most cases, and consequently we do not cannulate the

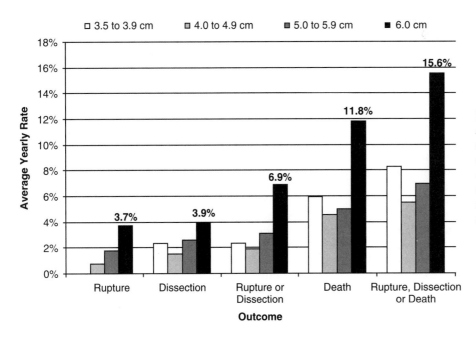

Figure 1
Average yearly rates of negative outcomes (rupture, dissection, and death). *(Used with permission from Davies RR, et al: Yearly rupture or dissection rates for thoracic aortic aneurysms: simple prediction based on size, Ann Thorac Surg 73:17, 2002.)*

Table 1 Current Guidelines for Surgery*

	Diameter	Ratio[†]
Marfan's (+ family history)	>4.3	1.3
Chronic dissections	>4.3	1.3
Degenerative without AI	>4.8	1.5
Degenerative with AI (degree)	>4.8	1.5
Bicuspid valve with dysfunction	>4.5	1.4
Other cardiac surgery	>4.8	1.5
Surgeon's experience	+0.5	0.15

*Adult age <40 yr, body surface area 2 m².
[†]Measured diameter/predicted diameter.
AI, aortic insufficiency.
Used with permission from Ergin MA, et al: Surgical treatment of the dilated ascending aorta: when and how? *Ann Thorac Surg* 67:1834, 1999.

aorta too high on the arch in order to facilitate excision of the cannulation site at the time of hemiarch reconstruction. Venous cannulation is achieved with an angled, dual-staged right atrial cannula and a smaller (e.g., 26 Fr) soft, right-angled cannula in the superior vena cava with its tip well cephalad to the azygous vein for retrograde cerebral perfusion (RCP) during HCA. A left ventricular (LV) vent is placed via the right superior pulmonary vein. Induction antegrade followed by continuous or intermittent low-flow retrograde blood cardioplegia is delivered. Patients are cooled until a flat EEG is obtained (usually below 16°C) when HCA is planned. During emergent cases when EEG monitoring is not practical patients should be cooled for a minimum of 45 minutes because we have demonstrated that this correlates with EEG silence in greater than 90% of patients.

When replacing the ascending aorta for aneurysm disease, dissection, rupture, or calcification, we prefer to replace its entire extent with hemiarch reconstruction and an open distal anastomosis. This approach eliminates the chance for recurrent or progressive aneurysmal disease of residual ascending aorta, ensures unobstructed antegrade flow through all arch vessels in cases of dissection, and facilitates optimal conditions for construction of the distal anastomosis (i.e., no clamp abutting the aortic suture line.)

Once cardiopulmonary bypass is initiated and the LV appropriately vented, systemic cooling is initiated. At the time of ventricular fibrillation or if LV vent flow is too high resulting in LV dilation, the aorta is clamped and induction antegrade cardioplegia delivered. Great caution should be exercised when placing an aortic clamp on a dissected or an atheromatous aorta to avoid disruption or embolization. During the period of cooling, dissection of the pulmonary artery off the aorta is completed, and the dissection of the aortic root/valve and any distal coronary arterial bypasses is completed. Once EEG silence is achieved, attention is immediately shifted toward completing the hemiarch reconstruction. Cardiopulmonary bypass is halted, and continuous RCP initiated maintaining a jugular venous pressure of 20 to 25 mm Hg (usual flows, 200 to 300 ml/min). The ascending aorta is excised to the level of the hemiarch including the cannulation site, and a Dacron graft is cut in a beveled fashion for hemiarch reconstruction. The distal anastomosis is often sparingly reinforced with bioglue in cases of acute dissection, friable aortic tissue, or elderly patients in whom

subsequent cardiac surgery is not contemplated. After completion of the anastomosis, the graft itself is cannulated distally, and cardiopulmonary bypass instituted again.

Rewarming is begun, and attention is focused on root replacement, valve repair or replacement, and the proximal aortic anastomosis as appropriate. Root replacement techniques are discussed at length elsewhere. There are several options available, and several factors should weigh into the decision for which type of root reconstruction. The modified Bentall method of composite replacement of the aortic valve and ascending aorta has offered excellent long-term results in most all patients. This is the only reconstruction technique that has extensive long-term follow-up. The technique's predominant disadvantage is the need for long-term anticoagulation. Several other techniques have sought to eliminate this need by either repairing the native valve or replacing it with another biologic valve (i.e., autograft, homograft, or xenograft). The main disadvantages of the biologic techniques are the lack of extensive long-term follow-up, concerns of progressive aortic insufficiency with both autograft and valve repair techniques and progressive calcification of homograft and xenograft roots. The age and comorbidities of the patient, pathology of the aorta, surgeon experience, and patient willingness to consent to long-term anticoagulation should all be considered when conduit choices are made.

After root replacement the final aortic graft-to-graft anastomosis is completed. Care must be taken when fashioning this anastomosis to cut both proximal and distal ends in a beveled fashion from lateral to medial to achieve slightly more length on the lateral aspect or greater curve and less length on the medial aspect or lesser curve to avoid both posterior and medial kinking. Upon completion and weaning off cardiopulmonary bypass, meticulous hemostasis is achieved prior to closure.

Postoperative management should include appropriate afterload reduction to maintain normal mean systolic blood pressure (70 to 85 mm Hg) and reduce stress on the aortic anastomoses. Early extubation, aggressive pulmonary toilet, and early ambulation are encouraged when appropriate. Anticoagulation for prosthetic valves is initiated on postoperative day one or two. A follow-up echocardiogram is scheduled for 3 months postoperatively.

Consensus among thoracic aortic surgeons of the optimal aortic root reconstruction has not yet been realized. Our approach has been to offer the modified Bentall composite root to most younger patients because of its long-term durability. Patients older than 70 are good candidates for biologic graft root reconstruction or valve-sparing root replacement. The newer porcine roots may offer better long-term durability than homografts with purported improvements in preservation techniques. Younger patients who do not want to be anticoagulated long-term may be offered aortic valve reimplantation with ascending aortic replacement if feasible, pulmonary autograft reconstruction or porcine root replacement with the understanding that they will likely require reoperation at some point in their adult lives.

Marfan patients may be less suited for pulmonary autograft replacement or valve-sparing replacement due to a higher incidence of delayed valve failure. These patients should undergo ascending aortic replacement earlier when their aortic index (measured/predicted aortic diameter) exceeds 1.3. Similarly, patients with bicuspid aortic valve and dilated ascending aorta or chronic type A dissection should be repaired earlier (aortic index 1.4) as long as comorbidity does not predict adverse outcome.

■ RESULTS

From January 1997 to June 2002 there were over 600 ascending aortic replacements and/or root replacements performed at the University of Pennsylvania. The average age was 58.8 years (range, 14 to 88 years). The majority of ascending aortic replacements were completed using HCA for hemiarch reconstruction with an open distal anastomosis. The overall hospital mortality of these patients was 5.2% (31 patients). Excluding patients with acute type A dissection yielded a 4.1% mortality rate (19 deaths, 10 of which were in patients who had undergone at least one prior cardiac operation, and one patient presented in cardiac arrest with an ascending aneurysm and presumptive rupture). The remaining 147 ascending aortic repairs were for acute type A dissection, and the hospital mortality rate for these surgically treated patients was 8.2% (12 patients). When the dissection patients who presented neurologically unresponsive or with ongoing CPR are excluded the mortality rate was less than 5%. Including only patients less than 70 years old who underwent elective repair of degenerative ascending aneurysms with or without root reconstruction yields a mortality rate of 1%.

These mortality rates are acceptably low and justify prophylactic intervention of ascending aortic aneurysms when they exceed 4.5 to 4.9 cm. A careful and consistent perioperative and intraoperative strategy should be used. Surgeon, perfusionist, and anesthesiologist must have a clear understanding of the orchestration of ascending aortic replacement, its nuances, and its pitfalls to achieve optimal outcomes.

SUGGESTED READING

Bavaria JE, Pochettino A: Retrograde cerebral perfusion (RCP) in aortic arch surgery: efficacy and possible mechanisms of brain protection, *Semin Thorac Cardiovasc Surg* 9:222, 1997.

David TE, et al: Results of aortic valve-sparing operations, *J Thorac Cardiovasc Surg* 122:39, 2001.

Davies RR, et al: Yearly rupture or dissection rates for thoracic aortic aneurysms: simple prediction based on size, *Ann Thorac Surg* 73:17, 2002; discussion 27.

Ergin MA, et al: Surgical treatment of the dilated ascending aorta: when and how? *Ann Thorac Surg* 67:1834, 1999; discussion 1853.

Kon ND, et al: Eight-year results of aortic root replacement with the freestyle stentless porcine aortic root bioprosthesis, *Ann Thorac Surg* 73:1817, 2002; discussion 1821.

Yacoub MH, et al: Late results of a valve-preserving operation in patients with aneurysms of the ascending aorta and root, *J Thorac Cardiovasc Surg* 115:1080, 1998.

Yun KL, et al: Composite valve graft versus separate aortic valve and ascending aortic replacement: is there still a role for the separate procedure? *Circulation* 96 (Suppl II):II-368, 1997.

DESCENDING THORACIC AORTIC ANEURYSMS

Joseph S. Coselli
Daniel J. DiBardino

■ HISTORY

The first successful experimentation using a prosthetic graft for the replacement of the descending thoracic aorta was reported by Hufnagel in 1947. Shortly thereafter, the modern era of repair for descending thoracic aortic aneurysms began when Lam and Aram reported the use of an aortic homograft in 1951. Although Bahnson presented lateral resection and aortorrhaphy in 1953, it was the pioneering work of DeBakey and Cooley at the Baylor College of Medicine that led to the first successful series of prosthetic graft replacement of the descending thoracic aorta.

■ ETIOLOGY

The majority (>60%) of descending aortic aneurysms are due to degenerative pathology, which includes both medial degenerative disease and atherosclerosis. Specifically, medial degeneration is the primary pathology responsible for most fusiform dilation of the thoracic aorta, whereas arteriosclerosis usually results in saccular dilation. In 2% to 5% of descending aneurysms, Marfan syndrome is accountable for the medial degeneration; in this subset of patients, an alteration in the gene that codes for fibrillin (chromosome 15, long arm) results in a connective tissue weakness and an especially severe degeneration of the tunica media of the aorta. Progressive dilation of the false lumen after dissection of the distal aorta is another important cause of descending aortic aneurysms. Less common causes include infection, trauma, and congenital disease (Table 1).

Acute aortic dissection results from an intimal tear in the aortic wall, after which the high pulsatile pressure of the

Table 1 Etiology of Descending Aortic Aneurysms According to Frequency

PATHOLOGY	FREQUENCY (%)
Degenerative pathology (medial degenerative disease and atherosclerosis)	>60
Chronic aortic dissection	25 to 30
Traumatic aneurysm	1 to 5
Infection (mycotic)	2
Coarctation	<1

aorta causes blood to tract through the medial layer. Only the thin adventitia and a small, outer portion of the tunica media contain this potentially lethal flow of blood within a "false lumen." By convention, a dissection is termed *chronic* after 14 days pass from the initial dissection event. Progressive dilation of a chronic dissection is responsible for 25% to 30% of descending aortic aneurysms.

Mycotic aneurysms are usually saccular and multiple and result from or are secondarily infected by bacteria arising in a distant site of infection. The primary infection, classically endocarditis, can also be from the urinary tract, pneumonia, ear and throat infection, salmonellosis, dental procedures, line sepsis, and even cellulitis. The pathogenesis of these aneurysms is embolization of infectious material from one of these sources into normal aortic wall, infection of defects in the aorta or atherosclerotic aortic segments, or the infection of intraluminal clot in a preexisting atherosclerotic aneurysm.

Traumatic aortic aneurysm begins with a severe decelerating trauma causing a laceration of the aorta and the containment of blood by periaortic/mediastinal tissues. If an aneurysm of this type is not repaired and remains stable for 14 days, it is termed a chronic traumatic aneurysm. In the chronic setting, the injured segment will continue to dilate and becomes calcified in many instances.

Coarctation of the aorta is occasionally responsible for descending thoracic aneurysms (<1%). The aortic wall in patients with coarctation is frequently abnormal and appears especially vulnerable to medial degeneration. These aneurysms may occur either in association or long after the correction of the coarctation and are susceptible to laceration, dissection, and rupture.

■ PRESENTATION, WORKUP, AND INDICATIONS FOR OPERATION

Descending aortic aneurysms are asymptomatic in as many as half of the patient population and are discovered serendipitously (Table 2). The only reliable symptom in the remainder is pain, occurring in the chest or back depending on the exact anatomy of the aneurysm. In the setting of acute dissection or rupture, chest pain may be sudden and severe. Hoarseness and pulmonary symptoms from recurrent laryngeal nerve involvement, tracheal deviation, and local airway compression each occur in less than 10% of patients. Physical examination alone is not reliable for the diagnosis of descending aortic aneurysms. As a result, imaging is an important component of the surgical algorithm.

Although previous recommendations would have stressed reliance on the aortogram in preoperative assessment, computed tomography (CT) scan and echocardiography together provide a complete noninvasive preoperative assessment of the aorta and the aortic valve. In fact, an aortogram can be misleading in the face of a luminal clot, because contrast will not demonstrate the full diameter of the aneurysm. CT scan provides aneurysm dimensions, delineates the existence and extent of aortic dissection, addresses luminal clot, and provides information about the relationship of the aneurysm to other structures. Signs suggesting a contained aortic rupture on CT scan include indistinct borders, the apparent extension of the aneurysm beyond a calcified wall, and left pleural fluid. Magnetic resonance imaging possesses the same sensitivity and accuracy as CT scan but is more expensive and not available at all centers.

The radiographic results and the clinical situation are taken together to assess the need for surgical intervention. Indications for aortic replacement include the following.

Aneurysm more than twice the size the adjacent, normal aorta
Aneurysm greater than 5 to 6 cm in diameter
Documented rate of expansion greater than 1 cm/yr in diameter
Presence of symptoms

These findings alone or in combination are all associated with an increased risk of rupture and generally mandate surgical repair in acceptable operative candidates.

Table 2 Symptoms of Descending Aortic Aneurysms According to Cause and Frequency

SYMPTOMS	CAUSE	FREQUENCY (%)
Back or chest pain	Local pressure	<50
Respiratory (shortness of breath, hemoptysis)	Tracheal deviating and local airway compression	8 to 10
Hoarseness	Stretching or compression of the left recurrent laryngeal nerve	8 to 10
Dysphagia	Esophageal compression	5
Hypotension and hemothorax	Aneurysm leak or rupture	3
Neurologic deficits	Spinal cord ischemia	3

■ PREOPERATIVE ASSESSMENT

Once an indication for operation is present, the ability of the patient to undergo a major thoracic procedure must be assessed. All patients require pulmonary function tests before elective thoracic aneurysm repair and all patients with a forced expiratory volume in 1 second of greater than 1.0 and a PCO_2 of less than 45 mm Hg are considered surgical candidates. Similarly, all elective patients require a cardiac evaluation, the extent of which depends on the presence of risk factors. Patients without risk factors can be cleared for surgery based on the results of physical examination, electrocardiography, and transthoracic echocardiography. Patients with signs or symptoms of coronary artery disease should undergo more rigorous evaluation, such as a dobutamine stress test or persantine thallium scan, and patients can be selected for cardiac catheterization based on the results of these studies.

Whenever possible, coronary artery disease should be addressed before operation on the thoracic aorta. In patients who have had previous coronary surgery, care should be taken not to place a cross-clamp on the aorta proximal to the subclavian artery if there is a patent left internal mammary graft to the left anterior descending coronary artery. In such situations, a carotid-subclavian bypass must be considered to protect blood flow to the left ventricle. In patients with known or suspected valvular disease, transthoracic and transesophageal echocardiography should be used to assess the specifics of valve and ventricular function.

Patients with known diffuse peripheral arterial disease, a history of cerebrovascular disease, or a carotid bruit on examination require duplex ultrasonography of the carotid arteries. If a 75% or greater stenosis is discovered, an arteriogram and surgical treatment of the affected carotid artery are considered before the elective repair of the thoracic aorta.

Each surgical candidate should have a blood cell count, electrolyte evaluation, and a coagulation profile, as well as a type and cross for packed red blood cells, platelets, and fresh frozen plasma. Preoperative elevations in blood urea nitrogen and creatinine may be secondary to intrinsic renal disease, hypertensive nephropathy, obstructive/anatomic phenomena, or the use of radiographic contrast material. This can be further investigated with noninvasive techniques such as renal ultrasound and CT scan or with more invasive techniques such as magnetic resonance angiography or angiography of the abdominal aorta. A contrast-associated rise in creatinine should ideally be allowed to return to baseline before operation.

■ OPERATIVE MANAGEMENT

A rapid sequence endobroncheal intubation is performed with a double-lumen tube, allowing for selective right lung ventilation during the operation. A pulmonary artery catheter, central venous line, and left and right radial arterial lines are placed, as are a Foley catheter and a nasogastric tube. Rectal, bladder, or esophageal probes are used to monitor core temperature. Patients are placed in the thoracoabdominal position with the pelvis rotated to the left to allow access to the left femoral vessels. The placement of the incision and entry into the chest depends on the anatomy of the aneurysm. The fifth intercostal space is adequate for exposure of the proximal descending aorta, whereas the sixth intercostal space allows exposure to the entire descending aorta. A cell-saver system and rapid infusion device are used in all patients.

Although active cooling is not routinely performed in our practice, the concept of "passive hypothermia" is used to protect against ischemic complications. Body temperature is allowed to drift downward to 32° to 33°C during the operation, and no rewarming is performed until the graft is in place and the chest is hemostatic. Cerebrospinal fluid (CSF) drainage should be considered in patients when a complex repair requiring prolonged ischemia is anticipated (>30 to 40 minutes). When used, CSF drainage to a pressure of 8 to 10 mm Hg is desirable. Heparin (1 mg/kg) is administered before the placement of the aortic cross-clamp. Depending on the extent of the aneurysm, the cross-clamp may be applied either proximal to or distal to the left subclavian artery. In the former setting, a separate clamp is applied to the left subclavian artery.

Once the aneurysm is opened, any chronic thrombus should be removed from the lumen and intimal calcification should be carefully débrided to ensure the aortic wall is suitable for anastomosis. Care must be taken to separate the proximal aorta from the esophagus and to transect the aortic wall completely, allowing for an end-to-end anastomosis with no injury to the esophageal wall. We do not routinely apply a cross-clamp to the distal aorta. The preferred aortic substitute in our practice is a gelatin or collagen sealed woven Dacron graft, usually 20 to 24 mm in diameter depending on the size of the native, nonaneurysmal aorta. The graft is then sewn in place beginning with the proximal anastomosis using running polypropylene suture, typically 3-0 suture on an SH needle. Often, the proximal suture line is reinforced with several strategically placed pledgetted mattress sutures to reduce the risk of bleeding once the anastomosis faces systemic arterial pressure. Intercostal arteries in the T8-12 region can then be selectively anastomosed to openings in the graft with running polypropylene suture in an inclusion anastomosis technique. Before the completion of the distal anastomosis, the patient is placed in deep Trendelenburg and the graft is cleared of air and debris.

Spinal Protection

If the aneurysm can be repaired in less than 30 minutes, no further spinal protection is required during the operation. Longer cross-clamp times, often associated with more complex aneurysms, have been shown to be an independent predictor of paraplegia and mandate the need for additional spinal protection. Bypass techniques to provide spinal cord protection represent a continuum of increasingly complicated maneuvers including placement of a Gott shunt, descending aortic bypass with partial heparinization, femoral-femoral cardiopulmonary bypass with complete heparinization, and hypothermic circulatory arrest.

No method of spinal cord protection can guarantee freedom from paraplegia. We believe that the selected use of descending aortic bypass (i.e., "left heart bypass") from the left atrium to either the distal aorta or femoral artery has contributed to a reduced overall paraplegia rate in our experience. This adjunct should be considered in complex aneurysm repair, acute aortic dissection, or aneurysm rupture. We do not use intrathecal cooling techniques, nor do we use intrathecal papaverine to protect against spinal cord ischemia.

The inability to safely apply a proximal cross-clamp on the aorta may occur in such cases as a proximal extent that involves the arch, severe atherosclerosis of the aorta with the threat of embolization, contained aortic rupture, the severely calcified "porcelain" aorta, or the occasional redo case with extensive mediastinal fibrosis and adhesions. In these situations, descending aortic repair may be performed under hypothermic circulatory arrest with femoral-femoral bypass. We generally restrict the use of circulatory arrest to avoid the potential adverse consequences, which include possible cerebral ischemia, effects on intellect and psychomotor performance, occasional postoperative seizures, and the effects of retracting the lung in a fully heparinized patient.

Dissection

In the presence of an acute aortic dissection involving the descending aorta, initial medical management with sodium nitroprusside and β-blockade in the intensive care unit setting is mandatory. Controversy still exists concerning the timing of surgical intervention for dissection of the descending aorta. Surgical repair for dissection should generally be carried out under the following conditions.

1. The presence of an aortic rupture
2. Failed medical management—this includes continued pain, hypertension that cannot be controlled, and expansion of the dissection despite medical management
3. Organ or limb ischemia that is refractory to other forms of treatment—aortic operation is a last resort in these cases, usually after failed endovascular techniques or other surgical options such as axillary-femoral or femoral-femoral bypass

Once the decision is made to repair a descending aortic aneurysm secondary to dissection, several specific technical principles apply. In the presence of dissection, a slightly finer suture is utilized (4-0 or 5-0 monofilament polypropylene) on an RB needle. This is done to improve hemostasis by preventing large needle holes in a thin and friable aorta. In the setting of an acute dissection, the false lumen should be obliterated at the distal suture line. Chronic dissecting membranes should be resected and adequately fenestrated at the distal aortic suture line to allow flow to both lumina.

Mycotic Aneurysms

The surgical approach to mycotic thoracic aneurysm requires additional measures that superimpose infection control and management on established aneurysm repair. The following principles apply.

1. These patients require aggressive débridement of the aneurysm wall and surrounding tissue before placement of the graft.
2. The amount of graft material should be as limited as much as possible, and the use of a gelatin-sealed, rifampin-soaked graft could be considered. The use of felt pledgets and braided sutures should be avoided.

3. The aneurysm wall should be left open.
4. Inpatient intravenous antibiotic therapy is initiated and continued as an outpatient via a tunneled central venous catheter. We have previously recommended 4 weeks for gram-negative rods and streptococci and 6 weeks for staphylococci. After this time, we recommend that the patient remain on oral antibiotics for a lifetime.
5. Consideration can be given to using an omental flap or other tissues to cover the graft in the setting of infection.

■ POSTOPERATIVE MANAGEMENT

Achieving and maintaining strict blood pressure control are extremely important in the immediate postoperative period to protect a fragile suture line. β-blockers, nitroprusside, and other drugs administered as a drip can be used to maintain a mean arterial pressure (MAP) between 80 and 90 mm Hg in the first 48 hours. Peripheral vascular exams are performed regularly. Chest tube output should be monitored closely in the initial postoperative period, because a leaking anastomosis will become evident in a bloody, high-volume output. Chest tubes are removed when the output falls to less than 100 ml/24 hr. If a preoperative CSF drain is placed and no adverse neurologic events occur, this catheter should be removed within 24 to 48 hours.

Neurologic examination should be performed regularly beginning as soon as the patient is alert enough to participate in a rudimentary examination. At the first sign of paraplegia or paraparesis of the lower extremities, a spinal fluid drain is placed and intravenous mannitol and steroids are given. The goal of spinal drainage should be a CSF pressure of 8 to 10 mm Hg; it is our practice to maintain an MAP of 90 to 100 mm Hg when lower extremity deficits are suspected. Any episodes of hypotension, arrhythmia, low oxygen saturation, and postoperative hypovolemia should be avoided at all costs, because these can initiate or exacerbate delayed paraplegia or paraparesis.

Because of the morbidity associated with an infected thoracic aortic graft, an aggressive stance on infection prophylaxis, surveillance, and control is preferred. Patients are maintained on broad-spectrum intravenous antibiotics until all lines, tubes, and drains are removed and oral antibiotics are maintained until after discharge from the hospital. Blood, sputum, and urine cultures should be obtained at the first signs or symptoms of infection, and antibiotics are liberally administered while taking into account the local hospital pathogen and sensitivity reports.

■ CONTEMPORARY SURGICAL RESULTS

With the application of the contemporary surgical approach, modern anesthesia, and critical care technology, the results of resection and repair of descending aortic aneurysms are excellent. A review of our experience in over 350 successive repairs of descending aortic aneurysms reveals an operative mortality of 5.1%. Factors independently associated with postoperative death include renal failure, pulmonary complications, and paraplegia. The rate of stroke in our series is 2.5%, and the incidence of renal failure and pulmonary failure is 8% and 33%, respectively. Fewer than half of the patients developing postoperative renal failure required dialysis. The only predictor of postoperative renal failure is aortic rupture.

Spinal cord dysfunction occurred in 2.2% of patients, most of whom presented with aortic dissection. In this retrospective analysis, the use of left heart bypass was not associated with a decreased rate of adverse spinal cord events. In fact, the only reliable predictor of paraplegia was aortic cross-clamp time. The mean clamp time of patients with no adverse neurologic outcomes was 29.7 minutes versus 48.6 minutes when a spinal cord event resulted ($p = .002$). Every effort must be used to minimize the cord ischemic time by keeping the aortic clamp time as short as possible. In addition, the routine reattachment of the lower intercostal

arteries and the judicious use of left heart bypass have contributed to an effective operative strategy.

SELECTED READING

Chan FY, et al: In situ prosthetic graft replacement for mycotic aneurysm of the aorta, *Ann Thorac Surg* 47:193-203, 1989.

Cooley DA, et al: Single-clamp technique for aneurysms of the descending thoracic aorta: report of 132 consecutive cases, *Eur J Cardio-Thorac Surg* 18:162-167, 2000.

Coselli JS, et al: Thoracic aortic anastomoses: operative techniques, *Thorac Cardiovasc Surg* 5:259-276, 2000.

Coselli JS, et al: Results of contemporary surgical treatment of descending thoracic aortic aneurysms: experience in 198 patients, *Ann Vasc Surg* 10:131-37, 1996.

Svensson LG, et al: Variables predictive of outcome in 832 patients undergoing repairs of the descending thoracic aorta, *Chest* 104:1248-53, 1993.

RECONSTRUCTION OF AORTIC ARCH ANEURYSMS

David Spielvogel
Randall Griep

Despite recent advancements in reconstruction of the aortic arch, cerebral protection, and prevention of cerebral embolization during cardiopulmonary bypass, the severely calcified and atherosclerotic aorta remains a challenge during repair. Modification of original techniques, from main arch graft implantation (Figure 1A-E) to separate brachiocephalic graft exclusion (Figure 2A-B) to our current technique, has shortened deep hypothermic circulatory arrest times considerably and therefore diminished associated temporary neurologic dysfunction and stroke.

Cerebral protection has evolved based on laboratory studies, so that periods of deep hypothermic cardiac arrest (DHCA) less than 30 minutes are well tolerated even in elderly patients when sufficient periods of core cooling are used (>30 minutes). Esophageal temperatures are lowered to 11° to 14°C until jugular bulb saturations are consistently greater than 95%. Additional adjuncts include packing the head in ice to prevent warming during the ischemic period, and high-dose steroids added to the original pump prime.

Prevention of cerebral embolization requires constant vigilance. Cannulation for arterial perfusion is via the right

or the left axillary arteries and rarely the ascending aorta. The femoral artery is avoided because the atherosclerotic process is often diffuse, and retrograde embolization is a constant threat.

■ TECHNIQUE

A median sternotomy is performed with extension of the incision superiorly along the medial border of the sternocleidomastoid muscle. The innominate vein may or may not be preserved. Ligation is of little consequence. Care is taken to preserve the recurrent laryngeal nerves as the aortic arch and brachiocephalic branches are exposed. A "no-touch" technique of surgical dissection is utilized, particularly when heavy atherosclerotic disease is present. The tissues are dissected away from the aneurysm.

The right axillary artery is exposed via a small infraclavicular incision that separates a portion of the pectoralis major from the clavicle. The axillary vein is mobilized and retracted inferiorly, exposing the axillary artery. Great care is taken in mobilizing the axillary artery as the brachial plexus may be intimately related. After exposure of 2 to 3 cm of the artery, vessel loops are placed and the artery is readied for cannulation. Heparin is administered. The axillary artery is cannulated with a right angle wire-reinforced arterial catheter and secured. The right atrium is cannulated with a standard two-stage atrial catheter. After appropriate connections are made to the cardiopulmonary bypass circuit, extracorporeal perfusion and cooling is begun. The temperature of the perfusate is lowered to 10°C. Examination of aortic arch perfusion with transesophageal echocardiography confirms retrograde flow and monitors for localized dissection.

When the heart fibrillates, the aorta is cross-clamped, and cardioplegic solution is infused into the root; alternatively, with aortic insufficiency, the aorta is opened, and cardioplegia

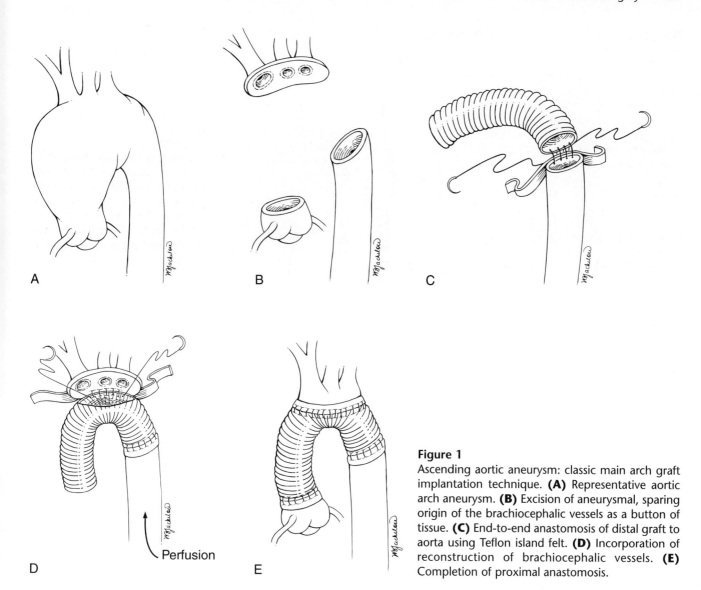

A

B

C

D   ⌐ Perfusion

E

Figure 1

Ascending aortic aneurysm: classic main arch graft implantation technique. **(A)** Representative aortic arch aneurysm. **(B)** Excision of aneurysmal, sparing origin of the brachiocephalic vessels as a button of tissue. **(C)** End-to-end anastomosis of distal graft to aorta using Teflon island felt. **(D)** Incorporation of reconstruction of brachiocephalic vessels. **(E)** Completion of proximal anastomosis.

solution is administered directly into the coronary ostia. A left ventricular vent from the right superior pulmonary vein or ventricular apex is placed. Cardioplegia solution is supplemented with topical hypothermia during the period of myocardial ischemia. If the ascending aorta is heavily calcified or atherosclerotic, no attempt at cross-clamping is made. The patient is cooled with the heart vented as described earlier. Just before the period of circulatory arrest, 60 mEq of KCl added to the venous reservoir and circulated, producing diastolic arrest of the heart.

Even patients with severe atherosclerotic disease of the aortic arch, the brachiocephalic vessels just beyond their origins are usually spared. This location is ideal for subsequent anastomoses. After carefully sizing the innominate, left carotid, and left subclavian arteries, a trifurcation graft is constructed. Generally, a 14- and 10-mm Hemashield graft or a 12- and 8-mm Hemashield is selected. The smaller graft is divided and beveled, and it is sewn to openings constructed in the side of the large graft in a sequential manner with a 3-0 or 4-0 polypropylene suture (Figure 3A).

The completion of this phase of the operation usually coincides with the end of core cooling. When the esophageal temperature drops to 12° to 15°C, the head is packed in ice. Jugular bulb oxygen saturation is measured throughout the period of cooling. When the saturation rises above 95%, maximum metabolic suppression is achieved and the patient is readied for circulatory arrest. The patient is placed in slight Trendelenburg position to prevent air entrapment during the period of circulatory arrest.

At the beginning of circulatory arrest, the innominate artery is transected just distal to its origin or at the level where atherosclerosis is minimal (Figure 3B). The end of the 12- or 14-mm graft previously constructed is trimmed and anastomosed with a 5-0 polypropylene suture. Great care is taken when tightening the suture line as the brachiocephalic vessels can easily tear. Next, the first of the 8- or 10-mm limbs is trimmed to the appropriate length and anastomosed in a similar fashion to the transected left common carotid artery. Finally, the second side branch of the trifurcation graft is sutured to the left subclavian artery. Each anastomosis

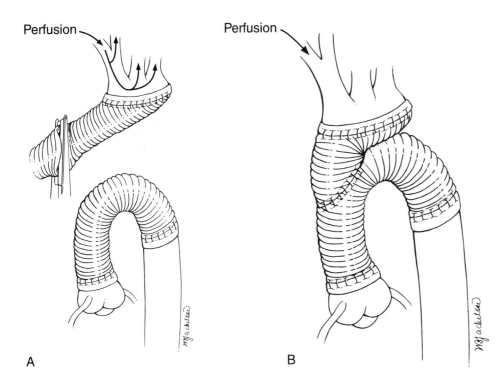

Figure 2
Ascending aortic aneurysm repair using separate brachiocephalic graft. **(A)** Graft to brachiocephalic trunk is used for antegrade perfusion during proximal and distal aortic anastomoses. **(B)** Completed anastomosis to aortic arch graft.

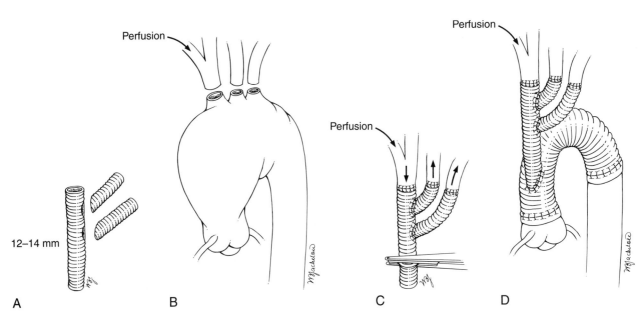

Figure 3
Technique for severe calcific disease of the aortic arch. **(A)** Construction of trifurcated Hemashield graft. **(B)** Transection of proximal great vessels. **(C)** Construction of graft limbs to individual great vessels. Perfusion is via the right axillary artery. **(D)** Completed reconstruction.

takes between 6 to 10 minutes, depending on exposure. The order of the reconstruction can be reversed as in some patients this may provide better exposure to the left subclavian artery.

The graft limbs are anastomosed to the individual brachiocephalic vessels. Perfusion via the right axillary artery is temporarily resumed at 500 ml/min, flushing air and any possible embolic material retrograde. Perfusion is

again stopped, aspiration is repeated, and flow is resumed. The trifurcation graft is carefully deaired, and the proximal portion (the 12- to 14-mm portion) is clamped, restoring perfusion to the head and upper extremities (Figure 3C). Perfusion pressure is maintained at about 50 mm Hg, requiring flows of 600 to 1000 ml/min. Blood temperature is allowed to drift upward.

The aortic arch is reconstructed in a variety of ways depending on the pathology. For ascending and arch disease with aortic valve involvement, a Bentall or Yacoub procedure precedes arch reconstruction. If the aortic valve is spared, arch repair begins at the proximal descending thoracic aorta, mobilizing the recurrent laryngeal nerve as necessary to obtain a suitable cuff of aortic tissue. If aneurysmal disease involves additional aortic segments, an "elephant trunk" may be constructed in either the distal or the more proximal aortic arch or the distal ascending aorta when aortic caliber permits a modified repair. This maneuver, as described by Kuki and Taniguchi, avoids the potential for nerve injury. The anastomosis is constructed with running 3-0 polypropylene reinforced with a strip of Teflon felt, taking great care to place the Dacron graft within the native aorta and the felt on the outside. This sandwich technique is extraordinarily hemostatic. The graft is stretched, measured to the appropriate length, and sutured to the sinotubular junction or previous graft used for aortic root reconstruction. Graft-to-graft anastomoses are performed with 2-0 polypropylene.

At this point, the Dacron graft is distended with a cardioplegic solution to facilitate choosing the ideal site for the brachiocephalic graft end-to-side anastomosis to the ascending portion of the aortic reconstruction. An elliptical opening is fashioned with an ophthalmic electrocautery, and the trifurcation graft is beveled and trimmed (Figure 3D). Cerebral and upper extremity perfusion is not interrupted. On completion of this final anastomosis, the patient is actively rewarmed. During rewarming, the anastomoses are carefully examined, and any bleeding points are controlled with individual sutures. The operating table is placed in the Trendelenburg position; active venting of the ascending aortic graft is performed with a 20-gauge slit angiocath before defibrillation. The left ventricular apex is aspirated. After a period of rewarming and resuscitation, the patient is temporarily weaned from cardiopulmonary bypass, removing any remaining air from the cardiac chambers. Vents in the right superior pulmonary vein and ascending aortic graft are removed and repaired in the usual fashion.

Once the patient's esophageal temperature reaches 37°C, cardiopulmonary bypass is discontinued. Protamine sulfate is administered along with fresh frozen plasma and platelets as required. The arterial perfusion cannula in the axillary artery is removed, and the artery is repaired with a running 6-0 polypropylene suture. Adequate hemostasis is achieved, and the chest is closed in the usual way.

■ THORACOSTERNOTOMY

For patients with prior ascending aortic replacement presenting with arch and proximal descending aortic pathology (Figure 4) or patients with distal arch and proximal descending aortic disease alone, an alternative approach can facilitate a one-stage repair.

Using an oblique transverse thoracosternotomy beginning over the anterolateral left chest below the nipple, the incision is extended across the midline into the contralateral interspace (Figure 4B). Both internal mammary arteries are ligated. Exposure to the transverse aortic arch and proximal descending thoracic aorta is outstanding.

Again, the options for brachiocephalic arterial reconstruction include a large Carrel patch, a separate graft, or a trifurcation graft to the individual vessels, depending on the degree of atherosclerotic disease and/or scarring from previous surgery (Figure 4C).

Patients tolerate the incision well, and exposure of the phrenic and recurrent laryngeal nerves allows easy preservation. The only drawback involves sternal union of the transverse incision. Secure stabilization of the sternal tables at the end of the procedure is imperative.

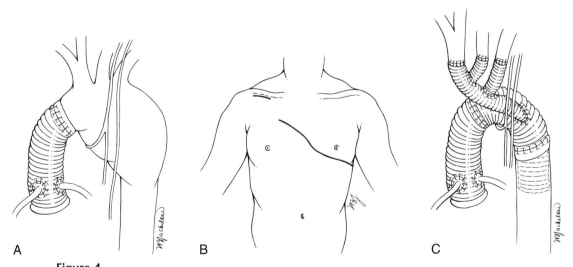

A   B   C

Figure 4
Aortic arch replacement with prior ascending aortic repair. **(A)** Aneurysmal aortic arch with previous ascending arch replacement. **(B)** Oblique transverse thoracosternotomy approach. **(C)** Completed repair with trifurcated graft to the individual tracheocephalic arteries anastomatosed to reconstructed arch.

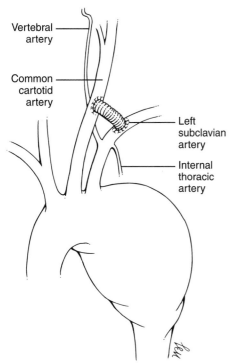

Figure 5
Adjunctive preoperative approach for left subclavian to common carotid bypass with Dacron graft. Left subclavian artery is ligated proximally.

Arterial perfusion is the same, through the right axillary artery. Venting of the left ventricle during systemic cooling and cardiac fibrillation occurs either via the right superior pulmonary vein or via a small separate thoracotomy overlying the left ventricular apex.

One additional adjunctive procedure for aortic arch repair that is worth mentioning is a preoperative left subclavian to common carotid bypass using either an 8- or 10-mm Dacron graft. The left subclavian artery is then ligated as it exits the mediastinum below the vertebral and internal mammary arteries (Figure 5). This small surgical procedure reduces the circulatory arrest time during arch reconstruction, reduces dissection of the left subclavian artery in the mediastinum in close proximity to the vagus and phrenic nerves, and, finally, may lower the risk of posterior cerebral circulation embolic stroke, if the origin is heavily involved in the atherosclerotic process. This adjunctive procedure is used selectively.

■ CONCLUSION

The described standard method of profound hypothermia and circulatory arrest is the cornerstone of aortic arch reconstruction. The actual methodology has changed to minimize the period of circulatory arrest and ischemic brain injury and to reduce the risk of embolic stroke and increase flexibility for varied surgical anatomy and clinical scenarios. Currently, we believe that the creation of bifurcation and trifurcation grafts to the brachiocephalic vessels, to be implanted into the main aortic arch graft at the conclusion of the repair, fulfills these goals. Undoubtedly, current techniques will continue to evolve as they have since their inception.

SUGGESTED READING

Borst HG, et al: *Surgical treatment of aortic dissection,* New York, 1996, Churchill Livingstone.

Crawford ES, et al: Surgical treatment of aneurysm and/or dissection of the ascending aorta and transverse aortic arch: factors influencing survival in 717 patients, *J Thorac Cardiovasc Surg* 98:659, 1989.

Ergin M, et al: Hypothermic circulatory arrest in operations on the thoracic aorta: determinants of operative mortality and neurologic outcome, *J Thorac Cardiovasc Surg* 107:788, 1994.

Griepp RB, Ergin MA. Aneurysms of the aortic arch. In Edmunds LH Jr, editor: *Cardiac surgery in the adult,* New York, 1997, McGraw-Hill, p 1197.

Griepp RB, et al: Prosthetic replacement of the aortic arch, *J Thorac Cardiovasc Surg* 70:1051, 1975.

Kuki S, et al: A novel modification of the elephant trunk technique using a single four branched arch graft for extensive thoracic aortic aneurysm, *Eur J Cardiothorac Surg* 18:246, 2000.

INTRAOPERATIVE CEREBRAL MONITORING

Harvey L. Edmonds, Jr.
Brian L. Ganzel

The 1 million cardiac surgical procedures performed annually worldwide represent a major source of neurologic injury. Experience with neurophysiologic monitoring during these procedures now challenges the widespread perception that these injuries are primarily macroembolic in origin and unavoidable. Simultaneous monitoring of cerebral blood flow, oxygenation, and synaptic activity shows a multifactorial etiology that is often amenable to therapeutic intervention. This chapter describes current techniques available for brain injury detection/prevention and summarizes results of more recent outcome studies.

■ RATIONALE FOR MULTIMODALITY NEUROMONITORING

Electroencephalography

Noninvasive electrophysiologic assessment of cerebral cortical synaptic function by electroencephalography (EEG) is the longest established method of brain monitoring during cardiac surgery. It has been used sporadically since the first application of cardiopulmonary bypass more than 50 years ago. EEG is exquisitely sensitive to change in cortical synaptic activity. Moderate synaptic depression leads to a loss of high-frequency EEG activity, whereas greater depression reduces the amplitude of all EEG waveforms, ultimately resulting in electrocerebral silence (i.e., flat-line EEG). Traditionally, these changes were monitored through continuous examination of the conventional multilead EEG waveforms. Current computer-processed numeric descriptors and trends greatly simplify the process, however.

The controversy surrounding EEG monitoring involves its role in injury prevention. In contrast to its standard-of-care status for carotid surgery, EEG monitoring has yet to achieve acceptance among many cardiac surgeons. Lack of EEG acceptance seems to be due primarily to its low specificity. There may be numerous causes of EEG suppression during cardiac surgery, but only some of them signify a brain at risk. Hypothermia, residual effects of cardioplegia, and high-dose anesthesia all can depress cortical function without causing harm. In the absence of other forms of neuromonitoring, attempting distinction between injurious and benign causes for EEG suppression becomes conjecture.

Transcranial Doppler Ultrasound

Noninvasive transcranial Doppler (TCD) measures the erythrocyte velocity in large cerebral arteries and veins. Because velocity is influenced by small changes in vessel diameter,

TCD cannot provide an absolute measure of blood flow. Instead, TCD is the only available method to assess continuously *change* in cerebral blood flow or its direction. In addition, the acoustic impedance (i.e., reflectivity) of gaseous and particulate emboli is much greater than that of erythrocytes. Most modern TCD devices also produce a semiquantitative estimate of the aggregate embolic echoes, or high-intensity transient signals. Devices currently available for routine clinical application are not able to determine, however, either the size or the composition of the highly reflective material.

Similar to EEG, TCD has become a standard of care for carotid surgery because of its ability to detect sudden flow change and its sensitivity to the presence of emboli. Also similar to EEG, TCD monitoring is not used often during or after cardiac surgery. Its limited application seems to be related to several practical issues. First, transcranial insonation of a major artery is possible only through several small, paper-thin cranial regions termed *ultrasonic windows.* In 10% to 15% of patients, temporal hyperostosis shuts these windows, making transcranial insonation difficult or impossible. Second, the clinical usefulness of the TCD signal is highly user dependent. Considerable training and continual practice are necessary to obtain and interpret TCD signals reliably, especially in the complex environment of cardiac surgery. Third, hemodilution complicates velocity-based flow estimates by reducing viscosity. Peak velocity may increase, while the net passage of erythrocytes decreases. Fourth, the reduction in oxyhemoglobin dissociation by hypothermia and alkalosis complicates interpretation of flow velocity changes. These limitations notwithstanding, TCD greatly enhances the clinical utility of EEG monitoring by improving specificity. With instantaneous information of blood flow change and embolization, sudden EEG changes suggesting a high injury potential can be identified more quickly and reliably and the appropriate intervention instituted. In the case of cranial hyperostosis, probe placement over the extracranial internal carotid ensures that ultrasonic monitoring of cranial perfusion can be performed in every patient.

Transcranial Near-Infrared Spectroscopy

Oxyhemoglobin and deoxyhemoglobin can be measured noninvasively within cerebral cortical tissue using infrared light. The measurement of these chromophores is possible because the skull is transparent to infrared light. Cerebral oximetry is distinct from pulse oximetry because it measures all reflected infrared light, both pulsatile (arterial) and nonpulsatile (venous and capillary). This highly focal cortical measure also is distinct from jugular bulb oximetry, which represents a global average of cranial venous effluent. Because the transcranial measure does not require flowing blood, pulsatile or otherwise, it is the only technique that can measure cerebral oxygen balance continuously during cardiopulmonary bypass and circulatory arrest.

This device has been approved by the U.S. Food and Drug Administration only more recently and is not yet considered standard of care for any procedure. Nevertheless, several outcome studies document its clinical utility in cardiac surgery. When used in conjunction with the other neuromonitoring modalities, it further reduces uncertainty in identification and management of brain injury.

■ NEUROMONITORING STRATEGY FOR CARDIAC SURGERY

The objective of neuromonitoring is simple: prevent or reduce brain injury. To achieve this objective, it is desirable to initiate brain monitoring before induction of anesthesia. Characterization of perfusion, oxygenation, and neuronal function in the awake brain is important to establish a reference and identify preexisting abnormalities. Each of these measures may vary widely among individuals so that intraoperative monitoring typically defines abnormality as marked deviation from individualized baseline rather than from established absolute threshold. Documentation of preexisting irregularities is vital for detection of developing injury and patient response to corrective actions (summarized in Table 1). This intervention algorithm uses neuromonitoring and routine physiologic signals to identify potentially injurious events and their most likely cause. The success of interventions designed to correct the problem also can be documented. The detailed rationale for each notification and intervention is described in the Suggested Readings.

Figure 1 illustrates the range of information provided to the cardiac surgery team by multimodality neuromonitoring. In this case example, an uneventful repair of an ascending aortic aneurysm took place using deep hypothermic systemic circulatory arrest with selective cerebral perfusion. The four traces represent the duration of cardiopulmonary bypass. The top (mean arterial pressure) trace depicts the limit of information relative to cerebral perfusion that is normally available without neuromonitoring. Comparison with the trace immediately below (peak blood flow velocity in the left middle cerebral artery) illustrates the lack of correlation between the two. During induction of deep hypothermia, cerebral blood flow decreased due to flow-metabolism

coupling, whereas systemic perfusion pressure was unchanged. Selective antegrade perfusion through the carotids maintained cerebral flow during systemic circulatory arrest. Without direct measurement of brain perfusion, there is no way to document selective antegrade or retrograde cerebral blood flow. During attempted retrograde perfusion through the superior vena cava, dark blood may efflux from the carotids without detectable flow in the basal cerebral arteries. The flow path is uncertain in this circumstance, but it does not involve the cerebral cortex.

The repair also was aided by measurement of regional brain oxygen saturation (rSO_2), which helped to define the adequacy of the Doppler-quantified cerebral flow velocity. During cooling, rSO_2 increased, while brain flow decreased. Reduction in cerebral metabolic demand was greater than the decrease in blood flow, resulting in a net improvement in oxygen balance. During selective cerebral perfusion, the slight decrease in rSO_2 suggested that brain blood flow was suboptimal but adequate. Greater desaturation during the late stages of rewarming documented that cerebral blood flow, although increasing, was still insufficient to meet the needs of a hypermetabolic brain.

Modern EEG monitoring also can be an asset during repair. We use the bispectral index (BIS) as an EEG-based multivariate quantitative descriptor of cerebral cortical synaptic activity. It has been used successfully in more than 1.5 million operations to measure anesthetic adequacy. BIS values greater than 70 signify a high probability of patient responsiveness, whereas values less than 40 indicate excessive anesthesia. Careful anesthetic titration within these limits facilitates fast-track cardiac anesthesia while guarding against patient recall. BIS has an additional benefit for cardiac procedures using deep hypothermia: Near-abolition of the BIS by cooling confirms optimal hypothermia. Individualized management

Table 1 Intervention Algorithm Initiated by Electroencephalography Slowing or Cerebral Oxygen Desaturation

TEMP	BP	TCD	NOTIFICATION	INTERVENTION
Pre-CPB				
0	0	– Peak velocity	Aorta obstructed	Reposition head; adjust aortic cannula
0	0	– Diastolic velocity	Cava obstructed	Reposition head or pulmonary artery catheter; adjust venous cannula
CPB				
0	0	+ Peak velocity	Hyperemia	– Pump flow
0	0	Gas emboli	Gas emboli	Repair circuit; deair; cool; hypertension; fosphenytoin; hyperbaric chamber
0	0	Particulates	Particulate emboli	Cool; fosphenytoin; retrograde perfusion
+	0	– Peak velocity	Flow-metabolic uncoupling	+ BP; – metabolic demand
0	0	– Peak	Cerebral flow low	+ Pump flow; reposition aortic cannula
Post-CPB				
0	0	– Diastolic velocity	Cerebral edema	Ultrafiltration; mannitol
Anytime				
0	–	– Peak velocity	Dysautoregulation	+ BP; fosphenytoin
0	0	0	Excess anesthetic	– Anesthetic
With + EEG Frequency or Bispectral Index				
0	0, +	0, + Peak velocity	Insufficient anesthetic	+ Anesthetic

0 = no change; + = increase; – = decrease; Temp, tympanic or nasopharyngeal temperature; BP, blood pressure; TCD, transcranial Doppler; CPB, cardiopulmonary bypass; EEG, electroencephalography.

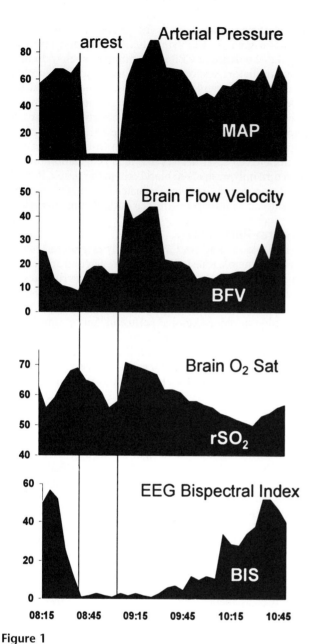

Figure 1

Changes in mean arterial pressure (MAP) *(top trace)*, left middle cerebral artery blood flow velocity (BFV) *(second trace)*, left frontal cerebral cortical oxygen saturation (regional oxygen saturation [rSO$_2$]) *(third trace)*, and electroencephalography (EEG) bispectral index *(bottom trace)* during cardiopulmonary bypass support for repair of an ascending aortic aneurysm. The period of deep hypothermic systemic circulatory arrest (21°C) is bounded by the two vertical lines. Brain blood flow and oxygenation are preserved during systemic arrest by selective antegrade perfusion of the carotid arteries. EEG silence (i.e., a bispectral index [BIS] of 0) was used to determine the optimal nasopharyngeal temperature for systemic circulatory arrest.

is important because the tympanic or nasopharyngeal temperature associated with obliteration of EEG activity varies among patients by more than 10°C. The benefit of cooling seems to derive from cessation of synaptic activity. Further unnecessary cooling is of questionable value but may increase coagulopathy and cardiopulmonary bypass time. After a period of deep hypothermic circulatory arrest, it is reassuring to note that the EEG has returned to its prebypass appearance.

The information provided by these neuromonitoring techniques enables the surgeon to minimize imbalance in cerebral perfusion and oxygenation. Partially as a result of this additional monitoring, our surgical morbidity for repair of aortic arch aneurysms is now similar to that for routine valve replacement. This experience is not unique to our center; the Utrecht group have stated that "adequate cerebral monitoring is mandatory for safe realization of selective antegrade cerebral perfusion."

■ INFLUENCE OF NEUROMONITORING ON OUTCOME

Unequivocal proof of therapeutic benefit comes only from adequately powered prospective randomized controlled studies. Because these studies are complex and expensive, only a limited number of widely used therapies have had such scientific validation. Most therapies are supported primarily by retrospective observational studies that show association between therapy and outcome, not absolute proof of cause and effect. Such is the case for all forms of neuromonitoring. Insurers often accept some associational studies as evidence of benefit (i.e., carotid endarterectomy), while denying others (i.e., cardiac surgery). Nevertheless, since the 1990s, there have been many retrospective controlled studies using one or more neuromonitoring modalities during cardiac surgery that suggest improved clinical outcome. Clinical benefit is not limited to stroke rate reduction. Monitoring also has improved subtle signs of cognitive function and nonneurologic end points, such as renal and pulmonary function, readmission, and death rates. These unexpected benefits apparently derive from enhanced perfusion and oxygenation of all vital organs, not just the brain. Several of the more recent studies also show reduced hospital charges. Because (1) the current weight of evidence indicates clinical benefit of neuromonitoring for cardiac surgery, (2) the risks of neuromonitoring are nil, and (3) its modest costs are overshadowed by larger savings, its use in cardiac surgery is strongly encouraged, particularly in higher risk cardiac patients.

SUGGESTED READING

Austin EH III, et al: Benefit of neuromonitoring for pediatric cardiac surgery, *J Thorac Cardiovasc Surg* 114:707, 1997.

Edmonds HL Jr: Advances in neuromonitoring for cardiothoracic and vascular surgery, *J Cardiothorac Vasc Anesth* 15:241, 2001.

Edmonds HL Jr: Detection and treatment of cerebral hypoxia key to avoiding intraoperative brain injuries, *J Clin Monit Comput* 16:69, 2000.

Ganzel BL, et al: Neurophysiological monitoring to assure delivery of retrograde cerebral perfusion, *J Thorac Cardiovasc Surg* 113:748, 1997.

NEUROPROTECTIVE STRATEGIES DURING CARDIAC SURGERY

Stephen M. Cattaneo II

William A. Baumgartner

Neurologic injury is a significant complication of cardiac surgery despite new strategies and techniques to avoid neurologic complications. Frank stroke occurs infrequently (1% to 6%), whereas neuropsychologic changes, including deficits in memory, attention, learning, and concentration, complicate 25% to 65% of cardiac operations. Although these psychomotor deficits are most pronounced early after surgery, they persist in 30% of patients after 1 year. Atherosclerotic emboli in the aorta and great arteries and hypoperfusion to watershed regions of the brain are the predominant causes of focal deficits. In contrast, mechanisms responsible for neuropsychologic deficits and changes in level of consciousness are likely multifactorial and include hypoperfusion, microemboli, metabolic derangements, general anesthesia, and initiation of a proinflammatory state. As a result, various intraoperative strategies and techniques have been employed to prevent these neurologic complications.

■ NEUROLOGIC INJURY RISK

Efforts to prevent cerebral injury begin with determining a patient's risk of experiencing a neurologic event. A study from our institution identified five criteria predictive of stroke in cardiac surgery patients: age greater than 70, hypertension, diabetes mellitus, previous stroke, and asymptomatic carotid bruits. Additionally the incidence of postoperative neurobehavioral deficits has been correlated significantly with older age, more than 100 perioperative microemboli (as estimated by continuous-wave carotid Doppler transducer), and palpable aortic plaque. When a patient's neurologic risk is assessed, a combination of strategies can be used to improve neurologic outcome.

■ NEUROPROTECTIVE STRATEGIES

Systemic Inflammatory State

The well-documented proinflammatory state induced by cardiopulmonary bypass (CPB) occurs due to activation of the complement and fibrinolysis systems and the intrinsic and extrinsic coagulation cascades. These elements contribute to bleeding and thromboembolism during CPB. Numerous cellular aggregates and debris are formed in the circuit that are capable of embolizing to capillaries throughout the body's vascular bed. The net effect is a significant systemic inflammatory response that is the presumed cause of global cerebral edema shown by post-CPB magnetic resonance imaging. Avoidance of CPB in off-pump cases may diminish the inflammatory response and the incidence of neurologic dysfunction, but randomized studies are not yet available. A more recent publication showed no relationship, however, between inflammatory mediators and objective neuropsychologic changes. Attempts to decrease the activation of inflammatory cascades have included heparin-coated perfusion circuits and cell-saver devices that filter coagulation proteins and return only washed red blood cells to the circuit. Protease inhibitors currently are being evaluated for benefit in preventing neurologic injury through their antiinflammatory effects.

Cerebral Perfusion

Cerebral blood flow on CPB typically is maintained well above an ischemic threshold as intrinsic cerebral autoregulation maintains flow over a wide systemic arterial pressure ranging from 50 to 120 mm Hg. Cerebral compromise still may occur, however, within boundary zones particularly susceptible to reduced global perfusion. Specifically, hypertensive patients are susceptible to ischemia because their cerebral autoregulatory curve is shifted to a higher pressure. Higher mean perfusion pressures are necessary in hypertensive patients to avoid a pressure-passive condition of cerebral perfusion.

Autoregulation of cerebral blood flow also is maintained in deep hypothermia for perfusion pressures of 30 to 100 mm Hg. At 15°C, cerebral oxygen consumption is a fraction of that during normothermia due to significantly decreased metabolism. Also, the oxygen dissociation curve is shifted leftward so that delivered oxygen is primarily in the dissolved form. Continuous cerebral perfusion in a pressure range that permits autoregulation should prevent ischemia and hypoperfusion during hypothermic circulatory arrest (HCA).

The technique of HCA is used widely for procedures to repair or replace the aortic arch. Efficient neurologic protection occurs at core body temperatures of 18°C if the period of circulatory arrest is less than 40 minutes. This technique alone may be inadequate for longer periods, however, and requires extended cooling and rewarming periods on CPB.

Retrograde cerebral perfusion (RCP) has been shown to be a safe adjunct to deep hypothermia but does not unequivocally improve outcome. RCP may augment the protective effect of hypothermia alone permitting longer periods of HCA. Also, RCP may flush out debris, air, and other emboli. Despite these proposed advantages, no clear benefit of RCP exists. Most reported retrospective series using RCP as an adjunct to HCA have arrest times less than 45 minutes, so it is unclear whether additional benefit is conferred by RCP over hypothermia alone. Also, well-documented valves in the human jugular system likely impede retrograde flow. Experimental studies show that some blood is shunted away from the brain during RCP due to venovenous anastomoses.

Cold blood antegrade cerebral perfusion (ACP) has been shown to prevent ischemic cerebral injury during prolonged hypothermic arrest and may be a useful adjunct to HCA when longer arrest times are needed. A significantly lower incidence of temporary neurologic dysfunction has been reported with ACP during prolonged HCA. Postulated mechanisms include enhanced delivery of oxygen to the brain and improved cerebral cooling. A major downside to ACP is that it requires more complex cannulation techniques with the possibility of accidental atheromatous embolization.

Although some surgeons continue to cool patients systemically to 10°C to 13°C in the setting of selective cerebral perfusion, ACP allows a higher core body temperature without sacrificing cerebral protection and shortens rewarming time. Packing the head in ice is used routinely in circulatory arrest to prevent warming of the scalp and head.

pH Management Technique

Following an α-stat protocol allows cerebral blood flow to be maintained in a normal autoregulatory range because blood gases are not temperature corrected. A pH stat protocol artificially maintains pH. During systemic hypothermia, the addition of carbon dioxide to the bypass circuit is necessary to maintain pH. This leads to a loss of autoregulation as cerebral blood flow becomes pressure-passive. Also, cerebral vasodilation due to hypercarbia increases the cerebral flow-to-metabolism ratio significantly. Although this increase ensures adequate oxygenation, unnecessarily high flow can lead to higher rates of cerebral embolization (see later). Clinical investigative work by Jonas et al at Boston Children's Hospital has shown less neurologic injury in infants using a pH stat protocol.

Cerebral Monitoring

Monitoring cerebral perfusion, especially for high-risk patients, during CPB can provide evidence of adequate cerebral oxygenation. Several methods have been developed, including near-infrared cerebral oximetry, which roughly estimates brain tissue oxygenation. Also, jugular bulb saturation can be used as an index of cerebral arterial-venous oxygen difference. Arteriovenous pressure differences are vital to provide adequate organ perfusion. For example, if superior vena cava return is obstructed, cerebral perfusion rapidly becomes compromised. Significant attention must be paid to heart and cannula manipulation, especially when attempting exposure on the posterior aspects of the heart. Additionally, diligent monitoring has shown a 5% to 10% incidence of malperfusion after CPB initiation in acute type A dissection. As a result, neurocerebral monitoring allows for expeditious correction of malperfusion by cannula repositioning or direct surgical fenestration.

Neurocerebral monitoring also may improve neurologic outcome for patients requiring hypothermic circulatory arrest. Methods include monitoring for greater than 95% jugular venous saturation or for the disappearance of subcortical somatosensory evoked potentials. Data suggest, however, that EEG silence is an optimal marker for minimal cerebral metabolic activity. Performing EEG monitoring until the occurrence of EEG silence may improve neurologic outcome compared with waiting a specific length of time for cooling or attempting to obtain a predetermined temperature. Bavaria et al at the University of Pennsylvania advocated neuromonitoring and cooling of patients until EEG silence. If monitoring is unavailable, cooling for 45 minutes should be adequate because less than 10% of patients still have demonstrable cerebral activity at this point. Terminating cooling at EEG silence potentially can shorten the cooling and the rewarming phases.

Embolization Avoidance

As stated previously, cardiac surgery–related strokes commonly occur secondary to embolization of atheromatous material from established aortic and great artery plaques. Careful placement of cannulae within atherosclerotic vessels is important to avoid dislodging plaque. Also, the placement of aortic cannulae at the takeoff of great vessels should be avoided because flow may disrupt established plaques. Transesophageal echocardiography (TEE) and epiaortic ultrasound scanning can serve as adjuncts to palpation for detection of the precise location and type of aortic plaques. Although TEE has limitations in detecting atherosclerotic plaque in the distal ascending aorta and arch, epiaortic ultrasound allows adequate visualization. The use of routine epiaortic scanning is expensive but has been shown to be beneficial for patients with documented neurologic risk factors, such as advanced age, significantly palpable plaque, or a history of stroke. TEE also allows for improved deairing after an intracardiac procedure. Insufflation of carbon dioxide into the pericardial well has decreased the incidence of postoperative air as detected by TEE.

Excessive aortic plaque near the innominate artery takeoff may prevent cross-clamp application and necessitate other maneuvers, such as moderate hypothermia and fibrillatory arrest, for selected operative procedures. This technique generally requires cannulation of the common femoral artery with placement of a left ventricular vent through the right superior pulmonary vein for adequate left ventricular decompression.

A single occlusion clamp applied to the ascending aorta for placement of proximal vein graft anastomoses has proved beneficial compared with a two-clamp technique, although there is a brief incremental period of myocardial ischemia using the former technique. The single-clamp technique lengthens cross-clamp time and delays myocardial rewarming. This reduces the degree of aortic manipulation, however, and avoids the application of a partial occluding clamp, which is probably the most traumatic aortic manipulation because the total clamping force is applied over a small area. A greater proportion of emboli are a result of partial clamp application (>25%) than cross-clamp application (<10%). A prospective analysis at our institution showed that adverse neurologic events are more common with the double-clamp technique compared with a single-clamp technique. Several other studies corroborate this benefit and show stroke rates of only about 1%. The single clamp technique also results in a decreased release of S-100 protein. This serum protein is a potential marker for increased cerebral embolization and increased clinically evident neurologic injury.

Off-pump coronary artery bypass graft (OPCAB) surgery should reduce atherosclerotic emboli by avoiding aortic manipulation and cannulation, while avoiding full heparinization and systemic inflammation associated with CPB. Nonrandomized studies reported a significantly decreased stroke rate with OPCAB procedures compared with conventional on-pump coronary artery bypass graft procedures, especially in patients with preexisting cerebrovascular disease. Other studies have not shown such clear neurologic benefit, however. The VA cardiac surgery programs are initiating a randomized, controlled study to estimate the efficacy of the OPCAB procedure compared with standard coronary artery bypass graft procedures.

Additionally, cerebral fat emboli may result from mediastinal fat aspiration into the CPB circuit by the cardiotomy suction. When cardiotomy suction is not used during CPB, serum S-100 protein levels are demonstrably decreased. Cell-saver devices that separate red blood cells from other cellular elements and debris can negate this complication.

Temperature Concerns

Various studies have produced conflicting results as to the neurologic benefits of normothermic versus hypothermic CPB. Normothermic CPB avoids the deleterious effects of hypothermia, while shortening CPB and total operating room times. A randomized trial showed no difference in neurologic and neurocognitive outcomes between normothermic and hypothermic (28°C to 30°C) CPB at a 6-week postoperative evaluation. Proponents of mild hypothermia (28°C to 32°C) counter that decreases in cerebral metabolism allow for lower flow rates, decreasing embolization rates. Additionally, cerebral embolization is associated most often with warm periods, such as initiation of CPB, aortic cannulation, and cross-clamp application and removal, so hypothermia provides no added benefit during these more critical maneuvers. Studies have shown no change in neurologic events by varying CPB temperature, but ischemic lesions have significantly greater extension with poorer clinical neurologic outcome with normothermic CPB. Even this conclusion has mixed opinions, however, as a follow-up study with similar design refuted this conclusion and found no difference in volume of cerebral infarct.

The rate of rewarming from mildly hypothermic CPB (28°C to 32°C) also may affect neurologic injury. Traditional rewarming protocols have suggested keeping the difference between nasopharyngeal temperature and perfusate temperature less than 4°C to 6°C. Slower rewarming (2°C temperature difference) allows for a lower peak temperature so that the target temperature is not overshot with a resultant hyperthermic period. Hyperthermia is associated with an altered balance of cerebral oxygen supply and demand with demonstrable declines in jugular venous saturation leading to a likely increased risk of cognitive dysfunction. Using this method of slower rewarming has been shown to have significantly better postoperative cognitive performance. Additionally, diabetic patients have impaired cerebral autoregulation during CPB and may have an increased benefit from slower rewarming.

Pharmacologic Therapy

Pharmacologic therapy potentially may decrease the incidence of neurologic injury. Previously, laboratory and clinical reports have shown minimal neuroprotective effects with barbiturates, propofol (Diprivan), and N-methyl-D-aspartate antagonists, but all have downsides, such as delayed emergence from anesthesia, delayed extubation, and varied neurologic side effects. Neurologic dysfunction is most exaggerated after HCA. Elucidation of the mechanism of injury may provide pertinent information that is generic to brain injury after all cardiac surgery procedures. Our laboratory experience suggests that neurocognitive deficits arising during HCA are the result of glutamate excitotoxicity leading to increased nitric oxide production and precipitating a cascade resulting in eventual neuronal cell death (Figure 1). Specific pharmacologic agents with actions at particular points in this pathway (i.e., glutamate receptor antagonists and neuronal nitric oxide synthase inhibitors) have shown benefit in our

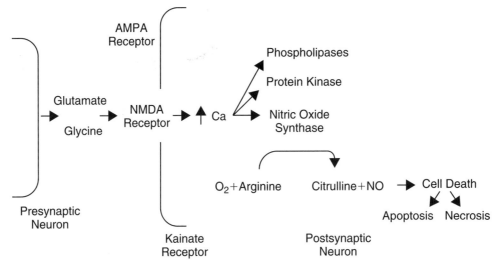

Figure 1
Proposed mechanism of neuronal cell injury and death after hypoxia and ischemia. An excessive amount of glutamate overactivates N-methyl-D-aspartate (NMDA) receptors. This causes an intracellular influx of calcium, resulting in the production of a variety of agents, including nitric oxide synthase. This leads to the production of nitric oxide, which acts as a neurotoxin, resulting in cellular death. *(From Baumgartner WA, et al: Ann Thorac Surg 67:1871, 1999.)*

laboratory canine model. Diazoxide, a potassium-dependent adenosine triphosphate channel opener, currently is being investigated clinically to determine its efficacy in reducing neurologic injury.

■ CONCLUSION

After identification of a patient's risk of neurologic injury during cardiac surgery, a myriad of options exists for reducing this complication. Although significant controversies remain, various more recent techniques have been employed resulting in a generalized improvement in the incidence of stroke and neuropsychologic changes. Several pharmacologic therapies show significant promise and likely will be added to the neuroprotective armamentarium in the future.

SUGGESTED READING

Baumgartner WA, et al: Assessing the impact of cerebral injury after cardiac surgery: will determining the mechanism reduce this injury? *Ann Thorac Surg* 67:1871, 1999.

Edmunds LH Jr: Inflammatory response to cardiopulmonary bypass, *Ann Thorac Surg* 66:S12, 1998.

Grigore AM, et al; Neurological Outcome Research Group and CARE Investigators of the Duke Heart Center: Prospective randomized trial of normothermic versus hypothermic cardiopulmonary bypass on cognitive function after coronary artery bypass graft surgery, *Anesthesiology* 95:1110, 2001.

Hammon JW Jr, et al: Approaches to reduce neurologic complications during cardiac surgery, *Semin Thorac Cardiovasc Surg* 13:184, 2001.

Hammon JW Jr, et al: Risk factors and solutions for the development of neurobehavioral changes after coronary artery bypass grafting, *Ann Thorac Surg* 63:1613, 1997.

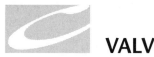

SELECTION OF A CARDIAC VALVE PROSTHESIS

Robert D. Riley
Neal D. Kon

Cardiac valve prostheses have evolved considerably since the first prosthetic valve implant in September 1952 by Hufnagel in a patient with severe aortic valve insufficiency. This landmark operation was performed without cardiopulmonary bypass and the prosthetic valve was inserted into the descending thoracic aorta. With the advent of cardiopulmonary bypass in 1954, valve operations became much more feasible. The first mitral valve replacement occurred in March 1960. Braunwald and Morrow inserted a polyurethane and Dacron prosthesis in the mitral position. By May 1960, Harken performed the first successful orthotopic aortic valve replacement (AVR) when he implanted a ball and cage device within the aortic annulus. Early operations were complicated by high mortality rates and numerous prosthesis-related problems as well as infection and endocarditis.

Technological development over the next 30 to 40 years resulted in an explosion of ideas for development of mechanical prostheses designed specifically for implantation in the mitral or aortic positions. Over the same time, advances were made in bioprosthetic implants. Xenograft tissue, both porcine valve and bovine pericardium, were attached to stents to support their structure and ensure valve competence. Stentless tissue designs were also developed to improve hemodynamics and avoid premature tissue failure. Similarly, allograft and autograft valves have been used with improved outcomes. All bioprosthetic valve development relies heavily on innovation in tissue preservation and anticalcification technology.

However, there is still no single ideal valve suitable for implantation in every location for all patients. A discussion of the potential considerations in selecting a heart valve replacement follows. These include patient lifestyle and life expectancy. The ideal valve closely resembles the normal aortic or mitral valve in function but not necessarily structure. Valve replacement should return the patient to a normal lifestyle and confer normal life expectancy for aged matched controls. These characteristics require different designs for mitral and aortic valves. The tricuspid and pulmonary valves are probably well suited for replacement with valves designed for mitral or aortic positions, respectively.

The ideal valve should (1) be hemodynamically efficient with laminar flow patterns and low transvalvular gradients; (2) be competent with unobstructed moving parts; (3) withstand the natural opening and closing forces on the valve without deterioration over time; (4) maintain normal myocardial function by preserving natural coordinated contraction and blood flow; (5) be 100% viable with the ability for self-repair, resistance to infection, and ability to grow as the patient grows; (6) be functionally inert with respect to interaction with the blood without hemolysis or thrombosis; (7) be durable enough to outlive the patient; and (8) be convenient in availability and ease of implantation.

Initial considerations for valve prosthesis selection usually involve two basic issues: anticoagulation and longevity. *Longevity* refers to both valve durability and patient life expectancy. The need for anticoagulation sets mechanical valves apart from tissue valves. Not all valves behave the same in all patients. In general, the younger the patient, the greater is the demand on the valve prosthesis and the more difficult is the choice. Younger patients have the potential to outlive or outgrow their prosthesis, have a higher metabolic rate, and destroy tissue valves more quickly. Older age, renal failure, concomitant coronary disease, and severe left ventricular dysfunction are all independently associated with decreased survival after valve replacement. In a patient with a limited life expectancy, valve selection may depend on other factors such as surgeon familiarity/comfort, availability, ease of implantation, and patient ability to take anticoagulants. All other factors being equal, the nuances of valve performance or implant technique will then guide the surgeon to choose a prosthesis.

■ INHERENT PROSTHETIC VALVE PROPERTIES

Some general statements can be broadly applied to the classes of prosthetic valves. Mechanical valves are structurally more durable than bioprosthetic valves and have a lower profile, causing less interference with subvalvular structures. They are made with rigid materials and do not flex or conform to the heart. This may limit or obstruct blood flow and alter hemodynamic function. The mechanical surfaces are not natural and their interaction with blood components may damage the blood, activate cells, or initiate thrombosis. The valves are biologically inert and cannot heal or repair themselves. They lack resistance to infection. Typically, mechanical valves require some regurgitation to wash the valve to prevent thrombosis. Mechanical valves also tend to be noisy. Some patients are sensitive to this and find the noise irritating. In summary, currently available mechanical valves have great durability but at the price of relative obstructive nature and need for anticoagulation.

Bioprosthetic valves come in several varieties: porcine, pericardial, allograft, autograft, stented, and stentless. The only generalization among this class of valves is the lack of need for anticoagulation, but structural deterioration is higher than that of mechanical valves. Stented biologic valves create similar hemodynamic and functional alterations as mechanical valves. The stent–hinge interface may create a stress point and contribute to structural valve-related deterioration. Stentless valves were developed to improve hydraulic dysfunction and subsequent durability.

ANTICOAGULATION

One critical decision regarding valve replacement to be addressed early is whether the patient will take or tolerate anticoagulants. Anticoagulation is not benign; there is substantial morbidity and mortality associated with blood thinners. Hemorrhagic complications leading to neurologic events, gastrointestinal hemorrhage, and hospitalization and blood transfusion have been reported. Anticoagulant management around the time of noncardiac surgery, dental procedures, and endoscopy, to name a few, is cumbersome and can increase morbidity. The desire to participate in contact sports, some lifestyle choices, or hobbies or predisposition to falls may contraindicate anticoagulation. Some oral anticoagulants, such as warfarin, are contraindicated in pregnancy, although intravenous heparin therapy and subcutaneous low-molecular-weight heparins are available as alternatives. Medical noncompliance and limited availability of INR testing are also relative contraindications to mechanical valves. Some patients have other indications for chronic anticoagulant therapy such as chronic atrial fibrillation, cardiomyopathy, and cerebrovascular diseases; in these cases, the mechanical valve may be preferred. One caveat is that usually a higher INR is maintained for valve prostheses than for most medical conditions. It should also be noted that some authors (although we do not) recommend 1 to 2 months of anticoagulant therapy for patients with bioprosthetic valves as well, until the sewing ring is endothelialized. This practice is not universal.

LIFE EXPECTANCY

Expected patient survival affects choice of a valve prosthesis as much as any other factor. Closely tied to this is the patient's chronologic age. Predicting the patient's natural history is difficult at best. Initially it may appear that mechanical valves are best suited for the young patient who would outlive the average bioprosthetic heart valve; however, there are numerous other factors to consider. Children requiring valve replacement still need to grow. A valve that would accommodate a child's growth would be ideal. Younger patients tend to be more active and more prone to injury and to take medicines less reliably. Pregnancy is also a possibility for the young female. Some surgeons argue that redo valve replacement is a safe procedure that can be accomplished with minimal risk that rivals the alternative risk of anticoagulation. Finally, comorbid conditions that affect patient life expectancy need to be considered. Some coexisting diseases also limit valve durability, such as renal failure and dialysis dependency. Patient preoperative condition may influence the choice of operation depending on surgeon comfort and skill. A simpler, quicker operation may be indicated in the extremely ill patient who may not tolerate a longer time on cardiopulmonary bypass or whose disease requires significant concomitant procedures necessitating longer cross-clamp times.

VALVULAR PATHOPHYSIOLOGY

Incompetent valves and stenotic valves create different anatomic pathologic changes that also directly influence prosthetic valve choice. Rheumatic disease of the mitral valve significantly affects the subvalvular structures and may require complete excision of the valve with subsequent altered myocardial function. This may be a limitation to mechanical and stented tissue prostheses. However, this presents a better opportunity for stentless mitral valve replacement with either allograft or the quadrileaflet pericardial mitral prostheses. These implants recreate the subvalvular structure and maintain near-normal myocardial function and annular mechanics. Another situation is the difficult aortic root. Significant root pathology or annular calcification, which requires extensive débridement to ensure adequate seating of the valve, is most effectively treated with a total root replacement. Mechanical valved conduits as well as stentless porcine roots and allograft roots are available to use in this situation. Similarly, infective endocarditis may require the same radical débridement and valve choice. Concomitant ascending aortic pathology or annuloaortic ectasia should be addressed during valve replacement operations. Some prosthetic valves require precise anatomic symmetry for implantation, such as the subcoronary stentless aortic valves. If the sinotubular ridge is substantially larger than the aortic annulus, this tends to predict future valvular incompetence. Patient prosthesis mismatch is also a concern. Particularly for the aortic position, implanting a small valve in a large person may leave the patient with persistent aortic stenosis.

MITRAL VALVE REPLACEMENT

The structure and function of the mitral valve are unique and difficult to duplicate. The valve opens as the pressure lowers during ventricular diastole. Flow across the valve is fairly slow until atrial systole. The force of ventricular systole acts to close the valve, which places the valve under considerable stress. Because of this, a mitral prosthesis is more prone to both thrombosis and structural deterioration. The mitral annulus is a pliable structure that participates in normal myocardial function. Leaflet coaptation and the subvalvular structures such as chordae tendineae and papillary muscles are important in maintaining competency under these extreme forces. These same structures are important in preserving ventricular geometry and function. Removal of these structures or limitation of the natural movements of any part of the apparatus (valve leaflets, annulus, subvalvular connections) may alter function of the valve or myocardium. Conversely, alterations in myocardial function and/or geometry may also affect valve function and competency. The complex anatomy and function of the mitral apparatus has precluded ideal mitral valve substitutes.

Because patients and surgeons were experiencing difficulty related to mitral valve prostheses, a renewed interest in repair techniques evolved. Mitral valve repair is preferred to replacement if feasible. The efficacy of mitral repair has been proved durable over time and remains the best option for many mitral valve pathologies. For most patients with mitral insufficiency secondary to degenerative disease, repair can be accomplished. Repair is also an excellent option for rheumatic disease in which the subvalvular apparatus is not destroyed and calcification is minimal. Many patients with ischemic mitral insufficiency can be repaired with a combination of an annuloplasty ring and myocardial revascularization. A large percentage of cases of mitral valve endocarditis can be handled with débridement and repair of the diseased tissue.

For valves that are not amenable to the various repair techniques, replacement is warranted. Most current mechanical mitral valves are bileaflet or tilting disk mechanisms. The older cage-and-ball or sliding disk variants are still available but are less popular. Tissue valves created for implantation into the mitral position generally are based on the structure of an upside-down aortic valve. The available bioprosthetic tissues are either xenograft porcine valve or bovine pericardial. Competency requires a stent. None of these configurations support normal annular or subvalvular mechanics. Stentless mitral valves are available as cryopreserved allografts or the quadrileaflet pericardial valve. These stentless valves are the only type of prostheses designed to function like the native mitral valve and withstand the innate forces of this position. Experience is limited with this technology, but, as they become more readily available and results are followed, we expect that they will find a niche in mitral replacement surgery.

It has been recommended that to best preserve the mitral annular and ventricular interaction as well as long-term myocardial function, whenever possible, subvalvular structures should be preserved. This usually entails saving at least the posterior leaflet and chords by plicating the leaflet to the posterior annulus with the valve sutures. The anterior leaflet may also be transposed to the posterior annulus. Polytetrafluoroethylene (PTFE) chords may be used when subvalvular structures are destroyed as in the severely rheumatic valve. Diligent care must be taken to ensure that the prosthetic valve leaflets (especially a mechanical disk or ball) are not impinged by this retained tissue and may require repositioning or excision of the subvalvular support. The surgeon must properly orient any prosthetic valve to obtain optimal hemodynamics. The prosthetic valve structure may itself obstruct left ventricular outflow. In the instance of bileaflet mechanical valves, it is best to place the leaflets in a position perpendicular to the ventricular septum. Stent-mounted tissue valves are oriented with the largest sinus facing the ventricular septum to limit left ventricular outflow obstruction.

Choice of prosthetic mitral valve has many algorithms. The following is a synopsis of our decision-making: Stented tissue valves are best suited for patients who will not outlive the durability of the prosthesis. Renal failure, concomitant coronary bypass, poor left ventricular function, and advanced age have all independently been shown to limit life expectancy. Mechanical prostheses are reserved for those patients without contraindication to anticoagulation. Younger patients, who outlive tissue valves, and those already requiring anticoagulants for other conditions receive mechanical valves preferentially. Calcium turnover and tissue destruction limit the usefulness of tissue valves in young patients. Stentless mitral valves (allografts and the quadrileaflet pericardial valves) are best suited for middle-aged patients who desire to avoid or have a contraindication to life-long anticoagulation. The best candidates are in normal sinus rhythm, with rheumatic (not calcified) pathology, and are aged 30 to 50 years. With anticalcification treatment and cryopreservation, it is hoped that these valves will last longer than the typical stented bioprostheses. These are designed with the mitral function in mind; they maintain a flexible annulus and have a subvalvular structure that maintains continuity with the ventricle. Although this most closely approximates the ideal mitral substitute, the implant technique is less familiar and more detailed, requiring longer operative times, which may discourage some surgeons from this technology.

■ AORTIC VALVE REPLACEMENT

AVR is truly one of the great contributions of cardiac surgery. The natural life expectancy of someone diagnosed with severe aortic valve stenosis or insufficiency is markedly diminished. Close to 80% of medically managed patients die within 2 years of this diagnosis. AVR has improved the quality of life and life expectancy substantially for these patients. Even with today's advanced biotechnology, AVR does not always result in normal life expectancy. Patients die from valve related complications, as well as from non–valve-related problems, at a faster rate than their age-matched controls. As with mitral valve surgery, myocardial function and remodeling are also altered after AVR. Left ventricular hypertrophy with resultant subendocardial ischemia, as well as ventricular irritability and dysrhythmias, are all of concern. Hemodynamic flow pattern, effective orifice areas, and transvalvular gradients affect valve performance, durability, and overall patient survival. The goal of a natural heart valve that lives and grows and is universally appropriate for implant in all circumstances is not yet available, but advances in that direction have occurred. AVR dilemmas include mechanical versus biologic, stented versus stentless, and subcoronary implant versus root replacement. An autograft aortic valve substitute that grows as a patient grows is also available.

Mechanical Valves

Mechanical aortic valve prostheses are durable substitutes for the diseased aortic valve. Nonstructural valve related complications such as thromboembolic or bleeding complications are issues of consideration. These have all the inherent issues of anticoagulation that were discussed earlier. However, in the aortic position, some authors have raised the possibility of replacing standard warfarin-based anticoagulation therapy with one that has less potential for bleeding complications while still offering protection from thrombosis. This is still a debated topic. The basic configurations of the commonly used mechanical prostheses use a single or double tilting disk technology. The disk may pivot in a hinge mechanism or on a strut. Single-disk valves create an eccentric flow pattern, and hemodynamics are different depending on valve orientation. The most natural flow patterns and hemodynamic patterns are achieved with the greater orifice of the valve opening toward the patient's right. This directs the jet of blood flow along the greater curve of the aorta. One criticism of single disk valves is the relatively easy opportunity to obstruct leaflet motion with a suture tag or pannus ingrowth. A frozen or impinged leaflet in this type of patient is poorly tolerated. Bileaflet aortic valves offer some protection against this while providing the same other advantages. Hemodynamics are affected by valve orientation as well but not to the same extent. Optimal flow characteristics are achieved with the leaflets oriented perpendicular to the ventricular septum. This also directs the flow of blood along the greater curve of the aorta in a more natural pattern. Although the mechanical aortic valve choices are durable and have minimal structural deterioration, they still may fail as a result of obstruction from tissue ingrowth, infection, intolerance to anticoagulants, or perivalvular leak. These valves may be the best option for a person who already requires anticoagulants (although an increased dosage may be required) or who wants the most durable valve option available. This includes young patients who are otherwise not candidates for a pulmonary autograft. There is no guarantee that a mechanical valve will be the last valve operation that the patient will require.

Tissue Valves

Biological aortic valve prostheses have traditionally been porcine aortic valve leaflets mounted on semi rigid stents. Various modifications have been made by using leaflets from several valves to create larger orifice areas and lower profiles. Another popular biomaterial is pericardium, also mounted to a stent. These stented aortic prostheses all have the advantage of ease of implantation. These are inserted into the annulus with a single suture line, and competency is ensured by the stent. The exposure and implant technique for the stented aortic valves is the same as for the mechanical prostheses. An aortotomy is created above the sinotubular junction and can be extended into the non-coronary sinus to enhance exposure. These are typically implanted in a supraannular position to implant a larger size but may also be placed intraannular. This is generally the easiest way to implant a valve and the least time consuming. Most surgeons are comfortable performing this operation in even the sickest of patients. The stented aortic tissue valves lack the long-term durability of the mechanical valves but, again, avoid the issue of anticoagulation. The average life expectancy of any of these stented tissue valves is approximately 8 to 12 years; they then tend to fail from structural valve deterioration. Valve preservation techniques, anticalcification advances, and better myocardial preservation and operative techniques have been used to improve on the natural tissue valves. The choice of a stented tissue valve for AVR is a good option in elderly patients whose aortic annulus is of sufficient size and when the surgeon prefers a quicker operation.

Stentless Tissue Aortic Valves

The most significant improvement in the use of natural valves for aortic replacement may be in the lack of a rigid stent. Stentless aortic bioprostheses are available in a variety of forms. The manufactured stentless valves are typically porcine and are available in configurations ranging from scalloped subcoronary implants to full aortic root replacements. Allograft tissue is less available but may also be tailored in any of the ways that their porcine counterparts can. The same is true for a pulmonary autograft, which has some advantages that are discussed later. The absence of a rigid stent allows for a larger effective orifice area that can otherwise be achieved and hence a lower transvalvular gradient. This tends to produce a more laminar flow pattern and more natural hemodynamics. It has been shown that this translates into more left ventricular mass regression, which may prolong survival by decreasing valve- and myocardium-related deaths. Another advantage of stentless technology is avoidance of abnormal stress and wear points on the prosthesis, which may improve durability.

Subcoronary Stentless Bioprosthesis

The St. Jude Toronto SPV is manufactured as a scalloped porcine aortic root that is covered in Dacron. This is placed in the subcoronary position using a freehand technique. Implantation requires two suture rows—one that fixes the inflow to the aortic annulus, and the second along the scallops and posts of the valve. This second row is the hemostatic layer, which is also responsible for the orientation of the valve commissures. Considerable care must be taken to orient this type of valve implant so that the commissure posts are 120 degrees apart and avoid obstruction of the native coronary ostia. Valve sizing is also different from the typical stented, subcoronary prosthesis. The relationship of the sinotubular ridge to the annulus is important. Therefore, the normal geometry and dimensions of the root need to be retained. Sinuses of Valsalva pathology or dilatation as well as heavy calcification of the aortic annulus or coronary ostia are relative contraindications to using this type of valve. Imprecise implant results in early valve insufficiency and late valve failure. The stentless subcoronary AVR requires a considerable learning curve as well as additional operative time compared with stented counterparts. These valves result in more normal hemodynamics than the bulkier stent mounted valves.

■ AORTIC ROOT REPLACEMENT

Cryopreserved allograft aortic valves and the Medtronic Freestyle stentless xenograft may be tailored for subcoronary implant as mentioned earlier but may also be used as a total aortic root replacement. The Freestyle valve is a skeletonized porcine aortic root with Dacron attached to the inflow cuff to aid in the handling characteristics and act as a sewing ring. The implant procedure is basically modified from Bentall. The aorta is transected at the sinotubular ridge. The non-coronary sinus and valve leaflets are excised. The native coronary ostia are mobilized on generous buttons of aortic wall and are reimplanted later. The radical removal of tissue is possible because the entire root is being replaced. It is this process that is responsible for improved outcomes in these situations. The root replacement technique also maintains the ideal environment for the newly implants cusps. The relationships between the tubular aorta, sinuses of Valsalva, and aortic root are natural and not distorted. Keeping the normal valve conduit architecture results in a more perfect valve that is less prone to insufficiency and exposes it to only natural wear and tear. A larger prosthesis may be implanted because this is not an inclusion technique that requires the valve to be stuffed within the lumen of the native aorta. All of these facts create a more natural hemodynamic flow pattern with unobstructed and laminar blood flow.

For the xenograft roots, this is generally considered a larger, longer, and more difficult operation than a typical subcoronary AVR. We have shown that, in experienced hands, morbidity and mortality with this procedure are comparable and in some circumstances improved. This is the ideal valve procedure after extensive annular débridement for calcification or infection. The allograft is generally preferred in cases of infection. Patients with a small aortic annulus, generally less than 21 millimeters, benefit most with an aortic root replacement. In patients over 65 years old, with reasonable life expectancy, we choose to use stentless xenograft valves. For younger patients, those aged 50 to 65, there is more literature support for use of a cryopreserved allograft root, and currently this is our choice as well. And for even younger patients, those less than 50 years old, and especially in the very young who are still growing, we recommend the Ross procedure.

The Ross procedure or pulmonary autograft is a two-valve operation for aortic valve disease. The native pulmonary valve is harvested and freshly implanted as a root into the aortic position. The pulmonary valve is typically replaced with a cryopreserved pulmonic allograft valve. The autograft valve is the only available tissue for AVR that grows with a child after implantation. This is a natural living valve that also has the ability for self-repair and natural defense against infection. There also is no rejection of foreign tissue in the aortic position to generate structural degeneration. The technique still has limitations pertaining to the pulmonary allograft rejection manifested early as pulmonary stenosis. This is the largest and longest operation for AVR; it requires multiple suture lines and places both valves at jeopardy. With the highest risk comes the potential for the highest benefit. To date, this operation comes the closest to replacing the aortic valve with an ideal substitute. In the future, tissue engineering and decellularization techniques may further improve aortic valve prostheses and are already in the early phases of development and testing.

■ CONCLUSION

Many tissue prostheses exist for patients requiring AVR who have a small aortic root or desire not to take anticoagulants. In patients younger than 50 years, we prefer to use the Ross operation. Between the ages of 50 and 65, a cryopreserved aortic allograft offers an excellent option. In those patients older than 65 years, we use a stentless porcine bioprosthesis. In AVR when patients have a contraindication to warfarin (Coumadin), the surgeon prefers a quicker operation, and the aortic annulus is of sufficient size, a stented tissue valve is the best option. In those patients who already take anticoagulants for atrial fibrillation or have a mechanical prosthesis in another position, a mechanical prosthesis is the best option.

SUGGESTED READING

Carpentier A: Cardiac valve surgery: the "French correction," *J Thorac Cardiovasc Surg* 86:323, 1983.

David TE: Mitral valve replacement with preservation of chordae tendineae: rationale and technical consideration, *Ann Thorac Surg* 41:680, 1988.

David TE, et al: Aortic valve replacement with stentless porcine bioprosthesis, *J Thorac Cardiovasc Surg* 99:113, 1990.

Kon ND, et al: Comparison of implant techniques using the Freestyle stentless porcine aortic valve, *Ann Thorac Surg* 59:857, 1995.

Zellner JL, et al: Long-term experience with the St. Jude medical valve prosthesis, *Ann Thorac Surg* 68:1210, 1999.

AORTIC VALVE REPLACEMENT

A. Marc Gillinov

Aortic valve disease is the most common indication for valvular heart surgery. A dysfunctional aortic valve may be stenotic, regurgitant, or both. Aortic stenosis is caused by degenerative disease or rheumatic disease. Causes of aortic regurgitation include degenerative disease; rheumatic disease; endocarditis; and primary aortic diseases, such as atherosclerotic aortic aneurysm, annuloaortic ectasia, and aortic dissection. Whether a valve is bicuspid or tricuspid has little impact on treatment except that bicuspid aortic valves with prolapse occasionally are amenable to repair. Echocardiography is the diagnostic modality of choice for characterization of aortic valve disease. Before aortic valve surgery, patients 40 years old or older should have coronary angiography to determine the need for coronary artery bypass graft (CABG) surgery. With the advent of echocardiography, direct catheter-based measurement of aortic valve gradients is rarely necessary.

■ INDICATIONS FOR OPERATION

The indications for surgery in patients with aortic stenosis are the presence of symptoms or hemodynamically severe aortic stenosis shown at echocardiography. Symptoms attributable to aortic stenosis include angina, syncope, and congestive heart failure. When symptoms develop in patients with aortic stenosis, life expectancy is limited. Surgery is indicated in virtually all symptomatic patients with aortic stenosis. Although criteria for hemodynamically important aortic stenosis vary, it generally is accepted that an aortic valve area less than or equal to 0.75 cm^2 or a peak transvalvular gradient greater than or equal to 50 mm Hg constitutes severe aortic stenosis. These values are typical in patients with symptoms. In asymptomatic patients, these hemodynamic values are an indication for surgery. In patients with moderate aortic stenosis (aortic valve area <1 cm^2) undergoing cardiac surgery for other indications, we favor concomitant aortic valve replacement.

As in aortic stenosis, surgery for aortic regurgitation surgery is indicated based on symptoms and findings at echocardiography. Patients with acute severe aortic regurgitation develop intractable heart failure and require urgent surgery. In most patients with chronic aortic regurgitation, surgery is performed for symptoms of congestive heart failure or decreased exercise capacity. In asymptomatic patients, surgery should be offered when there is evidence of left ventricular decompensation, manifest by ejection fraction less than 55%, left ventricular end-diastolic dimension 75 mm or greater, or left ventricular end-systolic dimension 50 mm or greater. Surgery for active endocarditis is indicated for intractable heart failure, persistent sepsis, embolic events, or extension of infection into adjacent cardiac structures. There is no benefit to delaying surgery in patients with active endocarditis who have one or more of these indications. When aortic regurgitation is caused by ascending aortic pathology, it is generally the aortic disease that dictates the indications and timing of surgery.

There are no absolute contraindications to surgery for aortic stenosis or aortic regurgitation. Operative risk is increased in patients with depressed left ventricular function; a low transvalvular gradient in patients with aortic stenosis and poor left ventricular dysfunction is an ominous sign. Surgical risk also is increased substantially in patients with a calcified ascending aorta because these patients frequently require ascending aortic replacement under hypothermic circulatory arrest to enable aortic valve replacement. There is no effective medical or catheter-based therapy for aortic valve disease. Nearly all patients with severe aortic valve disease are offered surgery. In rare instances, percutaneous aortic balloon valvotomy is used to provide temporary relief of aortic stenosis; this therapy has substantial risk and rarely provides a durable result.

■ SURGICAL TECHNIQUE

The ascending aorta and aortic valve may be approached through a variety of chest wall incisions. Although median sternotomy is standard, excellent results have been obtained using a partial upper sternotomy and a right thoracotomy approach to the aortic valve. A median sternotomy is mandatory if a CABG procedure is necessary. Aortic valve surgery requires cardiopulmonary bypass. Arterial cannulation is achieved via the ascending aorta; if ascending aortic pathology precludes aortic cannulation, the axillary artery is the preferred alternative site. Femoral artery cannulation has the risk of propelling embolic material retrograde toward the brain. Venous cannulation is achieved via the right atrium. A left ventricular vent may be placed via the right superior pulmonary vein, and this is particularly useful to improve visualization when the aortic annulus is small or complex aortic root procedures are necessary. In routine cases, a left ventricular vent is unnecessary. In aortic stenosis, the heart is arrested with antegrade cardioplegia given via the aortic root, and intermittent retrograde cardioplegia is used for the remainder of the procedure. In aortic regurgitation, antegrade cardioplegia is given directly down the coronary ostia after aortotomy, and retrograde cardioplegia is used thereafter. Cold blood cardioplegia is given retrograde every 15 minutes. If a particularly long operative procedure is anticipated, this is supplemented with antegrade cardioplegia down the coronary ostia every 30 minutes.

Distal CABG procedures are completed before aortic valve replacement, and cardioplegia subsequently is given down vein grafts. Similarly, mitral valve surgery is performed before aortic valve replacement because a rigid aortic prosthesis obstructs visualization of the mitral valve. An oblique aortotomy is constructed, and stay sutures are placed at each aortic commissure. Tacking these sutures to the drapes under tension elevates the valve toward the surgeon (Figure 1). The valve is excised sharply, and the annulus is débrided of

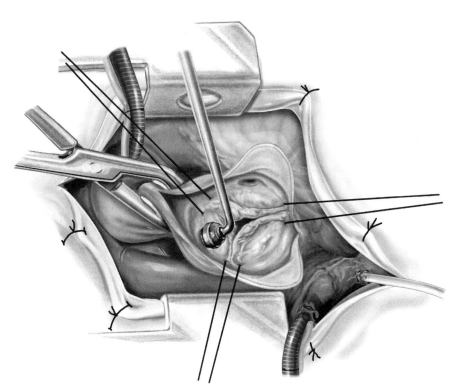

Figure 1
Aortic valve exposure via partial upper sternotomy. After aortotomy, sutures are placed at each commissure and tacked to the drapes under tension. This elevates the valve toward the surgeon.

calcium using rongeurs. Most of the calcium deposits should be removed from the annulus to ensure good seating of the prosthetic valve. Calcified deposits in the aortic sinuses or surrounding the coronary ostia should be removed only if absolutely necessary because aggressive débridement in these areas may damage the aorta or the coronary arteries.

Stented bioprostheses and mechanical valves are implanted with pledgeted horizontal mattress sutures. For stented bioprostheses, pledgets are placed on the ventricular aspect of the annulus. For mechanical valves, site of pledget placement varies with the type of prosthesis. When allograft valves are placed as an entire aortic root, the lower suture line is performed with either running 3-0 polypropylene suture or interrupted 4-0 polypropylene suture tied over a washer of autologous pericardium. In the Ross procedure, the pulmonary autograft is placed in a similar fashion to an allograft valve. Techniques for implantation of stentless bioprostheses vary depending on whether the valve is implanted as a full root, partial root, or subcoronary prosthesis.

There has been considerable discussion concerning surgical management of the patient with a small aortic annulus. It is widely held that larger and more hemodynamically efficient aortic prostheses result in superior patient outcomes. Patients with a small aortic annulus tend to be small and elderly, however. In many of these patients, a prosthetic valve of labeled size 19 mm provides excellent relief of aortic stenosis. Within reasonable limits, small aortic prosthesis size does not influence survival after aortic valve replacement. Special techniques, such as aortic root enlargement, rarely are indicated. In most of these patients, after

valve excision and complete débridement, the aortic annulus admits a valve that is adequate for the patient.

After the prosthesis is secured, the aortotomy is closed with running 4-0 polypropylene suture. If the aorta is thin-walled, the closure is reinforced with felt; however, if the aortotomy closure creates excessive tension, a pericardial patch is used to facilitate the closure. Any proximal saphenous vein graft anastomoses are completed after aortotomy closure. Prosthetic aortic valve function is assessed by intraoperative transesophageal echocardiography.

Occasionally, ascending aortic replacement is indicated at the time of aortic valve surgery. When the aorta is dilated to more than 4.5 cm in a patient younger than 70 years of age, we recommend ascending aortic replacement with a supracoronary graft. In more elderly patients, we replace the ascending aorta when the diameter is 5 cm or greater. Although supracoronary grafting is adequate for most of these patients, dilation of the sinuses to 5 cm or more is an indication for a Bentall procedure.

Some regurgitant aortic valves are amenable to repair. Bicuspid regurgitant valves are repaired by triangular resection of the prolapsing cusp and commissuroplasty. This repair is reasonably durable, with a 7-year freedom from reoperation of 84%. Trileaflet aortic valves with prolapse are difficult to repair and should be replaced in most instances. Aortic regurgitation caused by ascending aortic pathology frequently can be corrected by treatment of the primary aortic disease with preservation of the native aortic valve. Valve-sparing aortic root procedures as described by Yacoub and David are used in patients with aortic root aneurysm and normal aortic valve leaflets.

■ PROSTHESIS CHOICE

Options for aortic valve replacement include mechanical valves, stented and stentless bioprostheses, allograft valves, and the pulmonary autograft or Ross procedure. The primary choice is between mechanical and tissue valves. Choice of valve depends primarily on life expectancy, willingness to undergo a reoperation for structural dysfunction of tissue valves, and ability and desire to take warfarin (Coumadin) for mechanical valves. Mechanical valves carry the highest freedom from late aortic valve reoperation. Many patients younger than age 60 years who do not wish to undergo late reoperation choose to receive mechanical valves and take warfarin. In most patients older than 60, a stented bioprosthesis would not deteriorate in the patient's lifetime. With stented pericardial valves, the 15-year actuarial freedom from explant for structural valve dysfunction is 85% in 65-year-old patients and 93% in 75-year-old patients.

Allograft and pulmonary autograft procedures provide tissue valves with excellent hemodynamic profiles. These surgical procedures are more complicated than standard aortic valve replacement, however, requiring longer periods of cardiac arrest. In general, both of these valves entail aortic root replacement with coronary artery transfer. Occasionally, coronary artery transfer is hazardous or unsuccessful, resulting in the need for unanticipated bypass grafts. Allograft valves have an advantage in patients with endocarditis, with a lower risk of reinfection than standard prosthetic valves. The Ross procedure also may be useful in some patients with endocarditis, but its primary benefit probably is realized in children, in whom the autograft is expected to grow with the patient.

Similar to allograft valves, stentless bioprostheses have excellent hemodynamics. There is a great deal of interest in these valves, and many centers report excellent results in varying groups of patients. Implantation of stentless valves is more demanding, however, than implantation of stented prostheses, requiring greater surgical expertise and more time. The durability of stentless bioprostheses is unknown.

A conclusive advantage to stentless bioprostheses has not been shown.

Choice of valvular prosthesis does not influence patient survival. More than a decade of experience with modern mechanical valves, stented bioprostheses, and allograft valves has shown that the most important factor affecting survival is relief of severe aortic stenosis by aortic valve replacement. After that, patient factors, particularly age and presence of coronary artery disease, are key determinants of long-term survival. The specific choice of prosthesis and the size of the prosthesis do not influence survival. The extent to which prosthesis type and size influence other indices of clinical well-being, such as exercise capacity, is unknown.

■ RESULTS

Surgery increases life expectancy in patients with significant aortic valve disease. Operative mortality for isolated aortic valve replacement is less than 3%, and 10-year survival is generally about 60%. Risk factors for early death include older age, concomitant CABG surgery, higher New York Heart Association functional class, and aortic regurgitation alone. Important risk factors for late death include older age and presence of coronary artery disease. After surgery, most patients return to New York Heart Association functional class I or II.

SUGGESTED READING

Blackstone EH, et al: Prosthesis size and long term mortality after aortic valve replacement: a multi-institutional study, *J Thorac Cardiovasc Surg* 126:783, 2003.

He GW, et al: Up to thirty-year survival after aortic valve replacement in the small aortic root, *Ann Thorac Surg* 59:1056, 1995.

McGiffin DC, et al: An analysis of risk factors for death and mode-specific death after aortic valve replacement with allografts, xenografts, and mechanical valves, *J Thorac Cardiovasc Surg* 106:895, 1993.

Medalion B, et al: Aortic valve replacement: is valve size important? *J Thorac Cardiovasc Surg* 119:963, 2000.

AORTIC ROOT REPLACEMENT

Duke Cameron

Luca A. Vricella

Table 1 Indications for Aortic Root Replacement
Aortic aneurysm involving sinuses
Endocarditis involving root
Prosthetic valve endocarditis
Complex root dissection
Aortic valve disease in a small aortic root
Recurrent periprosthetic leak

The aortic root is a functional unit consisting of the aortic valve, the sinus segment of the ascending aorta, the aortic annulus, and the origin of the coronary arteries (Figure 1). The relationships among these subunits and how they contribute to the functional unit known as the aortic root are currently under investigative study. With better understanding of these relationships and growing experience with surgery of the aorta, aortic root replacement (ARR) is being performed with greater frequency. This increase is due to several factors: earlier recognition of asymptomatic aneurysms on screening examinations, widespread acceptance of pulmonary root autotransplantation (the Ross procedure), greater availability of various biologic root prostheses, and growing surgical confidence in attempting challenging root reconstructions, such as seen in endocarditis and dissection.

■ INDICATIONS

The most common indication for ARR is aneurysm of the sinuses; endocarditis, dissection, and aortic valve replacement in the small root constitute other relatively common indications (Table 1). Ascending aortic aneurysms may be localized to the sinuses, as in Marfan's syndrome and other connective tissue disorders, or may be part of more extensive aortic dilation, as in bicuspid aortic valve syndrome, atherosclerosis, Takayasu's and giant cell arteritides, mega-aorta syndromes, and postdissection aneurysmal dilation. For most ascending aortic aneurysms, dilation beyond 5.5 cm is considered an indication for surgery because the risk of rupture or dissection exceeds operative risk. This recommendation is based on several natural history studies that relate aneurysm size to risk of aortic catastrophe. Size is an imperfect predictor of such events, however, and must serve only as a guideline. Furthermore, patient comorbidity may raise the threshold for intervention because of greater operative risk. Similarly, other factors may lower the threshold: family history of rupture or dissection, rapid or symptomatic expansion of the aneurysm, presence of dissection in the ascending aorta, concomitant aortic valve or coronary disease, or the desire to preserve the aortic valve before distortion of the leaflets results from further dilation.

In the majority of cases of aortic endocarditis, infection is limited to the aortic valve leaflets; here, simple excision of the leaflets and placement of a common prosthesis will suffice. When infection involves the aortic annulus or perforates the aortic wall or left ventricular outflow tract (LVOT), however, it is considered a root infection. Although commonly termed root abscess, the term *abscess* is best avoided, at least preoperatively, because a frankly purulent cavity is not usually seen at operation. Root infections may be treated with radical débridement and reconstruction with autologous or bovine pericardium and even Dacron patches along with replacement of the valve with conventional prostheses. The best results are achieved with cryopreserved aortic homografts and avoidance of prosthetic material other than monofilament nonabsorbable sutures.

Dissections involving the ascending aorta (Stanford type A and DeBakey types I and II) frequently extend into the aortic root, compromising valve and coronary integrity, but never extend proximally to the aortic annulus. In more than 75% of cases, it is possible to reapproximate the dissected layers of the aortic sinus wall and to "resuspend" the commissural attachments of the valve to restore aortic valve competence and coronary perfusion, thus avoiding root replacement. Teflon felt and various biologic glues are useful adjuncts in these reconstructions. If the aortic valve is diseased (e.g., bicuspid or calcific stenotic disease), however, or if the sinuses are dilated (>4 cm), ARR is preferable.

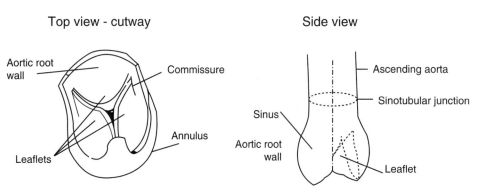

Top view - cutway

Side view

Aortic root wall
Commissure
Leaflets
Annulus

Ascending aorta
Sinotubular junction
Sinus
Aortic root wall
Leaflet

Figure 1
Anatomy of the aortic root. (*From Cochran RP, Kunzelman KS: Aortic valve sparing in aortic root disease. In Karp D, et al, editors:* Advances in Cardiac Surgery, *vol 8, St. Louis, 1996, Mosby–Year Book, p 81.*)

Some complex and extensive dissections leave the root tissue too friable to repair, making ARR inevitable.

Some patients needing aortic valve replacement, usually for stenosis, may have a small aortic root that cannot comfortably accommodate an adequate-sized prosthesis. Although there is controversy over what constitutes a minimally adequate size for a prosthesis for a given patient (the problem of patient-prosthesis mismatch), in general, a 70-kg active adult requires at least a 21-mm prosthesis and preferably a 23-mm one, whereas small, sedentary, or elderly patients may be adequately served by a 19-mm prosthesis. When it is not possible to place such a prosthesis in a small root, the surgeon either must consider a root-enlarging procedure (e.g., patch enlargement of the noncoronary sinus, a Manouguian annular enlargement procedure, or a modified Konno aortoventriculoplasty) or proceed with a total ARR, which allows a larger prosthesis to sit atop the annulus without the restrictions of the aortic diameter. A prosthesis at least one size larger, and often two sizes larger, can be placed when the root rather than the valve alone is replaced.

■ TECHNIQUE OF AORTIC ROOT REPLACEMENT

The first complete ARR is credited to Bentall and De Bono, who emergently fashioned a composite graft at the operating table by hand-sewing a mechanical valve to a tubular prosthetic conduit in a young patient with aortic dissection. The graft was sewn proximally to the aortic annulus and distally to the distal ascending aorta using an inclusion technique rather than a full-thickness, end-to-end anastomosis. The coronary arteries were left attached to the aneurysm wall and were approximated side-to-side to holes made in the side of the graft. The aneurysm wall was then wrapped around the conduit for hemostasis. This classic Bentall procedure is rarely performed today because of a disturbing incidence of late pseudoaneurysm development at the coronary and distal aortic anastomoses from failure to assure full-thickness anastomoses. It is also unwise to rely on the aneurysm wrap to achieve hemostasis, because the collection of blood between the aneurysm wall and the wrap expands over time and dehisces the coronary anastomoses. Instead, the currently favored modified Bentall procedure entails complete dissection and mobilization of the coronary arteries and full-thickness anastomoses (Figure 2).

Sternotomy and total cardiopulmonary bypass are employed. Minimally invasive approaches have been described, but, in our practice, the precision required for coronary anastomoses and the challenge of hemostasis have discouraged these approaches. We prefer bicaval venous cannulation so that the cannulae angle caudally and improve exposure of the root. Standard cardioplegic techniques are used; our preference is to give antegrade cold blood cardioplegia every 30 minutes directly into the coronary ostia and to supplement myocardial protection with continuous topical cold saline solution. The aorta is transected at least 1 cm proximal to the aortic cross-clamp, and the aortic root is reflected anteriorly. Dividing the tissue between the posterior aorta and the proximal right pulmonary artery allows the root to come forward considerably. The coronary arteries

are excised with generous collars of sinus tissue, which can always be trimmed later, and are retracted with stay sutures that maintain proper orientation of the buttons. Wide mobilization of both coronary arteries is recommended. Next, stay sutures at the top of the three commissures are placed on traction to deliver the root up and keep it splayed out. The sinus tissue and the valve are excised. We prefer to place pledgeted everting horizontal mattress sutures of 2-0 braided polyester around the annulus, usually 12 to 15 in total. Next, these sutures are passed through the base of the prosthetic root. We use the same technique whether employing a mechanical valved conduit, homograft, porcine bioprosthesis, or pulmonary autograft (Ross procedure). If the operation is for root infection or prosthetic valve endocarditis, polypropylene sutures without Teflon pledgets are used. Frequently in prosthetic valve endocarditis, there is separation of the aorta from the LVOT, which can be corrected by including both with the mattress sutures. Alternatively, the root prosthesis can be secured only to the LVOT. The prosthesis is then lowered and tied in place; if a homograft is used, it is important to check inside the graft to be certain that no sutures have caught the valve leaflets. It is also useful to use strips of pericardium or homograft to reinforce and "sandwich" the proximal aortic suture line for hemostasis.

The left coronary anastomosis is performed with 4-0 polypropylene and is usually directly posterior in the root, just a few millimeters above the annulus. In the absence of infection, the coronary artery button is encircled with a ring of Teflon felt, a so-called lifesaver for obvious reasons, to encourage hemostasis and prevent late pseudoaneurysm formation. This is particularly important in Marfan's syndrome and acute aortic dissection. The right coronary artery button is implanted almost 180 degrees away from the left coronary anastomosis, nearly directly anterior, and slightly more distal on the graft. A common technical error is to place the right coronary artery too far to the left and too low on the graft, leading to tension and distortion of the artery when the heart fills. Alternatively, one can perform the distal graft-to-aorta anastomosis, briefly release the cross-clamp, and select the optimal site of implantation for the right coronary artery. If this technique is used with a homograft, an external suture marking the anterior commissure should be placed to prevent valve injury when the hole is created for the right coronary anastomosis.

The graft-to-aorta anastomosis is performed end-to-end with 3-0 or 4-0 polypropylene. Choosing the proper length of the graft is important to prevent tension or kinking of the anastomosis; the natural tendency is to make the graft too long. We try to select an ideal length of graft and then make it 1 cm shorter. If the distal aortic aorta is thin or friable, external reinforcement with a felt strip is helpful.

There are several technical variations of the modified Bentall procedure. Some authors prefer to use continuous suture for the proximal aortic suture line. Others do not mobilize the coronary arteries much. In reoperations on the root when the coronary arteries are frozen and difficult to mobilize, an interposition polytetrafluoroethylene graft can bridge the distance from the graft to the coronary ostia. If there is extensive root destruction due to endocarditis, patch repair of defects in the aortoventricular connection may be necessary, or the homograft can be lowered deep into the

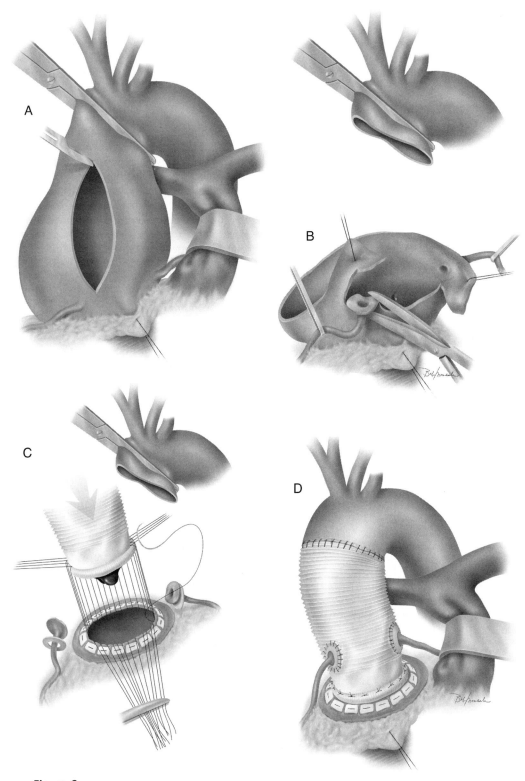

Figure 2
Aortic root replacement using a modified Bentall technique. **A** and **B**, After aortic cross-clamping, the aneurysm is opened, the aortic wall is excised, and the coronary arteries are mobilized with a collar of aortic wall. **C**, Everting interrupted mattress sutures are placed through the annulus and the sewing ring of the valved conduit. **D**, The coronary arteries are implanted on the side of the graft, and the distal graft-to-aorta anastomosis is completed.

LVOT and sewn directly to stronger, noninfected tissue. Heart block is a not infrequent complication, but permanent pacemaker placement is deferred until sepsis has resolved. If the coronary arteries cannot be reimplanted, bypass grafts may be necessary; as a rule, saphenous vein grafts are preferred because internal mammary grafts do not reliably provide total coronary blood flow in the early postoperative period. Endocarditic ventricular septal defects can usually be closed within the LVOT but sometimes are better approached through the tricuspid or pulmonary valves. The authors believe that it is prudent to routinely explore the right atrium and to close foramen ovales and atrial septal defects because they may contribute to the pathogenesis of left heart endocarditis.

■ ROOT PROSTHESES

Several prosthetic options exist for replacement of the aortic root: composite grafts with mechanical valves, cryopreserved human aortic allografts (homografts), glutaraldehyde-preserved porcine aortic roots, and porcine or pericardial stented xenografts attached to Dacron conduits, either commercially fashioned or constructed by hand in the operating room. The patient's own pulmonary root can also serve as an aortic root prosthesis, as described elsewhere in this book (Ross procedure).

The selection of an appropriate root prosthesis mirrors the selection of an isolated aortic valve prosthesis. Mechanical valves (composite grafts or combined valve-graft conduits) offer durability but mandate chronic anticoagulation and tempt recurrence of endocarditis. Bioprosthetic roots (homografts and xenograft roots) need no anticoagulation but lack durability, which may depend on patient age, size of the graft, and, in the case of cryopreserved homografts, an unpredictable immunologic reaction between graft and host. Homografts enjoy a clear advantage in the setting of invasive endocarditis, particularly when resistant or highly virulent organisms are present, such as gram-negative species and fungi. All these root prostheses are superior in hemodynamic performance to stented xenografts and mechanical prostheses. The Ross procedure is the only durable procedure in small children and offers some chance for growth.

■ VALVE-SPARING PROCEDURES

Many patients with aneurysm or dissection of the aortic root have normal aortic valves; traditionally, these patients have undergone complete root replacement, including the aortic valve, because this is technically more straightforward. As confidence improved and safety of root replacement increased, pioneers such as Professor Sir Magdi Yacoub and Tirone David explored ways to replace the aortic root while preserving the patient's aortic valve. Their modifications promised to avoid the limitations of valve prostheses, namely the need for anticoagulation and loss of durability, and also to lower the rates of endocarditis and thromboembolism. These procedures are still in evolution, and reports of long-term results are scant.

The David classification of valve-sparing operations (David I to David V) has become the established standard. David I and II represent two fundamentally different approaches, known as the reimplantation and remodeling procedures, respectively. In the reimplantation procedure (David I, Figure 3), a Dacron graft is placed around the

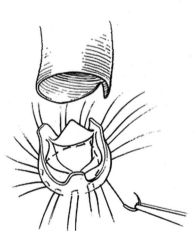
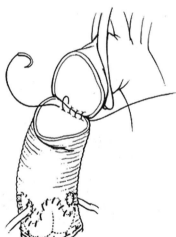
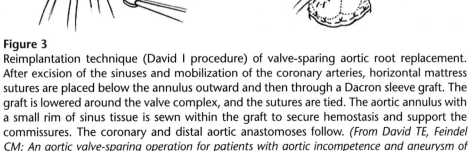

Figure 3
Reimplantation technique (David I procedure) of valve-sparing aortic root replacement. After excision of the sinuses and mobilization of the coronary arteries, horizontal mattress sutures are placed below the annulus outward and then through a Dacron sleeve graft. The graft is lowered around the valve complex, and the sutures are tied. The aortic annulus with a small rim of sinus tissue is sewn within the graft to secure hemostasis and support the commissures. The coronary and distal aortic anastomoses follow. *(From David TE, Feindel CM: An aortic valve-sparing operation for patients with aortic incompetence and aneurysm of the ascending aorta,* J Thorac Cardiovasc Surg *103: 617, 1992.)*

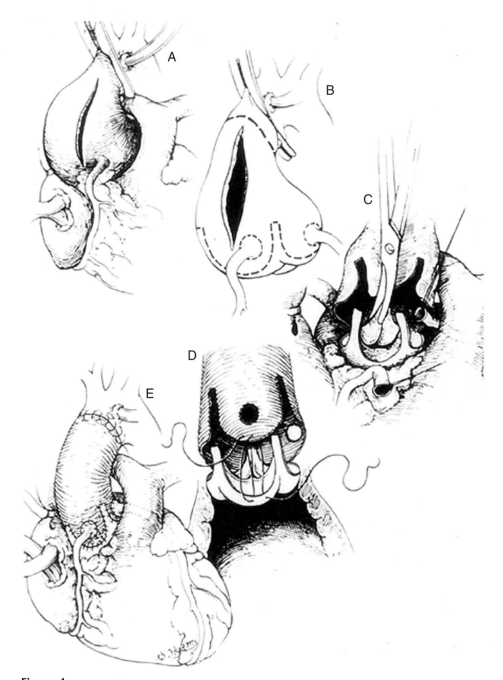

Figure 4
Remodeling technique (David II or Yacoub procedure) of valve-sparing aortic root replacement. **A,** Aneurysm is opened after aortic cross-clamping. **B** and **C,** The ascending aorta and sinus segments are excised, and the coronary arteries are widely mobilized. **D,** A Dacron graft tailored to produce three tongues to replace the sinuses is sewn to the aortic annulus. Coronary arteries are sewn to circular defects in the graft (not shown). *(From Yacoub MH, et al: Late results of a valve-preserving operation in patients with aneurysms of the ascending aorta and root,* J Thorac Cardiovasc Surg *115:1080, 1998.)*

skeletonized aortic valve and is secured below the annulus. The annulus and a rim of remnant sinus tissue are sutured to the inside of the graft for hemostasis and to support the valve commissures. The coronary artery and distal aortic anastomoses are then completed. This procedure stabilizes the annulus and prevents late annular dilation but in its early forms occasionally caused leaflet damage, late aortic insufficiency, and the need for reoperation for valve replacement. The remodeling procedure, also known as the David II or Yacoub procedure (Figure 4), replaces the sinuses and ascending aorta using a Dacron tube graft with three tongues to simulate the normal sinuses. The tongues are sewn to the scalloped, "king's crown" contour of the aortic annulus. Although this technique recreates sinuses and theoretically reduces leaflet stress, it does not stabilize the annulus diameter. In Marfan's syndrome, this can lead to late annular dilation due to splaying of the three tongues, stretching of the subcommissural triangles, and poor central coaptation of the leaflets. Later iterations of the David procedure attempted to stabilize the annulus while recreating sinuses and are essentially modifications of the reimplantation technique. A commercially available graft now has a preformed sinus segment to facilitate restoration of a more physiologic root. In general, these operations are less reproducible than standard root replacement with conventional valve prostheses, but with refinement and more widespread application they will probably find a prominent role in aortic root surgery.

■ RESULTS

Elective isolated aortic root replacement currently has an operative mortality rate of less than 5%, and several centers have reported series with a rate of less than 1%. Emergent operation for dissection, concomitant coronary or carotid disease, reoperation, and infection all increase the risk substantially. Prosthetic endocarditis still carries a 10% to 20% operative risk, but with use of cryopreserved homografts, the risk of recurrent infection is less than 5%. These results compare favorably with a natural history mortality rate of nearly 100% for medically treated prosthetic valve endocarditis. Late anastomotic or coronary problems are rare

with current techniques. Valve-sparing operations are still plagued by a 5% to 10% late reoperation rate, usually for progressive aortic valve insufficiency; however, these results are steadily improving.

Several authors have observed an unexpectedly low rate of endocarditis and thromboembolism in patients with aortic root prostheses as compared with patients with conventional stented bioprostheses or mechanical valves. It is possible that the more laminar flow through prosthetic roots and the absence of suture material, knots, and pledgets in the patients undergoing the root procedure may lead to less turbulence and hence lower rates of infection and thrombosis, but this awaits further investigation and confirmation.

■ SUMMARY

Aortic root replacement has evolved from a high-risk, emergent, and, at one time, desperate surgical effort to a low-risk routine surgical procedure when employed prophylactically in the treatment of aortic sinus aneurysms. Significant mortality still attends those operations performed for acute dissection or extensive root infection, however, as well as for patients with significant comorbidities. Valve-sparing operations are the focus of current interest in an effort to avoid the problems inherent with all prosthetic valves.

SUGGESTED READING

Bentall HH, De Bono A: A technique for complete replacement of the ascending aorta, *Thorax* 23:338, 1968.

David TE, Feindel CM: An aortic valve-sparing operation for patients with aortic incompetence and aneurysm of the ascending aorta, *J Thorac Cardiovasc Surg* 103:617, 1992.

David TE, et al: Results of aortic valve-sparing operations, *J Thorac Cardiovasc Surg* 122:39, 2001.

Gott VL, et al: Aortic root replacement. Risk factor analysis of a seventeen-year experience with 270 patients, *J Thorac Cardiovasc Surg* 111(1):28, 1996.

Yacoub MH, et al: Results of a valve-preserving operation in patients with aneurysms of the ascending aorta and root, *J Thorac Cardiovasc Surg* 115:1080, 1998.

AORTIC VALVE REPAIR

Charles D. Fraser, Jr

Despite tremendous progress and significant ongoing experimental and clinical investigation, the goal of an ideal replacement for the human aortic valve remains elusive. In counseling patients with aortic valve pathology, the cardiac surgeon must present numerous options, all of which represent a less than perfect solution. Patient age, gender, size, and comorbid conditions all have an impact on the selection of a valve prosthesis. In every case, the potential for repeat surgery and prosthesis dysfunction remain. Many centers have strong opinions about the "ideal" valve substitute. Recently, adult patients seem to be shifting toward heterograft, stentless valves because of purported superior hemodynamics, improved durability, the lack of need for chronic anticoagulation, and ready availability. However, such valves ultimately degenerate and require replacement. Mechanical prostheses theoretically resist structural deterioration but expose the patient to the life-long risk of anticoagulation, which becomes significant over time. Pulmonary autograft aortic root replacement (Ross operation) has achieved widespread application in a variety of clinical settings. Although results are encouraging, the Ross procedure remains a formidable surgical procedure that is not routinely practiced by most cardiac surgeons. Further, it is well recognized that the pulmonary autograft is not immune from structural deterioration. In addition, because the pulmonary valve is replaced with either a heterograft or homograft prosthesis, most patients undergoing the Ross procedure ultimately require reoperation. Finally, homograft aortic roots, although attractive in some patients, deteriorate at unpredictable rates, again exposing the patient to the challenging need of repeat root replacement.

In children, the considerations mentioned have become even more problematic. Infants and small children requiring aortic valve surgery are rarely of sufficient size for mechanical aortic prostheses. In those children who receive such valves, the challenge of chronic oral anticoagulation is enormous—changing body size, diet, gender, activity level, and psychologic maturity all affect the safety margin of chronic anticoagulation. These concerns make use of mechanical prostheses in some children highly inadvisable. Human allograft valves are notoriously unpredictable in durability, particularly in very young or preadolescent patients. It is well recognized that previous exposure to heterologous blood products may affect durability of homograft aortic valves. Recently, homograft valve availability has decreased as more centers use these scarce conduits for various indications. Another concern raised by the U.S. Food and Drug Administration has been the antiseptic processing by a large supplier of homograft tissue. Heterograft aortic valve replacement in children has been largely abandoned by most centers because of the poor durability of these valves in children. The Ross procedure has become the procedure of choice in small children requiring aortic valve replacement. However, as noted earlier, the Ross operation is challenging and not practiced by all surgeons or at all centers. Furthermore, ongoing concerns about need for multiple reoperations on the pulmonary valve patient limit enthusiasm for autograft root replacement. In addition, recent evidence suggests the pulmonary autograft may be structurally abnormal in patients with congenitally bicuspid aortic valves, predisposing to early autograft failure.

Aortic valve repair remains a controversial option for the patient with significant aortic valve disease. Nonetheless, because of the limitation of prostheses already enumerated, many surgeons believe that for certain forms of aortic valve pathology, strong consideration should be given to valve repair. In children, this may be an even more compelling option. Theoretical benefits of successful aortic valve repair include freedom from anticoagulation, potential for normal somatic growth (particularly of the aortic root), potentially superior hemodynamics, and improved durability. An additional attractive feature is the preservation of future options when reoperation is required. For example, we have frequently performed aortic valve repair in active adolescents with suitable valve pathology based on the premise that valve repair allows the patient to grow into adulthood before additional surgery is required. If repeat aortic valve operation becomes necessary, the patient has the option of choosing between mechanical and biologic valves.

In this review, a variety of methods are reviewed for repair of aortic valves, with emphasis on such repairs in children, the population in whom there is the most benefit from successful repair. Furthermore, children and young adults are more likely to have pathologic conditions amenable to successful repair.

■ INFANTS AND SMALL CHILDREN

In this age range, patients most commonly fall into one of three categories: congenitally stenotic aortic valves, congenitally insufficient aortic valves; and iatrogenically insufficient aortic valves.

Congenital Aortic Stenosis

Much has been written about management of critical aortic stenosis, particularly in the newborn. In current practice, the majority of these patients can be managed by balloon aortic valvotomy in the cardiac catheterization laboratory. It is a rare exception that such a patient goes for primary surgical valvotomy; this is most common in the setting of coexisting cardiac pathology. Surgical (open) valvotomy in infants is a straightforward procedure, best accomplished with cardiopulmonary bypass support. In the majority of cases, the surgeon encounters rudimentary commissures that are either partially or completely fused. Direct incision to the level of the aortic annulus often provides adequate relief but may result in significant insufficiency. If insufficiency is predicted, the surgeon may place a temporary suture ("Frater" stitch) through the corresponding nodules of Arantius. This ensures valve competence at the time of crossclamp removal. The suture is then removed after a stable rhythm is established.

Congenital Aortic Insufficiency

A large percentage of patients presenting with severe aortic insufficiency early in life have aortic valve pathology associated with persistent arterial trunk (truncus arteriosus). In these patients, the surgeon may encounter extremely dysmorphic aortic valve tissue with several (up to six) valve cusps. In some cases, inspection of the valve may demonstrate that one cusp is more severely affected than the others. In such cases, the surgeon may resect this cusp and the associated sinus. The aortic root is then primarily reconstructed, affecting a relative reduction in root diameter. The adjoining cusps typically need to be buttressed with a subcommissural suture.

Iatrogenic Aortic Insufficiency

Most patients undergoing neonatal or infant balloon aortic valvotomy develop some iatrogenic aortic insufficiency. In the majority, this is well tolerated. However, over the course of time, the insufficiency may increase, particularly if additional balloon dilation becomes necessary.

Valve repair in these patients may be challenging. The surgeon may encounter a grossly damaged aortic valve with cusp laceration, avulsion, or perforation. In many of these patients, there is insignificant tissue for repair. In others, repair may be considered. An avulsed cusp may be otherwise intact and suitable for reapproximation. Cusp extension with autologous or heterogeneous material may also be added. A recent study from Boston Children's Hospital, reported by Bacha and colleagues, documented no operative mortality and acceptable early valve performance in a small group of patients with aortic insufficiency after balloon aortic valvotomy. Although not likely to confer lifelong freedom from aortic valve replacement, such repair may delay the ultimate valve replacement.

■ AORTIC INSUFFICIENCY IN OLDER CHILDREN AND YOUNG ADULTS

Congenitally Bicuspid Aortic Valves

Patients presenting with insufficient congenitally bicuspid aortic valves are often good candidates for aortic valve repair. Valvar pathology includes elongation of the leading edge of one cusp (typically the conjoined left-right cusp) and significant leaflet prolapse. This results in poor leaflet coaptation and insufficiency. Even competent bicuspid aortic valves have a reduced zone of leaflet coaptation (lanula) compared with normal trileaflet aortic valves.

In insufficient bicuspid aortic valves, there may also be annular dilation, commissural fusion with some degree of stenosis, or leaflet calcification. Valve repair may be accomplished by creating cusp symmetry, usually by means of triangular resection of the prolapsing cusp segment (often with release or resection of the associated rudimentary commissure or raphe). Repair of the cusp is then performed with a continuous double-layered suture. In the majority of cases, subcommissural sutures are then placed to achieve a more narrow intercommissural angle and thereby increase the zone of coaptation or lanula. Using these techniques, we have achieved acceptable intermediate-term results in selected children and young adults.

Leaflet Perforation

Chronic leaflet perforation may be one of the best indications for aortic valve repair. This may result from previous, remote endocarditis, but in some cases, there is no definite history of infection. The leaflet perforation is simply repaired by a patch, preferably autologous pericardium. This is a very reproducible and durable repair.

A less attractive situation occurs in the setting of acute leaflet perforation in active endocarditis. Although some surgeons have reported successful cusp repair in this setting, we believe attempting repair in an actively infected valve is unpredictable and generally not advisable.

A challenging problem occurs when a perforation develops from chronic leaflet prolapse through an associated ventricular septal defect. In these cases, there is usually significant cusp distortion and elongation (windsock effect), with a perforation at the most dependent point. Repair is this setting may be much more challenging and less predictable.

Cusp Distortion With Associated Ventricular Septal Defect

All congenital heart surgeons struggle with the difficult problem of aortic insufficiency associated with a ventricular septal defect (VSD). This may occur with subarterial or supracristal VSDs in which the right coronary cusp is most commonly involved or perimembranous VSDs in which the right or noncoronary cusp may be affected. A typical clinical scenario is one in which a VSD previously thought to be relatively large starts to "close." This closure is related to cusp prolapse and is often associated with development of new aortic insufficiency. In our opinion, all such cases should undergo surgery to close the VSD, although whether an aortic valve repair should be attempted for mild degrees of aortic insufficiency is more controversial. Unfortunately, in the majority of cases, closure of the VSD alone does not rectify the aortic insufficiency.

The precise cause of aortic cusp distortion in patients with subarterial VSDs is not known, but most surgeons believe that it is related to chronic turbulent flow through the VSD with cusp prolapse and ultimate central incompetence through poor coaptation (Venturi effect). Unfortunately, longstanding cusp distortion can become severe and lead to an irreparable valve.

Several techniques have been described to achieve aortic valve competence in cases of cusp prolapse associated with VSD. The most widely applied, as initially performed and reported by Trusler, involves measured leaflet plication at the commissure to achieve cusp symmetry. Alternative techniques have been described that include triangular resection of the prolapsing cusp along with leaflet suspension with subcommissural sutures to improve the intercommissural triangle and thereby increase the zone of coaptation. We have found the latter technique to be more reproducible. An alternate technique described by Yacoub involves primary closure of the VSD with simultaneous plication of the associated sinus.

■ AORTIC INSUFFICIENCY IN PATIENTS WITH RHEUMATIC VALVE DISEASE

These patients are relatively rare today, although it may become more prevalent with recent resurgence of rheumatic fever.

Worldwide, rheumatic valve disease remains a significant cause of aortic insufficiency in children and young adults. In most of these patients, there is also mitral pathology, amenable to repair. Therefore, achieving aortic valvar competence through repair becomes a much more attractive possibility. Recent reports have documented acceptable mid-term results in patients with rheumatic aortic insufficiency undergoing pericardial extension of all three aortic cusps. This method is a slight modification of the cusp extension method previously described by Duran and involves three rectangular strips of autologous, glutaraldehyde treated pericardium to extend the deficient, retracted aortic valve cusps. At 5- and 7-year follow-up, actuarial freedom from reoperative valvular surgery was 92.1% and 90%, respectively. This technique is relatively straightforward and should be familiar to all surgeons treating children and adults with aortic valve pathology.

■ SUMMARY

Aortic valve reparative procedures exist to address a variety of aortic valve pathology. Although not considered "curative," these techniques may offer selected patients a reasonable alternative to aortic valve replacement. Methods discussed herein are straightforward and reproducible; they are particularly applicable to children and young adults. Surgeons treating patients in these age categories should know these methods and give strong consideration to valve repair during preoperative counseling of patient or family.

SUGGESTED READING

Bacha EA, et al: Valve-sparing operation for balloon-induced aortic regurgitation in congenital aortic stenosis, *J Thorac Cardiovasc Surg* 122:162, 2001.

Fraser CD, et al: Repair of insufficient bicuspid aortic valves, *Ann Thoracic Surg* 58:386, 1994.

Grinda JM, et al: Aortic cusp extension valvuloplasty for rheumatic aortic valve disease: mid term results, *Ann Thorac Surg* 74:434, 2002.

Thubrikar M: Diseases of the aortic valve. In: Thubrikar M, editor. *The aortic valve*, Boca Raton, FL, 1990, CRC Press, p 157.

Trusler GA, et al: Repair of ventricular septal defect with aortic insufficiency, *J Thorac Cardiovasc Surg* 66:394, 1973.

Yacoub MH, et al: Anatomic correction of the syndrome of prolapsing right coronary aortic cusp, dilation of the sinus, of Valsalva and ventricular septal defect, *J Thorac Cardiovasc Surg* 113:253, 1997.

THE SMALL AORTIC ROOT

John R. Doty
Donald B. Doty

Although the collective experience with aortic valve replacement spans more than 35 years, there is no single valve that is clearly superior for all patients. The surgeon can select from a variety of valves, including mechanical prostheses, bioprosthetic xenografts, homografts, and autografts. Device hemodynamic performance, risk of thromboembolism and infection, need for anticoagulation, long-term durability, patient preference, and patient reliability all play a role in proper valve selection.

In patients with morphologic narrowing of the aortic root, the choice of valve has greater implications. The surgeon often is limited in the size of the replacement device, and the obstructive nature of the various valves is compounded in the small aortic root. Aortic root enlargement and replacement procedures are key components of the proper treatment of these patients, in whom operative technique directly influences long-term results.

The aortic root is considered small when the diameter of the aortic annulus measures 21 mm or less in adult patients. Depending on the age and clinical status of the patient, the surgeon must make the appropriate decisions regarding type of valve for implantation and the need for aortic root enlargement. A wide range of valves is now available, including mechanical prostheses, stented and stentless bioprostheses, homografts, and autografts. The techniques for enlargement or replacement of the aortic root also vary and must be tailored to the individual patient.

■ RELEVANT AORTIC ROOT ANATOMY

The aortic valve normally has a three-cusp architecture, and the leaflets coapt centrally to achieve competence. The three highest points of attachment around the annulus are termed the *commissures* and are situated well above the ventriculoaortic junction. The lowest point of attachment for each leaflet rests below the ventriculoaortic junction, however. The triangular space directly inferior to each commissure is called the *interleaflet triangle,* and the tissue in this area is pliable and flexible. The posterior triangle, which is located between the left and noncoronary sinuses of Valsalva, is aligned directly over the midpoint of the anterior leaflet of the mitral valve. There are no chordae tendineae at this portion of the anterior leaflet of the mitral valve, allowing safe incision during posterior root enlargement.

The anterior relationships of the aortic valve also are important, particularly when removal of the pulmonary trunk for autografting is planned. The conduction system courses below the anterior commissure and the midpoint of the right coronary sinus, on the posterior rim of the membranous septum, before traveling down the ventricular septum to the right of the septal papillary muscle (of the conus). Anterior incision of the aortic root to the right of the septal papillary muscle can interrupt the conduction system.

The first septal branch of the left anterior descending coronary artery runs directly below the posterior cusp of the pulmonary valve, near the medial posterior commissure. The septal branch crosses the infundibular septum to supply the septal papillary muscle. Injury to the first septal branch can result in a septal myocardial infarction and heart block from interruption of the blood supply to the bundle of His.

■ AORTIC ROOT SIZING

Several authors have studied the dimensions of the normal aortic root and determined ratios for measuring or calculating the diameter of the root at various levels. Generally, surgeons consider the aortic annulus to be at the level of the ventriculoaortic junction, which is the same diameter measured to determine the size of a prosthetic valve. Normal dimensions (diameter) of the aortic annulus related to body size (surface area) have been determined, and nomograms have been established by Capps et al. The diameter of the sinotubular junction is normally about 90% of the diameter of the annulus in younger patients, becoming equal to that of the annulus in older patients. The diameter of the sinotubular junction is always abnormal when it exceeds that of the aortic annulus.

■ MECHANICAL VALVES

Replacement of the aortic valve with any mechanical valve that is 23 mm or larger (manufacturer's size) should provide an actual orifice that is hemodynamically suitable for most adult patients. The 21-mm mechanical valve can create significant flow obstruction and should be used only for patients with a body surface area less than 1.5 m^2 and who are sedentary. Any mechanical valve that is 19 mm or smaller may have a prohibitive pressure gradient across the valve and cause severe outflow tract obstruction. This gradient should be considered in its relationship to the long-term resolution of left ventricular hypertrophy that results from chronic aortic stenosis.

All of the mechanical prostheses that have been designed for aortic valve replacement and are available for implantation may be considered equivalent. All require long-term anticoagulation and have equivalent performance for thromboembolic events, valve thrombosis, and anticoagulant-related hemorrhage. All have excellent long-term durability and by the nature of design introduce some amount of turbulent flow. The sewing ring and housing for each valve create a fixed physical obstruction, reducing the diameter of the actual orifice of the valve 5 to 8 mm compared with the outside diameter of the device.

The Medtronic-Hall valve is offered as an even-sized valve, so that a 20-mm valve represents a 21-mm device inside a thinner sewing ring sized for a 19-mm annulus. The St. Jude Hemodynamic Plus valve retains the odd number–sized device within a thinner sewing ring so that a 21-mm Hemodynamic Plus valve is sized for a 19-mm annulus. The Carbomedics Top Hat valve is intended for insertion in a supraannular position to allow for a 2-mm larger valve placement.

We believe that a 19-mm mechanical prosthesis has a prohibitive pressure gradient and that the aortic root should be enlarged in such patients to accommodate a larger prosthesis. The 21-mm valve should be reserved for small patients with a sedentary lifestyle; otherwise, the root should be enlarged. Insertion of a 23-mm or larger mechanical prosthesis should be satisfactory for any patient.

■ BIOPROSTHETIC VALVES

An ever-widening range of bioprosthetic valves is available for aortic valve replacement, and some are more useful in the patient with small aortic root. Several centers now have long-term experience with porcine and bovine pericardial valves in the aortic position. Bioprostheses are limited by durability but do not require anticoagulation. The bovine pericardial valve in particular has been shown to have good long-term hemodynamic performance in the small aortic root. The support structure of a stented bioprosthetic valve results, however, in a 5- to 8-mm reduction in the outflow tract. Our recommendation for bioprosthetic valve replacement in the small aortic root is similar to that for mechanical valves.

The stentless valves offer an additional option because these valves show good hemodynamic performance even in small size when placed in a subcoronary position. When same-size external bioprosthetic valves are compared, stentless valves have a considerably larger internal diameter than stented valves. Stentless valves inserted within the intact aortic root using a freehand technique reduce the size of the outflow tract by about 2 mm, the thickness of the aorta of the bioprosthesis. Studies comparing stentless bioprostheses, stented bioprostheses, and mechanical valves have shown better regression of left ventricular hypertrophy with the stentless valves.

Currently, four stentless bioprostheses have been used on a fairly widespread clinical basis. The St. Jude Toronto SPV valve is fashioned from a porcine aortic valve and fixed at low pressure in glutaraldehyde without anticalcification treatment. The Toronto SPV valve can be implanted only in the subcoronary position. The Medtronic Freestyle valve is derived from a porcine aortic root preserved in glutaraldehyde with 0 net pressure on the valve and α amino-oleic acid to retard anticalcification of the valve. This device can be implanted using the subcoronary technique, the root inclusion technique, or as a freestanding aortic root replacement. The Edwards Prima Plus device is similar to the Freestyle valve except that fixation of the valve is at low pressure and Tween-80 is the anticalcification agent. The Cryolife-O'Brien valve is a composite valve fashioned from three noncoronary porcine leaflets fixed at low pressure with glutaraldehyde without anticalcification. This device can be implanted only in the subcoronary position, but it is designed to be attached in aortic sinus tissue above the annulus of the aortic valve.

The Toronto SPV valve and the Cryolife-O'Brien valve are pretrimmed and ready for implantation using the subcoronary technique. The Freestyle valve and the Prima Plus valve must be tailored by removing the sinus aorta from the right and left coronary sinuses of the bioprosthesis to implant the device in the subcoronary position. The preservation techniques of the stentless bioprostheses aid in proper implantation because even the trimmed graft holds its shape well, and the patient's native aorta may be conformed to the graft aorta in a reproducible fashion.

Full root replacement is possible only with the Freestyle and the Prima Plus bioprostheses and is particularly applicable to patients with a small aortic root. The aorta is divided above the sinotubular junction, and both coronary ostia are mobilized on generous buttons of aortic wall. The remaining sinus aorta is removed, the aortic valve is excised, and the annulus is débrided. A larger prosthesis may be employed because the device stands by itself and is not enclosed within the aorta. The bioprosthesis is implanted as a complete aortic root using multiple interrupted braided sutures or continuous monofilament sutures to attach the inflow sewing ring to the aortic annulus. A strip of polytetrafluoroethylene (Teflon) felt or pericardium may be incorporated for hemostasis. The coronary buttons are reimplanted in the appropriate position, and an end-to-end anastomosis of the distal end of the graft is constructed to the ascending aorta. Abnormally dilated or aneurysmal ascending aorta may be resected and replaced with a tubular prosthesis.

We do not recommend the root inclusion technique for implantation of a stentless bioprosthesis in patients with a small aortic root. These devices are stiff and are subject to distortion when the aorta is closed over them. In addition, the hemodynamic advantages of aortic valve replacement by aortic root techniques are lost when the device is within the aorta of the patient.

■ AORTIC HOMOGRAFT

As with stentless bioprostheses, aortic homografts are versatile, flexible tissue that has excellent hemodynamic performance in the aortic position. The homograft can be preserved with various techniques; the cryopreservation method appears best. Homografts are particularly well suited for use in the small aortic annulus, often without root enlargement, and can be used to enlarge the root when necessary. These valves do not require anticoagulation and are resistant to thromboembolism and endocarditis.

Originally, aortic homografts were implanted in a subcoronary position after removal of all aortic sinus tissue. Modification of this technique by retaining the noncoronary sinus, as described by Ross, ensures more reliable valve implantation by fixing the position of two of the three commissures. The entire aortic root also can be replaced using a freestanding root technique. Miniroot or cylinder inclusion techniques are, in our opinion, a less desirable approach for homograft implantation. If the patient requires only valve replacement and has a normal aorta, the noncoronary sinus technique allows for the smallest amount of homograft tissue to be implanted. More extensive root pathology, such as that with root abscess or poststenotic root dilation, requires the freestanding homograft root technique.

Root enlargement with aortic homograft is a useful technique that can be tailored to the severity of outflow tract obstruction. The posterior interleaflet triangle can be incised and a portion of the noncoronary sinus removed for isolated annular stenosis. A larger homograft can be used, attaching the proximal end to the mitral annulus and the roof of the left atrium. In patients with subvalvular obstruction, the incision is carried down onto the midportion of the anterior leaflet of the mitral valve. The homograft mitral valve is used to repair the defect in the recipient mitral valve, and the homograft noncoronary sinus is used to close the aorta after valve implantation.

Our experience with the cryopreserved aortic homograft has shown excellent freedom from thromboembolism and endocarditis in long-term analysis. Death from valve-related causes is infrequent, and the homograft seems to have good long-term durability. The noncoronary sinus technique or its variant with root enlargement was superior to other methods in our experience in offering the best chance for freedom from valve explantation. Late degeneration of the valve probably is related to a combination of technical and immunologic factors.

■ PULMONARY AUTOGRAFT

The pulmonary autograft operation, or Ross procedure, offers some advantages for aortic valve replacement. It is particularly applicable to patients with the small aortic root because the native pulmonary annulus is normally about 2 mm larger than the native aortic annulus, and pulmonary autografting results in a small valve upsize. Long-term performance of the pulmonary valve in the aortic position is currently unknown, but because the autograft is the patient's own tissue, the accelerated calcification and degeneration seen with homografts and porcine bioprostheses is unlikely. Patients do not require anticoagulation, and studies using this procedure in the setting of endocarditis underscore the autograft's inherent resistance to infection.

In the operation, the aortic valve and root are excised, retaining only the fibrous annulus and coronary ostia with sinus aortic buttons. The patient's own pulmonary trunk is excised, including the pulmonary valve. The pulmonary trunk is attached to the fibrous annulus of the aortic root using interrupted stitches. A polytetrafluoroethylene felt or pericardial strip is incorporated by tying the sutures around this strip. This is known as the *supported root technique* and helps prevent late dilation and valve incompetence by fixing the size of the outflow tract at the level of the pulmonary valve. The coronary arteries are reimplanted, and the distal end of the pulmonary trunk is attached to the ascending aorta. The diameter of the sinotubular junction also is fixed by prosthetic material to prevent dilation. The right ventricular outflow tract is reconstructed with a homograft pulmonary trunk. Devascularized pulmonary homografts may be used and may achieve better immunologic tolerance.

Root enlargement techniques may be combined with the pulmonary autograft operation. We believe that the left ventricular outflow tract (LVOT) should be altered to match the size of the native pulmonary trunk. Attempting to place a large pulmonary trunk into the small aortic root may cause distortion or stenosis of the pulmonary valve, as would deliberate narrowing of the autograft before implantation, and ultimately would result in valve failure. Similarly an enlarged aortic root should be reduced to appropriate anatomic dimensions.

After removal of the pulmonary trunk, the ventricular septum can be incised to widen the LVOT, known as the *Ross-Konno operation*. This incision is not as deep as the classic Konno operation and prevents injury to the first septal branch. Total relief of outflow tract obstruction can be achieved by progressive shaving of myocardium from the left side of the septum. The pulmonary autograft is seated deeply in the outflow tract by attaching it to the ventricular septum, and any septal defect may be filled with attached myocardium on the autograft. This approach allows perfect matching of the diameter of the outflow tract to the diameter of the autograft.

The pulmonary autograft operation is more complex than simple aortic valve replacement and at this time is best applied to younger patients. The pulmonary autograft has superior hemodynamic performance and is a good choice for valve replacement in athletic patients. The aortic valve disease may be cured permanently by using autogenous tissue, but the pulmonary homograft in the right ventricular outflow tract probably will require replacement.

OPERATIONS FOR AORTIC ROOT ENLARGEMENT

In addition to enlargement of the aortic root by aortic homograft or pulmonary autograft, there are three techniques generally employed for enlargement of the LVOT when mechanical or biologic prostheses are employed—the Nicks-Nunez operation, the Rittenhouse-Manouguian operation, and the Konno-Rastan aortoventriculoplasty. A variant of the last operation, the Ross-Konno operation, already has been described. Most root enlargement procedures in adult patients are performed best by a posterior aortic root approach.

The Nicks-Nunez operation for posterior enlargement of the LVOT involves extension of the aortotomy incision into the posterior commissure and the underlying interleaflet triangle. This incision allows separation of the compliant tissues in the interleaflet triangle and enlarges the outflow tract by 2 to 3 mm. A prosthetic patch is placed in the posterior commissure, and a larger prosthetic valve can be inserted; the prosthetic patch is tapered to close the noncoronary sinus and aortotomy.

Additional enlargement of the aortic root can be obtained by extending the incision into the midportion of the anterior leaflet of the mitral valve. Enlargement of 4 or 5 mm can be achieved in this manner, and the defect in the anterior leaflet is repaired with a prosthetic patch. The patch repair is continued across the defect in the roof of the left atrium. A larger prosthetic valve is inserted, and the noncoronary sinus and aortotomy are reconstructed in a similar fashion.

The Rittenhouse-Manouguian operation, also for posterior enlargement, involves extension of the aortotomy into the noncoronary sinus. The left atrium is opened laterally to the aortic incision, and the aortotomy incision is extended into the anterior leaflet of the mitral valve. This incision is slightly off-center in the anterior leaflet and must be shifted to the exact midposition of the leaflet. A prosthetic patch is used to reconstruct the defect in the anterior leaflet of the mitral valve and the left atrium, and a larger prosthetic valve is inserted. Enlargement of 2 to 4 mm can be obtained by this operation.

The Konno-Rastan aortoventriculoplasty for anterior enlargement of the LVOT is used when extensive enlargement is required of more than 2 to 4 mm in diameter. It traditionally was used in small children for placement of a large prosthesis that would accommodate growth, but it also can be useful in patients with subaortic tunnel stenosis. A vertical incision is made in the aorta into the right coronary sinus and extended into the right ventricular outflow tract anteriorly. The ventricular septum is incised at the aortic annulus, extending to the left of the conduction system. The first septal branch is at risk of injury during this portion of the procedure. The annulus of the aortic valve is widened greatly, and the valve cusps are removed. A diamond-shaped patch is used to repair the defect in the ventricular septum to the level of the annulus, a large prosthetic valve is inserted, and the patch repair is continued to close the aortotomy. A second patch is used to repair the right ventricular outflow tract. This procedure has been nearly abandoned in favor of the Ross-Konno modification because the pulmonary autograft should grow in proportion to patient growth.

CONCLUSION

The surgeon must be prepared to use a range of valve replacement devices in combination with aortic root enlargement techniques for patients with small aortic root. Regardless of the choice for valve replacement, all of the currently available valves carry an inherent risk for late failure and need for rereplacement. Mechanical prostheses may thrombose, become infected, or suffer excessive wear. Bioprosthetic and homograft tissues degenerate and calcify over time, rendering the valve stenotic, incompetent, or both. Aortic valve rereplacement is associated with increased operative risk and represents a unique surgical challenge when required in the patient with small aortic root.

Our current recommendations for choice of valve prostheses in this patient population are based primarily on patient age and activity (Table 1). For patients younger than age 55, we prefer the pulmonary autograft operation with root enlargement or reduction as necessary to match the LVOT perfectly to the pulmonary trunk. Mechanical prostheses generally are used for patients age 55 to 70 years, and the root is enlarged to accommodate at least a 23-mm prosthesis. A 21-mm prosthesis may be used in a small, sedentary patient. In patients older than age 70, we prefer to use a stentless bioprosthesis because these valves seem to have the best hemodynamic performance of the xenografts in the smaller sizes. Aortic homografts are reserved for patients with active infection and younger patients with contraindications to anticoagulation.

Table 1 Recommendations for Valve Replacement in Small Aortic Root

VALVE	AGE GROUP	COMMENT
Mechanical prosthesis	55-70	Enlarge root to accommodate 23-mm device; use 21-mm device only in small, sedentary patients
Bioprosthesis	>70	Stentless xenograft has best hemodynamic profile; consider aortic root replacement; long-term durability is key factor
Pulmonary autograft	<55	Well suited for athletic patients; use Ross-Konno modification to match outflow tract to autograft
Homograft	Any	Reserved for infection and in patients with contraindication to anticoagulation

SUGGESTED READING

Anderson RH, et al: Anatomy of the aortic root with particular emphasis on options for its surgical enlargement, *J Heart Valve Dis* 5(Suppl 3):S249, 1996.

Barratt-Boyes BG, Christie GW: What is the best bioprosthetic operation for the small aortic root? Homograft, autograft, porcine, pericardial? Stented or unstented? *J Card Surg* 9(2 Suppl):185, 1994.

Doty DB: Aortic valve replacement with homograft and autograft, *Semin Thorac Cardiovasc Surg* 8:249, 1996.

Doty JR, et al: Aortic valve replacement with cryopreserved aortic allograft: ten-year experience, *J Thorac Cardiovasc Surg* 115:371, 1998.

Gonzalez-Juanatey JR, et al: Influence of the size of aortic valve prostheses on hemodynamics and change in left ventricular mass: implications for the surgical management of aortic stenosis, *J Thorac Cardiovasc Surg* 112:273, 1996.

THE ROSS OPERATION

Ronald C. Elkins

Pulmonary autograft replacement of the aortic valve first was described in 1967 by Ross, and his pioneering efforts over 35 years have led to the identification of this operative procedure as the *Ross operation*. It is the only valve replacement in which the new valve is viable autogenous tissue and has growth potential. These unique characteristics provide the patient with an aortic valve that has normal flow characteristics and hemodynamics, limited risk of thromboembolism, resistance to infection, and the possibility of a permanent valve replacement. The operation was developed following the early experience with homograft replacement of the aortic valve and was performed as a scalloped subcoronary implant. The Ross operation proved to be technically demanding, and its use was hindered by the limited availability of homograft valves to reconstruct the right ventricular outflow tract (RVOT). The root replacement first was performed by Ross in 1974 and was introduced in the United States in 1986. This technique along with an increasing availability of homograft valves for right ventricular reconstruction has led to increasing popularity of the operation. The root replacement allowed the use of the operation in young children, and modifications have been developed for most abnormalities of the aortic valve and the aortic root.

■ INDICATIONS

The Ross operation can be used in patients ranging in age from newborn to the 50s and 60s who have an active lifestyle or who have medical reasons to avoid anticoagulation. Because the operation involves replacement of the aortic valve and the pulmonary valve, most surgeons restrict this operation to patients who do not have alternatives for aortic valve replacement with a tissue valve with similar hemodynamics and durability and do not require anticoagulation. The Ross operation has proved to be an excellent choice for patients with active aortic valve endocarditis requiring valve replacement for progressive congestive heart failure or thromboembolism. In patients with aortic and mitral valve disease, the Ross operation is indicated when the mitral valve can be repaired. The Ross operation would be the operation of choice if the patient did not have mitral valve disease. When the mitral valve is likely to require replacement, however, one of the benefits of the Ross operation (i.e., freedom from anticoagulation) would be lost, and the Ross operation rarely is indicated except in young children in whom the anticipated growth of the autograft valve warrants its use.

The operation is contraindicated in patients with significant abnormality of the pulmonary valve. I do not recommend use of a bicuspid pulmonary valve or a valve with multiple large fenestrations, particularly if they extend to the coaptive surface of the valve. Patients with a known genetic defect that involves fibrillin (Marfan syndrome) or other components of collagen or elastin are not candidates for this operation. Patients with immune complex disease, such as active rheumatic heart disease, systemic lupus erythematosus, or rheumatoid disease, when the aortic valve disease is secondary to the immune complex disease, are not candidates for a Ross operation. Patients with significant comorbid conditions that limit life expectancy are rarely candidates.

■ OPERATIVE TECHNIQUE

Since the 1980s, full root replacement has become the most common operative technique. This technique allows implantation of the pulmonary root as an anatomic unit and is not associated with early technical failure despite significant mismatch between the aortic annulus and the pulmonary annulus. Mismatch between the aorta and the pulmonary sinotubular junction still must be avoided, however. Operative techniques to deal with these variances are discussed. Root replacement allows the surgeon to deal not only with valvular abnormalities, but also subvalvular outflow tract obstruction and root pathology.

Most surgeons use full sternotomy; this should be the choice for surgeons with limited experience. Cardiopulmonary bypass (CPB) with aortic cannulation near the innominate artery is indicated, if the ascending aorta is normal; however, if it is dilated, cannulation of the transverse aortic arch between the innominate artery and the left carotid artery is preferred. I routinely use bicaval cannulation. Moderate systemic hypothermia with cold retrograde blood cardioplegia and protection of the right ventricle with ice slush is my routine.

In adult patients or patients of adult size, after institution of cardiac arrest, the aorta is opened, the aortic valve is inspected, and the appropriateness of performing a Ross operation is determined. The pulmonary artery is opened proximal to the origin of the right pulmonary artery. The pulmonary valve is inspected, and, if normal, the pulmonary artery and its contained valve are enucleated from the RVOT, protecting the left main coronary artery, the left anterior descending coronary artery, and the first septal perforator (Figure 1). The autograft root is trimmed so that 3 to 4 mm of right ventricular muscle remains proximal to the pulmonary valve annulus in the nadir of the valve sinuses. The remaining aortic root, to within a few millimeters of the aortic annulus, is excised. The right and left coronary ostia are mobilized with generous cuffs of aorta. After removal of the aortic valve and careful débridement of the aortic annulus, the aortic annulus is measured, then is adjusted to an appropriate size estimated for the patient based on the patient's body surface area.

Because the pulmonary annulus is variable in size depending on right ventricular volume, I do not use the pulmonary annulus size to determine the expected size of the aortic annulus. I reduce the aortic annulus size if it is more than 2 mm greater than the expected aortic annulus size based on the patient's body surface area. The aortic annulus is reduced with a double purse-string suture of 2-0 polypropylene placed at the level of the aortic annulus in the nadir of the

coronary sinuses and below the aortic annulus in the inter-leaflet triangle. These sutures are brought outside the aortic annulus in the midpoint of the noncoronary sinus, passed through a felt pledget, and tied with the appropriate size uterine dilator (Hegar) in the left ventricular outflow tract (Figure 2). This reproducibly reduces the aortic annulus to the appropriate size. The proximal anastomosis of the autograft root to the aortic annulus is performed with interrupted 4-0 polypropylene suture in adult patients and children of adult size. These sutures are tied over a thin Dacron strip to allow "fixation" of this anastomosis and to prevent late dilation (Figure 3). In patients requiring aortic annulus reduction, the proximal sutures encompass the annular reduction sutures. In the middle of the neo–left coronary sinus, a 5-mm hole is made with an aortic punch, and after trimming of the aorta around the left coronary ostium, the left coronary artery is sewn to this opening with 5-0 or 6-0 polypropylene. This anastomosis must be positioned and performed with care so that the left coronary artery is not kinked when the autograft is distended. The autograft is trimmed distally so that the distal anastomosis can be made at or near the sinotubular junction of the pulmonary autograft. If the ascending aorta is dilated or aneurysmal, it should be reduced in size by resection or by reduction aortoplasty.

Dacron tube graft placement of the aneurysmal aorta or markedly dilated ascending aorta may be appropriate. A graft that is the size of the aortic annulus or 10% smaller (the normal diameter of the sinotubular junction of the pulmonary root is 10% to 15% smaller than the pulmonary valve annulus) should be used. The distal anastomosis is completed with a running suture of 4-0 polypropylene, and the autograft root is distended so that an appropriate site for implanting the right coronary can be selected. It is important to select this site carefully so that distention of the autograft does not cause the right coronary artery to kink and produce severe right ventricular dysfunction after discontinuation of CPB. A 5-mm opening is made in the neo–right coronary sinus, and the right coronary artery is sewn to this opening. Reperfusion of the heart and rewarming can be instituted at this time.

A pulmonary homograft selected by size and age of the donor to match the recipient is implanted with a running suture line for the proximal and the distal anastomoses. I usually perform the proximal suture line first, then obtain good hemostasis in the bed of the pulmonary autograft. Placement of posterior sutures in the RVOT must be only in the cut edge of the right ventricular septum to avoid occlusion of a septal perforator. The distal anastomosis is completed being careful to avoid narrowing the anastomosis.

With rewarming and deairing of the left ventricle, the heart can be defibrillated, and CPB can be discontinued. Transesophageal echocardiography is done to verify function of both valves. Both valves should have a minimal outflow gradient and no more than trivial or mild insufficiency. Flow into both coronary arteries should be normal. Hemostasis should be secure before attempts at weaning from CPB. If additional sutures are needed in any of the autograft anastomoses, these should be placed during CPB so that systemic pressure can be lowered to avoid additional tears or holes.

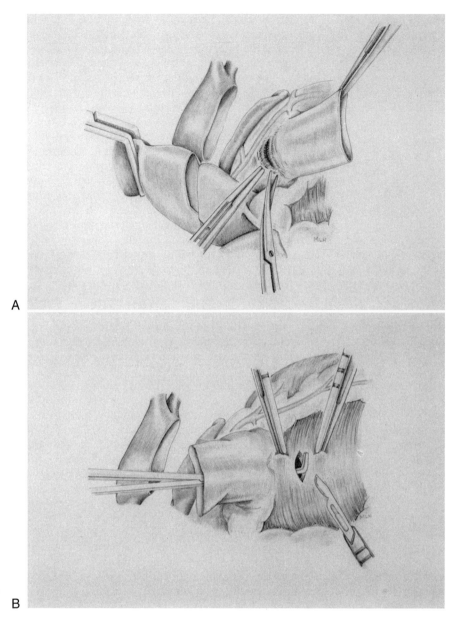

A

B

Figure 1
A, Dissection of the pulmonary autograft is initiated on the posterior aspect of the proximal pulmonary artery. Dissection is continued in this plane, adjacent to the pulmonary artery, until septal myocardium is encountered. The left main coronary artery and left anterior descending coronary artery are protected. **B,** Identification of the anterior right ventriculotomy is facilitated by placing a right-angled clamp through the pulmonary valve and indenting the myocardium 3 to 4 mm below the pulmonary valve annulus.

The operative procedure in children is modified to ensure opportunity for growth. Additionally, management of complex left ventricular outflow tract obstruction may be required. The suture lines are accomplished with fine absorbable sutures (PDS or Maxon). The proximal suture line is usually a continuous 5-0 PDS. Three sutures are placed near the nadir of the coronary sinuses to position the autograft root properly. This triangulates the aortic annulus, but these must be adjusted if the coronary arteries are malpositioned. The suture in the left coronary sinus is tied and is run to the midpoint of the right coronary sinus and tied. Then a suture is run from the left coronary sinus to the midpoint of the noncoronary sinus and tied. These sutures are run to the commissure between the right and noncoronary sinus so that the last sutures placed in the autograft are placed in the interleaflet triangle where injury to the autograft

valve is least likely. Before placement of the proximal suture line, subvalve aortic obstruction may be treated by resection or by left ventricular myomectomy if indicated.

If an inadequate aortic annulus is present, an aortoventriculoplasty (Ross-Konno) may be required. If aortic annulus dilation is present, I have used annular reduction with an absorbable suture without annular fixation so that future growth would not be restricted. The coronary anastomoses are made to small, 4-mm openings in the autograft sinuses and are completed with fine absorbable sutures. None of the suture lines are reinforced to avoid any inhibition of appropriate growth of the autograft root. Particularly in patients with prior aortic surgery, it is important to position the coronary arteries on the autograft root so that distention of the autograft root does not produce angulation or kinking of the coronary arteries.

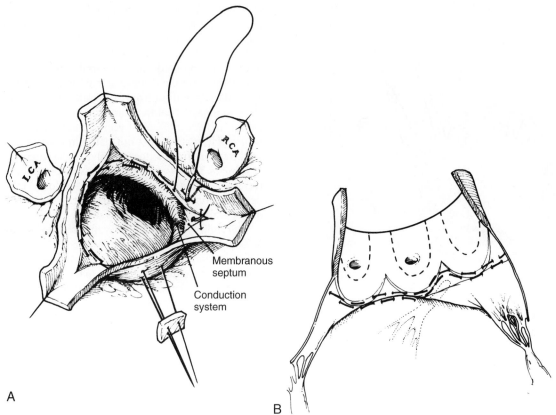

A

B

Figure 2
A, Two purse-string sutures of 2-0 polypropylene are placed at the aortic annulus in the nadir of the coronary sinuses, in the lateral fibrous trigone in the interleaflet triangle between the left and noncoronary sinus, in the muscle of the ventricular septum at the commissure between the left and right coronary sinuses, and in the membranous septum between the right and noncoronary sinus. The sutures are brought through the aortic annulus external to the aorta in the midpoint of the noncoronary sinus and passed through a felt pledget. **B,** An opened view of the aortic annulus shows the exact placement of the sutures. Notice the placement of the sutures in the membranous septum to avoid the conduction system.

■ RESULTS AND COMMENTS

The operative risk for an elective Ross operation is currently 2%. In patients who are unstable, have endocarditis, or have severe ventricular dysfunction, risk is slightly higher. Acute autograft valve dysfunction does not occur as long as the principles related to annulus size and size of the ascending aorta at the site of the distal anastomosis are followed. The most common problem is bleeding at the suture lines. The pulmonary autograft root is less resistant to bleeding from suture holes, and its tensile strength is less than the aorta. Tension on the distal suture line must be avoided and the sutures carefully placed. Pledgets should be avoided because they tend to tear when the autograft is pressurized. Significant hypertension must be avoided, and all repairs to the suture lines or to bleeding points should be made while the systemic pressure can be controlled easily by CPB.

Bleeding from the proximal suture line is difficult to identify and control after completion of the operation. To decrease the likelihood of bleeding from this suture line, I use a buttress for this suture line in all patients except children with anticipated growth. I use a woven Dacron strip in patients who require annular reduction, autologous pericardium in patients with a normal size annulus, and glutaraldehyde-fixed bovine pericardium in patients with endocarditis. If bleeding is noted from this suture line, it is best to reinstitute CPB for repair. Sometimes it is necessary to take down the distal suture line of the homograft or the right coronary anastomosis to obtain adequate exposure. Bleeding from the left coronary anastomosis is exposed more easily after taking down the distal homograft suture line. A short period of aortic cross-clamp and cardiac arrest may be required to control bleeding from the right or left coronary suture lines.

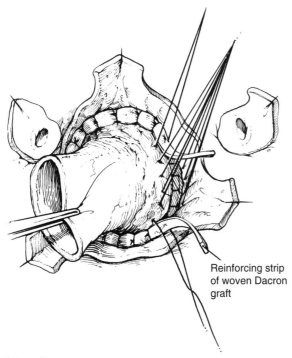

Reinforcing strip
of woven Dacron
graft

Figure 3
The proximal suture line is tied over a thin strip of woven
Dacron graft, being careful to keep the Dacron material
external to the autograft and not between the apposition
line of the aortic annulus and the autograft. The two ends of
the Dacron graft are tied together with the last two sutures
to complete the fixation of the aortic annulus.

Inotropic support rarely is needed after a Ross operation.
During the first 24 postoperative hours, systemic blood pressure must be controlled carefully. In general, systemic blood
pressure should be maintained at less than 130 mm Hg
systolic. Significant late postoperative bleeding has been
associated with significant postoperative hypertension.
Bleeding rarely is seen after the first 24 hours.

Late results after the Ross operation have been excellent.
At 10 years, actuarial survival is 94% ± 2%, actuarial freedom
from autograft degeneration in root replacements is

86% ± 5%, and actuarial freedom from all valve-related complications in root replacements is 70% ± 8%. Freedom from
operation for homograft failure (usually obstruction) is
90% ± 3% at 10 years. Results in children (≤17 years old)
have been reviewed and are similar to the entire patient
population. Actuarial survival is 92% ± 3% at 12 years with
an actuarial freedom from autograft degeneration of 90% ±
4% and an actuarial freedom from all valve-related complications of 79% ± 5% at 11 years. In children who have had a
root replacement with a normal pulmonary valve, the actuarial freedom from autograft valve replacement is 93% ± 5%
at 12 years. Two patients had a bicuspid pulmonary valve that
was used as an autograft valve and developed relatively early
degeneration requiring replacement. I do not recommend
use of a bicuspid pulmonary valve.

Durability of the homograft used to reconstruct the
RVOT is a significant problem. Accelerated degeneration with
early obstruction of the conduit (sometimes within 1 year of
implant) is extremely distressing to the patient and physician.
Although unproved, many surgeons believe that early
homograft degeneration is a result of the patient's immunologic response to the valve. Advances in reducing homograft
antigenicity and elimination of the humoral antibody
response may reduce the occurrence of homograft valve
degeneration and decrease the incidence of reoperation for
this complication.

Late dilation of the autograft root replacement also is a
concern. This has occurred in some of our patients but rarely
has required reoperation and autograft replacement in our
patient series. The preoperative diagnosis of a bicuspid
aortic valve has not been a risk factor for the development of
autograft degeneration in our patients.

SUGGESTED READING

Elkins RC, et al: Pulmonary autograft root replacement: mid-term results,
    J Heart Valve Dis 8:499, 1999.
Elkins RC, et al: Ross operation and aneurysm or dilation of the ascending
    aorta, *Semin Thorac Cardiovasc Surg* 11:50, 1999.
Oswalt JD, Dewan SJ: Aortic infective endocarditis managed by the Ross
    procedure, *J Heart Valve Dis* 2:380, 1993.
Ross D, et al: The pulmonary autograft—a permanent aortic valve, *Eur J
    Cardiothorac Surg* 6:113, 1992.

MITRAL VALVE REPLACEMENT

Harold M. Burkhart

Kenton J. Zehr

Since the first mitral valve replacement was performed by Starr more than 4 decades ago, the operative technique has remained largely the same. Differences in surgical technique have more to do with surgeon's preference than difference in long-term outcome. Indications for intervention on the mitral valve have become more clearly defined, however, the appropriateness of repair versus replacement remains an issue. The most significant change in treatment of patients with advanced mitral valve pathology has resulted from the realization that most degenerative mitral valves with severe regurgitation can be repaired with precision and durability. Replacement remains the standard of care for patients with rheumatic mitral pathology and elderly patients with severe ischemic mitral regurgitation (MR). Important technical issues regarding mitral valve replacement concern the surgical approach, method and extent of subvalvular apparatus preservation, and management of an extensively calcified annulus.

■ INDICATIONS FOR SURGERY

The timing for surgical intervention for severe MR is controversial. There is little argument that patients with severe acute MR secondary to papillary muscle rupture or endocarditis should undergo urgent mitral valve surgery. In patients with progressively worsening chronic MR, the timing of surgical intervention is less clear. The symptoms of chronic MR are typically that of dyspnea and fatigue. Patients with New York Heart Association (NYHA) functional class II through IV symptoms, with or without normal left ventricular (LV) function, should undergo mitral valve surgery. Asymptomatic patients who have chronic severe MR with LV dysfunction should undergo surgery. The findings of an ejection fraction less than or equal to 0.60 or LV end-systolic dimension equal to or greater than 45 mm on echocardiography are diagnostic indicators of LV dysfunction. Whether or not a patient with significantly decreased LV function (ejection fraction <0.30) would be helped by surgery is debatable. The best surgical outcome is obtained, however, in patients with a normal functioning left ventricle and no or minimal symptoms. Data from the Mayo Clinic confirmed the improved 10-year survival afforded by repair in patients with normal LV function (70% ± 3%) compared with patients undergoing mitral repair with less than 60% ejection fraction (41% ± 4%). These results imply that repair should be performed in repairable patients before a decrease in LV function. This implication pertains to many patients who are asymptomatic or with

NYHA class I symptoms. This approach is in significant contrast to the previous practice of awaiting debilitating symptoms or LV dysfunction.

Results from the Mayo Clinic also show significantly lower morbidity and mortality rates at early and late follow-up in patients undergoing mitral repair versus mitral replacement. Overall survival at 10 years in 195 patients undergoing valve repair was 68% ± 6% compared with 52% ± 4% (p = .0004) in 214 patients undergoing valve replacement. These findings suggest that the standard of care should be early repair if there is a high probability of success of repair in patients with severe MR despite symptoms. In these patients and patients with recent onset of atrial fibrillation, surgery is recommended if the likelihood of mitral valve repair is high.

When to intervene with mitral valve repair or replacement in patients with ischemic MR is not clear. These patients are at significant risk for morbidity and mortality due to decreased LV function and other comorbidities. It is not clear whether or not the risk of valve surgery outweighs the long-term benefit. Ischemic MR is associated with higher mortality, independent of baseline characteristics and the degree of LV dysfunction.

In a study from the Mayo Clinic analyzing 303 patients with a previous Q wave myocardial infarction by electrocardiogram, 194 were found to have ischemic MR and were compared with 109 without ischemic MR. The patients were matched for age, sex, and ejection fraction. After 5 years, the total mortality and cardiac mortality for patients with ischemic MR were 62% ± 5% and 50% ± 6%. These rates were significantly higher than for patients without ischemic MR (39% ± 6% and 30% ± 5%). In a multivariant analysis, the adjusted relative risk of total and cardiac mortality was associated with the presence of ischemic MR. The mortality risk was related directly to the degree of ischemic MR as defined by the effective regurgitant orifice and the regurgitant volume. Despite the excess mortality associated with even moderate regurgitant volumes, these patients generally are not operated on due to the risk of mortality and morbidity. We recommend valve intervention, however, if the MR is in 2 to 3+, 3+, or 4+ range when undergoing concomitant cardiac procedures.

If replacement is anticipated, surgery is delayed until symptoms develop or ventricular function begins to decline. According to the Society of Thoracic Surgeons database, patients undergoing combined mitral valve replacement and coronary artery bypass graft (CABG) surgery had a mortality of 12% to 13%. These high mortality rates also were found in patients undergoing mitral valve repair plus CABG surgery (7.5% to 9%). This is in contrast to patients undergoing isolated mitral valve repair for degenerative pathology, who had 2% mortality. Because of these mortality figures, most patients with ischemic MR await surgery until they reach NYHA class III or IV with anginal symptoms.

Symptoms of mitral stenosis include dyspnea on exertion and hemoptysis. In patients with moderate or severe mitral stenosis (mitral valve area ≤1.5 cm^2) and NYHA functional class III to IV symptoms, mitral valve replacement is recommended if they are not considered candidates for balloon valvotomy or repair. Surgery also generally is recommended for patients with minimal symptoms but who have severe stenosis (mitral valve area ≤1 cm^2) and severe pulmonary hypertension (pulmonary artery systolic pressure ≥60 to 80 mm Hg) if they are not valvotomy candidates.

■ SURGICAL ANATOMY

An understanding of the mitral valve anatomy and its anatomic proximity to the aortic valve, tricuspid valve, atrioventricular node, and circumflex coronary artery is essential for successful mitral valve replacement. The mitral valve components include the annulus, anterior and posterior leaflets, anterolateral and posteromedial papillary muscles, and chordae tendineae. The left atrium is a relatively unrelated inflow chamber. The left ventricle is an important subunit of the mitral valve structure, however. The fibroskeleton of the heart is a relatively fixed collagenous framework to which the valvular tissue and the atrial and ventricular muscle are attached. The skeleton itself appears as several adjoining rings around a central fibrous body. The fibrous mitral annulus is D-shaped, with the straight portion representing the area of continuity between the mitral and aortic valves. This anterior third of the mitral annulus' continuity is limited by the right and left fibrous trigones. It is adjacent to the left coronary aortic cusp and a portion of the noncoronary aortic cusp. Because of these associations, this fibrous tissue is relatively fixed and does not dilate pathologically. Maintenance of its flexibility is important for normal human dynamics because this portion of the mitral annulus deforms away from the LV outflow tract during systole and toward the LV outflow tract during diastole. This flexibility allows for a maximal, effective orifice area for blood entering the left ventricle and leaving the left ventricle. An oversized prosthetic valve impedes blood flow within the LV outflow tract. Posteriorly, between the left and the right fibrous trigones, lies the posterior mitral annulus. This completes the posterior circumference of the atrioventricular orifice. The posterior mitral leaflet is affixed to this portion of the annulus.

The annulus is a dynamic structure whose circumference changes from 9 or 10 cm in diastole to 8 cm in systole. The circumference of the annulus in a normal adult measures 8 to 12 cm. The anterior annulus is thicker and more complete than the posterior annulus, which may be incomplete or poorly defined. This portion of the annulus pathologically dilates as the left ventricle and the left atrium enlarge in patients with moderate or severe MR. As in all patients with MR, as the regurgitant volume increases, the LV size must increase to maintain the same cardiac output. In addition, the left atrium becomes volume and pressure overloaded. This overload ultimately allows for mitral annular dilation, which uniformly occurs posteriorly between the left and the right trigone. Normal systolic reduction of the annular diameter does not occur; this increases further the regurgitant volume and advances the pathologic state.

Important anatomic relationships exist between the mitral valve and other structures (Figure 1). The anterior leaflet is in direct continuity with the aortic valve, specifically a portion of the left and noncoronary aortic cusps. This situation puts the aortic valve at risk during mitral valve surgery. The conduction bundle is susceptible to damage in the area of the right fibrous trigone. Vascular structures vulnerable to damage during mitral valve surgery include the circumflex

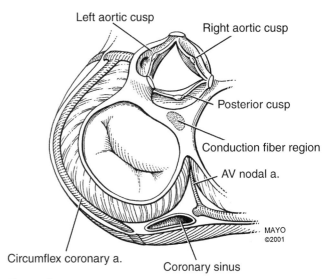

Figure 1
Surgical anatomy of the mitral valve. AV, atrioventricular.

coronary artery, whose course parallels the posterior annulus on the left, and the coronary sinus, which is superficial to the posterior annulus on the right. In a left dominant coronary artery system, the circumflex coronary artery is at risk for damage along the entire length of the posterior annulus.

■ SURGICAL TECHNIQUE

Surgical Approach

The standard approach to mitral valve surgery is via a median sternotomy. It allows the surgeon complete access to all the cardiac chambers and the great vessels. Placing the patient on cardiopulmonary bypass (CPB), managing aortic insufficiency, monitoring the left ventricle for distention, and evacuating air all are easier to do with this incision. In addition, the exposure allows for other cardiac procedures, such as CABG surgery, if necessary. Median sternotomy is associated with less postoperative pain than thoracotomy.

After the standard median sternotomy is performed, attention is turned to placing the patient on CPB and obtaining optimal mitral valve exposure. A single two-staged venous atrial cannula can be used as long as venous return is good and the mitral valve is well seen; this is usually possible, especially in the presence of a large left atrium. If the left atrium is small or if one anticipates that the single cannula would obstruct view of the mitral valve, two venous cannulae should be used. Typically, this includes a right-angle superior vena cava cannula and a straight or right-angle inferior vena cava cannula. Other maneuvers that may improve mitral valve exposure include lifting up on the right pericardial sutures, letting down the left pericardial traction sutures, dissecting the right-sided pulmonary vein to pericardial attachments and superior vena cava and inferior vena cava to pericardial attachments, and opening the left pleural space to allow the heart to fall and to bring the mitral valve into view.

Occasionally a right anterolateral thoracotomy is preferred for mitral valve surgery, such as in a patient with previous median sternotomy and anatomic considerations that make redo median sternotomy risky. Typical patients include patients with patent arterial CABGs, especially if they cross the midline, and patients with other potential hazards, such as an enlarged right ventricle. Female patients may prefer thoracotomy for cosmetic reasons.

For the right anterolateral approach, the patient is positioned at a 30-degree tilt, right side up, on a bean bag. The patient's right arm is positioned overhead. The chest is entered through the fifth interspace via an incision made from just right of the sternum to the anterior axillary line. One-lung ventilation is preferred. Pulling the diaphragm down with stay sutures brought through the inferior intercostal spaces and tagged on traction enhances exposure of the atria. The nonventilated lung is retracted out of the way, and CPB cannulae (two venous, one arterial) are placed. The aortic cannula may be difficult to insert, necessitating use of the femoral artery for arterial cannulation. Venous drainage via a femoral vein long cannula passed into the right atrium usually provides adequate flow. Vacuum assist is a helpful adjunct for venous drainage.

Atriotomy

After CPB is established, the patient is cooled to 34°C. The aortic cross-clamp is placed, and cold blood cardioplegia is administered for complete cardiac arrest. There are three atrial incisions to consider for mitral valve access—the right lateral, transseptal, and superior septal incisions.

The right lateral incision into the left atrium is used most commonly. Before making the atriotomy, the interatrial groove can be developed several centimeters with sharp dissection. The incision starts on the anterior lateral left atrium medial to the junction of the right superior pulmonary vein with the left atrium and continues inferiorly between the right inferior pulmonary vein and the inferior vena cava. By developing the interatrial plane, the left atrial incision can be made approximately 2 to 4 cm from the right pulmonary veins, giving closer exposure of the mitral valve.

The biatrial transseptal incision, known as the *Dubost incision*, is helpful in the case of a small left atrium or if there is right-sided cardiac pathology (atrial septal defect, tricuspid valve regurgitation) that should be addressed. The incision is started on the superior pulmonary vein and continues in a perpendicular fashion onto the right atrium. Next the incision is carried transversely across the interatrial septum/fossa ovalis.

The superior septal incision consists of a longitudinal right atriotomy that extends into the right atrial appendage. The incision is extended in a vertical fashion through the fossa ovalis and into the left atrial dome between the superior vena cava and ascending aorta. This incision opens both atria like a book, giving excellent mitral valve exposure. Disadvantages include that it is a more complex incision to close, and it is associated with a greater risk of loss of sinus rhythm due to sacrifice of the sinus node coronary artery branch.

Valve Replacement

When the heart is arrested and the atriotomy is performed, the mitral valve is inspected. Exposure of the mitral valve is facilitated by a hand-held retractor lifting up on the right atrium. Many commercial retractors are available to assist in retraction. The mitral valve is inspected for signs of infection or significant calcification. The inspection should include not only the leaflets and annulus, but also the chordae and papillary muscles.

When the mitral valve is evaluated and replacement is deemed necessary, a decision with regard to the fate of the subvalvular apparatus should be made. Generally the posterior leaflet and its subvalvular apparatus should be preserved if not involved by infection or calcification. Preservation of the posterior leaflet is relatively easy because it can be pinned posteriorly out of the way of mechanical valve leaflets and hinge. An issue is whether saving thickened leaflets and chordae results in placement of a significantly smaller valve. Preservation of the chordae helps maintain ventricular geometry and normal function of the papillary muscles. Maintaining the posterior leaflet and subvalvular apparatus allows suture placement within the posterior leaflet tissue and minimizes risk of placing sutures deep into the atrioventicular groove, reducing risk of atrioventricular groove disruption.

We typically excise the anterior leaflet and chordae, while leaving the posterior leaflet intact. If a tissue valve is being placed and the mitral orifice is large, we favor leaving the anterior leaflet and subvalvular mechanism intact. If a mechanical valve is being placed, it is difficult to tether the anterior leaflet and chordae out of the way of the valvular mechanism. To remove the anterior leaflet, an incision is made along the anterior leaflet parallel to and approximately 5 mm from the annulus. This leaves a ridge of anterior leaflet to anchor the prosthesis. The incision is carried to each commissure, freeing the anterior leaflet from the annulus. The anterior leaflet chordae are cut where they attach to the papillary muscles. If the posterior leaflet is too diseased to preserve, it is removed in similar fashion. The left ventricle is irrigated with cold saline to remove debris.

The annulus is sized, and the appropriate prosthetic valve is selected. We prefer pledgeted 2-0 braided polyester horizontal mattress sutures with pledgets on the ventricular side of the valve. This practice inverts the annulus and leaflet tissue. Many centers favor the eversion technique with the pledgets on the left atrial side. We find that a valve size can be gained by the inversion technique. All sutures are placed evenly along the annulus and secured sequentially on suture guides. When preserving leaflet tissue while placing a mechanical valve, the sutures should be placed first in and out of the leaflet, then through the annulus. This technique plicates the leaflet tissue out of the way of the valve mechanism, keeping any redundant leaflet tissue from interfering with prosthetic valve function. The sutures are passed through the prosthetic valve sewing cuff, and the valve is tied into position.

The left atriotomy is closed with a single layer of running 3-0 polypropylene suture starting at each end of the incision. A vent is placed into the left atrium through the atriotomy incision where the two running sutures meet. These sutures are brought through a Rumel tourniquet to secure the vent. If the patient has known mild aortic regurgitation, the valve can be stented open with a vent or Foley catheter to avoid LV distention after releasing the cross-clamp. This vent and the one in the ascending aorta help with evacuating air. It is standard of care to evaluate the prosthetic valve function by intraoperative transesophageal echocardiography.

Calcified Annulus

Valve replacement in the face of a heavily calcified mitral annulus presents a challenge. Calcification can be severe, involving the entire posterior annulus. Usually the anterior annulus is spared. Aggressive débridement of the posterior calcium is risky. Possible complications include circumflex coronary artery damage and atrioventricular disruption.

With mild to moderate calcification, the sutures usually can be placed in the usual fashion, taking generous tissue and avoiding the calcium. It is helpful to choose a valve with a generous sewing cuff. This serves to fill the crevices between the calcium with cloth. If calcification is severe, it is futile to attempt to force sutures through the annulus. Safer options exist. If the mitral leaflets are not involved in the calcification, the prosthesis can be anchored to the leaflets. An eversion technique involves placing pledgeted sutures from the left atrial side down through the leaflet at the outer edge of the leaflet. The suture is passed back up through the leaflet and into the prosthetic ring. One has to downsize the valve a size or two. Another option is to place the mitral valve prosthesis in a supraannular position. This option involves seating the prosthesis by placing mattress sutures within the left atrium, just above the calcified annulus. Everted pledgeted sutures are best using this technique. If the heavy calcification precluding suture placement is localized, one can locally débride the calcium and repair the defect before mitral valve prosthesis placement. If the defect is not too large, felt or pericardial strips can be placed along the atrial and the ventricular sides of the annular defect. Horizontal mattress sutures can be passed through the strips, atrium, and ventricle, creating a new portion of annulus. The prosthesis can be sutured into the annulus in the usual fashion.

If the defect created by annular débridement is larger, it can be patched before prosthesis insertion. This technique involves cutting a patch of autologous pericardium or glutaraldehyde-fixed bovine pericardium approximately 2 cm larger than the mitral annulus defect. The lower edge of the patch is secured with a running suture to the LV endocardium. The patch is secured with a running suture to the left atrial endocardium. The pledgeted sutures for the prosthesis are placed through the patch. The prosthesis is sutured in the usual fashion.

■ RESULTS

Operative mortality for elective mitral valve replacement has been reported to be 4% to 9%. Currently, operative mortality at the Mayo Clinic is 1% in patients younger than age 75 years undergoing mitral valve replacement. Survival rates in patients undergoing mitral valve surgery are 77%, 56%, and 44% at 5, 10, and 14 years. These are the results of 576 operative survivors (288 mitral valve replacements and 288 mitral valve repairs). CABG surgery was performed concomitantly in 211 patients. Independent predictors of survival were younger age, ejection fraction equal to or greater than 0.60, absence of coronary artery disease, and NYHA functional class I or II versus III or IV. These results suggest that coronary artery disease and LV dysfunction are major determinants of morbidity and mortality after surgical correction of mitral valve regurgitation.

SUGGESTED READING

Cohn LH, et al: Early and late risk of mitral valve replacement, *J Thorac Cardiovasc Surg* 90:872, 1985.

David TE, et al: Reconstruction of the mitral annulus, *J Thorac Cardiovasc Surg* 110:1323, 1995.

Dujardin KS, et al: Outcome after surgery for mitral regurgitation: determinants of postoperative morbidity and mortality, *J Heart Valve Dis* 6:17, 1997.

Enriquez-Sarano M, et al: Congestive heart failure after surgical correction of mitral regurgitation, *Circulation* 92:2496, 1995.

Grigioni F, et al: Ischemic mitral regurgitation: long-term outcome and prognostic implications with quantitative doppler assessment, *Circulation* 103:1759, 2001.

Yau TM, et al: Mitral valve repair and replacement for rheumatic disease, *J Thorac Cardiovasc Surg* 119:53, 2000.

MITRAL VALVE RECONSTRUCTION

Charles F. Schwartz

Eugene A. Grossi

Stephen B. Colvin

Aubrey C. Galloway

Patients undergoing mitral valve reconstruction had fewer late valve-related complications than patients having mitral valve replacement. Therefore, mitral valve repair has become the preferred treatment for patients with mitral insufficiency from degenerative disease.

With such excellent freedom from long-term complications, mitral reconstruction is now considered earlier in the course of the disease. With mitral insufficiency, significant, irreversible ventricular injury, including left ventricular dilatation and a fall in the ejection fraction, can insidiously evolve with few or no symptoms. Prompt operation is recommended for virtually all patients with significant symptoms due to mitral insufficiency, but in the current era operative repair is also recommended for asymptomatic patients with progressive ventricular dilatation or with the first sign of left ventricular systolic dysfunction. Given the 20% to 40% late mortality rates over 5 years postoperatively after mitral valve replacement in New York Heart Association class 4 patients, early mitral reconstruction is clearly attractive.

During the last several years, several important innovations in mitral valve reconstruction have been introduced. When Lillehei reported the first case of mitral valve repair in 1957, he used femoral artery cannulation for cardiopulmonary bypass (CPB) and approached the mitral valve through a right thoracotomy. New technology now allows us to revisit a minimally invasive version of this original operative approach. Recent innovations also include newer techniques for redundant posterior leaflet repair, improvements in repairing anterior leaflet pathology, better results after repair of ischemic mitral insufficiency, and better understanding of the role and function of annuloplasty devices.

■ EVALUATION OF MITRAL VALVE APPARATUS

Preoperatively, a comprehensive medical history and physical examination are essential. Coronary catheterization is indicated in patients with angina, prior myocardial infarction, or significant risk factors for coronary artery disease and for most patients over 55 years of age. Intraoperative transesophageal echocardiography (TEE) is a sine qua non for every case of mitral valve repair. Left atrial dimension, presence of thrombus, and left ventricular function are assessed,

as well as the aorta for atheromatous disease. A precise echocardiographic evaluation of the mitral apparatus, including leaflet motion, annular dilatation, and chordal pathology should be performed. The location, direction, and degree of insufficiency should be noted, as this helps the surgeon interpret the significance of any leaflet pathology present. In addition, cardiac function and wall motion abnormalities are ascertained.

Once the heart is opened, all components of the valve should be carefully examined. The endocardium around the annulus is inspected for the presence of a "jet lesion," represented by a roughening and thickening of the atrial endocardium from the regurgitant jet. Dilatation of the annulus is principally an increase in the anteroposterior diameter of the valve and may be markedly asymmetric in the inferolateral region after inferior wall myocardial infarction. Leaflet anatomy nomenclature specifies P1, P2, and P3 for the three typical scallops of the posterior leaflet and A1 and A2 for the major sections of the anterior leaflet. Pathologic changes in valve leaflets and subvalvular apparatus are detected by elevating different leaflet sections with a nerve hook. Commissural chordae are seldom elongated, providing a reference point to detect significant chordal elongation. Generally, if leaflet tissue prolapses more than 1 cm above the normal plane of the annulus when gently elongated intraoperatively with a nerve hook, the prolapse is considered significant. This invariably correlates with TEE evidence of significant mitral insufficiency. Periodic distention of the valve leaflets by injecting saline through a bulb syringe into the ventricle to check leaflet coaptation is a valuable technique to assess both valvular pathology and the adequacy of repair.

■ SURGICAL APPROACHES

Median sternotomy with conventional CPB remains the most popular approach in most centers. This technique has been well established for over three decades. CPB is initiated with cannulation of the ascending aorta and bicaval venous drainage. The aorta is cross-clamped, and the heart is arrested with cardioplegic solution given antegrade into the aortic root, or retrograde into the coronary sinus.

The most commonly used technique for exposure of the mitral valve is a left atriotomy, posterior and parallel to the interatrial groove. The mitral valve is exposed by elevating and rotating the septum superiorly and leftward, using self-retaining retractor blades. If this exposure is not optimal, such as in patients with a small left atrium, a deep chest, or an aortic prosthesis in place or in reoperations, alternative incisions such as transseptal, a superior approach through the dome of the left atrium, or the biatrial transseptal approach may be used. Good exposure, with a still, bloodless operative field, is critical for precise mitral valve repair; it permits a systematic, unhurried evaluation of the mitral valve pathology and a step-by-step evaluation of leaflet coaptation as the repair is performed.

Minimally invasive techniques for the surgical treatment of valvular heart disease have proved to be an important advance over the last 8 to 10 years. Beginning in 1994, experimental work performed at Stanford University and at

New York University (NYU) led to the introduction of a minimally invasive technique termed port access. At NYU, arterial cannulation may be achieved peripherally or centrally. Before selecting the cannulation technique, intraoperative TEE is used to evaluate the degree of atheromatous disease in the thoracic aorta and aortic arch. Severe peripheral vascular disease, abdominal aortic aneurysm, or central aortic atherosclerosis is considered relative contraindication to femoral cannulation and retrograde perfusion. Severe peripheral or central aortic atherosclerotic disease was diagnosed in 9.2% of the patients considered for minimally invasive cardiac surgery over 6 years at NYU, thus excluding these patients from approaches requiring peripheral cannulation.

At NYU, the operative incision most often used is a right anterolateral minithoracotomy. Alternative surgical approaches have been suggested such as a minithoracotomy or partial sternotomy incision. At the Cleveland Clinic, a parasternal incision was initially used, but a partial sternotomy approach was subsequently adopted in the majority of patients.

The patient is positioned supine and intubated with a single-lumen endotracheal tube. A 5-cm skin incision is made in the right inframammary groove and the fourth intercostal space is entered. Alternatively, a right third intercostal space incision may be used, with the skin incision above the breast. The third interspace approach allows good access to the ascending aorta for direct arterial cannulation, which is particularly useful in patients with peripheral vascular disease in whom peripheral perfusion may not be desirable. A soft tissue retractor is inserted, and the interspace is gently spread with a retractor. After systemic heparinization, the femoral artery is cannulated through a transverse arteriotomy with an arterial cannula. Alternatively, the ascending aorta may be cannulated directly using an aortic cannula placed through a small miniport in the right anterior second interspace or directly through the right third intercostal incision. The aorta is then occluded internally by a balloon, which is introduced via a side limb of the arterial cannula and positioned in the ascending aorta, or externally by direct cross-clamping.

A long venous cannula is introduced from the femoral vein and positioned in the right atrium under TEE guidance with the distal tip just into the superior vena cava. Vacuum-assisted venous drainage has been extremely important in keeping the heart empty and the field dry. Cardiopulmonary bypass is initiated, and the patient is cooled to 25° to 30°C. Cardioplegia may be administered in an antegrade or retrograde fashion. For retrograde cardioplegia, a transatrial coronary sinus catheter may be placed either directly by the surgeon or percutaneously by the anesthesiologist through an introducer sheath in the right internal jugular vein, with TEE assistance. Fluoroscopy may be used if difficulty is encountered, although it is seldom necessary.

Mitral valve repair can then be performed under direct vision, using standard techniques with specially designed, long-shafted instruments. A knot pusher is often necessary for knot tying.

The use of robotics to enhance minimally invasive surgery is an investigative approach in a few centers. Although this is an exciting use of new operative technology, there is as yet no

evidence that the additional operative time and cost with this procedure provide any enhanced patient outcome compared with a standard minimally invasive technique.

■ RECONSTRUCTIVE TECHNIQUES

Basic techniques of valve reconstruction include the use of an annuloplasty ring, quadrangular resection of the posterior leaflet, chordal transposition, chordal shortening, artificial chordae, and triangular resection for repair of the anterior leaflet. The remodeling ring annuloplasty concept was based on Carpentier's finding that the deformity resulting from mitral insufficiency was dilation of the annulus.

Posterior Leaflet Procedures

Quadrangular resection of the posterior leaflet has become the mainstay of mitral valve reconstruction. Diseased leaflet tissue in the posterior leaflet is excised with a quadrangular excision, usually removing 2 to 4 cm of tissue and, occasionally, over 50% of the posterior leaflet. Strong chordae of proper lengths are identified on each side of the excised leaflet and encircled with retraction sutures. A rectangular excision is performed cutting directly down to the mitral annulus but not excising the annulus. After leaflet excision, the gap of the posterior leaflet is corrected either by annular plication or by folding plasty or combination of both. The folding plasty technique involves folding down the cut vertical edges of the posterior leaflet to the annulus and closing the ensuing cleft (Figures 1A and 1B). With this technique, the central height of the posterior leaflet is reduced, the edge of leaflet coaptation is moved posteriorly, and annular plication is either eliminated or reduced. This elimination of annular plication avoids the serious complication of circumflex artery kinking, which may occur in the setting of a left dominant coronary artery circulation and a large posterior leaflet resection. Although the sliding plasty technique is also

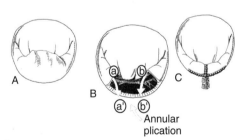

Figure 1a

Posterior symmetric folding plasty to reduce posterior leaflet height and minimize or eliminate posterior annular plication **A,** Large prolapsing posterior mitral leaflet with excessive leaflet height. **B,** Quadrangular resection of prolapsing posterior segment involving most of posterior annulus. Point a is brought to a' and b, to b'. Annular plication is performed between points a' and b'. **C,** Resultant reconstruction of symmetric folding plasty with small posterior annulus plication.

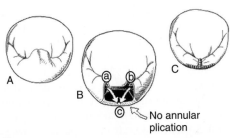

No annular plication

Figure 1b
Posterior symmetric folding plasty to reduce posterior leaflet height and minimize or eliminate posterior annular plication. **A,** Prolapsing posterior mitral leaflet with excessive leaflet height. **B,** Quadrangular resection of prolapsing posterior segment. Points a and b will be brought down to common point c on posterior annulus. Note that no annular plication is required. **C,** Result of symmetric folding plasty with cut edges of posterior leaflet sutured down to annulus and suture closure of posterior "neocleft."

successful in reducing posterior leaflet height in the setting of a "generous" anterior leaflet and also moving the edge of leaflet coaptation posteriorly, it is predicated on a substantial posterior annular placation, which is not always possible or preferable.

Anterior Leaflet Procedures

Reconstruction of the anterior leaflet involves different approaches. Although earlier reports predominantly involved patients with posterior leaflet pathology, it became evident that anterior leaflet pathology was present in approximately one third of the patients. Thus, to more effectively offer valve repair to this complex group of patients with anterior leaflet disease, several innovative approaches were suggested; these include chordal transposition, chordal shortening, artificial chordae replacement, and triangular resection of redundant anterior leaflet tissue. Hence, surgeons have become more confident in offering valve repair to patients with anterior leaflet disease. At NYU, in 374 patients requiring anterior leaflet procedures over the past two decades, repairs included triangular resection (54.1%), chordal shortening (22.2%), chordal resuspension (14.7%), and chordal transposition (9%). The incidence of anterior leaflet repair techniques has varied over this experience, with chordal transfer, shortening, and resuspension being favored for the first half of this period and triangular resection being the preferred procedure for the latter half.

Originally, Carpentier proposed chordal transposition with the free edge of the flail segment of the anterior leaflet resupported by intact chordae taken from the posterior leaflet as the primary method for anterior leaflet repair. Opposite to the diseased segment of anterior leaflet, a quadrangular resection (3 or 4 mm) of the free edge of the posterior leaflet with its supporting chordae is performed. This segment is reattached to the free edge of the anterior leaflet. The defect in the posterior leaflet is then corrected. Additionally, artificial chordae have been successfully used to resupport a prolapsing segment of anterior leaflet with reliable results.

These first two techniques are more rarely used now in our center, in preference to triangular anterior leaflet resection. This alternative method for treating anterior leaflet prolapse involves a triangular resection of the involved segment when there is redundant anterior leaflet tissue as is most often encountered. Adjacent, intact supporting chordae are identified and a triangular resection is then performed between them with the apex of resection positioned in the mid body of the anterior leaflet (Figure 2). This technique not only eliminates the prolapsing or flail segment, but additionally "debulks" the anterior leaflet, which may limit the incidence of postoperative systolic anterior motion.

A new technique—the "double-orifice" or "edge-to-edge" repair—has been proposed by Alfieri as an alternative, simple, option in mitral valve repair of mitral valve insufficiency. While used by many as a "bail-out" procedure for incomplete elimination of regurgitation, the proponents of this technique have advocated its use not only for anterior leaflet pathology but also for complex anatomic lesions, including endocarditis, in patients with impaired left ventricular function, and as adjunct procedure with partial left ventriculectomy in patients with dilated cardiomyopathy.

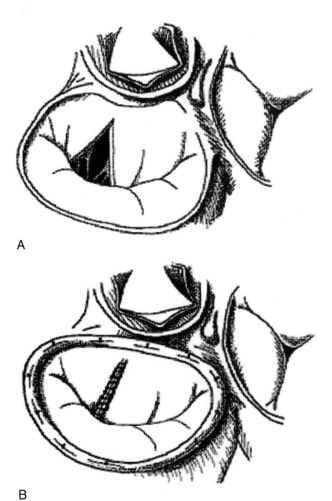

Figure 2
Triangular resection of the anterior mitral leaflet.

Annuloplasty

Prosthetic ring annuloplasty is one of the major steps of valve reconstruction and is mandatory in most cases of mitral valve insufficiency. The basic principle of ring annuloplasty is to restore the shape of the mitral orifice. The device both corrects insufficiency by elevating the posterior annulus and stabilizes the annular repair by reducing the stress on the plication sutures. Although controversy exists regarding the best type of annuloplasty device to use, it is clear that repair without using an annuloplasty device contributes to the incidence of later repair failure. This observation has also been made where autologous tissue was used for annular reinforcement.

Traditional mitral annuloplasty devices include both rigid rings, which maintain fixed annular geometry and restrict annular motion, and soft rings and bands, which can locally deform. The mitral annulus is a dynamic cardiac structure that undergoes alterations in size and shape throughout the cardiac cycle, and it has been suggested that annular motion has an impact on left ventricular function. Contradictory reports exist regarding annular dynamics following annuloplasty.

At NYU we are currently using a semirigid annuloplasty band (Future Band; Medtronic, Minneapolis, MN) designed to provide annular remodeling and physiologic flexibility. Initial clinical results have been excellent in more than 350 patients. Postoperative echocardiographic studies after repair with the semirigid band revealed a significant, physiologic reduction of orifice area (10.2%) and intertrigonal distance (6.3%) during systole. Significantly, the end-systolic anterior–posterior distance decreased by 8.5% compared with end diastole. This is in contrast to experience with earlier devices, which did not allow for reduction of orifice area during the cardiac cycle. Additionally, postoperative echocardiography revealed mean and peak mitral gradients were significantly lower with a semirigid band compared with a rigid ring.

Results of Mitral Reconstruction

Mitral repair provides excellent long-term durability in nonrheumatic patients. Patients with degenerative posterior leaflet pathology have 89% freedom from reoperation for valvular dysfunction at 15 years and 36% freedom from any endocarditis, thromboembolism, or anticoagulant-related complication. Posterior leaflet disease comprises the majority of leaflet disease in degenerative patients. The more challenging procedures are those that involve a predominance of anterior leaflet pathology. Initial outcomes in anterior leaflet repair with a reliance on chordal shortening were suboptimal, with an increased late failure rate. The results using artificial chordae reported by David and others are excellent, and this technique is a viable option for repair of anterior leaflet pathology.

In a recent study from NYU, 374 patients with degenerative etiology (31.3%) had an anterior leaflet repair; they were compared with 821 patients who did not. The techniques used for anterior leaflet repair included chordal transposition in 32 patients, chordal resuspension in 51 patients, chordal shortening in 80 patients, and anterior leaflet resection in 211 patients. The increasing use of anterior leaflet resection by year is illustrated in Figure 3. Interestingly, the late durability after anterior leaflet repair was not influenced by the technique used (chordal shortening, chordal reimplantation, chordal transposition, or anterior leaflet resection). In the patients with anterior leaflet repair, the 5-year survival from late cardiac death was 93%, the 5-year freedom from reoperation was 94%, and the 5-year freedom from valve-related complications was 90%. In the patients without anterior leaflet procedures, the 5-year survival from cardiac death was 91%, the 5-year freedom from reoperation was 92%, and the 5-year freedom from valve-related complications was 91%.

Multiple centers have shown excellent in-hospital results with minimally invasive approaches for mitral reconstruction. The question of compromising exposure with such techniques on long-term repair with such techniques remained. We studied this question by evaluating the early and intermediate-term results of 100 consecutive patients undergoing minimally invasive mitral valve repair with the last 100 patients who had mitral valve repair via sternotomy. The groups were similar in age and ejection fraction. There was a 1.0% hospital mortality with the sternotomy approach and no deaths with the minimally invasive approach. Freedom from any hospital morbidity was 88% for the sternotomy approach group and 91% for the minimally invasive approach group ($p > .05$). Additionally, the cumulative freedom from all valve-related complications and reoperation was not significantly different, and the late improvement in NYHA functional classification was equivalent between the two groups. Echocardiographic follow-up (mean, 33 months) revealed that residual mitral insufficiency was similar in both groups. Subsequent late follow-up studies on the 376 patients undergoing minimally invasive valve repair in the NYU series demonstrated that 5-year results were similar after minimally invasive and conventional mitral valve repair.

Repair for Ischemic Mitral Valve Disease

Of patients with mitral insufficiency, none is more challenging for the surgeon than those with ischemic valvular disease. Whether their ominous prognosis is due to the segmental or global injury of their ventricle or to associated comorbidities, 5-year survival in such patients rarely exceeds 50%. Until recently, it was uncertain whether mitral replacement was preferable due to increased procedural reliability. Controversy was fueled when Cohn reported that mitral reconstruction in ischemic patients was associated with a 5-year mortality 5 times higher than after replacement. It was hypothesized that decreased late survival of the repair patients was due to the high prevalence of annular dilation in the repair cohort, which functioned as a surrogate for poor ventricular function.

In addition to poor ventricular function, the outcome analysis of ischemic repairs was complicated by the heterogeneity of ischemic pathophysiologies. Ischemic etiology can produce annular dilatation, leaflet prolapse or chordal rupture/elongation, and leaflet restriction due to ventricular–papillary muscle displacement. Patients with "functional" mitral insufficiency are a more homogeneous subset of ischemic pathology due to the underlying damage to their ventricles and/or ventricular-papillary muscle units. Similarly, these patients benefit from surgical treatment with a similar procedure: a reduction annuloplasty to correct the insufficiency.

Type of Anterior Leaflet Repair

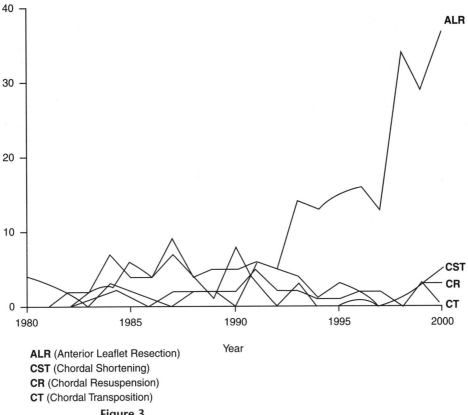

ALR (Anterior Leaflet Resection)
CST (Chordal Shortening)
CR (Chordal Resuspension)
CT (Chordal Transposition)

Figure 3
Type of anterior leaflet procedure by year of operation.

Recent studies have demonstrated that in the majority of patients, there is a survival benefit and superior long-term freedom from valve-related complications with reconstruction. At NYU, our recent review of 223 consecutive mitral valve operations for ischemic mitral insufficiency included 152 mitral valve reconstructions compared with 71 prosthetic mitral valve replacements. Coronary artery bypass graft surgery was performed in 89% of repair and 80% of replacement patients, with a 30-day mortality of 10% and 20%, respectively. This short-term mortality was higher for New York Heart Association functional class IV patients (odds ratio, 5.75; confidence interval, 1.25 to 26.5) and was reduced for patients with angina compared with those without angina (odds ratio, 0.26; confidence interval, 0.05 to 1.2). Repair patients had lower short-term death or complication rates than replacement patients (odds ratio, 0.43; confidence interval, 0.20 to 0.90). Eighty-two percent of repair patients had minimal insufficiency during long-term follow-up. Five-year complication-free survival was significantly superior for repair patients (64% versus 47%). Poor survival outcome was primarily related to preexisting comorbidities and ventricular dysfunction.

The primary reconstructive strategy for these "functional" ischemic patients is remodeling annuloplasty. Our preferred annuloplasty device is the Future Band, which was specially designed to produce annular remodeling in the anterior–posterior dimension. This has proved annular to be extremely important in patients with ischemic mitral insufficiency and in patients with increased left ventricular end-diastolic pressures from other causes. Repair of ischemic insufficiency is performed by inserting a device that is one size smaller than what would normally be dictated by the size of the anterior leaflet. This produces a degree of annular remodeling that reliably eliminates insufficiency due to carpentier Types 1 or 3b pathology and has resulted in excellent late durability after repair of ischemic mitral insufficiency.

■ **SUMMARY**

The excellent results with mitral valve repair that have been reported for more than 20 years have been expanded over the last 5 to 10 years due to important technical advances, such as the advent of minimally invasive techniques, more aggressive and refined techniques for anterior leaflet or bi-leaflet repair, improved results after repair of ischemic mitral insufficiency, and a better understanding of the role and function of annuloplasty devices. These advances have increased the number of candidates suitable for mitral repair, improved the late results, and lowered the morbidity after valve reconstruction. It is important that the practicing surgeon continue to evolve by adopting many of these new concepts into his or her day-to-day practice in order to offer patients the best immediate- and long-term results.

SUGGESTED READING

Galloway AC, et al: A comparison of mitral valve reconstruction with mitral valve replacement: intermediate-term results, *Ann Thorac Surg* 47:655, 1989.

Gillinov AM, et al: Hemisternotomy approach for aortic and mitral valve surgery, *J Card Surg.* 15:15, 2000.

Grossi EA, et al: Ischemic mitral valve reconstruction and replacement: comparison of long-term survival and complications, *J Thorac Cardiovasc Surg* 122:1107, 2001.

Grossi EA, et al: Late results of isolated mitral annuloplasty for "functional" ischemic mitral insufficiency, *J Card Surg* 16:328, 2001.

Grossi EA, et al: Minimally invasive mitral valve surgery: a 6-year experience with 714 patients, *Ann Thorac Surg* 74:660, 2002; discussion 663.

SURGICAL MANAGEMENT OF ENDOCARDITIS

David D. Yuh

■ BACKGROUND

Infective endocarditis generally results from bacterial or fungal seeding of compromised endocardial and valvular surfaces of the heart. Predisposing conditions for development of endocarditis include bacteremia, endothelial or endocardial damage, turbulence, and impaired host defenses. Bacteremia commonly originates from oropharyngeal, gastrointestinal, or genitourinary sources, secondary to active infections (e.g., diverticulitis, urosepsis) or traumatic manipulation (e.g., dental extraction, esophageal dilation). Intracardiac valves and other endocardial structures with damaged endothelial surfaces are vulnerable to infection during even transient bacteremias. Endothelial damage may arise from instrumental trauma, repetitive turbulent blood flow, and native destructive processes (e.g., rheumatic fever, degenerative disease). Turbulent blood flow often imparts shear stresses onto tissue surfaces, resulting in direct endothelial damage or local activation of tissue factors, both of which can result in bacterial seeding and vegetative formation. Finally, immunosuppressed individuals are at a heightened risk for bacteremia not only due to impaired host-defense mechanisms, but also due to long-term indwelling catheters (e.g., dialysis access, central venous lines). Complications from active endocarditis include congestive heart failure (CHF) due to valvular dysfunction, extravalvular extension of the infective process (e.g., abscess), systemic emboli, renal failure, and persistent sepsis.

■ INDICATIONS FOR SURGICAL THERAPY

Surgical intervention for endocarditis generally takes the form of valve replacement or repair, aortic root replacement, and débridement. Absolute indications for surgical treatment include CHF due to valvular dysfunction, peripheral or cerebral embolization, extravalvular extension of the infective process, persistent sepsis, and progressive renal dysfunction.

Congestive Heart Failure

CHF is a common sequela of endocarditis and usually results from severe mitral or aortic valvular insufficiency. In a retrospective review, Mills et al at the University of California San Francisco found that CHF developed in 79 of 144 patients with infective endocarditis within 6 months of admission. CHF was mild and moderate to severe in 40% and 60% of these patients. CHF developed in 80% of patients with aortic insufficiency compared with 50% in patients with mitral insufficiency. A higher proportion of patients with aortic insufficiency (two thirds) developed severe CHF compared with patients with mitral insufficiency (one half). Subjectively, these patients are often hemodynamically stable on initial presentation, but rapidly decompensate shortly thereafter. Most importantly, this and other studies have shown that surgical therapy for endocarditis complicated by severe CHF significantly improves survival over medical management.

Early valve replacement in endocarditis patients with CHF also leads to higher survival rates than with delayed, elective operation. Early operation should be undertaken in patients with endocarditis complicated by CHF, particularly if aortic insufficiency is present. Left ventricular end-diastolic pressure and wall stresses are substantially greater in patients with aortic insufficiency compared with patients with mitral insufficiency because the left ventricle is less compliant than the left atrium. CHF due to mitral insufficiency may be stabilized with medical therapy, including afterload-reducing agents, digoxin, and diuretics, but acute severe aortic insufficiency usually does not respond favorably to these conservative measures.

Peripheral Embolization

Embolic events commonly are observed in endocarditis, occurring in about 30% to 40% of cases, and are usually from vegetations on the infected valve leaflets or annulus. Clinical manifestations of peripheral embolization include Osler's nodes, hematuria from renal infarction, retinal hemorrhage, lung abscesses, and hepatic/splenic abscesses. The relative size and mobility of these vegetations seems to influence the incidence of clinical embolic events. Although there are no distinct embolic size thresholds from which one can predict embolic events accurately, it generally is accepted that vegetations greater than 1 cm in diameter have a propensity to embolize and are refractory to medical therapy. In a retrospective review, Rohmann et al found that patients whose vegetations increased significantly despite appropriate antibiotic therapy (36% of patients) were at higher risk to sustain embolic complications than patients whose vegetations decreased in size (64% of patients). In another review, Vuille et al found that endocarditis patients who were clinically cured but with persistence of a vegetation were not at an increased risk for late embolic complications. Taken together, these observations have led to a general consensus that small asymptomatic vegetations can be treated with antibiotic therapy alone. Large (>1 cm), mobile, symptomatic vegetations or vegetations that increase in size despite appropriate antibiotic therapy warrant surgical intervention.

Cerebral Embolization

Cerebral embolization due to endocarditis deserves special discussion as a subset of peripheral embolization because of the substantial morbidity and mortality associated with its presentation and surgical treatment. Pruitt et al found that central nervous system complications of endocarditis increased the mortality from 20% to 50%. Surgical intervention for endocarditis complicated by cerebral embolization is associated with an increased risk of extending cerebral infarction or converting a bland infarct into a hemorrhagic cerebral infarct due to anticoagulation required for cardiopulmonary bypass. In a retrospective review of 145 endocarditis patients sustaining a cerebral complication who subsequently underwent valve replacement, Eishi et al found that 50% of patients who underwent valve replacement within 24 hours of the cerebral event had an exacerbation or extension of their cerebral complication with 67% mortality. The neurologic exacerbation and mortality rates decreased to 10% and 20% if operative intervention was delayed at least 2 weeks.

The incidence of recurrent cerebral embolization seems to increase with uncontrolled sepsis. Ideally, surgical intervention for endocarditis complicated by central nervous system injury should be performed after sepsis has been controlled with antimicrobials and the neurologic injury has been characterized and stabilized. Early surgical intervention is warranted after cerebral embolization if a large, mobile vegetation has been identified, because additional embolic injury would lead to further neurologic debilitation. It is reasonable to delay valve repair or replacement due to endocarditis for 2 to 3 weeks after a bland cerebral infarct to allow for healing and to minimize further brain injury. After a hemorrhagic brain infarction, surgery should be delayed until sepsis is controlled with a full course of antibiotic therapy and when neurologic stabilization has been achieved.

Extravalvular Extension

Extravalvular extension of endocarditis typically takes the form of an annular abscess. Annular abscesses are much more common with prosthetic valvular endocarditis versus native valvular infection. Generally refractory to medical therapy, extravalvular spread of endocarditis is an indication for early surgical intervention and commonly manifests as structural injury to the interventricular septum, conduction pathways, and fibrous structure of the heart. Other less common manifestations include pseudoaneurysm and rupture producing intracardiac shunt or aortocavitary fistula and coronary artery embolization. In native valve endocarditis, extravalvular extension is associated more commonly with aortic than mitral disease. Transesophageal echocardiography should be performed in endocarditis patients deemed at high risk for extravalvular extension. These patients include those with staphylococcal or fungal endocarditis, prosthetic valvular endocarditis, or new conduction disturbances (i.e., persistent heart block). Several echocardiographic criteria have been established to identify extravalvular extension abscesses accurately: (1) anterior or posterior aortic root wall thickness 10 mm or greater; (2) perivalvular density of 14 mm or greater in the interventricular septum; (3) sinus of Valsalva defect or aneurysm; and (4) prosthetic valve "rocking" motion.

Progressive Renal Dysfunction

Renal failure is a recognized consequence of endocarditis in 5% to 10% of patients and may result from several mechanisms: (1) prerenal failure resulting from CHF, (2) immune complex glomerulonephritis, or (3) renal arterial embolization. Renal failure, particularly immune complex glomerulonephritis, is often a manifestation of persistent sepsis and represents failure of medical therapy. In these cases, prompt surgical eradication of the septic focus is indicated. Useful perioperative measures that should be considered for patients with renal failure secondary to endocarditis include perioperative hemodialysis, modified ultrafiltration for volume-overloaded patients, and use of aprotinin to reduce coagulopathic hemorrhage (i.e., platelet dysfunction).

Sepsis Refractory to Antimicrobial Therapy

Persistent sepsis is defined as failure to clear bacteremia after 3 to 5 days of directed antimicrobial therapy or the lack of a clinical improvement in symptoms after 1 week of antibiotic treatment. Surgical treatment for persistent sepsis secondary to endocarditis is directed toward eradication of the septic focus. Persistent sepsis from endocarditis may result from an antibiotic-resistant organism and intracardiac or extracardiac abscesses (e.g., splenic, renal, hepatic, cerebral). D'Agostino et al at Stanford found that a positive intraoperative valve culture or Gram stain is a strong predictor of adverse late outcome. Of 108 patients with native valve endocarditis, 87 patients with negative intraoperative cultures had a 1-year complication-free survival estimate exceeding 90% compared with less than 70% for 19 patients who had positive intraoperative cultures. Early operation for patients with uncontrolled sepsis is associated with a lower operative mortality.

Identification of the infecting organism is an important component of endocarditis therapy. α-Hemolytic or group D streptococcus and *Staphylococcus aureus* are the most common organisms identified in native valve endocarditis, whereas gram-negative and fungal infections are identified less frequently. *S. aureus* endocarditis deserves special mention because of its aggressive and destructive characteristics. Severe tissue necrosis and annular abscesses leading to rapidly progressive CHF and failure of medical therapy are seen commonly with this organism and should prompt consideration of expedient surgical intervention. Fungal endocarditis is an absolute indication for surgical therapy because of the dismal clinical response to antifungal agents. In contrast, streptococcal native valve endocarditis is usually responsive to medical therapy; cure rates exceed 90%. Regardless of the offending organism, there is a substantial risk of recurrent endocarditis after valve repair or replacement in active endocarditis. Alsip et al showed that the risk for developing prosthetic valve endocarditis after valve replacement for active native endocarditis is about 10% and has a mortality rate of 50%.

Prosthetic valve endocarditis generally is thought to be due to contamination at the time of surgery or subsequent infection in the setting of persistent bacteremia or fungemia. Infection often originates on the prosthetic sewing ring or, in the case of bioprosthetic valves, the valve leaflets. Sewing ring infections predispose to annular abscess formation. Annular abscesses and leaflet infections appear less common with homografts. Mechanical or bioprosthetic valvular endocarditis involving the sewing ring or annulus mandates valve rereplacement; early surgical intervention is associated with better survival. Reoperation should be undertaken when there is echocardiographic evidence of valvular dysfunction, large vegetations, or annular extension. Limited infections of bioprosthetic valve leaflets, particularly by streptococci, can often be treated successfully with antibiotics alone as long as valve function is preserved.

■ OPERATIVE TECHNIQUES FOR ENDOCARDITIS

Patient Evaluation and Preoperative Preparation

Echocardiography is the primary diagnostic mode for detecting and characterizing endocarditis. Transthoracic echocardiography is an excellent screening examination, but transesophageal echocardiography affords a more thorough evaluation of the intracardiac structures commonly affected by endocarditis. When a commitment to surgical intervention

has been made, hemodynamic optimization should be pursued expeditiously. When a diagnosis of endocarditis has been made by echocardiography, few, if any, other diagnostic tests are required. Coronary angiography should be reserved for patients with clinical evidence of ischemic heart disease or for older patients (> 50 years old) with strong risk factors for coronary artery disease.

Mitral Valve Endocarditis

For operations on the mitral valve, bicaval venous drainage and a pulmonary artery vent are recommended to minimize systemic venous and bronchial blood return to the right and left atria during cardiopulmonary bypass. As with any potentially prolonged, complex cardiac operation, myocardial protection is crucial. Protective measures include moderate systemic cooling to 28°C to 30°C, topical myocardial cooling (Daly cooling jacket or continuous application of topical cold saline), and intermittent antegrade or retrograde cold blood cardioplegia. Aminocaproic acid (Amicar) or, in cases of renal or hepatic dysfunction, aprotinin is recommended to reduce postoperative coagulopathy. Optimal mitral valve exposure can be challenging, but the use of a self-retaining retractor and one of several different left atrial incisions usually can afford adequate exposure. These incisions include the standard horizontal left atriotomy just anterior to the right superior and inferior pulmonary veins, an extended horizontal transseptal approach, Khonsari's biatrial transseptal approach, and Guiraudon's vertical biatriotomy; the latter three approaches are particularly well suited for the small left atrium.

The extended transseptal approach involves a right atriotomy made parallel to Sondergaard's groove followed by a transverse incision into the fossa ovalis and onto the roof of the left atrium. Khonsari's approach involves two parallel oblique incisions originating from the right superior pulmonary vein and taken inferiorly and to the left: The ventralmost incision crosses the right atrial free wall, whereas the deeper incision opens the interatrial septum. In Guiraudon's approach, a vertical right atriotomy is extended superiorly across the sulcus terminalis and across the left atrial dome; the interatrial septum also is opened.

Mitral valve repair, when technically feasible, is a preferred approach for native valve endocarditis. Generally, more than 50% of the valve tissue must be spared from destruction to permit repair. First, thorough débridement of all infected tissue must be performed, leaving a 2-mm margin of normal valvular tissue with the specimen. Depending on the remaining defect, valve repair may consist of patch closure of leaflet perforations, quadrangular resection and repair of posterior leaflet perforations, and chordal transposition. Defects in the anterior mitral valve leaflet can be repaired with a patch of autologous pericardium (Figure 1); excessive fixation of the pericardium with glutaraldehyde may render the patch too stiff for the otherwise pliable valve leaflet and should be avoided. Quadrangular resection of infected portions of the posterior mitral valve leaflet can be performed in a manner similar to repairs for myxomatous disease. After the specimen has been resected, 2-0 Ethibond sutures with autologous pericardial pledgets can be used to plicate the posterior annulus, and the leading edges of the remaining posterior leaflet are reapproximated with a 4-0 polypropylene suture.

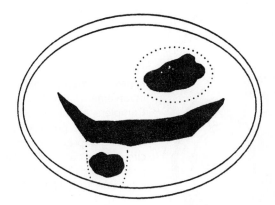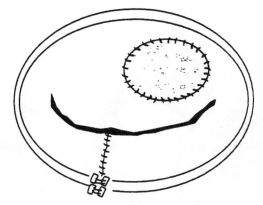

Figure 1
Repair of mitral valve leaflets. After complete débridement, posterior leaflet defects can be repaired via a quadrangular resection. Anterior defects can be closed with a pericardial patch. *(From Moon MR, et al:* Prog Cardiovas Dis *40:239, 1997.)*

If preexistent degenerative mitral disease or annular dilation is evident at the time of repair, annuloplasty of the posterior annulus can be performed with a strip of fixed autologous or bovine pericardium. Alternatively a prosthetic annuloplasty ring can be used, but in the setting of active infection avoidance of prosthetic materials is prudent. Infected primary chordae tendineae can be replaced by chordal transposition from the posterior leaflet or transposing secondary chordae to the leaflet free edge. Alternatively, Gore-Tex sutures can be used as substitutes for damaged but functionally critical chordae.

In the case of a critically ill, unstable patient or in the face of nonrepairable damage to the mitral valve, prosthetic mitral valve replacement should be performed expediently. A chordal-sparing approach should be taken, as with standard mitral valve replacement for degenerative disease, but thorough débridement of infected tissue should not be compromised. In general, the choice between a mechanical and bioprosthetic valve should be made according to the usual criteria, including age, risk of bleeding during long-term anticoagulation, patient preference and reliability, and coexistent disease (e.g., renal failure, hypercalcemia).

Small annular abscesses (<5 mm) often can be unroofed, débrided, and left open or primarily closed (Figure 2). Larger residual defects can be repaired with a pericardial buttressing strip. Extensive annular defects should be reconstructed using a large pericardial strip secured to a healthy rim of left ventricular endocardium using continuous 4-0 polypropylene suture (Figure 3). The valve sutures are placed through the pericardial patch. Rarely, intraatrial placement of a mitral valve prosthesis is required for extensive mitral annular destruction. In the so-called top-hat technique, a Dacron collar is attached to the prosthetic sewing ring, which is secured to the left atrial wall above the level of the native annulus (Figure 4).

Aortic Valve Endocarditis

The operative approach for aortic valve endocarditis is similar to that for mitral endocarditis. Alternatively a single two-stage cannula can be used for venous drainage. After an oblique aortotomy has been performed and the aortic valve and root inspected, thorough débridement of all infected tissue must be performed. Small abscess cavities can be débrided and left open. Larger abscess cavities or contiguous small cavities generally require patch repair with autologous pericardium or glutaraldehyde-fixed bovine pericardium. If less than 50% of the aortic annulus is involved with infection, a prosthetic valve can be inserted after annular débridement and repair. If more than 50% of the annulus has been damaged, however, formal aortic root replacement is recommended. It is widely held that homograft root replacement is less prone to recurrent endocarditis than root replacement with composite valve grafts. Alternatively the Ross procedure has been described as a surgical option for aortic valve endocarditis under optimal circumstances.

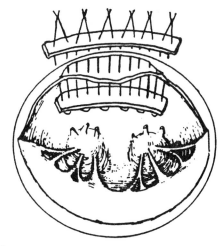

Figure 2
Repair of small mitral annular abscesses. After complete débridement, small mitral annular abscess cavities (<5 mm) can be repaired with a pericardial buttressing strip. *(From Moon MR, et al:* Prog Cardiovas Dis *40:239, 1997.)*

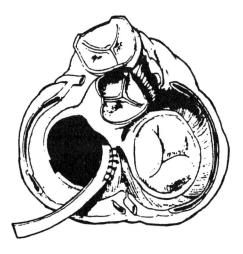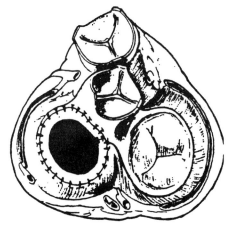

Figure 3
Repair of extensive mitral annular involvement with endocarditis. Complete mitral annular replacement may be performed by constructing a pseudoannulus with a circumferential pericardial strip. *(From David TE, et al: J Thorac Cardiovas Surg 110:1323, 1995.)*

Tricuspid Valve Endocarditis

Tricuspid endocarditis is observed most commonly in cases of intravenous drug use. *S. aureus* is the most common infecting agent, although polymicrobial sepsis is common. For isolated tricuspid valve disease, operative intervention is indicated for functional cardiopulmonary impairment or persistent bacteremia beyond 2 weeks of antimicrobial therapy. Fever, leukocytosis, and pulmonary emboli alone are not indications for operation. Operative options for tricuspid endocarditis include valve excision, repair, and replacement.

Complete tricuspid valve excision is reserved for critically ill, unstable patients. Valve excision removes all infected tissue and can be performed quickly in a beating heart. A substantial portion of these patients eventually develop CHF and require valve replacement. Some surgeons believe that tricuspid valve replacement generally requires a bioprosthesis because there is a higher incidence of valve thrombosis associated with mechanical valve prostheses in the tricuspid position. Many surgeons hesitate to place a bioprosthetic tricuspid valve in intravenous drug addicts because resumption of their drug habit generally leads to death from recurrent endocarditis or other drug-related causes. Early experience with tricuspid valve repair for endocarditis has shown promising results. With valve repair, competence is restored at least partially without prosthetic material. Repair of the anterior leaflet is crucial to a successful repair. Small perforations in the anterior leaflet can be repaired primarily. Tricuspid annuloplasty (e.g., DeVega annuloplasty) can be performed without prosthetic material to establish valve competence.

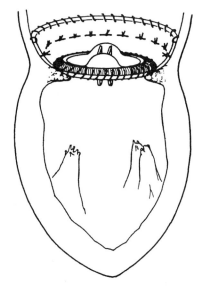

Figure 4
"Top-hat" technique for intraatrial mitral valve replacement. For extensive mitral annular destruction, a mitral prosthesis can be anchored to the left atrial wall in a supraannular position using a Dacron gusset. *(From Moon MR, et al: Prog Cardiovas Dis 40:239, 1997.)*

■ POSTOPERATIVE CONSIDERATIONS AND RESULTS

It generally is recommended that after surgical intervention for native valve endocarditis, directed intravenous antimicrobial therapy be continued. If intraoperative cultures prove negative after a full preoperative course of antibiotics, only 1 week of postoperative antibiotics is recommended. If a full preoperative course of antibiotics was not given and the intraoperative cultures are negative, the full 4- to 6-week course of antibiotics should be completed. Positive intraoperative cultures mandate an additional 4- to 6-week course of intravenous antibiotics postoperatively, regardless of preoperative antibiotic therapy. A similar postoperative course of intravenous antibiotic therapy is recommended in cases of prosthetic valve endocarditis.

Postoperative hospital mortality varies between 5% and 20%. Risk factors for mortality include perivalvular infection, staphylococcal infection, renal failure, multisystem organ failure, preoperative neurologic injury, and preoperative cardiogenic shock. There is a higher incidence of perivalvular leak for valve replacement in endocarditis (3% to 7%).

SUGGESTED READING

D'Agostino RS, et al: Valve replacement in patients with native valve endocarditis: what really determines operative outcome? *Ann Thorac Surg* 40:429, 1985.

Mills J, et al: Heart failure in infective endocarditis: predisposing factors, course, and treatment, *Chest* 66:151, 1974.

Moon MR, et al: Surgical treatment of endocarditis, *Prog Cardiovas Dis* 40:239, 1997.

Oswalt JD, et al: Highlights of a ten-year experience with the Ross procedure, *Ann Thorac Surg* 71(5 Suppl):S332, 2001.

Stinson EB: Surgical treatment of infective endocarditis, *Prog Cardiovasc Dis* 22:145, 1979.

TRICUSPID VALVE OPERATIONS

Duke Cameron

Luca A. Vricella

Sometimes called the "forgotten valve" and a "second-class structure" in cardiac surgery, the tricuspid valve is nonetheless a vital participant in normal cardiovascular function; it can be a potential source of considerable morbidity and mortality, both when it is the primary site of disease and when it is secondarily involved in left heart or pulmonary vascular disease ("functional tricuspid insufficiency"). As with the mitral valve, a thorough understanding of its anatomy and function is critical to successful surgical management.

■ ANATOMY

The three leaflets (Figure 1) are the *septal*, which is semicircular in shape, abuts the fibrous skeleton of the heart, and thus cannot dilate or stretch; the *anterior*, which is the largest and nearly quadrangular; and the *posterior*, which is usually the smallest, somewhat triangular, and rightward and lateral when the valve is inspected from within the right atrium. The valve resembles an inverted mitral valve, except that the septal leaflet is much smaller than the mitral valve septal (anterior) leaflet, and of course, there are three rather than two leaflets. The tricuspid valve is usually 2 to 3 mm larger than the mitral valve and has papillary muscle and chordal attachments to the ventricular septum, which the mitral

Figure 1
Surgical anatomy of tricuspid valve. *(From Doty DB: Cardiac surgery: operative technique, St Louis, 1997, Mosby, p 271.)*

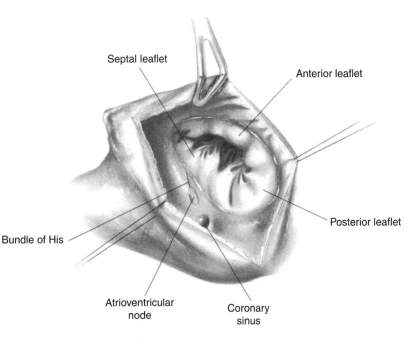

valve does not. Of particular surgical significance, the conduction system, in particular the atrioventricular node, lies just posterior to the commissure between the septal and anterior leaflets and is vulnerable to injury when sutures are passed through the annulus in the medial half of the septal leaflet. Also, just as the circumflex coronary artery is at risk lying in the atrioventricular groove on the left side of the heart, so is the right coronary artery vulnerable on the right side, particularly during suture placement near the annuli of the posterior leaflet.

ETIOLOGY

Tricuspid valve dysfunction is usually the result of annular dilatation and poor central coaptation of the leaflets with subsequent insufficiency. Less commonly, the leaflets themselves may be involved primarily by processes such as rheumatic fever, endocarditis, or scarring from carcinoid heart disease. Injury from previous congenital heart surgery, chest trauma, or indwelling pacemaker leads can also lead to a mixed pattern of regurgitation and stenosis. Many young adults who underwent repair of membranous or malignant ventricular septal defects in childhood have tricuspid regurgitation due to distortion of the anteroseptal commissure and subsequent annular dilatation from chronic right ventricular volume overload. Atrioventricular septal defect ("AV canal") repairs may also leave the tricuspid valve regurgitant, which usually progresses over the years. Some diet drugs ("phen-fen") and methysergide derivatives may cause a carcinoid-like valvulopathy.

CLINICAL MANIFESTATIONS

Tricuspid disease is usually evident as jugular venous distention, hepatic congestion, ascites, and peripheral edema. Frequently, the associated left heart valvar lesions such as mitral stenosis or regurgitation tend to dominate the clinical picture. Isolated tricuspid disease may also present as effort intolerance or dyspnea; the mechanism is limited cardiac output rather than pulmonary venous congestion. Longstanding tricuspid disease usually leads to severe atrial distention and atrial fibrillation. Some patients with chronic severe tricuspid disease may present with advanced liver disease from chronic congestion ("cardiac cirrhosis"); their hepatic dysfunction and coagulopathy in this setting present a significant surgical challenge and high operative morbidity.

DIAGNOSIS

The diagnosis is most often confirmed by transthoracic echocardiography, which provides additional important information such as mechanism of tricuspid regurgitation (TR) (annular dilatation, poor leaflet coaptation, destroyed or perforated leaflets), right ventricular dysfunction, concomitant mitral and/or aortic valve disease, and pulmonary hypertension. Cardiac catheterization is rarely required to establish or confirm tricuspid disease but is still useful for assessment of pulmonary artery pressure, left heart hemodynamics, and coronary artery disease. In some situations, transesophageal echocardiography (TEE) may be necessary for optimal preoperative imaging of the tricuspid valve, but this is unusual. TEE has become a standard intraoperative tool for valve surgery and, despite its limitations, provides the best intraoperative assessment of results of repair.

INDICATIONS FOR SURGERY

In primary tricuspid valve disease, surgery should be considered for medically refractory right heart failure, imminent or existing atrial fibrillation, or progressive right ventricular dilatation and dysfunction. More often, the decision is whether to address moderate or severe tricuspid disease during surgery for mitral or aortic valve disease. Persistent sepsis with large vegetations posing embolic risk constitute another indication, seen most often in intravenous substance abusers.

SURGICAL TREATMENT

The vast majority of tricuspid operations are repairs for secondary (functional) tricuspid insufficiency. The decision to repair or replace the tricuspid valve depends on the degree of leaflet and chordal destruction or distortion, as a dilated annulus is nearly always treatable with reduction techniques.

Repair

Rheumatic tricuspid stenosis is now a rare condition. It is amenable to commissurotomy if the leaflets have preserved pliability; commissurotomy can be combined with reduction annuloplasty if there is concomitant regurgitation. Endocarditic perforations can be treated by débridement and pericardial patch repair or by exclusion of a large portion of the affected leaflet by annular plication, with or without a reduction annuloplasty ring, band, or suture.

The most common operations do not involve leaflet or chordal manipulation but rather reduce the circumference of the annulus associated with the anterior and posterior leaflets. The annulus of the septal leaflet is part of the fibrous skeleton of the heart and neither stretches nor is amenable to reduction. The simplest method of annular reduction is a double-layer purse-string of polypropylene with pledgets at each end (Figure 2), known as a DeVega annuloplasty. The purse-string can be tightened around a plastic valve sizer or obturator, usually of 26 to 30 mm; a rule of thumb is to make the tricuspid one size smaller than the mitral prosthesis. It is difficult to create tricuspid stenosis as long as the annular diameter is greater than 25 mm. Localized plication of the posterior leaflet annulus (Kay annuloplasty) is sometimes used but runs a greater risk of kinking the right coronary artery.

Because pulmonary artery (and hence right ventricular) pressure are frequently elevated in TR, many surgeons now recommend routine use of an annuloplasty band or ring to stabilize the repair. Several prostheses of varying flexibility are available; most leave a gap in the region of the atrioventricular node to discourage suture placement that could create

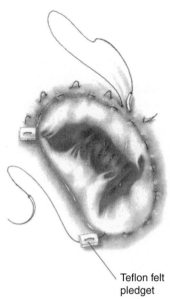

Teflon felt
pledget

Figure 2
DeVega tricuspid anuloplasty. (*From Doty DB:* Cardiac surgery:
operative technique, *St Louis, 1997, Mosby, p 273.*)

heart block. These rings or bands should be secured with
interrupted mattress sutures carefully placed in the annulus,
which is often thinner and more friable than the mitral
annulus.

Replacement

Replacement of the tricuspid valve is rarely indicated,
because repair techniques are generally successful, and even
moderate tricuspid regurgitation is well tolerated in the
absence of pulmonary hypertension or severe right ventricular dysfunction. The usual scenarios for tricuspid replacement include carcinoid heart disease, marked leaflet
destruction by endocarditis, Ebstein's malformation, or
severe right ventricular dilatation and dysfunction (Figure 3).

As with repair, tricuspid valve replacement can be done in
the beating, warm heart using bicaval cannulation and
snares on the cavae. Right anterior thoracotomy can provide
good exposure and may be preferable in reoperations, particularly if there are patent left-sided coronary artery bypass
grafts. If a beating heart technique is used, venting of the left
heart may still be advisable to prevent ventricular ejection,
and early inspection of the atrial septum for identification
and closure of a patent foramen ovale or atrial septal defect
is important to prevent paradoxical air embolism. Our preference is to perform the procedure during cardioplegic
arrest of the heart, as current methods of myocardial protection allow more than enough time for these relatively short
procedures, even when they are combined with aortic and
mitral surgery; the quiet heart remains the ideal setting for
precise suture placement. The key technical step in tricuspid
valve replacement is avoidance of the conduction when placing sutures along the medial half of the septal leaflet. In this
region, the septal leaflet should be preserved, folded onto
itself, and used to secure interrupted mattress sutures, placed
either from below upward or in an everting technique, and
then through the prosthetic sewing ring.

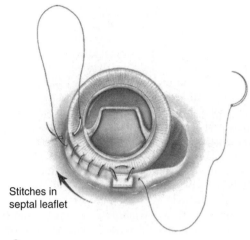

Stitches in
septal leaflet

Figure 3
Technique for tricuspid valve replacement. (*From Doty DB:*
Cardiac surgery: operative technique, *St Louis, 1997, Mosby,
p 275.*)

Many surgeons advocate routine placement of epicardial
ventricular pacing leads, as heart block may occur in about
5% of patients and even more late postoperatively. A tricuspid prosthesis makes transvenous pacing problematic
(bioprostheses) or impossible (mechanical valves). The rate
of heart block is twice as high (10%) when the mitral valve
is replaced concomitantly, and doubles again by 10 years
after surgery. Retention of the native valve tissue should
follow the same principles as with mitral prostheses: leaflet
tissue that could interfere with closing of mechanical valve
leaflets should be excised. Also, a large billowing anterior
leaflet may obstruct the right ventricular outflow tract if left
in place when stented bioprostheses are used.

The decision of whether a bioprosthesis or mechanical
valve should be placed must be individualized. Bioprostheses
do not require long-term anticoagulation and have a very
low incidence of endocarditis and thromboembolism. Their
shortcoming is limited durability, especially in young
patients (< 35 to 40 years), although durability is significantly
better than similar-sized prostheses in the mitral position.

A common misconception is that mechanical valves perform poorly in the tricuspid position, but this is not supported by current literature and contemporary prostheses.
Reoperations for degenerated bioprostheses have a low,
acceptable mortality rate, and may be facilitated by right
anterior thoracotomy approach when sternotomy was used
at the first operation.

■ RESULTS

Meaningful interpretation of the results of tricuspid valve
surgery is difficult because of the heterogeneity of the
patient population and frequent association of tricuspid disease with other diseases that are stronger determinants of
survival, such as endocarditis from intravenous drug abuse
or severe pulmonary hypertension. Isolated primary tricuspid repair in general carries a low operative risk (< 5% operative mortality rate), whereas the other end of the spectrum,

namely reoperative tricuspid valve surgery in conjunction with mitral and/or aortic valve surgery, may impart a risk exceeding 20% to 30%. Ebstein's anomaly, discussed elsewhere in this text, is often associated with varying degrees of right ventricular dysplasia and dysfunction, left ventricular dysfunction, and arrhythmia; repair in this setting has significant operative risk, particularly in younger patients.

Patients who undergo a successful repair have a 70% to 80% chance of freedom from significant residual TR 6 to 10 years postoperatively. Risk factors for late recurrence include omission of a stabilizing annuloplasty band or ring, progressive mitral disease, or persistent pulmonary hypertension. Early mortality rate after tricuspid valve replacement is approximately 5%. In a large series of patients, late survival rate was 70% at 5 years, 45% at 10 years, and 13% at 20 years. There was no difference in late survival between repair and replacement groups.

■ CONCLUSIONS

Most surgical tricuspid disease is functional TR in the setting of mitral or aortic disease. Severe TR is not a benign clinical condition because of its effect on right ventricular function,

atrial rhythm, and system venous congestion. Repair is usually possible by annuloplasty techniques, preferably with a ring or band to reduce and stabilize the annular diameter. Long-term results are good. Valve replacement is occasionally necessary when there is irreparable leaflet destruction; either mechanical or biologic prostheses can be used. Special consideration should be given to placing pacemaker leads at the time of tricuspid valve replacement because of a significant incidence of early and late heart block.

■ SUGGESTED READING

Abe T, et al: DeVega's annuloplasty for acquired tricuspid disease: early and late results in 110 patients, *Ann Thorac Surg* 48:670, 1989.

Carpentier A, et al: Surgical management of acquired tricuspid valve disease, *J Thorac Cardiovasc Surg* 67:53, 1974.

Duran CMG, et al: Is tricuspid valve repair necessary? *J Thorac Cardiovasc Surg* 80:849, 1980.

McGrath LB, et al: Tricuspid valve operations in 530 patients: twenty-five year assessment of early and late phase events, *J Thorac Cardiovasc Surg* 99:124, 1990.

Scully HE, Armstrong CS: Tricuspid valve replacement. Fifteen years of experience with mechanical prostheses and bioprostheses, *J Thorac Cardiovasc Surg* 109:1035, 1995.

PROSTHETIC VALVE ENDOCARDITIS

Christopher J. Knott-Craig
Timothy H. Trotter

Prosthetic valve endocarditis (PVE) demands an aggressive management strategy and optimal timing of surgical reoperation. PVE is a significant challenge to most cardiothoracic surgeons and is the most common reason surgeons refer patients to a "more experienced center" for treatment. In the UK Heart Valve registry for patients with PVE, 30-day mortality was 20%, and freedom from reoperation or death at 1, 5, and 10 years was 61%, 50%, and 34%. There is a persistent excess mortality associated with endocarditis that is 40 times the mortality rate for the general population at 1 year and more than double the mortality rate for the general population 10 to 12 years after the diagnosis. The incidence of PVE is estimated at 0.5% per patient-year for mitral valves and 1% per patient-year for other valves. Recurrent PVE

rates are reported at about 3% per patient-year. The symptoms of PVE can be protean. The diagnosis is based most often on strong clinical suspicion associated with fever, echocardiographic evidence of prosthetic valvular dysfunction, recent-onset heart failure, and new cardiac murmurs.

■ EARLY AND LATE PVE

PVE is classified practically into early-onset PVE and late-onset PVE. Reasons for this distinction include different management algorithms, pathogens, and prognosis. Early PVE occurs within 6 months of the prosthetic valve replacement (often within 60 days) and results from contamination of the prosthetic valve during the perioperative period, often at the time of operation, from a breach in sterile technique. Methicillin-resistant *Staphylococcus epidermidis,* diphtheroids, fungi, and gram-negative organisms are frequent pathogens in early PVE. The onset of early PVE peaks around 2 months postoperatively and decreases to a nearly constant rate at 6 months. The pathologic process is usually more fulminating, is much less likely to be treated successfully medically, and is associated with significantly higher mortality. Late PVE usually occurs beyond 1 year of operation. Late PVE results from bacteremia from a host of possible sources, including dental procedures, surgical procedures, gastrointestinal endoscopy, de novo infections, or drug abuse. The spectrum of organisms recovered in late PVE resembles that of native valve endocarditis. These most often are streptococci, enterococci, and *Staphylococcus aureus*. When *S. epidermidis* is cultured, it is usually methicillin sensitive; this generally translates to a less virulent clinical course, a better chance of early blood sterilization, and a better prognosis.

■ PREOPERATIVE EVALUATION AND TREATMENT

Preoperative evaluation of patients with PVE includes blood cultures and echocardiography. Use of coronary angiography usually is limited to patients older than age 40 or patients who have symptoms of coronary insufficiency. Preoperative computed tomography of the head cannot be overemphasized in the unconscious or focally impaired patient. Liberal use of abdominal computed tomography is encouraged to identify embolic abscesses to abdominal organs, such as the spleen or liver, because these infections potentially may reinfect the newly replaced valve.

Although the presence of PVE per se has been considered an indication for surgery, some patients may be able to be treated safely by medical management alone. Patients with nonstaphylococcal PVE, without evidence of significant left heart failure, and without echocardiographic evidence of annular abscess or significant vegetations (>1 cm, or pedunculated) in whom the blood is sterilized easily (within 72 hours) may be managed with antibiotics alone without an increase in the rate of reinfection, reoperation, or death. This is particularly relevant when the infected valve is a bioprosthesis, rather than a mechanical prosthesis. These patients need weekly surveillance echocardiograms to identify early extension of the disease process.

The decision to reoperate for PVE is influenced by the following factors: (1) the valve involved, (2) the extent of the infection, (3) the organism involved, and (4) patient comorbidity. Timing of surgical intervention is affected by the same factors and by the clinical course of the patient. Dedication to a prolonged course of antibiotic therapy in the face of clinical status deterioration is ill advised. PVE involving the tricuspid and pulmonary valves generally is treated conservatively unless there is extension of the pathologic process, recurrent pulmonary emboli, or relapse of infection. When the aortic valve prosthesis is involved, there should be a low threshold to operate early, particularly if there is significant aortic incompetence or extension of the infection or arrhythmias. PVE involving the mitral valve is best treated medically initially, particularly when bioprostheses are involved. Surgical intervention often can be avoided, unless structural deterioration of the valve has occurred.

The presence of congestive heart failure makes nonoperative therapy unlikely to succeed. Similarly, extension of the infective process into the annular structure of the heart makes prolonged medical management ill advised. Staphylococcus, fungus, and other organisms resistant to antibiotics make surgical intervention more urgent. Delaying surgery to administer antibiotics does not lessen the rate of reinfection of the prosthesis and may increase surgical risk. Indications for operation in the presence of PVE are shown in Table 1.

Neurologic dysfunction occurs in 40% of patients with endocarditis. Embolic cerebrovascular accident is the most

Table 1 Prosthetic Valve Endocarditis: Indications for Operation

Ongoing bacteremia (>72 hr) despite adequate antibiotic treatment
Large (>1 cm) or pedunculated vegetations
Congestive heart failure
Staphylococcal or fungal endocarditis
Early postoperative prosthetic valve endocarditis
Extravalvular extension
Arterial embolization

common complication in these patients. The presence of neurologic deficit significantly increases the mortality from endocarditis. A focal deficit is associated with a 22% mortality rate, whereas nonfocal findings have a 60% mortality rate. Cerebral mycotic aneurysms can occur in 1% to 12% and have an incidence of rupture of about 10%. Nearly half of mycotic aneurysms resolve with simple antibiotic therapy. Delay of surgery in the face of an acute cerebrovascular accident seems prudent, but early surgery may be required to avoid additional emboli. In patients with initially "bland" cerebral infarcts, the risk of extension of the infarct decreases to 10% at 2 weeks and 2% at 4 weeks. After an acute focal neurologic injury, we recommend waiting 7 to 10 days before operative intervention. Antibiotics remain the primary treatment for PVE. Specific agents and usual duration are listed in Table 2.

■ OPERATIVE MANAGEMENT

The approach to PVE at the University of Oklahoma has been an aggressive one in which patients are treated initially with antibiotics if clinically stable and free of heart failure, followed by surgical intervention.

General Considerations

Several special considerations regarding the surgery for PVE warrant mention. We believe it is important to maintain a high hematocrit (>28 to 30) throughout cardiopulmonary bypass and to maintain normal oncotic pressure by adding albumin to the perfusate. This allows ultrafiltration throughout bypass, decreases edema at the conclusion of operation, and improves tissue perfusion during and after operation. We usually use aprotinin and maintain a pump flow of at least 2.4 liters/min/m², adjusting systemic resistance to maintain mean blood pressure equal to the patient's age. We believe this practice minimizes the risk of new or recurrent brain injury, ensures good organ perfusion, and improves overall outcome. We usually do not cool to less than 30°C on cardiopulmonary bypass and usually perfuse the heart in a retrograde fashion continuously with cold blood during the cross-clamp period, essentially eliminating cardiac ischemia.

The use of warfarin (Coumadin) postoperatively in endocarditis patients has been associated with increased mortality due to neurologic events. Aspirin may decrease the incidence of cerebral emboli and hasten dissolution of vegetations. We do not recommend routine anticoagulation

Table 2 Antibiotic Treatment of Infective Endocarditis by Organism

DISEASE	ORGANISM	AGENT	DOSE	DURATION
Prosthetic valve endocarditis, empirical therapy				
Early (<6 mo postoperatively)	*Staphylococcus epidermidis, Staphylococcus aureus*	Vancomycin +	15 mg/kg IV q 12 hr	Early surgery
		Gentamicin +	1 mg/kg IV q 8 hr	
		Rifampin	600 mg orally q day	
Late (>6 mo postoperatively)	*S. epidermidis, Streptococcus viridans, Enterococcus, S. aureus*	Same as above		Same as above
Prosthetic valve endocarditis, positive cultures	*S. epidermidis*	Vancomycin +	15 mg/kg IV q 12 hr	6 wk
		Rifampin +	600 mg orally q day	6 wk
		Gentamicin	1 mg/kg IV q 8 hr	14 days
	S. aureus	Methicillin-sensitive:		
		Nafcillin +	2 g IV q 4 hr	6 wk
		Rifampin +	600 mg orally q day	6 wk
		Gentamicin	1 mg/kg IV q 8 hr	14 days
		MRSA:		
		Vancomycin +	1 g IV q 12 hr	6 wk
		Rifampin +	600 mg orally q day	6 wk
		Gentamicin	1 mg/kg IV q 8 hr	14 days
	S. viridans	As above		
	Streptococcus pneumoniae	Penicillin G	18-20 million U IV q day	4-6 wk
	Enterobacteriaceae	Aminoglycoside + Third- or fourth- generation cephalosporin		
	Proteus mirabilis	Gentamicin +	1 mg/kg IV q 8 hr	4-6 wk
		Ampicillin	1-2 g IV q 6 hr	4-6 wk
	Aspergillus	Amphotericin B +		
		Fluconazole	400 mg orally q day	
	Candida	Amphotericin B +	1-3 g preoperatively	?Lifetime
		Fluconazole	400 mg orally q day	?Lifetime

MRSA, methicillin-resistant *S. aureus. From Gilbert DN et al: Sanford guide to antimicrobial therapy, Hyde Park, VT, 2001, Antimicrobial Therapy, Inc.*

unless a mechanical valve is used, or unless other indications for anticoagulation exist. We initially maintain an international normalized ratio of 2.0 to 2.5.

Aortic Valve PVE

Our prosthesis of choice for aortic valve PVE is the cryopreserved aortic homograft implanted as a freestanding root. If there is minimal annular involvement and the patient is young, we use the pulmonary autograft operation (Ross operation). Homografts and autografts have a lower risk of early recurrent PVE, and there seems to be little difference in outcome 5 to 8 years after operation. The aortic homograft has excellent hemodynamic performance; is resistant to infection; and provides additional tissue with which the aortic root, the interventricular septum, and the mitral valve may be reconstructed. It is particularly helpful to use the homograft anterior mitral valve leaflet to reconstruct the roof of the left atrium, mitral valve annulus, or VSD. The muscular cuff attached to the homograft is not removed; its presence allows débrided areas to be "filled" and

improves hemostasis. The ability of the aortic homograft to replace the aortic root completely facilitates complete débridement of all infected tissues and minimizes difficulty of reconstruction. We believe that aggressive débridement of the infected tissue is responsible for our low rate of recurrent PVE. Hospital mortality is about 10%. In our experience, actuarial survival at 5 years was 88% for the Ross operation and 69% for homografts. Recurrent PVE occurred in 3% of the patients who underwent either Ross or homograft operations.

Implantation of the aortic homograft is undertaken after complete débridement of all infected tissues. The proximal suture line of the homograft is constructed with either interrupted or continuous 4-0 polypropylene suture. If significantly dilated, the aortic annulus is reduced to normal size with an annular cerclage suture of 2-0 polypropylene; this also permits use of smaller aortic homografts, which are in greater supply. A 2-mm-thick strip of pericardium can be used to reinforce the proximal suture line for hemostasis. The coronary artery is reimplanted using a running 5-0 polypropylene suture, and the distal suture line is completed with 4-0 suture.

Table 3 Endocarditis Prophylaxis for Dental, Oral, Respiratory Tract, or Esophageal Procedures

SITUATION	ANTIBIOTIC AGENT	REGIMEN
Standard general prophylaxis	Amoxicillin	Adult: 2 g orally 1 hr before Child: 50 mg/kg orally 1 hr before
Allergic to penicillin	Clindamycin	Adult: 600 mg orally 1 hr before Child: 20 mg/kg orally 1 hr before
	Cephalexin or cefadroxil	Adult: 2 g orally 1 hr before Child: 50 mg/kg orally 1 hr before

The pulmonary autograft procedure has been well described in several publications from this institution.

If homografts are unavailable, one of the stentless tissue valves can be used. We would not recommend use of a stented bioprosthesis or mechanical valve for PVE. At least 6 weeks of antibiotics are given postoperatively; this regimen is extended longer in cases of fungal and resistant organisms. Use of mechanical or bioprosthetic valves for native valve endocarditis is associated with a fivefold increase in incidence of PVE and is a risk factor for death.

Mitral Valve PVE

Surgery for PVE involving the mitral valve requires complete débridement of the annulus and subvalvular apparatus and rereplacement. Although either mechanical or bioprosthetic valves may be used, we prefer porcine or pericardial valves. Both have a large sewing cuff, which fits better in a well-débrided annulus, has less hemolysis postoperatively from small paravalvular leaks, and has a lower incidence of early reoperation should bacteremia persist early postoperatively. The option to avoid warfarin (Coumadin) anticoagulation postoperatively may improve outcome, particularly in patients with neurologic deficits. As more experience is gained with homografts in the mitral position, this may become an additional option in the future. Mortality rate for mitral valve replacement in PVE is 15% to 20%, and freedom from recurrent endocarditis at 5 years is 75%.

PVE Involving Right-Sided Valves

PVE of right-sided valves is less common and usually associated with congenital heart disease (before and after repair) or intravenous drug abuse. We strongly recommend replacement of the tricuspid prosthesis with a bioprosthesis rather than a mechanical valve. Simple excision of the prosthesis is another option. If this is done, narrowing the annulus with an annuloplasty stitch may reduce regurgitation.

Pulmonary vasodilation also is helpful early postoperatively. PVE involving a prosthesis in the pulmonary position is managed best by replacing the valve with a homograft, preferably a pulmonary homograft. In patients with a competent tricuspid valve and a normally functioning right ventricle, the prosthesis may be excised from the pulmonary artery and the pulmonary artery roofed with a patch of pericardium, creating a nonvalved conduit between the right ventricle and the pulmonary artery. Hospital mortality for operation for tricuspid or pulmonary PVE should be less than 10% and relates more to patient comorbidity than the operation itself.

■ PREVENTION

Dental evaluation before placement of a prosthetic heart valve is an important aspect of preoperative evaluation. If teeth extractions are required, we prefer to wait at least 72 hours before valve surgery. A similar delay is prudent if major dental work is needed.

Systemic antibiotics are given routinely at the time of prosthetic valve implantation and is usually a broad-spectrum agent, such as a cephalosporin particularly active against gram-positive organisms. This is continued for 48 hours postoperatively or until chest tubes and central lines have been removed. Any patient with a prosthetic valve is at risk for PVE from any procedure associated with bacteremia. All prosthetic valve patients should be advised about the need for antibiotic prophylaxis. A good rule is to encourage patients with prosthetic valves to insist on receiving intravenous antibiotics before invasive procedures, including major dental work and endoscopy. This practice is more cost-effective and safer than reoperation. Some recommendations for prophylaxis are listed in Tables 3 and 4; contact the American Heart Association for the latest recommendations.

Table 4 Endocarditis Prophylaxis for Genitourinary and Gastrointestinal Procedures

SITUATION	ANTIBIOTIC AGENT	REGIMEN
High-risk patient	Amp + Gent	Adult: Amp 2 g IM/IV + Gent 1.5 mg/kg within 30 min of procedure, then 6 hr later Amp 1 g IM/IV or Amoxicillin 1g orally Child: Amp 50 mg/kg IM/IV + Gent 1.5 mg/kg within 30 min of procedure, then 6 hr later Amp 25 mg/kg IM/IV or Amoxicillin 25 mg/kg orally
High-risk patient allergic to ampicillin/amoxicillin	Vanco + Gent	Adult: Vanco 1 g IV over 1-2 hr + Gent 1.5 mg/kg to be completed within 30 min of procedure Child: Vanco 20 mg/kg IV over 1-2 hr + Gent 1.5 mg/kg to be completed within 30 min of procedure

Amp, ampicillin; Gent, gentamicin; Vanco, vancomycin.

SUGGESTED READING

Dajani AS, et al: Prevention of bacterial endocarditis. Recommendations by the American Heart Association, *Circulation* 96:358, 1997.

Gilbert DN, et al: *The Sanford guide to antimicrobial therapy,* 2001, Antimicrobial Therapy, Inc, Hyde Park, VT p 19.

Gillinov AM, et al: Valve replacement in patients with endocarditis and acute neurologic deficit, *Ann Thorac Surg* 61:1125, 1996.

Miller DC: Predictors of outcome in patients with prosthetic valve endocarditis (PVE) and potential advantages of homograft aortic root replacement for prosthetic ascending aortic valve-graft infections, *J Card Surg* 5:53, 1990.

Niwaya K, et al: Advantage of autograft and homograft valve replacement for complex aortic valve endocarditis, *Ann Thorac Surg* 67:1603, 1999.

Vlessis AA, et al: Risk, diagnosis and management of prosthetic valve endocarditis: a review, *J Heart Valve Dis* 6:443, 1997.

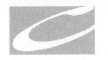

CORONARY ARTERY DISEASE

CARDIAC CATHETERIZATION

Alan W. Heldman

An ever-widening range of cardiovascular diagnostic and therapeutic maneuvers can be performed via transluminal catheters. Of particular relevance to the cardiothoracic surgeon are principles of diagnostic angiography, particularly of the coronary arteries, cardiac chambers, and great vessels. The interpretation of hemodynamic measurements also is important and often guides surgical decision making. Patients having surgery may have had prior coronary interventions or cardiac valvuloplasty; these procedures also are reviewed here. Emergency surgery for the management of angioplasty complications has become less frequent with the advent of modern coronary stents, but surgical emergencies still arise in the catheterization laboratory. Other special catheterization techniques are discussed in this chapter as they relate to the adult cardiothoracic surgical patient.

■ CORONARY AND CARDIAC ANGIOGRAPHY

Coronary Angiography and Intervention

Coronary angiography remains the definitive diagnostic technique to assess ischemic heart disease due to coronary artery atherosclerosis. A broad range of clinical presentations of ischemic heart disease may lead to catheterization. Coronary angiography is performed for elective outpatient evaluation of coronary anatomy and for emergency evaluation and management of acute cardiovascular events, often in critically ill and hemodynamically unstable patients. Angiography is done using hollow preshaped catheters, which are placed retrograde into the aorta and engaged into the ostia of the coronary arteries and coronary bypass grafts using x-ray fluoroscopic guidance. A solution of radiographic contrast material is injected through the catheter with sufficient force and volume to mix with or replace blood and to opacify the full dimensions of the arterial lumen. Still images are recorded in rapid succession (usually at 15 to 30 frames/sec) onto film or a digital format. The resulting cineangiographic moving pictures of the beating heart are a two-dimensional projection of a complex three-dimensional array of vessels. Images in multiple radiographic projections are required for adequate evaluation of the coronary arterial tree.

Coronary interventional techniques in current use include balloon dilation; stent-supported dilation; atherectomy and plaque ablation with a variety of devices; thrombectomy with aspiration devices; specialized methods of imaging and physiologic assessment with intracoronary devices; and application of local therapies to the diseased arterial wall with brachytherapy irradiation systems, drug delivery catheters, and drug eluting stents. Vasodilators and other drugs may be infused directly into the coronary arteries. In addition to narrowed coronary arteries, intervention can be performed on acutely occluded infarct vessels, chronic total occulusions, and diseased coronary bypass grafts and anastomoses.

Vascular Access and Vascular Complications

Cardiac catheterization commonly is performed by percutaneous insertion of a short self-sealing vascular sheath into either femoral artery and into the adjacent vein if needed. Vascular access also may be via brachial artery (percutaneous or cutdown) or radial artery. Catheterization by the radial approach should be attempted only when an intact palmar arch circulation has been shown. Artificial femoral bypass grafts usually can be entered percutaneously, and descending aortic aneurysms or repairs usually can be passed retrograde. Problems at the access site are the most common complications of cardiac catheterization and are more likely with anticoagulation, peripheral vascular disease, advanced age, small stature, and female gender. Complications include external bleeding, expanding hematoma, retroperitoneal bleeding, pseudoaneurysm, arteriovenous fistula, ischemia of the limb distal to the catheter insertion site, and embolization of atheromatous material into the distal circulation.

Bleeding at the femoral catheterization site is usually obvious, but even rapid and life-threatening bleeding may be missed when it occurs into the retroperitoneal space or a large thigh. Initial management should consist of application of firm pressure with the fingertips directly over the common femoral artery, *just proximal* to the site of catheter entry. Compression devices are no substitute for well-applied manual pressure. Bleeding that cannot be controlled by compression may require an emergency operation. Measurement of vital signs, hematocrit, and coagulation parameters should be done while compression is being applied and guides the need for volume resuscitation, transfusion, and surgery. Retroperitoneal bleeding may require a computed tomography scan to establish the diagnosis.

A discrete mass over the femoral artery catheterization site (particularly when associated with bruit) may be a pseudoaneurysm; the diagnosis is established by ultrasonography with Doppler flow mapping. Surgical repair, ultrasound-guided compression of the pseudoaneurysm, and ultrasound-guided thrombin injection may be used to treat the lesion and reduce the risk of late rupture or rebleeding. Femoral artery closure devices, including plugging, tamponading, thrombosing, and suture-mediated systems, commonly are used; when successful, they may improve patient comfort and hasten ambulation. Although generally safe, femoral artery closure devices do not eliminate the risk of bleeding and other complications and may be associated with more complex problems requiring surgical repair; the repair may be more complicated after unsuccessful deployment of these devices than after failure of manual compression because infection may be associated with the foreign body.

Distal ischemia caused by an occlusive arterial catheter may threaten a limb. If possible, the catheter should be removed. Hemostasis should be achieved with careful manual compression, while monitoring for return of distal pulses, using a vascular Doppler transducer if needed.

Distal embolism of atherosclerotic (cholesterol embolization) or thrombotic debris can appear after catheterization or any other arterial manipulation but may not appear until days or weeks later. Manifestations of arteriolar obstruction and of inflammation around cholesterol crystals include leg pains, "blue toes," cutaneous splinter hemorrhages, and organ involvement downstream from the source, resulting in gastrointestinal pain, infarction, pancreatitis, and renal failure. The same phenomena may occur after cardiac surgery and is associated with poor outcome. Identification of patients with severe aortic disease warrants consideration of a brachial or radial approach for left heart catheterization. Treatment options for this rare but protean syndrome are limited; anticoagulants generally are thought to be avoided.

Interpretation of a Coronary Angiorgram

Careful examination of the coronary angiogram is essential for evaluation of patients for coronary bypass operation. Significant coronary narrowings must be recognized and localized so that graft anastomoses can be placed in the correct segments of the localized coronary arteries. It is equally important to assess adequacy of the angiogram to *exclude* important disease. Some coronary arterial segments are difficult to image; if after reviewing an angiogram, questions remain about a potentially important segment, it may be worthwhile to obtain an additional angiographic study, possibly with intracoronary ultrasound. When considering a repeat bypass operation, an angiogram must account for all previously constructed grafts.

Critical assessment of the coronary angiogram includes the degree of lumen opacification by contrast material; injection should be sufficient to delineate the lumen–vessel wall interface with a distinct boundary. Smaller volume or less forceful injections may give the false appearance of narrowings or may fail to delineate significant abnormalities. Particularly important is the opacification of the coronary ostia. Adequate assessment of the coronary (and graft) ostia requires the angiographer to find a radiographic projection that places the ostium free of overlap by the coronary cusps of the aorta or by other vessel segments and free of foreshortening. The injection should be sufficient to reflux contrast material out of the coronary into the aorta, delineating the ostium even when the catheter is engaged into the body of the artery. An additional clue to the presence of a significant ostial coronary narrowing is found not in the angiogram itself, but in the hemodynamic monitoring through the end-hole angiographic catheter. Dampening (reduced peak systolic pressure) or ventricularization (having the appearance of a ventricular pressure recording with wide pulse pressure) of the waveform suggests that the catheter is partially occlusive in the coronary ostium.

Vessel Size

Knowing the lumen diameter of a coronary segment is important for planning bypass, just as it is for planning angioplasty. The catheter itself can serve as a reference. Catheter outer diameter is designated in French units. One Fr is $1/3$ mm; a 6 Fr catheter is 2 mm in diameter, and vessel size is measured against this calibration, either by visual estimation or by manual or automated calipers. Most diagnostic coronary angiograms currently are performed with 5 Fr or 6 Fr catheters. Sources of error in this measurement include nonuniformity of the background, measurement from a contrast-filled catheter, and magnification error when the coronary segment is not in the same plane as the reference catheter. The object that is farther away from the x-ray detector appears magnified.

A coronary artery may appear smaller than its true caliber if severe proximal disease causes underfilling of the distal vessel. This is particularly true when the vessel in question is occluded and is filled via collaterals from another coronary. Constriction of the epicardial coronaries can be severe, even in the absence of angiographically impressive atherosclerosis, and measurement of the true potential diameter requires administration of a vasodilator, generally nitroglycerin.

Coronary Flow and Myocardial Perfusion

Coronary flow is assessed angiographically as the velocity of contrast material passing to the distal segments of the epicardial vessels. In acute myocardial infarction, flow may be severely reduced or absent, generally because of thrombotic occlusion of a ruptured atherosclerotic plaque. Flow is graded according to the TIMI (Thrombolysis in Myocardial Infarction trials) grading system (Table 1). Timely restoration of infarct-artery patency is essential for the optimal treatment of an acute myocardial infarction. A meta-analysis of five large thrombolytic therapy trials confirmed the association between death and failure to achieve brisk epicardial coronary flow in 90 minutes, with increased 30-day mortality in patients having TIMI 0/1 flow (8.8% death) versus

Table 1 TIMI Angiographic Grading of Epicardial Coronary Flow

TIMI FLOW GRADE	DEFINITION
0	Contrast does not penetrate beyond total occlusion site
1	Contrast does not reach the distal vessel
2	Contrast reaches the distal segments of the infarct vessel, but more slowly then normal (relative to unaffected vessel.)
3	Normal epicardial flow

TIMI 2 (7.0%) versus TIMI 3 (3.7%). Grade 3 flow was associated with improved outcome measures (myocyte enzyme release, infarct size, and left ventricular function) whereas for many outcome measures grade 2 flow was not much better than an occluded infarct artery.

Even among patients with TIMI 3 flow in the epicardial coronary, the TIMI myocardial perfusion (TMP) grading system of tissue contrast blush can predict further clinical outcomes in acute myocardial infarction. According to this angiographic assessment of tissue-level microvascular flow, TMP grade 0 has no ground-glass myocardial blush, TMP grade 1 has myocardial blush that does not clear, TMP grade 2 blush clears slowly, and TMP grade 3 blush largely clears after three cardiac cycles of washout phase. In the TIMI 10b angiographic study, even among patients with normal-appearing TIMI grade 3 epicardial coronary flow after thrombolysis, TMP grade 0 or 1 was associated with 5% mortality at 30 days, TMP grade 2 with 2.9% mortality, and TMP grade 3 with 0.7% mortality. Despite restoration of early epicardial coronary patency, microvascular damage can occur during the acute ischemic event and during reperfusion. Pharmacologic strategies being investigated to prevent and to treat microvascular obstruction during percutaneous coronary interventions include inhibitors of platelet aggregation and vasodilator drugs given via the intracoronary route, including nitroglycerin, calcium channel blockers, adenosine, and nitroprusside.

Vascular Calcification and Nonangiographic Details

Besides the information conveyed by the contrast injections, other details of the images may reveal clinically important processes. Calcification or mineralization of cardiovascular structures is often a sign of significant disease and is detected by fluoroscopy and radiographic imaging. Calcification of the aorta suggests significant aortic atherosclerosis. Calcification of the coronary arteries is seen as a radiodense shadow that moves with the cardiac cycle. Coronary calcification is a major risk factor for complications during coronary angioplasty, often indicating noncompliant plaque prone to separate and dissect from the surrounding arterial wall when dilated. Calcification of the aortic valve often is associated with hemodynamically significant valvular stenosis, whereas calcification of the mitral valve annulus often is seen without hemodynamically important valve disease. Chronic left ventricular aneurysms may contain calcified mural thrombi. Calcification of the pericardium sometimes is detected, although this is not a sensitive test for pericardial disease. Also seen are sternal wires and vascular clips. The motion of mechanical prosthetic valve leaflets is noted. The presence, arrangement, and motion of implanted devices, such as valve annulus rings, pacemakers, and defibrillators, and their intracardiac leads are significant findings.

Coronary Anatomy

Understanding the anatomy of the coronary tree requires reconstructing a three-dimensional structure from a two-dimensional projection. A variety of schemes have been used, and one of the most helpful is to imagine two perpendicular loops, one representing the atrioventricular groove at the base of the heart and the other the interventricular septal groove dividing the right and left ventricles. These virtual structures are not seen on the angiograms but define a general course for the normal coronary arteries that may aid orientation when viewing different radiographic projections. The coronary sinus is a venous structure running in the atrioventricular groove. The coronary sinus gives one clue to the location of the atrioventricular groove and can be seen adjacent to the circumflex coronary during the venous phase, several cardiac cycles after contrast injection of the left coronary system.

Angiographers use right and left anterior oblique (RAO and LAO) x-ray projections, with more or less craniocaudal or caudal-cranial angulation, to obtain images of coronaries free of overlap or foreshortening. Accurate assessment of coronary narrowing requires at least two views, made in two orthogonal planes. RAO projection indicates that the x-ray source is underneath the patient and on his or her left and that x-rays are penetrating from the source through the body and encountering the detector above the patient on his or her right. More simply, an RAO view is from the patient's anterior right side, viewing obliquely through the body.

Figure 1 shows representations of two fundamental views of the coronary trees. Two perpendicular loops are defined. The planar loop of the atrioventricular groove includes the left circumflex coronary (LCx) wrapping around the posterior aspect of the groove and the right coronary artery (RCA) making up the other half of the loop. The loop of the interventricular septum includes the left anterior descending coronary artery (LAD), descending from base to apex on the anterior surface, and the posterior descending coronary artery (PDA), making up the posterior part of this loop. Branches arise from each of the major coronary trunks.

The major branches of the coronaries are named according to their appearance in the LAO projection. Anterior and posterior descending arteries descend from top to bottom of the image. Diagonal branches of the LAD run diagonally, from the upper left to the lower right of the image. Obtuse marginal branches of the LCx run along the obtuse, or more rounded, border of the heart in this projection on the right side of the image, whereas the acute marginal branch of the RCA (often a small branch) originates from the more angulated margin of the heart, on the lower left corner of the image. The left side of the image as viewed represents the right side of the patient's heart and vice versa.

Other clues to the identification of the vessels on a coronary angiogram include the morphology of the arteries and their branches. Because of their course along the edge of the loop of the interventricular septum, the LAD and PDA coronaries give off branches that penetrate into the septum. Because it loops around the back side of the heart, the LCx is the left coronary branch closer to the spine. This is particularly evident in a left lateral or cross-table projection, a view that may be especially valuable when planning repeat sternotomy. In this view, the proximity of the heart to the sternum can be appreciated.

Considerable variation exists in the normal range of coronary anatomy. *Dominance* of the coronary circulation is defined by whether the RCA or the LCx gives off the PDA branch that supplies the posterior septum (and with it generally the atrioventricular node). Of normal human hearts, 85% are right dominant, 8% are left dominant, and 7% are

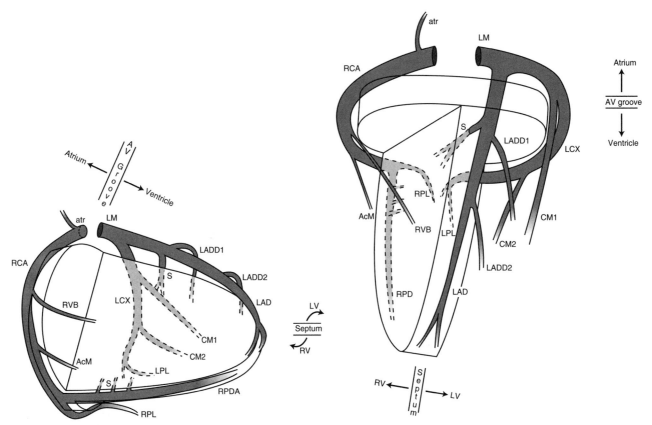

Figure 1

A; Viewed from the right anterior oblique projection, the anterior and posterior descending coronaries course from the base of the heart on the left of the image, toward the apex of the heart on the right of the image, while the left circumflex and right coronary arteries are captured running from top to bottom of the image, more or less in parallel with the loop they define at the base the heart. (LM, left main coronary; LAD, left anterior descending; LADD, diagonal branches; LCx, left circumflex; CM, marginal branches; LPL, left posterolateral branch; RCA, right coronary artery; RVB, right ventricular branch; AcM, acute marginal branch; RPDA, right posterior descending; RPL, right posterolateral branch. **B;** Viewed from a left anterior oblique perspective, the anterior (LAD) and posterior (RPD) descending arteries run from top to bottom of the image, and the loop of the septum is seen edge-on. The atrioventricular groove loop is opened and seen face-on; the RCA forms a C, and the LCx forms a backward C.

codominant (i.e., the right and the left coronaries contribute to the posterior septum). Anomalies of coronary anatomy are common. Most frequently seen are separate ostia of the LAD and LCx directly from the aorta ("double ostium left coronary") and anomalous origin of the circumflex from the RCA.

Atherosclerosis and Coronary Stenosis

Cardiac catheterization is performed most commonly to evaluate patients with known or suspected coronary artery disease. Examination of each coronary segment for narrowings requires that each segment be visualized free of overlap from other vessels and from foreshortening artifact. Despite its sensitivity for the detection of coronary narrowings, angiography may appear normal or nearly normal despite extensive atherosclerotic disease because the technique does not reveal details of the arterial wall. Vessel remodeling and dilation

may compensate completely for thickening of the vessel wall so that the lumen appears normal by angiography. Only when the arterial lumen contains a discrete space-occupying lesion that projects perpendicular to the plane of the x-ray imaging system does an angiographic narrowing appear.

Angiographic assessment of coronary artery stenosis is expressed as diameter stenosis (Figure 2), the reduction of the lumen relative to a (presumably nondiseased) adjacent reference segment. Visual estimation commonly is used, although when automated edge-detection quantitative coronary angiography systems are used, measured diameter stenoses are often less severe than estimated. An eccentric narrowing may appear more or less narrowed depending on the projection, and the "worst" view appearing as the greatest narrowing is the one used. Because intimal thickening and remodeling may be present in the reference segment, quantification of diameter stenosis is imperfect.

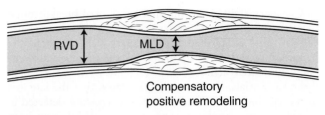

Compensatory
positive remodeling

Figure 2

Angiographic quantification of coronary diameter stenosis is based on minimum lumen diameter (MLD) and reference vessel diameter (RVD) and is expressed as a percentage stenosis (RVD-MLD/RVD). As shown, compensatory positive remodeling may obscure even large plaque volumes from the angiogram.

The significance of a coronary narrowing relates to its resistance to tissue perfusion, either at rest or with increased demand conditions such as exercise. The interpretation of the angiogram should integrate knowledge of the patient's symptoms and the results of stress tests or other examinations for ischemia. It is important to recognize the limitations of angiography. The most angiographically severe narrowings are not the ones that cause infarction; rather, milder narrowings associated with lipid-rich, crescent-shaped plaques (so-called vulnerable plaque) are prone to rupture and thrombose, causing acute coronary syndromes and infarction. Although these may not appear significant on an angiogram, the mild narrowing that ruptures and causes infarction is more significant to the patient than a severe narrowing that is stable and that causes exertional angina.

Intravascular Ultrasound (IVUS), Doppler Flow Wire, Pressure Wire

The development of coronary interventional techniques has been accompanied by engineering of imaginative devices for further understanding coronary pathophysiology in real time during catheterization procedures. Among these, three deserve mention for their value in preoperative assessment of the patient with coronary artery disease. Intravascular ultrasound (IVUS) is a special technique that can resolve anatomic details of the vessel wall outside the lumen. Flexible IVUS catheters less than 1 mm in diameter often are inserted over a guidewire into the coronary artery. These provide a 360-degree view from the inside of the vessel. Details of the vessel wall not apparent from the angiographic projection of the lumen are revealed, and quantification of lumen size and disease severity is possible. Coronary wires with Doppler flow sensor tips or with pressure-sensing micromanometer tips can be used to gain additional information about the hemodynamic significance of coronary narrowings.

Catheterization of Coronary Bypass Grafts

Just as a high-quality angiogram is crucial for coronary bypass surgery, the operative report is required to perform a catheterization study in a patient with prior bypass graft surgery. When each graft is identified and described, selective catheter engagement of grafts generally can be done quickly.

When this information is not available, the catheterization procedure may be more difficult, and ascending aortography may be needed to identify each patent graft and to ensure that one has not been missed.

Total Occlusions

Total occlusions may be suspected in error if the catheter is subselective (e.g., the left coronary catheter seats directly into the LAD so that the LCx is not opacified) or if an anomalous circulation is not recognized. Conversely, total occlusions may be missed if there is not an obvious "stump" of the proximal vessel and if the absence of the branch is not recognized. An explanation should be sought for a wall motion abnormality in any given territory, and careful study for a missing vessel may be required.

Coronary Collaterals

Coronaries that are totally occluded nonetheless may be opacified by contrast injection through collateral circulation. Coronary collaterals may be too small to resolve by angiography or may be large and well developed and may cause faint or dense opacification of the target vessel. Even without total occlusion, a severely narrowed artery may receive flow from the antegrade direction and from collaterals. Because collateral filling may appear only late in the cineangiographic injection run and may appear at a distance from the primary focus of that run, conscious searching for collaterals may be required for their identification.

Coronary collateral perfusion of a diseased artery is described as ipsilateral ("left to left" or "right to right") or contralateral ("right to left" or "left to right"). If the RCA is totally occluded, the distal right coronary branches may not be seen at all on RCA injection. Assessment of the suitability of the distal vessel for bypass depends on seeing it at the end of a left coronary injection run. If the distal RCA appears only faintly, limited conclusions can be drawn, but if it is well seen through dense collateralization the resulting image of the distal RCA is helpful in planning bypass. Even then, the vessel size may appear smaller than its true potential.

Coronary Angioplasty

Since its invention by Gruntzig in the late 1970s, coronary angioplasty has grown to eclipse coronary bypass surgery in volume of procedures. These two approaches to myocardial revascularization are complementary; selection of patients for one or the other treatment generally is guided by anatomic and clinical circumstances.

Techniques

Angioplasty is done with angiographic guidance; the aortocoronary ostium is engaged with a "guiding" catheter, and the segment of artery to be treated is defined by angiography. Anticoagulant and antiplatelet aggregation medications are given. The lesion to be treated is crossed with a guidewire, over which the angioplasty device is advanced into position. Although dilating balloons alone generally were successful, current interventional technique relies much more heavily on the implantation of coronary stents.

Percutaneous interventions can be performed on diseased coronary bypass grafts. The risk of complications, particularly embolization of friable graft atherosclerosis into the distal coronary bed, is increased compared with native coronary interventions. Temporary distal occluders or filters are in development as protection systems against this problem.

Angioplasty Complications and Coronary Stents

Because of the potential for causing coronary complications, angioplasty generally is performed in hospitals with a cardiac surgical program, with arrangements for the availability of emergency surgery. Dilation of the coronary artery can result in dissection of the vessel wall, and this has the potential to cause mechanical or thrombotic occlusion and resulting infarction. Emergency coronary bypass can limit the extent of myocardial damage. The need for such operations has been reduced dramatically by technical improvements, particularly stents. Stents are metal, most often 316-L stainless steel, and when expanded they cover approximately 15% to 25% of the surface area of the arterial segment with struts that scaffold the diseased vessel into an open conformation. In cases in which stents are used to treat dissection, they scaffold open the lumen and seal the dissection. The major reason for the widespread use of stents (in many centers close to 100% of angioplasties involve stenting) is, however, that by scaffolding against elastic recoil or constrictive remodeling of the arterial wall, stents reduce the incidence of restenosis and recurrence of the coronary narrowing. Most coronary stents are balloon expandable; that is, they are positioned at a lesion, then expanded by balloon inflation. The corollary characteristic is that these stents can be recompressed. At operation, stented coronaries may be pinched or compressed either intentionally or unintentionally by handling the decompressed heart. Some stents are self-expanding, and if compressed they return to their open configuration.

Despite advances in equipment, some surgical emergencies do arise. Perforation of the coronary artery occurs most often with the use of cutting or ablative angioplasty devices, and if the perforation is large with free flow into the pericardial space, it can cause pericardial tamponade and arrest within seconds. Treatment includes covering the perforation with an inflated angioplasty balloon to stop the leak, pericardiocentesis if needed, and other resuscitative measures. Smaller leaks sometimes can be managed by prolonged balloon inflation and reversal of anticoagulation. Larger leaks require a mechanical approach; stents covered with a membrane or with autologous vein or artery segments sometimes can be implanted to seal a perforation. Perforation remains a significant cause for emergency coronary bypass. A membrane-covered stent has been approved by the U.S. Food and Drug Administration for treating perforation. Other modes of acute angioplasty failure that may require surgery include dissection and closure of a vessel by the guidewire and damage to the left main coronary, often as a result of dissection by the guiding catheter.

Restenosis occurs within stented segments principally because of neointimal proliferation. In response to injury and to a variety of growth factors, vascular wall cells migrate from outside the stent to within, where proliferation of fibroblastic smooth muscle cells narrows the lumen available for blood flow. Certain factors predict the risk of restenosis, including vessel diameter and length of stent, but we are far from being able to identify in advance the one out of four or five patients who will require repeat intervention.

Coronary stents were the first substantial breakthrough in attempts to prevent restenosis after angioplasty. Early clinical trials established that coronary stents reduced the incidence of restenosis by increasing the lumen gain compared with that achieved with angioplasty alone. Even in those early trials, it was evident, however, that the late loss of lumen diameter (the degree of renarrowing detected at follow-up angiography) was greater in stented than in nonstented arteries. Although stent recoil or compression is not completely insignificant, by far the greatest cause of this lumen loss in stents is neointimal hyperplasia. This is the principal mechanism of in-stent restenosis, and as a disease of inappropriate cell proliferation, its treatment may draw on what oncologists already know about arresting cell growth. Vascular brachytherapy, the transcatheter application of radiation to the diseased segment of artery, inhibits neointimal proliferation. In-stent restenosis can be treated by redilation with a balloon (with or without a stent) or by ablation or removal of the neointimal tissue with laser or atherectomy catheters. After reopening, a measured radiation dose is applied, and this has proved effective at limiting the risk of recurrence. Increased rates of late stent thrombosis after brachytherapy (particularly when a new stent is implanted at the time of radiation treatment), suggest that healing and reendothelialization are impaired after brachytherapy. Long-term treatment with combination antiplatelet therapy (aspirin plus ticlopidine or clopidogrel) markedly reduces this risk.

Pharmacologic Agents Used in Angioplasty

Anticoagulants.   Until more recently, almost all patients undergoing coronary intervention were treated with unfractionated heparin and anticoagulation monitored by the activated clotting time.

Platelet Inhibitors.   Coronary inverventions expose tissue factors and thrombogenic plaque components to the circulating elements of the blood; platelet-mediated thrombosis can result, and antiplatelet therapy is always used. Aspirin is a relatively weak inhibitor of platelet aggregation. A thienopyridine antiplatelet drug (ticlopidine or clopidogrel) is given in combination with aspirin, and this combination is superior to aspirin alone or to aspirin plus warfarin in the prevention of coronary stent thrombosis.

Parenteral inhibitors of platelet aggregation are used for two coronary applications—for the prevention of complications of acute coronary syndromes and for prevention of angioplasty complications. These drugs inhibit the association of fibrinogen with its receptor on the platelet surface, the integrin glycoprotein IIb/IIIa. Three drugs are in current use: Abciximab is a large molecule, a monoclonal antibody fragment; eptifibatide is a cyclic heptapeptide; and tirofiban is a tyrosine analogue. The effect of the large molecule abciximab is believed to persist for hours or days after infusion; platelet function can be restored by platelet transfusion.

■ LEFT VENTRICULAR ANGIOGRAPHY

In patients with coronary artery disease, left ventricular (LV) function is a potent predictor of long-term outcome.

LV function can be assessed noninvasively with echocardiographic, nuclear, or magnetic resonance imaging techniques; however, LV angiography generally is performed with diagnostic coronary catheterization and allows the motion of each coronary vascular territory to be observed (Figure 3). In addition, overall LV volume, ejection fraction, and contractility can be assessed. Myocardial hypertrophy can be detected, although echocardiography may be more sensitive for measuring LV wall thickness. Ventricular septal defect is documented as contrast material crossing the ventricular septum to the right ventricle.

Coronary Vascular Territories

The two radiographic projections most commonly used for LV angiography are RAO and LAO (or LAO-cranial). Taken together, these two views allow observation of each LV segment.

Left Ventricular Function

Normal LV function appears uniform, with systolic contraction of each segment of the left ventricle. Regional wall motion is assessed as the contraction of each coronary vascular territory and designated as follows:

Hypokinetic—decreased but not absent inward motion during systole; may be mild, moderate, or severe
Akinetic—no motion
Dyskinetic—paradoxical motion, outward bulging during systole

The ejection fraction is calculated by:

$$\frac{EDV - ESV}{EDV} = \frac{SV}{EDV}$$

where *EDV* is the end-diastolic volume, *ESV* is the end-systolic volume, and *SV* is the stroke volume. Calculation of the volume of a complex three-dimensional shape (the LV chamber) from a planar projection (the ventriculographic image) depends on certain assumptions about the shape of the ventricular chamber. Many formulas can be used to quantify the LV ejection fraction.

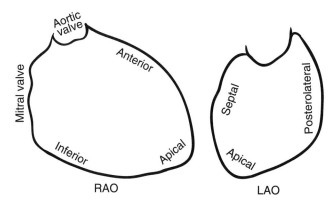

Figure 3
Coronary vascular territories assessed by left ventricular angiography. RAO, right anterior oblique; LAO, left anterior oblique.

Myocardial Viability

Myocardial viability may remain even in the presence of coronary total occlusion, and even the complete absence of motion of a LV territory need not imply irreversible necrosis and scarring. Viable myocardium may cause angina, which would be expected to improve with revascularization. An akinetic but viable territory similarly would be expected to resume contracting after revascularization. For these reasons, the identification of viable myocardium has important implications for the decision to perform a revascularization procedure, particularly when overall LV function is significantly impaired.

Assessment of Mitral Regurgitation

Mitral valve regurgitation is observed as reflux of contrast material into the left atrium, particularly in RAO projection. Mitral regurgitation is graded angiographically as 0 to 4+:

0	No Regurgitation
+	Mild contrast opacification of the left atrium, which clears rapidly
++	Contrast opacification of the left atrium to a lesser degree than of the left ventricle
+++	Left atrium fully opacified, becoming as dense as the left ventricle
++++	Left atrium opacification as dense or more than the left ventricle within one cardiac cycle; pulmonary vein filling with contrast material

or as mild, moderate, and severe. Artifactual causes of mitral regurgitation are ventricular ectopy resulting from the rapid injection of contrast material or from contact with the catheter and catheter interference with the mitral valve apparatus.

■ ANGIOGRAPHY OF THE AORTA AND GREAT VESSELS

Aneurysm and Dissection

Aortic diseases can be diagnosed by many imaging techniques, including magnetic resonance imaging, computed tomography, echocardiography, and angiography. Aortic angiography (*aortography*) can be used to diagnose aortic aneurysm or dissection, although in many centers one of the noninvasive imaging modalities is also highly sensitive and may be preferred. Careful manipulation of wires and catheters is required when aortic dissection is suspected. In the LAO projection, the arch of the aorta is opened, and the origins of the neck vessels can be delineated.

Assessment of Aortic Regurgitation

In the RAO projection, the aortic valve is viewed on edge, and aortic valve regurgitation can be assessed by injection through a catheter positioned in the aortic root, just above the valve. Contrast reflux across the valve from the aortic root into the left ventricle is graded as mild, moderate, or severe, or as 1+ to 4+ depending on the density of contrast material in the left ventricle after three cardiac cycles.

■ HEMODYNAMIC MEASUREMENTS

Catheterization of the Right Heart and Pulmonary Arteries
Vascular Access for Right Heart Catheterization

Catheterization of the right-sided chambers of the heart provides information for diagnosis of a variety of cardiovascular and pulmonary diseases and is done to allow monitoring of a variety of cardiovascular physiologic parameters during operation or during critical illness. When done in conjunction with femoral left heart catheterization, venous access most often is gained via the adjacent femoral vein. Right heart catheterization also can be accomplished from the arm, subclavian, or jugular veins. Right heart catheterization from the femoral approach requires fluoroscopic guidance to manipulate the catheter. Other approaches, particularly from the right internal jugular or left subclavian vein, can be used without the need for fluoroscopy.

Right heart catheterization has risks, including vascular complications, pneumothorax (with jugular or subclavian access), and precipitation of arrhythmias. Catheters touching the endocardium (particularly at the right ventricular outflow tract) can initiate ventricular tachycardia. During right heart catheterization, patients with left bundle-branch block on electrocardiogram are at risk of developing complete heart block as the catheter interacts with the right bundle branch along the right side of the interventricular septum. When used in the intensive care setting for long-term monitoring, catheter-associated infection is common.

Assessment of Valvular Heart Disease
Measuring a Pressure Gradient

If the pressure before a narrowing is P1, and the pressure after a narrowing is P2, the pressure gradient across the stenosis is the difference between P1 and P2. The gradient may be expressed as *peak-to-peak*, the difference between peak systolic pressures, or as *mean* gradient, the area between the two pressure tracings during systole (for the aortic valve) or during diastole (for the mitral valve). The mean gradient is measured by planimetry or integration of the area between the two pressure tracings on the chart recorder. Particularly when there is atrial fibrillation, significant beat-to-beat variation exists, and 10 cardiac cycles should be measured and averaged. "Peak instantaneous" gradients are measured during Doppler echocardiography and generally are not used in catheterization.

The pressure gradient across a valve can be measured by recording from two catheters simultaneously on either side of the stenosis or by pulling back a catheter through the valve while continuously recording. As noted earlier, the pulmonary capillary wedge pressure often is substituted instead of a direct measurement of left atrial pressure; however, the most accurate measurement of left atrial pressure is obtained by transseptal catheterization across the interatrial septum.

Calculating Stenotic Valve Area

Because the pressure gradient across a stenotic valve depends on blood flow (i.e., cardiac output), resistance to flow before or after the obstruction, and the pressure developed in the proximal chamber, calculation of the *valve area* is helpful to determine the contribution of the valve in a given physiologic state.

A common situation is aortic stenosis with a low pressure gradient, low cardiac output, and reduced LV function: Despite the low pressure gradient, the valve orifice may be severely narrowed. This circumstance in particular deserves careful hemodynamic and clinical assessment because the risk of valve replacement may be high, particularly if the LV pressure does not improve after relief of the obstruction.

The valve area is calculated by the method of Gorlin and Gorlin as:

$$Area\,(cm^2) = \frac{valve\ flow\,(\text{ml/sec})}{K \times C \times \sqrt{MVC}}$$

where *MVG* is the mean valvular gradient (mm Hg), *K* is a derived constant (44.3), *C* is an empirical constant that is 1 for aortic valves and is 0.85 for mitral valves, and valve flow (ml/sec) is measured during the systolic ejection period or the diastolic filling period.

Aortic value flow is:

$$\frac{CO\,(\text{ml/min})}{SEP\,(\text{sec/beat}) \times HR}$$

where *CO* is cardiac output (ml/min); *SEP* is systolic ejection period, the duration of the period during which there is flow across the valve (i.e., from the beginning of the measured gradient at aortic valve opening to the end of the gradient at the dicrotic notch of aortic valve closure); and *HR* is heart rate (beats/min).

Mitral valve flow is:

$$\frac{CO\,(\text{ml/min})}{DFP\,(\text{sec/beat}) \times HR}$$

where *DEP* is diastolic filling period, the duration flow across the valve (i.e., from mitral valve opening to end diastole).

Aortic valve areas less than 0.7 cm² are usually clinically important cause of angina, syncope, or heart failure. Mitral valve areas less than 1.0 cm² are often clinically important causes of pulmonary congestion and dyspnea. Some allowances must be made for body size, and larger valve areas still may be clinically important in larger patients. As with any test, the hemodynamic assessment of a stenotic valve must be integrated with the rest of the clinical situation and other data, including the patient's history, physical examination, and often echocardiographic findings.

SUGGESTED READING

Smith SC Jr, et al: ACC/AHA guidelines of percutaneous coronary interventions, *J Am Coll Cardiol* 15;37(8):2215-39, 2001.

Bashore TM, et al: Cardiac catheterization laboratory standards, *J Am Coll Cardiol* 37:2170-214, 2001.

Gibbons RJ, et al: ACC/AHA 2002 guideline update for exercise testing *Circulation*, 106:1883-1892, 2002.

Singh M, Ting HH, Berger PB, et al: Rationale for on-site cardiac surgery for primary angioplasty: a time for reappraisal. *J Am Coll Cardiol* 19;39(12):1881-9, 2002.

Rihal CS, Raco DL, Gersh BJ, Yusuf S. Indications for coronary artery bypass surgery and percutaneous coronary intervention in chronic stable angina, *Circulation* 108(20):2439-45, 2003.

CONDUIT OPTIONS FOR CORONARY ARTERY BYPASS SURGERY

Hendrick B. Barner

The worldwide standard operation for coronary artery bypass is use of the left internal thoracic artery (ITA) for the left anterior descending (LAD) artery and saphenous vein for other vessels. Lytle's report in 1999 on bilateral ITA grafting supported the increased use of arterial conduit, which has expanded slowly because of increased complexity, additional time for conduit harvest, and a probable increase in sternal infection that is definite in diabetics. There is now another conduit option that is measuring up to the right ITA in more recent reports. Use of the radial artery has expanded more rapidly than any other conduit, and current experience is beyond 10 years.

■ LEFT INTERNAL THORACIC ARTERY

The left ITA should be used for at least 95% of operations. It is rejected for diminutive size in 1% or less, for severe subclavian stenosis, for ITA ostial stenosis, for previous ligation, for iatrogenic conduit injury, and during emergency operations for cardiogenic shock or acute vessel closure after coronary angioplasty with ongoing ischemia. Age is rarely a contraindication, and early benefit has been reported in patients after age 80. Obesity, chronic obstructive pulmonary disease, diabetes, and prior thoracotomy are not contraindications. The left ITA usually is directed to the LAD, but it is appropriately directed to the circumflex system when the LAD does not require grafting or is small or the anterior wall is nonviable.

My practice is to routinely use sequential grafting to one or sometimes two diagonal branches or to two sites on the LAD; this was accomplished in 35% of the last 1000 patients. If the diagonal branch arises proximal or must be grafted lateral to the LAD, sequential grafting may not be feasible, and the diagonal must be grafted with a separate graft. These anastomoses are almost always in parallel and rarely crossing. This usage is more complex, and many surgeons are uncomfortable with this technique for fear of jeopardizing distal ITA flow and should not use it. Patency is excellent, however, in our experience and that of Dion and others who practice this configuration routinely.

■ MULTIPLE ARTERIAL CONDUITS

Although the left ITA grafted to the LAD is appropriate in most patients and situations, use of more than one arterial conduit increases the complexity of the operation. I focused on two arterial conduits (both ITAs) for less than a decade (1984-1990), when my interest became that of three to six arterial conduits (one for most targets) for complete revascularization, which was also the approach Calafiore championed. I have abandoned the use of more than three conduits, as I believe that sequential anastomosis obviates this need. Use of this (extreme) approach is reasonable if the patient's life expectancy is the 8 or 10 years necessary to show benefit for arterial conduits. Considerations are the patient's age, adequate ventricular function (>35% ejection fraction), freedom from other life-threatening disease, and absence of valvular heart disease.

I and others have found that the inferior epigastric artery is variable in size and length and frequently does not reach a distal site from the aorta. It is best used as a Y-graft from another arterial conduit. If both inferior epigastric arteries and both ITAs are harvested, abdominal wall necrosis is a potential complication. The right gastroepiploic artery has 10-year patency rates no better than saphenous vein in Suma's experience. It is also more sensitive to competitive flow and may provide inadequate flow if the right coronary artery is large. Its variability in size and length mandates preoperative angiography for assessment if it is to be an important component of the operation.

Important data now are accumulating on the radial artery. Patency to the LAD system or to the circumflex marginal branches is the same and equal to ITA patency. Patency decreases, however, when it is grafted to posterior descending or posterolateral branches, which is also true for the ITA. In addition, radial artery patency is more sensitive to competitive flow, so it should not be used if the coronary stenosis is less than 70% to 80%, which compares with 50% to 60% coronary stenosis for the ITA. Based on a report from this institution, I have stopped grafting arteries with less than 70% stenosis with the radial artery, but I continue to use it for all distal targets. The optimal conduit for the ungrafted arteries (<70% stenosis) is debatable and includes the right ITA, saphenous vein, and gastroepiploic artery.

■ BILATERAL INTERNAL THORACIC ARTERY

Bilateral ITA grafting is appropriate on a routine basis in patients up to age 70 and in selected patients older than 70. The risk of sternal infection is greater in patients with diabetes mellitus, but some data suggest that skeletonization of the conduit reduces the incidence of this complication and provides a longer conduit. There are several techniques for skeletonization; I have begun using the Harmonic scalpel for skeletonization of the right ITA. Some reports indicate that obesity and chronic pulmonary disease are additional risk factors for mediastinal infection with bilateral ITA harvest. Mediastinal infection is a devastating complication, and there is now an option to avoid bilateral ITA harvesting in patients at increased risk for infection, as discussed subsequently. I have stopped using both ITAs in diabetic and morbidly obese patients.

Data from multiple sources support placement of both ITAs to the left coronary circulation. Patency is better than when the right coronary is grafted with the right ITA. Several options exist for directing the right ITA to the left side of the heart. Historically, my choice has been to use it as a free graft from the aorta with a vein hood as an intermediary if present; if not, a pericardial patch should be used. Direct ITA-to-aortic anastomosis is associated with a 10% loss of patency. Other equivalent options include placement of the right ITA anterior to the aorta or through the transverse sinus; equally acceptable is placing it to the LAD and directing the left ITA to the circumflex system. I have used and am comfortable with all of these options. I now believe the best patency of the free right ITA is obtained by grafting it to the in situ left ITA. This has become my preferred usage and that of Calafiore and Dion. I also believe in the strategy of placing the ITAs to the most important coronaries (based on size and viable myocardium), but I believe this strategy now is challenged by the radial artery, which is becoming an equal conduit.

A variation of bilateral ITA grafting is the ITA T-graft, which Tector has espoused. The T-graft is the ultimate in complexity, not because of the T-anastomosis, but because of the need for sequential grafting to achieve complete revascularization. Adequate data from our experience and from Calafiore and Tector support the high success of arterial conduit-to-conduit anastomosis when performed end-to-side. Reaching the posterior circulation may be problematic for the skeletonized right ITA in this configuration. Also, diamond-shaped sequential anastomoses are often necessary to conserve conduit length. These are technically more demanding with an associated 10% loss of patency compared with parallel anastomoses. Intermediate patency data for the ITA T-graft are not yet available. Personal experience with this operation is limited because of my focus on the radial artery T-graft.

■ THREE ARTERIAL CONDUITS

With the availability of the radial artery, it is feasible to revascularize the heart with both ITAs, usually directed to the left coronary system, and the radial artery for the right, based on either an ITA graft (my preference) or the aorta. I now believe that patency is better for any free arterial conduit placed on another arterial conduit rather than the aorta. Calafiore has shown the reliability of arterial conduit Y-grafting with angiographic follow-up; we have shown the same with the radial artery T-graft. Failure of an end-to-side artery-to-artery anastomosis is rare. In this configuration, no grafts are placed on the aorta, reducing the likelihood of cerebral embolization from the aortic wall. Reoperation for any reason is simplified by having all grafts placed away from the aorta on the left side. The only disadvantage is the need for sequential grafting if more than three targets are needed. I believe that this is a better choice than three in situ arterial conduits because the radial artery is a consistent conduit (if the Allen test is negative) and provides more reliable results than the gastroepiploic artery. For the surgeon who wants three arterial conduits and is comfortable with two sources of in-flow, I believe this is the best option.

■ RADIAL ARTERY T-GRAFT

My current interest (80% of patients) continues to be the radial artery T-graft, which has allowed complete revascularization without the use of vein grafts (but with 10 gastroepiploic arteries) in 900 patients. Many surgeons do not use this configuration because of its complexity and the potential for hypoperfusion. This configuration is attractive because only two conduits are needed and can be harvested simultaneously. Patency (see "Multiple Arterial Conduits") has proved to be acceptable except for the issue of competitive flow and grafting distal branches of the right coronary and circumflex. Hypoperfusion has been present in less than 1% of cases and is usually secondary to intraoperative spasm or technical errors, both of which are correctable. In our series, there were no deaths in the intensive care unit from conduit spasm or closure, and no patient required emergent regrafting. In my experience or that of Dion, sequential ITA anastomoses are not associated with loss of patency (if they are in parallel), and it is logical to believe that similar results can be obtained with the radial artery. If the radial artery is grafted to two sites, the side-to-side anastomosis is always parallel. If three or more anastomoses are needed, one or more of them may need to be diamond or crossing anastomoses to have adequate radial artery length.

Our only assessment of collateral circulation to the hand is with the Allen test with a cutoff greater than 12 seconds. The test is positive unilaterally in 12% and bilaterally in 4% of patients; in more than 100 patients, we have had no reluctance to harvest from the dominant arm. At 1 year, about 10% have sensory loss in the superficial radial nerve that supplies the dorsolateral aspect of the thenar eminence and the base of the thumb, but rarely extends further into the thumb. We have not seen evidence of median nerve involvement, which would be manifested by weakness of thumb flexion or palmar sensory loss, as described by others.

Surgical Technique

We do not use the cautery beneath the fascia. Initially, we divided all branches with hemoclips, but subsequently using the Harmonic scalpel they are not required. The full length of the radial artery is harvested (20 to 24 cm in men and 2 cm less in women). Radial artery spasm is treated with intraluminal papaverine and blood (2 mg/ml) after performing the proximal anastomosis and exposure to arterial pressure. Visible spasm during conduit harvesting is treated with topical papaverine in lactated Ringer's solution (6 mg/ml). All patients receive an intravenous infusion of nitroglycerin or nicardipine for 6 to 24 hours postoperatively, which obviates the need for oral calcium antagonists.

The T-anastomosis or Y-anastomosis is performed to the posterior aspect of the ITA pedicle at its entry into the pericardium (incise across at the level of the pulmonic valve to the phrenic nerve) after giving heparin but before cannulation. Radial artery grafting to the lateral and posterior circulation is performed first (proximal to distal) followed by anastomosis of the ITA to the LAD and its branches. Occasionally, these routes are reversed with the ITA directed to one or two marginal branches and the radial artery to one or two diagonals, the LAD, and sometimes over the acute margin to the posterior descending artery.

■ REOPERATION

I strive to use all arterial conduits in reoperations, assuming there is reasonable life expectancy and the ejection fraction is greater than 35%, because reoperation frequently is indicated for vein graft failure due to accelerated atherosclerosis. Radial artery has been used in more than 100 reoperations. If one or both ITAs were not used, they would be the first and second conduit choices, followed by the radial artery if the target coronary artery was beyond reach of the ITA. We preferentially would attach the radial graft to an in situ ITA (usually the left, but also the right) or occasionally to the aorta via the old or new vein graft hood. I have recycled the previously used left ITA (if patent) 20% of the time by grafting the radial artery to it. Since using the radial artery, it rarely has been necessary to use the gastroepiploic artery. The option of bilateral radial artery harvest rarely is required. When replacing a diseased but patent vein graft with an arterial conduit, some surgeons leave the vein graft as it is to avoid hypoperfusion. Although I have followed this dictum on occasion, I also have deviated from it, particularly when the radial artery is used because of the greater sensitivity to competitive flow. To evaluate the severity of competition, I proceed first by coming off bypass and achieving a stable state followed by clamp occlusion (in the healthiest area) of the vein graft. Myocardial reperfusion is monitored for 10 minutes using hemodynamics, the electrocardiogram, and wall motion assessment by transesophageal echocardiography. If there is no evidence of hypoperfusion, the vein graft is definitively ligated, and protamine is given.

SUGGESTED READING

Buxton BF, et al: The right internal thoracic artery graft—benefits of grafting the left coronary system in native vessels with a high grade stenosis, *Eur J Cardiothorac Surg* 18:255, 2000.

Calafiore AM, et al: Revascularization of the lateral wall: radial artery versus right internal mammary artery: long term angiographic and clinical results, *J Thorac Cardiovasc Surg* (in press).

Dion R, et al: Long-term clinical and angiographic follow-up of sequential internal thoracic artery grafting, *Eur J Cardiothorac Surg* 17:407, 2000.

Lytle BW, et al: Two internal thoracic artery grafts are better than one, *J Thorac Cardiovasc Surg* 117:855, 1999.

Maniar H, et al: Effect of target stenosis and location on radial artery graft patency, *J Thorac Cardiovasc Surg* 123(1):45, 2002.

CONVENTIONAL CORONARY ARTERY BYPASS GRAFT SURGERY

Farzan Filsoufi
David H. Adams

In the 1980s and 1990s, clinical studies showed that coronary artery bypass graft (CABG) surgery is the gold standard therapy for patients with multivessel coronary artery disease. The procedure is safe, provides reliable relief of angina, and is associated with improved long-term survival. Indications for CABG surgery have changed with continued growth of interventional cardiology capabilities. Primary indications for CABG surgery currently include left main stenosis greater than 50%, multivessel coronary disease (particularly in patients with left ventricular dysfunction or insulin-dependent diabetes), and percutaneous coronary intervention failures.

In more recent years, much attention has been focused on the development of minimally invasive CABG techniques, particularly off-pump coronary artery bypass surgery. Stabilizing platforms, coronary shunts, and positioning devices have contributed to the adoption of these techniques. Nonetheless, conventional CABG surgery using cardiopulmonary bypass (CPB) under cardioplegic arrest remains the preferred approach in most centers today. The key points regarding the performance of conventional CABG surgery are emphasized here.

■ CONDUITS

A variety of conduit options are now available to the surgeon for CABG surgery. The most commonly used conduits include the left internal mammary artery (LIMA) and greater saphenous vein. Total arterial revascularization (TAR) may be facilitated by additional harvest of the right internal mammary artery (RIMA), radial artery, or right gastroepiploic artery.

Internal Mammary Artery

It is well established that use of the LIMA is associated with excellent long-term patency (95% at 15 years), improved survival, and decreased late cardiac events after CABG surgery. In conventional CABG surgery, the LIMA is harvested through a full sternotomy after opening the left pleural space. The LIMA is mobilized with a 2-cm pedicle containing the mammary veins, transversus thoracis muscle, and fascia. The endothoracic fascia is divided with the cautery, and side branches are clipped as encountered. The LIMA is taken down from its bifurcation distally to the subclavian vein proximally. Topical and intraluminal papaverine is used to dilate the artery. If the LIMA is not long enough to reach the site of anastomosis, its length is increased by performing several fasciotomies combined with ligation and division of mammary veins. Harvesting a skeletonized LIMA by leaving most of the endothoracic fascia in situ is justified when the need for a long LIMA graft is anticipated or when bilateral mammary harvesting is performed, in an attempt to preserve sternal vascularization. Although the LIMA is used in most patients, relative contraindications include (1) proximal left subclavian artery stenosis, (2) history of chest wall radiation or radical mastectomy, (3) iatrogenic fascial hematoma during harvesting, (4) emergency operation in the setting of hemodynamic decompensation, and (5) insufficient flow due to small size or persistent spasm.

Right Internal Mammary Artery

We employ a similar harvesting strategy for the RIMA. We prefer a skeletonized harvest of the RIMA and are careful to divide the mammary veins proximally. The benefit of a second internal mammary artery in bypass surgery is controversial. There is accumulating evidence, however, that patients who receive two internal mammary arteries have less risk of recurrent angina, late myocardial infarction, angioplasty, reoperation, and death. Several clinical studies have shown that the long-term patency of the pedicled RIMA is comparable to that of the LIMA. The patency rate of the free RIMA has been reported to be lower, however, mainly due to difficulty of the anastomosis between the thin-walled RIMA and the ascending thoracic aorta. A skeletonized RIMA often can reach distal coronary arteries (e.g., the posterior descending artery or an obtuse marginal artery through the transverse sinus).

Radial Artery

The use of the radial artery for CABG surgery first was reported in 1973 and was abandoned quickly because of a high rate of early failure. More recent progress in surgical technique and the prevention of arterial vasospasm by new classes of drugs have increased the use of radial artery conduits. The midterm patency rates are encouraging (85% to 90% at 5 years). Our protocol for the use of the radial artery in bypass surgery is described briefly.

The nondominant arm is checked for the presence of an intact palmar arch (Allen's test) by placing a pulse oximeter on the thumb and compressing the ulnar and radial arteries until loss of signal. The ulnar artery is released, and one looks for the presence of the pulse oximetry waveform. If Allen's test is negative, the arm is prepared circumferentially with povidone-iodine (Betadine) and draped. An incision is made over the radial artery just proximal to the wrist crease extending in a curvilinear fashion to the proximal forearm slightly lateral to midline. The pedicle is identified, and an intraoperative Allen's test is performed. This is done by occluding the proximal radial artery and feeling for a retro-

grade pulse distally. The pedicle is exposed moving distal to proximal using scissors and cautery. Arterial and venous branches are ligated with surgical clips. Special care is taken to avoid the lateral antebrachial and superficial radial nerves, which provide sensory innervation to the mid to distal radial aspect of the forearm and to the thumb, index finger, and part of the middle finger. During the harvest, the pedicle is sprayed with a solution consisting of verapamil, 5 mg; nitroglycerin, 2.5 mg; heparin 500 U; sodium bicarbonate (8.4%), 0.2 ml; and lactated Ringer's solution, 300 ml. After harvest, the artery is flushed and soaked with this solution. Verapamil, 0.5 mg/hr, is given to patients intravenously if they are hemodynamically stable. Postoperatively the patient is started on amlodipine, 5 mg/day, after discontinuing intravenous verapamil. Currently, TAR can be achieved using bilateral internal mammary artery combined with other arterial conduits, such as the radial artery. TAR may decrease significantly the incidence of graft atherosclerosis and reduce late cardiac related events, such as angioplasty or reoperation. It should be considered in all young patients (<50 to 60 years old) with critical stenosis (greater than 70%).

Right Gastroepiploic Artery and Inferior Epigastric Artery

The right gastroepiploic artery and inferior epigastric artery have been used clinically, but their application is limited. Several reports have presented a good patency rate in the early postoperative period. A patency rate of 80% has been reported for the right gastroepiploic artery at 5 years. We rarely use either the gastroepiploic artery or the inferior epigastric artery in our practice.

Saphenous Vein

The greater saphenous vein was the first conduit used for CABG surgery. Despite the broadening application of TAR, 95% of current procedures employ the use of at least one venous conduit. Advantages of venous conduits include simplicity, flexibility for sequential anastomoses, and reliable high early flow (not prone to spasm). In the long-term, development of atherosclerotic lesions in saphenous venous conduits adversely affects patency. Studies have reported a patency rate of 50% at 10 to 12 years for saphenous venous conduit. In our experience, most diseased vein grafts now can be managed by repeat interventional procedures.

Since the 1990s, one of the major advances in cardiac surgery has been the application of endoscopic techniques to harvest saphenous vein. A 2-cm incision is made at the medial aspect of the knee. The vein is located and encircled with a vessel loop. The Vasoview dissector (Guidant Corp., Indianapolis, IN) with a conical tip is placed in the leg, and the adventitia is dissected away from the vein on all surfaces. The vein branches are isolated with the dissector as well. The tunnel space is insufflated with carbon dioxide. The dissector is removed, and the bipolar cautery bisector is placed in the leg. The vein branches are cauterized and cut with the bisector. When all branches are cut, a no. 11 surgical blade is used to make a small incision over the proximal and distal ends of the vein. A mosquito clamp is placed through the incision, and the vein is clamped and cut. The residual vein is ligated. The vein is removed from the leg, and the side branches are double clipped. The use of endoscopic harvesting has reduced significantly the morbidity of leg wounds. Reduced leg wound infection rate (<1%) and early patient mobilization are the two major benefits of this technique.

In the reoperative setting or after vein stripping, the greater saphenous vein may not be available. In these cases, we favor arterial revascularization. We use the lesser saphenous vein or an allograft vein in certain circumstances, however.

■ OPERATIVE PRINCIPLES

Management of the Ascending Aorta

Embolization of atheroma from the ascending aorta or the proximal aortic arch is the principal cause of stroke after CABG surgery. Because of the aging population and rising incidence of severe atherosclerotic lesions of the ascending aorta, safe cannulation techniques have become increasingly important. Digital palpation of the ascending aorta and transesophageal echocardiography are insensitive methods for detection of ascending aortic atherosclerosis. Intraoperative epiaortic scanning using a surface probe is a safe, rapid, and precise method for detection of atherosclerotic disease. Epiaortic scanning is now our standard of care in all patients undergoing CABG surgery. Surgical strategy should be defined when the results of this examination have been analyzed carefully. If aortic disease is absent or minimal, conventional CABG surgery using CPB and cardioplegic arrest can be performed safely (see later). A single-clamp technique for distal and proximal anastomoses always is used to minimize aortic manipulation. If significant aortic disease (multiple or circumferential calcification, significant luminal thickening, mobile plaque) is documented on epiaortic scanning, alternative procedures to conventional CABG surgery that avoid aortic clamping must be considered. Currently, we prefer off-pump CABG surgery with the use of a proximal anastomotic device system (St. Jude Medical, St. Paul, MN), which allows mechanical proximal anastomoses without aortic clamping. Alternatively, we carefully select a disease-free site for aortic cannulation, and after cooling to 15°C on CPB, we replace the ascending aorta with a tube graft under total circulatory arrest, then clamp the graft and proceed with conventional CABG surgery. Another surgical option we employ involves careful aortic cannulation and institution of CPB with distal coronary anastomoses performed under cold fibrillatory arrest, followed by proximal anastomoses constructed on the aorta during brief periods of circulatory arrest.

Cardiopulmonary Bypass

After the selection of cannulation sites, an appropriate dose of heparin is administered. Coagulation management is facilitated by the HMS Plus System (Medtronic/Hemotec Inc., Minneapolis, MN) Target activated clotting time is 400 seconds. Kaolin is the medium used for the activated clotting time. Otherwise the machine performs heparin/protamine titration to detect the amount of heparin or protamine needed. This technology has allowed us to decrease overall heparin doses due to the precision of the device. More importantly, it has allowed us to decrease the protamine reversal dose by almost 50% over an empirical dosing regimen.

CPB is instituted between the ascending aorta and right atrium using a single dual-stage cannula. A Soft Flow aortic cannula (Sarns, Inc., Ann Arbor, MI) is used in every case to minimize disruptions of plaques in the ascending aorta and the arch. CPB is conducted with nonpulsatile flow of 1.6 to 2.2 liters/min/m² with a target mean arterial pressure greater than 50 mm Hg, which we increase to greater than 65 mm Hg in patients with increased risks for peripheral vascular disease. Systemic temperature is allowed to drift, then is maintained at 34°C. In primary elective CABG procedures, pump suction is not used. The principal reasons are (1) the blood aspirated from the surgical field and retransfused to the patient is incriminated as a source of brain lipid emboli during CPB, and (2) the fibrinolytic system of blood contained in the pericardium is highly active, and its reinfusion can have a considerable effect on hemostasis during CPB. Cell salvage is used for any shed mediastinal blood.

Myocardial Protection

Myocardial protection is achieved with intermittent infusion of cold blood cardioplegia (4°C) given in an antegrade and a retrograde fashion. Cardioplegia is four parts blood to one part crystalloid. The arresting dose includes potassium at an end concentration of 30 mEq/liter; $MgSO_4$, 3.4 mEq/liter; and $NaHCO_3$, 5 mEq/liter. The maintenance dose is 11 mEq/L of potassium with the other constituents at the same concentration. A double-lumen catheter is used for the administration of antegrade cardioplegia and for venting the heart through the aortic root during cross-clamping. A coronary sinus catheter allows the retrograde administration of cardioplegia. Cardiac arrest is accomplished first with the antegrade delivery of approximately 1200 ml of blood cardioplegia via the ascending aorta followed by retrograde cardioplegia. The aortic root and coronary sinus pressures are checked during the infusion. The coronary sinus pressure during the infusion of cardioplegia is maintained at less than 40 mm Hg. Supplemental doses of cardioplegia are delivered every 20 minutes (500 ml). Cardioplegia also can be delivered antegrade after the completion of distal saphenous vein graft anastomoses to ensure better distribution of cardioplegic solution. In patients with acute evolving myocardial infarction, preoperative cardiogenic shock, and severe left ventricular dysfunction, a solution of antegrade warm maintenance blood cardioplegia is administered before the removal of the aortic clamp ("hot shot" cardioplegia). Systemic rewarming usually is started during construction of the last distal anastomosis (LIMA to left anterior descending coronary artery).

Grafting Technique

We complete distal anastomoses followed by proximal anastomoses under a single aortic cross-clamp. In patients with three-vessel disease, we graft in the sequence of right coronary artery, circumflex artery, and left anterior descending coronary artery territories. We use 7 or 8-0 polypropylene, usually starting at the heel of the graft working toward the toe. Small bites should be taken around the toe and heel to prevent constriction of the anastomoses. While tying the anastomosis, we inject heparinized saline into the graft for deairing purposes and to distend the anastomoses to minimize the purse-string effect. This also allows for confirmation of distal runoff. Generally, we prefer end-to-side anastomoses with separate grafts. Sequential grafting of more than one artery with the same conduit is used when there is a shortage of conduits, a significant mismatch exists between the venous conduit and coronary artery caliber, and access to the proximal aorta is limited due to previous surgery or atherosclerotic disease.

Before performing proximal anastomoses, conduit length should be determined accurately to avoid tension or kinking. Proximal anastomoses are constructed onto a 4-mm hole in the ascending aorta and are sewn with 6-0 polypropylene for venous conduits and 7-0 polypropylene for radial arteries. After removal of the aortic clamp, the vein grafts are deaired with a small needle to prevent air embolization. Then proximal and distal anastomoses and the entire length of each conduit are inspected for hemostasis. After a brief period of reperfusion, most patients separate easily from CPB. If difficulty in weaning is encountered, return to full CPB and increasing systemic perfusion pressure with the heart fully decompressed is often useful. Inotropic support and intraaortic balloon counterpulsation are used liberally in patients with low cardiac output after conventional CABG surgery.

■ RESULTS

Operative mortality after conventional CABG surgery declined steadily during the 1990s. Current mortality rates typically are 1% to 3%. This is despite the fact that the patient population referred for CABG surgery is increasingly more challenging because of advanced age; diffuse coronary artery disease; late referral secondary to prior management with percutaneous transluminal coronary angioplasty; and increased comorbidities, including left ventricular dysfunction. Morbidity and mortality related to ascending aortic manipulation during conventional CABG surgery now can be prevented in most patients by careful epiaortic scanning before cannulation and clamping of the aorta. In patients presenting with ascending aortic atherosclerotic disease, alternatives to conventional CABG surgery, including off-pump CABG surgery with proximal mechanical anastomotic technology or revascularization using CPB without aortic clamping, should be performed. Technologic advances will offer patients additional revascularization options in the future, but we predict conventional CABG surgery will remain an important therapeutic option for patients with advanced coronary artery disease.

SUGGESTED READING

Aranki SF, et al: Single-clamp technique: an important adjunct to myocardial and cerebral protection in coronary operations, *Ann Thorac Surg* 58:296, 1994.

Leavitt BJ, et al: Use of the internal mammary artery graft and in-hospital mortality and other adverse outcomes associated with coronary artery bypass surgery, *Circulation* 103:507, 2001.

Lytle BW, et al: Two internal thoracic artery grafts are better than one, *J Thorac Cardiovasc Surg* 117:855, 1999.

Tatoulis J, et al: Total arterial coronary revascularization: techniques and results in 3,220 patients, *Ann Thorac Surg* 68:2093, 1999.

Wareing TH, et al: Management of the severely atherosclerotic ascending aorta during cardiac operations, *J Thorac Cardiovasc Surg* 103:453, 1992.

OFF-PUMP CORONARY ARTERY BYPASS GRAFT SURGERY

Michael J. Mack

Although coronary artery bypass graft (CABG) surgery initially was performed on a beating heart, the introduction of cardiopulmonary bypass (CPB) and ischemic cardioplegic arrest made efforts at expanding beating heart surgery moot. Although more than 10 million CABG operations have been performed, mostly on an arrested heart, since the late 1960s, only a few isolated centers (Benetti, Buffolo, Pfister) continued to perform beating heart surgery on selected patients, mostly for socioeconomic reasons or for associated medical conditions.

After minimally invasive thrusts in general surgery and other surgical subspecialties in the late 1980s and early 1990s, efforts in cardiac surgery were directed toward less invasive approaches. Initial attempts were focused on limited access surgery, either on an arrested heart (Heartport approach) or on a beating heart (minimally invasive direct coronary artery bypass). It became apparent to some investigators that the use of CPB was a more invasive aspect of performing CABG surgery than was the median sternotomy incision. Building on the work of the early investigators in the field, minimally invasive cardiac surgery rapidly expanded to wide access (median sternotomy) beating heart surgery (off-pump coronary artery bypass [OPCAB]). Although there still are isolated applications for the minimally invasive direct coronary artery bypass procedure (<2% of all CABG procedures, e.g., recurrent in-stent restenosis of the left anterior descending coronary artery [LAD] and investigative work in the field of robotics), beating heart surgery now is performed mainly as the OPCAB procedure. As of late 2001, the OPCAB procedure comprised an estimated 23% of all CABG procedures performed. This chapter focuses on current indications for beating heart surgery, techniques to facilitate its performance, and current results.

■ INDICATIONS

Although some centers perform virtually all CABG procedures on a beating heart, most centers still perform most procedures on an arrested heart. The indications for beating heart bypass surgery change based on the experience of the surgeon and the institution. Patients in whom the operation is technically easier to perform may not be the patients who benefit most from the procedure. Early in a surgeon's experience, appropriate selection of patients is based on the list in Table 1. Selection of patients who need one to three bypasses with large, minimally diseased target vessels on the anterior surface of the heart with good left ventricular function can optimize the early success rate in surgeons with little experience. When a surgeon is familiar with beating heart techniques, beating heart surgery can be an important option in the surgery armamentarium to address difficult operative challenges. Candidates for bypass surgery in whom there is evidence of benefit from the elimination of CPB and ischemic cardiac arrest are listed in Table 2. Elderly patients; patients with diminished ejection fraction; patients with significant comorbidities, including renal dysfunction, chronic obstructive pulmonary disease, cerebrovascular disease, and peripheral vascular disease; and reoperative patients are likely to benefit from beating heart approaches.

Contraindications to beating heart surgery also are relative and based on surgeon experience. Patients who need more bypasses, patients with small and diffusely diseased distal vessels, patients who need multiple bypasses on the posterior surface of the heart, patients with left ventricular hypertrophy, and reoperative patients with open grafts all are technically more challenging. Techniques have been described and technology has been introduced to allow beating heart surgery to be performed successfully in these patients, but the relative indications and contraindications are based on surgeon experience and comfort level. Patients who are hemodynamically unstable or acutely ischemic may be managed optimally by an "on-pump" beating heart approach.

Table 1 OPCAB Patient Selection in Early Experience

1-3 bypasses
Anterior surface of the heart
Large target vessels
Minimal distal disease
Good left ventricular function
Hemodynamically stable

Table 2 Patients Most Likely to Benefit from Beating Heart Surgery

Age ≥75 years
Low ejection fraction
Cerebrovascular disease
Peripheral vascular disease
Renal dysfunction
Chronic lung disease
Reoperative surgery

■ OPERATIVE TECHNIQUE

We first describe the operative technique for OPCAB. At the end of this section, specific modifications for limited access procedures, including lateral thoracotomy for revascularization of the circumflex artery, are described.

Anesthesia

For OPCAB procedures, some modifications of the standard technique for coronary artery bypass with CPB are necessary. In general, because immediate or early extubation is standard with this technique, short-acting agents, including sufentanil and propofol, are used so that immediate extubation is possible. It is our standard technique to use Swan-Ganz catheters and transesophageal echocardiography for hemodynamic monitoring. Because right heart function is crucial for hemodynamic stability in beating heart surgery, we find both of these monitoring tools to be helpful. Fluid management is directed toward optimizing right heart function, which includes volume loading with an average of 3 to 4 liters of crystalloid given during the procedure and liberal use of intravenous nitroglycerin to optimize right ventricular preload.

Surgical Technique

Standard median sternotomy incision is performed with the exception that the skin incision can be made shorter. Because access to the ascending aorta for cannulation is not necessary, and with the use of anastomotic connectors for placement of grafts on the ascending aorta without clamping, beginning the skin incision below the level of the sternal manubrium junction is sufficient for access. We have found it helpful to use an oscillating saw when the skin incision is shortened to divide the most superior and inferior portions of the sternum. After internal mammary artery (IMA) grafts are harvested in the standard manner, a sternal retractor is placed. Specific retractors for off-pump surgery are helpful to allow adjustment of pericardial stay sutures and placement of stabilizer and suction exposure devices on them. On completion of conduit harvest, the pericardium is opened. Wider opening of the pericardium along the diaphragmatic surface laterally is helpful. Extension of the pericardial incision to the left side toward the apex of the pericardium facilitates subluxation of the heart for posterior access. Opening the pericardium at the refection of the diaphragmatic surface on the right side down to just anterior to the phrenic nerve creates room for the right ventricle during displacement. We commonly place three pericardial stay sutures on each side and do not tie them. Traction or slackening of these stay sutures is performed multiple times during the procedure, either to enhance exposure or to improve hemodynamics. During this period, the operative choreography is strategized, and all graft preparation is performed so that the absolute minimum time possible is spent with the heart in the displaced access position. The patient is heparinized with 2 to 3 mg/kg of heparin.

Our standard practice is to revascularize the LAD with the left IMA first. This is the easiest vessel to access and expose and allows revascularization of the anterior wall and the septum before further maneuvers that may create myocardial ischemia are performed. If care is taken to be aware of the IMA pedicle, it is possible to perform all subsequent maneuvers without excessive traction or torsion of the graft. Before revascularizing the LAD, the slack on the pericardial stay sutures on the right side is loosened.

Hemodynamic Instability

Hemodynamic instability during OPCAB can be minimized by taking appropriate preparatory maneuvers (Table 3). The major cause of hypotension and decreased cardiac output is impairment of blood flow through the right ventricle. Minimizing distortion and compression of the right ventricular chamber during cardiac displacement and maximizing preload of the right side of the heart attenuate hemodynamic changes. Decrease of the pulmonary artery systolic pressure, increase in central venous pressure, and decreased mixed venous oxygen saturation are early clues as to whether right ventricular compromise has occurred. Volume loading to a central venous pressure of 8 to 10 cm H_2O with the addition of intravenous nitroglycerin helps to maximize preload of the ventricle. Placement of the operating table for the Trendelenburg position in preload augmentation and rotation of the operating table toward the surgeon to improve visualization are desirable maneuvers. Recognition of the state of the right ventricle during all aspects of the procedure is the most important aspect of the operative approach to maintain hemodynamic stability. Loosening the slack on the pericardial stay sutures on the right side and even opening the right pleural cavity to allow a portion of the heart to fall into the pleural space create room so that compression of the right ventricle does not occur. The use of suction exposure devices on the apex of the heart additionally minimizes right ventricular compression by causing elongation of the right ventricular cavity. If the hemodynamics are not optimal,

when the heart has been positioned for target vessel access, minor readjustments often are sufficient to improve the hemodynamics. If these minor adjustments are not effective, resetting and starting again usually results in hemodynamic stability.

Operative Choreography

Our practice is to revascularize the LAD first for reasons mentioned earlier. The exception to this is if there is a totally occluded right coronary artery (RCA), and the LAD supplies two zones of myocardium by collateral flow. In that case, the RCA is revascularized first. We have not found preconditioning to be necessary, and we do not routinely use intravascular shunts. There are two circumstances in which shunts are helpful. First, when a large dominant RCA that is not totally occluded is to be bypassed before the bifurcation, ischemia to the atrioventricular node can cause heart block and bradycardia. Placement of a shunt and maintenance of perfusion of the atrioventricular node while the revascularization procedure is performed can maintain sinus rhythm. Temporary atrial and ventricular pacemaker wires also can be placed in patients with open, dominant RCAs during vessel occlusion. Shunts also are helpful in situations in which there is an excessive flow through the arteriotomy, usually when there is heavy calcification of a coronary artery and a proximal snare is not sufficient to cause vessel occlusion.

When the LAD is to be bypassed, the right pericardial stays are loosened. A wet lap sponge is placed behind the heart to bring the LAD into view. A proximal Silastic snare is placed around the LAD with a blunt needle. A stabilization device is placed around the target vessel. We do not dissect out the target vessel until it has been stabilized. Although intramyocardial vessels are more problematic, successful revascularization still can be performed. With stabilization *before* attempting to expose the vessel and the use of a carbon dioxide blower to maintain a bloodless field, intramyocardial LAD vessels can be exposed routinely and bypassed.

When hemodynamic stability is ascertained, the arteriotomy is performed. The conduit already has been prepared so that immediately after opening the vessel, suturing can begin. We routinely use a single 7-0 polypropylene (Prolene) with three sutures placed in the heel before bringing the vessels into approximation. We then continue suturing around on the near side first, then the toe followed by the far side of the anastomosis. Liberal use of misted carbon dioxide helps maintain a bloodless field and allows optimal exposure of the edges of the vessels without the necessity for instrument traction. With optimization of these maneuvers, it is possible to perform a distal anastomosis routinely with an ischemic time of 5 to 7 minutes. On completion of this anastomosis, the heart is placed back in the normal position and allowed to recover hemodynamically before performing the remaining bypasses.

We have incorporated into our technique performance of the proximal anastomosis next for two reasons. First, performance of the proximal anastomosis first allows immediate perfusion of ischemic myocardium on completion of the distal anastomosis. Second, we now routinely use clampless proximal anastomotic connectors, which require the proximal anastomosis to be performed first. Although this is a significant change in operative technique for most

---

Table 3 Measures to Maintain Hemodynamic Stability during Cardiac Displacement

Volume loading to central venous pressure 8-10 cm H_2O
Nitroglycerin
Swan-Ganz, transesophageal echocardiography monitoring
Trendelenburg position
Table rotation toward the surgeon
Slackened right pericardium/open right pleura
Prevention of right ventricular compression/distortion
Apical suction exposure device
Left anterior descending revascularization first
Minimize heat loss

surgeons (ourselves included), one can adapt rapidly to this change in technique and develop a comfortable method of optimizing graft length. On completion of the proximal anastomosis, the remaining distal anastomoses are performed. As a general philosophy, we tend to proceed from the easier bypasses to the more difficult. The order in which the bypasses commonly are performed is listed in Table 4.

For access to the posterior circulation, a suction exposure device is employed routinely on the apex of the heart. As mentioned earlier, this device causes less distortion and compression of the left and the right ventricular cavities and allows better exposure with less hemodynamic compromise. An alternative method is placement of posterior pericardial traction sutures (as described by Lima) to allow traction on the base of the heart without significant ventricular compression. With the principles of hemodynamic stability as outlined earlier maintained, routine successful revascularization of the posterior portion of the heart can be performed. We also use the suction positioning device for exposure of the distal main RCA and branches beyond the bifurcation. Placement of the suction exposure device on the acute margin of the heart allows exposure without right ventricular compression. We reset the heart in its natural position between each distal anastomosis to allow total hemodynamic recovery before proceeding to the next anastomosis. Because we use no distal snares, we routinely use a cell saver, as a fair amount of shed blood can be salvaged.

On completion of the last anastomosis, heparinization is reversed with protamine. We do not routinely use any method of graft assessment, having performed an angiographic study early in our experience and being satisfied with the results. If any electrocardiogram changes or local wall motion abnormalities exist, further assessment of the graft by Doppler transit time measurement or intraoperative angiography is performed. We do not routinely use pacemaker wires, unless they have been placed during the bypass of the RCA. We use only small (19 Fr Blake or Jackson-Pratt) soft drains. After closure, extubation in the operating room is routine. If careful attention is paid to this operative strategy, a conversion rate to CPB of less than 2% should be attainable.

■ ON-PUMP BEATING HEART SURGERY

In instances of hemodynamic instability due to acute myocardial infarction, acute vessel occlusion in the cardiac catheterization laboratory, or severe depression of left ventricular function, the technique of on-pump beating heart surgery can be helpful. The greater risk of coronary bypass in these situations is global ischemic arrest rather than the use of CPB. Cannulation of the heart in the standard manner and use of stabilization with standard beating heart techniques allows hemodynamic stability but minimizes myocardial ischemia.

■ LATERAL THORACOTOMY FOR BEATING HEART CIRCUMFLEX REVASCULARIZATION

Frequently, revascularization of the circumflex system is necessary in instances of reoperation when catheter-based therapy is unsuccessful. Total occlusion of the circumflex coronary system or recurrent in-stent restenosis in patients with previous bypass surgery and patent left IMA grafts presents a revascularization challenge. Employment of a limited lateral thoracotomy (6 to 7 cm) in the seventh intercostal space with a short conduit of saphenous vein graft or radial artery from the descending aorta can simplify revascularization. The pericardium posterior to the phrenic nerve is opened to expose the circumflex vessels. The area is usually remarkably free of adhesions, and frequently a previous saphenous vein graft serves as a locator for the target vessel. The new conduit is brought from the descending aorta, which can be difficult at times because of atherosclerotic disease in the descending aorta. Use of recently introduced anastomotic connectors can facilitate performance of this portion of the procedure.

■ POSTOPERATIVE CARE

Patients routinely are extubated in the operating room, and a 3-day clinical care pathway is initiated. Attention to management of early postoperative pain by the use of epidural or local analgesia and liberal use of central α-agonists and intravenous antiinflammatory agents is extremely helpful. Early mobilization is encouraged and performed within 3 to 6 hours of surgery. Excessive postoperative bleeding is unusual, and monitoring lines usually are removed within 4 hours of surgery if the course remains stable to facilitate mobilization.

Because of loss of "postpump coagulopathy," aggressive use of antiplatelet agents is employed. We administer aspirin preoperatively and maintain it postoperatively. We also use clopidogrel (Plavix) in a loading dose of 300 mg on arrival in the intensive care unit and a maintenance dose of 75 mg/day for 30 days after surgery.

■ RESULTS

Since 2001, we have performed coronary revascularization with beating heart techniques in approximately 35% of our patients. This ranges up to 100% in the experience of some surgeons in our group. We now have experience with more than 2500 OPCAB procedures, and analysis of our results by

Table 4 Order of Anastomoses—Easiest to Hardest
Left anterior descending (unless RCA totally occluded, then RCA)
Diagonal
Distal circumflex, second, third obtuse marginals
Posterior ventricular RCA branches
Posterior descending
Higher obtuse marginals
Ramus
Main RCA

RCA, right coronary artery.

multiple logistic regression analysis indicates that the use of CPB is an independent risk factor for mortality with an odds ratio of 2.1:1. Further analysis of our results and those of the Washington Hospital Center by propensity score computer matching show the use of CPB to be an independent risk factor for mortality. Analysis of our results and published literature also indicates that there is a statistically significant lower incidence of postoperative bleeding, need for blood transfusion, intraaortic balloon use, postoperative inotrope use, atrial fibrillation, new-onset renal failure, and need for prolonged ventilation. There also is a trend toward a decreased incidence of stroke and neurocognitive dysfunction; however, this has not yet proved to be statistically significant.

■ CONCLUSIONS

Since the late 1990s, enormous strides have been made to facilitate the technique of beating heart surgery. The use of standard principles of hemodynamic monitoring and management, stabilization, exposure devices, and proper patient selection can lead to a valuable additional technique in the cardiac surgeon's armamentarium. With further advancements in facilitating technology and operative technique, optimization of educational avenues to disseminate these procedures, and clinical validation by further large series analyses, it is anticipated that off-pump techniques will continue to become the preferred method for coronary revascularization in more patients by more surgeons.

SUGGESTED READING

Mack MJ, et al: Improved outcomes in coronary artery bypass grafting with beating heart techniques, *J Thorac Cardiovas Surg* 124:598, 2002.

Magee MJ, et al: Elimination of cardiopulmonary bypass improves early survival in multivessel coronary artery bypass patients, *Ann Thorac Surg* 73:1196, 2002.

Mathison M, et al: Analysis of hemodynamic changes during beating heart surgical procedures, *Ann Thorac Surg* 70:1355, 2000.

Plomondon ME, et al: Off pump coronary artery bypass is associated with improved risk adjusted outcomes, *Ann Thorac Surg* 72:114, 2001.

Puskas JD, et al: Clinical outcomes, angiographic patency, and resource utilization in 200 consecutive off pump coronary bypass patients, *Ann Thorac Surg* 71:1477, 2001.

CORONARY ARTERY BYPASS GRAFT SURGERY DURING HYPOTHERMIC VENTRICULAR FIBRILLATION WITHOUT AORTIC OCCLUSION

Cary W. Akins

Despite the rapid growth of interventional cardiology, surgical myocardial revascularization remains the cornerstone treatment of symptomatic patients with multivessel coronary artery disease, left main coronary disease, and failure of interventional cardiologic procedures. Continued improvements in the operative management of patients having coronary artery bypass graft (CABG) surgery have led to reproducible success in most centers characterized by low mortality and complication rates and excellent, durable symptomatic results. Although most cardiac surgeons have converted to some form of cardioplegic arrest for myocardial protection during myocardial revascularization, modified hypothermic ventricular fibrillation without aortic occlusion, one of the earliest methods of myocardial preservation, remains an efficacious and reproducible alternative.

■ INDICATIONS AND CONTRAINDICATIONS

Hypothermic ventricular fibrillation without aortic occlusion can and has been used successfully for all types of primary and reoperative myocardial revascularization procedures and resection of left ventricular aneurysms. Only two pathologic situations truly can compromise this approach: significant aortic regurgitation and conditions that make the establishment of cardiopulmonary bypass (CPB) impossible.

Because the aorta is not cross-clamped during the procedure, aortic valve insufficiency can lead to ventricular distention. Usually this distention can be managed adequately with a left ventricular vent. If aortic regurgitation is severe enough to compromise this method of myocardial preservation, it is usually severe enough to warrant aortic valve repair or replacement.

Hypothermic ventricular fibrillation requires institution of CPB. Conditions that make CPB difficult, such as extensive calcification of the ascending aorta, can compromise this approach. In practice, however, this is rarely so serious that a site for arterial cannulation cannot be found.

In addition, using one proximal anastomosis or basing all bypass grafts on in situ arterial conduits is usually feasible.

TECHNIQUE OF HYPOTHERMIC VENTRICULAR FIBRILLATION

The underlying principle behind hypothermic ventricular fibrillation without aortic occlusion is a simple hydraulic argument—providing a continuous, adequate perfusion gradient of moderately cooled, oxygenated blood across the myocardium. The perfusion gradient is achieved by maintaining aortic perfusion pressure between 80 and 100 mm Hg, while keeping intracavitary left ventricular pressure low. Moderate systemic hypothermia is used to lower global myocardial oxygen demand to provide an increment of myocardial protection during the local occlusion of the coronary arteries required for performance of the distal anastomoses. The lowering of total body oxygen requirements also provides an element of security for perfusion complications.

The basic steps in the use of hypothermic ventricular fibrillation without aortic occlusion are as follows:

1. Initiation of intravenous nitroglycerin either during or just after the induction of anesthesia up to a dose of 1 mcg/kg/min, as tolerated by the patient.
2. Administration of β-blocking agents after the induction of anesthesia to lower the heart rate to less than 60 beats/min, as tolerated by the patient, if the patient is not adequately β-blocked preoperatively.
3. Early administration of the full heparin dose for CPB during harvesting and division of the internal mammary artery and before aortic cannulation.
4. Performance of proximal saphenous vein-to-aorta anastomoses before atrial cannulation and institution of CPB so that as each distal anastomosis is completed, that portion of the myocardium served by the bypassed coronary artery is perfused with oxygenated blood at an adequate perfusion pressure. Proximal anastomoses can be performed on CPB, however, before or after each distal anastomosis, if the situation warrants that approach.
5. Addition of mannitol to the crystalloid CPB priming solution for its osmotic and free radical scavenging effects.
6. Systemic hypothermia on CPB to about 30°C.
7. Maintenance of arterial perfusion pressure on CPB of 80 to 100 mm Hg, first by adjusting CPB pump flow, or if necessary, with pharmacologic agents, such as phenylephrine, to increase peripheral vascular resistance or nitroprusside to lower vascular resistance. (The accuracy of measuring and displaying the true arterial pressure is improved with use of an aortic perfusion cannula with an integral pressure-monitoring channel.)
8. Elective, but not electrically sustained, initiation of ventricular fibrillation if the heart does not fibrillate spontaneously during cooling.
9. Venting of the left ventricle through the right superior pulmonary vein. (The accuracy of measuring and displaying the true intracavitary left ventricular pressure is facilitated by use of a ventricular vent with an integral pressure-monitoring channel.)
10. Avoidance of cross-clamping the aorta. *Brief* periods of aortic occlusion are tolerable if necessary. (In my practice, this has been required fewer than five times in >5000 cases.)
11. Local vessel isolation with vinyl tapes for the performance of the distal anastomoses. (I try not to snare the artery circumferentially if possible.)
12. Initial grafting of the most ischemic zone first, if this can be identified preoperatively. If not, I usually first revascularize occluded vessels that are collateralized by other patent but diseased arteries so that when the patent, diseased arteries are grafted, blood flows retrograde through the collateral channels to limit ischemia in the myocardial distributions.
13. Grafting of diseased left circumflex coronary arteries before internal mammary grafting of the left anterior descending system to avoid excessive traction on the mammary pedicle, although mammary grafting can be performed at any time during the revascularization procedure.
14. Complete revascularization, whenever possible. (By this I mean any artery ≥1 mm in diameter that is judged to be significantly obstructed.)
15. Initiate rewarming on CPB during the last distal anastomosis.
16. Maintenance of good coronary perfusion and continuation of the intravenous nitroglycerin in the early postperfusion period.
17. If this technique is to be used for resection of a left ventricular aneurysm in conjunction with CABG surgery, I begin by opening the aneurysm and removing any intracavitary thrombus that could be dislodged with manipulation of the heart, then fully revascularize the diseased arteries, and finally close the aneurysm during rewarming on CPB.

Other than the above-listed steps in the performance of hypothermic ventricular fibrillation without aortic occlusion, most of the aspects of CABG surgery are similar to those used by many other surgeons, but some deserve emphasis.

PREOPERATIVE ASSESSMENT

Preoperatively, every effort should be made to bring the patient to the operating room in a nonischemic state. Intravenous nitroglycerin, antiplatelet agents, β-blockade, and calcium channel blockers may be required. If these agents fail to control ischemia, intraaortic balloon counterpulsation is indicated. In our institution's long-standing experience with acute ischemic syndromes, the most important lesson learned is that preoperative control of ischemia is a primary determinant of good outcome. We rarely are forced to perform truly emergent myocardial revascularization. Our results have been achieved with the cooperation and understanding of our cardiology colleagues. As a result, we rarely have to insert an intra-aortic balloon pump after myocardial revascularization has been performed.

Careful review of a current coronary angiogram (one performed within the preceding 6 months or sooner if the patient has had a significant change in his or her ischemic state) should be done preoperatively to delineate status of blood supply to all portions of the myocardium that are contractile. In virtually all cases, the revascularization procedure should be determined and planned before induction of anesthesia.

The available conduits should be evaluated carefully and completely preoperatively, especially when there has been previous removal of significant lengths of greater saphenous vein. Occasionally, angiographic visualization of the mammary arteries, noninvasive saphenous vein mapping, and preoperative radial artery assessment may be warranted.

■ PRIMARY MYOCARDIAL REVASCULARIZATION

Virtually all primary CABG operations use the left internal mammary artery to bypass branches of the left anterior descending system. More compete arterial revascularization is reserved for special indications. Supplemental grafting of other arterial distributions usually is performed with reversed greater saphenous vein. During the last several years at our institution, there has been gradual, but almost total conversion to endoscopic harvest of saphenous vein. This conversion has been associated with preservation of quality of the saphenous vein conduits, a significantly decreased incidence of saphenous vein harvest complications, and greater patient satisfaction. Endoscopic vein harvest by experienced operators usually can be completed in the time it takes the primary surgeon to open the chest, harvest the left internal mammary artery, and cannulate the ascending aorta.

My usual preference is to revascularize each of the three major coronary artery distributions—anterior descending, left circumflex, and right—with one piece of conduit if possible. This usually means that the left anterior descending and any of its diseased diagonal branches are grafted with the left internal mammary artery. I usually need only two segments of vein, one to graft the circumflex branches and one for the right coronary artery and its branches. Because I average about five bypass grafts per patient, many of the anastomoses are portions of sequential grafts.

Heparinization is initiated before division of the mammary pedicle distally and before opening of the pericardium. After the aortic cannula is inserted, some of the patient's heparinized blood is used to distend and prepare the saphenous vein.

Proximal vein-to-aorta anastomoses usually are performed over a side-biting clamp before atrial cannulation and institution of CPB. Proximal anastomoses may be done at any time, however. If I am concerned over the quality of the ascending aorta, I perform the proximal anastomoses on CPB when the quality of the aorta can be assessed more easily with a brief interruption of CPB. Left-sided grafts usually are placed on the left side of the aorta, and right-sided grafts are placed on the right side.

Distal anastomoses are performed with the local area of the coronary artery isolated with hollow vinyl loops. I prefer

to have at least two interrupted sutures at each end of the distal anastomosis to avoid any possibility of purse-string sutures. I always pass the suture needle from the lumen to the adventitia of the coronary artery and try to minimize handling of the artery. Minimal manipulation is particularly important when one also is manipulating the internal mammary artery.

Rewarming is initiated during the last distal anastomosis. Defibrillation is performed, if necessary, when systemic temperature is about 34°C. During rewarming, I routinely place two atrial and two ventricular temporary pacing wires.

■ REOPERATIVE REVASCULARIZATION

Patent arterial bypass grafts do not pose a myocardial protection problem with the technique of hypothermic ventricular fibrillation. Patent but diseased vein grafts are sequentially removed and replaced in a sequence that minimizes manipulation of diseased conduits.

Proximal anastomoses often can be performed before CPB on the hoods of old occluded vein grafts or on previously unused portions of the aorta. Then the sequence of revascularization becomes one of alternating proximal and distal anastomoses.

■ POST–CARDIOPULMONARY BYPASS MANAGEMENT

Management after CPB focuses on preservation of adequate coronary arterial perfusion by maintenance of good arterial perfusion pressure and continuation of intravenous nitroglycerin. Pure inotropic agents rarely are needed, but vasopressor agents may be useful to keep arterial pressure at appropriate levels.

Removal of excess fluid accumulated on CPB is achieved by aggressive diuresis. All organ systems, including myocardium, function better in a nonedematous state. Low-dose dopamine can be useful in some patients with preoperative renal failure or resistance to diuretics. For patients who are refractory to diuretics, a continuous drip of furosemide and mannitol can be useful.

Anticoagulation with aspirin is initiated on the evening of the CPB procedure. Intravenous nitroglycerin usually is discontinued when the patient is fully rewarmed and extubated.

■ SUMMARY

Hypothermic ventricular fibrillation without aortic occlusion is a proven method of myocardial protection for all forms of surgical myocardial revascularization and left ventricular aneurysm resection. Compared with cardioplegic methods of protection, this method (1) avoids aortic cross-clamping; (2) eliminates global myocardial ischemia; (3) avoids the cannulation and fluid administration for cardioplegia delivery; and (4) is generally simpler, less cumbersome, quicker, and cheaper. Some aspects of the technique may seem, however, to be potential disadvantages: (1) Coronary arteries must be isolated and locally occluded during distal anastomoses, (2) partial aortic occlusion is necessary for proximal vein anastomoses, (3) retraction of the heart may be more difficult, and (4) the operative field is not bloodless.

SUGGESTED READING

Akins CW: Noncardioplegic myocardial preservation for coronary revascularization, *J Thorac Cardiovasc Surg* 88:174, 1984.

Akins CW: Early and late results following emergency isolated myocardial revascularization during hypothermic fibrillatory arrest, *Ann Thorac Surg* 43:131, 1987.

Akins CW: Resection of left ventricular aneurysm during hypothermic fibrillatory arrest without aortic occlusion, *J Thorac Cardiovasc Surg* 91:610, 1986.

Akins CW: Myocardial preservation with hypothermic fibrillatory arrest for coronary grafting, *J Mol Cell Cardiol* 22:S44, 1990.

Akins CW, Carroll DL: Event-free survival following nonemergency myocardial revascularization during hypothermic fibrillatory arrest, *Ann Thorac Surg* 43:628, 1987.

REOPERATION FOR CORONARY ARTERY DISEASE

Bruce W. Lytle

Coronary reoperations are the result of the success of coronary artery bypass graft surgery in prolonging life expectancy and the inability to arrest completely the progression of atherosclerosis in bypass grafts (particularly in saphenous vein grafts [SVGs]) and native coronary arteries. The number of coronary reoperations performed in the United States has continued to increase, but the exponential rise in coronary reoperations that occurred during the 1980s has slowed. Current data from the Society of Thoracic Surgeons (STS) database (1997-2000) indicate that 9.3% of operations for isolated bypass surgery reported to the registry were reoperations.

■ BACKGROUND

The anatomic indications for coronary reoperations are progression of atherosclerosis in native coronary arteries, graft failure, or a combination of the two. In the early years of bypass surgery, primary operations often were performed for limited coronary artery disease, and many reoperations were needed solely because of new disease occurring in previously ungrafted arteries. That indication is rare today because most patients undergoing primary operation have multivessel disease. The anatomic indications for reoperation almost always include graft failure, usually SVG atherosclerosis. When progression of native vessel disease contributes to the need for reoperation, it is often distal progression of disease in grafted vessels. The interval between first and second operations has lengthened with time, and today most reoperations occur more than 10 years after primary surgery.

Candidates for reoperation are different than patients undergoing primary surgery. Problems of sternal reentry are unique to reoperations. Also unique to reoperations are situations in which areas of myocardium are graft dependent, either on internal thoracic artery (ITA) grafts that are at risk for damage during a repeat procedure or on SVGs with stenoses caused by pathologies that are different from native vessel coronary artery disease (intimal fibroplasia and vein graft atherosclerosis).

Vein graft atherosclerosis is a dangerous lesion and underlies many of the difficulties in dealing with patients with previous bypass surgery. Although native vessel atherosclerosis tends to be proximal, eccentric, based on the media, and encapsulated, vein graft atherosclerosis is diffuse, circumferential, superficial, and extremely friable. Vein graft atherosclerosis is an active lesion that seems to incite thrombosis and embolization. Embolization of atherosclerotic debris from SVGs has been a significant cause of myocardial infarction during reoperation and percutaneous interventions and probably accounts for the unfavorable natural history of patients with late stenoses in vein grafts.

Other challenges may not be unique to reoperative patients but are more common in that setting. In general, cardiac and noncardiac atherosclerosis and their sequelae are more common during repeat surgery. Aortic atherosclerosis makes arterial cannulation for cardiopulmonary bypass (CPB) more problematic and, along with cerebrovascular disease, creates a risk of stroke. Coronary atherosclerosis is often extremely distal and diffuse in reoperative candidates, much more so than is seen during primary operation. Shortage of bypass conduits is a common problem during reoperation, particularly for patients who have undergone multiple previous procedures.

One of the difficulties in the management of patients with previous surgery is the lack of comparative studies of treatment or even natural history studies of patients with previous surgery who have recurrent ischemic syndromes. We conducted two nonrandomized retrospective studies of patients who underwent repeat angiography after bypass surgery to identify the impact of stenotic vein grafts on outcomes with and without reoperation. We found that patients with early stenoses in vein grafts (usually caused by intimal fibroplasia) had relatively favorable survival outcomes even without reoperation, although reoperation did improve symptom status. Patients with late (≥5 years after operation) stenoses in vein grafts (usually caused by vein graft atherosclerosis) had a relatively unfavorable survival outcome without surgery, however, that was improved by reoperation. The improvement in survival with reoperation was particularly dramatic if the SVG subtended the left anterior descending coronary artery (LAD). Reoperation to improve prognosis is indicated for patients with an atherosclerotic vein graft subtending the LAD or other major areas of viable myocardium. For patients without any patent grafts, reoperation to improve prognosis is indicated by the same criteria that indicate primary operation—left main stenosis, multivessel disease including a proximal LAD lesion, and a positive stress test. Reoperation for symptom relief is indicated for patients with consistently limiting symptoms, jeopardized but graftable coronary arteries that supply areas of viable myocardium, and a positive stress test.

What role do percutaneous treatments play in the management of patients with previous surgery? The percutaneous treatment of vein graft stenoses has not been effective over time. Although the use of stents has improved a formerly dismal rate of restenosis, the combination of in-stent restenosis and new stenoses in nonstented portions of vein grafts still produces a high rate of treatment failure, particularly if the follow-up period is longer than 6 months after the procedure. Percutaneous treatment rarely is indicated as a treatment for diffusely atherosclerotic important vein grafts. For patients with early vein graft stenoses, limited late stenoses in noncritical vein grafts, and native vessel stenoses that are accessible to angioplasty, percutaneous treatments can offer effective relief of angina. Also, there are situations in which the treatment of acute vein graft occlusion is best approached percutaneously.

■ PREOPERATIVE MANAGEMENT

Reoperations may be indicated for patients who have life-threatening anatomy or symptoms that are caused by ischemia, combined with graftable vessels subtending areas of viable myocardium and the presence of bypass conduits that would allow grafting. The preoperative evaluation should establish those points.

A complete preoperative angiogram is essential for accurate decision making. Coronary arteries may receive their blood supply from patent or stenotic arterial or venous bypass grafts arising from multiple locations, including the ascending aorta, descending aorta, and in situ arterial grafts. Coronary or noncoronary collaterals may contribute to myocardial blood supply. The failure to identify coronary vessels at angiography does not mean that graftable vessels are not present if all the proper contrast injections have not been made or the angiographer did not allow time for filling by collaterals. Previous angiograms and operative notes are helpful to the cardiologist in performing the angiogram and

to the surgeon in interpreting it. Viable myocardium almost always has an identifiable blood supply.

Multiple imaging strategies are available for establishing myocardial viability, including positron emission tomography and stress echocardiography, the imaging techniques we most often employ. We have found positron emission tomography to be the most sensitive measurement of viability (although not 100% specific) and stress echocardiography to be our best assessment of contractile reserve.

Preoperative conduit assessment is important. It is not wise to discover in the operating room that conduits are not available to graft critical vessels. Greater and lesser saphenous veins are studied with Doppler studies, as are the inferior epigastric arteries. Ideally the ITAs should be studied during the preoperative angiogram, but if they are not, Doppler studies may identify ITA abnormalities. Doppler studies may not identify correctly a severe subclavian stenosis, however, in which case ITA angiography is better. Radial arteries should be studied with perfusion indices or Allen's test to establish adequate ulnar collateral flow. These radial artery studies do not establish that the arteries are without stenoses, however, and in many patients with previous surgery one or both of the radial arteries have been damaged by radial artery arterial pressure monitoring catheters at a previous operation.

Preoperative echocardiography helps to establish ventricular and valvular function and may identify ascending aortic atherosclerosis. The preoperative posteroanterior and lateral chest x-ray gives clues to the route of patent ITA grafts and the proximity of mediastinal structures to the sternum. In questionable cases, a computed tomography scan may give a more accurate picture of substernal structures, although we do not routinely obtain a preoperative computed tomography scan.

■ OPERATIVE MANAGEMENT

Safe sternal reentry and conduit preparation may take time, and anesthetic management needs to maintain hemodynamic stability while the operation proceeds. Maintenance of hemodynamics is aided by pulmonary artery pressure monitoring with a Swan-Ganz catheter and often with transesophageal echocardiography.

The greatest cause of death during or after reoperation is perioperative myocardial infarction, which is often anatomically related. Anatomic causes of myocardial infarction include damage to preexisting patent or stenotic bypass grafts, embolization of atherosclerotic debris from the aorta or vein grafts, bypass graft failure due to thrombosis or technical error, incomplete revascularization, and failure to deliver cardioplegia to major myocardial areas. Our operative strategies are designed to avoid those events.

Sternal reentry is accomplished with an oscillating saw, leaving the posterior aspect of the sternal wires intact until the bone has been completely divided. If a problem with reentry is anticipated, arterial access via the femoral or axillary artery is obtained along with femoral venous access. Radial artery and venous conduits are prepared before the sternotomy. In some cases, a small anterior right thoracotomy can be performed to allow dissection of the right ventricle and aorta, away from the sternum. When the sternum is opened, the mediastinal structures are dissected away, the pleurae are opened on both sides, and any ITAs to be used for grafts are dissected from the chest wall. If the left ITA graft is patent, it is not dissected out until the new bypass conduits are prepared and when the aorta and the right atrium are dissected out and available for cannulation. Isolation of the left ITA is delayed until cannulation is accomplished so that if the graft does get injured, CPB can be instituted immediately for subsequent repair.

Cannulation of the aorta may be a problem because of a combination of aortic atherosclerosis, aortic scarring, the presence of sutures and pledgets, and the presence of patent or stenotic vein grafts. The femoral artery is a common alternative arterial cannulation site, but many reoperative patients have significant aortic iliac disease or severe aortic atherosclerosis, situations in which we would rather not use retrograde perfusion. We often use the right axillary artery as an alternative arterial cannulation site. After that vessel is prepared, heparin is given, and an 8-mm collagen-coated graft is sewn to the axillary artery in an end-to-side fashion, placing the arterial cannula within the graft. During decannulation at the end of the procedure, the graft is cut off a few millimeters above the level of the axillary artery and oversewn. For venous return, a two-stage venous cannula is placed in the right atrium. A stylet is used to place a retrograde cardioplegia cannula with a self-inflating balloon through a purse-string suture in the right atrium into the coronary sinus. A needle for antegrade cardioplegia delivery and aortic venting is placed along the surface of the aorta.

When cannulation is accomplished, CPB is established, the aorta is cross-clamped, and antegrade and retrograde cold blood cardioplegia are given. With the heart arrested, the left side of the heart is dissected out by incising along the diaphragm to the left of the apex of the heart, then proceeding in a superior direction to the left side of the LAD. This strategy avoids an ITA graft or a vein graft to the LAD. If a patent left ITA graft has not been controlled before this point, it now is dissected out, and an atraumatic clamp is placed across it. If retrograde cardioplegia delivery is adequate as judged by coronary sinus pressure, myocardial cooling, and return of deoxygenated blood through the coronary arteries when they are opened, doses of retrograde cardioplegia are repeated every 15 minutes, and further antegrade delivery is avoided or minimized.

Grafting strategies are related to the details of the coronary anatomy. In a simpler era, our general rule was to replace all vein grafts more than 5 years old. Today that is often not possible due to a lack of bypass conduits and multiple prior vein grafts. If possible, we still prefer to replace completely severely atherosclerotic vein grafts to remove the possibility of atherosclerotic embolization. This is accomplished by replacing vein grafts with vein grafts. If adequate vein is not available, it sometimes is necessary to leave old vein grafts in place. When arterial conduits are used to bypass vessels supplied by stenotic vein grafts, the old vein grafts are not removed, but rather arterial grafts are added to the vessel. Removing a vein graft (even a stenotic vein graft) to a large vessel and replacing it with only an arterial graft is a strategy that risks hypoperfusion. Although leaving any atherosclerotic vein graft in place risks embolization, using

care in dissecting the heart along with retrograde cardioplegia minimizes that danger, and it is less than the danger of hypoperfusion associated with removing stenotic grafts and replacing with smaller arterial grafts.

In reoperative patients, the atherosclerotic disease often has extended far distally. Often the intramyocardial coronary segments are the best to graft. These characteristics may make sequential grafts difficult, particularly using arterial conduits. Performing sequential arterial grafts to intramyocardial vessels risks kinking the graft as it extends out of the plane of the epicardium. We sometimes compensate for this problem by using short Y-grafts to graft intramyocardial vessels.

Multiple strategies are used for inflow (proximal) anastomoses. Aortic anastomoses of vein grafts usually are carried out at the site of a previously placed vein graft. There are multiple possible sites for proximal anastomoses of arterial grafts. One effective proximal site is a new or previously placed in situ left ITA graft. If the left ITA has been used previously for a graft, it is often a large vessel, and construction of a T- or a Y-type anastomosis with the right ITA or a radial artery is relatively straightforward. This strategy provides plenty of length for the new artery to graft the left side of the heart and may reach the posterior descending branch of the right coronary artery. If a composite arterial graft is not possible due to damage to the left ITA in the past, or if the left ITA is encased in scar, the proximal anastomosis of the arterial grafts often is made to the hood of a new or old vein graft off of the aorta. The "bubble" on the hood of a vein graft appears to be relatively protected with regard to atherosclerosis, and the thinner vein is a more favorable site than the reoperative aorta for a proximal arterial graft. If a new left ITA is being used at the reoperation, that vessel can be the site of a proximal anastomosis of a radial, ITA, or even a vein graft.

When all anastomoses are constructed under a single period of aortic cross-clamping, a reperfusion "hot-shot" dose of cardioplegia is given, and the cross-clamp is removed from the aorta. When ventricular function has returned and is documented by transesophageal echocardiography, the patient is weaned from CPB, decannulation is accomplished, and protamine is given.

■ ALTERNATIVE REOPERATIONS

Most patients undergoing reoperation have diffuse and distal coronary artery disease and may need grafts performed to multiple vessels. Because of these characteristics, we usually choose to perform reoperations through a median sternotomy with the use of CPB instead of employing a small incision or off-pump surgery. In specific circumstances, however, alternative surgical approaches and beating heart surgery can be useful during reoperation.

Our most common alternative incision is a left lateral thoracotomy, which provides excellent exposure to graft the vessels of the lateral wall. A saphenous vein or radial artery graft is anastomosed to the descending aorta or subclavian artery with the use of a partial occluding clamp after heparinization. Then the distal coronary graft is performed without CPB using a suction-type stabilizer. A second alternative is a left anterior thoracotomy to access the distal LAD. In this setting, the left ITA or a vein graft (anastomosed to the axillary artery through a separate incision) is used to graft the LAD without CPB.

Off-pump (beating heart) surgery through a median sternotomy is the most common alternative strategy for CABG surgery being used for primary operations today and can be used in the reoperative setting. There are disadvantages to this approach at reoperation, however. First are the dangers of atherosclerotic embolization from patent vein grafts during the dissection of the beating heart. Although not all reoperative candidates have atherosclerotic vein grafts, many do. Second, the need to use a partial occluding clamp on the aorta for the construction of proximal vein or arterial anastomoses is a disadvantage. The use of newly developed aortic "connectors" for the construction of vein-to-aortic anastomoses may lessen the impact of this problem. Third, the diffuse distal disease and the need to graft intramyocardial vessels in many reoperations make off-pump surgery more difficult, particularly if lateral wall vessels need to be grafted through a median sternotomy.

The advantages of beating heart surgery at reoperation are most evident if patients have extensive, noncardiac (particularly aortic) atherosclerosis and need only a few grafts. We employ this approach most commonly when using ITA conduits to graft an anterior or anterolateral vessel concomitant with grafts to right coronary branches.

■ RESULTS

In general, the short-term and long-term results of reoperation are less favorable than the results of primary procedures. In-hospital risks of reoperations are increased when compared with primary procedures. The STS database documented a mortality rate of 1.91% for 340,458 primary elective isolated bypass operations and a 5.2% risk for 35,768 elective reoperations between 1997 and 2000.

A nonelective or "emergency" status dramatically increases the risk of reoperation. The same STS database noted a 9.14% risk for reoperations for patients classified as *urgent/emergent/salvage*. The absolute risk of emergency reoperations depends on the definition of *emergency*. In the STS database, 19% of patients were in this nonelective category, indicating a broad definition. All authors who have examined this problem have noted, however, a substantial risk for emergency reoperations, with the absolute numbers being related to the definition of emergency. Other variables that increase risk include congestive heart failure, female gender, abnormal left ventricular function, and the number of patent but atherosclerotic vein grafts present.

Diffuse disease or "bad vessels" are a determinant of risk during reoperation. Because *bad vessels* is a concept that is hard to quantify, it usually is not examined in studies. Bad vessels are the most common reasons patients are not considered for reoperation, however. When reoperation is undertaken, bad vessels often compromise the effectiveness of the revascularization that can be achieved. Few reoperative candidates are truly completely revascularized.

The long-term outcomes of reoperation are influenced by the far advanced state of cardiac and noncardiac atherosclerosis at the time of the reoperation and the fact that many patients are not made perfect by reoperation. Our most recent detailed studies of long-term follow-up showed that by 5 years after reoperation, 35% to 50% of patients had some symptoms, although few had severe symptoms. Late survival of hospital survivors was 69% at 10 years after reoperation. These data are not as favorable as data for primary operation, but they do not indicate that reoperation is futile.

Patients presenting for third or fourth operations are becoming more common and have the same characteristics as patients undergoing second operations, but only more complex. Conduit availability is often a problem at a third operation. These are difficult reoperations and are carried out at increased cost and risk. Age has influenced the long-term outcome of these patients. The 5-year survival rate after a third operation was 82% for patients younger than 70 years old but only 52% for patients older than 70.

Many factors seem to be slowing the time-related incidence of coronary reoperation. The use of arterial grafts, increased surgical experience, postoperative treatment with cholesterol-lowering medications, and increased use of interventional catheter procedures all may play a role. Reoperations are still prevalent, however, and provide coronary surgeons with their greatest challenges.

SUGGESTED READING

Loop FD, et al: Reoperation for coronary atherosclerosis: changing practice in 2509 consecutive patients, *Ann Surg* 212:378, 1990.

Lytle BW, et al: The effect of coronary reoperation on the survival of patients with stenoses in saphenous vein bypass grafts to coronary arteries, *J Thorac Cardiovasc Surg* 105:605, 1993.

Lytle BW, et al: The influence of arterial coronary bypass grafts on the mortality in coronary reoperations, *J Thorac Cardiovasc Surg* 107:675, 1994.

Lytle BW, et al: Fifteen hundred coronary reoperations: results and determinants of early and late survival, *J Thorac Cardiovasc Surg* 93:847, 1987.

Lytle BW, et al: Third coronary artery bypass operations: risks and costs, *Ann Thorac Surg* 64:1287, 1997.

POSTINFARCTION VENTRICULAR SEPTAL DEFECT

Christopher M. Feindel

Left ventricular rupture is the cause of death in almost one third of patients who have a fatal myocardial infarction (MI). Although most of these ruptures occur in the free wall and result in immediate death, 15% to 20% occur in the interventricular septum and are amenable to surgical repair. The first successful surgical repair of a ventricular septal rupture was performed in 1957 by Cooley. Daggett introduced the infarctectomy and patch technique in 1977, and until more recently this was the standard approach used by most surgeons. Operative mortality remained high in most reports, however, frequently greater than 50%. In 1995, David introduced a simplified endocardial patch technique with infarct exclusion, which, considering 19% operative mortality, represented a significant improvement in technique. Despite advances in the surgical management of these patients, repair of postinfarction ventricular septal defect (VSD) remains one of the most challenging operations for cardiac surgeons today. Cardiogenic shock and early rupture after initial infarction are grave prognostic signs. Following is a brief description of our surgical approach to the postinfarction VSD.

■ DIAGNOSIS

The diagnosis of postinfarction VSD is suggested by the history of a recent MI along with the development of a new pansystolic murmur, often in the setting of hemodynamic compromise. In more recent years, thrombolytic therapy has been administered routinely to patients at the time of initial presentation of MI. Thrombolytic therapy may have led to an increased incidence of this mechanical complication after MI. The main differential diagnosis is a ruptured papillary muscle with mitral regurgitation. An oxygen saturation step-up in the right side of the heart indicates the presence of a left-to-right shunt, and the diagnosis is confirmed with transthoracic and, if necessary, transesophageal echocardiography. Ventriculography, performed at the time of coronary angiography, also is diagnostic. Defects are located in the anterior septum in patients who have occluded left anterior descending artery. Posterior defects occur in patients in whom either the right coronary artery or a dominant circumflex artery occlude. Noninfarcted areas of the left ventricle are typically hyperdynamic due to unloading of volume into the lower pressure right side. By contrast, right ventricular function usually is severely compromised by volume overload and, if the right coronary artery is occluded, by muscle damage. In a small percentage of patients, VSDs are detected late after the original MI as a result of

investigations for a pansystolic murmur discovered incidentally on examination. In these patients, the defects are usually small and rarely cause hemodynamic compromise. This discussion focuses only on the management of acute postinfarction VSD.

■ SURGICAL CONSULT

Without surgical intervention, the natural history of patients with postinfarction VSD is poor. Mortality ranges from 60% to 70% in the first 2 weeks, with less than 10% of patients alive after 3 months. Cardiologists are aware of this dismal natural history and request the surgeon operate as soon as possible. However, few patients taken to the operating room in profound shock and in fulminate pulmonary edema survive. Therefore, it is important for the surgeon to evaluate carefully and optimize the patient's cardiopulmonary status before proceeding to the operating room.

■ PREOPERATIVE MANAGEMENT

When the diagnosis of postinfarction VSD is suspected, we recommend inserting an intraaortic balloon pump in all patients, with the exception only of the few patients who are completely stable. The intraaortic balloon pump helps to stabilize the patient, improves coronary perfusion, enhances forward cardiac output, and makes it safer to perform coronary angiography. Inotropic agents and vasodilator agents should be given to maintain organ perfusion and urine output. If right ventricular failure is severe, efforts to minimize pulmonary afterload must be made and include ensuring adequate ventilation to avoid respiratory acidosis. If ventilation is required, it is important to remember that positive pressure and aggressive positive end-expiratory pressure increase right ventricular afterload, which further compromise right ventricular function. Nitric oxide may be useful in this setting to reduce pulmonary resistance. With this regimen, patients often improve over 6 to 24 hours. During this time, coronary angiography should be performed to delineate coronary anatomy. We proceed to surgery within this 24-hour window after the diagnosis, preferably within 12 hours.

While providing emotional support to the patient and family, it is equally important to be realistic about expected outcomes. We explain to the conscious patient that the surgery is risky, but that without the procedure there is no realistic chance of survival. We are especially careful to emphasize to the family the severity of the operation.

If the patient fails to improve despite the aforementioned aggressive medical management and deteriorates further, we carefully reevaluate the situation. These patients rarely survive operation. The decision for surgery then becomes an ethical issue and is influenced by the patient's age and overall medical status, especially in the presence of severe multivessel coronary artery disease. It is important that the surgeon, family members, and referring cardiologist are aligned in this decision. In some cases, the expectations and insight of family members and possibly the cardiologist may influence the surgeon to proceed even though there is little chance of survival.

■ OPERATIVE MANAGEMENT

The anesthetic management of the patient with postinfarction VSD is similar to any cardiac surgery patient who is compromised hemodynamically or is in cardiogenic shock. The surgical team must be in the operating room at the time of anesthetic induction. The loss of sympathetic tone when the patient is asleep often heralds sudden cardiac compromise, if not cardiac arrest. Tachycardia is common and should be recognized as the patient's natural effort to maintain forward blood flow. Well-intended efforts to treat sinus tachycardia are likely to be disastrous and should be avoided. Because individual anesthesiologists rarely have a large experience with these patients, the surgeon must be present to assist and advise during anesthetic induction.

The legs should be prepared and saphenous vein harvested as necessary. We do not recommend using arterial grafts in these patients for two reasons. First, time is often of the essence, and, second, the need for postoperative inotropes may cause spasm in arterial grafts. We consider using internal thoracic artery grafts only when vein conduits are not available. The occluded artery responsible for the VSD should not be grafted.

The sternotomy should be performed, but the pericardiotomy should be delayed until sternal bleeding is controlled and heparin is given. Particular caution must be exercised if blood is seen under the pericardium. We recommend that the surgeon wait until the activated clotting time exceeds 200 seconds before opening the pericardium in case rapid establishment of cardiopulmonary bypass (CPB) is necessary. Rapid establishment of CPB will likely be needed if, in addition to the VSD, there is a partial free wall rupture that is tamponaded by the pericardium. Even in the absence of obvious rupture, the surgeon can expect to find old or fresh blood in the pericardium because there is often some leakage through the infarcted myocardium.

Standard aortic cannulation is used, and both vena cavae are cannulated either directly or via the right atrium. An enlarged right ventricle may make direct caval cannulation difficult. Tapes should be placed around the superior vena cava and inferior vena cava. We routinely allow the patient's systemic temperature to drift down to 34°C but do not actively cool. We use antegrade cold blood cardioplegia for myocardial protection. Retrograde coronary sinus cardioplegia is avoided because it may lead to severe hemorrhage into the infarcted and friable muscle. While establishing CPB, a bovine glutaraldehyde-fixed pericardial patch is washed and prepared.

We prefer to repair the septal defect first, then proceed with any necessary coronary artery bypasses. Because the infarcted area in the heart is extremely friable, lifting the heart and retracting it to perform bypasses first before the repair may dislodge pieces of necrotic muscle inside the heart resulting in a cerebral embolus. Only major stenotic coronary arteries are bypassed to avoid prolonged cross-clamp times.

When CPB is established, the heart is arrested with antegrade cold blood cardioplegia. We do not attempt to repair the defect with the heart beating, which in our opinion, greatly reduces visualization and impedes the chance of a successful repair. We do not routinely insert a left ventricular sump drain.

The approach to repair depends on the location of the VSD, specifically whether it is anterior or posterior. Anterior defects are easier to repair than posterior defects, the latter being difficult because of their location and proximity to the mitral valve. Each repair is described separately.

■ OPERATIVE TECHNIQUE

Anterior VSD

In patients with anterior VSD, the heart is lifted carefully by placing sponges behind it. The area of the anterior wall infarction is identified, and an incision is made into the center of the necrotic area 1 to 2 cm to the left and parallel to the left anterior descending artery. The incision is extended proximally and distally to within 0.5 cm of viable muscle. The VSD and the margins of the infarcted muscle are located inside the ventricle. Loose muscle is removed, but no attempt is made to excise infarcted tissue. A glutaraldehyde-fixed bovine pericardial patch is cut in an oval shape to a size slightly larger than the size of the infarcted area. The patch can be trimmed as necessary and in most cases is about 4 cm × 6 cm. The pericardial patch is sutured to the lower part of the noninfarcted endocardium of the interventricular septum using continuous 4-0 polypropylene with a large needle. The suture bites must be taken deep into the muscle and pulled taut, yet gentle enough so as not to tear out. In some cases in which the muscle appears particularly fragile, a second suture line of 4-0 polypropylene can be run to secure the patch in the septal area, this time with a small needle. In the uppermost and lowermost ends, the sutures are passed through the patch, then through the ventricle wall and buttressed with another thin strip of bovine pericardium on the epicardial surface. One or two separate interrupted sutures may help secure the corners. The patch is flipped over and sutured to the noninfarcted endocardium of the anterolateral free ventricular wall. Each bite of this suture line should pass through the entire ventricular wall, be secured through a strip of pericardium on the epicardial surface, and passed back through the wall to the endocardial patch. This is especially important in cases in which the infarct involves the base of the anterior papillary muscle.

Residual air is removed easily from the left ventricular cavity by running cardioplegia while compressing the aortic annulus to render the aortic valve incompetent. Significant leaks through the patch–to–left ventricle suture line can be repaired at this time. With the patch completely secured to the endocardium of the left ventricle, the infarcted area and the VSD now are excluded from the left ventricular cavity. The ventriculotomy is closed over two strips of bovine pericardium, one for the right side of the suture line and the other being the same strip that was used to secure the endocardial patch on the left free wall.

Posterior VSD

The repair principles for posterior VSDs are the same as for anterior VSDs. The awkward angle and proximity of the mitral valve make this repair more difficult, however. An assistant or device is needed to gently retract the heart superiorly. Placing the patient in the Trendelenburg position improves exposure. The cardiomyotomy is made along the inferior wall of the left ventricle, approximately 1 to 2 cm to the left and parallel to the posterior descending artery. Similar to anterior VSD, this incision is extended proximally and distally to within 0.5 cm of the viable myocardium, that is, proximally toward the mitral annulus and distally toward the apex of the ventricle. Stay sutures, passed through the fat pad of the apex of the ventricle and margins of the ventriculotomy, further aid in the exposure of the ventricular cavity. A bovine pericardial patch is prepared and shaped as a triangular ellipse approximately 4 cm × 7 cm. The patch is sutured using 4-0 polypropylene with a large needle starting at the level of the fibrous annulus of the mitral valve. The suture line is brought medially first to the level of the posteromedial papillary muscle, then further medially toward the septum until the noninfarcted endocardium is reached. At this point, the suture is secured with several interrupted bites, trimming off any excess patch material. The medial margin of the triangular-shaped patch is sewn to healthy septal endocardium with continuous suture and reinforced with a second suture of 4-0 polypropylene using a fine needle in the septal area. As in the anterior VSD repair, the lateral side of the patch is flipped over and sutured to the posterior wall of the left ventricle using through-and-through sutures reinforced with a strip of bovine pericardium on the epicardial surface. The patch is tested by running cardioplegia as described in the anterior VSD repair, with additional sutures placed to correct leaks.

The ventriculotomy is closed in two layers of sutures buttressed on strips of pericardium. If the head of the posteromedial papillary muscle is ruptured, repair can be accomplished by reattaching it with a 5-0 expanded polytetrafluoroethylene (Gore-Tex) suture, first securing it to the remaining papillary muscle stump, then anchoring it to a pledget on the epicardial surface of the posterior wall.

■ SEPARATING FROM CARDIOPULMONARY BYPASS

After a period of myocardial reperfusion, the patient is weaned from CPB. Inotropes and vasodilators are usually necessary. Right ventricular function usually is improved as the volume overload has been corrected. Nitric oxide may be a valuable adjunct, in cases of severe right ventricular failure. Sinus tachycardia is not treated, and atrioventricular pacing is used if the heart rate is too slow. With a reduced ventricular volume, patients increase cardiac output by increasing heart rate rather than increasing ventricular volume. A heart rate of 90 to 100 beats/min is acceptable.

■ POSTOPERATIVE CARE

Management in the intensive care unit is similar to any patient with severely compromised ventricular function. The intraaortic balloon should remain in place for at least an additional 24 hours and longer if necessary.

■ SUMMARY

Although patients with postinfarction VSD represent one of the most challenging problems facing cardiac surgeons today, careful attention to appropriate selection of patients and to the details of the operation provides the best possible chance of survival with surgical repair.

SUGGESTED READING

David TE, et al: Postinfarction ventricular septal rupture: repair by endocardial patch with infarct exclusion, *J Thorac Cardiovasc Surg* 110:1315, 1995.

De Boer HD, de Boer WJ: Early repair of postinfarction ventricular septal rupture: infarct exclusion, septal stabilization, and left ventricular remodeling, *Ann Thorac Surg* 65:853, 1998.

Pretre R, et al: Role of myocardial revascularization in postinfarction ventricular septal rupture, *Ann Thorac Surg* 69:51, 2000.

MITRAL REGURGITATION AND THE ISCHEMIC HEART

Vinay Badhwar
Steven F. Bolling

The management of ischemic mitral regurgitation (MR) continues to be one of the last enigmas in cardiac surgery. Historical fears of prohibitive operative risk and poor understanding of the insidious dysfunction associated with the ischemic mitral apparatus have resulted in some patients with ischemic MR being managed without mitral reconstruction. It now is appreciated, however, that ischemic patients with uncorrected MR, numbering more than 2 million in the United States, have a truly bleak outlook due to the swift development of refractory heart failure. The 1-year mortality of these patients is greater than 50%. Patients who do not die rapidly have progressive heart failure that severely limits quality of life and necessitates frequent hospitalizations. With improved knowledge of the natural history and pathophysiology of ischemic MR, there has been renewed interest in the effective surgical management of these high-risk patients.

Fundamental to the management of ischemic MR is a firm understanding of the functional anatomy of the mitral valve. The mitral valve apparatus consists of the annulus, leaflets, chordae tendineae, papillary muscles, and the entire left ventricle. The maintenance of chordal, annular, and subvalvular continuity is essential for the preservation of mitral geometric relationships and overall ventricular function.

The existence of ischemic MR is defined by a direct causal relationship between ischemic insults due to coronary artery disease and the development of MR due to geometric distortion of the mitral apparatus. Patients with incidental coronary disease in association with primary anatomic valvular pathology, such as rheumatic or myxomatous degeneration, should be excluded from the definition of ischemic MR. Although ischemic MR can be classified crudely into acute or chronic, these are essentially two different pathophysiologic entities with two different management strategies.

The presentation of acute postinfarction MR is rare, representing only about 1% to 2% of ischemic MR patients. Because it is a complication of a large transmural infarction in continuity with a papillary muscle, this occasionally results in partial or subtotal papillary rupture, florid MR, and cardiogenic shock unresponsive to inotropic or intraaortic balloon pump therapy. The mortality of these moribund patients is 10% to 40% with surgery, but it is virtually assured without surgery. Repeated attempts at complex mitral repair in this setting are imprudent and not tolerated by these critically ill patients with acutely stunned ventricles. A rapidly performed apparatus-preserving prosthetic replacement provides for the highest likelihood for success in this rare setting.

Chronic ischemic MR is preceded by either prolonged global ischemia or a precise coronary event. These patients constitute most cases that present for surgical consideration. After an ischemic event, the entire left ventricle, but particularly the lateral and posterior walls, undergo adaptive remodeling. These geometric changes include regional myocardial thinning, annular distortion, reduced leaflet closing force, papillary muscle foreshortening, and increased tethering of the posterior leaflet relative to the anterior leaflet resulting in an eccentric jet of MR (Figure 1). This follows the restrictive pathophysiology outlined by Carpentier's classification type IIIB. These perturbations to the annular-ventricular apparatus and ventricular geometry combine to result in loss of the zone of coaptation and the development of progressive regurgitation and, eventually, heart failure. Reconstructing this geometry and restoring the zone of coaptation is the basis for any effective surgical strategy for ischemic MR.

◼ SURGICAL CONSIDERATIONS

Essential to the effective surgical management of these high-risk patients is a thorough preoperative medical management. Myocardial function and systemic end-organ perfusion should be optimized with adequate antianginal therapy, β-blockade, diuresis, and afterload reduction as tolerated. Whenever possible, patients with ischemic MR should be brought to the operating room in a euvolemic state and free of evolving myocardial ischemia. Information from preoperative transesophageal echocardiography is important to identify the pathoanatomy of the mitral apparatus and formulate the operative plan before the induction of anesthesia.

After bicaval cannulation, complete exposure of the mitral valve can be achieved, even in patients with a small left atrium. Mobilization of the superior vena cava and inferior vena cava followed by complete dissection of the interatrial groove permits entry into the roof of the left atrium at the level of the septum and full visualization of anterior and posterior leaflets. Patients who are not undergoing redo procedures and patients requiring concomitant coronary revascularization are approached through a conventional sternotomy using a comprehensive strategy of myocardial protection. Patients with previous cardiac surgery not requiring revascularization or aortic valve replacement can undergo mitral surgery with the heart beating on cardiopulmonary bypass via a right thoracotomy approach.

◼ MITRAL REPLACEMENT

Although rare, the presence of acute valvular disruption as a complication of myocardial infarction is a surgical emergency. Patients are often in cardiogenic shock that is unresponsive to inotropic support, intraaortic balloon pump implantation, and percutaneous coronary interventions. It is essential to recognize early on that these patients will not improve without surgery. Attempts should be made to perform surgery before the manifestation of end-organ dysfunction because this significantly increases mortality and operative risk.

The surgical goals are to provide the patient with complete revascularization and mitral competency with the least

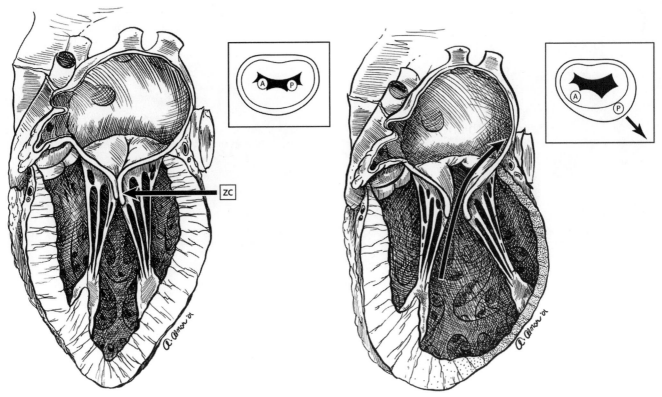

Figure 1
Note the geometric changes that occur from the normal (left) to the ischemic left ventricle (right). With the myocardial scarring and thinning of the lateral wall, the restricted posterior (P) mitral leaflet cannot meet adequately with the extended anterior (A) leaflet, resulting in a loss of the zone of coaptation (ZC). Geometric mitral regurgitation results from a combination of annular dilation (right inset) papillary muscle foreshortening, increased leaflet-tethering forces, and weakened leaflet-closing forces.

anoxic time to the ventricle. The key problem in acute ischemic MR is the inability for the myocardium to handle the sudden marked elevation in left ventricular (LV) wall stress and volume overload in conjunction with the severe impairment of coronary perfusion pressure. Any effective surgical approach must involve adequate LV venting to minimize wall stress and a comprehensive strategy of myocardial protection that may include retrograde blood cardioplegia. When the heart is vented, distal coronary anastomoses first are completed with vein grafts because these can be used for effective antegrade delivery of cardioplegia and resuscitation of the stunned myocardium.

With the understanding that the mitral apparatus is anatomically and functionally contiguous with the ventricle, preservation of subvalvular integrity is essential for optimal ventricular recovery after mitral valve replacement. Excision of the subvalvular structures at the time of mitral valve replacement, as performed historically, results in a series of mechanical and geometric perturbations leading to changes in myocardial wall thickness, loss of normal systolic torsional deformation, and increased regional wall stress. After chordal transection, the depression of ventricular function at the defunct papillary muscle base also results in slowed relaxation that contributes to diastolic dysfunction. Conversely, chordal preservation at the time of mitral valve

replacement renders significant hemodynamic benefits, especially in the setting of depressed LV function. The improved ventricular geometry with chordal preservation results in a reduction of ventricular wall stress, enhanced regional wall motion, superior LV performance, and, perhaps most importantly, improved long-term survival over patients without chordal preservation.

For acute ischemic MR, attempts at total preservation should be made during mitral valve replacement. This can be achieved without leaflet excision by the circumferential placement of imbricating pledgeted valve stitches from the atrial side of the annulus to the zone of coaptation on both leaflets. If the anterior leaflet is redundant, concerns of subvalvular obstruction of the prosthesis are avoided by simple elliptical excision of the body of the anterior leaflet followed by placement of the annular sutures to preserve the attachments to the anterior papillary muscle.

Because the LV cavity is often small in acute ischemic MR, the implantation of a low-profile prosthesis is paramount. Although mechanical valves have the lowest profile, the durability of anticoagulation-avoiding bioprostheses is sufficient for these patients with limited long-term survival. Should a bioprosthesis be chosen, close attention should be paid to avoid the pitfall of strut impingement against the LV wall of these small ventricles resulting in difficulty weaning

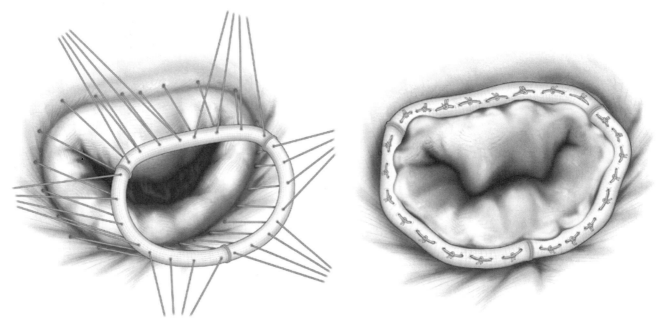

Figure 2
Successful augmentation of the zone of coaptation and prevention of recurrent mitral regurgitation can be achieved by implanting an undersized circumferential annuloplasty ring.

from cardiopulmonary bypass and potential LV outflow tract obstruction. In this situation, if a bioprosthesis is selected, implantation of a pericardial valve may be preferable due to the low profile of the struts.

■ MITRAL RECONSTRUCTION

The most common presentation of ischemic MR occurs as a result of ventricular remodeling after myocardial ischemia. This geometric distortion of the mitral apparatus results in a tethering of the posterior leaflet relative to the extended anterior leaflet and a loss of the zone of coaptation. The term *papillary muscle dysfunction* is inaccurate because it is actually *lateral wall dysfunction* that is the culprit of ischemic MR. Most often the chronic geometric alterations that occur as a result of postischemic remodeling of the mitral apparatus do not recover completely with revascularization, as previously was believed. A more aggressive approach is needed to restore this geometry to interrupt the vicious cycle of MR, annular dilation, and ventricular remodeling that eventually results in heart failure.

Geometric mitral reconstruction involves the implantation of an undersized circumferential annuloplasty ring (Figure 2). In treating patients with ischemic MR, the most significant determinant of leaflet coaptation and MR is the diameter of the distorted mitral valve annulus. Undersizing and overcorrecting the mitral annulus during reconstruction restores the zone of coaptation and prevents progressive annular dilation. The acute internal remodeling of the base of the heart that occurs with this reparative technique reestablishes the normal geometry and ellipsoid shape of the left ventricle, which may explain its effective application in ischemic patients with diminished ejection fractions.

At the University of Michigan, 100 ischemic patients with a mean age of 73, ejection fraction of 32%, New York Heart Association class III or IV symptoms, and severe MR underwent primary coronary artery bypass graft surgery in combination with geometric mitral reconstruction. The 30-day mortality was 4%, and the 1-year survival was 90%, with all patients being in New York Heart Association class I or II. This straightforward technique of geometric mitral remodeling can be performed independent of or in combination with coronary artery bypass graft surgery without a prohibitive increase in mortality.

As surgeons have gained a renewed appreciation of the geometric alterations involved in ischemic MR and the principles of its correction, the surgical reconstruction of these patients now is being performed with mortality rates of 3% to 6% in selected series. The resulting marked improvements in survival and quality of life after reconstruction compared with ischemic patients with uncorrected MR provide us with the edict to repair ischemic MR aggressively whenever possible.

SUGGESTED READING

Aklog L, et al: Does coronary artery bypass grafting alone correct moderate ischemic mitral regurgitation? *Circulation* 104(12 Suppl I):I-68, 2001.

Bolling SF, et al: Mitral valve reconstruction in elderly, ischemic patients, *Chest* 109:35, 1996.

Grigioni F, et al: Ischemic mitral regurgitation: long-term outcome and prognostic implications with quantitative Doppler assessment, *Circulation* 103:1759, 2001.

Lamas GA, et al: Clinical significance of mitral regurgitation after acute myocardial infarction, *Circulation* 96:827, 1997.

Sheikh KH, et al: Intraoperative transesophageal Doppler color flow imaging used to guide patient selection and operative treatment of ischemic mitral regurgitation, *Circulation* 84:594, 1991.

VENTRICULAR ANEURYSMS

Igor D. Gregoric

Denton A. Cooley

V*entricular aneurysm* commonly denotes a left ventricular (LV) aneurysm that complicates a myocardial infarction related to coronary artery disease, usually of the left anterior descending coronary artery (LAD). The ischemic injury causes expansion and thinning of the infarcted area, resulting in paradoxical motion of the ventricle: As the ventricle contracts, the aneurysm expands, reducing the ejection fraction and possibly leading to LV failure. Aneurysms most commonly affect the anterolateral and anteroseptal portions of the left ventricle.

Definitive treatment of these lesions dates from 1958, when the senior author (D.A.C.) used a linear technique to repair an LV aneurysm with the aid of cardiopulmonary bypass. This technique consisted of an incision and ventriculorrhaphy, followed by buttressing of the repair with felt strips. A similar method customarily was used in that era for repairing aortic aneurysms. Although linear LV aneurysm repair remained the standard until the mid-1980s, its results were suboptimal because the geometry of the repaired ventricle was unnatural. Ventricular function improved only modestly, and some patients required intraaortic balloon support during the early postoperative period.

To obtain better results, surgeons tried various other methods, including excision, plication, septoplasty/plication, patch placement, and overlap techniques. In the mid-1980s, several surgeons, each working separately, pioneered patch repairs that were more physiologic. Jatene and Dor devised a repair that yielded a circular suture line. Cooley introduced a similar but less complex technique, known as *endoaneurysmorrhaphy* (intracavitary repair), a concept proposed in 1888 by Matas. The Cooley repair excludes the noncontractile portion of the left ventricle and restores the normal filling volume and geometric chamber configuration. This approach is the focus of this chapter because it has been used for all LV aneurysm repairs at our institution since 1989.

■ INDICATIONS AND PATIENT SELECTION FOR REPAIR

Ventricular aneurysms may lead to congestive heart failure (with or without angina), thromboembolism, and tachyarrhythmias. In weighing the advantages of medical versus surgical treatment, the deciding factors include the extent and characteristics of the involved tissue, the degree of LV function, and the severity of symptoms. For asymptomatic aneurysms that appear small on angiography, surgery is not indicated. In contrast, large asymptomatic aneurysms

should be monitored closely, and surgery should be performed if the aneurysms begin to cause symptoms. For any patient with severe symptoms and medically intractable heart failure or angina, repair is indicated.

If ventriculography or ultrasonography shows a contractile area at the base of the ventricle, repair should be successful even if the aneurysm is massive; if ventricular impairment appears global, successful repair may not be possible. The primary relative contraindication to aneurysm repair is severe LV dysfunction (a nonaneurysmal wall ejection fraction of <30%). In these cases, cardiac transplantation or cardiomyoplasty may be the only surgical option.

■ OPERATIVE TECHNIQUE

The ventricular endoaneurysmorrhaphy is performed through a median sternotomy with the aid of cardiopulmonary bypass and moderate (26°C to 28°C) hypothermia, with or without aortic cross-clamping. For venous and arterial flows, single cannulae are inserted into the ascending aorta and the right atrium; the latter structure requires a large-bore cannula. If a mitral repair is to be performed, bicaval cannulation may be preferred. Asystole and myocardial relaxation are induced with a cold crystalloid cardioplegic solution containing potassium chloride. Approximately 500 ml of this solution is delivered antegrade at 4°C via a large-bore needle in the ascending aorta. This needle is retained in the aorta to allow venting throughout the repair.

Pericardial adhesions are dissected, and the left ventricle is exposed. To verify presence of an aneurysm, the ventricle is decompressed via the cardioplegia needle; if an aneurysm is present, it collapses. For anteroseptal aneurysms, a ventriculotomy is performed 2 cm lateral and parallel to the LAD. For posterior wall aneurysms, the lesion is incised posteriorly. In all cases, the incision is made over the apex and thinnest portion of the aneurysm (Figure 1A). Before the repair is undertaken, any thrombi (which are present in about half of cases) must be removed to prevent fragments from entering the ventricular cavity. Unless a thrombus is suspected, however, one should refrain from incising small areas that have akinesia, dyskinesia, or paradoxical motion and whose surfaces have normal myocardium.

When blood has been evacuated from the operative field, the surgeon can identify the site of transition between the scarred, white aneurysmal tissue and the viable, maroon-colored myocardium. This transition site is where the patch should be applied. Although we prefer a woven Dacron patch, we occasionally use glutaraldehyde-treated bovine pericardium. The patch is tailored carefully to conform to the normal LV volume; in most cases, 2 cm × 4 cm is a sufficient size. After being positioned under (but not into) the ventriculotomy, the patch is secured with a continuous 2-0 or 3-0 polypropylene suture (Figure 1B-C). The surgeon should take care to avoid the papillary muscles and to preserve the interventricular groove on the epicardial surface because the distal LAD still may be patent. If the mitral valve is dysfunctional, it may be repaired or replaced through the ventriculotomy.

At the end of the repair, the ventriculotomy is closed with a double row of continuous 2-0 or 3-0 polypropylene sutures.

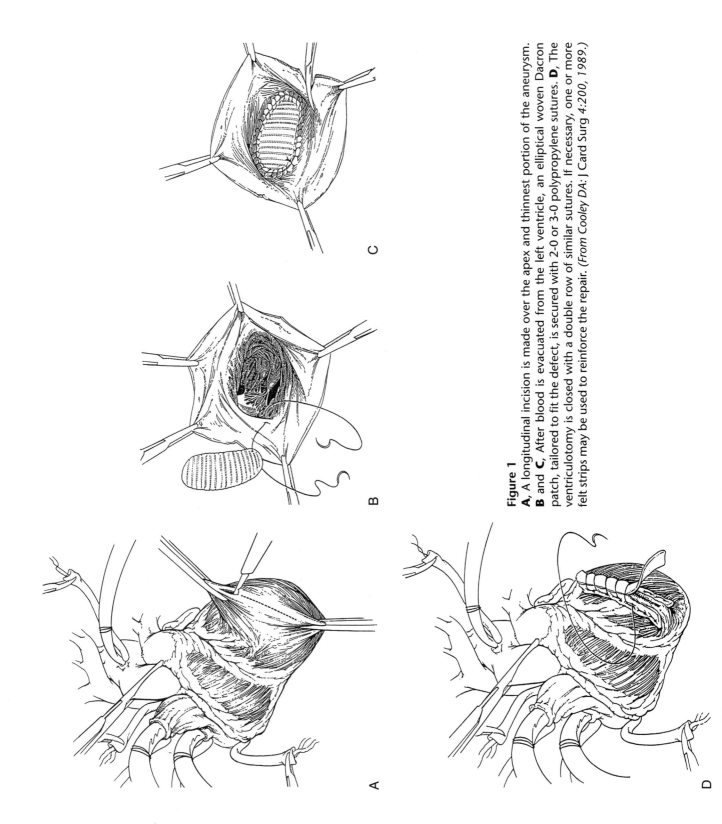

Figure 1

A, A longitudinal incision is made over the apex and thinnest portion of the aneurysm. **B** and **C,** After blood is evacuated from the left ventricle, an elliptical woven Dacron patch, tailored to fit the defect, is secured with 2-0 or 3-0 polypropylene sutures. **D,** The ventriculotomy is closed with a double row of similar sutures. If necessary, one or more felt strips may be used to reinforce the repair. *(From Cooley DA: J Card Surg 4:200, 1989.)*

If necessary, felt strips may be used to reinforce the repair (Figure 1D). These strips later may become a site of infection or pseudoaneurysm formation, so we usually omit them. This omission is acceptable because the Dacron patch stabilizes the ventricle, and the suture line is not exposed to intracardiac pressure.

In all cases, the LAD should be bypassed with an internal mammary artery. Other coronary vessels also should be bypassed, if necessary, with reversed saphenous vein grafts. When all of the required procedures have been performed, protamine is given to reverse the effects of heparin, and the rest of the operation is completed in a routine fashion.

■ POSTOPERATIVE CARE

Postoperatively, repair of an LV aneurysm entails a clinical course similar to that of other cardiac operations. The following conditions indicate a particularly poor prognosis: congestive heart failure, LV dysfunction, poor cardiac output, elevated LV end-diastolic pressure, impaired septal systolic function, and arrhythmias. In the presence of severe heart failure or an acute myocardial infarction, an intraaortic balloon pump or a temporary LV assist device may be required.

■ RESULTS

In the literature, the mortality of LV aneurysm repair ranges from 3% to 7%. At our institution, ventricular endoaneurysmorrhaphy yields a low mortality and morbidity rate. Postoperatively, our patients usually have a significant improvement in LV function, especially in cases involving large aneurysms, when the ejection fraction may increase twofold to threefold. This excellent result persists into the late postoperative period. Most of our patients have a substantially improved postoperative quality of life, as reflected by the return of New York Heart Association functional status to class I or II. The risk of postoperative arrhythmias is lower in endoaneurysmorrhaphy patients than in patients who have had a linear repair.

■ CONCLUSION

Since the 1950s, when modern surgical therapy for LV aneurysms became possible, operative treatment of these lesions has undergone various modifications designed to restore the left ventricle's normal configuration. Today the emphasis is on repair, rather than excision, of the diseased tissue. We have long used a ventricular endoaneurysmorrhaphy for all of our LV aneurysm cases. In concept, this approach is similar to the methods of Jatene and Dor. The Jatene procedure is done on the beating heart, however, and involves placement of an internal purse-string suture at the transition site between the healthy and aneurysmal tissue. This purse-string, which is tightened before the ventricular cavity is reconstructed, later may give way if subjected to undue stress. Likewise, Dor also places sutures in the epicardial surface, possibly opening the way for postoperative hemorrhage. In his approach, the aneurysm is excised, and the resulting defect is patched. The Jatene and Dor procedures tend to distort the outer surface of the ventricle.

In contrast, our technique excludes the noncontractile, scarred tissue, compartmentalizing the left ventricle and restoring its normal contour, contractility, and volume. The patch graft stabilizes ventricular contraction during systole, taking stress off the ventriculotomy and preventing suture-line hemorrhage. This approach is suitable for repairing not only anterolateral or anteroseptal aneurysms, but also lesions involving the posterior ventricular wall. The technique also may be modified slightly to allow repair of pseudoaneurysms (in these cases, cardiac rupture has occurred, and the resulting hemorrhage is contained by previous pericardial adhesions). Endoaneurysmorrhaphy is especially valuable for calcified lesions, aneurysms on the posterior ventricular surface, and regions of diffuse dyskinesia. Without this procedure, high-risk patients with these lesions might be inoperable. In patients with ventricular tachycardia, endoaneurysmorrhaphy may be particularly beneficial because it addresses the arrhythmogenic focus, which often is located at the transition between aneurysmal and normal tissue. Even in cases involving massive or otherwise inoperable LV aneurysms, endoaneurysmorrhaphy yields excellent immediate and long-term results, restoring most patients to normal, active lives.

SUGGESTED READING

Cooley DA: Ventricular endoaneurysmorrhaphy: a simplified repair for extensive postinfarction aneurysm, *J Card Surg* 4:200, 1989.

Cooley DA, et al: Intracavitary repair of ventricular aneurysm and regional dyskinesia, *Ann Surg* 215:417, 1992.

Cox JL: Left ventricular aneurysms: pathophysiologic observations and standard resection, *Semin Thorac Cardiovasc Surg* 9:113, 1997.

Cox JL: Surgical management of left ventricular aneurysms: a clarification of the similarities and differences between the Jatene and Dor techniques, *Semin Thorac Cardiovasc Surg* 9:131, 1997.

Doss M, et al: Long term follow up of left ventricular function after repair of left ventricular aneurysm: a comparison of linear closure versus patch plasty, *Eur J Cardiothorac Surg* 20:783, 2001.

CORONARY ENDARTERECTOMY

Arun K. Singhal

Thoralf M. Sundt

■ BACKGROUND

Coronary endarterectomy (CE) for the treatment of coronary occlusive disease was introduced by Bailey and Longmire in the 1950s and was popularized by Johnson and others in subsequent decades. The procedure demanded meticulous care in the removal of plaque, and the sometimes tedious reconstruction entailing prolonged ischemic time in an age before routine use of cardioplegic arrest. The remarkable results achieved under these circumstances are a tribute to the courage and expertise of the pioneers of coronary artery surgery. The technique of endarterectomy was largely overshadowed by the introduction of coronary artery bypass graft (CABG) surgery with saphenous vein in the mid-1960s. CABG surgery rapidly proved a technically more straightforward procedure with reproducibly excellent results. Since that time, however, CE has been championed by a cadre of loyal enthusiasts as a complement to CABG surgery when target vessels are extensively diseased. Originally carried out over the entire length of the vessel, endarterectomy today is used most often to prepare a distal target site for placement of a CABG.

As a result of the widespread application of percutaneous techniques and the success with which primary CABG surgery has prolonged the survival of patients with coronary occlusive disease, cardiac surgeons are challenged more frequently to treat patients with more advanced and diffuse coronary artery disease. New technologies, such as transmyocardial laser revascularization or the direct delivery of angiogenic growth factors, are being introduced. These new technologies may be effective in such cases. Until this effectiveness is proven, however, we believe that CE will continue to have a place in the armamentarium of the coronary surgeon.

■ INDICATIONS

Opinions differ regarding the threshold for application of CE. Presently, most surgeons reserve CE as an adjuvant technique to primary CABG surgery. The general consensus is that multiple anastomoses to more distal targets are preferable to endarterectomy of a more proximal vessel. In the case of the right coronary artery (RCA), separate anastomoses to the posterior descending artery and posterior left ventricular artery are preferable to CE of the distal RCA at the crux. Similarly, if technically feasible, multiple anastomoses to several sites on the left anterior descending artery (LAD) are probably preferable to endarterectomy of this vessel.

The frequency with which CE is performed varies widely in the literature. At our institution, CE is applied in slightly more than 2% of patients undergoing CABG surgery. This rate is not dissimilar to 4.1% reported by Asimakopoulos et al, but it is far short of the rate reported from Johnson's institution, where Brenowitz et al reported CE in 50% of patients requiring revascularization. Most surgeons believe that CE is technically more difficult and provides less reliable results than primary CABG surgery (see later). Consequently, in more recent years, opinion leaders such as Goldstein et al have reduced their use of CE from 11% to 3% in favor of grafting more distal targets when feasible.

In our view, CE is indicated when coronary disease is sufficiently diffuse to prohibit satisfactory primary CABG surgery with effective runoff or when the vessels distal to the disease are small in diameter and threaten graft patency (<1 mm). This may be the case in patients having undergone previous surgery and is seen occasionally in young patients with severe dyslipidemias or long-standing insulin-dependent diabetes. In the interest of complete revascularization, we have employed this technique whenever a vascular territory cannot be grafted otherwise, without regard to previous infarction or function of the region in question.

■ TECHNIQUE

The most important principle of endarterectomy is the establishment of adequate outflow via the removal of disease at the origins of branch vessels and distal to the arteriotomy. As in the endarterectomy of other arteries, the distal plaque specimen should be "feathered," ensuring that no shelf of distal plaque is left behind. Premature fracture of the plaque necessitates distal arteriotomy to complete the endarterectomy. Meticulous technique and steadfast adherence to this principle are crucial to success with CE. We prefer to perform this operation with cardioplegic arrest rather than intermittent cross-clamp, fibrillatory arrest, or "off-pump" techniques. When CE is anticipated, we make arrangements for retrograde delivery of cardioplegia.

Endarterectomy may be anticipated in many instances on the basis of the preoperative angiogram, particularly when extensive calcification of the vessel wall is apparent, or may be an unexpected necessity when coronary arteriotomy reveals an atheromatous core rather than a lumen. In the latter instance, the adventitia often separates spontaneously from the core, initiating an endarterectomy plane. The surgeon must choose between continuing the endarterectomy or closing the arteriotomy and searching distally for a more appropriate grafting site.

Endarterectomy of the RCA system typically is performed via limited arteriotomy just proximal to the crux. The specimen usually can be extracted using an eversion technique, taking care to remove material from the origin of the posterior descending artery and the continuation of the RCA. We have used only manual extraction techniques, although forceful injection of carbon dioxide or cardioplegia in the endarterectomy plane has been described. Care must be taken to hold the specimen firmly and exert only modest traction, while pushing the distal vessel off the core. In contrast, attempting to pull the core out of the vessel usually results in premature fracture of the core and an unsatisfactory, inadequately feathered endarterectomy.

We do not attempt retrograde endarterectomy of the proximal vessel because, in our experience, this may not open the origins of the acute marginal vessels adequately and risks thrombosis of the proximal segment and worsening of right ventricle perfusion. We have seen this occur with sudden development of ventricular tachyarrhythmias. Retrograde thrombosis was confirmed angiographically.

In contrast to eversion endarterectomy of the RCA, endarterectomy of the LAD typically is performed "open" via an extended arteriotomy that may be 8 to 10 cm or more in length. Because patch reconstruction is straightforward on the front of the heart, we extend the arteriotomy as far distally as may be required to achieve adequate plaque removal. This exposure also permits meticulous removal of material from the origins of the septal perforators and diagonal branches.

Obtuse marginal branches of the circumflex are difficult to endarterectomize, in part because of the difficulty in visualizing this surface of the heart and in part because they tend to arborize extensively. We avoid endarterectomy of this territory as much as possible. In our experience disease of this type may be the best indication for transmyocardial laser revascularization.

Reconstruction of the RCA is most often via an extended saphenous vein hood. The LAD may be repaired in a similar manner if the decision has been to use saphenous vein to this target. If the internal thoracic artery (ITA) is to be used, reconstruction may be accomplished either by opening the ITA itself sufficiently to patch the vessel or by placing a saphenous vein patch to which the ITA can be anastomosed.

■ POSTOPERATIVE CARE

If endarterectomy is performed, we prefer not to use antifibrinolytics intraoperatively or postoperatively. If these agents have been initiated intraoperatively before the decision to carry out CE, we simply discontinue their use at that point. A heparin infusion is initiated 6 hours postoperatively, provided that bleeding has been controlled; this practice is based on evidence from the CE literature. Despite the lack of prospective randomized data on the subject, we routinely anticoagulate patients with warfarin (Coumadin) for 3 to 6 months postoperatively. The target international normalized ratio is 2.0 to 3.0. Aspirin is administered routinely to all patients undergoing coronary revascularization. We have not studied use of clopidogrel, although it may be a superior alternative to aspirin. We also routinely administer lidocaine for 12 to 24 hours to reduce the risk of life-threatening arrhythmias in the event of acute thrombosis.

■ RESULTS

In most comparative studies, the risk of perioperative death after CE exceeds that after CABG surgery alone (Table 1). Because none of these studies are prospectively randomized, it is impossible to know whether this increased risk is due to

Table 1 Perioperative Mortality				
AUTHOR	CABG	CE	1 CE	>1 CE
Brenowitz	4%	6.2%	5.9%	14%
Asimakopoulous	0%	3.6%		
Goldstein		8%		
Beretta		5.2%		
Sundt	4.5%	6.2%	5.9%	14%

CABG, coronary artery bypass graft; CE, coronary endarterectomy.

patient selection or the procedure itself. Even with comparable demographics between groups, it is intuitively obvious that patients undergoing endarterectomy have more severe coronary artery disease and may be at higher risk for perioperative death. Patients requiring endarterectomy of multiple vessels seem to be at incrementally higher risk of death than patients requiring endarterectomy of only a single vessel. Similarly the risk of perioperative myocardial infarction is widely held to be higher among patients undergoing CE (Table 2). Early evidence suggested that the risks of infarction and death were higher for endarterectomy of the LAD than of the RCA, although the results of our study and those of others more recently have refuted that position.

Graft Patency

Early and late graft patency after coronary endarterectomy have been addressed in the literature. Brenowitz et al published their CE experience from 1978 to 1986, including 2501 patients and 2504 controls. They observed similar 30-day patency rates for saphenous vein grafts to targets with (88.9%) and without (89.9%) endarterectomy. Late study of symptomatic patients revealed similar patency rates: 71.7% at 31.4 months for endarterectomized vessels versus 75.8% at 38.8 months for conventional bypass grafts.

Other investigators have confirmed these results. In 1991, Goldstein et al reported patency data for 51 consecutive patients undergoing CE from 1985 to 1987. They performed early angiographic studies on 40 patients 6 to 259 days (mean 19 days) postoperatively. Of the cohort, one patient died, nine refused to participate, and one had documented thrombosis at reexploration. Documented early patency was 90%. Additionally, 27 of the patients participated in late follow-up (range 11 to 40 months [mean 19 months]). Of the 12 patients who were not studied, 4 had previously documented occlusion, 5 refused to participate, 2 had significant other illnesses prohibiting control angiography,

Table 2 Perioperative Myocardial Infarction				
AUTHOR	CABG	CE	1 CE	>1 CE
Brenowitz	5.6%	9.8%	6.5%	13.1%
Asimakopoulous	0%	5.4%		
Goldstein		8%		
Beretta		6.3%		
Sundt	3%	5.6%	5.9%	0%

CABG, coronary artery bypass graft; CE, coronary endarterectomy.

and 1 had severe obesity and could not be studied. Late patency was 64%.

Ferraris et al carried out a retrospective, controlled study comparing the results of angiograms performed on 97 symptomatic patients who had undergone endarterectomy to 154 symptomatic patients who had standard surgical revascularization. Using Kaplan-Meier survival estimates, they estimated "graft survival time" for saphenous grafts in the control group to be 152 months (range 142 to 160 months) compared with 102 months (range 98 to 106 months) for saphenous grafts to endarterectomized vessels ($p<.001$). They noted a graft survival time of 127 months (range 119 to 135 months, $p<.001$) for conventional grafts to nonendarterectomized vessels among study patients requiring endarterectomy of at least one other vessel. This finding supports the argument that the atherosclerotic process was more severe in patients undergoing endarterectomy. The most appropriate control in the evaluation of graft patency after endarterectomy may not be grafts among nonendarterectomy patients, but rather grafts to nonendarterectomized vessels among endarterectomy patients.

As is the case for other target vessels, graft patency for endarterectomized vessels may be influenced by conduit choice as well. In their study of 96 patients requiring endarterectomy, Beretta et al compared early and late patency of grafts among 50 patients reconstructed with saphenous vein and 46 undergoing revascularization with either the right or the left ITA. In the early postoperative period, patency rates were 85% and 93% for venous and arterial conduits. Follow-up angiograms at 30 to 36 months revealed patency rates of 67% and 82%. Additional follow-up at 54 to 60 months revealed no additional occlusion in either cohort.

Early patency rates in the literature generally are greater than 85%, and rates greater than 90% have been reported. Long-term patency rates range from 60% to 75% at 3 to 5 years. The use of ITA for revascularization probably improves short-term and long-term patency. Overall, late patency may not be equivalent to conventional grafts, but it is sufficient to warrant endarterectomy as an alternative to leaving a territory ungrafted.

Long-Term Results

A review of the literature suggests that at 5 years freedom from angina is 65% to 75%, inferior to freedom from angina after standard CABG surgery. The 5-year actuarial survival is variable and depends most on left ventricular dysfunction and choice of conduit for revascularization. Presuming normal left ventricular function and use of venous revascularization, the expected 5-year survival after CE is probably approximately 80%.

■ CONCLUSIONS

CE remains a useful technique for surgical management of diffuse coronary artery disease. CE should be avoided, however, in preference to conventional CABG surgery to more distal branches of the coronary tree whenever possible. Perioperative risk of death and infarction may be increased and graft patency decreased in endarterectomized vessels, but they are not prohibitive. Late survival and angina relief with this technique are acceptable. After endarterectomy, it is appropriate to reconstruct the LAD with an ITA graft, although other considerations may favor direction of this valuable conduit to other territories. The success of endarterectomy depends on meticulous technique.

SUGGESTED READING

Asimakopoulos G, et al: Outcome of coronary endarterectomy: a case control study, *Ann Thorac Surg* 67:989, 1999.

Beretta L, et al: Coronary "open" endarterectomy and reconstruction: short- and long-term results of the revascularization with saphenous vein versus ITA graft, *Eur J Cardiothorac Surg* 6:382, 1992.

Brenowitz JB, et al: Results of coronary endarterectomy and reconstruction, *J Thorac Cardiovasc Surg* 95:1, 1988.

Ferraris VA, et al: Long-term angiographic results of coronary endarterectomy, *Ann Thorac Surg* 69:1737, 2000.

Goldstein J, et al: Angiographic assessment of graft patency after coronary endarterectomy, *J Thorac Cardiovasc Surg* 102:539, 1991.

Sundt TM, et al: Reappraisal of coronary endarterectomy for the treatment of diffuse coronary artery disease, *Ann Thorac Surg* 68:1272, 1999.

TRANSMYOCARDIAL REVASCULARIZATION

Rachel H. Cohn
Todd K. Rosengart

A new era of direct transmyocardial revascularization (TMR) began in the 1990s based on the use of laser energy to create myocardial channels to perfuse the heart. Since then, more than 6000 patients have undergone some form of TMR-based technique, alone or in combination with synergistic drug therapy or traditional interventional approaches. The administration of growth factors to stimulate new blood vessel growth (therapeutic angiogenesis) represents a corollary of this strategy. In reality, these "new" therapies actually represent modifications, and perhaps enhancements, of the old needle acupuncture and poudrage techniques of Beck, Vineberg, and Pifarré.

TMR uses laser energy to create channels in the myocardium that direct oxygenated blood from the left ventricular cavity into ischemic myocardium, bypassing the coronary vasculature altogether. Therapeutic angiogenesis describes the strategy of administering growth factors via a variety of delivery techniques to enhance myocardial revascularization. Controversy exists, however, in regard to whether TMR actually induces the formation of patent channels or whether the injury induced by TMR causes an increase in endogenous growth factors, a natural response to injury, and thereby induces angiogenesis, much like the exogenous delivery strategies.

■ MECHANISMS OF ACTION

There are currently two theories on the mechanism of action for TMR: (1) induction of angiogenesis causing increased myocardial collateral circulation and (2) myocardial denervation.

Increased Myocardial Perfusion

Recent studies have suggested that there is an increase in vascular endothelial cell growth factor and other angiogenic growth factors in the ischemic zone of laser-treated animals. Perfusion and function studies in these animal models have also suggested that TMR enhances myocardial blood flow. In clinical trials, patients who underwent TMR demonstrated greater angina relief compared with patients who were medically managed, although a placebo effect could not be ruled out. More important, several studies using sestamibi–single-photon emission computed tomography and other similar techniques have indicated there is significant improvement in perfusion to laser–treated sections of the ventricle after TMR.

Myocardial Denervation

This hypothesis suggests that anginal symptoms decrease after TMR due to the destruction of cardiac nerve fibers. There is some controversy, however, whether myocardial denervation can explain long-term benefits of TMR or if neuronal damage better explains the immediate improvement in angina than does an angiogenesis mechanism, which would be expected to produce relatively delayed symtomatic improvement.

■ INDICATIONS

Indications for TMR vary and are not standardized. In general, patients considered for TMR should be Canadian Cardiovascular Society (CCS) class III or IV, have angina refractory to medical therapy (usually on more than two antianginal drugs), demonstrate reversible ischemia by thallium scan, have failed previous conventional procedures, or have coronary disease not amenable to bypass or angioplasty.

■ TECHNIQUE

Both of the clinically approved TMR devices—the holmium:YAG laser and the CO_2 laser—use infrared light to thermally ablate myocardial tissue to create transmyocardial channels. The energy per pulse of the CO_2 laser is about 40 J, whereas the energy per pulse of the holmium: YAG laser is 2 to 5 J. The CO_2 laser is more efficiently absorbed by water molecules than the holmium:YAG laser. Due to these characteristics, a series of pulses are required by the holmium:YAG laser to generate transmural channels, therefore, the holmium:YAG laser requires multiple cardiac cycles to create a single channel, whereas the CO_2 laser creates a transmural channel with a single pulse.

The fiberoptic holmium:YAG laser device is easier to manipulate than the bulkier CO_2 device, which requires mirrors to generate the laser beam. A targeted area of ischemia, identified by preoperative studies, is accessed via sternotomy when TMR is an adjunct to coronary artery bypass graft surgery or by thoracotomy or thoracoscopy. A series of 1-mm channels undergo laser treatment through the ischemic myocardium at approximately 1-cm intervals, for a total of 30 to 50 channels. Echo is used to confirm transmural penetration by the presence of air bubbles in the left ventricle. The entire TMR procedure takes approximately 1 hour, and the actual laser treatment takes about 10 to 20 minutes.

■ RESULTS

In early reports of high-risk groups of patients, operative morbidity and mortality have approached 25% and 10%, respectively, but recently reported outcomes have been more favorable. Complications of bleeding, myocardial compromise, and ischemia-related deaths have been encountered. Recent clinical trials have indicated that patients who undergo TMR have anginal relief postoperatively and through 1-5 year follow-up. Generally, more than 70% of TMR patients can expect an improvement in angina of at least 1 CCS class through the first year postoperatively. As noted, evidence suggests that most of these patients will sustain anginal relief for longer intervals. Furthermore, exercise tolerance, freedom from cardiac-related hospitalizations, and survival free of cardiac events up to 1 year postoperatively have been reported to be significantly better in TMR-treated patients compared with medically managed patients. Although one-year cardiac-related mortality rate can be expected to be approximately 15%. Between 3 and 5 years postoperatively, TMR-treated patients have continued to report freedom from severe angina or no anginal symptoms at all. Factors that can adversely affect long-term survival include age, diabetes, hypercholesterolemia, and lower body mass index.

Newer methods that avoid general anesthesia and open-chest surgery include endoscopic techniques and catheters for percutaneous myocardial revascularization (PMR). Using a femoral artery approach, these PMR catheters can be advanced into the left ventricle in the catheterization laboratory, creating channels from the endocardial surface. With the pericardium intact, the risk of myocardial perforation and subsequent pericardial tamponade is minimal (<1%). Studies assessing the efficacy of this alternative approach have, however, not been compelling.

SUGGESTED READING

Allen KB, et al: Comparison of transmyocardial revascularization with medical therapy in patients with refractory angina, *N Engl J Med* 341:1029, 1999.

Bridges CR: Myocardial laser revascularization: the controversy and the data, *Ann Thorac Surg* 69:655, 2000.

Frazier OH, et al: Transmyocardial revascularization with a carbon dioxide laser in patients with end-stage coronary artery disease, *N Engl J Med* 341:1021, 1999.

Hughes GC, et al: Induction of angiogenesis after TMR: a comparison of holmium:YAG, CO_2, and excimer lasers, *Ann Thorac Surg* 70:504, 2000.

Krabatsch T, et al: Factors influencing results and outcome after transmyocardial laser revascularization, *Ann Thorac Surg* 73:1888, 2002.

Lee LY, Rosengart TK: Transmyocardial laser revascularization and angiogenesis: the potential for therapeutic benefit, *Semin Thorac Cardiovasc Surg* 11:29, 1999.

COMBINED CAROTID AND CORONARY DISEASE

Alan Dardik
Bruce A. Perler

Carotid endarterectomy (CEA) is the most common non-cardiac vascular operation in the United States today, with more than 130,000 procedures performed annually. Several randomized prospective clinical trials have confirmed the safety and efficacy of CEA and its superiority in long-term stroke prevention compared with optimal medical management of patients with significant carotid artery disease. There is less agreement, however, even among cardiovascular surgical specialists, with respect to the most appropriate management of patients with coexistent significant carotid and coronary artery disease (CAD). This chapter provides a rational approach to these patients.

■ EPIDEMIOLOGY

The close association between carotid atherosclerosis and CAD is well established. Approximately 50% of patients with significant carotid disease have clinical evidence of CAD. In a large study performed at the Cleveland Clinic, coronary angiography confirmed severe disease in 73%, mild to moderate disease in 22%, and completely normal coronary arteries in only 5% of patients with significant carotid disease. Although the risk of operative mortality after CEA is now less than 1% in many large series, most of these deaths in contemporary practice are secondary to cardiac events. Nonfatal myocardial infarction is a much more common perioperative complication of CEA than stroke in many contemporary reports. CAD also accounts for 50% to 70% of late deaths after CEA.

Conversely, it has been reported that at least 6% to 16% of patients with significant CAD also have significant carotid disease. Although the incidence of perioperative stroke among patients undergoing cardiac surgery has declined, this remains a potentially devastating complication that occurs in at least 2% of patients who undergo a coronary artery bypass graft (CABG) procedure. The incidence is higher among the very elderly. In addition to uncorrected significant carotid stenoses, there are many other potential causes of perioperative stroke, including embolization of atheromatous debris or thrombus from the aorta, air emboli, aortic dissection, intracerebral hemorrhage, and low cardiac output. Hemodynamically significant carotid stenoses may predispose to cerebral ischemia during the period of cardiopulmonary bypass and during the early postoperative period when intermittent arrhythmias and depressed cardiac output are most likely to occur.

Patients with bilateral or symptomatic carotid disease incur the greatest risk of neurologic morbidity after CABG surgery.

In a series of 4000 CABG cases, perioperative stroke occurred in 6.1% of patients with a unilateral significant stenosis, 14% of patients with a unilateral carotid occlusion, 20% of patients with a significant stenosis contralateral to an occlusion, 33% of patients with bilateral internal carotid occlusions, but in only 1.9% of individuals without significant carotid disease. In another study, the incidence of perioperative stroke was 9% among CABG surgery patients with symptomatic carotid disease versus 3% among asymptomatic patients. Although the cause of perioperative stroke among cardiac surgical patients is clearly multifactorial, and although clinically significant carotid disease occurs in a minority of patients who are candidates for coronary revascularization, significant carotid artery disease is nevertheless one potentially preventable etiology.

DIAGNOSTIC EVALUATION

Among patients who present primarily for CEA, evaluation of possible CAD should progress in a logical fashion along three planes of increasing invasiveness: careful analysis of the clinical history, radionuclide imaging, and coronary angiography. Essentially, analysis of several clinical factors identifies a subset of patients who should undergo radionuclide imaging, and a subset of these patients requires coronary angiography.

Several clinical factors historically have been found to be highly predictive of cardiac morbidity after CEA, including Q waves on the electrocardiogram, a history of exertional angina, recent myocardial infarction, a history of ventricular arrhythmia, congestive heart failure, diabetes mellitus, and age greater than 70 years. If none of these markers is identified, and the patient is reasonably active so that absence of angina is a valid observation, the patient may proceed to CEA. If one or more factors are present, especially if the patient leads a fairly sedentary lifestyle, further evaluation by radionuclide imaging is indicated. Stress thallium-201 scintigraphy and intravenous dipyridamole-thallium scanning are relatively noninvasive and highly sensitive methods of identifying the patient with significant underlying coronary disease. If the results are negative, the patient may undergo CEA with a low risk of experiencing cardiac morbidity. Among patients in whom a significant redistribution of thallium is noted, suggestive of significant CAD and an increased risk of perioperative cardiac morbidity, formal coronary arteriography should be performed if the carotid disease is stable. With objective documentation of the severity of the coronary disease provided by angiography, an informed clinical judgment may be made concerning proper therapy and its timing.

Conversely, among patients who present primarily with CAD for myocardial revascularization, carotid duplex examination is the most important diagnostic modality. We believe a duplex study should be performed on all patients scheduled for a CABG procedure if there is a history of stroke or transient ischemic attacks or if a carotid bruit is identified. In addition, in view of the documented incidence of asymptomatic carotid disease among older individuals with evidence of atherosclerotic occlusive disease in other beds, such as the coronary or peripheral circulations,

we believe a baseline duplex scan is appropriate in individuals older than age 70 scheduled for elective CABG surgery. In our practice, the decision to recommend a CEA is based on the results of the duplex scan and the clinical history in most cases. If the patient is referred with a scan that was performed in an unaccredited vascular laboratory, we repeat the study in our facility. If the findings are in conflict; if the severity of the stenosis in an asymptomatic patient is of borderline hemodynamic significance; or if there are confounding issues, such as a suspected high carotid bifurcation, proximal great vessel occlusive disease, or a previous CEA, we obtain a conventional arteriogram. In our practice, contrast angiography is required in only a few patients, however. In some cases, we confirm the findings of the duplex scan with magnetic resonance angiography.

MANAGEMENT

Carotid Endarterectomy Patient

With the current methods of anesthetic management and hemodynamic monitoring, the patient with significant carotid disease and mild CAD may undergo CEA safely without coronary revascularization. If moderate coronary disease is identified angiographically, and if it is treatable by percutaneous transluminal coronary angioplasty (PTCA), it seems most reasonable to proceed with this intervention. If the extent of the CAD is beyond the scope of PTCA, and the patient has experienced stable angina, we believe the patient still may undergo CEA safely if medical management is maximized preoperatively, including aggressive use of β-blockade, and if careful attention is paid to intraoperative and postoperative hemodynamic monitoring and blood pressure control. Some would recommend, however, a CABG procedure, to be followed by the CEA, if the carotid disease is stable. We have not favored this so-called reverse staged approach in this clinical scenario. Rather, if the patient presents primarily with symptomatic or severe asymptomatic carotid disease and stable CAD, we perform the CEA, observe the patient in a monitored unit for 24 to 48 hours postoperatively, then proceed with CABG surgery if clinically indicated in a staged manner.

Coronary Artery Bypass Graft Surgery Patient

The decision to proceed with CEA in a patient presenting primarily with CAD depends on the hemodynamic significance of the carotid artery disease, the presence or absence of neurologic symptoms, the severity of the CAD, and the patient's overall medical condition. This is a relatively subjective decision that must be individualized on a case-by-case basis, and there is no consensus among specialists in this area. In general, we approach the carotid issue as if there were not a confounding element of CAD. How would the patient be managed if he or she simply presented in the office for evaluation and possible treatment of carotid disease in the absence of CAD? With rare exception, we believe a patient with CAD and a history of symptomatic carotid disease should have the disease process in both systems addressed. We favor a relatively conservative course, however, with respect to surgical intervention for asymptomatic carotid disease, and in general we do not perform CEA in the setting of a unilateral moderate (60% to 70%) asymptomatic stenosis. If the patient presents with severe CAD requiring coronary revascularization and has a unilateral moderate carotid stenosis, we would recommend proceeding with CABG surgery. We reserve CEA for patients who require a CABG procedure and who also have bilateral significant carotid stenoses (operating on the side with the most severe stenosis) or patients with a high-grade (>80%) unilateral stenosis and otherwise good medical risk. The timing of the two procedures (staged versus synchronous) depends on the urgency of the CEA and coronary revascularization procedures.

Staged Repair

Although some have advocated performing CEA with the patient awake under cervical block anesthesia, there are no conclusive scientific data to support this approach. In the ACAS randomized trial, the incidence of cardiac complications was higher among patients in whom the operation was performed by this method. Although performing CEA and CABG surgery synchronously during the same period of anesthesia has theoretical appeal, there are clinical advantages to staging the two procedures. The general anesthetic technique employed for CEA is different from that used in patients undergoing coronary revascularization. In addition, immediately after completion of the endarterectomy the patient is awakened in the operating room, allowing assessment of neurologic status. Any neurologic abnormality suggestive of a technical problem with the carotid procedure allows the surgeon to reexplore the carotid artery immediately and if a defect is identified to repair it before a permanent ischemic insult has been sustained by the patient. In a combined procedure, after completion of the endarterectomy, the myocardial revascularization proceeds for several hours, and the patient remains asleep for several hours postoperatively. If the patient eventually awakens with a neurologic deficit, the opportunity for the vascular surgeon to correct any technical fault with the endarterectomy has been lost.

Today in many patients with coexistent significant CAD and carotid disease, we favor staging the two procedures, with the CEA preceding the CABG procedure. Acute cardiac decompensation requiring immediate institution of cardiopulmonary bypass has never occurred during CEA in our experience. It is well recognized that most cardiac complications in the CEA patient do not occur intraoperatively, but rather 24 to 48 hours after surgery. After CEA, the patient is kept in a monitored unit, with a radial artery catheter in place for systemic blood pressure monitoring. Strict blood pressure control is maintained with intravenous nitroprusside or phenylephrine and nitroglycerin as necessary. We routinely administer β-blockers, if tolerated. If unstable angina develops, we are prepared to proceed with emergent CABG surgery, although this has occurred rarely in our experience.

Patients with a unilateral asymptomatic carotid stenosis undergoing CABG surgery as an isolated procedure, as noted earlier, incur a slightly increased risk of perioperative stroke. Nevertheless, it seems that this incremental increase in risk at least is balanced or exceeded by the risk of cardiac morbidity inherent in performing CEA in patients with severe CAD or by the risks of a combined procedure. In patients with an asymptomatic unilateral carotid stenosis and severe CAD, the reversed staged approach seems most logical—performing the CABG procedure first, using pulsatile cardiopulmonary bypass, and performing the CEA later, after recovery from CABG surgery, if the procedure is clinically indicated.

Synchronous Repair

Combined CEA and CABG surgery is indicated for patients with the most severe CAD and carotid artery disease. In our practice, we recommend synchronous CEA/CABG surgery for patients with significant carotid disease and severe three-vessel CAD, left main disease, unstable angina, or poor left ventricular function or for patients who are being managed with an intravenous heparin or nitroglycerin infusion or intraaortic balloon pump support. In patients undergoing synchronous repair, there are several ways in which to sequence the intraoperative events. Some recommend performing the median sternotomy simultaneously with or before the neck incision so that the surgeon can be prepared fully for any sudden cardiac decompensation that might occur during CEA. Perhaps the most aggressive approach involves opening the chest, cannulating, and placing the patient on cardiopulmonary bypass before proceeding with the carotid repair. This option seems illogical to us because it negates the rationale for performing the combined procedure. In our institution, CEA is performed before median sternotomy. This provides a quiet field for the vascular surgeon, and because the saphenous vein may be harvested simultaneously, it imposes at most a slight delay on the coronary procedure. At the conclusion of the carotid procedure, a drain is placed, and the neck is closed in the usual fashion except for the skin. We have found that this strategy minimizes the risk of developing a neck hematoma during cardiopulmonary bypass and maximum anticoagulation. The skin simply is closed at the completion of the cardiac surgical procedure, with any hematoma evacuated before skin closure.

Carotid Percutaneous Transluminal Angioplasty/Stent Placement

Carotid PTA/stent placement is another option for treating carotid disease among patients with severe concomitant CAD. Although there is considerable and growing enthusiasm for this endovascular modality, particularly among interventional cardiologists and radiologists, it cannot be overstated that carotid angioplasty must be viewed as an investigational procedure at present. There is considerable variability in reported results from center to center, including some reports documenting prohibitively high rates of periprocedural neurologic complications; only a fraction of these series have been reported in full-length articles in the peer-reviewed literature; almost no long-term follow-up data are currently available on the durability of carotid stenting and clinical outcome; and the technology is rapidly evolving, including the more recent introduction of a variety of carotid artery–specific stents and cerebral protection devices. CEA remains the gold standard treatment for most patients with significant carotid artery disease and should remain so until completion of randomized prospective clinical trials comparing the conventional operation with carotid PTA/stent placement. Nevertheless, carotid PTA/stent placement may be appropriate in high-risk patients with coexistent CAD and carotid artery disease. Specifically, if an experienced interventionalist is available, carotid PTA/stent placement should be considered in patients with severe carotid disease and end-stage CAD without options for PTCA or CABG surgery, assuming the patient has sufficient life expectancy to justify the carotid procedure. In addition, carotid PTA/stent placement may be appropriate for patients with significant coexistent CAD and carotid disease in whom the risk of conventional CEA may be increased, such as patients with a high-grade recurrent carotid stenosis, an anatomically high carotid bifurcation/lesion, or a history of previous radical neck surgery and irradiation. Until further data become available with respect to the safety and durability of carotid PTA/stent placement, however, we still favor performing a combined CEA/CABG procedure in patients with severe coexistent carotid disease and CAD, rather than a carotid PTA/stent procedure followed by CABG surgery.

■ SUMMARY

In view of the dramatic aging of the population, cardiovascular specialists will encounter an unprecedented number of patients with significant coexistent carotid disease and CAD in the future. The most appropriate management of these patients involves individualized clinical judgment. Although dozens of articles have been published on this subject over three decades, almost all of these series are retrospective or anecdotal in nature, and analysis of these data is confounded by the heterogeneity of the patient populations reported, different therapeutic strategies undertaken, varying indications for intervention, and other factors. There is no consensus among specialists with respect to the optimal therapeutic strategy, and it is unlikely that one will evolve until a multicenter randomized clinical trial addresses this important clinical problem. Although we, as others, have observed the highest incidence of perioperative morbidity among patients who undergo combined CEA and CABG surgery, this observation reflects the fact that because we increasingly have elected to stage CEA and CABG surgery in our institution in more recent years, the patients with the most severe coexistent carotid disease and CAD are selected for the synchronous approach. Nevertheless, until completion of randomized clinical trials comparing conventional CEA with carotid PTA/stent placement, we believe combined CEA/CABG surgery is preferable to treating the carotid disease by angioplasty and stent placement in all but the most exceptional patient with significant coexistent carotid disease and CAD.

SUGGESTED READING

Bilfinger TV, et al: Coronary and carotid operations under prospective standardized conditions: incidence and outcome, *Ann Thorac Surg* 69:1792, 2000.

Das SK, et al: Continuing controversy in the management of concomitant coronary and carotid disease: an overview, *Int J Cardiol* 74:47, 2000.

Hertzer NR, et al: Surgical staging for simultaneous coronary and carotid disease: a study including prospective randomization, *J Vasc Surg* 9:455, 1989.

Perler BA, et al: The safety of carotid endarterectomy at the time of coronary artery bypass surgery: analysis of results in a high risk patient population, *J Vasc Surg* 2:558, 1985.

Perler BA, et al: Should we perform carotid endarterectomy synchronously with cardiac surgical procedures? *J Vasc Surg* 8:402, 1988.

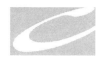

SURGERY FOR MYOCARDIAL DISEASE

HYPERTROPHIC CARDIOMYOPATHY

Frank G. Scholl
Walter H. Merrill

The spectrum of disease known as *hypertrophic cardiomyopathy* (HCM) is manifest as left ventricular myocardial hypertrophy, which frequently is asymmetric and is associated with histologic evidence of myocardial fiber disarray. Typically, patients with this disorder have supranormal systolic function and impaired diastolic relaxation and compliance. The cause of HCM is currently unknown. Patients can present with either a familial form, which follows an autosomal dominant pattern of inheritance with variable penetrance, or a sporadic form. Ventricular hypertrophy in HCM occurs most commonly at the level of the basal septum, with midventricular, apical, and symmetric forms being less common. The location and severity of the hypertrophied muscle mass have important effects on the pathophysiology of the lesion. Septal hypertrophy accompanied by anterior displacement of the papillary muscle and anterior mitral leaflet may lead to subaortic obstruction at rest or on provocation. The obstruction is thought to be due to Venturi forces that pull the anterior mitral leaflet into the ventricular outflow tract during systole. The elongated and thickened anterior mitral leaflet moves abnormally and may lead to varying degrees of posteriorly directed mitral regurgitation. Over time, this may cause left atrial dilation and atrial arrhythmias. In some patients, subaortic obstruction exists without systolic anterior motion of the mitral valve; this is thought to be due to anterior displacement of the hypertrophied papillary muscles that narrow the outflow tract. Approximately 20% to 25% of patients with HCM have significant ventricular outflow tract obstruction. Many of these patients develop significant free wall hypertrophy as a result of outflow obstruction.

Coronary artery diameter in this condition may be abnormally large, and approximately 5% of patients have significant atherosclerotic disease. Additionally, ventricular wall thickening and systolic compression of coronary arteries may result in obliteration of intramuscular branches. These findings, in addition to the abnormal myocardial relaxation and elevated ventricular diastolic filling pressures, may lead to ischemia and infarction despite absence of significant obstructive atherosclerotic lesions.

Symptoms associated with HCM are dyspnea on exertion, fatigue, angina, presyncope, syncope, and palpitations related to atrial fibrillation or ventricular arrhythmias. Sudden death may occur at a rate of 2% to 3% per patient-year and is related to atrial or ventricular arrhythmias.

Signs on physical examination usually include a prominent left ventricular apical pulsation, a systolic left ventricular outflow tract murmur of variable intensity and duration, and a bifid pulse. Surface echocardiography can be helpful in establishing an anatomic diagnosis and defining the nature of the associated physiologic changes. Additional preoperative assessment should include coronary angiography in adults and left heart catheterization. Right heart catheterization should be considered to assess pulmonary artery pressure and to rule out rare instances of right ventricular outflow tract obstruction. Intraoperative assessment with transesophageal echocardiography has been a valuable adjunct to determine septal thickness and shape, to determine the point of mitral valve contact with the septum, to evaluate the adequacy of surgical resection and degree of residual outflow gradient, and to detect the presence of systolic anterior motion and mitral regurgitation.

■ TREATMENT OPTIONS

Treatment of hypertrophic obstructive cardiomyopathy is based on symptoms. Medical management provides symptomatic relief for most patients and consists of negative inotropes, mainly β-blockers and calcium channel blockers, to decrease outflow tract obstruction. Medical management with β-blockers aims to reduce myocardial oxygen demand, decrease ventricular contractility, and lower heart rate. These mechanisms may reduce left ventricular outflow gradients. Calcium channel blockers, in addition to decreasing heart rate and contractility, improve diastolic relaxation, which enhances ventricular filling and alleviates the diastolic dysfunction in patients with HCM. In patients who fail to obtain significant improvement despite medical therapies, due to either intolerance of side effects or incomplete resolution of symptoms, further efforts to reduce left ventricular outflow gradient and alleviate symptoms must be sought.

Dual-chamber cardiac pacing, percutaneous transluminal myocardial ablation, mitral valve replacement, and transaortic septal myomectomy all have been proposed to provide relief of outflow tract gradient and resolution of symptoms. The indications for individual treatment options have not been well defined, tend to be controversial, and seem to be based at least in part on the discretion and experience of the treating center.

Dual-chamber DDD pacing has been proposed by some as a nonoperative method of treatment for symptomatic HCM patients who fail medical management.

The mechanism by which DDD pacing helps to relieve outflow tract obstruction is poorly understood. It may be related to decreased septal motion, delayed activation of the base of the septum relative to the apex, or altered ventricular contractility. This treatment option is a poor choice for patients in atrial fibrillation and is not as well tolerated in younger, more active patients. In a nonrandomized, concurrent cohort series comparing dual-chamber pacing with septal myomectomy, the latter offered a greater reduction in left ventricular outflow gradients and more improvement in objective measures of patients' symptoms and functional status. The complication rates in another series of pacing in patients with HCM were unacceptably high.

Percutaneous transcatheter myocardial ablation has been described as a technique to alleviate left ventricular outflow obstruction in patients with HCM. It consists of an intracoronary dose of ethanol to induce a controlled septal myocardial infarction. There have been reports of successful short-term reduction in outflow tract gradients, but no long-term follow-up studies are available yet; the technique was described initially in 1995. The reported incidence of atrioventricular conduction delay and complete heart block requiring a permanent pacemaker after ethanol-induced septal ablation is of some concern. Additionally the development of further myocardial fibrosis over the long term may worsen ventricular arrhythmias in this group of patients who already are at a greater risk of life-threatening dysrhythmia.

Numerous surgical techniques and operative approaches for relief of left ventricular outflow tract obstruction have been described. The most commonly employed techniques include mitral valve replacement and transaortic septal myectomy. Replacement of the mitral valve with a low-profile mechanical prosthesis removes the anterior mitral leaflet and prevents systolic anterior motion, with consequent relief of outflow tract obstruction. Some authors have used this technique routinely in patients with a relatively thin septum on echocardiographic assessment. In patients with a septal thickness less than 18 mm, adequate septal resection might be difficult and pose a greater risk of postresection ventricular septal defect. The mechanical prosthesis exposes the patient to the inherent risks of a valvar prosthesis and to the continuous risk of anticoagulation. Patients who are not candidates for long-term anticoagulation should receive a biologic prosthesis if mitral valve replacement is required. Mitral valve replacement also is indicated in patients who continue to have systolic anterior motion with significant outflow obstruction measured by intraoperative transesophageal echocardiography after myectomy.

Surgical myectomy for relief of symptomatic subaortic obstruction was refined by Morrow and has been used successfully in many centers. Myectomy remains the procedure of choice for long-lasting symptomatic relief in patients who have failed medical therapy and have documented outflow tract obstruction at rest or on provocation.

The operation currently is performed with the routine use of intraoperative transesophageal echocardiography to map out the area of the proposed surgical resection and to provide real-time intraoperative measurement of residual gradient across the outflow tract and the degree of mitral regurgitation after myectomy. Median sternotomy, single venous cannulation, and antegrade and retrograde cardioplegia are used routinely. The aortic cannula is placed just inferior to the pericardial reflection, and the ventricle is vented through the right superior pulmonary vein.

The heart is arrested with cold blood cardioplegia, and a generous oblique aortotomy is made with care to avoid injury to the right coronary artery and aortic valve. The aorta is inspected, and the aortic valve leaflets are retracted and protected carefully throughout the procedure. The interventricular septum is rotated into the surgeon's field of view by gentle retraction and counterpressure on the anterior surface of the heart (Figure 1). A narrow ribbon retractor is placed through the aortic valve to protect the anterior mitral leaflet and chordal apparatus. The location of the thick and obstructing septum and the fibrotic contact point of the anterior mitral leaflet are noted beneath the right aortic leaflet. This should be the area of maximum resection. Septal hypertrophy may be delineated further by palpation with the left index finger through the valve. The septal myectomy is begun by making a longitudinal incision in the septum 2 to 3 mm to the right of the nadir of the right aortic leaflet beginning several millimeters below the valve. An angled knife handle with a no. 10 or no. 15 blade facilitates this incision. The incision is carried distally several centimeters toward the apex of the heart. A second incision is made parallel to the first, to the left of it as far as is practical, leaving a 2.0- to 2.5-cm-wide, 4.5- to 5.0-cm-long area to be removed (Figure 2). The third incision joins these two longitudinal incisions and carves out the rectangular segment,

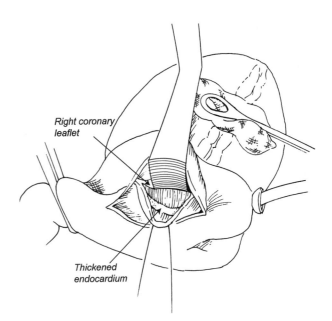

Figure 1
Through an oblique aortotomy, the bulging hypertrophied interventricular septum is visible below the right coronary leaflet. A ridge of thickened endocardium is seen on the most prominent portion of the septum. Exposure is facilitated by careful traction on the right coronary leaflet and by counterpressure on the left ventricle. *(Redrawn from Morrow AG: J Thorac Cardiovasc Surg 76:423, 1978.)*

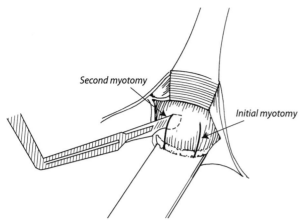

Figure 2
Initial myotomy incision is performed 1 to 3 mm to the right of the nadir of the right coronary leaflet. The second incision is made parallel to the first one and about 1 cm to the left. *(Redrawn from Morrow AG: J Thorac Cardiovasc Surg 76:423, 1978.)*

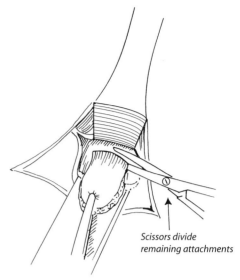

Figure 4
Using scissors, the remaining muscular attachments between the resected specimen and the septum are divided under direct vision. *(Redrawn from Morrow AG: J Thorac Cardiovasc Surg 76:423, 1978.)*

leaving a wide trough through the previously obstructing hypertrophied tissue (Figure 3). Frequently, it is necessary to divide remaining small muscle attachments with scissors (Figure 4). After the removal of the rectangular piece of septum, additional trimming by further deepening or widening of the trough can be done using scissors or a scalpel as necessary. The thickness of the remaining septum should be 6 to 8 mm at the completion of the myectomy as measured by intraoperative transesophageal echocardiography. The ventricular cavity is irrigated with cold saline after protecting the coronary ostia or while giving retrograde cardioplegia,

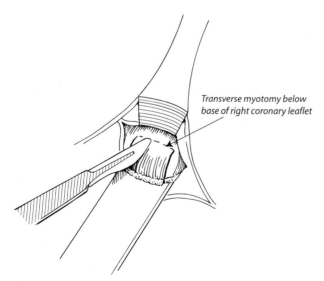

Figure 3
A transverse myotomy below the base of the right coronary leaflet connects the two vertical incisions. *(Redrawn from Morrow AG: J Thorac Cardiovasc Surg 76:423, 1978.)*

and the retractors are removed. The aortic valve is inspected carefully for evidence of injury.

The aortotomy is closed, and the patient is weaned from cardiopulmonary bypass on minimal inotropic support. Intraoperative transesophageal echocardiography can be used to assess the outflow tract and may provide valuable data on the presence of residual outflow tract gradient, systolic anterior motion, mitral valve regurgitation, or ventricular septal defect.

Several potential pitfalls must be kept in mind while performing a septal myectomy for HCM. The aortic valve must be kept out of harm's way from retractor injury and injury while performing the myectomy. The mitral valve and chordae tendineae must be protected so as to avoid possible injury. Injury to the conduction system and membranous septum can occur, particularly if the resection is begun too far rightward beneath the junction of the right and noncoronary commissure. A muscular ventricular septal defect may be created by excessive resection of ouflow tract musculature. The first attempt at resection is likely to give the best chance of achieving the goal of alleviating the outflow tract obstruction and avoiding these potential complications. To accomplish this goal, it is important to take adequate time to set up excellent exposure, carefully visualizing the aortic valve, the subvalvular area, and the proximal septum, allowing the safe performance of an adequate myectomy. Postoperatively, patients are maintained on little or no inotropic support because these agents exacerbate any residual outflow tract obstruction. Many of these patients are predisposed to atrial and ventricular arrhythmias, and appropriate antiarrhythmic agents are used as necessary. As a result of the abnormal diastolic relaxation and impaired ventricular filling, postoperative atrial fibrillation may be poorly tolerated and should be treated aggressively, including

Table 1 Results of Septal Myectomy for Hypertrophic Obstructive Cardiomyopathy

DATE	AUTHOR	YEARS	NO. PATIENTS	MEAN PREOPER-ATIVE RESTING GRADIENT	MEAN NYHA CLASS	% EARLY MORTALITY	% LATE MORTALITY	MEAN YEARS OF FOLLOW-UP	MEAN POSTOP-ERATIVE NYHA CLASS	MEAN POSTOP-ERATIVE RESTING GRADIENT
1992	ten Berg	1977-1992	38	72	3.0	0.0	0.0	6.8	1.5	6
1992	Cohn	1972-1991	31	96	3.10	0.0	16.0	6.5	2	4.5
1994	McCully	1986-1992	45	NA	3.20	0.0	2.0	2.2	1.5	NA
1996	Robbins	1972-1994	158	64	2.77	3.2	10.0	6.1	NA	8.2
2000	Merrill	1981-1999	22	78	NA	0.0	9.0	6.6	NA	12

NYHA, New York Heart Association; NA, not available.

the use of electrical cardioversion should any hemodynamic compromise occur. Two atrial and two ventricular temporary epicardial pacing wires are inserted routinely.

■ RESULTS

The results of transaortic septal myectomy for hypertrophic obstructive cardiomyopathy are excellent. Many centers have published data on medium-term and long-term outcomes that document substantial improvement in subjective and objective variables. Early and late mortality rates for patients undergoing the procedure at this institution have been comparable to those reported in the literature. In a study from this institution looking at 22 patients from 1981 to 1999, there were no early deaths and two late deaths with a mean follow-up of 6.6 years. All surviving patients had minimal to mild symptoms with a mean resting outflow gradient of 12 mm Hg by echocardiography. The symptomatic improvement seen in these patients has been sustained, and all have had improvement in functional class. Late complications were related to diastolic dysfunction rather than outflow obstruction. This observation also has been reported by others. In other studies, the need for concomitant coronary artery bypass graft surgery and advanced age at operation have been suggested as risk factors for late death but not for perioperative mortality. The results of several studies are summarized in Table 1. There were no patients reported who needed reoperation for residual or recurrent outflow obstruction in these series. The incidence of surgically created heart block and ventricular septal defect also was quite low. These reports show that septal myectomy for HCM can be done safely, with minimal morbidity and mortality, and that the procedure provides durable symptomatic improvement in patients with outflow obstruction due to HCM.

SUGGESTED READING

Erwin JP 3rd, et al: Dual chamber pacing for patients with hypertrophic obstructive cardiomyopathy: a clinical perspective in 2000, *Mayo Clin Proc* 75:173, 2000.

Lakkis N, et al: Hypertrophic obstructive cardiomyopathy: alternative therapeutic options, *Clin Cardiol* 20:417, 1997.

Merrill WH, et al: Long-lasting improvement after septal myectomy for hypertrophic obstructive cardiomyopathy, *Ann Thorac Surg* 69:1732, 2000.

Morrow AG: Hypertrophic subaortic stenosis: operative methods utilized to relieve left ventricular outflow obstruction, *J Thorac Cardiovasc Surg* 76:423, 1978.

Robbins RC, Stinson EB: Long-term results of left ventricular myotomy and myectomy for obstructive hypertrophic cardiomyopathy, *J Thorac Cardiovasc Surg* 111:586, 1996.

LEFT VENTRICULAR VOLUME REDUCTION

Mohammed A. Quader

Katherine J. Hoercher

Rick White

Patrick M. McCarthy

The prevalence and incidence of heart failure rapidly are reaching epidemic proportions with an estimated 4.8 million individuals with this syndrome; an additional 400,000 to 700,000 new cases are diagnosed annually. The magnitude of heart failure in the United States will continue to worsen as the population ages. Heart transplantation, although an effective treatment for the most critically ill patients, remains an option for only a small percentage of this population due to the limited supply of organ donors. The devastation wrought by heart failure and its economic burden have led to the development of innovative surgical therapies to address the problem of heart failure. Progressive left ventricular (LV) remodeling is related directly to the progression and the pathogenesis of heart failure with subsequent deterioration in LV performance and increased morbidity and mortality. As a greater understanding of the significance of LV remodeling in the disease process has evolved, the emergence of surgical reconstruction of the dysfunctional left ventricle to arrest or reverse remodeling is showing significant promise as a treatment option. This chapter focuses on two procedures: (1) reconstruction (modified Dor procedure) for postinfarction LV dysfunction and (2) partial left ventriculectomy (PLV) (Batista) for dilated cardiomyopathy.

■ PARTIAL LEFT VENTRICULECTOMY

Surgical LV reconstruction for dilated cardiomyopathy or PLV attempted to create a more normal LV volume, a more elliptical LV shape, and decreased LV wall tension. Popularized by Batista, this operation gained worldwide attention. The operative technique consists of excision of the lateral LV wall, usually between the papillary muscles or with papillary muscle transection and reimplantation. If needed, mitral valve repair also was performed. At the Cleveland Clinic Foundation, 62 patients with nonischemic cardiomyopathy underwent PLV between 1996 and 1998. Preoperatively, mean LV ejection fraction was 14%, and mean peak oxygen consumption was 10.8 ml/kg/min; 61% were in New York Heart Association (NYHA) class IV, indicating the disease severity of this cohort. Operative mortality was low (3.2%). Although some patients derived a significant benefit, we observed a high early failure rate and an event-free survival at 36 months of only 26%. Reports

from other centers cite perioperative mortality of 6% to 22% with most patients developing recurrent symptoms of heart failure. PLV was abandoned at the Cleveland Clinic Foundation because of the unpredictable early failures and late return to heart failure.

■ LEFT VENTRICULAR RECONSTRUCTION FOR ISCHEMIC CARDIOMYOPATHY

Ischemic cardiomyopathy is the most common cause of heart failure in the current era in the United States, ranging from 40% to 70% in different studies. In these patients, anterior myocardial infarction (left anterior descending coronary artery infarct) is a frequent initiating event resulting in LV scarring. Left untreated, this scar expands over time, resulting in akinesia—LV infarct with a thin rim of viable myocardium, leading to no movement during systole (but with enough myocardium to prevent paradoxical bulging) or dyskinesia/LV aneurysm—transmural LV infarct with subsequent wall thinning, leading to paradoxical segmental outward bulging during LV systole. Replacement of the anterior wall and septum with scar results in hypertrophy of the remote muscle (right coronary artery and circumflex territories), which produces an alteration of LV shape (remodeling) leading to the manifestations and consequences of heart failure. The development of heart failure after myocardial infarction is related to the volume and shape change of the LV. Studies have shown that regional infarction of more than 30% of LV circumference causes progressive dilation of remote viable muscle, which converts the normal elliptical LV shape to that of a sphere.

Surgical LV reconstruction for ischemic cardiomyopathy has existed since the first LV aneurysmectomy by Cooley in 1959. The standard operation for LV aneurysm, linear aneurysmectomy, has evolved to a more complicated repair that includes the infarcted septum and free wall. Although most patients undergoing this early linear repair had an improvement in symptoms of heart failure, clinical outcomes were less predictable than today with a reported perioperative mortality of 7% to 18%. This prompted the development of a newer approach, used for dyskinetic and akinetic regions.

Our current technique of LV reconstruction for ischemic cardiomyopathy is performed through a sternotomy incision on full cardiopulmonary bypass. During aortic cross-clamp, mitral valve repair and coronary artery bypass graft surgery are performed as needed. The aortic cross-clamp is removed, and the LV reconstruction is performed on the beating heart to help delineate the border zone between infarcted myocardium and the remote areas of contracting myocardium. Subendocardial resection of scar tissue and cryoablation of the border zone is performed for patients with a history of ventricular tachycardia. A purse-string suture is placed through the scar tissue at the border zone between infarcted and normal myocardium and, on tying the suture, effectively excludes the infarcted segment from the LV cavity. Additional purse-string sutures and felt closure of the scar tissue are done to complete the reconstruction (similar to the technique of Jatene). In our early experience, a patch was placed after the first purse-string suture was tied to exclude the infarcted segment (similar to the technique of Dor). More recently, patients rarely underwent patch reconstruction. Patch reconstruction still is indicated, however, for patients with a heavily calcified LV aneurysm that does not allow for reconstruction with only sutures or for patients in whom reconstruction without a patch would leave a small residual LV cavity.

■ RESULTS

From July 1997 to July 2001, 131 patients have undergone anterior LV reconstruction at the Cleveland Clinic Foundation, 49 for akinetic and 82 for dyskinetic regions. Additional procedures include coronary artery bypass graft surgery in 85% and mitral valve repair in 50%. There was a low perioperative mortality (1.5%), and survival at 36 months is 75% for the akinetic group and 89% for the dyskinetic group. There was an improvement in the mean ejection fraction from 20.7% to 27%; concurrently the end-systolic volume index decreased from a mean of 106 ml/m^2 to 74 ml/m^2, and end-diastolic volume index decreased from a mean of 144 ml/m^2 to 107 ml/m^2. The NYHA functional class changed from a preoperative mean of 2.91 to 1.7 at 12 months' follow-up, reflecting a simultaneous functional improvement. Survival of patients with severe LV dysfunction undergoing complicated operations, including coronary artery bypass graft surgery, valve surgery, and LV reconstruction, is excellent with improvements in LV function and NYHA functional class. These results stand in marked contrast to the reconstructions that were performed for idiopathic dilated cardiomyopathy.

SUGGESTED READING

Batista RJ, et al: Partial left ventriculectomy to improve left ventricular function in end-stage heart disease, *J Card Surg* 11:96, 1996.

Dor V: Reconstructive left ventricular surgery for post-ischemic akinetic dilatation, *Semin Thorac Cardiovasc Surg* 9:139, 1997.

Franco-Cereceda A, et al: Partial left ventriculectomy for dilated cardiomyopathy: is this an alternative to transplantation? *J Thorac Cardiovasc Surg* 121:879, 2001.

McCarthy JF, et al: Partial left ventriculectomy and mitral valve repair for end-stage congestive heart failure, *Eur J Cardiothorac Surg* 13:337, 1998.

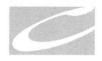

CONGENITAL AORTIC STENOSIS

John W. Brown
Mark D. Rodefeld
Mark W. Turrentine

Aortic stenosis (AS) is encountered in 5% of children with congenital heart disease. Left ventricular (LV) outflow tract (LVOT) obstruction may occur at the valvar, subvalvar, and/or supravalvar level. Although excellent clinical results may be initially achieved, surgical therapy in most cases is considered palliative; most children presenting with valvar AS (VAS) eventually present for valve replacement. We reviewed our 42-year experience with surgical treatment of congenital AS at the James Whitcomb Riley Hospital for Children in Indianapolis. Between 1960 and 2002, 668 operations were performed on 508 patients. Age at operation ranged from 1 day to 19 years (mean, 7.4 years). Ninety-three infants (18%) were less than 6 months of age. Preoperatively, the majority of patients (68%) were in New York Heart Association (NYHA) functional class III or IV. Single-level LVOT obstruction was present in 81% (supravalvar, 10%; valvar, 58%; subvalvar, 32%), and multilevel obstruction was present in 19%. The aortic valve was unicuspid in 6%, bicuspid in 73%, and tricuspid in 21%. All patients underwent preoperative cardiac echocardiography, catheterization, or both. Peak aortic gradient ranged from 0 to 200 mm Hg, with a mean value of 79.4 mm Hg. Patients with low aortic gradients (<35 mm Hg) underwent surgery because of symptoms (dyspnea, angina, syncope, and fatigue) or aortic regurgitation (13%). Patients with severe aortic incompetence underwent initial valve replacement. The majority of patients underwent median sternotomy and had repair using cardiopulmonary bypass. The exceptions were patients receiving an apical aortic conduit (AAC) or neonates who underwent closed transventricular valvotomy (CTV) via left thoracotomy and without the aid of cardiopulmonary bypass.

■ DIAGNOSIS AND SURGICAL MANAGEMENT

Valvar Aortic Stenosis

VAS is the most common cause of LVOT obstruction and is commonly accompanied by other left-sided cardiac lesions involving the mitral valve, left ventricle, subaortic region, and aortic arch and isthmus. Initial aortic valve replacement (AVR) was performed in only 26 patients (5%) in our 508-patient series. Mechanical prostheses were used in 10 patients. One patient had an aortic homograft inserted in 1993. Since 1993, all 15 initial AVRs were performed using a pulmonary autograft (Ross procedure). All patients undergoing the Ross procedure had right ventricular outflow tract reconstruction using a pulmonary homograft. One hundred nine (26 initial and 83 redo) AVRs have been performed in 98 children. Ten Ross-Konno procedures have been performed as redo procedures. The results of AVR in children comparing the Ross with mechanical and other bioprostheses have been previously reported.

Neonatal critical AS accounts for less than 10% of congenital AS cases. Without intervention, the prognosis in this subgroup is almost uniformly fatal. In the past, open valvotomy or CTV has been the preferred initial operative treatment at our institution. Since 2000, however, we have preferred balloon aortic valvulotomy. Sixty-four neonates and young infants younger than 6 months with critical VAS underwent CTV. The LV apex was elevated and an apical pledgeted mattress suture was placed. A balloon catheter or serial dilators were passed through a stab incision in the LV apex and across the stenotic aortic valve using digital palpation of the aortic root. Progressive dilation was carried out stopping at or 1 mm more than the aortic annulus estimate on preoperative echocardiogram (range, 5 to 8 mm). Since 1999, we have performed CTV under transesophageal echocardiographic guidance and we stop dilation when mild aortic regurgitation is produced.

Supravalvar Aortic Stenosis

Supravalvar aortic stenosis (SVAS) is repaired by patch aortoplasty. Recent reports advocate two or three sinus repair. Ninety-two patients with SVAS underwent the insertion of a simple, diamond-shaped Dacron or polytetrafluoroethylene patch extending from the base of the noncoronary sinus of Valsalva to a level above the obstruction. An inverted bifurcated patch extending into the right coronary sinus as well as the noncoronary sinus was inserted in 12 patients. Nine additional children had extensive patches for most of their entire aortic arch. These children required femoral artery cannulation and a brief period of circulatory arrest for arch reconstruction.

Subvalvar Aortic Stenosis

Subvalvar aortic stenosis (SAS) represents a spectrum of disease ranging from a discrete fibrous membrane to diffuse fibromuscular or tunnel LVOT obstruction. Children with discrete SAS had complete resection of the fibrous subaortic membrane, with an associated myotomy and/or myectomy in one third of these cases. The 22 patients between 1978 and 1992 who required insertion of an AAC for tunnel SAS had a porcine (n = 20) or St. Jude mechanical (n = 2) valved Dacron conduit placed between the LV apex and descending thoracic aorta by a closed technique. Since 1993, the Ross-Konno procedure has replaced the AAC operation in children at our institution.

■ OUTCOMES

Overall survival for the entire group was 89% at 5 years and 88% at 20, 30, and 40 years. Freedom from reoperation was 75% at 10 years, 65% at 20 years, 63% at 30 years, and 62% at 40 years.

Valvar Aortic Stenosis

Two hundred forty-two children underwent aortic valvotomy with an operative mortality rate of 13%. All except two of the early deaths occurred in neonates. Aortic valvotomy (<6 months of age) carried a operative mortality rate of 34% and was responsible for 73% of all early deaths. Conversely, children over 6 months of age with aortic valvotomy or AVR had a 1% operative mortality rate. Since 1986 the operative mortality rate for neonatal CTV has been 17%. There has not been a surgical death in a child over 2 months of age since 1975 regardless of operative technique. Bicuspid aortic valves represent a main cause of isolated aortic insufficiency (AI), which usually presents at a young age. Approximately one third of patients with a bicuspid aortic valve remain asymptomatic and have a normal life span. Therefore, it is reasonable to attempt valve repair in an effort to restore a competent aortic valve and return patients to a reasonable long-term outcome.

Less Than 6 Months of Age

Ninety-three patients less than 6 months of age have undergone surgical procedures for AS. Eight patients with multilevel obstruction were included in the multilevel LVOT obstruction group described in further detail later. There were 30 early deaths (30 of 85, 35%): 11 patients with open valvotomy and 19 patients with CTV. Seven of the 8 patients who were operated on before 1978 with open aortic valvotomy died. After 1978 we adopted the CTV approach in

patients younger than 8 weeks. The operative mortality rate during the same period with open valvotomy was 0%, but the mean age of the infants was 3 months, reflecting an older, more stable group with less dysplastic valves. Overall survival is shown (Figure 1). There have been six late deaths. Since 1985, survival has been 85% (62 of 85). Univariate risk factors for death include endocardial fibroelastosis, LV hypoplasia, disease complexity, aortic valve annulus less than 5.0 mm, and repair before 1978. Of these, only hypoplastic LV and repair before 1978 remain significant on multivariate analysis. AI was not documented before surgery; however, 34 of 45 patients (76%) had documented AI on late follow-up: it was mild in 47% (16 of 34), moderate in 32% (11 of 34), and severe in 21% (7 of 34) of patients.

Sixteen reoperations have been performed in 14 of 55 patients (26%). The predominant indication for reoperation was the presence of combined AS and AI (9 of 14, 64%), followed by restenosis (4 of 14, 29%) or pure AI (1 of 14, 7%). Nine patients eventually required a Ross procedure, two had AVR with mechanical valves, two had repeat open valvotomies, and one patient received a heart transplant. The mean time from initial surgery to first reoperation was 8.0 years. Overall freedom from reoperation was 91% at 5 years, 82% at 10 years, 77% at 15 years, and 71% at 20 years. Univariate and multivariate analyses showed the presence of CTV ($p = .02$) as the best preoperative predictor of late reoperation in survivors. Forty-five patients (100%) are currently in NYHA functional class I or II. None have atrioventricular block or have required pacemaker implantation.

Greater Than 6 Months of Age

One hundred fifty-seven children older than 6 months underwent surgery for isolated valvar AS: 141 patients (90%,) underwent a standard aortic valve commissurotomy and 16 patients (10%) underwent an initial AVR (10 patients with a pulmonary autograft [Ross procedure] and 6 with a mechanical prosthesis). An additional 65 patients with multilevel LVOT obstruction had open valvotomy (n = 50), CTV (n = 7), or AVR as part of their initial treatment. There were two early deaths (1%) that occurred before 1975 and were secondary to low cardiac output. There were two late deaths at 5 and 12 years after the initial procedure. Both of these patients required subsequent AVR; one died secondary to

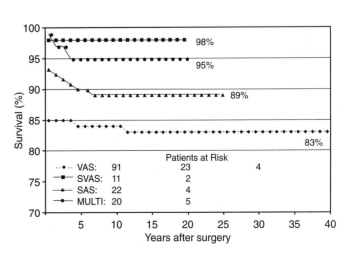

Figure 1
Actuarial survival (Kaplan-Meier) according to level of obstruction. VAS, valvar aortic stenosis; SVAS, supravalvar aortic stenosis; SAS, subvalvar aortic stenosis; MULTI, multilevel aortic stenosis.

end-stage renal disease and massive myocardial hypertrophy and the other died of a cardiac dysrhythmia 1 year after valve replacement surgery. Overall survival, including early mortality, is 97% at 40 years (see Figure 1). AI was documented in 32 of 157 patients (20%) before surgery; however, 103 of 155 patients (67%) had AI documented on late follow-up: mild in 56% (58 of 103), moderate in 27% (27 of 103), and severe in 17% (17 of 103).

Fifty-five reoperations were performed in 45 of 155 patients (29%). The indications for reoperation were recurrent stenosis with AI (58%), isolated stenosis (29%), or pure AI (9%). Two patients required reoperation (both with mechanical AVR). Eight patients required a third aortic procedure: Ross aortic root replacement in six and mechanical AVR in two. Both patients with mechanical AVR previously had undergone porcine valve insertion and were reoperated (2 and 16 years after the initial surgery) due to prosthesis degeneration. Two children had a fourth procedure: one for resection of ascending aortic aneurysm and the other for autograft valvuloplasty with resection of LV pseudoaneurysm. The mean time from initial surgery to first reoperation was 11.0 years, and from first to second reoperation, 6.7 years. A bicuspid valve was present in 36 patients (80%) who required reoperation; this did not differ significantly from the initial population (p > .05). Thirty-three patients (21%) followed for greater than 25 years and 15 patients (10%) followed for more than 15 years after their initial surgery have required AVR.

Overall freedom from reoperation estimated by the Kaplan-Meier method was 80% at 10 years, 67% at 20 years, 62% at 30 years, and 61% at 40 years (Figure 2). One hundred forty patients (93%) are currently in NYHA functional class I or II, and 11 patients (7%) are in class III. Comparing NYHA class of reoperated and nonreoperated patients, the latter were in a significantly better NYHA class (p = .02) at last follow-up. Among the patients who were NYHA class III, one had ventricular arrhythmia, one had a left anterior hemiblock, and two had atrioventricular block and pacemaker implantation.

Supravalvar Aortic Stenosis

Sixty-two patients with supravalvar AS had a patch aortoplasty as part of their initial surgical procedure (single-sinus repair, n = 50; two-sinus repair, n = 12). Three patients with single-sinus repair required reoperation at a later date. There was one hospital death (1 of 40, 2.5%) in patients who underwent repair of isolated SVAS. This resulted from postoperative cardiac failure early in the series (1962). In this patient, Dacron patch enlargement of the aorta had been confined to the aortic root. There have been no late deaths since 1987. Overall survival is excellent (see Figure 1). Univariate and multivariate analyses identified none of the tested variables as risk factors for death. AI was documented in 2 of 40 patients (5%) before initial operation, and 7 of 33 patients (21%) had AI documented on late follow-up: AI was mild in 86% (6 of 7), and moderate in 14% (1 of 7).

Three reoperations were performed in 3 of 39 patients (8%). Two patients with recurrent SVAS underwent redo patch aortoplasty (2 and 10 years after initial surgery), and the third patient with recurrent SVAS and moderate AI underwent a Ross procedure (11 years after initial surgery). Presence of late LV aortic gradient greater than 35 mm Hg was identified as a risk factor for reoperation by univariate analysis (p = .05). Overall freedom from reoperation was 97% at 5 years, 95% at 10 years, and 92% at 20 years (see Figure 2). Postoperatively, all patients were in NYHA class I or II. Recent echocardiographic follow-up showed persistence of mild stenosis of the pulmonary artery branches in two patients with initial severe pulmonary branch stenosis that were repaired by patch enlargement at the time of initial SVAS surgery.

Subvalvar Aortic Stenosis

One hundred thirty-two patients (132 of 508, 24%) with isolated SAS have undergone surgical procedures. There were 110 patients (83%) with discrete subaortic membrane and 22 patients (17%) with diffuse tunnel-like fibromuscular obstruction. An additional 73 patients had surgery for SAS as a part of their treatment for multilevel LVOT obstruction (fibrous resection [n = 37], fibromuscular resection [n = 29], and valve-sparing Konno [n = 7]). There were 5 early deaths (4%) that occurred in patients with isolated discrete SAS and one patient with tunnel SAS (0.8%). Three of the five deaths in patients with discrete membrane occurred in the early part of our experience (1960–1963).

There were eight late deaths (6%): two patients with discrete SAS and six patients with tunnel-like SAS. The two late deaths in patients with discrete SAS were of cardiac origin: one due to cerebrovascular accident (3 months after surgery) and one with congestive heart failure (7 years after surgery). Causes of the six late deaths in tunnel SAS group were as follows: three were from low cardiac output (1, 2, and 3 years after surgery, respectively) and one was sudden of unexplained cause 5 years after repair. Two deaths were noncardiac (one due to hemoptysis 4 years after operation and one due to aspiration and respiratory arrest 6 months after reoperation). Overall survival including early and late mortality was 90% at 5 years and 89% at 25 years (see Figure 1).

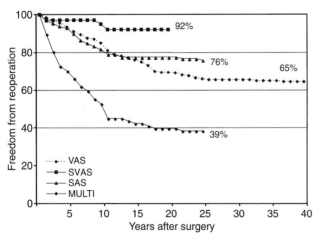

Figure 2

Actuarial freedom from reoperation (Kaplan-Meier) according to level of obstruction. VAS, valvar aortic stenosis; SVAS, supravalvar aortic stenosis; SAS, subvalvar aortic stenosis; MULTI, multilevel aortic stenosis.

Univariate and multivariate analyses identified date of operation (before 1975) as a risk factor for death ($p = .002$).

Late mean postoperative LV-aortic gradient was better for the patients with discrete SAS (26.8 mm Hg) than for patients with diffuse SAS (43.9 mm Hg; $p = .02$). Likewise, the proportion of patients with late postoperative LVOT gradients greater than 50 mm Hg was significantly greater in patients with tunnel obstruction (7 of 13, 54%) than for those with discrete obstruction (16 of 94, 16%, $p = .001$). Mild AI was documented in 20 patients (20 of 132, 15%) before surgery, and 31 patients had AI on late follow-up (31 of 107, 29%; $p = .055$). The AI was mild in 84% (26 of 31), moderate in 13% (4 of 31), and severe in 3% (1 of 31) of patients.

Thirty reoperations were performed in 25 surviving patients (25 of 120, 21%): 10 patients with discrete SAS required reoperations, as did 15 patients with diffuse SAS. The mean time from initial surgery to first reoperation was 7.5 years. Three patients underwent second reoperation (mean, 2.7 years), and two patients underwent third reoperation (mean, 2.5 years). The predominant indication for reoperation was the presence of recurrent SAS with AI (12 of 30, 40%) and isolated recurrent SAS (12 of 30, 40%) or pure AI (1 of 30, 3%). Two patients with cardiomyopathy required heart transplantation. Six patients who required an AAC initially underwent removal of the AAC due to stenosis or thrombosis (n = 4) or pseudoaneurysm at the LV anastomosis (n = 2). Two underwent late insertion of an AAC after an initial attempt to relieve SAS directly. An aortic valve replacement was performed with pulmonary autograft in five patients (one of them with Konno procedure), a mechanical prosthesis in two patients, and an aortic homograft in one patient. A repeat resection of subaortic membrane was performed in 10 patients (7 of them with myotomy and myectomy). Two patients required a valve-sparing Konno procedure.

Overall freedom from reoperation was 90% at 5 years, 79% at 10 years, and 76% at 25 years (see Figure 2). Univariate analysis of risk factors for recurrent SAS includes hypoplasia of aortic annulus less than 5 mm, presence of AAC, and higher preoperative LVOT gradient. Independent risk factors for reoperation by multivariate analysis were AAC insertion and late follow-up gradient greater than 40 mm Hg in patients specifically with tunnel SAS. Of the 120 patients with SAS in this study followed postoperatively, 100 patients had the discrete type of SAS and 20 patients had the diffuse type of SAS. There was no significant difference between the groups in preoperative functional class. However, postoperatively the patients with the discrete form of SAS were in better functional class (88 in class I and 12 in class II) than the patients with the tunnel type of SAS (12 in class I, 6 in class II, and 2 in class III; $p = .01$).

Multilevel Left Ventricular Outflow Tract Obstruction

The 94 patients with multilevel LVOT obstruction underwent 212 initial and redo procedures. Eight patients were neonates with critical AS as part of their LVOT obstruction. One early death (1.1%) occurred in a 1-month-old infant who underwent a Ross-Konno procedure with an extensive aortic arch patch and atrial and ventricular septal defect closure secondary to intracranial bleeding while weaning extracorporeal membrane oxygenation support 5 days repair. There were five late deaths. Overall survival was 95% at 5, 10, 15, and 20 years (see Figure 1). AI was documented in 6 of 94 patients (6%) before surgery, and 40 of 75 patients (53%) had documented AI on late follow-up. It was mild in 27 (67%), moderate in 9 (23%), and severe in 4 (10%) patients.

Reoperations were performed in 34 patients (37%). The mean time from initial surgery to first reoperation was 5.1 years. Nine patients underwent second reoperation (mean, 4.8 years), and four patients underwent a third reoperation (mean, 5.0 years). All patients with neonatal critical AS (n = 7) as part of their multilevel AS underwent reoperation 3.6 years after the initial procedure. The predominant indication for reoperation was presence of recurrent SAS with AI (32%), recurrent SAS (45%), or pure AI (6%). One patient with cardiomyopathy required heart transplantation. Six patients underwent insertion of an AAC and six additional patients with AAC underwent removal or revision of their AAC for the following reasons: two were revised for AAC valve regurgitation and four were removed or ligated for AAC thrombosis. In 17 patients, an AVR was performed by the following techniques: 13 Ross AVRs, 3 Ross-Konno AVRs, and 1 aortic homograft AVR. A repeat resection of a subaortic membrane was performed in six patients (one of them with myotomy and myectomy). Four patients underwent repeat open valvotomy, two patients underwent aortic valvuloplasty due to severe AI, one patient had resection of an LV pseudoaneurysm, and one patient underwent resection of an ascending aortic pseudoaneurysm. Three patients required a valve-sparing Konno procedure. Overall freedom from reoperation was 66% at 5 years, 53% at 10 years, 40% at 20 years, and 39% at 25 years (see Figure 2). Risk factors for reoperation in patients with multilevel LVOT obstruction were diagnosis of neonatal critical AS in infants less than 6 months of age ($p = .002$), history of valvotomy for neonatal critical AS ($p = .0015$), and AAC insertion ($p = .005$). All survivors (n = 92) are in NYHA functional class I or II and are leading normal or near-normal lives.

■ COMMENT

These results substantiate the general safety and efficacy of surgical therapy for congenital aortic stenosis. In most instances, the operation can be performed with a low mortality rate (8% in our entire series, 2% excluding neonates and infants less than 6 months of age) and a high probability of successful outcome. The palliative nature of operative intervention for VAS should be reemphasized. Over time, an increasing proportion of patients with VAS and multilevel AS present for reoperation. At 20 years after their initial operation, 27% of the surviving patients in our entire series had undergone a subsequent operative procedure (VAS, 59 of 242, 24%; multilevel AS, 34 of 94, 36%) (Table 1).

Two high-risk subgroups for recurrence and reoperation have been clearly identified. The group with the highest early mortality rate is the neonate and infant group less than 6 months of age. Neonatal repair is often more difficult and less precise than in older patients because the valves are

Table 1 Preoperative, Intraoperative, and Follow-up Aortic Valve Gradients

LEVEL	AORTIC VALVE GRADIENT (mm Hg)		
	Preoperative	Intraoperative	Follow-up
Valvar	78.8 ± 27.9	15.8 ± 11.9	29.7 ± 26.5
<6 mo	68.7 ± 27.6	22.8 ± 10.9	33.5 ± 27.8
>6 mo	82.4 ± 27.3	12.6 ± 10.9	30.7 ± 27.8
Supravalvar	86.5 ± 43.1	24.1 ± 13.1	19.4 ± 18.4
Subvalvar	74.7 ± 30.5	12.7 ± 9.1	29.9 ± 25.7
Discrete	72.6 ± 31.3	10.7 ± 7.9	26.8 ± 24.2
Tunnel	83.2 ± 23.3	17.1 ± 10.2	43.9 ± 28.8
Multiple	85.2 ± 30.9	20.7 ± 10.0	35.3 ± 37.2
Total	79.4 ± 30.8	16.3 ± 11.2	29.0 ± 25.9

frequently very dysplastic. Furthermore, the higher likelihood of associated cardiac anomalies, especially borderline LV hypoplasia and endocardial fibroelastosis, in this subgroup affects both early and late results. This group represents one of the most challenging facets of congenital AS, and a wide variety of surgical approaches have been advocated. We have found that transventricular closed aortic valvotomy without bypass has worked as well or better in our neonates with critical AS as any other surgical or balloon valvotomy method. Long-term survival and reoperative rates compare favorably with other forms of treatment for neonatal critical AS. These procedures are considered palliative and reintervention is usually required within 10 years. Neonates with evidence of severe aortic annulus hypoplasia, low ejection fraction, endocardial fibroelastosis, and small left ventricles are not good candidates for surgical valvotomy and should be considered for a univentricular repair (i.e., Norwood). Further long-term follow-up or perhaps a randomized trial is needed to determine accurately which therapy (transventricular valvotomy, open valvotomy, balloon aortic valvuloplasty, or even neonatal Ross-Konno procedure) will have the best long-term outcome for critical AS in the neonate and infants less than 6 months of age.

The other patient group at considerably higher risk for reoperation is the group with multilevel LVOT obstruction. The choice of the first or second surgical procedure is determined by the location and anatomy of the LVOT obstruction and by patient age and size. The Ross AVR, the Ross-Konno procedure, and the valve-sparing Konno procedure are techniques that appear to have the long-term ability to relieve LVOT pathology.

VAS can often be surgically palliated in children until they reach adolescence or adulthood. Valvotomy has several advantages over early valve replacement. It relieves most of the obstruction, preserves the native valve with low risk of thromboembolism and no need for anticoagulation, and offers 10 to 20 years with low reoperative risk. During this time, the aortic annulus grows sufficiently in most cases to accommodate a prosthesis of adequate size. When valve replacement is required, it is performed with low mortality and acceptable morbidity. A major problem encountered in

non-Ross AVRs in children has been the progressive restriction of prosthesis related to patient growth. The Ross AVR is the only AVR that has growth potential and is the only AVR where LV mass has returned to a normal range.

Some centers advocate the Ross procedure as the first procedure for LVOT obstruction. The LVOT gradient is completely relieved and there is regression of excess LV mass, which may improve the long-term prognosis and obviate the need for subsequent LVOT surgery. The immediate surgical risk is still high for the Ross procedure in infants, however. Risk factors for late mortality in Ross AVR are young age at operation and number of prior aortic operations. It has been suggested that selection of the first aortic valve procedure should be based on valvar anatomy, arguing in favor of valvuloplasty if the valve is trileaflet, but opting for insertion of the Ross pulmonary autograft in the presence of dysplastic bicuspid valves and after a failed surgical or balloon valvulotomy.

In conclusion, children with single-level obstruction have a low operative mortality and good hemodynamic benefit from standard surgical techniques. Neonates with critical AS have significantly higher mortality, reflecting severe symptomatic congestive heart failure and associated cardiac anomalies (hypoplastic left ventricle, endocardial fibroelastosis). Children with multilevel LVOT obstruction have higher reoperation rates. AVR with Ross pulmonary autograft has been performed with low mortality and morbidity but should be reserved for failed conservative attempts for relief of LVOT obstruction.

SUGGESTED READING

Brown JW, et al: Surgery for aortic stenosis in children: a forty-year experience, *Ann Thorac Surg* 76:1398, 2003.

Brown JW, et al: Surgical spectrum of aortic stenosis in children: a thirty-year experience with 257 children, *Ann Thorac Surg* 45:393, 1988.

Brown JW, et al: Surgical repair of congenital supravalvular aortic stenosis in children, *Eur J Cardiothorac Surg* 21:50, 2002.

Brown JW, et al: Clinical outcomes and indicators of normalization of left ventricular dimensions after Ross procedure in children, *Semin Thorac Cardiovasc Surg* 13(Suppl 1):28, 2001.

Brown JW, et al: Apicoaortic valved conduits for complex left ventricular outflow obstruction: technical considerations and current status, *Ann Thorac Surg* 38:162, 1984.

Chartrand CC, et al: Long-term results of surgical valvuloplasty for congenital valvar aortic stenosis in children, *Ann Thorac Surg* 68:1356, 1999.

Detter C, et al: Aortic valvotomy for congenital valvular aortic stenosis: a 37-year experience, *Ann Thorac Surg* 71:1564, 2001.

Gatzoulis MA, et al: Contemporary results of balloon valvuloplasty and surgical valvotomy for congenital aortic stenosis, *Arch Dis Child* 73:66, 1995.

Hawkins JA, et al: Late results and reintervention after aortic valvotomy for critical aortic stenosis in neonates and infants, *Ann Thorac Surg* 65:1758, 1998.

Karl TR, et al: Critical aortic stenosis in the first month of life: surgical results in 26 infants, *Ann Thorac Surg* 50:105, 1990.

Stamm C, et al: Forty-one years of surgical experience with congenital supravalvular aortic stenosis, *J Thorac Cardiovasc Surg* 118:874, 1999.

PERCUTANEOUS CATHETER INTERVENTIONS IN CONGENITAL HEART DISEASE

Jonathan J. Rome

Catheter interventions have become part of the standard treatment of most congenital cardiovascular defects. In some instances, these techniques have replaced surgery as the primary mode of therapy. In others, a combination of surgical and catheter interventions is used. Space prohibits an exhaustive discussion of all available catheter procedures. The purpose of this chapter is to give the surgeon some familiarity with current catheter treatments and the most common lesions to which they may be applied. Most catheter treatments are divided into procedures for relief of obstruction (dilation and stents) and vascular closure procedures (device closures and embolizations).

■ DILATIONS AND SEPTOSTOMY PROCEDURES

Catheter therapy for congenital defects began with balloon atrial septostomy by Rashkind in 1966. Inflation balloon angioplasty was developed in 1974 by Gruntzig for treatment of atherosclerotic peripheral arterial stenosis. Advances in equipment and technique have allowed application of balloon dilation to a variety of valvar and vascular stenoses in patients of all ages.

Atrial Septostomy Creation
Balloon atrial septostomy remains standard palliation for infants with transposition and inadequate atrial mixing. Catheter access is obtained via either the femoral or the umbilical veins. After the septostomy catheter is advanced through the patent foramen ovale to the left atrium, the balloon is inflated, and the catheter is pulled back rapidly to the right atrium, tearing the septum primum. Adequacy of the communication created can be assessed by measurement of saturations, pressures, and echocardiography. The procedure may be performed without fluoroscopy under transesophageal echocardiography guidance in the intensive care unit. Balloon septostomy is highly effective in most infants younger than 6 weeks of age. After this age, the atrial septum is too thick for this approach. In addition, infants with hypoplastic left heart syndrome and intact or virtually intact atrial septum have a thick septum not amenable to balloon septostomy. Other approaches (discussed later) are used in these cases.

Older patients may require creation of an atrial communication for a variety of indications. Examples include relief of left atrial outlet obstruction in patients with complete mixing lesions, left atrial decompression in patients c.. extracorporeal membrane oxygenator support for left heart failure, or augmentation of systemic output in the setting of right ventricular dysfunction (e.g., tetralogy repair). In these instances, the atrial septum is crossed with a transseptal needle, and the septum sequentially is dilated with static angioplasty balloons until a hole of the desired size is created. This method has the advantage of permitting control over the size of the intraatrial communication and minimizes risk of atrial perforation. It also is effective in thicker atrial septa. A similar strategy may be used for fenestration creation in patients after the Fontan procedure.

Valvuloplasty
Pulmonic Stenosis
Balloon valvuloplasty is the preferred treatment for pulmonary valve stenosis. After hemodynamic evaluation, a right ventricular angiogram is performed to assess anatomy and measure the pulmonary annulus dimension. An angioplasty balloon catheter is advanced over a guidewire that has been positioned in the distal pulmonary artery tree through the stenotic valve. For dilation of the pulmonary valve, an oversized balloon (120% to 140% that of the annulus diameter) is chosen. As the balloon is inflated, the stenotic valve creates a waist, which then disappears. Most cases result in excellent relief of obstruction—restenosis is uncommon. Patients with severe right ventricular hypertrophy may develop acute dynamic infundibular obstruction after dilation. This condition generally can be treated effectively with β-blockers. Although balloon valvuloplasty is less effective in cases of dysplastic pulmonary valves (commonly seen in patients with Noonan's syndrome), dilation still should be attempted as first-line treatment. Dilation is rarely effective in patients with infundibular stenosis, supravalvar pulmonic stenosis, or hypoplasia of the pulmonary valve annulus. These cases all require surgical intervention to enlarge the right ventricular outflow tract.

In newborns with critical pulmonic stenosis, moderate cyanosis is common after dilation from right-to-left shunting at the atrial level. Cyanosis diminishes as right ventricular compliance improves. Severe cyanosis after valvuloplasty should prompt further evaluation. In cases in which inadequate relief of right ventricular outflow obstruction is present after technically adequate balloon valve dilation, right ventricular outflow patch augmentation is required, usually in combination with a systemic-to-pulmonary artery shunt. Newborns with valvar pulmonary atresia can be treated by balloon dilation after perforation of the valve by radiofrequency or lasers. When the right ventricle is well developed, this approach yields similar results to dilation of critical pulmonic stenosis.

Aortic Stenosis
All current treatment of aortic stenosis, whether surgical (valvuloplasty, valve replacement, autograft) or transcatheter, must be considered palliative. Balloon dilation in infancy through young adulthood usually is effective for adequate gradient relief and creates only minimal aortic regurgitation in most instances. Reported failure rates vary from 0 to 10%, whereas significant increases in aortic regurgitation can occur in approximately 10% of patients.

The durability of the results varies from patient to patient, although reintervention is delayed for 5 years or more in most cases. These results are comparable to surgical valvuloplasty; balloon dilation is recommended as the first treatment for patients with aortic stenosis and little regurgitation. The procedure usually is performed via a retrograde approach from the femoral artery. After hemodynamic evaluation, including pressure pullback across the aortic valve, angiography is performed in the aortic root and left ventricle for valve anatomy, the degree of insufficiency, and annulus measurement. Valvuloplasty balloons are chosen to be equal or slightly less than annulus diameter. Aortic insufficiency is much more likely when the balloon-to-annulus ratio exceeds 110%.

Newborns with critical aortic stenosis are at high risk; outcome primarily depends on left ventricular function and anatomy. Balloon aortic valvuloplasty is probably the treatment of choice when left ventricular size (including mitral valve, ventricular volume, and aortic valve sizes) and function are deemed adequate to support systemic circulation. After successful valvuloplasty, ventricular function generally improves, allowing discontinuation of ventilatory and intravenous inotropic support within a few days. If clinical improvement fails to occur, it must be presumed that left heart size or function or both are inadequate. Repeat diagnostic catheterization should be performed, and efforts should be made to determine the cause of persistent symptoms. Adequate relief of valvar stenosis with inadequate left heart size typically manifests as diastolic dysfunction. In such instances, the Norwood procedure is the only approach likely to lead to long-term survival. If the left heart is of adequate size, repeat balloon dilation may be warranted. When significant aortic insufficiency or combined insufficiency and stenosis are present, aortic root replacement with a pulmonary autograft (Ross procedure) may be the best strategy.

Other Valves

Dilation has been used for congenital mitral and tricuspid and bioprosthetic valve stenosis. Although results have been disappointing, balloon valvuloplasty may be an appropriate first-line treatment in certain anatomic subtypes of congenital mitral stenosis ("typical" congenital mitral stenosis or multiple orifice mitral valve) because these lesions often respond poorly to surgical valvuloplasty. Dilation of bioprosthetic valves may be useful. Although restenosis is likely to occur, the procedure may increase significantly the longevity of the prosthesis. Subaortic stenosis is a surgical lesion.

Angioplasty and Stents

Techniques for balloon angioplasty of congenital or postoperative stenoses were adapted from approaches for atherosclerotic disease. Relief of obstruction generally is due to myointimal disruption at the site of stenosis. Vascular integrity after successful angioplasty may depend on intact adventitia and perivascular tissue; dilation should not be performed within 6 weeks to 2 months of surgical dissection. Endovascular stenting has proved useful for a wide range of stenotic vessels. Because overdilation is not necessary with stenting, the procedure is probably safer than dilation in treating vascular obstructions occurring early on after surgery.

Arch Obstructions

Balloon angioplasty commonly is used for native and recurrent coarctation occurring after surgery. Dilation is successful in 80% to 90% of cases. Restenosis is frequent after dilation of native coarctation in young infants, prompting most practitioners to advocate surgical treatment in this group. Aneurysm formation has been reported after dilation of coarctation; the true incidence is unclear but probably between 2% and 5%. In current practice, balloon angioplasty is the treatment of choice for postoperative arch obstructions and an acceptable alternative to surgery for native coarctation beyond early infancy.

Endovascular stenting has emerged as an effective therapy for native or postoperative coarctation in adolescents and adults, although follow-up is limited. Results of dilation for restenosis after interrupted aortic arch and hypoplastic left heart surgery are comparable to simple recoarctation, although risks tend to be higher, particularly in patients with palliated heart defects.

Pulmonary Artery Stenoses

Pulmonary artery stenosis, distortion, and hypoplasia are common in congenital cardiovascular disorders and remain therapeutic challenges. These abnormalities are a direct result of the underlying defect (elastin arteriopathy, Alagille's syndrome, tetralogy of Fallot with diminutive pulmonary arteries), are a result of surgical intervention (tetralogy of Fallot, truncus arteriosus, prior shunts), or both. Balloon angioplasty and stenting may be effective in treating these lesions. Distal stenoses usually are treated with angioplasty, whereas stents are effective in more proximal branch pulmonary artery stenoses. In patients with complex or multiple pulmonary artery narrowings, angioplasty procedures may be lengthy. Approximately 80% of dilations result in significant immediate improvement in vessel size; however, restenosis occurs with some frequency. Potential complications include vessel perforation, aneurysm formation, or dissection. Stents are deployed on angioplasty balloons advanced through long sheaths to the site of the stenosis. Limitations of endovascular stenting include the need for repeat dilation to accommodate growth and restenosis from neointima formation, which appears most significant in small-diameter stents.

Although branch pulmonary artery narrowings may occur in isolation, these lesions usually occur in association with other defects. Treatment often requires a combination of catheter and surgical intervention. Because early postoperative dilation and surgery that involves dissection of freshly dilated vessels may be risky, a thoughtful overall therapeutic strategy is essential for these problems. The patient in whom early postoperative hemodynamic compromise occurs from previously unrecognized or inadequately treated pulmonary artery distortion may be treated by interventional catheterization. These situations must be approached case by case comparing risks of surgical versus catheter approaches. Endovascular stenting is the preferred transcatheter treatment in these patients because the risk of vascular disruption is lower than with angioplasty.

Other Vascular Obstructions

Less common vascular obstructions are amenable to transcatheter treatment. Stents have been effective in patients with systemic venous pathway obstruction after Mustard or Senning operations, Fontan pathway obstructions, and obstructed conduits or homografts. Active investigation is under way to perfect catheter-delivered valved stents. These devices have been applied to stenotic and regurgitant conduits with encouraging early results.

In contrast to the advances noted previously, pulmonary vein stenosis remains a difficult-to-treat disease. Angioplasty or stents for congenital stenosis rarely result in long-term improvement. Restenosis occurs from neointimal proliferation within the stent or progressive vascular disease in the more peripheral pulmonary veins.

■ CLOSURE PROCEDURES

Transcatheter embolization procedures may be performed for the closure of unwanted vessels or prosthetic vascular connections, whereas occlusion devices are used to close intracardiac defects.

Embolizations

Pediatric cardiologists have adapted embolization techniques developed by interventional radiologists for treatment of superfluous vascular connections in congenital heart defects. These techniques rely on the transcatheter delivery of occlusive material, which results in thrombosis of the unwanted vessel, shunt, or connection. The most commonly used device is the Gianturco coil (Cook Inc., Bloomington, IN). The coil is a stainless steel wire with woven synthetic fibers. When pushed out of a catheter, the coil assumes a complex shape in the target vessel promoting thrombosis. Coils also are made of platinum (nonferromagnetic) and are available in many conformations. Some are detachable, allowing greater control over delivery. Embolizations also may be performed with particulate matter (polyvinyl alcohol). This armamentarium has permitted application of transcatheter embolization to a wide range of lesions.

Patent Ductus Arteriosus

Transcatheter occlusion of patent ductus arteriosus (PDA) first was performed by Porstmann using an Ivalon plug. Subsequently, Rashkind developed an occlusion device appropriate for closure of PDA in children. Although reasonably effective, the Rashkind occluder was never approved for use in the United States. After the successful treatment of PDA using these devices, coil embolization was described as a means of treating small PDA. The method has been enhanced over the years with many modifications in coils and technique. Coil embolization is probably the most common method used for closure of small and moderate-sized PDA (outside the newborn period) in the United States. One or more coils are delivered into the ductus via either a transpulmonary or a transarterial approach. Occlusion of the PDA is the result of thrombosis and tissue ingrowth; this may occur immediately or 18 months after coil placement. In more recent series, reported occlusion rates are approximately 95%. Patients with residual flow after previous embolization may undergo placement of an additional coil. Complications are rare after the procedure. Hemolysis rarely has been reported after incomplete closure, however, as well

as one case of endocarditis. Coil embolization is not well suited to larger PDA. The Amplatzer Duct Occluder (AGA Medical Corp., Golden Valley, MN) has been shown to be effective in moderate and large PDA. This device has completed U.S. trials; and is FDA approved.

Systemic-to-Pulmonary Collaterals

Systemic-to-pulmonary collateral arterial connections are ubiquitous in cyanotic congenital cardiac defects. Major aortopulmonary collaterals are encountered most frequently in tetralogy of Fallot with pulmonary atresia but may be seen in a variety of other lesions. When these collateral arteries are redundant with other sources of pulmonary blood flow, they are eliminated to minimize ventricular volume loading and to decrease the risk of pulmonary vascular obstructive disease. Coil embolization has proved effective in this setting. In patients with chronic cyanosis, particularly patients who have undergone previous chest surgery, multiple small systemic-to-pulmonary collateral vessels commonly are seen. These collaterals are usually a network of transpleural and transmediastinal, connections fed from internal mammary, thyrocervical trunk, and intercostal arteries, among others. Because of redundant connections, coil embolization of the feeding vessels alone may not suffice to eliminate collateral flow. The most effective strategy for dealing with this type of collateral flow is particle embolization: Feeder arteries are cannulated subselectively and 500- to 1000-μ particles are delivered through the catheter to occlude the small distal collateral vessels. The larger feeder arteries are coil occluded. This type of collateral is ubiquitous in patients with single-ventricle heart disease; indications for embolization are controversial. Our practice is to embolize these connections in cases in which evidence suggests they may be detrimental to the patient's hemodynamics.

Venous Connections

Decompressing veins may result in cyanosis after superior or total cavopulmonary connection. The most common among these is a persistent left superior vena cava; however, a large variety of others has been described. One of the indications for preoperative catheterization before cavopulmonary connection is the identification and embolization of decompressing veins. Patients with unexplained cyanosis after these operations undergo catheterization in part to identify and treat decompressing veins.

Other Embolizations

Other less common lesions are amenable to transcatheter embolization. Coronary cameral fistulas present at a variety of ages. Rarely, these lesions may result in heart failure in infancy from volume overload. More commonly, patients present with a continuous murmur. In either case, closure of significant fistulas is indicated. All patients should undergo angiography to delineate fistula anatomy. In most cases, the lesions can be treated safely by embolization using standard or detachable coils.

Hemoptysis is a well-described complication of cyanotic congenital cardiac defects. When blood loss is severe or chronic, angiography should be performed to identify the bleeding source. Often dilated bronchial arteries are identified that feed an extensive network of vessels in a peribronchial or parenchymal blush. The presumed mechanism of bleeding is erosion of the vessels into the bronchial lumen. Particle and coil embolization of these vessels is the most effective treatment for this type of hemoptysis and can be lifesaving.

Device Closures

Devices designed for closure of PDA, atrial septal defects, and ventricular septal defects (VSD) have been developed and tested sinced the 1960s. In more recent years, governmental regulatory agencies, such as the Food and Drug Administration in the United States, have approved a growing number of closure devices with a resultant geometric increase in their use throughout the world. Device designs differ greatly but fall into two groups: devices designed to cover holes and devices designed to stent them (Figure 1). The Helex (A.W. Gore, Flagstaff, AZ), and Cardioseal or Starflex (NMT Medical, Boston, MA) devices close defects by covering each side with overlapping occlusive disks or umbrellas, whereas the Amplatzer family of devices (AGA Medical Golden Valley, MN) is designed to stent defects with a central occlusive "plug." The method for device closure of defects is similar for most devices in most types of defects. Anatomy is defined angiographically and often echocardiographically (either transesophageal or intracardiac), and balloon sizing of the defect is performed. A large delivery catheter or sheath is advanced through the defect. The device is deployed, its position is confirmed, then it is released.

Defects in the Atrial Septum

The largest application of closure devices is for atrial communications. To date, 5000 to 10,000 devices have been placed worldwide. Device closure rapidly is becoming the dominant method for treatment of atrial septal defects in the fossa ovalis. The anatomy of the defect dictates which type of device is optimal; the Amplatzer Occluder is most effective in closing large holes, whereas the other type of device is optimal for multifenestrated defects. Very large defects, particularly in smaller patients, still are treated best surgically. Studies comparing transcatheter and surgical closure show that efficacy is equivalent or slightly higher for surgery, whereas hospital stay and complications are lower for device closure.

An association between patent foramen ovale (PFO) and embolic stroke emerged several years ago. It is presumed that stroke in these cases results from paradoxical embolus through the PFO, and closure has emerged as a treatment strategy. Because the prevalence of PFO is high in the general population, it is impossible to be certain that the PFO is responsible in most instances. Accumulated data on recurrence risk and treatment options in this group of patients do not help in determining optimal treatment. Risk of recurrent events usually is low, although some studies suggest patients with large PFO or patients with PFO and atrial septal aneurysm are a subset at high risk. Data show that device closure of PFO is a procedure with low morbidity, high efficacy (i.e., complete closure of the PFO), and a low rate of recurrent events after the procedure. No study has compared device closure with medical treatment of these patients in a controlled fashion; randomized trials are in the planning stage. Pending results of these trials, device closure should be individualized based on patient-specific risk factors and preferences.

Catheter-delivered closure devices have proved exceptionally versatile in a wide range of venous and intraatrial communications. They have been particularly useful in closing systemic-to-pulmonary venous communications after Fontan procedures. The concept of the intentionally created Fontan baffle fenestration was predicated on subsequent device closure; this strategy has had a dramatic effect on clinical course and outcome after Fontan surgery. Device closure also is useful in patients with residual leaks after Mustard or Senning procedures.

Ventricular Septal Defects

Application of closure devices to VSDs followed close on the heels of their use in the atrial septum. Some devices are applicable to atrial septal defects and VSDs (Starflex and Cardioseal), whereas others have been designed specifically for use in the ventricular septum (Amplatzer muscular and membranous VSD devices). Although fewer data have been accumulated on transcatheter closure of VSDs, results have been encouraging. Device closure has proved to be an effective means of dealing with defects in the apical and anterior muscular septum, which traditionally have been challenging

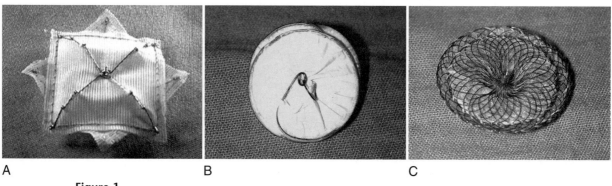

A B C

Figure 1
Closure devices. "Covering" type devices include Starflex (**A**) and Helex (**B**), whereas the Amplatzer (**C**) stents the hole.

surgical problems. Placement of multiple devices has allowed biventricular repair of patients with so-called Swiss cheese septa. Transcatheter device closure of remote muscular defects has been combined with surgical treatment of other lesions in patients with tetralogy, transposition, and other complex disease. Because of impingement on atrioventricular or semilunar valves can occur, the devices are not suited for closure of atrioventricular canal or malalignment defects. Early results with the more recently designed Amplatzer membranous VSD device have been encouraging, however.

■ SUMMARY AND CONCLUSIONS

Transcatheter treatments are now available for many cardiovascular lesions. For simple defects, interventional treatments have replaced surgery in some instances as the primary therapeutic modality. In other cases, catheter-based and surgical therapies are alternative or complementary modalities. Patients with complex lesions may require several operations and interventional catheterizations. In these cases, outcome is optimal when surgeon and cardiologist, both educated in the range of therapeutic options, work together to construct a comprehensive treatment strategy.

SUGGESTED READING

Bridges ND, et al: Baffle fenestration with subsequent transcatheter closure: modification of the Fontan operation for patients at increased risk, *Circulation* 82:1681, 1990.

Bush DM, et al: Frequency of restenosis after balloon pulmonary arterioplasty and its causes, *Am J Cardiol* 86:1205, 2000.

Du ZD, et al: Comparison between transcatheter and surgical closure of secundum atrial septal defect in children and adults: results of a multicenter nonrandomized trial, *J Am Coll Cardiol* 39:1836, 2002.

Magee AG, et al: Transcatheter coil occlusion of the arterial duct: results of the European Registry, *Eur Heart J* 22:1817, 2001.

McCrindle BW: Independent predictors of long-term results after balloon pulmonary valvuloplasty, *Circulation* 89:1751, 1994.

Moore P, et al: Midterm results of balloon dilation of congenital aortic stenosis: predictors of success, *J Am Coll Cardiol* 27:1257, 1996.

Perry SB, et al: Transcatheter closure of coronary artery fistulas, *J Am Coll Cardiol* 20:205, 1992.

Rothman A: Interventional therapy for coarctation of the aorta, *Curr Opin Cardiol* 13:66, 1998.

CARDIAC PACING IN CHILDREN

Jane E. Crosson
Richard E. Ringel

Although children account for only 1% to 2% of pacemaker patients, they often present more complex problems than their adult counterparts. Cardiologists and surgeons caring for these children must take into account the need for a lifetime of pacing, growth parameters, and often complex venous and intracardiac anatomy. New pacemaker technologies have mitigated but not eliminated these problems. Generators now are small enough to implant comfortably even in premature infants and have self-adjusting outputs to conserve battery drain. Steroid-eluting leads can reduce pacing thresholds. Despite these advances, we still must implant hardware that needs to be replaced multiple times during the child's life, necessitating careful selection of the pacing system and implantation technique.

■ INDICATIONS FOR PACING

Most pediatric patients requiring pacing for bradycardia have advanced atrioventricular (AV) block. Slightly less than half of these are due to isolated congenital AV block, and the remainder are due to congenital heart disease, in which heart block can occur de novo or secondary to surgical damage of the conduction system. Sinus bradycardia is seen most often after surgical correction of congenital heart disease but occasionally occurs as a primary arrhythmia and is a less common pacing indication. Rare indications for pacing include the long QT syndrome and pause-dependent ventricular tachycardia.

Indications for pediatric pacing were revised by the American Heart Association in 2002. In cases of congenital AV block, a pacemaker is indicated for any patient with congestive heart failure or low cardiac output, syncope, presyncope or exercise intolerance, heart rates less than 55 beats/min in an infant, a wide QRS escape rhythm, or coexisting structural congenital heart disease. Natural history studies suggest that permanent pacing should be considered strongly before adulthood in all patients with congenital AV block, owing to the risk of sudden death even in asymptomatic patients, but a consensus on these patients has not been reached. All patients with surgically induced AV block (advanced second-degree or third-degree block) persisting more than 7 to 10 days postoperatively should receive a permanent pacing system before hospital discharge. Patients with sinus bradycardia generally require pacing only for symptoms correlating with severe bradycardia. Sinus pauses greater than 3 seconds and sustained extreme bradycardia (<30 beats/min) are other indications for pacing in asymptomatic patients.

Indications for antitachycardia pacing systems are not well established in children. Automatic implantable defibrillators are used in cases of resuscitated sudden death and in patients with strong risk factors, such as severe heart disease or family history of malignant arrhythmia. Antitachycardia pacing for the atrium had fallen out of favor due to the risk of inducing more malignant arrhythmias, but newer dual-chamber devices may correct this problem. Detailed discussion of antitachycardia pacing is beyond the scope of this chapter.

■ CHOOSING THE PACING SYSTEM AND SURGICAL APPROACH

Of the two implantation techniques, transvenous (endocardial) systems generally are preferred over epicardial systems because they are less traumatic to implant and have fewer pacing problems. Historically, transvenous leads have better durability and lower chronic thresholds. Transvenous systems are contraindicated, however, in patients with a right-to-left shunt and in small children. Implanting physicians must understand that the functional life span of a pacemaker lead is no more than 10 to 20 years. When leads are replaced, the old leads can be left in the veins or can be extracted. Because both options carry risks, the epicardial approach usually is preferred in the very young patient.

If a transvenous approach is contemplated, patient size is an important consideration, correlating well with the risk of venous obstruction. Venous occlusion occurs commonly even in adults with transvenous leads and can wreak havoc with future pacing options. In the small child, preoperative evaluation of vessel size with ultrasound or venography may help establish suitability of a transvenous implant. The total cross-sectional area of pacemaker leads related to body surface area also is a strong predictor of venous occlusion and can determine whether one or two leads can be implanted safely. Most patients weighing more than 20 kg can receive a transvenous system safely. For patients weighing 10 to 20 kg, the transvenous approach is possible if epicardial pacing thresholds have been poor. When feasible, small, unipolar leads and single-lead systems should be chosen for these children.

In patients with congenital heart disease, the transvenous options are limited. A patient with "single-ventricle" physiology cannot receive an endocardial ventricular lead due to risk of systemic arterial embolus. Patients with an extracardiac Fontan procedure cannot have an endocardial atrial lead because no atrial myocardium is accessible within the venous circuit. Scarring in the atrium may limit good pacing sites as well. Careful preoperative evaluation of venous anatomy and size is essential.

Single-chamber versus dual-chamber pacing should be the next consideration. Dual-chamber pacing systems have become popular as generators and leads have decreased in size. Although more closely mimicking normal AV conduction, dual-chamber pacing is not clearly superior to single-chamber pacing in young children with good cardiac function. The need to preserve venous access for later in life may prevail. Patients with isolated congenital AV block usually do well with rate-responsive ventricular pacing for many years. In patients with sinus bradycardia, atrial pacing is sufficient if good lead parameters are obtained. Single-pass AV leads allow atrial sensing and ventricular pacing from a single lead. Some implanting physicians have had great success with these leads, whereas others have had difficulty finding good sites. The distance between the atrial and ventricular components precludes its use in smaller patients.

■ TRANSVENOUS IMPLANTATION

When the decision in favor of endocardial pacing is made, the next decision is whether the central veins can accommodate safely one or two endocardial leads and whether thinner, low-profile leads should be used. Figa et al developed a method based on body surface area for estimating subclavian vein capacity in children. It predicts the maximum cross-sectional area of pacing leads appropriate for placement in a subclavian vein. This formula is used to determine the feasibility of dual-chamber pacing and the need for smaller leads. We use active fixation, steroid-eluting screw-in leads with silicone (versus polyurethane) insulation.

Implantation is performed under general anesthesia. If the child has associated congenital heart abnormalities, hemodynamic cardiac catheterization may be performed as well. An angiographic, multipurpose catheter is advanced into the subclavian vein. For patients with normal cardiac situs, the left subclavian vein is preferred, but if the patient is left-handed and active in physical activities, right-sided implantation is appropriate. With the tip of the angiographic catheter in the proximal axillary vein, 5 to 10 ml of contrast material is injected by hand, and an anteroposterior cineangiogram is performed to delineate the anatomy of the venous return and to confirm adequate size of the veins for placement of the pacing leads.

Leaving the angiographic catheter as a landmark, a clamp may be placed on the skin to mark the proposed puncture site at the axillary vein as it enters the thorax, usually at the lateral margin of the second rib. A transverse skin incision is made medial to the puncture site in a region that allows the pulse generator to sit comfortably over the anterior surface of the pectoral muscle without extending into the axilla. The incision is placed one to two fingerbreadths below the clavicle so that the head of the pulse generator does not ride up into the clavicle. A subcutaneous pocket large enough to accommodate the pulse generator is created by blunt dissection. The pacemaker rarely is placed below the pectoral muscle because there generally is adequate space and tissue thickness to accommodate current pulse generators in the subcutaneous tissue.

After the pocket has been created, the catheter in the axillary vein is used to guide vessel puncture. The needle is advanced through the lateral-most margin of the pocket toward the catheter under fluoroscopic guidance. When the vessel is entered, a J-tipped 0.018-inch flexible guidewire is advanced through the axillary vein and into the subclavian vein. Over the guidewire, a 4 Fr micropuncture coaxial catheter set (Cook, Inc., Bloomington, IN) is inserted. Dilators are used to enlarge the tract and prepare it for insertion of the sheath. A peel-away SafeSheath (Pressure Products, Inc., Rancheros Palos Altos, CA) of 6 Fr to 10.5 Fr in diameter is selected based on the lead choices. For most children, lead insertion into the right ventricle is straightforward, although shaping of the lead stylet usually is required. After threshold measurements confirm appropriate lead placement, the helix is screwed into place, and threshold measurements are repeated. This process is repeated until optimal pacing and sensing thresholds are recorded. A retaining wire is inserted through the sheath alongside the ventricular lead if an atrial lead is to be inserted. Positioning of an atrial lead can be more challenging, as described subsequently.

When the sheath has been peeled away and removed, the leads are advanced to give adequate redundancy within the heart to allow for downward displacement of the heart with standing and future growth. An additional half to two thirds loop of ventricular lead is left in the atrium. For the atrial lead, extra length is inserted to create a generous loop, while avoiding the tricuspid valve. After hemostasis is obtained, and the pocket is dry, it is irrigated with antibiotic solution. The leads are attached to the pacemaker, and the pocket is closed in standard fashion.

Special Considerations

When inserting pacing leads into patients who have had prior repair of congenital heart disease, venography is crucial before lead insertion to rule out venous stenoses or occlusion. Although less commonly used today, right atrial appendage cannulation for cardiopulmonary bypass and postbypass ligation was performed routinely years ago. This procedure limits usefulness of the appendage for atrial lead fixation. Mustard or Senning palliation for complete transposition of the great arteries presents additional obstacles. These patients often require pacemaker insertion for sinus node dysfunction. A concern specific to these "atrial switch" patients is possible narrowing in the upper limb of the venous pathway that "tunnels" systemic venous return from the superior vena cava to the mitral valve. This pathway can become critically narrowed by pacing leads. Pressure measurements in the atrium and superior vena cava and venography are essential before implantation.

Also of concern in any patient after extensive atrial surgery is fibrosis and prosthetic material within the atrium; these can make P wave sensing and atrial pacing difficult and sometimes impossible. In atrial switch patients, the systemic venous pathway channels blood flow through the left atrium. If the atrial pacing lead is positioned within the left atrial appendage, pacing of the diaphragm may result due to proximity of the left phrenic nerve. It is important in these patients to assess the effect of high-output pacing on diaphragm contraction before securing the atrial lead. In some patients, it may not be possible to find an appropriate site within the left atrium that would sense and pace adequately, but not stimulate the diaphragm. In this circumstance, rate-responsive ventricular pacing may be required. If sensing and pacing thresholds are suboptimal,

placement of a (left) ventricular lead may be desirable as a backup should atrial undersensing or exit block develop over time.

■ EPICARDIAL IMPLANTATION

When epicardial pacing is necessary because of patient size or anatomy, the approach to the heart is usually subxyphoid, and the generator is placed in the abdominal wall. A left thoracotomy is used by some surgeons, but this technique is not discussed here. Epicardial leads also may be implanted via sternotomy at the time of corrective surgery. Whenever possible, steroid-eluting leads should be used, as should some form of automatic threshold control. The Medtronic Inc. (Minneapolis, MN) CapSure Epi lead is the only currently available epicardial steroid-eluting lead, but if thick scar tissue is present from previous surgery, these leads may not provide adequate thresholds. Screw-on leads that penetrate deeply into the myocardial wall may be preferable. For programmability of automatic thresholds, the best system at present is AutoCapture available in the late-model St. Jude Medical Inc. (Sylmar, CA) generators.

Subxyphoid Approach

After induction of general anesthesia, a short vertical incision is made in the midline inferior to the sternum. The anterior fascia of the left rectus muscle is divided, and the rectus muscle is split or retracted to reach the posterior fascia. Division of the fascia at the xyphoid exposes the pericardium. A lead may be placed on the right ventricular surface, taking care to avoid the right coronary artery and its branches. Fixation of the CapSure Epi requires suturing of the sleeve, whereas screw-on leads require two or three turns. Exposure of the lateral wall of the right atrium is possible if dual-chamber pacing is desired. A fishhook or suture-on lead is used here due to the thin atrial wall. Thresholds for sensing and pacing are evaluated, and if necessary the lead is relocated. A pocket is created posterior to the rectus muscle but anterior to the posterior rectus sheath; in older children, it can be made subcutaneously. The lead wires are connected to the generator and gently coiled into the pocket, avoiding torque on the lead at its attachment. Standard closure techniques are employed for the rectus sheath, subcutaneous tissue, and skin. Antibiotics are administered intravenously perioperatively and for 1 postoperative day, then continued orally for 2 days for the epicardial and the endocardial approach.

■ RESULTS

Older studies of long-term functioning of pacing leads and generators in children have shown a higher rate of failure of epicardial systems, most owing to high pacing thresholds (exit block). More recent studies suggest, however, that epicardial systems using steroid-eluting leads and automatic capture algorithms may perform as well as transvenous systems. Other lead-related complications often result from insulation breaks, including failure of sensing or capture, loss of current causing rapid battery drain, and possible exposed wire that can perforate a chamber or venous structure. Modern steroid-eluting lead failure rates are approximately 10% over 2 years for either approach and are higher than in adult patients. Infection of the pocket or lead, chamber or vessel perforation, venous occlusion, and strangulation of the heart by an epicardial lead also have been reported.

Advances in threshold management have extended generator longevity, but this effect has been offset substantially by the use of smaller generators and batteries. Although smaller systems provide obvious benefits for pediatric patients, battery depletion occurs more rapidly in this population. In smaller patients with faster heart rates, a generator can be expected to require replacement every 5 years or sooner; in contrast, a generator may last 10 years in older patients with good pacing thresholds. Other factors influencing generator longevity include lead impedance and percent of time pacing in each chamber. Nominal longevity quoted by the manufacturer refers to adult applications and cannot be used to predict results in children.

SUGGESTED READING

Dodge-Khatami A, et al: A comparison of steroid-eluting epicardial versus transvenous pacing leads in children, *J Card Surg* 15:323, 2000.

Figa FH, et al: Risk factors for venous obstruction in children with transvenous pacing leads, *Pacing Clin Electrophysiol* 20:1902, 1997.

Gregoratos G, et al: ACC/AHA/NASPE 2002 guideline update for implantation of cardiac pacemakers and antiarrhythmia devices: summary article: a report of the American College of Cardiology/American Heart Association Task Force on Practice Guidelines, *Circulation* 106:2145, 2002.

Sachweh JS, et al: Twenty years experience with pediatric pacing: epicardial and transvenous stimulation, *Eur J Cardiothorac Surg* 17:455, 2000.

CARDIOPULMONARY BYPASS AND HYPOTHERMIC CIRCULATORY ARREST

Irving Shen
Ross M. Ungerleider

■ CARDIOPULMONARY BYPASS

Cardiopulmonary bypass (CPB) is the extracorporeal apparatus that temporarily takes over the function of the heart and the lungs. CPB allows temporary cessation of the patient's native circulation through the heart and lungs and permits operations to be performed on these organs. Over the 5 decades of its existence, CPB has undergone dramatic improvements that make the application of CPB safer and yield more consistent results.

In the most simplified form, the basic components of the CPB circuit consist of at least one venous cannula that drains venous blood from the patient to a reservoir. The deoxygenated blood is pumped through an oxygenator/heat exchanger unit, an arterial filter, and an arterial cannula back into the arterial system of the patient. This chapter briefly discusses the components of the CPB circuit and the various strategies available to apply this technology to cardiac surgery.

Circuit Components
Venous Cannula

The size of the venous cannula must be large enough to adequately drain the systemic venous return to the venous reservoir of the oxygenator. This usually is done by gravity, although more recent modifications include applying a low-level vacuum to assist the venous drainage. Vacuum-assisted venous drainage allows the use of a smaller venous cannula, which can be advantageous in minimally invasive small incision surgery. One of the potential risks of using vacuum-assisted venous drainage is that it can increase the amount of trauma to the blood resulting in hemolysis.

For most operations on the aortic valve, left ventricular outflow tract, and ascending aorta as well as coronary artery bypass graft surgery, CPB can be established using a single-stage venous cannula placed in the right atrium. Alternatively a dual-stage venous cannula placed through the right atrium and extending into the inferior vena cava allows better venous drainage. In operations in which at least one of the cardiac chambers needs to be opened, separate venous cannulae placed into the superior vena cava (SVC) and inferior vena cava are necessary. If a left SVC also is present without a connecting left innominate vein, another venous cannula draining the left SVC may be needed. Direct cannulation of the SVC, especially in infants and young children, must be done carefully to minimize the risk of causing SVC injury. Occasionally, venous drainage is achieved through peripheral cannulation by using one or more of the large peripheral veins.

The size of venous cannula used depends on the number of venous cannulae, the size of the patient, and the anticipated CPB flow rate. A list of suggested venous cannula sizes based on patient weight is provided in Table 1.

Table 1 Cardiopulmonary Bypass Cannula Selection Guide

PATIENT WEIGHT (kg)	ARTERIAL (Fr)	VENOUS (Fr)	SVC (Fr)	IVC (Fr)
1-4	6-8	16-20	12	12-14
5-9	10	20-22	12	14-16
10-15	12	22-24	16	18-20
16-24	14	24-28	16	20
25-39	16	26-32 or 22/30; 32/40 (two stage)	16-18	20-24
40-80	20	34/46 (two stage)	22-24	28
>80	24	36/51 (two stage)	24	28

SVC, superior vena cava; IVC, inferior vena cava.

Pump

Two kinds of pumps are commonly available for CPB. The roller pump consists of two roller heads set at 180 degrees apart, which rotate inside a metal raceway. Tubing is placed between the roller heads and the raceway where the rollers partially occlude the tubing. Blood inside the tubing is propelled forward in the same direction as the rotation of the rollers. Pump output is proportional to the speed of rotation of the rollers, the degree of tubing compression by the rollers, and the diameter of the tubing. Alternatively a centrifugal pump has a rapidly rotating impeller within the blood compartment that propels blood forward. Flow is a function of outflow pressure, however, and can be determined only by a precalibrated flowmeter.

Oxygenator

The oxygenator is where carbon dioxide (CO_2) in the blood is exchanged for oxygen. Essentially all modern-day oxygenators are made from silicone or polypropylene, which separates the blood compartment from the gas compartment. Oxygen and CO_2 diffuse into and out of blood along concentration gradient. The oxygen content of the gas compartment is regulated by a blender that mixes oxygen with air to the desired partial pressure of oxygen. Inhalational anesthetic agents also can be delivered to the patient by placing a vaporizer in-line with the ventilating gas to the oxygenator.

Heat Exchanger

The heat exchanger and oxygenator usually are built together as an integral unit. The inclusion of a heat exchanger enables CPB to be an efficient method of cooling and warming the patient's core temperature. Cooling and rewarming the patient too rapidly must be avoided, however, to prevent formation of microbubbles in the circulation. Warming the blood to greater than 40°C to facilitate faster rewarming must be avoided to prevent destruction of enzymes and denaturing proteins in the blood.

Arterial Filters and Arterial Cannulae

Oxygenated blood is passed through an in-line arterial filter for trapping particulate and gaseous emboli before being pumped back into the arterial circulation of the patient. The oxygenated, temperature-regulated, and filtered blood is returned to the patient's arterial circulation via an arterial cannula, which usually is placed in the distal ascending aorta but can be placed in other major peripheral arteries in the body. The optimal size of the arterial cannula depends on the size of the patient and the anticipated CPB flow rate. A list of suggested arterial cannula sizes based on patient weight is presented in Table 1.

Priming the Circuit

In adults, most circuits usually are primed with a balanced electrolyte solution. Colloid, similar to albumin or plasma, seldom is used because it is expensive and has little benefit. Likewise, blood is rarely necessary to prime the circuit unless the patient is anemic before surgery or is small. Sometimes additional crystalloid may need to be added during CPB when the amount of perfusate in the venous reservoir is too low to sustain adequate bypass flow.

Priming the CPB circuit for neonates and small infants can pose a substantial challenge because the priming volume is often much larger than the patient's total blood volume. As a result, most neonates and small infants undergo significant hemodilution when placed on CPB if the prime is asanguineous. Currently the priming volume for most neonatal CPB circuits can be reduced to approximately 400 ml (including all components of the circuit, such as cardioplegia). Even at this small volume, some bank blood usually is required to be added to the priming fluid. Using bank blood to prime the circuit requires adding calcium to neutralize the citrate. Buffers such as sodium bicarbonate or tromethamine are used to adjust the pH of the prime.

Anticoagulation

Exposure of blood to the extracorporeal surface of the CPB circuit activates the clotting cascade. Without systemic anticoagulation, the blood clots quickly in the circuit and obstructs the oxygenator. Unfractionated heparin generally is used for anticoagulation during CPB. The initial dose of heparin (300 U/kg) usually is given either intravenously or directly into the right atrium before cannulation for CPB. Anticoagulation is regulated by following the activated clotting time, which is measured before the initiation of and approximately every 30 minutes during CPB. The goal is to maintain the activated clotting time greater than 400 seconds. Additional heparin may need to be added before or during CPB to prevent thrombosis. Currently, prepackaged commercial kits also are available to measure blood heparin concentration directly; this allows more accurate titration of heparin dose during CPB and decreases the amount of protamine needed to reverse the heparin afterward.

Heparin exerts its anticoagulation effect by activating the action of antithrombin III. Occasionally the patient is not anticoagulated adequately despite adequate heparin administration. This situation may be a result of antithrombin III deficiency and can be corrected by giving exogenous antithrombin III or fresh frozen plasma.

After weaning from CPB, protamine sulfate is used to reverse the effect of heparin and to facilitate postoperative hemostasis. The usual protamine dose is 1 mg for every 100 U of heparin used. The protamine/heparin complex can activate complement and stimulate mast cells to secrete histamine, both of which can cause vasodilation and cardiac dysfunction, leading to transient hypotension. Protamine can stimulate synthesis and secretion of thromboxane A_2 from platelets, leading to severe pulmonary vasoconstriction and systemic circulatory collapse. The surgical team must be prepared to treat severe systemic vascular collapse as protamine is administered. Resuscitation may necessitate immediate reheparinization and reinstitution of CPB.

Flow Rate and Pressure

An anesthetized adult at normothermic temperature requires a CPB flow rate of 2.2 to 2.4 liters/min/m^2 body surface area for adequate oxygen delivery to meet all of the body's metabolic needs. In neonates and infants, a higher flow rate (150 to 200 ml/kg body weight/min) is desirable due to their higher lean body mass and higher metabolic demand. Guidelines for desired CPB flow rate based on body weight at normothermic body temperature are shown in Table 2. With systemic hypothermia, overall metabolic demand is less, and CPB flow rate can be decreased safely without the risk of adverse complications. Minimum flow rates for body temperature of 13°C have been calculated; cooling to these temperatures can allow the flow rates to be reduced so that surgery can be performed with a dry operative field.

Even with adequate flow rates, minimal perfusion pressure is crucial for maintaining adequate perfusion to all vital organ systems. This is particularly true in older patients with atherosclerotic disease. For adults, a mean systemic blood pressure during CPB in the range of 50 to 70 mm Hg is considered safe at normothermic body temperature. A mean blood pressure less than 45 mm Hg for a prolonged period at normothermic temperature is associated with increased postoperative neurologic complications, although lower perfusion pressure is acceptable at moderate hypothermia.

Perfusion pressure during CPB can be manipulated by changing the flow rate or by administering intravenous vasoconstrictors or vasodilators.

Hematocrit Management

As blood viscosity increases with systemic cooling, blood flow through the microcirculation may become impaired. Hemodilution frequently is employed during hypothermic CPB to provide adequate oxygen delivery and to prevent sludging in the capillary beds. A hematocrit of approximately 20% is targeted for hypothermic CPB down to 18°C to 20°C. Data in children suggest, however, that the problem of blood viscosity is more theoretical than real and that a higher hematocrit (approximately 30%) may be more beneficial during hypothermia.

Temperature

Cardiac operations performed using CPB often are done under some degree of systemic hypothermia. Cooling the body temperature during CPB decreases the metabolic activity and overall total body oxygen consumption; this allows a reduction of CPB flow rate without compromising adequate oxygen delivery to vital end organs. Under deeply hypothermic conditions, bypass perfusion can be turned off safely for a short time to allow the surgeon to deal with a difficult portion of the repair when it would be beneficial to have a totally bloodless field. During aortic cross-clamping when the heart is arrested with cold cardioplegic solution, systemic hypothermia minimizes the rewarming of the heart tissue and decreases myocardial injury that otherwise might occur during the ischemic period. Systemic hypothermia is beneficial for operations that have a long projected duration of myocardial ischemia.

Weaning from CPB

The heart must regain sufficient function to provide adequate cardiac output, and the lungs must have satisfactory gas exchange before termination of CPB. An excessively slow heart rate can be increased with temporary pacing. Nonsinus rhythm may benefit from electric cardioversion. Patients who are anticipated to have inadequate myocardial contractility postoperatively should be started on an inotropic agent while still on CPB.

Factors that have an impact on cardiac and pulmonary function must be assessed and all abnormalities corrected before weaning. If hypothermia was used during CPB, the patient should be fully rewarmed to a core temperature of 36°C or greater. Inadequate rewarming, especially in infants, can lead to "rebound" hypothermia with subsequent deterioration of myocardial function. Inadequate rewarming can cause coagulopathy and bleeding because the coagulation system normally functions optimally at normal body temperature.

It is customary to check an arterial blood gas, potassium, ionized calcium, glucose, and hematocrit concentration before weaning from CPB. Any significant acidosis can influence cardiac contractility negatively and should be corrected. Hyperkalemia after cardioplegic arrest rarely occurs in patients with normal renal function, but hypokalemia is fairly common due to diuresis while on CPB. Ionized calcium may be low due to hemodilution or transfusion of

Table 2 Desired Cardiopulmonary Bypass Flow Rate at Normothermia	
PATIENT WEIGHT (kg)	**RECOMMENDED FLOW AT 37°C (ml/kg/min)**
0-7	120-200
7-10	100-150
10-20	80-120
>20	2.2-2.4 liters/min/m^2 BSA

BSA, body surface area.

citrate-containing blood products. This can be corrected easily by administering calcium intravenously. Hyperglycemia is common after CPB and should be treated with insulin. This is important in diabetic patients because even moderate hyperglycemia can increase significantly the risk of postoperative infection. A mild to moderate degree of anemia is usually not a problem in patients with normal ventricular function, but this may not be tolerated well in patients with marginal cardiac reserve or in pediatric patients who still have significant residual right-to-left shunting and abnormal arterial oxygen saturation.

During hypothermic CPB, the requirement for anesthetic agents and muscle relaxants is less as a result of the anesthetic effect of hypothermia and slower metabolism of these agents. During rewarming, the amount of these agents must be escalated, however, to prevent patient awareness and shivering. Before separation from CPB, the lungs are inflated manually to eliminate atelectasis. Slow expansion of the lungs suggests either bronchospasm, which should be treated with bronchodilators, or a mucous plug obstructing the endotracheal tube, which is treated by endotracheal suction. Passing a suction catheter down the airway must be done carefully to avoid mucosal trauma and bleeding in a fully anticoagulated patient. If the pleural space is violated during the operation, the pleural space should be aspirated to eliminate any significant amount of blood or effusion and to allow full expansion of the lung.

The weaning process starts by partial occlusion of the venous line. This occlusion decreases the amount of blood returning to the bypass reservoir, leaving more blood in the heart. This increase in preload encourages more blood ejecting from the heart. Arterial flow rate simultaneously is reduced gradually, and hemodynamic parameters are assessed. If they are adequate, the process of decreasing venous return and decreasing arterial flow rate is continued until the patient's heart is ejecting the entire cardiac output on its own and CPB is discontinued. When the patient is hemodynamically stable, the cannulae can be removed and the heparin reversed to help achieve hemostasis.

■ DEEP HYPOTHERMIA WITH CIRCULATORY ARREST

Deep hypothermia with circulatory arrest (DHCA) is a useful tool in the performance of certain cardiovascular surgical procedures. The patient's temperature is lowered gradually to 18°C to 20°C using CPB. Perfusion is stopped, the patient's blood volume is drained into the pump reservoir, and the cannulae can be removed, allowing surgery to be performed in a bloodless field that is unencumbered by cannulae.

Indications

There are certain situations for using DHCA in cardiac surgery (Table 3). When a period of DHCA is anticipated, CPB is used to cool the patient's core temperature down to 18°C to 20°C. The heart may fibrillate during cooling. Although this is not ordinarily a problem, left ventricular distention can occur in some instances (e.g., in patients with severe aortic valve insufficiency or in patients with excessive systemic-to-pulmonary collateral blood flow). Left ventricular

---

Table 3 Indications for Deep Hypothermia Circulatory Arrest

Any cardiopulmonary procedure or repair of complex congenital cardiac defects that requires an asanguineous field (e.g., repair of tiny pulmonary arteries in patients with excessive systemic-to-pulmonary collateral flow)

Repair of the distal ascending aorta or the aortic arch

Atherosclerotic disease or heavy calcification of the aorta that would make clamping of the aorta hazardous

Cardiac surgery in infants with complex systemic venous return

Control and repair of massive hemorrhage as a result of cardiac or aortic laceration from reopening prior median sternotomy

Surgery on tiny neonates (<1800 g)

Selected extracardiac vascular procedures that otherwise would be complicated by uncontrollable bleeding (e.g., excision of renal tumors invading the IVC)

IVC, inferior vena cava.

---

distention can be prevented by placement of a vent into the left ventricle. Alternatively the aorta can be cross-clamped and the heart arrested with cardioplegic solution when the ventricle fibrillates.

Rate and Duration of Cooling

The brain is the most sensitive organ with the lowest tolerance to ischemia during DHCA. Inadequate cooling can lead to cerebral rewarming during the circulatory arrest period, which can result in neurologic injury. In most cases, it is prudent to cool for at least 20 to 25 minutes before induction of DHCA to ensure adequate suppression of cerebral metabolic activity.

Neuroprotection and Monitoring

There is no direct way to monitor cerebral metabolism clinically, and indirect measures must be employed to determine the degree of cerebral protection during DHCA. Because cerebral metabolism is a direct function of brain temperature, nasopharyngeal or tympanic membrane temperature often is used clinically as an indirect measurement of cerebral cooling. Monitoring temperature at various sites in the body, including esophageal, blood, rectal, bladder, and nasopharyngeal, can reflect uniform cooling throughout the body.

Other ways to monitor cerebral metabolism during cooling include measuring internal jugular venous saturation (saturation >95% signifies minimal cerebral oxygen extraction) and monitoring electroencephalographic (EEG) activities. Using silent EEG activity as an end point for cooling is not always reliable because EEG activity does not always become silent at a consistent body temperature. More recently, some groups have used near-infrared spectroscopy to monitor cerebral metabolism during cooling and DHCA. Nevertheless, there is currently no definite correlation between any method of cerebral monitoring and eventual neurologic outcome after DHCA.

Various strategies can be used to minimize the deleterious effect of DHCA. Packing the patient's head with ice during the period of cooling and DHCA has the theoretical advantages of more rapid and uniform cooling and prevention of rewarming during the arrest period. This strategy seems to be more effective in neonates and infants than in adults presumably due to the larger surface area-to-volume ratio of the head. Drugs and additives given in the pump prime or given to the patient just before DHCA have not been shown consistently to be efficacious. Intravenous methylprednisolone (10 mg/kg) given at least 8 hours before DHCA seems to decrease the systemic inflammatory response and the deleterious effect of DHCA on cerebral metabolic recovery.

The acid-base management strategies used during cooling seem to have a significant effect on cerebral blood flow and metabolism. CO_2 solubility in blood decreases at low temperature, and this leads to alkalemia during cooling. The more commonly employed α-stat acid-base management allows blood to remain alkalemic during cooling. In pH-stat acid-base management, CO_2 is added to the bypass circuit to normalize the blood pH. CO_2 is a potent cerebral vasodilator, and using pH-stat acid-base management during cooling can increase blood flow to the brain significantly, leading to more rapid and homogeneous cooling. Excess CO_2 can cause an acidotic milieu in tissues at the time of DHCA and could result in significant impairment in cerebral metabolic recovery after DHCA using pH-stat cooling alone. There is now evidence, however, that if pH-stat acid-base management during cooling is changed to α-stat for a few minutes before the onset of DHCA, the acidotic effects of pH-stat with respect to cerebral metabolic recovery is avoided.

Safe Duration of DHCA

The possibility of brain injury seems to increase with the duration of the circulatory arrest period. The period of DHCA should be limited to time when circulatory arrest is absolutely necessary to achieve the surgical objectives. Usually 30 to 40 minutes of uninterrupted DHCA is considered safe at a nasopharyngeal temperature of 18°C to 20°C. Continuous low-flow cardiopulmonary bypass or DHCA interrupted by intermittent periods of low-flow reperfusion (50 ml/kg/min for 1 to 2 minutes) may provide better end-organ protection than a prolonged period of uninterrupted DHCA. In adults, using continuous retrograde or antegrade cerebral perfusion during DHCA can extend the length of "safe" arrest period with decreased postoperative neurologic complications.

Reperfusion and Rewarming

When CPB is reestablished after DHCA, a period of cold reperfusion for approximately 10 minutes before active rewarming may result in increased cerebral blood flow, but it is not known whether this alters neurologic outcome. Too-aggressive rewarming or overwarming the body core temperature to greater than 36°C can increase the risk of neurologic injury and must be avoided.

■ COMPLICATIONS OF CPB AND DHCA

All the major organ systems can be affected adversely by a period of CPB and DHCA. Coagulopathy and platelet dysfunction often result in excessive bleeding postoperatively requiring clotting factors and platelet transfusion. The systemic inflammatory response to hypothermic CPB and DHCA often results in capillary leak and profound tissue and total body edema. Various degrees of pulmonary, renal, and hepatic dysfunction also can occur, which may prolong the convalescent course in the hospital. The severity of these problems seems to be related to the duration of exposure to CPB, and there are data to suggest that using periods of DHCA to limit the time of CPB perfusion may ameliorate some of these complications.

The brain is the most sensitive organ with the greatest risk for injury after circulatory arrest. Neurologic symptoms usually are related to global cerebral ischemia or compromised perfusion. Seizures, when they occur, are usually temporary and do not require long-term antiseizure treatment. Seizures may be related more to air embolization in the arterial circulation rather than to the effects of ischemia. Choreoathetosis, although rare, can occur after DHCA. This most commonly occurs 2 to 6 days after surgery, and the symptom severity usually improves with time. In some severe cases, choreoathetoid movements or hypotonia can be permanent. The exact pathophysiology of choreoathetosis is unclear, but it is most likely due to ischemic injury to the basal ganglia. With the advent of pH-stat cooling and limiting the duration of DHCA exposure by employing intermittent or continuous low-flow perfusion, many of the clinically recognizable complications related to DHCA are disappearing.

SUGGESTED READING

Edmonds LH Jr: Inflammatory response to cardiopulmonary bypass, *Ann Thorac Surg* 66(5 Suppl):S12, 1998.

Greeley WJ, et al: Effect of deep hypothermia and circulatory arrest on cerebral blood flow and metabolism, *Ann Thorac Surg* 56:1464, 1993.

Jaggers J, et al: Cardiopulmonary bypass in infants and children. In Gravlee GP, et al, editors: *Cardiopulmonary bypass: principles and practice*, ed 2. Philadelphia, 2000, Lippincott Williams & Wilkins, p 633.

Janvier G, et al: Extracorporeal circulation, hemocompatibility, and biomaterials, *Ann Thorac Surg* 62:1926, 1996.

Jonas RA: Neurological protection during cardiopulmonary bypass/deep hypothermia, *Pediatr Cardiol* 19:321, 1998.

MYOCARDIAL PROTECTION IN CHILDREN

Ivan M. Rebeyka

The successful surgical repair of congenital heart malformations in infants and children depends on a technically accurate repair, which can be best achieved through optimal exposure in an immobile, bloodless field. To obtain these favorable conditions, it usually is necessary to employ cardioplegic arrest, which subjects the heart to an obligatory ischemic insult. After exposure to surgically induced global ischemia, myocardial function inevitably becomes impaired even when the ischemic conditions are optimized and the duration of ischemia is short. The heart generally has sufficient functional reserve to allow rapid recovery from minor insults as reflected in the surgical results of simple congenital heart lesions, in which mortality rates approach zero. When a longer duration of ischemic arrest is required to perform a complex reconstruction in a heart that may be compromised adversely by various preoperative conditions, the degree of postoperative myocardial dysfunction may become the primary determinant of surgical outcome and patient survival. Adequate myocardial protection is an essential requirement for safe and effective pediatric cardiac surgery.

Most experimental studies using various models and end points have indicated that the immature myocardium is more tolerant of global ischemia than mature myocardium, yet clinical experience suggests that pediatric patients have a higher incidence of postoperative low cardiac output than typically is seen in adults. This apparent paradox may be explained by several factors associated with clinical pediatric cardiac surgery. Numerous congenital heart lesions are characterized by cyanosis, which may make the myocardium more vulnerable to ventricular dysfunction after exposure to ischemia. Many congenital heart defects are associated with preoperative pressure or volume overload, and the resulting ventricular hypertrophy undoubtedly compromises the ability of these hearts to tolerate an ischemic insult. Optimal myocardial protection becomes particularly important in surgical repairs involving univentricular hearts in which the single ventricle may be required to maintain systemic and pulmonary blood flow while still recovering from surgically induced ischemia. Another factor that places the pediatric heart at a disadvantage compared with the adult heart is the inability to effectively use the intraaortic balloon pump for postoperative mechanical support with borderline ventricular function. These factors highlights the importance of myocardial protection in contributing to morbidity and mortality after technically successful intracardiac repair in infants and children.

■ PRINCIPLES OF MYOCARDIAL PROTECTION

The successful application of myocardial protection techniques in children and adults requires a background understanding of the pathophysiology relating to myocardial ischemia. Ischemic damage is essentially time dependent, and myocardial protective methods employ therapies aimed at delaying the injury process. Surgically induced ischemic injury is minimized by the reduction in metabolic rate achieved through diastolic arrest in combination with hypothermia. The protection afforded through hypothermia and arrest is conceptualized best by considering myocardial oxygen consumption rates. Oxygen consumption in the working heart averages about 10 ml/min/100 g and falls to roughly 5 ml/min/100 g in the empty beating state on bypass. Initiation of normothermic (37°C) arrest lowers the consumption rate to about 1 ml/min/100 g, and as the arrested heart is cooled to 10°C, oxygen consumption rate progressively falls to less than 0.2 ml/min/100 g. Hypothermic cardioplegic arrest is capable of lowering metabolic rate by a factor of approximately 50-fold, and this metabolic reduction delays the onset of injurious processes associated with global ischemia.

The basic principles of myocardial protection were studied extensively by Hearse et al in the 1970s in a large series of experimental studies that characterized the individual components of potassium-based cardioplegic solutions. These principles were studied primarily in relation to the adult heart but are in large part directly applicable to pediatric cardiac surgery. Hearse defined the three main principles or components of effective cardioplegic protection as (1) rapid and complete diastolic arrest; (2) slowing of metabolic rate by hypothermia; and (3) prevention of ischemic related damage with various other protective measures, such as pH buffering and the addition of blood and oxygenation to the cardioplegic solution. These studies led to the development of St. Thomas Hospital Solution (STHS), which is produced commercially as Plegisol and forms the basis of most cardioplegic formulations currently used in North America. Numerous experimental studies have found, however, that the degree of protection afforded by STHS cardioplegia is inferior in the neonatal heart compared with the adult heart. Studies by Watanabe et al showed a differential mechanical response to cardioplegic administration in the neonate suggesting potassium-induced contracture.

■ METHODOLOGY

The standard method of protecting the heart during pediatric cardiac surgery employs hypothermic cardioplegic arrest administered in an antegrade fashion via the aortic root. Since the 1970s, many experimental and clinical studies have been and continue to be reported describing a myriad of protective agents and techniques. Considering the numerous variables involved in myocardial protection, there are probably as many different cardioplegia solutions and techniques of administration as there are cardiac surgeons. Our incomplete understanding of ischemic pathophysiology combined with the many factors that interact in a complex fashion to influence postischemic myocardial function would preclude any claim that a specific myocardial protective technique is superior. Nonetheless, clinical experience supported by experimental data has provided the basis for the following recommendations.

Cardioplegic Formulation

Most cardioplegic solutions in current use have an "extracellular" ionic formulation as characterized by relatively normal concentrations of sodium and calcium. In contrast, "intracellular" solutions (e.g., Euro-Collins and University of Wisconsin solutions used for liver and kidney transplantation) have low sodium and zero or ultra-low calcium concentrations. Although intracellular-type solutions can provide excellent myocardial preservation, they are not used commonly in clinical pediatric cardiac surgery because their protective capabilities seem to be temperature dependent and are lost if profound hypothermia is not absolutely maintained during ischemia.

Potassium

Although there are numerous agents acting through various mechanisms that result in cardiac asystole, the conventional method used to induce diastolic arrest in cardiac surgery is through elevation of extracellular potassium levels with hyperkalemic solutions. It is important to understand the physiology of hyperkalemic arrest to prevent potential myocardial damage. Hyperkalemia acts to arrest the heart by depolarizing or raising the normal resting membrane potential (-85 mV) to levels where the voltage-dependent sodium channels become inactivated. This occurs when the membrane potential reaches -65 mV, which corresponds to an extracellular $[K^+]$ of 10 mM. At $[K^+]$ of 30 mM, the membrane potential becomes depolarized further to -40 mV, at which level the calcium channel becomes activated, and detrimental calcium influx can occur. There is a relatively narrow potassium window that is deemed safe. Cardioplegic potassium concentrations of 15 to 20 mM are considered optimal, and higher concentrations are potentially damaging, especially with solutions containing normalized calcium levels because potassium contractures are produced more easily in neonatal hearts.

Calcium

The optimal calcium content of pediatric cardioplegia solutions has received considerable attention because high cellular levels have been implicated as a major contributor to myocardial injury during ischemia and reperfusion. There are potential problems when either low or high calcium levels are used. Zero or ultra-low levels of calcium have the theoretical potential of causing a severe "calcium paradox" type of injury, whereas normal calcium levels seem to be associated with ventricular contraction even in the arrested heart and may exacerbate further the calcium overload of ischemia. In clinical practice, the ionized calcium concentration can be difficult to control precisely in blood cardioplegia because of variations primarily related to pH and temperature. The weight of experimental evidence suggests that cardioplegia calcium concentrations of 0.3 to 0.6 mM are advisable.

Magnesium

Magnesium has often been included as an additive to cardioplegic solutions based on numerous experimental studies in immature and mature animal models showing improved myocardial preservation. Magnesium is thought to displace calcium from sarcolemmal binding sites, which aids in arresting the heart and reducing the calcium influx associated with potassium arrest. The inclusion of magnesium seems to be particularly important when the solution contains calcium. Early studies by Hearse's group showed the protective effects of elevated magnesium with a dose-response curve indicating optimal levels of 16 mM. Other investigators in studies using blood cardioplegia formulations have confirmed these findings.

Lidocaine

Lidocaine is capable of arresting the heart by blocking sodium channels and reducing the sodium-induced depolarization of the action potential. Although it is debatable whether another arresting agent in addition to hyperkalemia is necessary, there may be several benefits to including lidocaine in the cardioplegic formulation. At $[K^+]$ greater than 20 mM and corresponding membrane potential of -55 mV, voltage-dependent sodium channels become activated resulting in potential transmembrane sodium influx. Sodium channel blockade by the addition of lidocaine may help to limit myocardial uptake of sodium. In addition, when cardioplegic infusion is initiated at room temperature, lidocaine-supplemented cardioplegia may facilitate rapid diastolic arrest before the cardioplegia solution is cooled. Dose-response studies have indicated that cardioplegia lidocaine concentrations less than 1 mM should be used.

Blood versus Crystalloid

Although crystalloid cardioplegia continues to be employed successfully in many centers, surveys have found that greater than 50% of congenital cardiac surgeons currently use formulations containing blood. In clinical practice, the cardioplegia blood content ranges from extremely dilute (1 part blood:5 parts crystalloid) to near-normal hematocrit (4 parts blood:1 part crystalloid). Reports suggesting a potential for sludging from red blood cell rouleau formation and impaired capillary perfusion have prompted us, however, to use a blood-to-crystalloid ratio of 2:1 with a resulting hematocrit level of 15% to 18%.

Although it is still not clearly established that blood cardioplegia is superior in the immature heart, the purported benefits of adding blood to the cardioplegic formulation include the provision of oxygen and buffering capacity to maintain a degree of aerobic metabolism during the ischemic period. In addition, the presence of erythrocytes may have a rheologic effect that improves capillary flow to the microcirculation compared with purely crystalloid solutions. Studies also have shown that the addition of blood to cardioplegic solutions may reduce the cytotoxic effects of hyperkalemia on endothelial cells, which are thought to be more susceptible to injury during ischemia and reperfusion than myocytes. As noted earlier, it is vital that the concentrations of the various ions are controlled precisely within the final solution after blood dilution to prevent inadvertent myocardial damage. The cardioplegia formulation used for

Table 1 Cardioplegic Solution Composition
Crystalloid base solution
1000 ml 0.9% normal saline
40 mM potassium chloride
40 mM magnesium sulfate
15 ml lidocaine 2%
Base solution is mixed with arterial blood from the
cardiopulmonary bypass circuit in 2 parts blood:1 part
crystalloid ratio

pediatric cardiac surgery at the University of Alberta Hospitals is listed in Table 1.

Cardioplegia Delivery

Commercially available blood cardioplegia delivery systems with low prime volumes are available that mix arterial blood from the oxygenator or arterial line with an asanguineous solution. The blood-to-crystalloid ratio can be controlled by varying the tubing size from the blood and crystalloid sources, and an integrated heat exchanger within the unit allows precise control of cardioplegia temperature. Cardioplegia usually is administered in an antegrade fashion through the aortic root using a plastic catheter. The presence of significant aortic regurgitation precludes effective cardioplegic administration via the aortic root and necessitates direct coronary ostial infusion. When the aortic root is open, repeat doses can be administered in a similar fashion. Another useful option is retrograde administration via the coronary sinus, which is possible even in a neonatal heart using a small balloon-tipped catheter facilitated by a purse-string suture around the coronary sinus ostium.

Temperature

In our protocol, cardioplegic infusion is initiated at a temperature of 20°C because we believe that the rapid induction of myocardial hypothermia before the heart is completely arrested can result in an increase in intracellular calcium and varying degrees of contracture. As the heart becomes flaccid in diastolic arrest, the cardioplegia is cooled to 10°C using the blood cardioplegia device. When profound hypothermia and circulatory arrest is used for aortic arch reconstruction, the initial cardioplegia temperature is 15°C. Unless the cross-clamp period is expected to be short (<15 minutes), myocardial hypothermia is maintained during the ischemic period with topical cooling. This may be particularly important in the neonate because small hearts have a higher ventricular surface area-to-mass ratio, making them more susceptible to rewarming. While recognizing the potential for phrenic nerve injury with topical ice, saline slush is placed within the pericardial cavity but separated from the heart by a small gauze square. Irrigation of the pericardial cavity with iced saline slowly dripping over the heart is another effective method of maintaining myocardial hypothermia.

Dosage and Interval

The standard dose volume of cardioplegia is 30 ml/kg body weight. This dose is based on studies by Hearse indicating that crystalloid cardioplegia volumes of 4 ml/g heart wet weight provided adequate protection, and higher volumes conferred no additional benefit. When secondary doses of cardioplegia are employed, repeat infusions of 10 to 15 ml/kg body weight are administered. The need for multidose cardioplegic administration in the neonatal heart remains controversial, however, with some studies suggesting that repeated infusion may be more harmful than beneficial by increasing myocardial edema. Conversely, periodic reinfusion may improve protection by maintaining hypothermia and washing out acid metabolites that might inhibit anaerobic metabolism. We prefer to readminister cardioplegia at 20- to 30-minute intervals with care to ensure low-pressure infusion.

Pressure

Although a sufficient cardioplegic infusion pressure is necessary to ensure adequate myocardial distribution, the infant heart seems especially prone to edema when exposed to excessively high pressures. Although we recognize the potential for a discrepancy between intraaortic and cardioplegia delivery line pressure depending on flow rate, we routinely monitor pressure from a side port on the delivery system and maintain line pressure less than 50 mm Hg during cardioplegic infusion in neonates and infants and less than 75 mm Hg in older children.

■ MECHANISMS OF INTRAOPERATIVE INJURY IN PEDIATRIC CARDIAC SURGERY

Although the extent of ischemic injury during the cardioplegic arrest interval is likely the major determinant of postoperative myocardial dysfunction, there is potential for damage to the immature heart from other factors introduced intraoperatively. Optimal myocardial protection does not simply involve keeping the heart arrested and cold during the ischemic interval. Rather, attention to numerous details of cardiopulmonary bypass (CPB) management is essential to avoid inadvertent injury to the heart. This is especially important in the neonatal heart, which is more likely to be sensitive to the unphysiologic conditions imposed during surgery. Injury may occur during the preischemic and postischemic stages of the procedure if careful attention is not paid to the overall management of CPB.

Preischemic Phase
Perfusion Pressure

The neonatal heart is considered to be susceptible to myocardial edema resulting from excessive perfusion pressure on CPB. The typical CPB flow rates of 150 ml/kg/min used for neonates usually maintain perfusion pressure between 30 and 35 mm Hg. Perfusion pressures greater than 40 mm Hg are not necessary and are potentially injurious.

Myocardial Distention

Significant injury is associated with distention of the heart on CPB, which can occur rapidly in the presence of either aortic valve insufficiency or excessive pulmonary venous return from a patent ductus arteriosus or patent Blalock-Taussig shunt.

Cyanotic patients are particularly prone to this problem from either major or diffuse aortopulmonary collaterals. Attention must be paid not only to ensuring the accurate placement of properly sized venous cannulae with no restriction of venous return to the bypass circuit, but also to adequate venting of the left ventricle and early control of extracardiac sources of pulmonary blood flow. In our experience, it is often difficult to achieve diastolic arrest, as indicated by a soft, flaccid heart when cardioplegia is administered to a distended and tense myocardium.

Reoxygenation on Bypass

In cyanotic patients, there is an abrupt reversal of hypoxemia that occurs with the initiation of CPB. Because there is some experimental evidence that hypoxia may jeopardize the myocardium's capacity to withstand oxygen-mediated injury, the conventional method of starting bypass with oxygen tension levels of 400 to 500 mm Hg may result in an inadvertent reoxygenation injury that adversely affects postoperative myocardial function. Despite the absence of strong clinical evidence to verify effectiveness, the simple maneuver of maintaining normoxia by keeping initial PO_2 levels less than 100 mm Hg can be adopted easily into pediatric bypass protocols and may be advisable. Conversely, studies have indicated that cerebral protection may be enhanced when hyperoxic perfusion is employed in the setting of deep hypothermia and circulatory arrest.

Hypothermic Perfusion

Although hypothermia remains the most potent and important protective measure available to protect the heart and other organs from ischemic damage, the reduction of metabolic rate itself can have adverse consequences if not applied carefully. Systemic perfusion cooling on bypass to profoundly hypothermic temperatures potentially can induce "cooling contracture" of the heart that results in severe myocardial injury, especially if combined with a period of ischemia. This occurrence is the clinical manifestation of a phenomenon well known to muscle physiologists. *Rapid cooling contracture* refers to a marked increase in resting tension in cardiac and skeletal muscle in response to a sudden decrease in temperature secondary to calcium release from intracellular stores. This cold-induced injury seems to be preventable by maintaining perfusate temperature at greater than 12°C and perfusion pressure less than 40 mm Hg on bypass.

Postischemic Phase
Intracardiac Air Removal

It is essential to evacuate carefully all air from the left side of the heart before myocardial reperfusion to prevent coronary and cerebral emboli. The risk of large air emboli is greatest during the initial ventricular ejections immediately after electrical defibrillation. Air easily becomes trapped within pulmonary veins in nondependent areas of the lung when the left heart is opened and must be removed before release of the cross-clamp. Forward flow is promoted repeatedly through partially inflated lungs while the ascending aorta is still vented and the left ventricular vent is clamped. Routine intraoperative echocardiography is useful in ensuring that air is no longer present within the left heart before full separation from CPB is completed and the aortic vent site is closed.

Reperfusion Pressure and Temperature

Although experimental studies showing the beneficial effects of hypothermic and low-pressure reperfusion have not been verified by clinical studies, we reduce bypass flow rate to 50% and maintain perfusate temperature at 25°C during the initial several minutes of reperfusion when hypothermic bypass is employed.

Calcium Administration

Reperfusion at normothermia in the presence of normal calcium levels has been shown experimentally to exacerbate ischemic injury. It has become common clinical practice to delay calcium administration until the heart is ready for separation from bypass.

◼ CARDIAC SURGERY WITHOUT CARDIOPLEGIC ARREST

If one accepts that even short periods of global ischemia are damaging and adversely affect postoperative myocardial function, the obvious way to ensure myocardial protection is to maintain coronary perfusion throughout the operation. Many congenital heart repairs can be performed safely without the need for cardioplegia ischemic arrest. It is possible to repair simple atrial septal defects and perform open atrial septectomies using electrically induced ventricular fibrillation, although great care must be taken to prevent coronary and cerebral emboli from air retained within the left heart. Similarly the Fontan procedure now is performed frequently using an extracardiac conduit that can be accomplished without arresting the heart, optimizing postoperative ventricular function by avoiding myocardial ischemia. Procedures limited to the right heart can be completed in the empty, beating heart on CPB, provided that no septal defects are present.

SUGGESTED READING

Allen BS, et al: Pediatric myocardial protection: an overview, *Semin Thorac Cardiovasc Surg* 13:56, 2001.

Chambers DJ, Hearse DJ: Cardioplegia and surgical ischemia. In Sperelakis N, et al, editors: *Heart physiology and pathophysiology.* San Diego, 2001, Academic Press, p 887.

Drinkwater DC, Laks H: Pediatric cardioplegic techniques, *Semin Thorac Cardiovasc Surg* 5:168, 1993.

Rebeyka IM: Intraoperative neonatal myocardial management: protection versus injury, *Adv Card Surg* 8:1, 1996.

Watanabe H, et al: Functional and metabolic protection of the neonatal myocardium from ischemia, *J Thorac Cardiovasc Surg* 97:50, 1989.

PEDIATRIC EXTRACORPOREAL MEMBRANE OXYGENATION AND MECHANICAL CIRCULATORY ASSIST DEVICES

James Fackler

Extracorporeal membrane oxygenation (ECMO) is a widely used form of short-term cardiorespiratory support for critically ill children with profound but reversible respiratory and/or cardiac failure. Although ECMO has a 40-year history for support of adults with the acute respiratory distress syndrome (ARDS), two randomized studies of ECMO for ARDS showed no benefit. In contrast, ECMO for severe persistent fetal circulation (PFC) in neonates has been shown remarkably efficacious both by overwhelming anecdotal experiences from as early as 1985 and in two randomized clinical trials. The most recent data from the Extracorporeal Life Support Organization (ELSO) show more than 8500 neonates with PFC have been treated with ECMO; approximately 90% survived. ECMO for cardiac support is a more recent development; efficacy data are strictly anecdotal.

ECMO is indicated for neonates with respiratory failure if the respiratory failure is caused by a reversible lesion and if the severity of the respiratory failure is profound. In addition, the neonate must be full term, free of significant intracranial hemorrhage, and free of congenital heart disease.

▪ EXTRACORPOREAL MEMBRANE OXYGENATION FOR RESPIRATORY FAILURE

PFC, primary pulmonary hypertension of the newborn (PPHN), and meconium aspiration syndrome are primarily vascular lesions of the newborn. That the lesion is reversible is supported by the fact that ECMO is successful most often in less than 5 days of support. Severity of illness is often estimated by the oxygenation index (OI).

$$OI = \frac{P_{AW} \times F_{IO_2} \times 100}{P_{aO_2}}$$

An OI 40 or greater should prompt consideration of ECMO. If high-frequency oscillatory ventilation (HFOV) is used, the threshold for ECMO should be OI of 60.

Pulmonary hypertension is associated with other newborn conditions; ECMO should be carefully considered in all of these circumstances. Sepsis in the newborn, even with a coagulopathy, is not a contraindication, although survival is 75% compared with 90% in isolated PFC. Congenital diaphragmatic hernia (CDH) has a significant component of pulmonary hypertension but is associated with significantly

worse outcomes than isolated PFC (50% mortality). Recent evidence suggests ECMO benefits newborns with CDH and moderately severe respiratory failure. CDH with congenital heart disease has been associated with poor survival, but recent evidence suggests outcomes are improving for infants with this combination of lesions.

ECMO is also occasionally used for respiratory failure in children beyond the neonatal age range. ECMO for ARDS in children is rarely indicated because most children survive with only mechanical ventilation as long as the child has no other comorbidities. Infants with *severe* respiratory syncytial virus (RSV) consistently respond favorably to ECMO. ECMO is relatively or absolutely contraindicated in the setting of ARDS and comorbid conditions (e.g., ARDS after bone marrow transplantation or with submersion injury and significant anoxic encephalopathy). A number of centers have published experiences with adults treated for ARDS by ECMO; the data are difficult to interpret because survival is also improving in adults with ARDS treated with conventional mechanical ventilation.

In summary, if ECMO is to be used in any child or adult with ARDS, the underlying lesion associated with ARDS must be reversible. Yet equal scrutiny must be applied to whether the underlying lesion is reversible *without* ECMO. In the setting of ARDS, remarkable improvements in survival have been demonstrated over the past few years. In the ECMO experience with ARDS, long courses (3 to 4 weeks) are commonplace; recovery from ARDS without ECMO often requires the same duration of mechanical ventilation with attendant need for perspective and patience.

If ECMO is to be used for ARDS, severity of illness must also be high (OI > 40) and mechanical ventilation must be failing. Contraindications for ECMO use are profound acute central nervous system (CNS) damage, significant immune suppression (e.g., congenital, acquired, or iatrogenic), and significant chronic lung disease.

ECMO for cardiac support also has a role in the setting of life-threatening cardiac failure. Decisions to invoke ECMO for cardiac failure are more complex than for neonatal respiratory failure, as there are no "definitive" indications for cardiac support. The only absolute prerequisite for consideration of ECMO for cardiac support is that the lesion responsible for cardiac failure must be reversible. Decisions about which lesions are reversible are judgment calls for which little data are useful. Practically, ECMO for cardiac support is most often invoked when "maximal" medical therapy "fails." Identifying that point in any individual's course differs among institutions, individuals within an institution, and by day for individual practitioners. Overall, survival of patients treated with ECMO for cardiac support is about 50%.

▪ EXTRACORPOREAL MEMBRANE OXYGENATION FOR CARDIAC FAILURE

Myocardial failure occurs most commonly in three settings: postcardiotomy, myocarditis, and cardiac arrest. Myocarditis is the most homogeneous of the three as these children usually have structurally normal hearts and global cardiac dysfunction. Dysrhythmias are variable. Escalating vasopressor support in the presence of ongoing shock and/or malignant dysrhythmia should trigger consideration of ECMO. Myocarditis resulting in a witnessed cardiac arrest should also trigger a rapid initiation of ECMO, as long as cardiopulmonary resuscitation (CPR) is effective and extracorporeal support can begin within 1 hour of the cardiac arrest. ELSO reports a 60% survival in children treated with ECMO for myocarditis. ECMO runs may be as long as 21 days. However, because data describing severity of illness in these 130 patients are not available, placing any particular patient in this context is difficult.

Most commonly, cardiac ECMO is used in 1% to 2% of children after open cardiac procedures. Failure to wean from bypass in the operating room is the most common indication (and is associated with 38% survival). Unlike in myocarditis, each child's preoperative lesion, operative procedure, anesthesia, and bypass techniques differ. Whether a particular combination of lesions is reversible is often uncertain. If ECMO is begun, 72 hours of support is usually a sufficient duration to detect improvement in cardiac function. Support should be continued until it is clear that there is no hope for further recovery or recovery occurs, rendering ECMO unnecessary.

CPR for any lesion should also prompt ECMO consideration, but there are little data to guide decisions. Paramount is predicting whether the cardiorespiratory failure and the underlying disease process(es) are reversible. Asthma, hypothermia, and drug intoxication are examples that are treatable with ECMO. Obviously, comorbid chronic conditions, adequacy of ongoing resuscitation, and ongoing organ damage must be carefully, albeit quickly, analyzed.

If ECMO is to be used in the setting of CPR, the rapidity of institution of ECMO is crucial. A variety of techniques have been devised to allow rapid initiation of ECMO. Preassembled ECMO circuits, if handled carefully, can be stored for weeks. There are no data on how long saline-primed ECMO circuits can be safely stored. Blood-primed circuits must be used within hours of their setup; as such, blood priming should be held until a firm decision to begin ECMO has been made. Other solutions for rapid circuit availability are "mini-cardiopulmonary bypass devices" generally with centrifugal pumps and short-term oxygenators. Most often the rate-limiting step for ECMO initiation is vascular access. In the best of hands, ECMO initiation lags 15 to 45 minutes behind the decision, so consideration of ECMO for cardiorespiratory arrest must be used only in a center well prepared with equipment, personnel, and protocols.

■ VENTRICULAR SUPPORT FOR CARDIAC FAILURE

A growing body of experience and literature supports use of ventricular assist devices (VADs) in the subset of children with isolated cardiac failure. Experiences in adults are far more extensive but do not easily translate to children because device size, relationship to body surface area, and physiology (the lack of isolated ventricular dysfunction) are quite different. VADs have a number of advantages over ECMO for cardiac support. Certainly if gas exchange is adequate, the introduction of a membrane oxygenator is unnecessary.

Further, the amount of heparinization for a VAD is less than with ECMO. VAD circuits are less complex than ECMO, making VAD setup easier. A downside of VAD is that cannulation must be through the chest, as cannulas are placed directly in the atrium and aorta or pulmonary artery. Biventricular support is technically possible with two VADs (or BiVAD). However, BiVAD requires cannulas in the right and left atria (RA and LA), the pulmonary artery, and the aorta; at times this is physically difficult in children. ECMO has advantages, even in the setting of isolated ventricular dysfunction, as familiarity with ECMO technique is far more ubiquitous and thus more consistently applied. Finally, ECMO provides biventricular support delivered with two cannulas (RA and aorta) placed through the neck. As such, full cardiac support can be delivered with a fully closed chest.

A difference between ECMO and a left ventricular (LV) assist device (LVAD) for isolated LV dysfunction worth special attention is the possibility of LA hypertension during ECMO. When LV dysfunction is worse than right ventricular (RV) dysfunction in a structurally normal heart (e.g., myocarditis, anomalous left coronary artery), blood in the RA is incompletely drained by the venous ECMO cannula. This blood traverses the pulmonary bed and enters the LA. With poor LV contractility, pulmonary edema and increased LV wall stress lead to hypoxia and an increased LV work (hindering myocardial recovery). Venting the LA is critical in this setting, either with a transthoracic LA cannula or by balloon septostomy.

■ TECHNIQUE—EXTRACORPOREAL MEMBRANE OXYGENATION

ECMO can be delivered via either venoarterial (VA) or venovenous (VV) routes. Most often, a roller pump is used to provide nonpulsatile flow. In neonates, the right jugular vein is identified through a cutdown incision (after fentanyl and local lidocaine anesthesia). A venous drainage cannula (usually between 12 Fr and 16 Fr) is placed if VA ECMO is anticipated or a double-lumen venous cannula is placed for VV ECMO. The right common carotid artery is cannulated in VA ECMO for placement of an 8 Fr to 12 Fr arterial cannula.

Blood drains via gravity into a small reservoir (bladder). The bladder is a tiny (50 ml) buffer available for balancing inflow and outflow. Some newer ECMO circuits use pressure differentials to balance flows. The circuits have no bladder. Blood is stripped through the roller head and forced through the oxygenator. Gas runs countercurrent and blends with both oxygen and carbon dioxide to maintain normal blood gases. From the oxygenator, blood flows to a heater and then to the arterial cannula.

The cannula of the VV double-lumen cannula requires special attention. Placement of the VV double-lumen cannula must be within the chamber of the RA. The venous port is on the proximal end of the cannula. The distal or "arterial" end of the VV cannula returns oxygenated blood across the tricuspid valve and through the pulmonary bed. The lumen of the arterial end cannula is small, increasing its velocity and further increasing the chance that oxygenated blood will proceed antegrade rather than recirculate back into the venous limb. Echocardiography is often useful to confirm positioning and blood flows. Measurement of the blood oxygen saturation in the venous limb is important, and a high oxygen saturation indicates significant recirculation and necessitates repositioning the cannula.

VV ECMO is appropriate only when respiratory failure is not associated with significant cardiac dysfunction. Systemic blood pressure with VV ECMO is dependent on a functioning left heart. Some dysfunction may be present at initiation of VV ECMO. Occasionally, there is a need to convert VV to VA ECMO.

Full support in a neonate requires flow of approximately 100 ml/kg/min. Estimates of the proportion of total cardiac output provided by ECMO (based on a "normal" neonatal cardiac output) can be misleading. Arterial catheters for pressure monitoring should be placed in all children on ECMO. A flat arterial waveform trace indicates systemic pressure is nonpulsatile and thus supplied completely by the ECMO pump. A pulsatile arterial waveform indicates myocardial recovery. Presence of end-tidal CO_2 can be achieved only (in VA ECMO) if RV function is adequate to deliver blood to the pulmonary capillary bed.

Mechanical ventilation during VA ECMO, strictly from a total gas exchange perspective, is unnecessary. However, the practice of "lung rest" must be carefully considered in each case as alveolar distention with high end-expiratory pressure and unnecessary atelectasis (from "subphysiologic" pressures) are both best avoided. An important caveat about mechanical ventilation during ECMO for cardiac support is that (because most coronary artery blood flow comes from the native circulation) the lungs should be ventilated with an FIO_2 of 0.4.

Anticoagulation during ECMO is necessary before cannulas are placed. The activated clotting time (ACT) is routinely monitored. Normal ACT is approximately 100 seconds. A heparin infusion is used to keep the ACT during ECMO at 180 to 200 seconds. With ECMO at full flow, ACT can be as low as 160 seconds if bleeding, or risk of serious bleeding, is present. If during weaning, ECMO flow is decreased significantly, the ACT should be kept at approximately 220 seconds. Vigilant attention for clots in the circuit must be maintained. If clots occur in a dangerous place (e.g., after the heater) or are large, the circuit must be replaced.

Weaning from ECMO is most often accomplished by slowing decreasing support as native function returns. For newborns with PFC, weaning typically begins on day 3 and separation from ECMO ("decannulation") occurs on day 4 or 5. Often the chest radiograph clears dramatically, the pulmonary compliance improves significantly, and gas exchange is accomplished with mechanical ventilation on reasonable settings with ECMO flow as low as is possible (without significant thrombotic complications). In marked contrast, if ECMO is being used for ARDS, improvement in native function may not begin to appear until day 20 of ECMO. Weaning may take an additional week. Some centers access the likelihood of successful decannulation with arterial blood gas measurement while the patient is "clamped off." In this scenario, the patient must be on relatively low-pressure ventilator settings. If the PaO_2 is 60 mm Hg or greater on an FIO_2 of 0.3 (and the pH is normal), newborns with PFC can be separated from ECMO. Newborns with CDH are more difficult as oxygenation criteria must be coupled with a ventilation criteria (often an estimation of total dead space).

■ MORBIDITY AND QUESTIONS

Short-term complications of ECMO (except the rare problems isolated to the circuit) are difficult to associate with ECMO, the underlying the disease process(es), or other therapies used before or during ECMO. Of ECMO-treated neonates, 9.4% have a CNS infarction identified by computed tomography or ultrasonography. CNS hemorrhages are reported in 5.3% of ECMO-treated neonates. As these newborns were profoundly hypoxic, variably hypotensive, hyperventilated, and/or coagulopathic, these CNS lesions may have no relationship with ECMO use. Further, it is generally recognized that ECMO-treated newborns with CDH have significant morbidity. Because the oldest survivor of neonatal ECMO is now about 24 years old, whether adulthood will bring untold problems is unknown. ECMO has also produced a generation of adults with ligated right carotid arteries. Only time will tell whether these ECMO survivors will fare better than their counterparts who have reconstructed carotid arteries at decannulation.

Much progress has been made, but much remains to be learned.

SUGGESTED READING

Bartlett RH, et al: Extracorporeal circulation in neonatal respiratory failure: a prospective randomized study, *Pediatrics* 76:479, 1985.

Chen YS, et al: Analysis and results of prolonged resuscitation in cardiac arrest patients rescued by extracorporeal membrane oxygenation, *J Am Coll Cardiol* 41:197, 2003.

Duncan BW: Mechanical circulatory support for infants and children with cardiac disease, *Ann Thorac Surg* 73:1670, 2002.

Lund DP, et al: Congenital diaphragmatic hernia: the hidden morbidity, *J Pediatr Surg* 29:258, 1994.

VALVE REPLACEMENT IN CHILDREN

R. Eric Lilly

Richard A. Hopkins

James D. St. Louis

Each year approximately 60,000 heart valves are implanted in the United States and nearly 170,000 are implanted worldwide. A small minority of these are placed in children, yet pediatric valve replacement remains technically challenging and the subject of continued evolution and refinement because of the inherent limitations of prostheses in children: lack of growth, unavailability and poor performance of some prostheses in smaller sizes, and the complications of anticoagulation in children. Fortunately, valve repair techniques have advanced, making use of prostheses less common, although perhaps only delayed. Pulmonary autografts for aortic and mitral valve replacement have also been used; of these, 40% are tissue valves.

The first clinical application of a tissue valve was by Gordon Murray in 1956 who implanted a fresh aortic homograft into the descending aorta of a patient with aortic insufficiency. In 1962, both Donald Ross in England and Sir Brian Barratt-Boyes in New Zealand reported their initial clinical use of aortic homografts in the aortic valve position. Since then, multiple clinical series have confirmed the advantages of homograft valves for reconstruction of both the left and right ventricular outflow tracts. Donor availability, the complexity of implantation, and limited durability have diminished the widespread clinical use of homografts. The recent introduction of stentless porcine tissue valves has sought to address this clinical void by providing a readily available supply of valve prostheses similar to homografts in terms of hemodynamic profile and available in multiple sizes with promising durability. This chapter provides an introduction to homograft prostheses and their clinical use and examines the potential role of the stentless porcine valve prosthesis.

Central to homograft valve durability are the initial procurement, sterilization, and storage of the allograft valve. Beginning in 1962, the first homografts used clinically were harvested from donor cadavers in an aseptic fashion with subsequent implantation within a few hours to days. These "fresh" homografts performed well both initially and long term. Since these initial efforts, homograft preparation methods have evolved from a clean harvest with harsh sterilization technique to gentle antibiotic sterilization and wet storage at 4°C ("fresh wet-stored") to the modern technique of antibiotic disinfection then cryopreservation in dimethylsulfoxide with storage at −196°C. This process of cryopreservation has allowed commercialization of allograft valves. Interpretation of clinical series examining homograft valves is largely dependent on the method of valve preparation and storage at least with respect to mid-term outcome.

At the time of implantation, modern valvular allografts do contain a significant number of viable cells. Data from O'Brien have demonstrated uptake of radioactive proline by 50% to 90% of fibroblasts within the allograft. At the time of explantation, however, few, if any, of these cells are viable. In one study, transmission electron microscopic examination of explanted long-term allograft valves (up to 9 years after implantation) demonstrated no viable cells, focal calcification centered around dead cell remnants, and distorted but largely preserved collagen. This lack of viable cells was primarily attributable to ischemia-induced apoptosis associated with harvesting, preservation, and implantation. Other reports have demonstrated survival of a few cellular elements in explanted valvular allografts but insufficient cells to render the allograft capable of active metabolic function, much less growth. The quality of the allograft therefore is related to the quality of the collagen from which it is composed.

Failure of transplanted allografts used for left ventricular outflow tract reconstructions typically occurs secondary to valvular incompetence either by cusp rupture, distortion of the allograft with cusp retraction, or cusp perforations. In contrast, failure of allografts when used for right ventricular outflow tract reconstructions most frequently occurs secondary to stenosis relative to somatic growth in children. The walls of these allografts typically exhibit extensive calcification while the cusp tissue remains relatively free of calcification. Despite the lack of a significant number of viable cells within cryopreserved transplanted allografts and recognized modes of clinical failure once transplanted, freedom from degeneration and/or replacement at 10 to 15 years is reported between 50% and 90%. This durability is equivalent to that of bioprosthetic valves.

The hemodynamic characteristics of allograft valves are clearly superior to either mechanical valves or stented bioprostheses. A 19- to 20-mm internal diameter allograft aortic valve is usually adequate for most adults and hemodynamically analogous to a much larger prosthetic valve.

■ LEFT VENTRICULAR OUTFLOW TRACT RECONSTRUCTIONS

Clinical situations in which an allograft valve should be considered for left ventricular outflow tract reconstruction are listed in Table 1. Of the indications listed, the most commonly accepted are in young to middle-aged patients with active endocarditis and contraindications to anticoagulation or in young females who desire to become pregnant.

O'Brien et al reported a series of 1022 patients who received aortic valvular allografts with follow-up to 29 years. Active endocarditis was the indication for valve operation in only 8.7% of the series patients. The overall 30-day or hospital mortality rate was 3%. This clinical experience encompassed three different preservation methods and three basic implant methods. For cryopreserved allograft root replacements, the total incidence of thromboembolic events (both transient and permanent) was 1.7% and the actuarial freedom from reoperation due to structural deterioration,

Table 1 Considerations for Aortic Valvular Allograft

Clinical situations in which chronic anticoagulation is undesirable (e.g., women of child-bearing age who desire to become pregnant, active adults, children)
Aortic root replacement
Aortoventriculoplasty
Small aortic annulus
Endocarditis
Reoperation for failed aortic prosthesis secondary to accelerated degeneration

endocarditis, and technical causes was 83% at 10 years. O'Brien et al also examined the impact of age of allograft recipient on freedom from reoperation and found that patients aged 0 to 20 years had a 47% freedom-from-reoperation rate at 10 years compared with 95% in those older than 20 years. Few patients in this series had primary allograft transplants in place beyond the second decade.

Relative contraindications to use of the aortic allograft are listed in Table 2. In general, contraindications relate to mechanical factors that would limit the surgeon's ability to implant the valve. There are no absolute contraindications. The presence of connective tissue or rheumatoid disorders is considered a contraindication to allograft use. Marfan syndrome patients require buttressing annulus and sinotubular junction with Dacron strips if an allograft is chosen.

Accurate matching of the aortic root size to the valvular allograft is crucial for successful long-term durability of the transplanted valve. Preoperative echocardiography in which the left ventricular outflow tract diameter is measured from a parasternal long-axis view of the left ventricle minus approximately 3 mm provides a good estimate of the annular diameter, thereby allowing for approximate-sized allografts to be made available. The actual annular diameter is determined directly in the operating room using rigid Hegar dilators after aortotomy and débridement of the aortic annulus. Because the average wall thickness of an allograft is 2 mm, it is necessary to subtract 4 mm from the directly measured internal annular diameter to obtain the appropriate external diameter of the allograft for implantation. If a significant amount of calcium remains within the annulus after débridement, an oversized allograft should be avoided. In this situation the allograft should be undersized by approximately 1 to 2 mm.

Table 2 Relative Contraindications to Aortic Valvular Allograft

Severe calcification of the annulus, septum, mitral valve, or fibrous trigones precluding smooth seating of the valve
Lack of valve availability
Unfavorable coronary anatomy
Aortic root ectasia with diameter >30 mm
Aortic valve replacement as a part of a complex total operation
Severe left ventricular dysfunction
Connective tissue disorders (e.g., Marfan syndrome or cystic medial necrosis)

Techniques for aortic valvular allograft implantation include a subcoronary or "free-hand" technique, the intraluminal cylinder technique, and total root replacement. In the subcoronary technique, varying amounts of the allograft aortic sinus wall are removed for reconstruction of the recipient aorta, which provides flexibility, allowing for annular enlargement or for dealing with a problem aorta. O'Brien et al detail experience with each of these basic implant methods and state that they have abandoned the other methods in favor of the total aortic root replacement method. When the aortic morphology is grossly distorted (such as in chronic severe aortic stenosis), total aortic root replacement is necessary when using allograft valves. Infective endocarditis may also mandate the technique of total root replacement. Routinely, aortic allografts come with the anterior leaflet of the mitral valve attached. This tissue is particularly helpful in the reconstruction of aortic annulus or interventricular septum after débridement for abscess. The "free-hand" and total aortic root replacement techniques are illustrated in Figures 1 and 2.

■ RIGHT VENTRICULAR OUTFLOW TRACT RECONSTRUCTIONS

Owing to accelerated calcification of bioprosthetic valves in younger patients and lack of durability of mechanical valves in the pulmonary position, allograft valves are the conduits of choice for right ventricular outflow tract reconstructions. The indications for right ventricular outflow tract reconstructions to ensure a competent pulmonary valve are largely related to congenital heart defects in children (e.g., tetralogy of Fallot, truncus arteriosus, pulmonary hypoplasia, and absent pulmonary valve syndrome). In adults, the most common indications relate to pulmonary insufficiency occurring late after right ventricular outflow tract reconstruction. Although extracardiac valveless prostheses have been used for right ventricular outflow tract reconstructions in children in the past with good clinical results, a significant number of these patients develop right ventricular dysfunction and require reoperation with a valved conduit.

Either aortic or pulmonary allografts may be used for right ventricular outflow tract reconstructions. Sizing of allografts in this regard is flexible with a broad tolerance of sizing that can be used. In general, allografts of 22 to 26 mm are used in adults, whereas in infants, the size varies according to the weight of the patient. The technique for right ventricular outflow tract reconstruction involves incision across the pulmonary valve with excision of any residual valvular tissue (Figure 3). The proximal anastomosis is then accomplished beginning posteriorly. The ventriculotomy is then closed with an additional piece of pericardium, Gore-Tex patch, or the anterior leaflet of the mitral valve if an aortic allograft was used.

In a review of 405 valved allografts placed in the subpulmonary position at Great Ormond Street Hospital from 1971 to 1993, the mean patient age at operation was 6.8 years (age range, 2 days to 28 years). Freedom from conduit replacement at 5, 10, and 15 years was 84%, 58%, and 31%, respectively. The age of the longest surviving conduit was 22.7 years. In a multivariate analysis of predictors of conduit

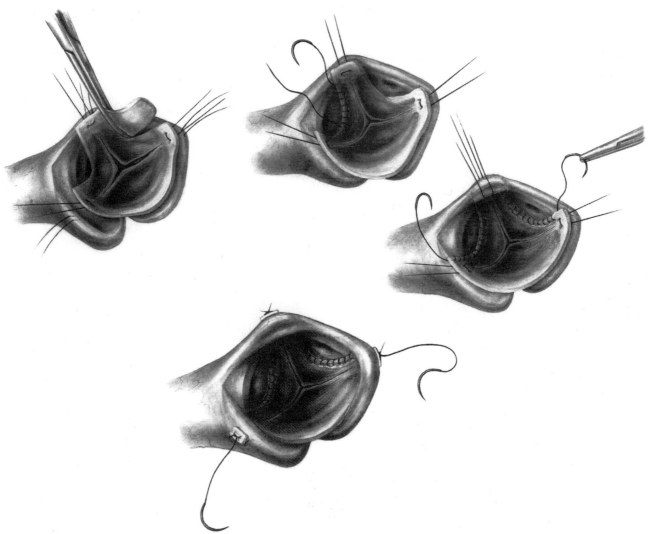

Figure 1
Subcoronary "free-hand" aortic valve replacement with allograft valve.

survival, only reoperation and order of conduit (i.e., relating to preservation method) were significant. Neither the type of allograft (i.e., aortic or pulmonary) nor the conduit size was associated with conduit survival.

■ STENTLESS PORCINE VALVES

Stent-mounted glutaraldehyde-preserved bioprosthetic valves have been used in clinical practice since the early 1970s. Follow-up echocardiography after implantation of these stent-mounted prostheses commonly demonstrates resting transvalvular gradients of 20 to 25 mm Hg. In contrast, valvular allografts in the aortic position have essentially no gradients. The scarcity of readily available aortic allografts stimulated the interest in stentless glutaraldehyde-preserved porcine valves in the 1990s. Two stentless valves were approved by the Food and Drug Administration in 1997 for insertion in the aortic position. They are similar in

overall configuration and contain a varying amount of Dacron cloth covering the proximal edge of the prosthesis, but they differ in terms of the anticalcification technology (Figure 4).

When compared with stent-mounted bioprostheses, stentless valves are clearly superior in hemodynamic performance. A study by David of 198 pairs of matched patients who underwent aortic valve replacement with either a stented Hancock II bioprosthesis or a stentless Toronto SPV demonstrated a significant reduction in cardiac mortality and valve-related morbidity in those who received the Toronto SPV. Actuarial survival at 8 years for the Hancock II group was 69% compared with 91% for the Toronto SPV. The authors attributed this improved survival to better resolution of left ventricular hypertrophy in the stentless group.

A small randomized trial compared left ventricular mass reduction in adult patients who underwent aortic valve replacement with an allograft aortic valve versus patients receiving stentless bioprostheses. No difference in

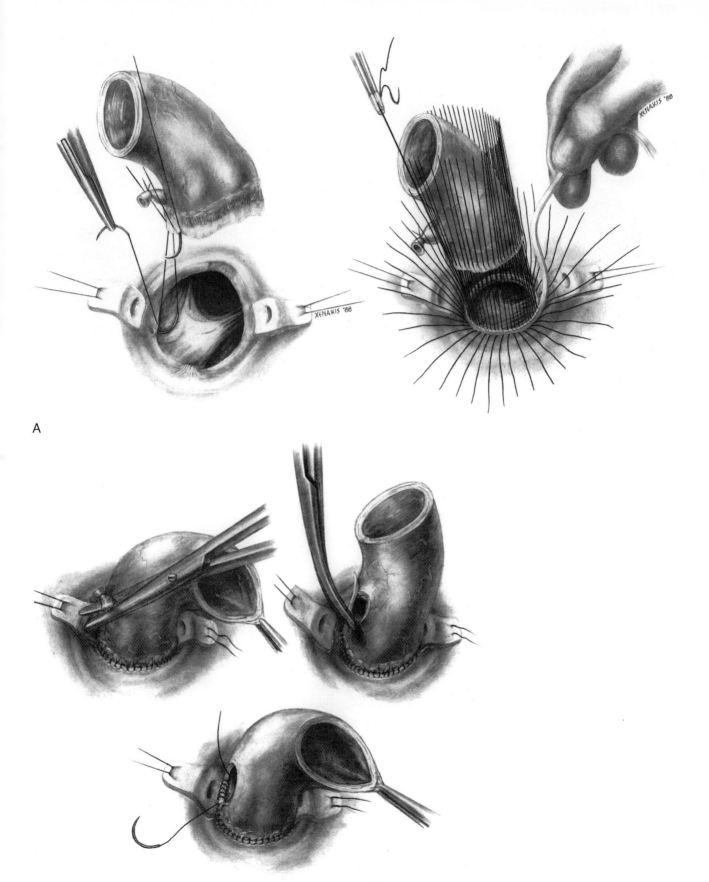

Figure 2
(A) Total aortic root replacement with aortic allograft. **(B)** Completion of total aortic root replacement with reimplantation of coronary arteries.

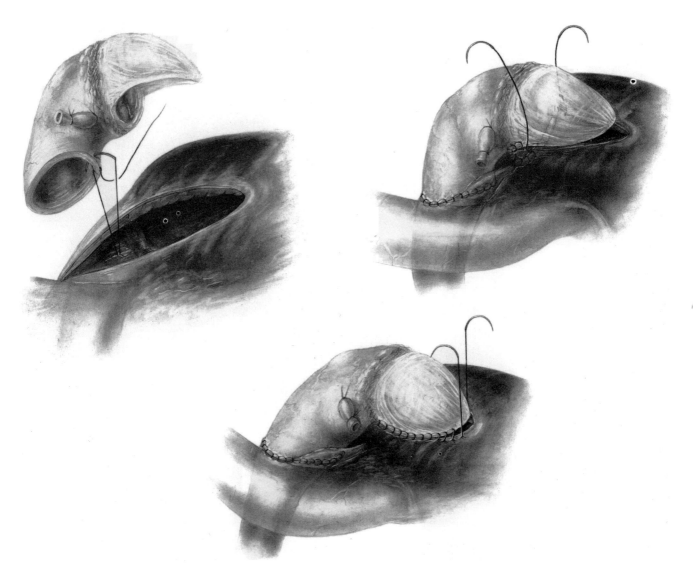

Figure 3
Right ventricular outflow tract reconstruction with aortic allograft.

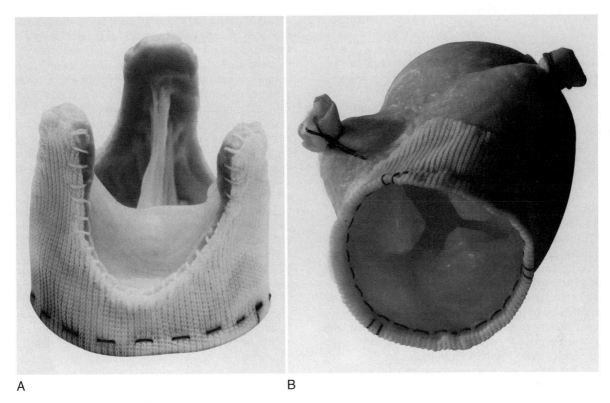

A   B

Figure 4
(A) Toronto SPV bioprosthesis. **(B)** Medtronic Freestyle stentless bioprosthesis.

left ventricular mass regression was detected between the groups. Long-term follow-up for stentless bioprosthetic valves is lacking; however, freedom from reoperation secondary to valvular failure for the Toronto SPV is reported to be 97.2% at 6 years in one series of 621 patients with freedom from prosthetic valve endocarditis of 98.6%.

The techniques for stentless bioprosthetic valve implantation are similar to those illustrated above for "free-hand" allograft aortic valve placement. Appropriate valve sizing of the stentless valves is crucial to adequate valve function. Both commercially available models require sizing of the valve at the sinotubular junction. If the sinotubular junction is much smaller than the aortic annulus, excessive coaptation of the leaflets will occur resulting in an increased transvalvular gradient. If the sinotubular is more than one size larger than the annulus, the valve may be splayed outward, resulting in valvular incompetence.

Clinical situations in which the stentless bioprosthetic valve should be considered include patients with a small aortic root who are being considered for bioprosthetic valve replacement. Relative contraindications to stentless valves include patient age less than 30 years and those with heavily calcified aortas.

■ MECHANICAL PROSTHESES

Mechanical prostheses have superior durability over bioprostheses in children, but they lack growth potential and necessitate chronic anticoagulation with sodium warfarin. Lesser anticoagulation regimens in general have not been successful. Repeated venipuncture for anticoagulation monitoring, hemmorrhagic complications, the inevitability of fibrous ingrowth in and about the prostheses, and the low but real risk of thromboembolism and endocarditis make mechanical prostheses unattractive for most infants and children, but nonetheless their use may be necessary, especially in severe mitral disease in early childhood.

SUGGESTED READING

Hopkins RA: Left ventricular outflow tract reconstructions. In *Cardiac reconstructions with allograft valves.* New York, 1989, Springer-Verlag, pp 98-99.

Ibawi MN, et al: Valve replacement in children: guidelines for selection of prosthesis and timing of surgical intervention, *Ann Thorac Surg* 44:398, 1987.

Jonas RA, et al: Long-term follow-up of patients with synthetic right heart conduits, *Circulation* 72(Suppl II):II-77, 1985.

PALLIATIVE OPERATIONS FOR CONGENITAL HEART DISEASE

Duke Cameron

Luca A. Vricella

Palliative operations for congenital heart disease still play a vital role in the management of congenital heart disease, even though early total correction surgery has really grown in acceptance and practice. There are several heart defects for which early palliation followed by delayed total correction is still optimal, and some defects such as single ventricle are not amenable to total correction. Although conceptually simple, palliative operations may be technically challenging, and the postoperative management of palliated children in some respects is more complex and higher risk than those after total correction. Incomplete separation of the circulations means that the surgeon, anesthesiologist, intensivist, and cardiologist must cooperatively manage the balance of systemic and pulmonary blood flow postoperatively.

Ligation of the patent ductus aside, most of the early operations performed for congenital heart disease were palliative procedures. In 1944, Blalock's construction of a systemic-to-pulmonary artery shunt to augment pulmonary blood flow for cyanosis heralded exciting possibilities for intervention in heart disease. Conversely, pulmonary artery banding to restrict excessive pulmonary blood flow was reported by Muller in the early 1950s and gave surgeons another means by which to balance the circulations. Blalock and Hanlon's atrial septectomy to improve mixing of oxygenated and desaturated blood added to the complement of surgical options.

The majority of palliative operations are designed to correct an imbalance between systemic and pulmonary blood flow and thus provide adequate oxygenation in the systemic circulation without excessive volume overload to the ventricles and without damage to the pulmonary vascular bed from excessive flow or pressure (Figure 1).

■ SYSTEMIC-TO-PULMONARY ARTERY SHUNTS

Most cyanotic heart lesions are characterized by inadequate pulmonary blood flow, the classic defect being tetralogy of Fallot (ventricular septal defect with infundibular or valvar pulmonic stenosis). Lesions such as simple tetralogy can be repaired at nearly any age and any weight above 1 to 1.5 kg. Early total correction is the preferred treatment. Small body size is not necessarily sufficient reason for a shunt rather than correction, as shunt construction in the very small infant is at least as problematic as intracardiac repair. At the other end of the spectrum of indications, lesions characterized by absence of two functionally adequate ventricles (such as

tricuspid atresia and hypoplastic left heart syndrome) must be managed in a staged approach because the high pulmonary vascular resistance of infancy precludes immediate establishment of the Fontan circulation. If such a lesion is associated with cyanosis due to inadequate pulmonary blood flow, a systemic-to-pulmonary artery shunt is indicated. Between simple tetralogy and single ventricle, there are a number of other lesions for which use of a shunt versus early correction is controversial and the decision must be individualized. Factors to consider include need for complex intracardiac repairs or baffles, other medical conditions, use of conduits (which are incapable of growth), and uncertainty about eventual two-ventricle repair. Examples of these lesions include tetralogy with pulmonary atresia or anomalous left anterior descending coronary artery across the right ventricular outflow tract, double-outlet right ventricle with pulmonic stenosis (unless the ventricular septal defect [VSD] is subaortic and the lesion is akin to simple tetralogy), and transposition with VSD and pulmonic stenosis.

Shunts have evolved significantly over the nearly 60 years of clinical experience. The classic Blalock-Taussig (BT) shunt (Figure 1, A) was performed via thoracotomy, typically on the side opposite the aortic arch (usually right thoracotomy), and used the divided and turned-down subclavian artery, which was anastomosed end-to-side to the pulmonary artery. Advantages are avoidance of prosthetic material and thus the possibility of growth, which was particularly important in the era before total correction. Disadvantages are arm ischemia in older children, tendency toward kinking of the shunt if performed on the side of the aortic arch, unpredictable results in small infants because of the diminutive arterial anastomoses, and sometimes uncontrollable late pulmonary overcirculation if the subclavian artery dilates. In large part, the classic BT shunt has been replaced by the

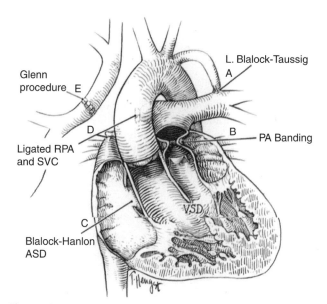

Figure 1

Palliative operations for congenital heart disease. (*From Hallman GL, et al, editors: Surgical treatment of congenital heart disease. Philadelphia, 1987, Lippincott Williams & Wilkins.*)

modified BT shunt (MBTS), in which a polytetrafluoroethylene (PTFE) graft is interposed between either subclavian artery and the pulmonary artery. The MBTS is technically easier to perform, does not sacrifice the subclavian artery, and is easier to take down later because the dissection plane around the graft is easier to enter. Late overcirculation does not occur; rather the converse is true: it has no potential for growth and therefore provides palliation of limited durability. However, this is no longer a significant concern because total correction (or conversion to a bidirectional cavopulmonary shunt or Fontan procedure) usually proceeds within the "life span" of the shunt. Increasingly, the MBTS is being performed via median sternotomy rather than thoracotomy; when coupled with complex cardiac or aortic reconstructions, the reason is obvious, but there are advantages to median sternotomy even in "closed" shunt procedures. These advantages include superior exposure of the systemic and pulmonary arteries without lung retraction, less injury to phrenic and recurrent laryngeal nerves at shunt construction and during shunt takedown, ability to institute cardiopulmonary bypass emergently for life-threatening hypoxia if necessary, and better access for ductus arteriosus ligation.

Several forms of "central" aortopulmonary shunts have had transient success but are rarely used today. The Potts shunt, in which the descending thoracic aorta is anastomosed side-to-side to the left pulmonary artery via left thoracotomy, was complicated by difficulty in controlling shunt flow and, in particular, the hazards of shunt takedown, namely hemorrhage and air embolism. Pulmonary artery scarring and distortion were also frequent and unfortunately difficult to treat where they occurred distally in the pulmonary artery. The counterpart of the Potts shunt in the ascending aorta, the Waterston shunt, anastomosed the ascending aorta side-to-side with the right pulmonary artery. It shared the limitations of the Potts shunt, although not as severely. Both shunts have been abandoned except that a "modified Waterston" is sometimes performed with a short PTFE graft. When a central shunt is preferred, particularly when the branch pulmonary arteries are very small (<3 mm), use of a short, small-caliber PTFE graft to the pulmonary artery confluence may be advisable. The proximal end of the shunt may arise from the ascending aorta, innominate, carotid, or subclavian arteries.

All systemic-to-pulmonary artery shunts improve oxygenation by improving pulmonary blood flow, but they do so at the expense of volume overload to the left (or systemic) ventricle. The improvement in oxygenation is small compared with the increase in ventricular volume work because of mixing of the systemic and pulmonary venous returns. These considerations conspire to make these shunts undesirable for long-term palliation, particularly when there is only one functional ventricle whose function must be well preserved over time. As a rule, it is optimal to move to a "venous shunt" as defined later within 6 months of age when there is one functioning ventricle and within 1 to 2 years of age, if not sooner, when there are two functioning ventricles.

■ VENOUS SHUNTS

"Venous" shunts improve oxygenation and pulmonary blood flow by directing part or all of the systemic venous return directly to the pulmonary bed. This is a highly efficient form of oxygenation but requires a low-resistance pulmonary vascular bed so that lung perfusion and thus cardiac output can be maintained at low central venous pressure. These conditions are not met until 3 to 4 months of age in the normal infant.

The first venous shunt was the classic Glenn procedure (Figure 1, E). The divided right superior vena cava (SVC) was anastomosed end-to-end with the divided right pulmonary artery. This shunt produced a substantial improvement in pulmonary blood flow and oxygenation and also conferred potential for growth, as it incorporated only viable autologous tissue. Many patients received decades of good palliation with classic Glenn shunts. Limitations of the classic Glenn are that it cannot be performed in the first 3 to 4 months of infancy because of elevated pulmonary vascular resistance, it augments blood flow to only one lung, and it is frequently complicated by late development of pulmonary arteriovenous fistulas, resulting in recurrent hypoxemia. The cause of the fistulas remains unclear, but two theories hold that either (1) the absence of an ill-defined "hepatic factor" created when hepatic venous blood no longer perfuses the lung or (2) loss of pulsatile pulmonary blood flow leads to emergence of the fistulas. Reversal of the fistulas after recruitment of hepatic blood flow by either a systemic shunt or diversion of inferior vena cava (IVC) flow to the pulmonary artery has been observed repeatedly and supports the former hypothesis.

Another limitation of the Glenn shunt is gradual hypoxemia resulting from development of venovenous collaterals (usually from SVC to IVC) that "decompress" the higher-pressure SVC and worsen the right-to-left shunt. This compounds the hypoxemia resulting from growth of the patient from an infant in whom SVC flow is a larger component of cardiac output than in adults, and thus the proportion of pulmonary blood flow decreases with age.

The bidirectional Glenn shunt (BDG) was introduced to allow blood to flow bidirectionally to both lungs and encourage symmetric pulmonary artery growth. Total pulmonary blood flow is not necessarily greater than with a classic Glenn, but if there is some antegrade blood flow from the right ventricle, development of pulmonary arteriovenous fistulas may be avoided because the right pulmonary artery is not divided. However, in the absence of antegrade pulmonary blood flow, these fistulas may occur in both lungs. The BDG and its modification, the hemi-Fontan, are part of the Fontan management pathway for various forms of single ventricle heart defects and are typically offered at about 6 months of age, when pulmonary vascular resistance is low enough to accept SVC flow without elevated central venous pressure (<15 mm Hg). They typically provide systemic arterial saturation of 80% to 85%, and sometimes even higher in the presence of some antegrade pulmonary blood flow.

Another advantage of the BDG is its ability to straddle and thereby correct pulmonary artery distortion and scarring when the BDG is placed at the site of a previous MBTS.

■ PULMONARY ARTERY BANDING

Some congenital heart defects result in excessive pulmonary blood flow and lead to congestive heart failure, poor growth, and eventual development of pulmonary vascular disease.

Most of these lesions have a VSD and little or no pulmonary outflow obstruction. Although the majority are conducive to early correction, several are not: multiple muscular VSDs, unbalanced atrioventricular canal (or atrioventricular septal defect), and a variety of single-ventricle lesions such as double-outlet right ventricle with mitral stenosis or atresia, double-inlet left ventricle, and even some forms of tricuspid atresia. In these settings, early control of excessive pulmonary blood flow is critical to protect the pulmonary vascular bed and ventricular mass until total correction or staged palliation with a cavopulmonary anastomosis can be performed. Rarely, some children with correctable lesions but with a severe intercurrent illness such as respiratory syncytial viral pneumonia are better managed with pulmonary artery banding and early definitive repair after resolution of the illness.

Pulmonary artery banding (Figure 1, B) limits pulmonary blood flow and attempts to balance systemic and pulmonary blood flow, but it does so at the risk of right ventricular hypertension and distortion of the branch pulmonary artery origins and even the pulmonary valve itself. Furthermore, in lesions in which the infundibular (or conal) septum is displaced posteriorly, such as interrupted aortic arch, pulmonary artery banding may aggravate the left ventricular outflow tract obstruction.

Although a pulmonary artery band should not stretch, some "loosening" of the band is often seen after surgery. Acute placement of the band causes infolding of the main pulmonary artery wall, but over the early months after banding, there is resorption of these folds and an increase in effective lumen at the band site. This, in addition to the natural fall in pulmonary vascular resistance that occurs in early infancy, may lead to recurrent pulmonary overcirculation.

■ MIXING PROCEDURES

Some cyanotic cardiac lesions have normal or even increased pulmonary blood flow but, because of atrioventricular or ventriculo-arterial discordance, have transposition physiology, that is, nearly parallel rather than serial pulmonary and systemic circulations. Of course, transposition of the great arteries with intact ventricular septum is this situation in the extreme. Palliation is achieved not by increasing or decreasing pulmonary blood flow but rather by encouraging mixing of the circulations to increase systemic arterial saturation. The Blalock-Hanlon septostomy (Figure 1, C) was the first surgical procedure to accomplish this; it was an ingenious procedure in which a side-biting clamp excluded the right lateral aspect of the right and left atria and enabled a right atriotomy and septal excision without use of cardiopulmonary bypass. Unfortunately, it carried a high operative mortality and was technically difficult in small infants. It gave way to catheter procedures (Rashkind septostomy, with or without a catheter blade incision in the septum). Today, catheter septostomy is most commonly performed in neonates with transposition of the great arteries and intact ventricular septum as a prelude and stabilizing maneuver before the arterial switch, although institutional preferences dictate whether this is a routine procedure. Open (on cardiopulmonary bypass) atrial septectomy is a routine component of the first-stage palliation for

hypoplastic left heart syndrome and is still occasionally required in the setting of mitral atresia or critical mitral stenosis and single ventricle when the atrial septum is intact or the atrial septal defect is restrictive.

When cyanosis is due to streaming at the ventricular level (double-outlet ventricle with subpulmonary VSD), early total correction is the best option, as improving atrial level mixing is unlikely to yield benefit.

■ TECHNICAL CONSIDERATIONS

As with all pediatric cardiac procedures, meticulous attention to detail and a thorough understanding of the patient's anatomy and physiology are the sine qua non of a successful operation. Administration of supplemental oxygen must be judicious; although it confers safety in cyanosis, it may drop pulmonary vascular resistance and lead to cardiovascular collapse when there is severe pulmonary overcirculation. An arterial monitoring catheter, a pulse oximeter, and a central venous line are useful; the latter may be placed directly into the right atrium in neonates and small infants who will eventually require cavopulmonary anastomoses, to avoid internal jugular or SVC thrombosis. In our practice, virtually all children undergo median sternotomy for these procedures, unless the pulmonary artery banding is concomitant with coarctation repair via thoracotomy.

Partial thymectomy and a limited upper pericardial incision provide adequate exposure yet minimize pericardial adhesions and risk of myocardial injury at subsequent sternal reentry. Shunts are typically placed at the undersurface of the right subclavian/innominate artery junction using a side-biting clamp. Most infants receive a 3.5-mm PTFE shunt. Very small infants (<3.5 kg) may be better served by 3-mm stents, and larger infants, a 4- or even a 5-mm stent. The optimal shunt size will also depend on alternate sources of pulmonary blood flow. It is our practice to administer heparin (50 units/kg), and not reverse it with protamine at the close of the procedure. It is useful to measure and cut the shunt before clamps are applied and to use fine polypropylene marking sutures on the proximal and distal extent of both the subclavian and pulmonary artery anastomotic sites to maintain proper orientation. After the subclavian clamp is applied, the anesthesiologist should be asked to palpate the contralateral carotid for pulsation, as the carotid origin can become kinked by the clamp and compromise cerebral perfusion. The cephalad anastomosis is performed with 7-0 polypropylene, and the clamp on the graft is briefly released to ensure good inflow before completing the pulmonary arterial anastomosis. If a large ductus arteriosus is present, consideration should be given to ligating it to avoid early postoperative overcirculation or worse, competitive flow, and shunt thrombosis. We administer heparin (10 units/kg/hr) for 72 hours beginning 12 hours postoperatively and continue aspirin until the shunt is taken down. Saturations in the low 80s (on room air or minimal FIO_2) are generally sought, although lower saturations may be preferable in HLHS.

The BDG shunt is usually performed via sternotomy and may be constructed without cardiopulmonary bypass if there are alternate sources of pulmonary blood flow. The ipsilateral MBTS must be sacrificed before placing the BDG. A central venous catheter is useful for postoperative monitoring but should be removed within 1 or 2 days to minimize risk of thrombosis. It is important to ligate and divide the azygous (or hemiazygous) vein to prevent hypoxemia from diversion of pulmonary blood flow to the IVC. The cavopulmonary anastomosis is prone toward purse-stringing, which can be avoided by use of interrupted sutures or by a continuous nonabsorbable suture with intermittent locking of the suture. We do not heparinize or treat BDG shunts with aspirin.

For pulmonary artery banding, the same anesthetic and monitoring considerations apply. Ligation of the ductus or its remnant should be routine in all patients under 6 months of age, as reopening of the ductus may occur after pulmonary artery pressure falls. The main pulmonary artery is encircled with a silicone-coated Teflon tape using the subtraction technique and dissection is limited to the area directly affected by the band. This is to reduce the potential for band migration as well as to simplify dissection at later operations. A useful guide for determining band tightness is Trusler's rule: the children's weight in kilograms plus 20 equals band circumference in millimeters. The band may be further tightened or loosened according to the patient's degree of mixing, right ventricular strain, or pulmonary congestion and vascular resistance. Physiologic end points include an arterial saturation approximately 80% on FiO_2 of 0.2-0.3 and pulmonary artery pressure less than half systemic. Systemic arterial blood pressure typically rises 10-15 mm Hg with band tightening. The band should be fixed to itself with a pledgeted horizontal mattress suture, as simple sutures may tear through the band material. The band should also be fixed to the proximal pulmonary adventitia to prevent distal migration. An aphorism states that all bands are perfect in the operating room and all are either too loose or too tight by the time the child returns to the intensive care unit.

■ ATRIAL SEPTECTOMY

The risks attending cardiopulmonary bypass are so low today that open septectomy is preferred over closed surgical procedures. The septum primum and secundum are excised completely; unroofing the coronary sinus into the left atrium may reduce the risk of recurrent restriction, but care must be taken to avoid the atrioventricular node. In some instances, a catheter septectomy may suffice.

■ RESULTS

Operative risk for palliative procedures is frequently higher than for total correction, reflecting not the complexity of the operative procedure but rather the precarious balance of circulation following palliation and sometimes the extenuating circumstances that raise perioperative risk, such as low birth weight, other concurrent illnesses, and ventricular hypoplasia. Risks are particularly high when complex cardiac repairs are coupled with palliative shunts, especially when the pulmonary blood flow is completely shunt dependent. Operative mortality rates for shunts and bands are frequently 5% to 10%, although for BDG procedures are usually well below 5%. Long-term results obviously depend more on the underlying cardiac malformation.

SUGGESTED READING

del Nido PJ, et al: Closed heart surgery for congenital heart disease in infancy, *Clin Perinatol* 15:681, 1988.

Gladman G, et al: The modified Blalock-Taussig shunt: clinical impact and morbidity in Fallot's tetralogy in the current era, *J Thorac Cardiovasc Surg* 114:25, 1997.

Perry SB, et al: Creation and maintenance of an adequate interatrial communication in left atrioventricular valve atresia or stenosis, *Am J Cardiol* 15:622, 1986.

Pizarro C, De Leval MR: Surgical variations and flow dynamics in cavopulmonary connections: a historical review, *Semin Thorac Cardiovasc Surg Pediatr Cardiac Surg Ann* 1:53, 1998.

Takayama H, et al: Mortality of pulmonary artery banding in the current era: recent mortality of PA banding, *Ann Thorac Surg* 74:1219, 2002.

CORONARY ARTERY DISEASE IN CHILDREN

Constantine Mavroudis
Carl L. Backer

Coronary artery disease in children can be congenital (anomalous origins of the coronary arteries, arteriovenous fistulas, and intramyocardial course) or acquired (Kawasaki disease or iatrogenic injury). The incidence of coronary anomalies in the general population is 0.2% to 1.2%. Although coronary anomalies are rare, they still present a diagnostic and surgical challenge to the cardiologist and congenital heart surgeon. This chapter describes the most common forms of coronary artery anomalies, the tools that are used to diagnose them, and surgical techniques that are recommended for repair.

■ ANOMALOUS LEFT CORONARY ARTERY FROM THE PULMONARY ARTERY

Anomalous left coronary artery from the pulmonary artery (ALCAPA) occurs in 1 out of 300,000 live births. It was described first by Brooks in 1885 and in greater detail by Bland et al in 1933. ALCAPA can cause myocardial ischemia, myocardial infarction, mitral insufficiency, congestive heart failure, and death in infancy. The degree to which cardiac signs and symptoms become manifest depends on intercoronary collaterals from the right coronary artery that provide adequate blood flow into the anomalous left coronary artery. In the past, two types of circulatory systems have been identified: an adult form and an infantile form. Patients with the adult type of circulation can be asymptomatic for many years. The infantile type of circulation has no collateral development, and symptoms can present within days to weeks after birth. In the current era, this classification no longer is used because operative intervention is recommended for all patients with ALCAPA.

Diagnostic Tools
Chest x-ray, electrocardiogram (ECG), two-dimensional echocardiography, and cardiac catheterization are considered to be the best diagnostic tools. Fast magnetic resonance angiography gives a more precise origin and proximal course in relation to the great vessels.

Surgical Technique
Our preferred surgical therapy was performed first in 1974 by Neches et al, when they reimplanted the anomalous left coronary artery into the aorta, establishing a two–coronary

artery anatomy. The conduct of the operation is by aortic and bicaval cardiopulmonary bypass followed quickly by antegrade or retrograde cardioplegia. Exposure is by pulmonary artery transection. A button of pulmonary artery is excised with the coronary artery for the implantation into the ascending aorta (Figure 1). The resulting defect in the pulmonary artery is reconstructed with a patch of pericardium.

Although patients with adult-type circulation may be asymptomatic for years, sudden death has been reported to occur at a mean age of 35 years. We recommend surgery as soon as ALCAPA is diagnosed. For patients who have unfavorable coronary anatomy, an operation was described by Takeuchi in 1979 in which a baffle of pulmonary artery tissue is used to reroute the ALCAPA into the aorta.

■ LEFT MAIN CORONARY ARTERY FROM RIGHT AORTIC SINUS OF VALSALVA

Left main coronary artery from right aortic sinus of Valsalva (LMCA from RASV) is the most serious anomaly of

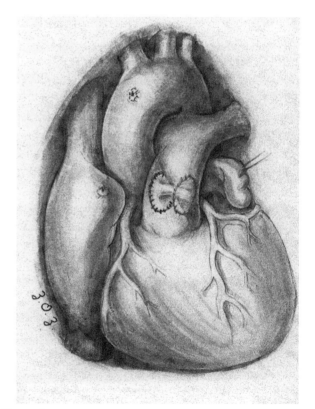

Figure 1
Aortic implantation of the anomalous left coronary artery from the pulmonary artery (ALCAPA) through a median sternotomy with extracorporeal circulation. The ALCAPA has been detached from the pulmonary artery with a button of pulmonary artery wall. This coronary button has been implanted into the left lateral side of the ascending aorta. (*From Backer CL, et al:* J Thorac Cardiovasc Surg 103:1049, 1992.)

coronary origin because it is associated with the highest incidence of sudden death. Symptoms include angina, congestive heart failure, syncope, and myocardial infarction. The rate of sudden death can be 30% in untreated patients, and 27.3% to 64% of deaths are related to exercise. The biggest dilemma that clinicians encounter is whether or not to operate on asymptomatic patients. Most authors agree, however, that because of the high incidence of sudden death even in asymptomatic patients, coronary surgery should be recommended.

Diagnostic Tool

Cardiac catheterization is considered to be the best diagnostic tool because it shows the right anterior oblique and lateral views.

Surgical Technique

The goal is to restore a normal anatomic position of the left coronary ostium or bypass an obstructed course using the internal thoracic artery. In 1982, Mustafa and Yacoub performed an anatomic ostial correction that consisted of opening the aortic root, incising the ostium of the LMCA, and unroofing it along the intramural segment to the midpoint of the LMCA sinus and detaching the intercoronary commissure. The intima of the LMCA is fixed to the aortic root, and the commissure is reattached to the aortic wall that brings the left main coronary ostium back to its natural position in the left aortic sinus of Valsalva. Alternatively, internal thoracic-to-coronary artery bypass can be performed. The long-term results of both these procedures have yet to be assessed.

■ RIGHT CORONARY ARTERY FROM LEFT AORTIC SINUS OF VALSALVA

Right coronary artery from left aortic sinus of Valsalva (RCA from LASV) represents 6% to 27% of all coronary anomalies. Although previously it was considered benign, it has been associated more recently with sudden death on exertion. Symptoms include angina, myocardial infarction, syncope, and high-grade atrioventricular block. Generally, ischemic symptoms should be present before surgery is advised.

Diagnostic Tool

Cardiac catheterization is considered to be the best diagnostic tool.

Surgical Technique

Bypass surgery is performed. If the right internal thoracic artery is used to bypass the aberrant right coronary artery, ligation of the right coronary artery at its origin is recommended.

■ ANOMALOUS CIRCUMFLEX CORONARY ARTERY FROM RIGHT AORTIC SINUS OF VALSALVA OR RIGHT CORONARY ARTERY

The occurrence of anomalous circumflex coronary artery from right aortic sinus of Valsalva or right coronary artery is 0.2% to 0.71%. Symptoms of sudden death are rare. In most cases, ischemic symptoms should be present before surgery is recommended.

Diagnostic Tool

Cardiac angiography in the right anterior oblique view is considered to be the best diagnostic tool.

Surgical Technique

Bypass surgery is performed with rotation of the proximal aorta to access the proximal circumflex artery and to perform the proximal anastomosis posteriorly on the aorta to avoid kinking.

■ SINGLE CORONARY ARTERY

The reported incidence of this anomaly is 0.04%. This is a rare anomaly that frequently is associated with complex congenital heart disease, such as transposition of the great arteries, tetralogy of Fallot, and truncus arteriosus. In 1950, Smith proposed the first classification of this anomaly: type 1—one artery supplying the entire heart, the other being absent, left or right in equal distribution; type 2—a single artery subdivides into two branches; type 3—other. Type 2 was subdivided further by Sharbaugh in 1974: type 2a—the branch that is the missing artery of origin passes anterior to the great vessels; type 2b—the branch that is the missing artery passes between the great vessels; type 2c—the branch that is the missing artery passes posterior to the great vessels. The most dangerous forms of single coronary artery are those in which the LMCA traverses between the aorta and pulmonary artery before it bifurcates. Under these circumstances, serious consideration should be given to coronary artery surgery to adjust the proximal course or to perform internal thoracic-to-coronary artery bypass.

Diagnostic Tool

Cardiac catheterization is considered to be the best diagnostic tool.

Surgical Technique

Surgery depends on the associated congenital defect and course of the single coronary artery.

■ CONGENITAL ATRESIA OF THE LEFT MAIN CORONARY ARTERY

A single right coronary artery feeds the entire heart, but flow into the left anterior descending coronary artery (LAD) and into the circumflex coronary artery is retrograde, depending on collaterals from the right coronary artery. The pathophysiology is similar to that seen in the most severe forms of anomalous coronary artery takeoff from the pulmonary artery.

Diagnostic Tools

Two-dimensional echocardiography and coronary angiography are considered to be the best diagnostic tools.

Surgical Techniques

Bypass graft surgery of the LAD is performed with internal thoracic artery or proximal LMCA arterioplasty with pericardium or harvested pulmonary artery patch autograft.

■ CORONARY ARTERIOVENOUS FISTULAS

Coronary arteriovenous fistulas (CAVF) can be isolated or associated with other congenital heart defects, such as tetralogy of Fallot, atrial septal defect, patent ductus arteriosus, and ventricular septal defects. Infants and young children can present with signs and symptoms of congestive heart failure based on a large left-to-right shunt. More often than not, patients are asymptomatic, presenting with a typical murmur and signs of a left-to-right shunt, such as cardiomegaly and ECG changes. The absence of symptoms can persist until the second decade of life, when angina, dyspnea, congestive heart failure, arrhythmias, and fatigue begin to occur.

Diagnostic Tools

Chest x-ray, color flow Doppler echocardiography, and cardiac catheterization (Figure 2) are considered to be the best diagnostic tools.

Surgical Techniques

More than 50% of CAVFs can be treated without the use of cardiopulmonary bypass by epicardial dissection and selective ligation using intraoperative transesophageal echocardiography. Cardiopulmonary bypass and intracavitary ligation may be necessary for inaccessible lesions. Special attention is required for lesions that might cause distal coronary artery occlusion when the fistula is ligated. Internal thoracic artery-to-coronary artery bypass may be required. Success with coil occlusion has changed operative indications. Even so, approximately 50% of all CAVFs require operative intervention based on location, proximity to distal coronary arteries, and patient size.

■ INTRAMYOCARDIAL COURSE OF CORONARY ARTERIES (BRIDGING)

The general estimated incidence of intramyocardial course of coronary arteries (bridging) in the general population is 5.4% to 85.7%. Symptoms begin to appear in individuals in their 30s. This anomaly is associated with hypertrophic cardiomyopathy, ischemic cardiomyopathy, idiopathic cardiomyopathy, mitral valve prolapse, and muscular subaortic stenosis. Rarely, coronary artery bridging can cause angina and myocardial infarction in children.

Diagnostic Tools

Four classification systems for coronary artery bridging have been proposed over 50 years. In 1951, Geringer proposed the first classification based on autopsy reports: type 1—LAD deep in the interventricular groove with a circumferential muscle bridge; type 2—muscle bridge from trigonum fibrosum "investing the LAD" as it passes toward the apex.

In 1976, Noble proposed an angiographic classification: group 1—less than 50% narrowing of the LAD; group 2—50% to 75% narrowing; group 3—more than 75% narrowing. Kramer devised a variation (also based on angiographic studies) of Noble's classification in 1982: group 1—less than 30% narrowing; group 2—31% to 50%; group 3—51% to 100% narrowing. The latest classification scheme (based on autopsy studies) was proposed in 1991 by Ferreira et al and is based on Geringer's classification: type 1 hearts—a superficial bridge crosses the artery transversely toward the apex of the heart; type 2 hearts—the bridge crosses the LAD, surrounds the vessel by a bundle, arises from the right ventricular apical trabeculae, crosses the vessel, and terminates in the interventricular septum.

Surgical Technique

Surgical myotomy is performed on cardiopulmonary bypass.

■ CORONARY ANEURYSMS

The incidence of coronary aneurysms has been reported to be 0.3% to 4.9%. Coronary aneurysms are more common in males. They can be acquired or congenital. Symptoms include angina, congestive heart failure, and myocardial infarction. There are two classification systems of aneurysms. Markis in 1976 devised the following angiographic classification: Type 1 has diffuse ectasia of two to three vessels, type 2 has diffuse ectasia in one vessel, and type 4 has localized ectasia in one vessel. The Coronary Artery Surgery Study proposed another classification in patients who have coronary artery disease. Group A patients have an aneurysm but no coronary artery disease. In group B patients, an aneurysm is present in association with coronary artery disease, but less than 70% stenosis. In group C patients, an aneurysm is present with coronary artery disease and more than 70% stenosis. Acquired coronary aneurysms frequently are caused by Kawasaki disease.

Diagnostic Tools

ECG, echocardiography, and angiography are considered to be the best diagnostic tools.

Surgical Technique

Coronary artery bypass graft surgery using the internal thoracic artery is used for symptomatic patients or in asymptomatic patients who have had documented progression of coronary artery stenotic lesions.

■ CORONARY ANEURYSMS IN KAWASAKI DISEASE

Kawasaki disease is one of the leading causes of acquired heart disease in infants, children, and teenagers. Kato et al divided patients with Kawasaki disease into four groups. Group I comprises Kawasaki patients who have regression of aneurysm, no symptoms, no ECG changes, and a negative thallium test; group II consists of patients with an unobstructed aneurysm; group III patients have an obstructed

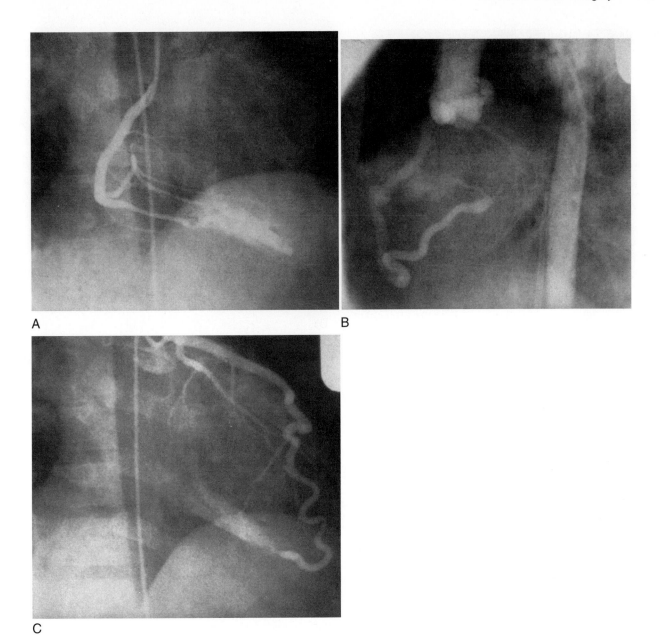

A

B

C

Figure 2

A and **B,** Selective right coronary artery angiogram (right anterior oblique/left anterior oblique view) shows drainage of the posterior descending coronary artery to the right ventricular apex through a coronary artery fistula. Note the enlarged right coronary artery. **C,** Selective left coronary artery angiogram (left anterior oblique view) shows drainage of the left anterior descending coronary artery to the right ventricular cavity through a coronary artery fistula. Note the enlarged left anterior descending coronary artery. (*From Zales VR, et al: In Mavroudis C, Backer CL, editors:* Pediatric cardiac surgery, *ed 2. St. Louis, 1994, Mosby-Year Book.*)

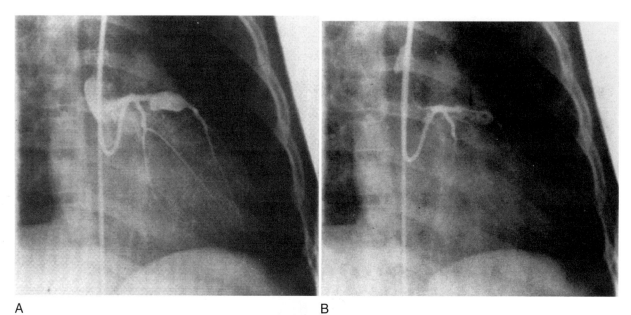

A   B

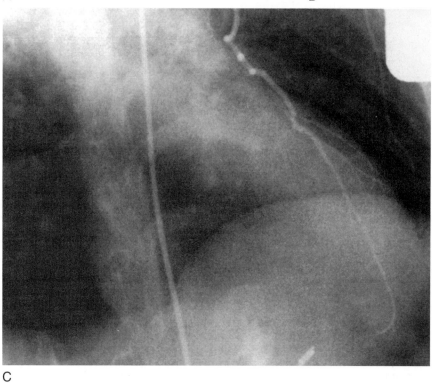

C

Figure 3
A, Selective left coronary artery angiogram in a patient with Kawasaki's disease shows a giant aneurysm of the left anterior descending coronary artery (LAD). **B,** Follow-up left coronary artery angiogram 2 years later shows thrombosis of the giant aneurysm with only a small jet of antegrade flow in the distal LAD *(arrow)*. **C,** Postoperative left subclavian artery angiogram shows a patent internal mammary artery bypass graft to the left coronary artery for the patient in Figure 2B, with near-occlusion of the LAD. (*From Zales VR, et al: In Mavroudis C, Backer CL, editors:* Pediatric cardiac surgery, *ed 2. St. Louis, 1994, Mosby-Year Book.*)

aneurysm; and group IV patients have a nonstenotic irregular arterial wall. Aneurysms develop in approximately 20% of patients; they can be treated with intravenous gamma globulin. Patients who develop giant aneurysms can be at risk for myocardial infarction, arrhythmia, and sudden death.

Diagnostic Tools
Echocardiography and cardiac catheterization (Figure 3) are considered to be the best diagnostic tools.

Surgical Techniques
Coronary artery bypass (internal thoracic artery to coronary artery), saphenous vein bypass, and angioplasty are performed.

SUGGESTED READING

Backer CL, et al: Anomalous origin of the left coronary artery: a twenty-year review of surgical management, *J Thorac Cardiovasc Surg* 103:1049, 1992.

Dodge-Khatami A, et al: Congenital Heart Surgery Nomenclature and Database Project: anomalies of the coronary arteries, *Ann Thorac Surg* 69(Suppl):S270, 2000.

Mavroudis C, et al: Coronary artery fistulas in infants and children: a surgical review and discussion of coil embolization, *Ann Thorac Surg* 63:1235, 1997.

Mavroudis C, et al: Expanding indications for pediatric coronary artery bypass, *J Thorac Cardiovasc Surg* 111:181, 1996.

ATRIAL SEPTAL DEFECTS

Mark W. Turrentine

The advent of open-heart repair for intracardiac defects dates back to 1953, when Gibbon first used a pump oxygenator to close an atrial septal defect (ASD). This novel approach became the foundation on which modern-day cardiac surgery evolved, and its use quickly outdated "closed" ASD repair techniques. ASDs were among the most straightforward and simple intracardiac defects to repair, and current surgical techniques vary little from those established decades ago. Evolutionary changes in the clinical practice of ASD repair focus on the use of less invasive surgical methods and catheter-based interventions.

■ ANATOMY AND EMBRYOLOGY

The atrial septum is developed from an infolding of the atrial roof, which develops into a thick superior atrial wall terminating as the superior limbus. The lower portion of the atrial septum is derived from the septum primum, which extends superiorly and leftward of the limbus. A patent foramen ovale allows right-to-left shunting but closes when the left atrial pressure rises to exceed right atrial pressure after birth. The lower edge of the septum primum normally fuses with the developing endocardial cushions to complete atrial septation in the embryo.

   Three basic types of defects occur in the atrial septum: ostium secundum (80%), sinus venosus (5% to 10%), and ostium primum (5%) (Figure 1). Ostium secundum defects

are among the most common cardiac malformations. They occur in 10% to 15% of all patients with congenital heart disease and present as isolated lesions in 3% to 5%. They occur twice as frequently in women than in men, and there are no known etiologic factors. Secundum defects are caused by developmental failure of the septum primum allowing for a range of sizes from the (1) small persistent foramen ovale, located superiorly; to (2) "typical" larger, 1- to 3-cm single or trabeculated defects, generally positioned centrally within the septum fossa ovalis; or (3) "inferior" defects extending down to the inferior vena cava (IVC). Sinus venosus defects occur at the junction of the superior vena cava (SVC) and right atrium, but may also extend inferiorly across the septum or present slightly remote to the atrial-caval junction. Typically, this defect is associated with anomalous drainage of the right upper and middle pulmonary veins. In most presentations, the SVC-atrial junction, pulmonary vein

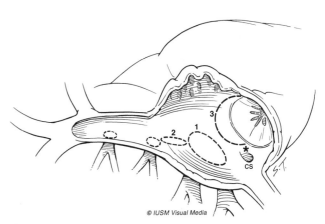
© IUSM Visual Media

Figure 1
Anatomic location of atrial septal defects and components: (1) secundum, (2) sinus venosus with typical location of anomalous pulmonary veins, (3) ostium primum. cs, coronary sinus. *Atrioventricular nodal area.

orifices, and ASD are intimately related. However, the location of the anomalous veins can be variable and may enter high in the SVC, or, less commonly, the right lower lobe pulmonary veins are anomalous and enter the IVC (scimitar syndrome). In rare cases, partial anomalous pulmonary venous return (PAPVR) can present as an isolated defect without an associated ASD.

The third basic type of ASD, the ostium primum defect (partial atrioventricular [AV] canal), is part of the spectrum of endocardial cushion defects. They account for approximately 5% of all ASDs and occur in 20% to 30% of children with trisomy 21. Other than this association with Down's syndrome, no other etiologic factors are known. This defect occurs as a result of incomplete development of the superior and inferior endocardial cushions resulting in a deficiency of atrial septum primum. It differs only from complete AV canal defects by the absence of an associated ventricular septal defect (VSD) and degree of valvar malformation. By definition, primum defects have an associated cleft (trileaflet) mitral valve, and 30% to 40% of patients exhibit moderate or severe insufficiency between the left superior and left inferior leaflets. Chordal attachments are to the leading edges of the valve leaflets and aid in determining landmarks for cleft repair. Anomalous chordae in partial AV canal and complete AV canal can attach to the ventricular septum, ultimately giving rise to left ventricular outflow tract obstruction. The defect can vary substantially in size and is crescent-shaped across the superior border. The inferior margin is defined by the annular demarcation between the tricuspid and mitral valves. The conduction system is displaced from its usual position in the triangle of Koch to a location bounded by the coronary sinus, the lower border of the septal defect, and the tricuspid valve, putting the AV node at risk during repair (see Figure 1).

A fourth category of ASDs includes two rare presentations: In one, the entire atrium septum fails to develop, giving rise to a "common atrium"; it often is associated with endocardial cushion defects. In the other, a small ASD may be present in the coronary sinus and is typically in the combination of a persistent left SVC and unroofed coronary sinus. The embryology and development of both unusual presentations are uncertain.

Although ASDs generally present as isolated lesions, associated defects include pulmonary stenosis, VSD, patent ductus arteriosus, mitral valve prolapse, and the spectrum of complex lesions dependent on interatrial shunting. Each type of isolated ASD possesses a distinct association with another specific cardiac defect: mitral stenosis (secundum ASD, Lutembacher's syndrome); PAPVR (sinus venosus ASD); and cleft mitral valve, with or without mitral insufficiency (primum defects).

■ PATHOPHYSIOLOGY

In the normal heart, left atrial pressure exceeds right atrial pressure, favoring a natural left-to-right shunt. In larger defects, the interatrial pressures equalize, and the direction of the shunt becomes dependent on compliance of the ventricles and pulmonary vascular resistance (PVR). Because of a difference in wall thickness (8 to 10 mm versus 4 to 5 mm),

the left ventricle (LV) is normally less compliant than the right ventricle (RV). This leads to left-to-right shunting when atrial pressures are otherwise similar. The ventricles are morphologically similar in the first 2 years of life, and the differences in compliance generally manifest beyond this age. Additionally, PVR is increased in the first year of life. As PVR drops, more interatrial shunting occurs. Both mechanisms account for limited atrial shunting early in life and delay clinical detection to a later age, generally beyond 1 to 2 years.

The natural history of ASDs shows they are relatively well-tolerated defects. But unlike VSDs, rarely close spontaneously. In contrast to intracardiac shunts that produce high pressure and volume pulmonary overcirculation (i.e., VSD, aortopulmonary window), ASDs rarely cause elevated PVR in the early years of life. Pulmonary hypertension is observed, however, in 15% to 20% of adult patients. In a third of these adult patients, pulmonary hypertension presents before age 20; in a third, it manifests in the 20s to 40s; and in the remaining third, beyond age 40 years. The increased PVR seems to be independent of age or shunt volume, but at its onset it rises rapidly and may not respond to surgical closure of the defect. In extreme cases, severe pulmonary hypertension results in irreversible pulmonary vasculopathy leading to "fixed" right-to-left shunting (Eisenmenger's syndrome). A form of "reversible" right-to-left shunting can occur transiently during exercise or in the third trimester of pregnancy, when there is increased intravascular volume and elevated right atrial pressures.

Most patients are asymptomatic, although pulmonary overcirculation may lead to dyspnea on extreme exertion and increased susceptibility to upper respiratory infection. Additionally, excessive pulmonary blood flow "steals" from the systemic circulation and may retard growth. Beyond 5 years of age, exercise capacity is decreased with a reduction in the ventilatory threshold. Undiagnosed secundum ASDs in adults reduce life expectancy to 50 years. Of patients, 75% die by age 50 and 90% by age 60. One mechanism of death is pulmonary hypertension (15% to 20%). Others die (15 to 20 years prematurely) of cardiac failure as a result of chronic right atrial and ventricular dilation, congestive heart failure, and dysrhythmia. Symptoms typically develop in individuals in their 20s to 30s. Patients with undiagnosed ostium primum defects die of severe mitral regurgitation or dysrhythmia at a mean age of 35 years.

Asymptomatic patients without cardiomegaly and who have pulmonary-to-systemic flow ratios 1.5 or less do not seem to be at risk for symptoms or pulmonary vascular obstructive disease. Development of elevated PVR, albeit rare, is unpredictable. Irreversible pulmonary vascular disease can occur in young patients with simple secundum ASDs and necessitate bilateral lung transplantation and ASD closure. As a result, all clinically significant ASDs are generally referred for elective surgical repair before 5 years of age or if patients exhibit signs and symptoms of pulmonary overcirculation or cardiomegaly. Patients diagnosed later in life undergo closure of the defect after evaluation of the pulmonary vascular bed. Adults presenting with embolic events but with otherwise small asymptomatic ASDs are a therapeutic dilemma. Although this is presumed to occur because of intermittent right-to-left shunting, ASD repair does not completely eliminate the risk of recurrent neurologic events.

■ CLINICAL FEATURES

Most patients can be diagnosed based on physical examination findings. Common symptoms are exertional dyspnea, fatigue, and palpitations. Infants are rarely symptomatic, but some may develop congestive heart failure, cardiomegaly, and failure to thrive. The defects may be large, with excessive left-to-right shunting, or be part of a complex of defects leading to early repair to control symptoms and improve growth. Dyspnea is more frequent in adults and results from either pulmonary hypertension or cardiac failure. Atrial dysrhythmias become frequent in the 30s secondary to right atrial hypertrophy or dilation and may complicate congestive heart failure. When established, these dysrhythmias may persist despite cardiac repair. Cyanosis, as a result of right-to-left shunting, is rare but can be the hallmark of irreversible pulmonary vasculopathy and hypertension.

The classic finding on physical examination is a soft systolic grade II/VI murmur along the left upper sternal border from increased flow across the pulmonary valve. In addition, prolonged emptying of a volume-overloaded right ventricle leads to asynchronous closure of the aortic and pulmonary valves and wide fixed splitting of the second heart sound.

Chest x-ray typically shows slight to moderate cardiac enlargement due to dilation of the right atrial and ventricular chambers and sometimes enlargement of the pulmonary artery. The lung fields may be relatively clear with prominence of the central pulmonary vasculature in simple defects, but primum ASDs show a dilated pulmonary artery with prominent pulmonary vascular markings. Patients with mitral insufficiency also may show left atrial enlargement.

Electrocardiogram (ECG) findings are right ventricular hypertrophy with right axis deviation and potential conduction abnormalities, such as a right bundle-branch block due to delayed right ventricular depolarization. Left axis deviation suggests an ostium primum defect. This ECG pattern is thought to be due to a primary abnormality of the conduction system because it persists after surgical repair.

Two-dimensional echocardiography has become the mainstay of diagnosis for virtually all forms of atrial septal anomalies. Findings include absence of echo in the septal region and right atrial or ventricular dilation and may include evidence of pulmonary venous drainage to an enlarged SVC or a cleft in the mitral valve, with or without regurgitation. Cardiac catheterization is important in patients with anomalous systemic or pulmonary venous return and in patients with suspected pulmonary hypertension or other lesions. One common finding on echocardiography and cardiac catheterization is a 10- to 30-mm Hg gradient across the right ventricular outflow tract due to the large volume of blood flow. After repair, these flow velocities return to normal.

■ SURGICAL TREATMENT

Indications and Contraindications

Surgery for uncomplicated secundum ASD generally is recommended for patients with defects 1 cm or larger in diameter or when the pulmonary-to-systemic blood flow (Qp:Qs) ratio exceeds 1.5:1. At our institution, we recommend repair of all sinus venosus and primum defects. When diagnosed in childhood, we prefer to repair the defect between ages 2 and 5 years, before development of exercise physiologic changes and before the start of school. Patients with delayed diagnosis generally are repaired as soon as practical, as are younger patients symptomatic from congestive heart failure or exhibiting growth failure. Studies have shown that repair before age 24 years results in long-term survival equal to that of age-matched and sex-matched controls. Patients who undergo repair later in life have significantly worse survival.

The single contraindication to repair is irreversible pulmonary hypertension, defined as PVR 8 to 12 U/m^2 and Qp:Qs less than 1.2:1. This rarely occurs before ages 40 to 50. Sporadic and unpredictable cases have been reported in younger patients, however. Patients who fall in the "gray area" of pulmonary hypertension and reversible/irreversible resistance have survived ASD repair, but the reduction in pulmonary pressure has been muted. Overall outcome in adults undergoing ASD repair depends on the degree of right heart chamber dilation or hypertrophy, pulmonary artery pressure, and presence of dysrhythmia.

Operative Technique

Cardiopulmonary bypass (CPB) is required for all types of ASD repair. The surgical approach varies, however. Standard techniques include median or transverse sternotomy, via vertical or bilateral inframammary incisions. Some surgeons favor right anterior lateral thoracotomy for cosmetic reasons, particularly in girls. One drawback is the difficulty in determining where the breast bud tissue is or will develop. Additionally, cardiac deairing procedures are more complicated compared with transsternal approaches. The selected technique should give adequate exposure of the defect.

My approach for these three standard defects is partial sternotomy except for high PAPVR defects. This allows for a short cosmetic vertical incision, which in most children is less than 2 inches in length. The sternum is divided in a caudad-to-cranial direction and generally does not extend into the manubrium. The sternum is pliable due to lack of ossification in the young, but adequate exposure is possible even in young teenagers. Avoiding division of the manubrium and leaving the thymus intact result in a hemostatic surgical field on completion of the procedure. The sternal retractor is placed with the blades at the low end of the sternum. The sternum is opened and the superior aspect of the skin incision can be retracted cephalad with a small retractor clamped to the cross member of the sternal retractor. The pericardium is opened longitudinally and reflected with stay sutures to the edges of the incision. General extracardiac inspection is performed to assess systemic and pulmonary venous return.

The right atrial appendage is used for IVC cannulation in all patients. After placement of this purse-string suture, the appendage can be reflected inferiorly and, along with retracting the aorta leftward, gives additional exposure to the SVC. A second venous purse-string suture is placed in the SVC near the atrial-caval junction for ostium primum defect repairs. For sinus venosus defects, the SVC is dissected to its junction with the innominate vein. Depending on the location of pulmonary veins entering into the cava, the SVC purse-string suture is positioned accordingly. For secundum defects, either the SVC or the atrial appendage can be used for the SVC venous drainage. A purse-string suture is placed in the ascending aorta, and after heparinization (400 U/kg), the patient undergoes aortic and bicaval cannulation. With a partial sternotomy approach, the patient occasionally is placed on CPB with one venous cannula to assist exposure of the SVC for cannulation. The patient is cooled (32°C for secundum defects; 28°C for all others), the heart is emptied, and either a left ventricular-apical or left atrial decompression line is inserted.

Hypothermic cardiac arrest is used with repeated doses of blood cardioplegia at 15- to 20-minute intervals. An insulation pad is placed posteriorly in most patients, and topical ice-cold saline is used for additional epicardial cooling. I prefer to use warm blood cardioplegia after the repair and transition to warm blood perfusion of the aortic root with the cross-clamp left in place. In combination with continuous nitroglycerin infusion initiated before CPB, this allows for improved regional coronary blood flow due to coronary vasodilation and controlled coronary perfusion pressure. After myocardial reanimation, the cross-clamp is released, and the coronary perfusion catheter is removed with the site left open for deairing. On rewarming to 35°C, the patient is weaned from CPB, and transesophageal echocardiography is performed to assess the repair in all but straightforward secundum ASD closures. All the patients undergo modified ultrafiltration followed by protamine reversal of heparin. Temporary epicardial pacing wires are applied when appropriate, and the mediastinum is drained with a single Blake drain unless the patient is coagulopathic. The lower portion of the sternum is closed with interrupted stainless steel wire, and the remainder of the incision is closed in multiple layers. Patients generally are extubated in the operating room, then taken to the intensive care unit. Initial pain control management is achieved in many patients with a caudal block and a parasternal 0.25% bupivacaine (Marcaine) regional block placed after sternal reapproximation.

Secundum Defect
After institution of CPB, the patient is cooled to 32°C, the left ventricle is decompressed, and the heart is arrested with cold blood cardioplegia after placement of the aortic cross-clamp. Caval tapes are applied, and an atriotomy is performed, extending from the atrial appendage toward the IVC parallel to the AV groove. I prefer to keep the incision high and limited in length to avoid extension into the midbody of the right atrium; this minimizes risk of injury to the sinoatrial node and crista terminalis and limits right atrial dysfunction and dysrhythmia postoperatively. Stay sutures are placed for exposure, and the intracardiac anatomy is assessed, including size and location of the secundum defect and coronary sinus, identification of the eustachian valve, presence of additional septal defects, and location of the pulmonary veins. If there is an indication of a gradient across the mitral valve by echocardiogram, inspection should include evaluation of the mitral valve.

Small defects and defects with redundant tissue can be closed primarily with 4-0 or 5-0 polypropylene suture for children and 3-0 suture for adults. Care is taken to avoid suture-line tension, which can lead to dehiscence of the closure. For most patients, the defect is closed with a pericardial

or Dacron felt patch using a continuous running suture technique with an appropriate size polypropylene suture (Figure 2). The decompression line is clamped, and left heart deairing occurs through the defect before completion of the suture line. A warm dose of cardioplegia is given followed by warm blood perfusion of the aortic root, during which time the atriotomy is closed with 4-0 or 5-0 absorbable monofilament suture.

Sinus Venosus Defect
After careful external cardiac evaluation and location of the anomalous pulmonary veins, the SVC cannula is positioned, and the patient is placed on CPB. For standard sinus venosus defects, I prefer to repair the defect via a transcaval approach. A longitudinal venotomy is performed along the superior aspect of the SVC extending from just inferior to the venous cannula down to, but not including, the atrial-caval junction. This avoids the sinoatrial node and its artery. Stay sutures are applied, and a small vein retractor is used inferiorly to gain exposure to the atrial septum. A 0.4-mm Gore-Tex cardiovascular patch is cut in an oblique teardrop fashion and sutured with 5-0 or 6-0 polytetrafluoroethylene (PTFE) suture around the inferior aspect of the associated ASD (Figure 3A). The suture line is brought up along the inferior aspect of the SVC and laterally around the ASD and pulmonary veins. The patch is made redundant to allow for adequate caliber of the pathway from the pulmonary vein orifices to the septal defect. Pericardium also can be used as the patch; however, Dacron should be avoided because it can develop a thick peel, narrowing the pathway and producing pulmonary venous obstruction.

If the ASD is remote to the pulmonary veins or is small, it can be enlarged so that the pathway is unrestrictive. In the rare circumstance when an associated ASD is not present, one can be created through the atrial septum near the septal-caval junction. The repair is finished with a teardrop 0.4-mm cardiovascular PTFE patch to augment the SVC (Figure 3B).

The same technique can be used for pulmonary veins that enter into the midportion of the SVC because the SVC generally has adequate caliber to accommodate an elongated tunnel patch. For patients exhibiting pulmonary veins entering into the high SVC, either a direct anastomosis of the

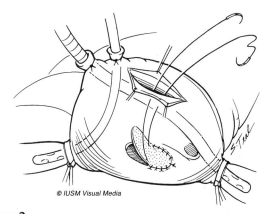

© IUSM Visual Media

Figure 2
Patch closure of secundum defect—bicaval cannulation with limited atriotomy.

Figure 3
Transcaval closure of sinus venosus defect: **A,** Polytetrafluoroethylene (or pericardial) baffle via anterior vena caval approach. **B,** Completed repair with superior vena cava augmentation.

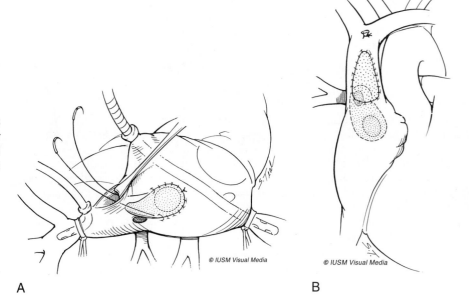

A   B

divided SVC to the atrial appendage is performed, or it is necessary to create a flap extension of the atrium to reach the inferior portion of the transected SVC (Figure 4A). The anterior wall is reconstructed with pericardium, creating a tunneled pathway to the body of the right atrium. In both cases, the SVC is oversewn, or patch-closed, just superior to the entry of the pulmonary veins. The intracardiac PTFE patch is positioned around the ASD and superolateral aspects of the SVC orifice to direct pulmonary blood flow from the SVC stump through the ASD (Figure 4B).

Ostium Primum Defects

For partial AV canals, extensive intracardiac inspection is carried out to confirm the anatomy as defined by echocardiography. The mitral valve is inspected carefully, and a small nerve hook is used to provide traction on the anterior leaflet to separate the left superior and inferior leaflets. The primary chordae attach to the leading edge of these two leaflets and help identify the extent and location of the cleft. The cleft is closed with multiple 5-0 or 6-0 PTFE sutures placed in horizontal mattress with pericardial pledgets (Figure 5A). I prefer PTFE suture because it is slightly elastic, soft, and easily covered with endothelium. Theoretically, this may allow some accommodation for mechanical and hemodynamic stresses, helping to protect the repair during cleft fibrosis. For most repairs, the cleft is completely closed, generally with three to four such sutures. If the mitral valve is hypoplastic and relatively competent, however, the cleft is not closed completely so as to avoid mitral stenosis. The valve can be tested for insufficiency by pressurizing the left ventricle with cold crystalloid solution through the apical decompression line. In adults, annular

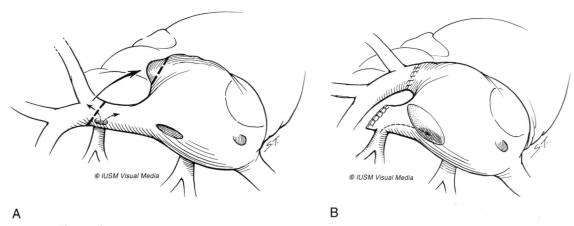

A   B

Figure 4
Cavoatrial repair of sinus venosus defect. **A,** Relationship of atrial septal defect and remote partial anomalous pulmonary venous return. **B,** Direct superior vena cava–atrial anastomosis with intracardiac baffle directing pulmonary venous blood flow *(arrow)* to the atrial septal defect.

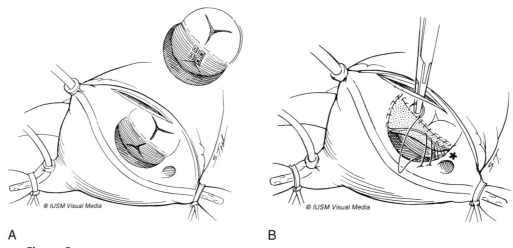

Figure 5
Ostium primum defect. **A,** Position of atriotomy and cleft closure. **B,** Orientation of intracardiac pericardial patch. *Location of coronary sinus and atrioventricular node.

dilation may have occurred requiring the addition of an annuloplasty ring.

A fresh pericardial patch is procured and cut to the general configuration of the septal defect. The leading edge is anchored to the base of the mitral cleft with a horizontal 4-0 or 5-0 polypropylene suture depending on the size of the patient. This suture is run in a simple continuous fashion along the annular interface between the tricuspid and mitral valves. As the suture line approaches the area of the AV node, the suture is passed through the base of the mitral leaflet in a horizontal mattress fashion paralleling the annulus. The pericardial patch is secured to the base of the mitral valve, then transitioned onto the left aspect of the septal wall before transitioning back into a full-thickness bite of the septum (Figure 5B). Superiorly the suture line continues along the annular interface and transitions onto the atrial septum. The suture line is completed after deairing of the left heart.

A more classic alternative technique is to extend the suture line along the base of the tricuspid lateral to the coronary sinus, then bring the patch over to the ridge of the septal defect, leaving the coronary sinus to drain to the left side of the heart. Our technique of leaving the coronary sinus on the right side of the heart has not resulted in a higher incidence of AV conduction abnormalities than the classic approach.

■ TECHNICAL PITFALLS

Persistent Intracardiac Shunting

Perioperative cyanosis can occur as a result of persistent intracardiac shunting after repair. A classic board examination question describes a patient who is cyanotic in the recovery room after ASD repair. This complication is the result of suturing the ASD patch to the eustachian valve and diverting IVC blood flow to the left atrium. In such occurrences, the lower edge of large or low-lying secundum ASDs may be difficult to visualize. It is imperative that the orifice of the IVC is fully identified and kept to the right side of the

septal repair. In patients with azygos continuation of the IVC, the degree of right-to-left shunting via the hepatic vein would be tolerable, but hepatic blood flow must remain in the pulmonary circuit to avoid development of pulmonary arteriovenous malformations. A combination of extracardiac and intracardiac inspection establishes the location of the hepatic vein confluence in relation to the pulmonary veins, and the repair proceeds accordingly. Transatrial cannulation of the IVC (or hepatic vein confluence) separates the ASD from the eustachian valve, maintains proper orientation, and prevents misinterpretation of the valve as the inferior rim of the defect. For patients who undergo direct IVC cannulation, one must be vigilant to identify the septal defect margins and associated intracardiac structures.

Multiple septal defects are another source of postoperative residual right-to-left shunts. The entire septal area must be inspected before repair, and if multiple defects are remote to one another, they are repaired individually. More commonly, there is a fenestrated thin tissue, however, septating the defect. This tissue should be removed and a single patch repair performed.

An additional cause of persistent intraatrial shunting is the "partially unroofed coronary sinus." This defect is suspected when no ASD or anomalous pulmonary vein can be found in a patient with a known oxygen step-up in the right atrium. To expose the defect, an incision is made in the intraatrial septum, then the repair proceeds, depending on the presence or absence of a corresponding left SVC draining to the coronary sinus.

Contraindications to Closure

ASD repair is contraindicated, or detrimental, in patients with unrecognized or unrepaired cor triatriatum because it creates pulmonary venous obstruction. Likewise, closure of a defect without addressing associated severe mitral stenosis (Lutembacher's syndrome) or severe mitral insufficiency results in an acute elevation of left atrial pressure and pulmonary edema. ASDs also should be kept open in patients with hypoplastic or poorly functioning right ventricles and critical pulmonary stenosis. After pulmonary valvotomy, the ASD allows right-to-left shunting and maintenance of cardiac output while the right ventricle is unable to handle the entire venous volume. As previously mentioned, ASDs should not be closed in patients with irreversible pulmonary vasculopathy.

Fenestrated Patch Repairs

A fenestrated ASD repair is useful to maintain left-sided filling and cardiac output in patients with moderate-to-severe PVR who are otherwise candidates for surgical closure and in patients undergoing cardiac repairs involving severely hypertrophied right ventricles. In patients with marginal hypoplasia of the left ventricle, we have promoted left ventricular growth by limiting left-to-right atrial shunting with a fenestrated atrial patch and forcing increased pulmonary venous return to the left ventricle. Adequate systemic cardiac output is maintained by leaving the VSD open in combination with a pulmonary artery band. This allows right ventricular function to contribute to pulmonary and systemic cardiac output while the left ventricle is developing an adequate chamber dimension. Complete cardiac repair is staged at a later date.

■ POSTOPERATIVE CARE

Patients generally require no special management other than continuous cardiac monitoring to identify perioperative dysrhythmias and usually are ready for discharge within 3 to 4 days after surgery. In patients with sinus venosus repairs, a chest x-ray is performed to ensure there is no pulmonary venous congestion of the right upper and middle lobes. Jugular venous distention on physical examination would suggest obstruction of the baffle or SVC.

Patients with partial AV canal defect repairs also require close monitoring due to the proximity of the conduction system to the suture line. These patients are prone to pulmonary hypertensive events. In children, we use a 3- to 5-day tapering course of chlorpromazine (Thorazine) for mild sedation and α-blockade to lower pulmonary artery pressures. Patients who present with moderate to severe pulmonary hypertension preoperatively and exhibit at least one-half systemic pulmonary artery pressures after repair in the operating room often remain intubated with pulmonary hypertension precautions, including mild hyperventilation and hyperoxia. They too are placed on a tapering chlorpromazine protocol and generally are extubated on the first postoperative day. Typically, these children are discharged home in 4 to 5 days.

■ RESULTS

ASDs can be repaired with low surgical risk. The reported risk for mortality in secundum and sinus venosum defects is 1%. No mortality is expected, however, with repair of either defect. Morbidity likewise is exceedingly low, reflecting the standard risks of CPB and general anesthesia and bleeding,

atelectasis, and wound infection. Cerebrovascular accidents are the most feared complication in straightforward procedures and are the result of air, particulate matter, or malposition of the aortic cannula. Sick sinus syndrome can result from injury to either the sinus node or nodal artery, both of which are at risk in patients undergoing repair of sinus venosum defects.

Ostium primum repairs have a higher morbidity and mortality. The reported incidence of complete heart block ranges from 0% to 7%. The mitral valve, although usually functionally normal after repair, remains anatomically deformed and prone to early degeneration. Postoperative residual mitral insufficiency is found in 5% to 10% of patients. If severe, it generally results in another operation within several years. Approximately 10% of patients require mitral valve replacement 10 years after repair, and additional patients may need valve replacement in early adulthood. The use of pericardium instead of a Dacron patch for septal reconstruction significantly reduces red blood cell mechanical stresses resulting from a cleft insufficiency jet hitting the patch and essentially has eliminated the risk of perioperative hemolytic anemia. The overall mortality risk ranges from 1% to 5% and is influenced by the degree of mitral insufficiency, presence of pulmonary vascular disease, and age at time of repair. As reported in the Mayo Clinic series, long-term survival is good; at 20 years after operation, survival rate is 96%, and freedom from reoperation is 86%. Nearly 90% of survivors were New York Heart Association functional class I or II.

■ FOLLOW-UP

Patients generally are discharged on a 2- to 4-week course of diuretics because of post-CPB sodium retention. Congestive heart failure symptoms resolve postoperatively in virtually all patients, and S_2 becomes more physiologic. In addition to the surgical postoperative visit, annual examinations by cardiology are scheduled, and echocardiograms are performed when indicated.

Right ventricular outflow tract systolic gradients are less than 10 mm Hg in all patients without pulmonary stenosis (PS). Elevated PVR, if present, usually does not change significantly after repair. Abnormal left ventricular performance, such as abnormal septal motion, decreased LVDD, and an abnormal ejection fraction response to exercise, has been observed in patients with secundum defects. These abnormalities revert to normal after repair, suggesting right ventricular volume overload rather than intrinsic left ventricular myocardial dysfunction.

Repair of ASDs in adults can be more complicated and carry an operative mortality of 3% to 6%. Patients are at higher risk for pulmonary hypertension, congestive heart failure, and dysrhythmias. Established supraventricular dysrhythmias are unlikely to improve, but patients are otherwise generally asymptomatic or improved. Anticoagulation of patients presenting with cerebral emboli is controversial but generally is recommended in patients with coexisting atrial fibrillation and pulmonary hypertension.

TOTAL ANOMALOUS PULMONARY VENOUS CONNECTION

Vincent Tam

Total anomalous pulmonary venous connection (TAPVC) is an uncommon heart defect characterized by abnormal return of all pulmonary venous blood to a chamber other than the left atrium. It represents approximately 1% to 3% of all congenital heart disease and, importantly, is one of the few heart defects that frequently demands immediate surgical correction.

There are four major types of TAPVC: supracardiac (45%), cardiac (25%), infracardiac (25%), and mixed (5%). They are distinguished by the route via which pulmonary venous blood returns to the right heart. In supracardiac TAPVC, all four pulmonary veins typically coalesce to a pulmonary venous confluence behind and outside the pericardium and subsequently drain via a left vertical vein to the innominate vein and thence to the right atrium. Intracardiac TAPVC drains to the right atrium or coronary sinus. In infracardiac TAPVC, the confluence drains via a common pulmonary vein below the diaphragm to a major systemic or hepatic vein. In mixed TAPVC, the four pulmonary veins do not all coalesce and may have multiple separate and distinct connections to the heart or systemic veins. The clinical presentation of these forms depends in large part on the degree of pulmonary venous obstruction, which is highest in infracardiac and lowest in supracardiac TAPVC.

Despite the widespread successful use of transthoracic echocardiography in the newborn, TAPVC is potentially a subtle echocardiographic diagnosis and may frequently be missed. A common scenario is a newborn admitted to the neonatal intensive care unit for possible extracorporeal circulation membrane oxygenation (ECMO). The pre-ECMO echocardiogram, however, shows the diagnosis to be TAPVC, accounting for the child's hypoxemia. The newborn with obstructed TAPVC constitutes one of the few remaining indications for emergent surgical intervention. Severe hypoxemia (Pao_2 <25 mm Hg), metabolic acidosis, pulmonary venous congestion, and excessive ventilator settings in an effort to improve gas exchange mandate early repair. Unfortunately, in the newborn with severe obstruction, even a good early hemodynamic surgical result does not ensure survival because respiratory failure may persist. The degree of lung abnormality may be so severe that these children are unable to be weaned from mechanical ventilation and they consequently linger in the intensive care unit and die from iatrogenic and infectious complication.

Another common presenting scenario is an infant who may be thriving but presents for murmur evaluation. These infants typically have the physiology of left-to-right shunting similar to that seen in children with atrial septal defects, although perhaps to a much greater magnitude. Surgical correction in this setting has been most gratifying.

Chest radiography often leads to the diagnosis. In the setting of obstructed TAPVC, the characteristic severe diffuse pulmonary venous congestion is difficult to mistake. Other characteristic images, for example, the "snowman" cardiac silhouette encountered in supracardiac TAPVC, are legion. Two-dimensional echocardiography with continuous-wave Doppler is the diagnostic test of choice. An effort should be made to identify all four pulmonary veins, and the surgeon must remain vigilant for the possibility of a mixed-type TAPVC at the time of surgery. As mentioned earlier, obstructed TAPVC should be dealt with on an emergent basis. Typically, these infants cannot be managed medically and require surgery within the first few hours of life. Once the diagnosis is made, most newborns, as well as older infants, should have surgery urgently, even if the veins are unobstructed.

When TAPVC occurs in conjunction with other complex heart defects, the prognosis becomes less favorable. Conventional surgery for hypoplastic left heart syndrome with TAPVC has generally had dismal results. In some lesions, staging the surgical corrections may be most sensible. TAPVC would be repaired first, in conjunction with pulmonary artery banding for the newborns with excessive pulmonary blood or placement of a systemic arterial-to-pulmonary artery shunt for infants with inadequate or ductal-dependent pulmonary blood flow. Alternatively, heart or heart-lung transplantation has been proposed.

■ SURGICAL REPAIR

Adequate exposure to the back of the heart is the key to repair. A standard median sternotomy incision is used. This heart defect is repaired using hypothermic cardiopulmonary bypass (CPB), without circulatory arrest. Before the institution of CPB, the ductus arteriosus is dissected free and doubly ligated. Some preliminary dissection may be done behind the right atrium to help define the pulmonary venous anatomy. In the case of supracardiac TAPVC, the common pulmonary vein should be identified and dissected free at this time. Frequently there are left upper lobe pulmonary vein branches that may enter the left vertical common pulmonary vein more cephalad than one would expect. Care should be taken to avoid ligating these branches. After the administration of heparin (400 units/kg), the distal ascending aorta is cannulated, followed by direct cannulation of the superior vena cava (SVC) and inferior vena cava (IVC). CPB is initiated and the patient cooled to 20° to 25°C. If exposure becomes problematic because of excessive pulmonary venous return, perfusion flow rates can be reduced transiently to facilitate the repair. The pulmonary venous anatomy is completely defined. The infracardiac common pulmonary vein is carefully identified as it penetrates the diaphragm. Depending on the pulmonary venous branch anatomy, this common pulmonary vein may be divided, to minimize distortion to the pulmonary vein and left atrium anastomosis. Frequently the pulmonary vein branches are more caudal than the left atrium and may distort the anastomosis with the left atrium. A purse-string suture is placed in the left atrial appendage, through which a vent will eventually be placed. This suture also provides the needed counter traction to properly locate and create the opening in the posterior left atrium.

The heart is now arrested with cold antegrade cardioplegia via the aortic root. Cardioplegia administration is repeated in 20 to 30 minutes, if needed. Continuous cold topical irrigation is impractical and generally not used for this repair. After the heart is arrested, in the case of supracardiac TAPVC, the left vertical vein may now be ligated or, alternatively, occluded with a Rumel tourniquet. For infracardiac TAPVC, the common pulmonary vein is now ligated or divided. To aid in the exposure of the pulmonary vein confluence, the tourniquets around the SVC and IVC are used to help rotate the heart to the left. Additional traction sutures may be helpful in maintaining rotation of the heart. The use of a retractor, such as a malleable retractor or an aortic root retractor, may be necessary to provide optimal exposure. However, these retractors should be used cautiously. Continued, excessive pressure on the crux of the heart by a retractor accounts for complete heart block that occasionally persists after repair, and as such should be avoidable.

With the heart arrested and rotated to the left, the incision in the pulmonary venous confluence is now made. This incision is limited to the confluence only and incision of the individual pulmonary vein branches is avoided. Of course, the exact location of this incision must take into account its relationship with the left atrium, to avoid distorting the anastomosis.

A conventional oblique right atriotomy incision is made and the intracardiac anatomy examined. Looking through the fossa ovalis, the left atrium is inspected and the appropriate site for the pulmonary vein anastomosis is selected. Care is taken to select the area directly anterior to the opening in the pulmonary vein confluence. In the cases of cardiac TAPVC, the repair would simply consist of excising the septum primum and baffling the pulmonary venous return from pulmonary venous confluence to the left atrium via the fossa ovalis. For supracardiac and infracardiac TAPVC, incision in the left atrium is made with the utmost care. Frequently the left atrium is small in these infants and the atrioventricular groove containing the circumflex coronary artery and coronary sinus is closer than one would expect while looking at the inside of the left atrium. A small right angle clamp is used to locate the left atrial incision, and the site is inspected from outside the heart, to avoid putting the incision too close to the atrioventricular groove.

The anastomosis is begun away from the surgeon, with the first few lateral sutures being simple sutures. A pump sucker, directed from right to left, may be placed in the pulmonary vein confluence to allow for optimal exposure at the commencement of the anastomosis. Absorbable monofilament suture, such as polydioxanone (Ethicon, Somerville, NJ), is used. Pathologic studies have suggested that absorbable monofilament sutures result in less inflammation than polypropylene suture material. Once the first few simple lateral sutures are placed, a vent may be positioned through the left atrial appendage, into the pulmonary venous confluence. A continuous suture technique is now used, taking meticulous care not to purse-string this anastomosis. Rewarming

may be commenced at this point. The rightwardmost portion of the anastomosis, near the insertion of the right pulmonary veins into the confluence, is completed with simple sutures. The anastomosis may now be inspected through the fossa ovalis, after which the atrial septal defect is closed, followed by closure of the right atriotomy. A terminal dose of warm cardioplegia is given during atriotomy closure.

After rewarming, the patient is separated from CPB. In the patients with supracardiac TAPVC, the vertical vein may be ligated before separation from CPB. The left atrial vent is replaced by a left atrial monitoring catheter. In some patients, left ventricular compliance initially may be poor, and elevated left atrial pressure may be necessary to achieve adequate cardiac output. Occasionally, leaving the left vertical vein open for the first several hours after repair may be helpful in avoiding excessively high left atrial pressure, provided that cardiac output is acceptable. Additional right atrial catheters may be placed as needed for central venous access. Because of the occasional patient with complete heart block, atrial and ventricular temporary epicardial pacing wires are secured with fine polypropylene.

Mixed TAPVC is handled using the above techniques in conjunction with direct anastomosis, for example, of the left vertical vein with the left atrial appendage. Division of the right SVC and baffling pulmonary venous flow to the left atrium via the fossa ovalis, then subsequently reconnecting the cephalad end of the SVC to the right atrial appendage, is a useful technique.

Intraoperative transesophageal echocardiography has become the standard of care. Doppler interrogation of pulmonary venous return along all four veins is performed. The pulmonary vein–to–left atrial anastomosis is visualized as well. Left ventricular performance is noted along with examination of the mitral valve. High-dose inotropic support is likely counterproductive. Given the decreased left ventricular compliance, a rapid heart rate will not result in improved cardiac output.

In newborns, the sternum is frequently not closed. Rather, the skin incision is closed with a Silastic patch. As in other neonates after complex open repairs, this approach greatly simplifies the initial postoperative care. While the underlying coagulopathy is being corrected, cardiac tamponade is largely avoided. This approach will also minimize ventilatory requirements when the lungs are edematous and may be quite sensitive to additional barotrauma from positive pressure mechanical ventilation. Diuretics are begun the morning of the first postoperative day. I favor use of continuous furosemide infusion, which provides more steady diuresis than bolus medication. Typically, urine output will pick up by the evening of the first postoperative day, such that, on average, delayed sternal closure is accomplished on the second postoperative day.

Although only a small proportion of patients develop postoperative pulmonary venous obstruction, this is nevertheless a lethal complication and should be mentioned as a possible outcome in the preoperative discussions with parents. Recurrent pulmonary venous obstruction will often manifest within weeks of the infant's initial surgery. The risk seems highest in infants after repair of obstructed infradiaphragmatic TAPVC. The progressive development of pulmonary venous obstruction is not subtle and is manifest by tachypnea, decreased cardiac output, and signs and symptoms of pulmonary edema. The characteristic radiographs are difficult to mistake. Echocardiography with Doppler interrogation typically show worsening accelerated and turbulent blood flow through the entrances of the individual pulmonary veins into the left atrium, along with the development of elevated pulmonary arterial pressure. Repeat surgery is the only viable solution and tends to take place at the peak of inflammation after the initial surgery.

At reoperation, the entire pulmonary venous confluence is sclerotic with the individual pulmonary vein entrances constricted to pinholes. Sutureless pericardial well repair offers the most rational approach, although is not, in the author's experience, uniformly successful. The left atrium is incised to expose the previous anastomosis with the pulmonary vein confluence. The pulmonary veins are opened widely through the narrowed orifices into the dilated portion of each pulmonary vein. The left atrium is then anastomosed to the posterior pericardium, without direct suturing of the pulmonary veins themselves. For older children, the use of intravascular stents has had only sporadic success, because of progressive intimal ingrowth.

Total anomalous pulmonary venous connection is a cyanotic heart defect most often diagnosed in early infancy. Surgical repair usually leads to a successful and gratifying result, with few surviving children having long-term sequelae. Late pulmonary venous obstruction is the most common postoperative complication; unfortunately, prognosis after this complication is poor.

SUGGESTED READING

Caldarone CA, et al: Relentless pulmonary vein stenosis after repair of total anomalous pulmonary venous drainage, *Ann Thorac Surg* 66:1514, 1998.

Gaynor JW, et al: Long-term outcome of infants with single ventricle and total anomalous pulmonary venous connection, *J Thorac Cardiovasc Surg* 117:506, 1999.

Lacour-Gayet F, et al: Surgical management of progressive pulmonary venous obstruction after repair of total anomalous pulmonary venous connection, *J Thorac Cardiovasc Surg* 117:679, 1999.

Serraf A, et al: Modified superior approach for repair of supracardiac and mixed total anomalous pulmonary venous drainage, *Ann Thorac Surg* 65:1391, 1998.

ISOLATED VENTRICULAR SEPTAL DEFECT

Michael D. Black

The ability to construct a Blalock-Taussig shunt successfully was considered necessary to be an effective congenital heart surgeon during the 1970s and the early 1980s. With the trends toward neonatal repair, the requirements for consideration of a "good" pediatric heart surgeon have changed. Adequate closure of a ventricular septal defect (VSD) remains such a required skill and a "foundation" for the successful repair of simple and complex neonatal abnormalities. VSDs remain one of the most frequent congenital heart lesions requiring repair in early life. This chapter discusses the treatment of isolated VSD.

The overall incidence of VSD of 1.5 to 2.5 per 1000 live births has not changed, but the timing of correction has. Pulmonary vascular resistance remains elevated after birth but soon drops, most dramatically during the neonatal transition period. This is followed by a secondary drop within the first 5 to 7 days and a third and more gradual decline during the first few months of life. Signs and symptoms of high-output congestive heart failure may develop according to (1) declining resistance of the pulmonary vascular bed and (2) the degree of mechanical restriction of the ventricular defect.

■ THERAPEUTIC GOALS AND ALTERNATIVES

VSDs are varied in size and location. When the defect is muscular or perimembranous in location, spontaneous closure may occur secondary to hypertrophied trabecular carinae and tricuspid valve adherence/fibrosis. When there is a pressure differential across the defect, the term *restrictive* can be applied. Unrestrictive defects require management before 18 to 24 months to prevent irreversible damage to the pulmonary vascular bed. These irreversible changes, known as *Eisenmenger syndrome*, rarely are seen now in children born and followed in North America. A different mechanism underlies spontaneous closure of supracristal defects (subaortic); these lesions must be followed carefully and repaired. A Venturi effect from blood flow across the defect ultimately distorts and "sucks" the right coronary cusp (sometimes with the noncoronary cusp) of the systemic semilunar valve (aortic) into the defect, limiting the degree of left-to-right shunting. This defect rarely is associated with high-output congestive heart failure. The natural history is one of progressive deterioration in aortic valve function and eventual development of aortic valve insufficiency.

Only 5% of children require closure during the first few weeks of life. The remaining children are followed and treated medically with diuretics, afterload-reducing agents, and digoxin. Approximately 80% of defects close during the first year of life. Indications for surgical closure include (1) failure to thrive (failure to meet expected growth curves in weight gain, height, and head circumference), (2) increased risk for premature and irreversible pulmonary hypertension (children with trisomy 21 and other genetic abnormalities and even moderate sized defects), (3) persistent left-to-right shunt with chamber enlargement in children and young adults with a restrictive VSD, (4) VSD in combination with right ventricular muscle bundles or a double chamber right ventricle, and (5) supracristal or subaortic defect.

The mortality rate for the closure of an isolated VSD should be less than 1% regardless of age, size, and location. The smaller the infant, the more technically demanding, especially if one avoids ventriculotomy. Only multiple muscular defects ("Swiss cheese" septum) remain associated with a higher degree of mortality and sometimes require a pulmonary arterial band for short-term palliation. New cardioscopic techniques have allowed even this lesion, however, to be addressed with low mortality and morbidity rates, approaching rates seen with clearly isolated defects. These may become the technique of choice in coming years.

■ SURGICAL APPROACH

The conduct of surgical repair for VSDs remains fairly uniform, with only slight exceptions depending on patient size. Advances include robotic video-assisted repairs that limit the size of the incision and shorten duration of hospitalization.

Venous return routinely is obtained via bicaval cannula (right-angled, metal-tipped). Exceptions include a left superior vena cava (or in the case of situs inversus/dextrocardia a right-sided superior vena cava), in which case a Y connector in concert with dual superior venae cavae cannulae may be used for drainage of the upper body. An alternative strategy includes drainage of the coronary sinus from within the right atrium.

Arterial inflow is established just proximal to the takeoff of the innominate artery. Only moderate hypothermia is used (nadir rectal temperature of 32°C). High flows are maintained throughout the case. Cardioplegia is administered antegrade with a blood/crystalloid combination. Arrest may be obtained with a "warm shot" followed by cold cardioplegia as the heart's electrical-mechanical activity ceases. Caval snares are placed but tightened only after the heart arrests. The inferior vena cava cannula is rotated down the inferior vena cava (and later returned to within the right atrium) during the cooling process to avoid inadvertent hepatic congestion during periods of normothermia.

Variables in the repair strategy include patch material and suture technique. These may depend in part on size of the patient. For neonates less than 3.0 kg, I prefer an autologous pericardial patch fixed in glutaraldehyde. Two 5-0 polypropylene sutures with felt pledgets are used; the first is placed at the inferior transition zone and the second just superior to the aortic valve.

With larger infants, I prefer a Sauvage Polyester patch (Impra, Inc., Tempe, AZ) with interrupted braided nonabsorbable polytetrafluoroethylene (Teflon)-coated pledgeted sutures. Using the above-mentioned techniques, heart block can be avoided regardless of the location of the VSD.

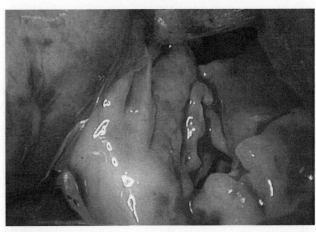

Figure 1
A restrictive ventricular septal defect (perimembranous in location). This frequently is associated with right ventricular muscle bundles.

Occasionally, primary suture closure of a small and restrictive defect can be carried out. Location of the conduction tracts is less obvious due to fibrosis, and one must take care with suture placement (Figure 1). In addition, a frequent occurrence is an obstructive right ventricular muscle bundle juxtaposed to the ventricular defect that requires resection or transection to relieve right ventricular outflow tract obstruction.

The various types of VSD are shown in Figure 2. Defects are approached via the right atrium; supracristal defects may

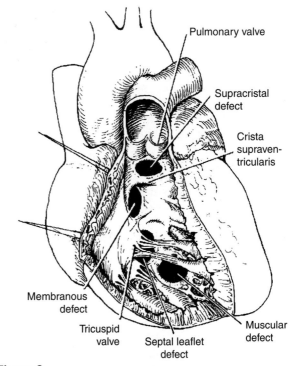

Figure 2
Anatomic types of ventricular septal defects. (*From Verrier ED: In:* Current surgical diagnosis and treatment. *Norwalk, CT, 1994, Appleton & Lange, p 395.*)

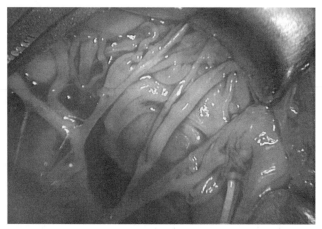

Figure 3
A perimembranous ventricular septal defect with inlet extension bridged by multiple chords emanating from the septal leaflet of the tricuspid valve.

be the exception. I prefer not to weave sutures through the chordal attachment of the septal leaflet of the right atrioventricular valve (tricuspid valve) but instead divide and reattach the chordal arrays after patch placement. A clear, uninhibited view is key to avoid damage to surrounding structures, such as the aortic and tricuspid valves and the conduction system (Figures 3 and 4).

Supracristal defects are approached routinely via a main pulmonary arteriotomy. Half of the sutures are placed

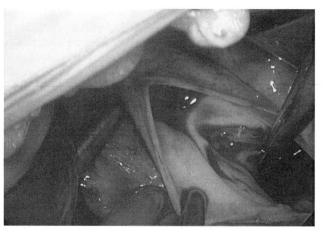

Figure 5
A supracristal ventricular septal defect located just proximal to the origin of the pulmonary valve leaflets.

within the pulmonary valve annulus (nonpledgeted braided polyester) and the other half via the muscular septum (pledgeted braided polyester). A Sauvage patch is chosen to "buttress" the prolapsing valve leaflet; deformation of a pericardial patch may recreate the situation favoring aortic valve regurgitation (Figure 5).

Concurrent presentation of coarctation and significant VSD deserves special mention. I prefer a one-stage repair from the front using selective cerebral perfusion to avoid circulatory arrest and deep hypothermia. The combination of left thoracotomy and temporary pulmonary artery band followed by a median sternotomy within a 2- to 3-week period still is used by some surgeons.

SUGGESTED READING

Black MD, Bissonnette B: Initial experience with selective cerebral perfusion: an alternative approach to cerebral protection in neonates/infants with complex cardiac procedures requiring aortic arch reconstruction. Canadian Cardiovascular Society, Ottawa, Ontario, *Can J Cardiol* 14 (Suppl F):87F, 1998.

Black MD, et al: Repair of isolated multiple muscular ventricular septal defects: the septal obliteration technique, *Ann Thorac Surg* 68:106, 2000.

Hoffman JIE, Rudolph AM: The natural history of ventricular septal defects with special reference to selection of patients for surgery, *Adv Pediatr* 17:57, 1970.

Soto B, et al: Classification of ventricular septal defects, *Br Heart J* 43: 332, 1980.

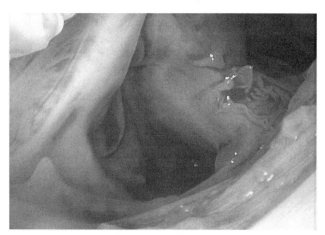

Figure 4
A large unrestrictive ventricular septal defect (perimembranous in location). Note the close proximity of the aortic valve.

PATENT DUCTUS ARTERIOSUS AND AORTOPULMONARY WINDOW

Redmond P. Burke

Robert L. Hannan

■ PATENT DUCTUS ARTERIOSUS

Patent ductus arteriosus (PDA) is one of the most common congenital heart defects and one of the first anomalies successfully addressed surgically, by Gross and Hubbard in 1938. Advances in surgical treatment and interventional catheterization have expanded options for treatment of PDA and have complicated the treatment algorithm for this straightforward lesion.

The ductus is a normal structure in utero originating from the left sixth aortic arch, connecting the pulmonary artery and the aorta. In utero, the normal ductus diverts right ventricular blood away from the high-resistance pulmonary vascular bed into the descending aorta. In full-term infants, the ductus starts closing in the first 24 hours of life by smooth muscle contraction and intimal protrusion of thickened intima. Permanent closure and obliteration concludes in most full-term infants by 3 weeks of age. Persistence of the ductus allows left-to-right shunting, causing an increase in pulmonary blood flow and subsequent increased volume load on the left ventricle, and may result in low diastolic blood pressure, reduced bowel perfusion (leading to necrotizing enterocolitis), and reduced myocardial perfusion. The magnitude of the shunt depends on the size of the ductus and the relative pulmonary and systemic vascular resistances.

In full-term, normal-birth-weight infants, the incidence of PDA is about 1 in 2000 live births, accounting for 5% to 10% of all congenital heart anomalies. In premature infants, physiologic developmental retardation and especially the decreased vasoconstrictor effect of oxygen lead to a high incidence of PDA. The incidence of PDA approaches 80% in infants weighing less than 1200 g.

Diagnosis

In premature, low-birth-weight infants the diagnosis of PDA is based on evidence of left-to-right shunt and left ventricular volume overload. Shunt and volume overload depend on pulmonary vascular resistance and presence of pulmonary disease. The diagnosis is confirmed by echocardiography.

In term infants and older children, a small ductus is usually asymptomatic and found by echocardiography during evaluation for murmur. A larger ductus with low pulmonary vascular resistance may lead to a large left-to-right shunt and heart failure, including failure to thrive and tachypnea. The diagnosis almost always can be made on clinical grounds and echocardiography. In rare cases, it may be difficult to determine if there is a coexisting coarctation of the aorta or arch hypoplasia; in these circumstances, diagnostic cardiac catheterization is indicated.

Indications for Closure

Premature infants with symptomatic left-to-right shunts should be treated. Typically the neonatologist pursues closing the ductus when the left-to-right shunt seems to be contributing to respiratory failure or to systemic hypoperfusion.

Infants born at term or older than age 3 to 6 months with a patent ductus are unlikely to undergo spontaneous closure. Typically, these infants are referred for signs or symptoms of heart failure (in the presence of a large ductus) or for closure of an asymptomatic ductus to prevent development of endocarditis and pulmonary vascular disease. The management of children with a small, asymptomatic ductus found on echocardiography without a heart murmur ("silent ductus") is controversial. Some cardiologists advocate closing all such lesions, others believe that they should be left entirely alone, and still others pursue closure only when interventional catheterization techniques are unavailable or fail.

Techniques of Closure

Multiple techniques are available for PDA closure. Medical treatment frequently is effective in low-birth-weight infants. Open surgical closure, video-assisted thoracic surgery (VATS) closure, and interventional catheterization all are effective in closing PDA.

Low-Birth-Weight Infants

Symptomatic premature low-birth-weight infants are treated with indomethacin, unless there are contraindications, such as renal failure, myocardial ischemia, or necrotizing enterocolitis. Three courses of indomethacin usually are attempted before children are referred for surgery.

Low-birth-weight infants who are unsuitable for or fail medical treatment may be treated successfully with VATS ductal ligation (see later). Our current practice is to close PDA in premature infants in the neonatal intensive care unit (ICU), however, via a limited left posterolateral thoracotomy. We find this practice minimizes anesthesia and operating time. Allowing the child to remain in the neonatal ICU may prevent temperature instability during transport to the operating room and reduces the complexity of transferring infants on the oscillator ventilator.

A limited left posterolateral thoracotomy is performed. Extreme caution is used while opening the pleura to prevent damage to lung parenchyma, even by transmitted electrocautery current. The descending aorta, ductus, left pulmonary artery, isthmus, left subclavian artery, and recurrent nerve all are identified, and the ductus is dissected carefully using the electrocautery and gentle blunt dissection. No attempt is made to encircle the ductus, and the greatest care is taken at the superior edge of the ductus and the underside of the aortic arch. A single titanium clip suffices in closing the ductus. No attempt should be made to reposition or remove a clip. An immediate rise in diastolic blood pressure and disappearance of the murmur in the esophageal stethoscope ensure that the ductus is closed. A steady pulse oximeter signal from the lower extremity is reassuring that the aorta is not obstructed. A single 12 Fr chest tube is placed in the pleural space and usually removed on the first postoperative day. In many cases, no chest tube is necessary.

Infants and Children
In full-term infants and children, VATS closure is our method of choice. This approach avoids the chest wall deformities and scoliosis associated with thoracotomy in children. It requires facility and experience with thoracoscopic techniques and patience and judgment to avoid iatrogenic mishaps.

We prefer a four-incision technique using the 4-mm, 30-degree video camera and the hockey-stick electrocautery (Figure 1). The ductus is interrupted with one or two titanium clips, and complete closure is verified by transesophageal echocardiography, disappearance of the murmur, and rise in diastolic blood pressure. In rare circumstances, it may be advisable or necessary to convert the VATS approach to an open procedure (by connecting the port sites) when uncontrollable bleeding occurs from the posterior aspect of the duct or when the duct is unexpectedly large.

In full-term infants and children, many surgeons use a left posterolateral thoracotomy. The conduct of the operation is similar to that in neonates, although many groups advocate obtaining complete proximal and distal control of the aorta and dividing the ductus rather than ligating it. The disadvantages of pediatric thoracotomy are well documented, including scoliosis, chest wall deformity, and increased trauma to the patient. We use a limited left thoracotomy in children who have large or calcified ducts. Using the video camera through the limited thoracotomy incision reduces the need to spread the ribs and subsequent chest wall trauma.

Interventional catheterization is used in many centers for closure of PDA in children. Several different types of devices are available, including Gianturco coils (especially useful for small ducts), the Grifka device (for larger ducts), and various atrial septal defect closure devices. The main advantage of interventional catheterization techniques is minimal trauma to the child. Disadvantages include potential prolonged radiation exposure, potential for endocarditis, obstruction of the left pulmonary artery, damage to the femoral vessels, potential for catastrophic device embolism, and the need for surgical coverage.

Adults
Adults with PDA, especially if the ductus is large and calcified, are a high-risk group. Several techniques currently are used. The ductus may be patched from inside the aorta via left thoracotomy and aortotomy. The ductus also may be approached through a median sternotomy and the left pulmonary artery with cardiopulmonary bypass (with control of the pulmonary arteries after the initiation of bypass to avoid pulmonary overcirculation). Adults with evidence of pulmonary hypertension should undergo cardiac catheterization to evaluate pulmonary vascular resistance before closure of the ductus. Several technical suggestions and avoidable pitfalls are listed in Table 1.

Outcome of PDA Closure
Morbidity and mortality after ductal closure should approach zero. Critically ill, low-birth-weight neonates may die from other causes, but ductal ligation is well tolerated even in these patients. Mortality is related primarily to surgical mishaps or embolization of devices placed in the catheterization laboratory. Morbidity includes transient vocal cord paralysis from recurrent nerve injury, chylothorax, and recanalization of a ligated ductus.

Maintaining Ductal Patency for Palliation of Congenital Heart Disease
Children with more complex forms of congenital heart disease may benefit from prolonged ductal patency. Children with coarctation of the aorta and ductal dependent pulmonary blood flow typically are treated with prostaglandin preoperatively to preserve ductal flow. Prostaglandin E also may improve mixing in infants with transposition of the great arteries. Long-term ductal patency for increased pulmonary blood flow as a palliative modality historically has been maintained by injection of the ductus with glutaraldehyde in

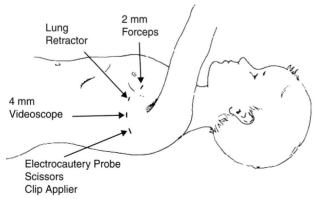

Figure 1
The four thoracoscopy incisions for VATS interruption of a PDA.

Table 1 Specific Technical Suggestions and Avoidable Problems with Patent Ductus Arteriosus Closure

An echocardiogram to confirm ductal patency should be obtained shortly before surgery (within 24 hr)

The recurrent laryngeal nerve is injured most commonly during dissection posterior to the ductus or using electrocautery to dissect

Clips on the ductus in a premature neonate should never be manipulated or moved once placed: uncontrollable hemorrhage may result

Aortic arch hypoplasia, hypoplasia of the isthmus, and coarctation of the aorta must be evaluated before PDA closure is considered

Children with small aortic arches and large PDA have had the ductus misidentified as the aortic arch (mistaking the isthmus for the left subclavian) and the left pulmonary artery ligated instead of the ductus

The ductus or both pulmonary arteries should be controlled before or immediately after initiation of cardiopulmonary bypass to prevent pulmonary overcirculation the operating room or more recently by stenting the ductus in the catheterization laboratory.

■ CONCLUSION

The focus at Miami Children's Hospital is to minimize the trauma to children with congenital heart disease. Our current therapeutic strategy varies depending on the size and age of the patient and the size of the patent ductus. All patients are evaluated by a multidisciplinary team that includes surgeons and interventional cardiologists. Premature infants in the newborn ICU have an extremely expeditious limited thoracotomy and PDA clip ligation to minimize lung trauma and anesthesia. Larger children with small PDA usually are treated with one or two coils in the catheterization laboratory. Children with larger ducts are evaluated for closure by VATS or percutaneous devices, depending on the exact anatomy and circumstances.

■ AORTOPULMONARY WINDOW

Aortopulmonary window (APW) is an uncommon lesion that occurs as a defect between the aorta and the main pulmonary artery just above the sinuses of Valsalva. APW may present as an isolated lesion or in association with coarctation of the aorta, interrupted aortic arch, and anomalous origin of the right pulmonary artery. Importantly, it may be associated with anomalies of the origin of the coronary arteries, with the coronaries originating on the edge of the window or from the pulmonary artery side of the window. APW also is an uncommon but important complication of interventional cardiac catheterization. It is seen in postoperative arterial switch patients with pulmonary stenosis who undergo balloon angioplasty of the main and branch pulmonary arteries.

AWP physiology is basically that of a large unrestrictive ductus. Children with APW have a left-to-right shunt that increases in the first weeks of life as pulmonary vascular resistance decreases. Signs and symptoms include congestive heart failure, tachypnea, failure to thrive, and other signs of pulmonary overcirculation. Some infants may present with severe congestive heart failure, pulmonary overcirculation, and systemic hypoperfusion that require preoperative stabilization, including measures to reduce pulmonary blood, such as hypoventilation or administration of nitrogen and carbon dioxide.

Diagnosis in most patients is made by echocardiography. Cardiac catheterization is reserved for patients with unclear anatomy on echocardiography or older patients to evaluate pulmonary vascular resistance. Repair is indicated in all patients with APW and should be done shortly after

diagnosis. In 1948, Gross was the first to ligate an APW successfully.

Repair of APW is undertaken via median sternotomy on cardiopulmonary bypass. The aorta should be cannulated distally and the branch pulmonary arteries controlled with snares before initiation of bypass. We use two venous cannulae and a left atrial vent to afford a completely dry operative field. No attempt is made to dissect out the APW. After inducing cardioplegic arrest, the APW may be approached through the aorta, the pulmonary artery, or the window itself. We preferentially approach mostly through an aortotomy. The aorta is opened above the APW, and the window is repaired from inside the aorta using an autologous glutaraldehyde-treated patch and running monofilament suture. Great care is taken to identify the origins of the coronary arteries. If the right pulmonary artery arises anomalously from the aorta, it is detached proximally and anastomosed to the main pulmonary artery; the aortic defect is closed with autologous pericardium. The use of an autologous pulmonary artery flap to close large defects in infants has been advocated by some to preserve growth potential in the aorta.

Technical pitfalls to avoid include pulmonary artery stenosis and injury to the coronary arteries. Patients with iatrogenic APW after pulmonary angioplasty for pulmonary artery stenosis after arterial switch for transposition present a technical challenge. Urgent recognition and repair are essential. We have found remarkable tension across the pulmonary arteries in these patients, who require extensive homograft reconstruction of the right ventricular outflow tract and patch aortoplasty to complete the repairs. Outcome after repair of APW should be excellent, with essentially no morbidity and no mortality. Follow-up echocardiography is done to rule out branch pulmonary artery stenosis.

SUGGESTED READING

Burke RP, Rosenfeld HM: Primary repair of aortopulmonary septal defect, interrupted aortic arch, and anomalous origin of the right pulmonary artery, *Ann Thorac Surg* 58:543, 1994.

Burke RP, et al: Video-assisted thoracoscopic surgery for congenital heart disease, *J Thorac Cardiovasc Surg* 109:499, 1995.

Gross RE, Hubbard JP: Surgical ligation of patent ductus arteriosus: report of first successful case, *JAMA* 112:729, 1984.

Gross RE: Surgical closure of an aortic septal defect, *Circulation* 5:858, 1952.

Laborde F, et al: A new video-assisted thoracoscopic surgical technique for interruption of patent ductus arteriosus in infants and children, *J Thorac Cardiovasc Surg* 105:278, 1993.

Matsuki O, et al: New surgical technique for total-defect aortopulmonary window, *Ann Thorac Surg* 54:991, 1992.

Pontius RG, et al: Illusions leading to surgical closure of the distal left pulmonary artery instead of the ductus arteriosus, *J Thorac Cardiovasc Surg* 82:107, 1981.

COARCTATION OF THE AORTA

John L. Myers

Edward R. Stephenson

Resection and end-to-end anastomosis for coarctation of the aorta first were performed in 1944 by Crafoord and Nylin and by Gross and Hufnagel. Surgical repair in an infant was not reported until 1950.

Hemodynamic molding is the process by which blood vessels grow and develop around a flowing column of blood. Anomalies that alter the flow of blood through the heart can result in differential growth and development of the cardiac chambers, valves, and great vessels. Any process that increases the ratio of right-to-left ventricular outputs can result in decreased left ventricular output and abnormal growth and development of the aortic valve, aortic isthmus, and juxtaductal region of the aorta.

Specific intracardiac anomalies that can cause coarctation of the aorta based on the hemodynamic molding concept are those that reduce output of the left side of the heart. Anomalies clinically associated with coarctation are ventricular septal defect, bicuspid aortic valve, congenital aortic stenosis, hypoplastic left ventricle, congenital mitral valve stenosis or atresia, restrictive interatrial communication, and Taussig-Bing double outlet right ventricle. As might be expected, coarctation is rare among the lesions that reduce output of the right side of the heart, such as tetralogy of Fallot, pulmonary stenosis, and pulmonary atresia.

Generally, there are two types of clinical manifestations. In infants, coarctation is usually preductal and is associated with isthmus hypoplasia as well as the above-described intracardiac anomalies. These infants have severe congestive heart failure and require intensive medical therapy before surgical correction. Coarctation of the aorta in older patients is associated infrequently with other cardiac anomalies and is usually a discrete coarctation membrane at or just beyond the level of the ligamentum arteriosum (juxtaductal coarctation). With time, the aorta may grow unequally and cause a greater downward displacement of the lateral wall and coarctation membrane compared with the medial wall that is held in place by the ligamentum arteriosum. This results in a "postductal" coarctation. In this latter group, consisting primarily of older children and young adults, the diagnosis usually is made incidentally when a patient is being evaluated for hypertension, headaches, epistaxis, lower extremity claudication, diminished femoral pulses, or heart failure.

■ PREFERRED APPROACH

Proper treatment of coarctation of the aorta is achieved by surgical procedures designed to eliminate the coarctation gradient. Aggressive medical management is essential for optimal preoperative preparation of these patients.

■ PREOPERATIVE MANAGEMENT

Newborns and Infants

Infants with coarctation of the aorta most frequently have severe congestive heart failure, signs of systemic hypoperfusion, and metabolic acidosis. During fetal life, the pulmonary arteries are in a parallel circuit with the ductus arteriosus and descending aorta. Closure of the ductus arteriosus in infants with coarctation of the aorta causes a marked increase in the pulmonary arterial blood flow and a decrease in lower body (abdominal viscera and extremities) blood flow. The resulting increase in pulmonary venous return is delivered to the left ventricle, which is already compromised by the severe afterload caused by the coarctation. The end result is severe congestive heart failure and hypoperfusion of the abdominal viscera and lower body, which leads to metabolic acidosis, oliguria, and further myocardial depression. Prompt, aggressive intervention is mandatory to improve systemic perfusion and to correct metabolic acidosis.

The use of prostaglandin E_1 (PGE_1) is imperative in the preoperative management of these infants. The infusion of PGE_1 is begun at 0.1 to 0.2 μg/kg/min. The dosage is tapered by decrements of 0.0025 μg/kg/min to a minimum of 0.005 μg/kg/min as long as ductal patency is maintained. Opening the ductus allows better perfusion of the abdominal viscera and lower body, decreasing the production of lactic acid by improved tissue perfusion and allowing excretion of acid by improved renal perfusion. The increased blood flow through the ductus arteriosus also lessens afterload on the left ventricle, improving left-sided congestive heart failure. Administration of dopamine sometimes is necessary for inotropic support of the compromised myocardium. An infusion of 3 to 5 μg/kg/min is usually sufficient. Sodium bicarbonate often is required initially to correct the acidemia while systemic hypoperfusion is being corrected.

Endotracheal intubation and mechanical ventilation are often helpful in infants with pulmonary edema. Hyperventilation is useful to eliminate acid further in the form of carbon dioxide. A low arterial P_{CO_2}, an elevated pH, and an increased P_{O_2} promote a decrease in pulmonary vascular resistance, however. With an open ductus arteriosus, the amount of blood flow through the lungs and lower body depends on the ratio of the vascular resistance in the respective vascular beds. When ductal patency is established and acid-base balance is optimized, the ventilatory support should be adjusted to maintain a P_{CO_2} of 35 to 40 mm Hg, and the fraction of inspired oxygen should be reduced to the lowest fraction permitting an arterial P_{O_2} of 25 to 35 mm Hg; this allows normalization of the pulmonary vascular resistance and reduction of pulmonary overperfusion. When an infant's medical condition is satisfactory, and a complete diagnostic assessment has been completed, prompt surgical intervention is mandatory.

■ SURGICAL TECHNIQUES

Infants Younger than 1 Year Old

In infants younger than 1 year old, we use one of two techniques depending on the individual infant's anatomy. We have used subclavian flap angioplasty in many infants, and based on our experience, this technique has provided excellent short-term and long-term results. The second technique includes resection of the coarctation and an extended end-to-end anastomosis. Subclavian flap angioplasty is performed via a left posterolateral thoracotomy through the fourth intercostal space with dissection of the aorta and its branches from the left carotid to about 2 cm beyond the ductus arteriosus. The recurrent nerve is protected, and the intercostal vessels are spared and controlled, if necessary, with Potts' ties. The subclavian artery is mobilized out to the origin of the vertebral artery, and both are ligated distal to this bifurcation. The duct is ligated with 2-0 silk, and the aortic cross-clamps are placed proximally between the left carotid and left subclavian arteries and distally approximately 2 cm distal to the ductus arteriosus.

The subclavian artery is divided at the origin of the vertebral artery. A longitudinal incision is made in the aorta opposite the ductus and extended proximally across the coarctation, across the isthmus, and into the subclavian artery. The aortotomy is extended distally for at least 1 cm beyond the ductus. The coarctation shelf is excised with scissors, taking care that all the excess tissue is removed without injury to the aortic wall. Trimming or tapering of the subclavian flap should not be done and is detrimental to the repair. A mattress suture of 6-0 or 7-0 monofilament suture material is placed at the apex of the subclavian flap and the distal extent of the aortotomy. The U-shaped repair is completed with a continuous suture. Air is evacuated, and the aortic cross-clamps are removed. It is important to extend the aortotomy well beyond the area of coarctation to avoid residual narrowing. The subclavian artery is not dissected beyond the origin of the vertebral artery because this may jeopardize collateral circulation to the arm. In our experience, no patient has had ischemic injury of the arm, and the subclavian artery always has been of adequate length to permit its use.

When the extended end-to-end technique is used, the aortic arch is dissected and mobilized proximally to the innominate artery and distally halfway down the descending aorta. The ductus arteriosus is ligated with a 2-0 silk suture. Cross-clamps are applied, and the aorta is transected proximal and distal to the coarctation site. All of the coarctation tissue is excised. The aorta is incised proximally on the "underside" of the aorta often to the level of the left carotid artery. The incision is extended proximal to any important narrowing in the aortic arch. A counterincision is made on the lateral aspect of the descending aorta. The isthmus tissue is not excised; it becomes a flap that is sewn into the counterincision in the distal aorta. This results in an oblique suture line, which has had a low incidence of recoarctation.

Older Children (>1 Year Old) and Adults

After 1 year of age, the technique depends on the individual patient. If the isthmus is small or if the coarctation is long in a 2- to 3-year-old child, the subclavian flap angioplasty still can be used. After 12 months of age, our standard operation consists of resection and end-to-end anastomosis, however. We avoid the use of synthetic graft material whenever possible. We perform resection of the coarctation and all juxtaductal tissue, while mobilizing the entire descending aorta and distal aortic arch. Repair is accomplished by end-to-end anastomosis using a continuous running monofilament suture. The end-to-end repair subsequently has evolved into a technique referred to as an *extended end-to-end repair* as

described earlier. This large anastomosis allows resection of all ductal tissue, avoids prosthetic material, preserves the subclavian artery, and is of particular use in patients who have narrowing of the aortic arch proximal to the ductus. We have managed a few patients with a short coarctation with direct aortoplasty (longitudinal incision, excision of membrane, and transverse closure).

■ OTHER SURGICAL APPROACHES

Prosthetic Patch Aortoplasty

The use of a patch of prosthetic material (Dacron or polytetrafluoroethylene) has been advocated by some as a method of coarctation repair. The proposed advantages are the ability to extend the patch to any length, the ability to produce a tension-free anastomosis, and the preservation of the subclavian artery. A significant concern about patch aortoplasty has been the demonstration of aneurysm formation of the aortic wall opposite the patch repair. The use of this technique may be employed for repair in recurrent coarctation not amenable to balloon angioplasty.

Graft Interposition

Prosthetic graft interposition has been used for long coarctations in which direct end-to-end anastomosis would result in excessive suture line tension. There are significant disadvantages associated with this technique, however. When prosthetic material is used as a tube graft, its main drawback has been the lack of growth and the potential for infection. Its use in repair of aortic coarctation is limited to adult patients in whom the aorta has completed full growth.

Patients with mild coarctation and minimal collateralization are probably at higher risk for spinal cord ischemia. We usually manage these patients with temporary left atrial-to-descending aortic bypass with a centrifugal pump.

■ POSTOPERATIVE CARE

Postoperative hypertension is relatively common and is treated with β-blockade, nitroprusside, and angiotensin-converting enzyme inhibitors. Abdominal pain requiring bowel rest and intravenous fluids occasionally occurs. The development of chylothorax from the disruption of the lymphatics may occur and initially is treated conservatively with a low-fat diet. Surgical exploration for a persistent chylous leak is occasionally necessary.

■ RESULTS

The results of aortic coarctation repair at our institution have been excellent, with a low mortality rate (≤2%). The perioperative mortality rate of older patients is 1%. The rate of recurrent coarctation is 5% to 20% in most series depending on the type of repair and the age of the patient at the time of repair.

From 1975 through 2000, 284 patients underwent repair of coarctation of the aorta at our institution. The associated cardiac anomalies and mortality in these patients are presented in Table 1. Table 2 presents the operative mortality as a function

Table 1 Associated Cardiac Anomalies and Morbidity: 1975-2000

ANOMALY	N	DEATHS (%)
Isolated coarctation	203	2 (1.0)
Coarctation and VSD	45	0 (0.0)
Coarctation and complex anomalies (DORV, AVC, TGA, and VSD)	36	2 (5.6)
Total	*284*	*4 (1.4)*

VSD, ventricular septal defect; DORV, double outlet right ventricle; AVC, atrioventricular canal defect; TGA, transposition of the great arteries.

of age at operation. There have been only 3 deaths in 133 infants operated on in the first year of life. Of the 284 patients operated on for coarctation of the aorta, 133 (47%) were less than 1 month old, 171 (60%) were less than 6 months old, and 182 (64%) were less than 1 year old.

Table 2 Age at Operation and Morbidity: 1975-2000

AGE	N	DEATHS (%)
1-30 days	133	3 (2.3)
31-180 days	38	0 (0.0)
180-365 days	11	0 (0.0)
>1 year	102	1 (1.0)
Total	*284*	*4 (1.4)*

Aggressive preoperative preparation with PGE_1 infusion has allowed stabilization of neonates with profound cardiovascular decompensation. The low operative mortality rate and excellent late results have led us to recommend that coarctation of the aorta should be repaired at the same time of diagnosis regardless of age or symptoms. Age is no longer a risk factor, and late hypertensive morbidity should be reduced by early successful repair.

PULMONARY VALVE AND INFUNDIBULAR STENOSIS

Neal Hillman

John Hawkins

Pulmonary stenosis with intact ventricular septum (PS/IVS) is one of the most common causes of right ventricular outflow tract (RVOT) obstruction and accounts for 8% to 10% of all congenital heart lesions. The etiology of pulmonary stenosis is unclear, but there is an increased incidence in siblings with pulmonary stenosis, a familial tendency, and an association with syndromes (Noonan's syndrome, Watson syndrome, neurofibromatosis) and chromosomal abnormalities (trisomy 18). These characteristics point to a genetic basis. Pulmonary stenosis presenting in the neonatal period is different from pulmonary stenosis presenting later in life, so the two are discussed separately.

■ NEONATAL CRITICAL VALVULAR PULMONARY STENOSIS

Morphology

Neonates with critical pulmonary stenosis typically are critically ill and cyanotic and present in the first week of life.

Gikonyo et al described six anatomic variants of pulmonary valve stenosis: tricuspid, bicuspid, unicommissural, domed, hypoplastic annulus and valve, and dysplastic. The typical morphology of the critically stenotic pulmonary valve is a doming, trileaflet valve with variable degrees of commissural fusion and central obstruction. Pulmonary valve dysplasia represents an important subgroup of patients with isolated pulmonary valve stenosis. Found in 10% to 20% of patients with isolated pulmonary valve stenosis, the incidence of valvular dysplasia is greatest among patients with Noonan's syndrome and cardiofacial syndrome. The dysplastic valve is characterized by subvalvular narrowing, annular hypoplasia, and thickened myxomatous leaflets with severe immobility despite well-formed commissures. These morphologic characteristics determine the initial management strategy.

The degree of right-sided morphologic change is related to the severity of the pulmonary stenosis. The right atrium typically is enlarged, and there is often right-to-left shunting at the atrial level leading to cyanosis. Right ventricular hypertrophy from the outflow obstruction reduces intraventricular volume. Right ventricular volume is mildly to moderately decreased in 49% and severely hypoplastic in 5%. Concentric hypertrophy may be associated with endocardial ischemia and endocardial fibrosis, further decreasing right ventricular compliance. Tricuspid valve incompetence is common. Right ventricular to coronary artery fistulas are uncommon, and right ventricle–dependent coronary blood flow is not seen. The proximal pulmonary arteries may appear hypoplastic due to underfilling from decreased pulmonary blood flow. Significant pulmonary artery hypoplasia occurs in less than 4%.

Pathophysiology and Natural History

During in utero development, severe right ventricular outflow obstruction leads to right ventricular hypertrophy, smaller right ventricular cavity size, and decreased endocardial blood flow in the face of increased oxygen demands leading to endocardial fibrosis. The resultant decrease in right ventricular compliance in combination with tricuspid regurgitation increases right atrial pressure. Consequently, right-to-left shunting at the atrial level results in cyanosis at birth. Pulmonary blood flow is maintained through the patent ductus arteriosus. Unless pharmacologic measures (prostaglandin E_1) are instituted to maintain ductal blood flow, hypoxemia progresses and leads to acidosis and hemodynamic demise. Essentially all neonates with critical pulmonary valve stenosis and hypoxemia die within days to weeks without intervention.

Presentation and Diagnosis

Neonates with PS/IVS present critically ill, cyanotic, and in respiratory distress. On auscultation, there is a loud systolic ejection murmur at the base of the heart. The physical findings of tricuspid insufficiency may be evident. The chest film usually shows cardiomegaly and a prominent right heart border. Pulmonary vascular markings may be diminished. The electrocardiogram may show diminished right ventricular forces due to a small right ventricle. Right axis deviation, right ventricular hypertrophy, and strain may be seen. The echocardiogram provides the definitive diagnosis and permits functional and anatomic evaluation of the cardiac lesion. Cardiac catheterization is performed frequently; it not only provides confirmatory information and additional hemodynamic data, but also shows important anatomic details necessary for percutaneous balloon valvuloplasty.

Management

The primary goal of treatment for PS/IVS is two-ventricle repair. Initial treatment is aimed at reestablishing hemodynamic stability and correction of acid-base abnormalities. Prostaglandin E_1 infusion is instituted to maintain ductal dependent blood flow. Intubation may be required to counteract prostaglandin E_1–induced apnea and aid correction of acid-base imbalance. Inotropic support is added as needed to maintain adequate cardiac output and tissue perfusion. When stabilization has been achieved, establishment of flow through the RVOT is undertaken.

Treatment of PS/IVS has evolved from a surgical approach to preferred percutaneous balloon valvuloplasty. McGoon and Kirklin introduced modern-era surgical treatment using open pulmonary valvotomy and cardiopulmonary bypass in 1958. Open surgical treatment lost favor with the development of percutaneous balloon valvuloplasty by Kan et al in 1982.

Percutaneous Balloon Valvuloplasty

After resuscitation, percutaneous right heart angiography is performed to determine the anatomy of the obstruction (e.g., valvar, infundibular, supravalvar). A guidewire is passed across the pulmonary valve, and balloons are passed over the guidewire across the valve and inflated. Incrementally larger balloons are used until no waist is seen when the balloon is inflated. Repeat right heart angiography is performed to confirm relief of the stenosis.

Surgical Valvotomy

Intraoperative transesophageal echocardiogram is useful to assess the adequacy of the valvotomy, postvalvotomy valve gradient, and degree of pulmonary insufficiency. After median sternotomy, aorto-bicaval cannulation is performed. The patent ductus arteriosus is isolated and temporarily occluded. Cardiopulmonary bypass is instituted with or without cardioplegic arrest of the heart. Through a transverse pulmonary arteriotomy, the valve and infundibulum are evaluated. Fused commissures are incised to the level of the pulmonary annulus. Thickened valve edges are excised. Obstructing infundibular muscle bundles are resected. In the unusual case in which the pulmonary annulus Z-score is less than −3 or the residual gradient is greater than 30 mm Hg, a transannular patch may be required. The arteriotomy is closed. After the heart is arrested with cold blood cardioplegia, or cardiac fibrillation with cooling occurs, the right atrium is opened, and the interatrial communication is closed. In cases of severe right ventricular dysfunction, the interatrial communication may be left open to allow right-to-left shunting, maintaining cardiac output in the postoperative period. The atriotomy is closed, and the patient is separated from cardiopulmonary bypass. If arterial Po_2 remains greater than 35 mm Hg, the ductus is permanently ligated. If the Po_2 is less than 35 mm Hg, the ductus is left open, and prostaglandin E_1 is reinstituted. If the Po_2 remains low despite these measures, a systemic-to-pulmonary artery shunt is required.

Outcomes

The success of balloon valvuloplasty in the modern era is 90% to 95%. Reported mortality rates are less than 5%, and morbidity rates are approximately 10%. Immediate failure to relieve RVOT obstruction may be due to inability to cross the obstruction with the balloon catheter, hypoplasia of the right ventricle, or muscular infundibular stenosis. High residual infundibular gradients immediately after balloon dilation do not preclude eventual relief of muscular obstruction. Balloon valvuloplasty may promote growth of the pulmonary valve and prevent subsequent surgical intervention. Of patients, 80% to 100% show mild pulmonary valve insufficiency after balloon valvuloplasty. Restenosis occurs in 5% to 20%. Suboptimal long-term results relate to level of stenosis, older age, dysplastic valve morphology, and higher pre–balloon dilation and post–balloon dilation gradients.

Early experiences with surgical valvotomy had a mortality rate of 0% to 20%. Excellent results usually are achieved with surgical valvotomy. Mild to moderate pulmonary insufficiency almost always is present. Open pulmonary valvotomy without inflow occlusion or cardiopulmonary bypass is a risk factor for early mortality. Restenosis after surgical valvotomy is 4%.

The only prospective study comparing surgical valvotomy with balloon valvuloplasty for neonates with PS/IVS was performed by the Congenital Heart Surgeons Society. This study group enrolled 101 neonates with critical pulmonary stenosis. Overall survival was 94% in the perioperative period, 89% at 1 month, and 81% at 4 years post intervention. After treatment, 81% of the patients had relief of obstruction. Of the patients, 26% required reintervention within 2 years due to residual or recurrent stenosis (>30 mm Hg). Reintervention was usually within the first week of initial treatment and was prompted most commonly by persistent hypoxemia necessitating a systemic-to-pulmonary artery shunt. In this study, 85% of patients went on to biventricular repair. The study concluded that balloon valvuloplasty is the initial treatment of choice, and surgical intervention is reserved for balloon valvuloplasty failures.

■ PULMONARY VALVE STENOSIS IN INFANTS, CHILDREN, AND ADULTS

Morphology

Pulmonary valve stenosis beyond the neonatal period is often less severe than in neonates. The pulmonary valve is typically more normally developed with partial commissural fusion accounting for the valve stenosis. Poststenotic dilation of the main pulmonary artery is common. Right ventricular hypertrophy is often progressive. When hypertrophy involves the infundibular septum, secondary RVOT obstruction may become a more important factor than valve stenosis. With time, decreased right ventricular compliance may increase right-to-left shunting at the atrial level, resulting in cyanosis as the clinical presentation. The progression of RVOT obstruction is variable, and regression can occur. Frequent follow-up is required to identify patients with progressive stenosis and to determine optimal timing of intervention.

Presentation and Diagnosis

The severity of pulmonary valve stenosis dictates the presenting symptoms and age of presentation. Of patients, 25% to 35% are asymptomatic and are identified during active physical examination by auscultation of a systolic murmur. When symptoms occur, exertional dyspnea and fatigue are typical. Cyanosis may result from poor right ventricular compliance and right-to-left atrial level shunting. During the second and third decades of life, clinical presentation may reflect right heart failure.

On physical examination, a harsh systolic ejection murmur and thrill are present over the second left intercostal space. S_2 may be split, diminished, or absent depending on the degree of valve stenosis. In most, the electrocardiogram shows right atrial enlargement and right ventricular hypertrophy. The amplitude of the R-wave in V1 correlates with the degree of right ventricular hypertension. The chest x-ray commonly reveals an enlarged main pulmonary artery resulting from poststenotic dilation. Peripheral lung vascular markings are typically normal.

Two-dimensional echocardiography confirms the diagnosis and identifies the anatomy and morphology of the obstructing valve. Additional cardiac defects may be identified. The velocity of flow across the valve is measured to calculate peak transvalvular gradient. Tricuspid valve regurgitation,

if present, can be used to estimate the right ventricular pressure. Interventional catheterization is performed in anticipation of transcatheter balloon valvuloplasty.

Management
Indications

Balloon valvuloplasty is the mainstay of initial management. Transvenous balloon valvuloplasty should be performed on all symptomatic patients. The more problematic patients are those who are asymptomatic. Only 15% of asymptomatic infants with mild pulmonary stenosis require intervention within 2 years, whereas most patients with gradients of 50 to 79 mm Hg have progression of the gradient and require intervention. Based on these findings, patients with a transvalvular gradient greater than 50 mm Hg should undergo intervention before developing sequelae of right ventricular hypertension.

Transvenous Balloon Valvuloplasty

The technique of balloon valvuloplasty is the same as described for the neonate. Results have been excellent, with immediate reduction in transvalvular gradient in most patients. Factors influencing the success of valvuloplasty include site of stenosis, residual gradient, and failure to oversize the balloon at the time of valvuloplasty. Despite high residual infundibular gradients immediately after valvuloplasty, significant reduction in infundibular gradients may occur late. Restenosis has been reported as low as 5% but occurs more frequently in patients with dysplastic valves.

Surgical Valvuloplasty

Surgical technique already has been described. In the current era, surgical treatment is limited to cases of failed balloon valvuloplasty or to centers where valvuloplasty is not performed. The mortality of surgical valvuloplasty approaches 0%. Results are excellent. Nearly all patients have some degree of residual valve insufficiency. Long-term insufficiency may lead to right ventricular overload and late pulmonary valve replacement.

SUGGESTED READING

Anand R, Mehta AV: Natural history of asymptomatic valvar pulmonary stenosis diagnosed in infancy, *Clin Cardiol* 20:377, 1997.

Hanley FL, et al: Outcomes in critically ill neonates with pulmonary stenosis and intact ventricular septum: a multiinstitutional study: Congenital Heart Surgeons Society, *J Am Coll Cardiol* 22:183, 1993.

Hayes CJ, et al: Second natural history study of congenital heart defects: results of treatment of patients with pulmonary valvar stenosis, *Circulation* 87:128, 1993.

Kan JS, et al: Percutaneous balloon valvuloplasty: a method for treating congenital pulmonary valve stenosis, *N Engl J Med* 307:540, 1982.

Kopecky SL, et al: Long-term outcome of patients undergoing surgical repair of isolated pulmonary valve stenosis: follow-up at 20 to 30 years, *Circulation* 78:1150, 1988.

McCrindle BW, Kan JS: Long-term results after balloon pulmonary valvuloplasty, *Circulation* 83:1915, 1991.

TRUNCUS ARTERIOSUS

Luca A. Vricella

Victor T. Tsang

Truncus arteriosus or common arterial trunk (CAT) is a rare cardiac malformation that constitutes 0.2% to 4% of all congenital cardiac anomalies. It is defined by common origin of pulmonary and coronary arteries from a single arterial trunk and represents the shared outflow tract of both ventricular chambers. CAT is associated with anomalies of the neural crest, DiGeorge syndrome, and in one third of neonates chromosome 22q11 deletions.

■ MORPHOLOGY

Perturbation in the normal development of the aorticopulmonary septum results in the wide spectrum of conotruncal anomalies observed in neonates with CAT. The defect in the normal process of cardiac septation involves both ventricular outflow tracts, arterial trunks, and semilunar valves. CAT (typically larger in diameter than the normal aorta) gives rise to pulmonary, systemic, and coronary circulations; the absence of continuity between the morphologic right ventricle and pulmonary arteries distinguishes this malformation from pulmonary atresia and its variants.

Two classifications have been used to describe the various features of CAT (Figure 1). In 1949, Collett and Edwards described four variations of truncal anomalies according to the origin of the pulmonary arterial vasculature.

In Collett-Edwards type 1 truncus (60% of cases), a common pulmonary artery arises from the supracoronary arterial trunk, bifurcating into right and left branch pulmonary arteries. Type II (20%) and type III (10%) are defined by separate pulmonary ostia. These are located in proximity to (type II) or 180 degrees apart from (type III) each other along the truncal circumference. Because CAT by definition should give origin to the pulmonary arterial supply, extrapericardial origin of the pulmonary arteries (type IV) no longer should be included in truncal anomalies. Instead, this anatomic variant should be described as a solitary arterial trunk with aorticopulmonary collaterals and absent intrapericardial pulmonary arteries. The classification scheme introduced by Van Praagh and Van Praagh in 1965 includes description of associated anomalous origin of one pulmonary artery (type 3), aortic arch anomalies (type 4), and ventricular septal defect (VSD) (A, present; B, absent).

CAT is associated with a large semilunar truncal valve. The valve is most frequently tricuspid (65%) and dysplastic but may be bicuspid. Up to six cusps have been described, and malfunction most frequently results in regurgitation rather than stenosis.

Atrioventricular connection is usually concordant. The arterial trunk typically overrides a nonrestrictive VSD. In 42% of cases, contribution of well-developed right and left ventricles to the outflow tract is equal. There is no right ventricular infundibulum, and the truncal valve typically straddles the continuum between the ventriculoinfundibular fold and trabecula septomarginalis. The truncal valve is the superior margin of the VSD. There is usually mitral-truncal continuity, and the atrioventricular conduction system lies posterior and to the left of the crest of the VSD. In one third of cases, there is continuity between tricuspid and truncal valves, which creates a greater challenge to preserve the integrity of the conduction system during VSD closure. A patent foramen ovale often is seen, and a true atrial septal defect is present in approximately 10% of patients.

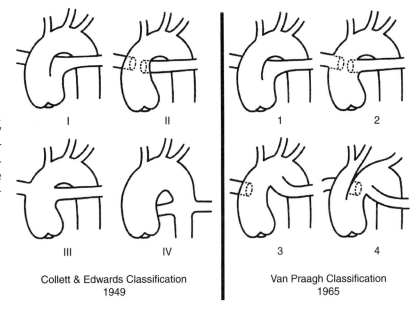

Figure 1

Morphologic classifications of truncus arteriosus. Collett-Edwards anatomic types I through IV are described according to pulmonary vascular origins, whereas the Van Praagh scheme concerns anomalies of the aortic arch and presence (subtype A) or absence (subtype B) of ventricular septal defect.

Collett & Edwards Classification
1949

Van Praagh Classification
1965

Associated coronary anomalies are found in nearly 50% of patients. Most frequently, the anomaly is either high takeoff of the left main coronary artery or anomalous origin of the left anterior descending coronary artery from the right coronary artery. Abnormal development of the fourth and sixth aortic arches is the embryologic basis for the association between truncus arteriosus and aortic arch anomalies (25%). Specifically, interrupted aortic arch type B (discontinuity of arch between left common carotid and left subclavian arteries) is the most common configuration associated with CAT; a right-sided aortic arch in seen in 18% to 36% of cases. Other associations (tricuspid stenosis or atresia, atrioventricular septal defect and vascular rings, among several others) also have been described.

PATHOPHYSIOLOGY

Neonates with CAT typically present with pulmonary over-circulation, pulmonary hypertension, and complete mixing across an unrestrictive subarterial VSD. Cyanosis usually is moderate (systemic arterial oxygen saturation 85% to 95%), and shunting largely depends on the balance between pulmonary and systemic vascular resistance. Immediately after birth, left-to-right shunting is reduced by elevated pulmonary vascular resistance. During the natural postnatal decrease in pulmonary resistance, left-to-right shunting increases at the expense of pulmonary congestion. If surgically untreated, late cyanosis and congestive heart failure supervene as a consequence of pulmonary vascular arteriolar changes, with late development of Eisenmenger's syndrome. The risk of developing severe early pulmonary hypertension is increased by the fact that pulmonary hypertension is systolic and diastolic, since the pulmonary ostia lie above the truncal valve.

When truncal valvular regurgitation is present, ventricular enlargement and coronary hypoperfusion may lead to rapid hemodynamic decompensation. Truncal valve stenosis is a rare clinical scenario, in which ventricular pressure overload, concentric hypertrophy, and dysfunction are predominant. When CAT is associated with aortic arch interruption, a large patent ductus arteriosus provides direct continuation of CAT into the descending aorta.

DIAGNOSTIC STUDIES

Neonates with conotruncal anomalies frequently have well-balanced intrauterine development and present shortly after birth with various degrees of cyanosis. Although mild-to-moderate cyanosis and pulmonary congestion are the typical clinical presentation, deep cyanosis should suggest shunt reversal and pulmonary hypertension. In rare cases, pulmonary edema can be attenuated by concomitant pulmonary branch arterial stenosis. Differential diagnosis is limited to Fallot-type pulmonary atresia and aortico-pulmonary window.

Chest radiographs disclose plethora or oligemia and ventricular enlargement. The electrocardiogram typically shows biventricular hypertrophy. Echocardiography is the diagnostic procedure of choice and enables the clinician to define truncal anatomy, intracardiac defects, coronary and aortic arch anatomy, and valvular function. Cardiac catheterization is rarely indicated and is reserved for patients in whom anatomy or valvular function cannot be assessed fully by echocardiography. In infants with marked cyanosis referred late for surgical correction, cardiac catheterization delineates pulmonary arterial anatomy and pulmonary vascular resistance.

NATURAL HISTORY

CAT was uniformly fatal before introduction of surgical treatment, as a consequence of accelerated onset of irreversible pulmonary hypertension. If untreated, one half of all patients die as a result of pulmonary hypertension and congestive heart failure during the first month of life. Approximately 75% die in the first year. Early postnatal diagnosis is followed by rapid surgical intervention, and complete intracardiac repair is currently the standard of care.

TREATMENT

Palliation by pulmonary arterial banding was introduced by Armer in 1961 and was followed in 1962 by the first successful complete repair by Behrendt. Initial right ventricular outflow tract (RVOT) reconstruction used a valveless conduit but gave way to the first allograft reconstruction by McGoon in 1967.

Medical treatment of CAT is limited to preoperative stabilization and infusion of prostaglandin E_1 in cases of aortic arch interruption. Improvement in neonatal critical care strategies has had a substantial impact on postoperative outcome in recent years. The goals of complete intracardiac repair of CAT are (1) disconnection of the pulmonary arterial trunk and its branches from the CAT, (2) VSD closure and reconstruction of right ventricle-to-pulmonary artery continuity, and (3) same-stage correction of associated anomalies.

Operative correction of the most common anatomic form of CAT (Van Praagh classification type A1) is illustrated schematically in Figure 2. The procedure is accomplished via a median sternotomy. The thymus is resected if present. The operation is performed on cardiopulmonary bypass, with aortic and bicaval cannulation and moderate hypothermia. The branch pulmonary arteries are mobilized extensively and occluded on initiation of extracorporeal circulation. After aortic cross-clamping and cardioplegic arrest, the main pulmonary artery is excised from the arterial trunk with a variable portion of truncal wall (Figure 2A). In a variation of the technique described, the CAT can be transected distally and proximally to the pulmonary arterial takeoff and the branch pulmonary arteries prepared as a "cylinder" of truncal tissue; continuity of the trunk is restored after this type of pulmonary-truncal separation by end-to-end anastomosis. During detachment of the pulmonary arterial origin from the trunk, great care is taken to avoid injury to the left and right coronary arteries. The truncal valve is inspected, and if preoperative truncal valve regurgitation is confirmed at operation by findings of a severely dysplastic valve, replacement of the truncal root with an allograft should be considered. Alternatively, truncal valve repair can be attempted. Mild or moderate regurgitation can be tolerated and expected to improve with the diminished volume loading of the outflow tract and afterload reduction after complete repair. The truncal defect created by excision of the trunk is repaired primarily or with a patch. A right-angle clamp is advanced carefully through the truncal valve to identify an ideal location for a longitudinal right ventriculotomy (Figure 2B). The subarterial VSD is closed with a prosthetic patch (Figure 2C). Careful placement of the suture is imperative to ensure avoidance of heart block, particularly in cases with tricuspid-truncal valve continuity. For this purpose, the suture is placed through the tricuspid valve, close to its annulus. The superior margin of the VSD closure is carried out along the uppermost margin of the right ventriculotomy and the anterior margin of the truncal valve annulus, avoiding injury to the semilunar valve leaflets. The RVOT is reconstructed with an allograft (appropriately sized aortic or pulmonary, 14 to18 mm in diameter). Alternatively, a Dacron prosthesis with xenograft porcine valve may be used. Reconstruction of the RVOT has also been accomplished with nonvalved conduits, autologous left atrial appendage interposition, and direct right ventricular-to-pulmonary artery connection. Alternatively, a monocusp valve can be inserted in the RVOT to preserve early diastolic competence of the reconstruction.

We firmly believe that RVOT reconstruction with a competent valve is beneficial and allows better hemodynamic tolerance of the transition from right ventricular volume to pressure overload in the early postoperative period. The posterior aspect of the proximal running suture line of the allograft is secured to the superior aspect of the VSD (Figure 2D). A patch of prosthetic material often is necessary to contour the hood of the RVOT reconstruction (Figure 2E). Alternatively, the retained anterior leaflet of the donor mitral valve can be used for this purpose when an aortic allograft has been chosen. We do not favor the latter technique because the curve of the RVOT reconstruction is distorted by the natural angulation between aortic homograft and anterior mitral valve leaflet. Through a right atriotomy, a fenestration is created across the atrial septum. The patient is rewarmed and weaned from cardiopulmonary bypass. Modified ultrafiltration is routinely performed. On chest closure, excessive bowing and angulation of the allograft is avoided by allowing leftward cardiac rotation through a generous pleuropericardial opening.

Coexistent aortic arch interruption is repaired at the same operation. In this case, arch repair is accomplished under profound hypothermic circulatory arrest or with moderate hypothermia and selective antegrade low-flow cerebral perfusion. End-to-end anastomosis or reverse subclavian flap arterioplasty can be used for aortic arch reconstruction.

■ POSTOPERATIVE CARE

Patients who have undergone repair of CAT are at significant risk for postoperative pulmonary hypertensive crises. This is

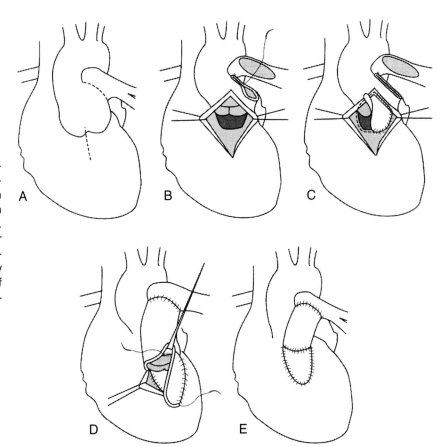

Figure 2
Operative correction of type I (Collett-Edwards) or 1A (Van Praagh) common arterial trunk. **A**, Line of incision. **B**, Inspection of truncal valve and separation of main pulmonary artery from the arterial trunk. **C**, Prosthetic path closure of the ventricular septal defect. Closure of subarterial ventricular defect. **D**, Right ventricular outflow tract reconstruction. Posterior aspect of graft sutured to the superior aspect of ventricular septal defect. **E**, Completed repair.

particularly true for patients who undergo correction after the neonatal period. Postoperative strategy to minimize pulmonary vascular resistance includes administration of nitric oxide, sedatives, narcotics, muscle relaxants and avoidance of hypercarbia and acidosis. Perioperative right ventricular hemodynamics are supported with inotropes and monitored carefully by indwelling pulmonary, left atrial, and central venous pressure lines.

RESULTS

The modern era of complete intracardiac repair in the neonatal period and during early infancy begins with the landmark report by Ebert et al of 77 patients repaired in the first 6 months of life with an unprecedented operative mortality of 9%. The report underscored the benefit of correcting the anomaly before severe pulmonary vascular changes ensue. Early intervention has nevertheless been challenged by some authors, who point to the disadvantages of intervening too early on patients with low operative weight. With modern techniques of improved myocardial protection, extracorporeal circulation and perioperative advances in critical care, operative survival of 5% to 21% has been reported, with 5-, 10-, and 15-year actuarial survival of 90, 85, and 83%.

In the Boston Children's Hospital experience, association of coronary anomalies or aortic arch interruption, age at repair greater than 100 days, and severe truncal valve insufficiency were major determinants of adverse outcome. Other predictors reported in the literature are operative weight less than 2.5 kg and need for intervention on the truncal valve.

Freedom from reintervention in children with CAT is related to the durability of the conduit for RVOT reconstruction. Neonates and infants undergoing early complete repair almost invariably require reoperation for structural conduit failure or relative somatic growth in the intermediate term. This reintervention rate can be as high as 43% at 3 years for neonates undergoing repair, and is associated with aortic or pulmonary allografts less than 15 mm in diameter. Median time to conduit replacement is approximately 5 years.

Although allografts are considered by most to be the gold standard for RVOT reconstruction, several alternatives exist. Dacron-xenograft valved conduits were favored initially, although endoluminal obstruction from progressive pseudointimal growth is the typical mode of late structural conduit failure. Valved bovine jugular vein xenografts have been used, whereas left atrial appendage interposition in the

reconstruction is believed to retain the potential for conduit growth. Some authors have observed decreased need for late reintervention with direct right ventricular-to-pulmonary artery anastomosis and advocate this technical variation if allografts are unavailable.

The other determinant of late outcome and reintervention is function of the truncal valve. Ten-year freedom from truncal valve repair or replacement is less in patients with preoperative mild or moderate insufficiency compared with patients with competent truncal valves at operation (63% versus 95%). Moderate to severe truncal valve regurgitation may warrant repair or replacement at initial correction; should important valve insufficiency develop postoperatively, similar consideration should be given to surgical reintervention. Although not reported extensively in the literature, some authors favor repair by leaflet excision and truncal reduction annuloplasty over valvular suture techniques.

SUMMARY

Neonates and infants with CAT are a small group of patients with a grim prognosis if untreated surgically. Severe pulmonary overcirculation and rapidly progressive pulmonary vascular changes lead to irreversible pulmonary hypertension and inoperability. Intervention shortly after birth with complete repair and RVOT reconstruction has evolved during recent years and is regarded by most authors as standard of care. Concomitant anomalies represent adverse outcome predictors in several clinical series and should be corrected simultaneously. Good operative survival should be expected, whereas intermediate and late outcomes are still largely influenced by the need for conduit exchange and progressive truncal valve dysfunction.

SUGGESTED READING

Common arterial trunk. In Anderson RH, Wilcox BR, editors: *Surgical anatomy of the heart.* London, 1992, Gower Medical Publishing, p 8.29.

Brizard CP, et al: Management strategy and long-term outcome for truncus arteriosus, *Eur J Cardiothorac Surg* 11:687, 1997.

Ebert PA, et al: Surgical treatment of truncus arteriosus in the first six months of life, *Ann Thorac Surg* 200:451, 1984.

Hanley FL, et al: Repair of truncus arteriosus in the neonate, *J Thorac Cardiovasc Surg* 105:1047, 1993.

Schreiber C, et al: Common arterial trunk associated with double aortic arch, *Ann Thorac Surg* 68:1850, 1999.

TRANSPOSITION OF THE GREAT ARTERIES

Brian W. Duncan

Roger B. B. Mee

Transposition of the great arteries (TGA) is one of the most common conditions causing significant cyanosis in newborns. In children with TGA, the aorta arises from the morphologically right ventricle anterior and usually to the right of the pulmonary artery origin from the morphologically left ventricle. The usual coronary artery pattern (approximately 70% of cases) consists of the left anterior descending and circumflex coronary arteries arising from the anterior/leftward sinus (sinus 1) with the right coronary artery arising from the posterior/rightward sinus (sinus 2). The next most common coronary artery pattern (approximately 20% of cases) has the right and circumflex coronary arteries arising from sinus 2 while the left anterior descending coronary artery arises from sinus 1. Other coronary artery patterns, including single right coronary, single left coronary, and intramural coronary arteries, are much less common. In approximately three-quarters of the cases there is an intact ventricular septum (TGA-IVS), whereas the remainder possess a hemodynamically significant ventricular septal defect (TGA-VSD). Other associated lesions such as left ventricular outflow tract obstruction and hypoplastic or interrupted aortic arch are uncommon but have major implications for the management of these children (see "Special Situations").

Systemic venous blood returns to the right ventricle and is ejected into the aorta while pulmonary venous return enters the left ventricle and is ejected into the pulmonary artery. The systemic and pulmonary circulations therefore function in parallel. Without a large communication between the systemic and pulmonary circulations at the atrial, ventricular, or great vessel level, effective pulmonary blood flow (the systemic venous return that enters the pulmonary arterial circulation) is low and cyanosis is intense. A patent ductus arteriosus, maintained by prostaglandin infusion, volume loads the left atrium and encourages left-to-right shunting (mixing) at the atrial level even though a restrictive atrial septal defect is often inadequate to alleviate severe cyanosis in children with TGA-IVS. To increase mixing between the systemic and pulmonary circulations sufficient to maintain systemic oxygen saturations at an acceptable level, a balloon atrial septostomy is often performed in infants with TGA-IVS. Children with TGA and an unrestrictive VSD often exhibit adequate systemic oxygen saturations without the administration of prostaglandin or the performance of a balloon atrial septostomy; however, occasionally streaming is pronounced and a balloon atrial septostomy aids mixing in these cases.

■ MANAGEMENT OF CHILDREN WITH TRANSPOSITION OF THE GREAT ARTERIES

Diagnosis

Echocardiography usually provides an accurate and complete diagnosis for this condition. The great vessel orientation, location and number of VSDs, semilunar valve anatomy, and presence of significant associated anomalies can be accurately determined with echocardiography. The coronary artery anatomy can often also be defined with a high degree of certainty; however, the ultimate determination is always made at the time of operative repair. Cardiac catheterization has little, if any, role in preoperative diagnosis for these neonates.

Historical Aspects of Operative Repair

The atrial level switch, which provides physiologic repair of TGA, was first reported by Mustard in 1964 and Senning in 1958. These procedures produced excellent operative survival and revolutionized the management of this condition. However, unsatisfactory long-term outcomes for these patients due to a significant incidence of arrhythmias and failure of the right ventricle and tricuspid valve on the systemic side of the circulation, particularly in patients with a large VSD, provided the impetus to perfect anatomic repair. Jatene first reported the successful performance of an arterial switch operation in 1975. Yacoub demonstrated that TGA-IVS in older patients could also be successfully treated with an arterial switch operation after conditioning the left ventricle to withstand systemic pressures by first performing pulmonary artery banding. Castenada first reported a series of newborns with TGA-IVS successfully treated by a primary arterial switch operation taking advantage of the fact that the left ventricle is conditioned to withstand systemic pressure loading during the neonatal period. The arterial switch operation is now considered the surgical treatment of choice for TGA-IVS, TGA-VSD, and other conditions with transposition physiology such as double outlet right ventricle with subpulmonary VSD.

Timing of Operative Repair

The timing of operative repair for TGA should be individualized based on the underlying anatomy and physiology. Patients with TGA-IVS should undergo an arterial switch operation within the first 2 weeks of life. However, if operation is delayed for some reason beyond this period, an arterial switch operation may still be safely performed for TGA-IVS in infants up to 2 months of age without preoperative conditioning of the left ventricle (see "Special Situations"). Individuals with TGA-IVS encountered beyond this period will likely require left ventricular conditioning by placement of a pulmonary artery band before the arterial switch operation or by postoperative support with a left ventricular assist device. Pulmonary artery banding usually intensifies cyanosis and a concomitant small systemic to arterial shunt is often required. Infants with TGA and a restrictive VSD may be expected to follow a similar clinical course as patients with TGA-IVS and should undergo early repair. Infants with TGA and prostaglandin-dependent circulations due to associated aortic arch abnormalities such as interruption of the aortic arch or aortic coarctation should undergo early arterial switch operation and concomitant arch reconstruction.

Children with TGA and an unrestrictive VSD should undergo individualized management based on the severity of congestive heart failure. Children with TGA-VSD who are ventilator bound due to severe congestive heart failure should undergo an early arterial switch operation. Children with TGA-VSD in whom symptoms of congestive heart failure are easily managed with oral medications may have repair deferred beyond the neonatal period. However, all of these children should undergo repair within the first 90 days of life, as the development of pulmonary vascular obstructive disease becomes an increasing risk beyond this period.

Technical Aspects of the Arterial Switch Operation

The pump is primed with fresh (less than 24 hours old) heparinized blood. Repair of TGA-IVS is performed at a nasopharyngeal temperature of 22°C, whereas for more complex forms of TGA requiring arch reconstruction, the temperature is lowered to 18°C. Phenoxybenzamine (1 mg/kg) is administered before or just as cardiopulmonary bypass is instituted. Pump flows are maintained at 150 to 220 ml/kg/min to attain a mean perfusion pressure of approximately 35 to 40 mm Hg.

The patient is positioned with a roll under the shoulders and the head extended. A median sternotomy is performed and a large piece of anterior pericardium is harvested for the reconstruction of the neopulmonary artery. It is important to carefully assess the coronary artery anatomy at this point. Marking sutures are placed on the pulmonary artery at the future sites of implantation of the coronary arteries. The coronary implantation sites are best determined at this point with the great vessels fully distended, in their native position, before institution of cardiopulmonary bypass. The aorta is cannulated as far cephalad as possible, opposite the take-off of the innominate artery. Bicaval cannulation is required for TGA-VSD, whereas single venous cannulation may be used for repair of TGA-IVS. As cardiopulmonary bypass is instituted the ductus arteriosus is ligated and divided, and the aortic end of the ductus oversewn with a second suture. The pulmonary arteries are skeletonized to the lobar branches in the hilum of the lung. The ascending aorta is cross-clamped as far distally as possible, and a single dose of cardioplegia is administered into the aortic root.

The ascending aorta is then transected approximately 2 to 3 mm above the upper edge of the coronary ostial bulge and inspected internally for the exact location of the coronary ostia before the transection is completed. The internal anatomy of the coronary sinuses is then carefully analyzed and corroborated with the external appearance of the coronary arteries. Coronary buttons are then fashioned by excising a D-shaped cuff of coronary sinus wall leaving only a 0.5- to 1-mm rim above the line of attachment of the valve leaflet. Ostia occupying an eccentric location in the sinus close to a leaflet commissure can be managed by dissecting the commissure off of the aortic wall to allow an adequate rim of aortic sinus to be obtained around the coronary ostium. The commissure can be resuspended later from the pericardial patch that is used to reconstruct the pulmonary artery.

The pulmonary artery is then transected approximately 2 to 3 mm above the previously placed coronary implantation marking sutures. The pulmonic valve is inspected to ensure that it has normal morphology. Medially hinged trapdoor flaps are then created in the main pulmonary artery at or above the sinotubular junction (Figure 1). The coronary artery cuffs are then sewn into the defects using 7-0 polypropylene suture, taking great care to avoid axial rotation of the buttons. At the completion of the suture line, the medially based flaps create a conical extension of the proximal neoaorta, which reduces the angle through which the transposed coronary artery must rotate after implantation (Figure 2).

The Lecompte maneuver, which is performed in all cases where the aorta arises anterior to the pulmonary artery, results in the reconstructed neopulmonary artery lying anterior to the reconstructed aorta. The Lecompte maneuver may be facilitated by anterior traction on Silastic vessel loops placed around the branch pulmonary arteries or by repositioning the aortic cross-clamp distal to the transected pulmonary artery to maintain the new relationship between the great vessels. The aortic reconstruction is then completed by suturing the distal aorta to the proximal neoaorta with 7-0 polypropylene sutures. The atrial septal defect is repaired primarily at this point with a brief period of circulatory arrest if only a single venous drainage cannula has been used. The aortic cross-clamp is then removed using the cardioplegia site for deairing. The myocardium should be carefully evaluated for adequate perfusion of all areas. Gradual resumption of

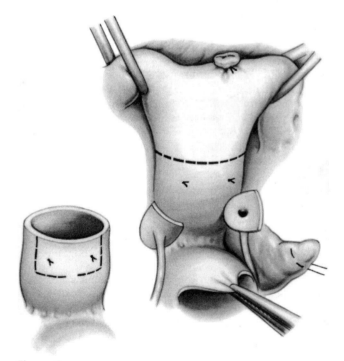

Figure 1
Medially hinged trapdoor flaps created in the main pulmonary artery for coronary artery implantation. (*From Mee RBB: The arterial switch operation. In Stark J, Pacifico AP, editors:* Surgery for congenital heart defects, *ed 2. Philadelphia, 1994, WB Saunders, p 489, reprinted with permission.*)

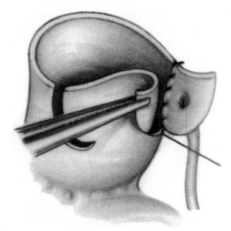

Figure 2
Medially based trapdoor flaps create conical extensions of the proximal neoaorta that reduce the angle through which each transposed coronary artery must rotate after implantation. (*From Mee RBB: The arterial switch operation. In Stark J, Pacifico AP, editors:* Surgery for congenital heart defects, *ed 2. Philadelphia, 1994, WB Saunders, p 491, reprinted with permission.*)

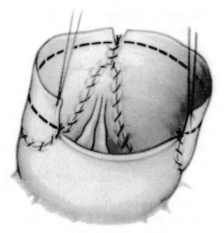

Figure 3
Reconstruction of the neopulmonary artery with patches of fresh, autologous pericardium, sewn together over their posterior extent. (*From Mee RBB: The arterial switch operation. In Stark J, Pacifico AP, editors:* Surgery for congenital heart defects, *ed 2. Philadelphia, 1994, WB Saunders, p 493, reprinted with permission.*)

normal sinus rhythm without ventricular ectopy is an important indication that myocardial blood supply is adequate. Prolonged ventricular arrhythmia or persistent bluish discoloration of the ventricular myocardium as warming occurs suggests that problems exist with the coronary transfer. Takedown and reimplantation of the coronary arteries or placement of horizontal mattress plication stitches to reduce kinking at the coronary suture lines may be necessary to improve coronary blood flow.

The neopulmonary artery reconstruction is performed after removal of the aortic cross-clamp with the heart perfused and beating. The coronary sinus defects may be filled with individual patches of fresh, autologous pericardium that are sewn together using 7-0 polypropylene suture over their posterior extent (Figure 3). Alternatively, a single pantaloon shaped patch of pericardium may be used for neopulmonary artery reconstruction. With either technique, it is important to create a significant posterior extension of the neopulmonary artery that reduces tension on the anastomosis to the distal pulmonary artery and places the pulmonary artery bifurcation well above the coronary implantation sites. The neopulmonary artery is then sewn to the distal pulmonary artery with a running suture of 7-0 polypropylene.

After completion of the repair, intracardiac monitoring lines are placed in the left atrium and pulmonary artery. Temporary atrial and epicardial pacing wires are also placed. Weaning from cardiopulmonary bypass is almost always achieved on 5 µg/kg/min of dopamine, which usually produces excellent hemodynamics. Mediastinal drainage and chest closure are performed as per routine for neonates. We routinely place peritoneal catheters after infant cardiac surgery to serve as a continuous drain of the abdominal cavity which may also be used for peritoneal minidialysis for

persistent low urinary output or hyperkalemia or to remove fluid. In the immediate postoperative period, systemic hypertension is avoided and left atrial pressure is ideally maintained at 10 mm Hg or less. Phenoxybenzamine is continued during the first several days after surgery.

■ SPECIAL SITUATIONS

Ventricular Septal Defect
If bicaval cannulation has been used, VSD closure is performed through a right atriotomy without interruption of cardiopulmonary bypass. VSD closure can be performed before or after the arterial switch operation with additional doses of cardioplegia.

Unusual Coronary Artery Patterns
As discussed previously, abnormal coronary artery patterns may be encountered in up to 30% of these patients. The circumflex coronary artery travels behind the pulmonary artery if the circumflex arises from the right coronary artery in sinus 2. In this setting, implantation of the right coronary artery in the usual location may result in kinking of the circumflex coronary artery. Placing the right coronary implantation 2 to 3 mm higher on the neoaorta may allow the circumflex to assume a less angulated course, thereby avoiding this problem.

Intramural coronary arteries often pass behind a commissure of the aortic valve with the sinus opening very close to the other coronary artery. In this situation, the commissure is taken down, the intramural coronary artery is unroofed on the aortic luminal side, the ostia are separated, and buttons are fashioned in the usual way. The commissure is then resuspended onto the pericardial patch used to repair the aortic sinus defects.

Left Ventricular Outflow Tract Obstruction

Subpulmonic or left ventricular outflow tract obstruction may take several forms. Preoperatively, dynamic subpulmonic narrowing may occur due to leftward septal shift arising from systemic pressure in the right ventricle. In this case, performance of the arterial switch operation reestablishes the normal septal orientation as the left ventricle is exposed to systemic arterial pressure. Obstructive muscle bands or accessory atrioventricular valve leaflet tissue may be resected through the pulmonary valve after transecting the pulmonary artery. Valvar pulmonic (neoaortic) stenosis may also be treated by a conservative valvotomy through the main pulmonary artery.

Aortic Coarctation or Interrupted Aortic Arch

If the arch is interrupted or very small, the ductus arteriosus and ascending aorta are cannulated. After cardiopulmonary bypass is established the duct is ligated proximal to the ductal cannula and the duct, the aortic arch and the upper descending aorta are fully mobilized. At a nasopharyngeal temperature of 18°C, isolated coronary perfusion may be instituted. Bypass flows are reduced to 10%, the arch vessel snares are tightened, the ductal cannula is removed, and a cross-clamp is placed obliquely just distal to the aortic cannula. Pump flows are adjusted to achieve an arterial bypass line pressure of 30 mm Hg, maintaining the heart perfused and beating. All ductal tissue is then excised, and the descending aorta is anastomosed to the underside of the proximal arch with running 7-0 polypropylene suture. The proximal end of this anastomosis should lie opposite the innominate artery origin. When aortic reconstruction is complete, the clamp is shifted proximal to the aortic cannula, cardioplegia is administered, full bypass is resumed, and the remainder of the operation is performed in a standard fashion.

Arterial Switch Operation in Patients Possessing a Deconditioned Left Ventricle

After an extended time in the pulmonary circulation, the left ventricle becomes deconditioned and incapable of supporting systemic blood pressure. Patients presenting for the arterial switch operation at an older age with a deconditioned left ventricle generally fall under three categories: (1) patients with congenitally corrected transposition possessing both atrioventricular and ventriculoarterial discordance, (2) patients who have previously undergone an atrial level switch but in whom the systemic right ventricle is failing or is at risk to fail, and (3) a few patients with TGA-IVS who present at an advanced age. We believe that a primary arterial switch operation can be safely performed up to 60 days of age in all patients with TGA-IVS or TGA with a restrictive VSD. Patients presenting beyond this age in whom the left ventricle–to–right ventricle pressure ratio is less than 0.65 for infants or less than 0.90 for adolescents, or in whom the left ventricular mass index is less than 80 g/m² in adolescents and older patients, require conditioning of the left ventricle prior to performance of the arterial switch operation. Left ventricular conditioning is accomplished by pulmonary artery banding (often with the addition of a small systemic to pulmonary arterial shunt) for late presenting uncorrected TGA-IVS, followed by interval repair. For patients with congenitally corrected transposition, complete repair entails the arterial switch operation combined with an atrial level switch after pulmonary artery banding. Patients with a failing atrial level switch undergo an arterial switch operation plus takedown of the atrial level switch and atrial resetation after left ventricular conditioning.

■ RESULTS

From July 1993 through April 2001, 117 consecutive infants less than 90 days of age underwent an arterial switch operation at our institution. Seventy-five (63%) had TGA-IVS, and the remainder had TGA-VSD (n = 33) (28%) or double outlet right ventricle (n = 9) (7.7%). Three double outlet right ventricle patients had associated aortic arch interruption (n = 2) or aortic coarctation (n = 1). Eight TGA-IVS patients underwent an arterial switch operation beyond 14 days of age (range, 17 to 46 days). Eighty-four (72%) had usual coronary artery patterns (left anterior descending and circumflex coronary arteries arising from sinus 1, right coronary artery arising from sinus 2). During a median follow-up of 8.4 months for this group (range, 0.2 to 73 months) one patient (0.8%) died during hospitalization due to renal failure, and one patient died 33 months after discharge in a crush accident (1.6% total mortality). A single patient (0.8%) has required further intervention for neopulmonary valvar stenosis. In this experience, arch abnormalities, delayed presentation for TGA-IVS (up to 60 days of age), and unusual coronary artery patterns did not impart additional risk.

From July 1993 through March 1997, we encountered 29 patients beyond 3 months of age who were treated by anatomic correction of TGA. Seventeen of these patients required preliminary pulmonary artery banding for low left ventricular pressure and inadequate left ventricular mass. Fourteen patients had a Senning operation plus an arterial switch operation or Rastelli procedure for congenitally corrected transposition, all of whom survived. Twelve patients with a failing atrial level switch underwent resetation of the atrium and an arterial switch operation resulting in eight survivors, one early death, and three late deaths. Three patients presented beyond 90 days with TGA-IVS who underwent an arterial switch operation; all three patients survived. Twenty-eight of these 29 patients (97%) were early survivors with 25 of 29 late survivors (86%).

■ SUMMARY

TGA is one of the most commonly encountered causes of cyanotic congenital heart disease. The arterial switch operation has emerged as the treatment of choice for this condition. With appropriate modification and management, excellent results for the arterial switch operation may be anticipated in even the most complex cases such as TGA accompanied by aortic arch abnormalities, atrioventricular discordance, and unusual coronary artery patterns.

SUGGESTED READING

Asou TT, et al: Arterial switch: translocation of the intramural coronary artery, *Ann Thorac Surg* 57:461, 1994.

Castenada A, et al: Transposition of the great arteries and intact ventricular septum: anatomical repair in the neonate, *Ann Thorac Surg* 38:438, 1984.

Davis AM, et al: Transposition of the great arteries with intact ventricular septum: arterial switch repair in patients 21 days of age or older, *J Thorac Cardiovasc Surg* 106:111, 1993.

Helvind MH, et al: Ventriculo-arterial discordance: switching the morphologically left ventricle into the systemic circulation after 3 months of age, *Eur J Cadiothorac Surg* 14:173, 1998.

Wilson NJ, et al: Long-term outcome after the Mustard repair for simple transposition of the great arteries, *J Am Coll Cardiol* 32:758, 1998.

CONGENITALLY CORRECTED TRANSPOSITION OF THE GREAT ARTERIES

Tom R. Karl
Andrew D. Cochrane

Congenitally corrected transposition of the great arteries (ccTGA) is a complex cardiac lesion involving abnormal (discordant) atrioventricular (AV) and ventriculoarterial (VA) connections. Alternate terms to describe ccTGA include corrected transposition, discordant transposition, AV and VA discordance, physiologically corrected transposition, double discordance, AV discordance with transposition, L-transposition (L-TGA), inverted transposition, mixed levocardia/mixed dextrocardia, and dextroversion. Segmental nomenclature (e.g., SLL, IDD) has also been applied. A full review of the nomenclature and a proposed classification recently have been adopted for the STS Database for Congenital Heart Surgery, and ccTGA has become a universally understood term.

The features common to all patients are (1) the systemic venous atrium (morphologic right atrium) is connected to the morphologic left ventricle (LV) through a mitral valve, (2) the LV is connected to the pulmonary artery (PA) through the pulmonary valve, (3) the pulmonary venous atrium (morphologic left atrium) is connected to the morphologic right ventricle (RV) by means of a tricuspid valve, which therefore functions as the systemic AV valve, and (4) the RV is then connected to the aorta via the aortic valve. As a result of the discordant connections at both levels, blood flows in a "congenitally corrected" physiologic pathway, despite the anatomic derangements (Figure 1).

Associated defects are the rule. The three major and common anomalies are ventricular septal defect (VSD), pulmonary valve or subpulmonary stenosis (resulting in LV outflow tract obstruction [LVOTO]), and tricuspid valve malformations (resulting in systemic AV valve regurgitation).

The anatomy of the conduction system and the coronary arteries are also abnormal. The associated conditions may affect the timing and mode of presentation, the severity of symptoms, and ultimately the management strategy. Features that distinguish ccTGA from the more commonly encountered concordant TGA are shown in Table 1.

■ NATURAL HISTORY AND CLINICAL PRESENTATION

The natural history of ccTGA is extremely variable. Infants with severe pulmonary stenosis or pulmonary atresia and those with severe left AV valve regurgitation may present early in life. At the other extreme, some individuals (usually the 1% to 2% with no associated defects) are asymptomatic for many years and are diagnosed only late in life or at postmortem. Symptoms are related to abnormal pulmonary blood flow, systemic AV valve regurgitation, bradycardia from heart block, or systemic ventricular dysfunction.

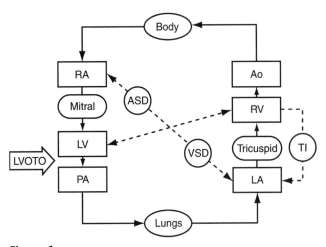

Figure 1
The circulation in ccTGA. The RA connects to the LV via a mitral valve, and the LA connects to the RV via a tricuspid valve. The VA connections are also discordant, with LV connecting to PA and RV connecting to Ao. There is a potential for both intraatrial and intraventricular shunting, as well as LVOTO and TI.

Table 1 Features that May Distinguish Discordant TGA (Congenitally Corrected Transposition of the Great Arteries) From the More Common Concordant TGA

FEATURE	DISCORDANT TRANSPOSITION (ccTGA)	CONCORDANT TRANSPOSITION (TGA)
AV connection	Discordant (RA-LV, LA-RV)	Concordant (RA-RV, LA-LV)
VA connection	Discordant (RV-Ao, LV-PA)	Discordant (RV-Ao, LV-PA)
LVOTO	Common (>50%)	Unusual (<20%)
VSD	Common (>75%)	Seen in minority (<30%)
AV valves	TV dysplastic and often incompetent	Structurally normal, usually competent
Coronary arteries	Many variants, 1R, 2LC$_x$ most common	Many variants, 1LC$_x$, 2R most common
Conduction system	Anterior AV node and His bundle, CHB (congenital, spontaneous, or surgical block is common)	Normal
Great arteries	Ao commonly anterior and to left of PA, in nearly side-by-side relation, many variations possible	Ao commonly anterior to PA, many variations possible

Ao, Aorta; TV, tricuspid valve; R, right; LC$_x$, left circumflex; CHB, complete heart block.

Severe pulmonary stenosis or atresia leads to cyanosis in the newborn period. These infants require prostaglandin infusion and an early systemic-pulmonary arterial shunt (see later). Children with severe tricuspid regurgitation or a large VSD with only mild LVOTO may present in the first few weeks of life with heart failure. The most common presentations during childhood or adolescence are exercise intolerance or poor growth due to a left-to-right shunt or increasing cyanosis and exercise intolerance due to pulmonary stenosis. Progressive systemic AV valve regurgitation may complicate these presentations or occur as an isolated finding. Some patients present with heart block and bradycardia. The proportion with spontaneous complete heart block increases by 2% per year to reach 30% by adult life.

Systemic RV function can deteriorate early after surgical repair or spontaneously during the second decade of life. There is a difference in survival between operated and unoperated patients, whereas RV dysfunction is almost always associated with long-standing tricuspid regurgitation. In general, for both definitively operated and palliated patients, survival is significantly less than the normal population from early infancy onward.

■ DIAGNOSIS

The diagnosis can usually be established accurately by two-dimensional echocardiography. Catheterization may provide important information about the hemodynamics, anatomic relationships, and PAs. The angiographic views should define the site and number of VSDs, the morphology of the ventricular chambers, the nature of the pulmonary stenosis, and other associated anomalies.

■ SURGERY

Repair of ccTGA began during the late 1950s, and a summary of currently used strategies is presented in Table 2. The potentially unfavorable natural history of children

Table 2 Surgical Options for Repair of the Various Anatomic Subsets of Congenitally Corrected Transposition of the Great Arteries, With Advantages and Disadvantages

ANATOMIC TYPE	PROCEDURE	COMMENT
VSD	Classic repair (VSD closure)	Leaves discordant AV and VA connections. Late TV and RV failure common. Technically straightforward.
	Senning-ASO (double switch)	Technically complex. Requires near-systemic LV pressure. Restores concordant AV and VA connection. TI and RV function may improve.
VSD and LVOTO	Classic repair (VSD closure and LV-PA conduit or direct connection)	Leaves discordant AV and VA connections. Late TV and RV failure common. High probability of reoperation.
	Senning-Rastelli	Technically complex, but restores concordant AV and VA connections. TI and RV function may improve. Conduit replacement may be required.
Unseptatable (straddling AV valves, hypoplasia of one ventricle, multiple VSDs)	Univentricular strategy (BCPS, TCPC-Fontan)	Good physiologic solution, low risk, technically straightforward. Susceptibility to late Fontan problems, as in other anatomic variants.

TCPC, total cavopulmonary connection.

with ccTGA and a systemic RV has been documented in numerous clinical reports. Over the past decade, many surgeons have moved toward anatomic repair (i.e., placing the RV in the pulmonary circuit and the LV in the systemic circuit), instead of the "classic" approach (i.e., leaving the RV in the systemic circuit and the LV in the pulmonary circuit).

Palliative Procedures

The main palliative operations used in ccTGA are systemic to PA (modified Blalock-Taussig) shunts and PA banding. The modified Blalock-Taussig shunt is a useful palliative strategy in the following circumstances.

1. Infants and neonates with severe LVOTO or pulmonary atresia who are expected to undergo classic or anatomic repair with an extracardiac conduit at a later date
2. Infants with ccTGA, LVOTO, and unseptatable hearts (unbalanced ventricles, straddling AV valves, or multiple unfavorable VSDs) who are being considered for a Fontan strategy

We prefer a transternal approach for all modified BT shunts, using a 4-mm polytetrafluoroethylene (PTFE) tube graft interposition from the innominate artery or right subclavian artery, regardless of arch anatomy. With this approach, subsequent takedown is facilitated, and PA distortion can be minimized.

As the majority of children with ccTGA have a natural limitation of pulmonary blood flow, banding is required only in a small subset. A PA band may be indicated under the following circumstances.

1. Children with pulmonary hypertension due to high pulmonary blood flow (from a large VSD), in whom a double switch operation is planned after early infancy
2. Selected patients who develop RV failure following a classic repair and who are under consideration for conversion using a double switch strategy

Definitive Procedures

The decision between classic and anatomic repair can be difficult. Features favoring the classic approach include competence of both AV valves, balanced ventricular size, and excellent RV function. Features favoring the anatomic approach include disparity in ventricular size, poor RV function, tricuspid insufficiency, and a nearly systemic LV pressure. In general, anatomic (as opposed to physiologic) correction requires a more complex surgical approach but has a better expected long-term outcome. Although the results of classic repair are well documented, at the time of this writing the results of anatomic repair are still under assessment, and the long-term relative benefit for patients who are suitable for either type of repair is still theoretical. However, there is no question that an anatomic approach is a better prospect for patients who already have problems with the RV and/or tricuspid valve and who are therefore poor candidates for classic repair.

The univentricular (Fontan or cardiopulmonary shunt) strategy should generally be reserved for patients in whom septation is difficult or inadvisable (severely unbalanced ventricular size, unfavorable VSD location and/or number, straddling atrioventricular valve [AVV]).

Classic Repair

Working through the mitral valve, the VSD in ccTGA can usually be well exposed and closed with a patch using interrupted pledgeted sutures. Along the anterior-superior rim of the VSD, sutures are placed on the RV aspect, working through the VSD. As the transition is made to territory away from nonconduction tissue, the sutures can be placed on the LV aspect, and through the base of the septal mitral leaflet.

The degree and nature of the LVOTO in ccTGA are highly variable, but annular, leaflet, and subvalvar components may all be present. Direct relief of the LVOT is usually unsatisfactory, due to the posterior position of the pulmonary outflow tract, which is wedged between the AV valves. A second major impediment is the presence of the penetrating bundle in the proposed area of resection. It may be possible to partially relieve the LVOTO (leaving a moderately elevated LV pressure) in some cases, in preference to placing an extracardiac conduit. This may be well tolerated physiologically due to the structure of the pulmonary ventricle.

The most reliable way to relieve LVOTO in ccTGA is with the use of an extraanatomic LV-to-PA valved conduit. We generally use cryopreserved pulmonary or aortic homografts, but there are alternatives (e.g., nonvalved tubes, pericardial valved tubes, xenograft valved tubes, direct connections).

Anatomic Correction

The Senning plus arterial switch operation (ASO) (double switch) strategy was first used by Imai in 1989 and subsequently by the Melbourne group (Figure 2). Candidates for this procedure generally must satisfy the following criteria.

1. No obstruction between either ventricle and its respective semilunar valve
2. Balanced ventricular size (RV volume >75% of LV)
3. Septatable heart with no major AVV straddling
4. LV pressure of 75% of RV pressure, with good function (this may be a consequence of a large VSD, PA band, or pulmonary hypertension related to RV failure)
5. Translocatable coronary arteries

Although we have used the double switch operation in neonates, it is perhaps technically and physiologically a better option later in life. For this reason a preliminary PA band may be justified in neonates with a large VSD and systemic PA pressure, with repair deferred to 12 months of age. Other candidates may require banding to induce systemic LV pressure for ventricular retraining.

Operative Technique

Incision, cannulation, and CPB strategy are as described for classic repair. The ASO is generally performed first, using a technique similar to that used for concordant TGA. The Lecompte maneuver is usually used, except for the rare case of a posterior aorta. VSD closure is performed via the right atrium and mitral valve or a trans–left atrial (transtricuspid valve) approach in patients with situs solitus and dextrocardia. As in classic repairs, the technique of de Leval and associates

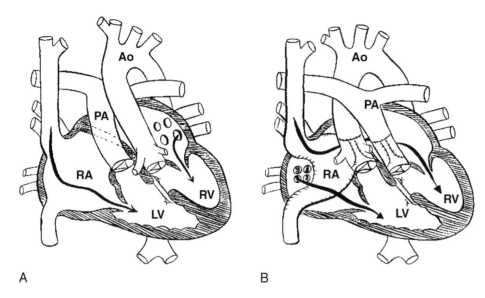

Figure 2
"Classic" versus anatomic repair of ccTGA. **(A)** "Classic" repair leaves a discordant AV and VA connection, and a TV functioning at systemic pressure. **(B)** Anatomic repair (Senning plus ASO) leaves both connections concordant, and the TV functioning at pulmonary pressure.

A

B

can be used to avoid injury to the anterosuperior conduction system. Closure via the transected aorta may also be a possibility.

We prefer the Senning over the Mustard technique for atrial reconstruction in combination with ASO. Our familiarity with this approach and its general superiority to the Mustard procedure in the long term in most published concordant TGA series are also considered.

Senning Plus Rastelli Operation

Patients not suitable for the Senning ASO option due to LVOTO may still be candidates for an anatomic repair, using a more complex strategy. The approach of an atrial level repair combined with intraventricular baffle and RV-PA conduit was proposed by Yagihara et al in 1989. In this combined Senning (or Mustard) and Rastelli approach, a baffle is placed within the RV (via right ventriculotomy) to connect the LV to the aorta, via the VSD, usually including the PA as well. The VSD may have to be enlarged to ensure a nonobstructed connection between LV and aorta, taking into account the location of the conduction system. RV-to-PA continuity is established with an extracardiac valved conduit or a direct REV (reparation a l'etage) type connection between RV and PA. In the latter case, the Lecompte maneuver may be useful, and the connection may be made with a monocusp-bearing patch placed anteriorly. AV concordance is established with a Senning (or Mustard) baffle, usually with concurrent enlargement of the pulmonary venous atrium, as described earlier.

■ OTHER PROCEDURES FOR CHILDREN

Children with nonseptatable hearts (those with severe straddling of an AV valve, unbalanced ventricular size, multiple unfavorable VSDs) are palliated with a bidirectional cavopulmonary shunt (BCPS) or primary Fontan operation, according to the usual hemodynamic criteria. We would generally employ an extracardiac conduit approach using normothermic CPB without aortic occlusion.

Further options for children with ccTGA and LVOTO have been suggested. Mavroudis et al have used a BCPS as an adjunct to pulmonary valvotomy. Recognizing that complete LVOTO relief would be anatomically unlikely without the use of an extracardiac conduit, LV pressure was reduced by diverting all superior vena cava blood to the confluent PAs. This is an attractive approach for selected patients with good tricuspid valve (TV) and RV function as well as a suitable LVOT.

Finally, cardiac transplantation will eventually be required in some patients with ccTGA. The techniques used in concordant hearts apply in ccTGA, and the abnormal great artery position does not preclude implantation using individual aortic, PA, and caval anastomoses. Prior surgical procedures present the main technical and physiologic challenges.

Results of Surgery
Classic Repairs

Mortality for classic repairs has ranged from 4% to 33%. In the Royal Children's Hospital series of operations leaving the RV in the systemic circuit (reported in 1995), 28 patients had VSD closure as an isolated procedure (n = 7), with direct relief of LVOTO (n = 5), or with placement of an LV-PA conduit (n = 16). Hospital mortality was 4% and actuarial survival at 10 years was 83%. Twenty of the 24 long-term survivors are in New York Heart Association (NYHA) class I and 3 are in class II. Sixteen of 24 had important tricuspid insufficiency, and 12 of 22 had deterioration of RV function. These changes were noted within 3 years of operation in 75% of cases, and Q_p/Q_s > 1 was a risk factor for both (related) problems ($p < .05$). These results led us to explore the possibility of anatomic correction for ccTGA, especially for patients with high pulmonary blood flow. Other groups have reported similar results.

Anatomic Repair

In 1997 we reported the Royal Children's Hospital results for the ASO plus Senning repair in a group of 14 patients, age range 0.5 to 120 months. All but one had an LV/RV pressure ratio of greater than 0.7 due to a large VSD (with or without prior PA band), severe congestive heart failure (CHF) due to

RV dysfunction and tricuspid insufficiency (TI), or PA band placed for ventricular conditioning following failed classic repair. Ten of 14 had strong contraindications to classic repair (RV hypoplasia, RV dysfunction, or TI). There was one hospital death (7%; confidence limit, 0% to 34%), and actuarial survival beyond 10 months was 81%, currently with (700) patient-month follow-up. The median grade of TI fell from 3/4 preoperatively to 1/4 postoperatively ($p = .003$). RV function remains normal in 11 of 12 survivors, all except 1 of whom is in NYHA class I. Three patients have required reoperation, for either revision of the Senning baffle, repeat tricuspid valve replacement, or revision of a coronary anastomosis. Imai reported 44 patients with ccTGA who had anatomic correction by Senning plus Rastelli (n = 35) or Senning plus ASO (n = 9), with 9.1% early mortality. Helvind et al reported 14 patients with ccTGA who had either Senning plus ASO or Senning plus Rastelli operations, with no deaths. Two patients required pacemaker insertion postoperatively. Sharma et al used a Senning/Rastelli (n = 7) or Senning/ASO (n = 7) approach, with 6 survivors in each group. Follow-up ranged from 1 to 48 months, with an LV ejection fraction of 65% after double switch and 52% after Senning/Rastelli. All patients were in sinus rhythm, and 10 of 12 in NYHA class I.

Imamura et al (Cleveland Clinic) most recently reported results for 22 patients undergoing anatomic repairs for ccTGA with no mortality. International results reported to date are summarized in Table 3. Importantly, tricuspid valve function improved significantly in the majority of patients who had dysfunction before operation, confirming earlier experience with fewer patients.

■ CONCLUSION

ccTGA remains a challenging lesion. It is likely that the anatomic approach to repair will improve long-term outlook.

Table 3 Metaanalysis of Outcome of Anatomic Repairs for Congenitally Corrected Transposition of the Great Arteries. The global mortality risk was 7.4% (confidence limit 3% to 14%).

AUTHORS	NUMBER	HOSPITAL MORTALITY
Imai 1997	44	4 (9%, CL = 3-21%)
Acar 1998	9	1 (11%, CL = .3-48%)
Reddy 1997	11	1 (9%, CL = .2-41%)
Imamura 2000	22	0 (0%, CL = 0-15%)
Metras 1997	8	0 (0%, CL = 0-37%)
Sharma 1999	14	2 (14%, CL = 2-42%)
Karl 1997	14	1 (7%, CL = .1-34%)

Understanding the complexities of this lesion is critical for strategic planning and optimal outcome.

SUGGESTED READING

Imai Y: Double-switch operation for congenitally corrected transposition, *Adv Cardiac Surg* 9:65, 1997.

Imamura M, et al: Results of the double switch operation in the current era, *Ann Thorac Surg* 70:100, 2000.

Karl TR, et al: Senning plus arterial switch operation for discordant (congenitally corrected transposition), *Ann Thorac Surg* 64:495, 1997.

Mavroudis C, et al. Bidirectional Glenn shunt in association with congenital heart repairs: the 1 (1/2) ventricular repair, *Ann Thorac Surg* 68:976, 1999.

Sano T, et al: Intermediate-term outcome after intracardiac repair of associated cardiac defects in patients with atrioventricular and ventriculoarterial discordance, *Circulation* 92 (Suppl II):II-272, 1995.

Wilkinson JL, et al: Congenital Heart Surgery Nomenclature and Database Project: corrected (discordant) transposition of the great arteries (and related malformations), *Ann Thorac Surg* 69S:236, 2000.

TETRALOGY OF FALLOT

Luca A. Vricella
Duke E. Cameron

Tetralogy of Fallot (ToF) occurs in approximately 10% of all patients born with congenital heart disease and is the most common cyanotic cardiac anomaly diagnosed in infancy. As originally described by Etienne-Louis Fallot in 1888, *la maladie bleue* associates a large subaortic ventricular septal defect (VSD) and biventricular aortic connection with right ventricular outflow tract (RVOT) obstruction and subsequent muscular hypertrophy. The morphologic spectrum of this pathology varies between this association and the more extreme forms of aortic override (such as tetralogy-type double-outlet right ventricle) and right ventricular obstruction (as in the case of pulmonary atresia with VSD). For the purpose of this chapter, we will focus mainly on the classic form of tetralogy, with normal ventriculoarterial connection and without pulmonary atresia.

■ MORPHOLOGY

ToF is believed to originate from underdevelopment of the right ventricular infundibulum during embryogenesis.

The hallmark of the lesion is anterior and cephalad deviation of the outlet septum, away from the ventriculoinfundibular fold. This results in RVOT obstruction and dextroposition of the aorta, which overrides the interventricular septum to form the superior margin of the VSD (Figure 1). The typically nonrestrictive VSD is classified as a malalignment type and is cradled by the two limbs of the septomarginal trabeculation. Additional muscular VSDs are rarely seen, and location and course of the atrioventricular conduction axis follow the same landmarks as for non–Fallot-type VSDs. Obstruction may be simultaneously present at various levels within the RVOT; subvalvar obstruction may be in the form of an internal muscular "os" and can be either isolated or associated with valvar or supravalvar stenosis. Although the pulmonary valve is typically dysplastic, bicuspid, and obstructive, various degrees of hypoplasia of the pulmonary trunk and branch pulmonary arteries may be present. Obstruction of the right ventricular outflow tract can range from mild stenosis to pulmonary atresia with ductus-dependent pulmonary circulation or systemic-to-pulmonary collaterals. Frequently associated anomalies include atrial septal defect, atrioventricular septal defects, patency of the arterial duct, and persistence of the left superior vena cava. A right-sided aortic arch and anomalous origin of the left anterior descending coronary artery (most commonly arising from the proximal right coronary artery) are observed in 25% and 3% of cases, respectively.

■ CLINICAL PRESENTATION

Signs and symptoms of ToF in infants and children without pulmonary atresia largely depend on the degree of RVOT obstruction and right-to-left shunting across the nonrestrictive VSD. Shunting is dictated by the balance between systemic and pulmonary resistance; this is particularly true in neonates and infants after closure of the arterial duct, when pulmonary perfusion comes to rely completely on antegrade flow from the right ventricle.

The typical clinical course is that of progressive cyanosis in infancy due to increasing RVOT obstruction and myocardial hypertrophy; patients with severe impediment to blood egression from the right ventricle into the pulmonary artery present earlier in life and require systemic-to-pulmonary shunting or complete intracardiac repair to avert prolonged cyanosis. On the other hand, children with limited obstruction are mostly acyanotic with varying episodes of cyanosis associated with transient or progressive increase in right ventricular afterload. These transient episodes (also known as cyanotic "spells") are associated with volume depletion, decreased systemic vascular resistance, or increased pulmonary impedance. Besides varying degrees of cyanosis, physical examination typically reveals a diminished second heart sound, a systolic murmur from RVOT obstruction, and digital clubbing if cyanosis persists beyond 6 months. Respiratory symptoms from extrinsic bronchial compression may be prominent in patients with ToF and absent pulmonary valve who typically have massively enlarged pulmonary arteries. Rarely, cerebrovascular accidents are the main mode of clinical presentation.

■ DIAGNOSIS

ToF should be strongly suspected in patients who present either at birth or in the postnatal period with cyanosis and a precordial systolic murmur. In older children, similar findings in association with the above-mentioned clinical features of chronic cyanosis may suggest the diagnosis. The appearance of the mediastinum on anteroposterior chest radiograph is classically described as *coeur en sabot* ("boot-shaped heart"); hypovascularity of the lung fields, elevation of the ventricular apex, and diminished prominence of the pulmonary arterial segment along the left mediastinal border are other typical findings observed on chest radiographs. Electrocardiographic findings are consistent with right ventricular hypertrophy.

In the current era, echocardiography is the mainstay of diagnosis and should be all that is required from a diagnostic standpoint before proceeding to palliative intervention or complete intracardiac repair in most cases. Location, number, and size of the VSDs should be identified, as well as the level of obstruction within the RVOT. The size and continuity of

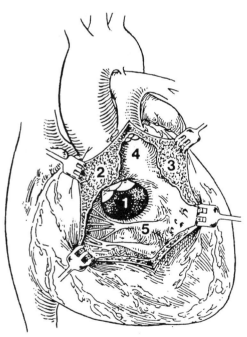

Figure 1
Schematic view of a heart with tetralogy of Fallot, as would be seen through a large right ventriculotomy. Unrestrictive ventricular septal defect (1) with overriding aorta (2) behind the ventriculoinfundibular fold. The hypertrophied septoparietal trabeculations (3) and deviated outlet septum (4) result in right ventricular outflow tract obstruction. The medial papillary muscle of Lancisi (5) supports the anteroseptal commissure of the tricuspid valve. (*Reproduced with permission from Bove EL, Lupinetti FM: Tetralogy of Fallot. In Mavroudis C, Backer CL, editors:* Pediatric cardiac surgery, *2nd ed. St Louis, 1994, Mosby, p 1107.*)

the pulmonary arterial trunk and branch pulmonary arteries are defined, as well as the morphology of the arterial duct and the position (right or left) of the aortic arch. In cases of tetralogy-type pulmonary atresia with VSD, additional systemic sources of pulmonary blood flow should be suspected and imaged; this is a common indication for cardiac catheterization. Of utmost importance in surgical planning is accurate preoperative definition of coronary anatomy and in particular, the detection of anomalous coronary branches crossing the RVOT. Most of the information can be accurately obtained by transthoracic echocardiography, relegating cardiac catheterization to those cases in which coronary anatomy, pulmonary runoff, and collateral supply need further definition. Cardiac catheterization should also be considered preoperatively in children who have had a systemic-to-pulmonary shunt in infancy and present for complete intracardiac repair, to define shunt-induced pulmonary distention.

■ SURGICAL INDICATIONS

The natural history of patients with untreated ToF (without pulmonary atresia) is poor: one third of nonoperated patients die in the first year. Nevertheless, most patients with ToF have adequate pulmonary perfusion at birth and do not require surgical management in the neonatal period. More than 70% of cases, however, meet criteria for operative intervention within the first year of life. The presence of severe cyanosis (systemic oxygen saturation <80%) is an indication for surgery regardless of patient age.

Even though the diagnosis per se is an indication for surgical intervention, controversy remains over the optimal therapeutic strategy. Early intracardiac repair is intuitively ideal, but the approach of initial staged palliation and delayed repair has achieved equally good results. For acyanotic patients, intervention with elective complete repair should be performed before 18 months of age, if not sooner.

■ THERAPEUTIC OPTIONS

The history of surgery for ToF parallels in many ways that of the early development of congenital cardiac surgery. The first palliation of a 15-month-old child with tetralogy and pulmonary stenosis was performed by Alfred Blalock at the Johns Hopkins Hospital in 1944. The pioneering work of C. Walton Lillehei culminated in the first complete intracardiac repair of ToF with parental cross-circulation at the University of Minnesota in 1954. John Kirklin at the Mayo Clinic carried out the first complete repair with conventional cardiopulmonary bypass in 1955. Over the ensuing years, evolution of extracorporeal perfusion techniques, myocardial protection, and refinement of anesthesiologic and critical care strategies have allowed performance of early complete repair with low morbidity and mortality in cyanotic newborns and infants. Nevertheless, the decision to proceed with palliation versus complete repair still largely relies on the individual surgeon's experience and the philosophy of the institution caring for the child.

Initial Palliation and Delayed Complete Intracardiac Repair

Systemic-to-pulmonary shunt achieves the goal of ameliorating cyanosis and encouraging pulmonary arterial growth. The procedure is currently performed mainly in patients with severe cyanosis in early infancy and in those with pulmonary atresia and tetralogy who are not candidates for early complete repair. This approach should be considered in patients with a large anomalous coronary artery traversing the RVOT or those with multiple VSDs. The classic Blalock-Taussig shunt is performed by anastomosing the subclavian artery to the pulmonary artery via a thoracotomy, typically on the side opposite the aortic arch. The classic shunt offers the advantage of using autologous tissue with potential for growth but sacrifices a major portion of brachial arterial inflow, and is rarely performed today. The procedure has evolved from its original description into the "modified" Blalock-Taussig shunt. In this technical variation, a polytetrafluoroethylene conduit (usually 1.2 mm/kg in diameter) is interposed between the subclavian artery and branch pulmonary artery. The shunt is easily taken down at reoperation and offers the advantage of regulating pulmonary perfusion by its diameter and length, as well as by the diameter of the subclavian or inordinate arteries. This is in contrast to central and other shunts (now mainly of historical interest and described elsewhere in this textbook) in which pulmonary overcirculation from poorly regulated shunting can easily occur. The surgical approach to systemic-to-pulmonary shunting has also evolved over recent years. Several authors currently advocate median sternotomy, which allows simultaneous ligation of the arterial duct and (although rarely required with confluent and unobstructed branch pulmonary arteries) the possibility of instituting cardiopulmonary bypass.

Early Intracardiac Repair

Early intracardiac repair of ToF-pulmonary stenosis is intuitively advantageous in that intervention is carried out before significant hypertrophy of septoparietal muscular bands has occurred, allowing normal antegrade perfusion of the pulmonary vascular tree. Early intervention in turn facilitates the procedure by limiting the amount of infundibular muscular resection required and the extent of the right ventriculotomy; this may reduce the incidence of late diastolic and systolic dysfunction, as well as the occurrence of arrhythmias.

If this management strategy is chosen, the principal goal is to obliterate the interventricular communication and relieve RVOT obstruction. The procedure is typically performed via median sternotomy with bicaval venous cannulation and moderate-to-profound hypothermia. Reduction in flow and left atrial venting are used to minimize collateral return during the procedure. The VSD can usually be repaired (with interrupted or continuous sutures) via right atriotomy. For those defects with prominent outlet septal extension and that require ventriculotomy to relieve right ventricular obstruction, a combined approach (via the atrium and the ventricle) may be used to close the VSD. The ventriculotomy can be extended across the pulmonary annulus in case of concomitant valvar stenosis and severe annular hypoplasia. Should a ventriculotomy not be necessary, the RVOT may be inspected through a pulmonary arteriotomy. Appropriate sizers are coupled with nomograms of pulmonary annular diameter by age. Should annular size be insufficient, a pulmonary valvotomy or, alternatively, a transannular incision into the ventricle can be performed. The length of the ventriculotomy should be kept to a minimum to minimize early postoperative and late ventricular dysfunction. The pulmonary arteriotomy may be carried distally into the left main pulmonary artery, to avoid branch pulmonary arterial stenosis commonly seen at the site of ductal insertion. A prosthetic or an autologous tissue patch is then sutured in place. Should an aberrant left anterior descending coronary artery be found or known to cross the RVOT, it may be bridged by a right ventricle–to–pulmonary artery conduit.

Concomitant cardiac anomalies are dealt with accordingly. A patent arterial duct is ligated on initiation of cardiopulmonary bypass. A coexisting atrioventricular septal defect should be repaired before pulmonary arteriotomy, to allow testing of the atrioventricular valve repair by saline instillation into the right ventricle. Atrial level communications are usually closed, although minimal residual defects may be left intentionally when severe postoperative diastolic dysfunction is anticipated, or in neonates with reactive pulmonary vasculature. In the latter group, a monocusp pulmonary valve can inserted to minimize right ventricular pressure and volume overload in the early postoperative period. Modified ultrafiltration is carried out routinely in patients weighing less than 20 kg. At completion of the repair, ratios of right to left ventricular pressure are directly measured, and persistent obstruction is addressed surgically when the ratio is greater than 0.70.

■ OUTCOMES

Early postoperative course varies according to the age of the patient, the intraoperative events and, most importantly, with the degree of early postoperative right ventricular diastolic dysfunction. The latter may require substantial inotropic support with adrenergic agonists and phosphodiesterase inhibitors, as well as aggressive fluid administration. Ventricular dysfunction may be aggravated by an extensive right ventriculotomy. The incidence of complete heart block after repair is less than 1%. Patients who develop junctional ectopic tachycardia (JET) can have a particularly troublesome postoperative course, requiring surface cooling and antiarrhythmic therapy and amiodarone infusion. Relief of long-standing pulmonary obstruction rarely results in pulmonary edema and prolonged ventilatory support.

In the current era and in appropriately selected patients, both single-stage repair and initial palliation followed by delayed intracardiac correction have achieved low morbidity and mortality. In the early Boston Children's Hospital experience, complete repair had a higher operative mortality when performed in the first month of life. In infants beyond the neonatal period, shunting and one-stage repair have similar hospital mortality (approximately 1% to 3%). Early intervention has been associated with smaller ventriculotomy and less need for transannular patching or extensive infundibular resection, as most of the ventricular hypertrophy and subendocardial fibrosis appears to develop in patients operated on beyond infancy. The challenge of complete repair in small infants balances well against the intermediate-term results and attrition of systemic-to-pulmonary shunts. Interim mortality for patients with "balanced ventricles" who undergo initial shunting has been reported in recent series to be as high as 7%. This is often secondary to shunt thrombosis and is a greater concern in patients with completely shunt-dependent pulmonary perfusion, such as those with ToF-pulmonary atresia without systemic-to-pulmonary collaterals.

In patients followed up for nearly two decades, 80% have good ventricular function and more than 90% are in sinus rhythm and have good functional capacity. Only 10% have evidence of severe pulmonary regurgitation, typically well tolerated for several decades.

Late sudden death rate has been reported as high as 6% and is most likely the result of an arrhythmic event in the setting of ventricular dysfunction. Late inducibility of monomorphic ventricular tachycardia can be as high as 28%; a QRS duration longer than 180 milliseconds or prolongation greater than 3.5 msec/yr is predictive of sustained ventricular tachycardia. Progression of QRS elongation can be halted by restoration of pulmonary valve competence. Patients who manifest ventricular irritability and QRS prolongation on Holter monitoring should be aggressively studied in the electrophysiology laboratory and undergo preoperative or intraoperative ablation of monomorphic foci.

Between 5% and 15% of patients with ToF pulmonary stenosis will require late reintervention. The most common indications for reoperation are the long-term sequelae of chronic pulmonary insufficiency or recurrent RVOT obstruction. In those cases in which RVOT reconstruction has been performed with a conduit (e.g., in patients with ToF-pulmonary atresia or in those who have undergone late conduit placement for pulmonary regurgitation), conduit failure with stenosis or insufficiency is a common indication for redo sternotomy or catheter-based reintervention. Other indications for late reintervention are residual VSD, tricuspid valve regurgitation and aneurysmal degeneration of the RVOT. Reoperation generally carries a low morbidity and mortality. When a competent pulmonary valve must be inserted, several predictable choices are available; an in-depth discussion of the options is beyond the scope of this chapter. Catheter-placed "stented valves" offer another promising alternative.

Considerable debate still surrounds the timing of operative reintervention. The advantage of early reintervention must be weighed against the limited durability of most conduits but should precede onset of severe and potentially irreversible right ventricular dysfunction. Widely accepted indications for pulmonary valve insertion are (1) exercise intolerance and symptom progression, (2) significant ventricular dysfunction or progressive tricuspid regurgitation, (3) sustained arrhythmias and/or increase in QRS duration, and (4) severe recurrent or residual RVOT stenosis.

SUGGESTED READINGS

Atallah-Yunes NH, et al: Postoperative assessment of a modified surgical approach to repair of tetralogy of Fallot. Long-term follow-up, *Circulation* 94(Suppl II):II-22, 1996.

Discigil B, et al: Late pulmonary valve replacement after repair of tetralogy of Fallot, *J Thorac Cardiovasc Surg* 121:344, 2001.

Owen AR, Gatzoulis MA: Tetralogy of Fallot: late outcome after repair and surgical implications, *Semin Thoracic Cardiovasc Surg Pediatr Card Surg Annual* 3:216, 2000.

Parry AJ, et al: Elective primary repair of acyanotic tetralogy of Fallot in early infancy: overall outcome and impact on the pulmonary valve, *J Am Coll Cardiol* 36:2279, 2000.

Reddy VM, et al: Routine primary repair of tetralogy of Fallot in neonates and infants less than three months of age, *Ann Thorac Surg* 60(Suppl):S592, 1995.

HYPOPLASTIC LEFT HEART SYNDROME

Paul M. Kirshbom
Thomas L. Spray

Hypoplastic left heart syndrome (HLHS) comprises between 7% and 9% of all congenital cardiac anomalies diagnosed within the first year of life. This constellation of cardiac and great vessel malformations is nearly uniformly fatal if not treated and accounts for 25% of all cardiac deaths in the first week of life. The defining features of HLHS are hypoplasia or absence of the left ventricle with an associated diminutive ascending aorta. Aortic valve atresia represents the most extreme form of HLHS in which the ascending aorta is typically smaller than 3 mm and serves as a common coronary artery, supplying the myocardium via retrograde flow from the arch. The single, morphologic right ventricle supplies the systemic circulation through the ductus arteriosus and the pulmonary circulation through the branch pulmonary arteries. Survival of the child is dependent on both mixing of systemic and pulmonary venous return and continued patency of the ductus arteriosus.

The surgical management of patients with HLHS has provided congenital cardiac surgeons with a physiologic and technical challenge since the first attempt at palliation was reported by Redo and associates in 1961. Over the subsequent two decades, numerous techniques and case series were reported; however, the first successful series of staged reconstruction for HLHS was reported by Norwood and colleagues in 1980. The surgical procedures subsequently developed and popularized by Norwood and colleagues provide the basic framework on which our current practice is based.

Primary infant heart transplantation has been proposed as an alternative to staged single ventricle palliation. Although there have been significant advances in infant and pediatric transplantation, with good intermediate term results, several difficult obstacles remain including donor organ shortages, chronic immunosuppression in growing children, and chronic rejection. This chapter will focus on the staged reconstructive approach to HLHS.

■ PRINCIPLES OF STAGED RECONSTRUCTION

As with other forms of single ventricle, the ultimate goal for most patients with HLHS is a Fontan-Kreutzer procedure. To successfully achieve this goal, certain intermediary requirements must be satisfied by the first-stage operation. First, an unobstructed pathway must be created for systemic perfusion by the single (right) ventricle. Because the ventricle must be subjected to a volume load while it supplies both the pulmonary and systemic circulations, any unnecessary additional pressure load must be eliminated. The second goal is provision of controlled pulmonary blood flow, which must be sufficient to encourage growth of the pulmonary vascular bed but limited so as to minimize development of pulmonary vascular obstructive disease. Finally, interatrial communication must be unrestrictive so as to ensure adequacy of venous mixing and unobstructed pulmonary venous drainage to the ventricle.

Tricuspid valve regurgitation can be a difficult problem in children with HLHS. Tricuspid regurgitation can be the result of either myocardial ischemia or the volume load to which the single ventricle is subjected. In either case, significant regurgitation may be an indication for attempted valve repair at either the first- or second-stage operation. In the case of severe regurgitation with ventricular dysfunction, consideration must be given to cardiac transplantation rather than continuation down the pathway of single ventricle palliation.

Early attempts at single-stage reconstruction with completion of the Fontan-Kreutzer procedure in infants were unsuccessful. High pulmonary vascular resistance combined with the prolonged surgical procedure resulted in a low cardiac output state. Subsequent attempts at staged reconstruction with aortic reconstruction and shunt-dependent pulmonary perfusion were successful. However, this first-stage procedure leaves the child with a volume-loaded right ventricle and requisite cyanosis due to complete mixing.

The second-stage procedure is usually performed at 3 to 6 months of age. This procedure decreases the volume load on the ventricle and improves effective pulmonary blood flow by directing fully desaturated superior vena caval blood flow directly into the pulmonary circuit. The final stage of the reconstruction, a modification of the Fontan-Kreutzer procedure, is performed between 1{1/2} and 2 years of age. Most commonly, a single fenestration is placed between the circuits, allowing right-to-left shunting at the atrial level during times of stress or increased pulmonary vascular resistance, thus maintaining ventricular preload and cardiac output.

There have been numerous modifications of the second and third stages of the reconstruction for HLHS. Most centers prefer one of two approaches: the bidirectional Glenn shunt followed by extracardiac Fontan completion or the hemi-Fontan procedure followed by a lateral tunnel Fontan. Each procedure has its advantages and disadvantages. The bidirectional Glenn shunt, which requires fewer atrial suture lines, was thought to decrease the incidence of atrial arrhythmias, although recent studies suggest that this is not the case. Also, in some patients this procedure can be performed without the use of cardiopulmonary bypass. The primary advantages of the hemi-Fontan procedure are the relative simplicity of the completion lateral tunnel Fontan procedure and the reliability of the fenestration in this final stage as opposed to the extracardiac Fontan. Another advantage of the hemi-Fontan procedure in patients with HLHS is the ability to widely patch the pulmonary arteries, which are often distorted or hypoplastic in these patients. Our institutional preference has been the hemi-Fontan procedure with lateral tunnel fenestrated Fontan completion, which will be described here.

■ PREOPERATIVE PREPARATION

Many patients with HLHS are relatively asymptomatic until the ductus arteriosus begins to close and systemic perfusion becomes compromised. At that point, metabolic acidosis and cardiovascular collapse can develop very rapidly. Infants who present in this manner will have better outcomes if they are resuscitated before surgical correction. Ductal patency is maintained or reestablished with prostaglandin E_1 (0.025 to 0.05 μg/kg/min). Patients who do not develop apnea secondary to the prostaglandin infusion can be allowed to breathe room air spontaneously. Those patients who require mechanical ventilation should be maintained on the lowest possible oxygen concentration so as to minimize pulmonary vasodilatation and pulmonary overcirculation. Metabolic acidosis is reversed with sodium bicarbonate. Ventricular dysfunction typically resolves after the initial metabolic acidosis is reversed and stable systemic perfusion is reestablished. Low-dose inotropic agents may be useful in some patients, but these agents must be used judiciously so as to avoid increasing systemic vascular resistance. Digoxin and careful diuresis can be helpful in dealing with the ventricular volume load before and after surgical correction. If possible, it is often best to allow several days for recovery of renal and hepatic function in patients who have had a period of significant hemodynamic instability. During this time, neurologic status and any noncardiac anomalies can be assessed.

Generally, surgery is performed electively after any organ system dysfunction has resolved. Rarely, the atrial septal

defect or patent foramen ovale is restrictive (2% to 5% of cases), which results in pulmonary congestion and severe hypoxemia. These patients may require either emergent balloon atrial septostomy or surgical septectomy, with or without completion of the first-stage procedure depending on the severity of the metabolic derangement at presentation.

■ OPERATIVE TECHNIQUE

Stage 1

After a standard median sternotomy, the thymus is removed for exposure and the pericardium is opened in the midline. Care must be taken throughout the preliminary dissection (Figure 1) as the volume-loaded ventricle can be very irritable and ventricular fibrillation is easily induced. The diminutive aorta is dissected away from the pulmonary artery down to the sinuses of Valsalva, proximal to the takeoff of the right pulmonary artery. The aorta is then dissected distally including the arch vessels and down to the descending aorta beyond the ductus arteriosus insertion. Care must be taken during the distal dissection to avoid damage to the ductus, which is friable and prone to hemorrhage. The pulmonary arteries are mobilized bilaterally. The arch vessels and pulmonary arteries are then encircled with snares and tourniquets for control later on. At this point purse-string sutures are placed in the proximal pulmonary artery and the

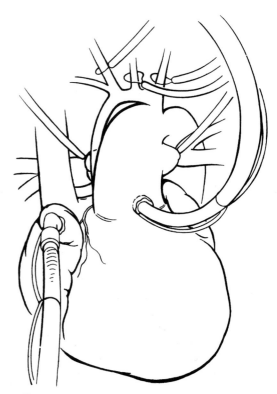

Figure 1

Initial dissection and mobilization of the aortic arch and arch vessels as well as the branch pulmonary arteries. (*Reprinted from Surgical repair of the hypoplastic heart syndrome. In Bove E, Mosca R, editors:* Progress in pediatric cardiology, *vol 5. Philadelphia, 1996, WB Saunders, p 23.*)

right atrial appendage for cannulation. It can be helpful to make the atrial purse-string larger than usual, allowing for later atrial septectomy through the purse-string. After heparin is administered, a polytetrafluoroethylene (PTFE) tube graft (typically 3.5 or 4 mm in diameter) is cut to appropriate length and beveled proximally for the innominate anastomosis. The pulmonary artery and right atrium are then cannulated, cardiopulmonary bypass is initiated, and the branch pulmonary artery tourniquets are tightened to prevent pulmonary run-off during cooling. The patient is cooled to a nasopharyngeal temperature of 18°C over 15 to 20 minutes.

During cooling, the proximal anastomosis of the modified Blalock-Taussig shunt can be fashioned. A partial occlusion vascular clamp is placed on the proximal innominate artery and the shunt is anastomosed to a longitudinal arteriotomy using 7-0 monofilament suture. Once the suture line is complete, shunt flow can be tested by removing the vascular clamp, after which the shunt is controlled with a hemoclip. If the alternative technique of selective cerebral perfusion is chosen, the shunt can be cannulated after cooling is complete, allowing continued low-flow bypass through the innominate artery rather than complete circulatory arrest.

When cooling is complete, cardiopulmonary bypass is discontinued, the snares on the arch vessels are tightened, and the descending aorta is clamped with a vascular clamp. Cardioplegia is then given through the arterial cannula with retrograde perfusion of the coronaries via the arch and ascending aorta. After cardioplegia, the cannulae and pulmonary artery tourniquets are removed. The ductus arteriosus is ligated on the pulmonary artery side and divided flush with the aorta. An atrial septectomy is performed through the venous purse-string.

The pulmonary artery is then divided transversely immediately proximal to the right pulmonary artery origin (Figure 2). The resulting defect in the distal main pulmonary artery is typically closed with a circular patch from the pulmonary homograft later used for the aortic reconstruction. Occasionally the pulmonary artery is large enough to allow for primary closure of the distal stump without impinging on the branch pulmonary artery orifices. After the pulmonary bifurcation is closed, the distal end of the Blalock-Taussig shunt is anastomosed to a longitudinal incision in the cephalad aspect of the right pulmonary artery using 7-0 monofilament suture. The shunt is completed at this time because of the excellent exposure available prior to creation of the neoaorta.

At this point the focus of the procedure turns to reconstruction of the aorta. An incision is made in the medial ascending aorta beginning at the level of the transected proximal main pulmonary artery and carried across the arch, through the ductal insertion site, and onto the descending aorta (Figure 3). A second dose of cardioplegia is typically delivered into the proximal ascending aorta using an olive-tipped cannula. As much ductal tissue as possible is débrided from the aorta. If a coarctation shelf is present opposite the ductal insertion, it is also removed. Several (three to five) interrupted 7-0 monofilament sutures are used to approximate the proximal end of the aortic incision to the adjacent pulmonary artery. A chevron-shaped patch of pulmonary homograft is then fashioned to widely

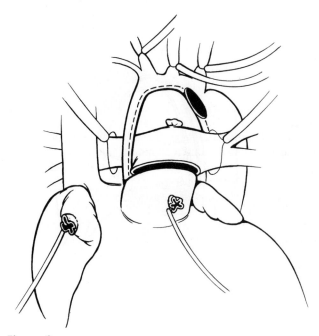

Figure 2
After an atrial septectomy is performed, the ductus arteriosus is ligated and divided, and the proximal pulmonary artery is divided. (*Reprinted from Surgical repair of the hypoplastic heart syndrome. In Bove E, Mosca R, editors:* Progress in pediatric cardiology, *vol 5. Philadelphia, 1996, WB Saunders, p 23.*)

augment the aorta, beginning distally and running the patch proximally to the pulmonary artery/aortic juncture (see Figure 3, inset, and Figure 4). The width of the patch should be tailored depending on the size of the ascending aorta, but care must be taken to avoid an excessively redundant patch, which can twist under systolic pressure, resulting in kinking of the innominate artery take-off proximally or the descending aorta distally. In general, it is better to err on the side of a narrow patch rather than a wide one. Also, care must be taken to avoid a patch that is too long, as this can cause proximal kinking of the pulmonary artery leading to ventricular outflow obstruction and neoaortic insufficiency.

Upon completion of the reconstruction, the atrial and aortic cannulation sites are filled with saline to evacuate air and the cannulae are replaced. Cardiopulmonary bypass is reinstituted slowly, the arch vessel tourniquets are removed, and the infant is rewarmed to 37°C. At this point, myocardial perfusion should be assessed and vigorous myocardial function should return. Final deairing can be accomplished through ventricular apical aspiration. Significant ventricular distention during rewarming should be assessed because if there is distortion and regurgitation of the pulmonary valve, it must be corrected.

Once rewarming is complete, transthoracic atrial lines are passed through the atrial purse-string suture next to the cannula. These lines are used both for pressure measurement and drug infusions. The majority of patients are placed on low-dose inotropic support consisting of dopamine at 3 μg/kg/min and milrinone at 0.5 μg/kg/min. A bolus of milrinone is commonly placed in the cardiopulmonary bypass

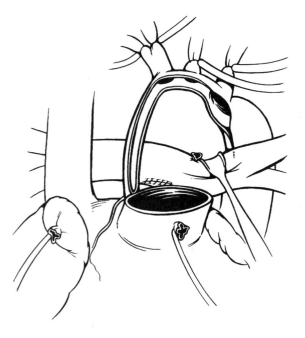

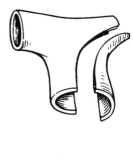

Figure 3
The aorta is incised from the level of the proximal pulmonary artery to beyond the ductal insertion. The aortic defect is then augmented with a patch of pulmonary homograft (inset). (*Reprinted from Surgical repair of the hypoplastic heart syndrome. In Bove E, Mosca R, editors: Progress in pediatric cardiology, vol 5. Philadelphia, 1996, WB Saunders, p 23.*)

circuit to decrease vasoconstriction and improve ventricular function. Other centers have used α-blocking agents such as phenoxybenzamine for this purpose. Ventilation is initiated using high tidal volumes (generally >25 ml/kg) to eliminate atelectasis and decrease pulmonary vascular resistance.

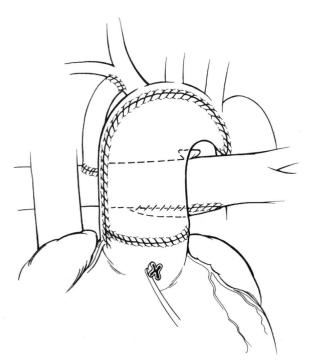

Figure 4
The aortic reconstruction is completed with a patch closure of the distal main pulmonary artery stump and placement of a modified Blalock-Taussig shunt. (*Reprinted from Surgical repair of the hypoplastic heart syndrome. In Bove E, Mosca R, editors: Progress in pediatric cardiology, vol 5. Philadelphia, 1996, WB Saunders, p 23.*)

If all appears well, the hemoclip is removed from the shunt and the patient is quickly weaned off of cardiopulmonary bypass. Modified ultrafiltration is routinely used for these patients in our center to decrease myocardial edema, improve ventricular performance, and minimize the intravascular volume load in the early postoperative period. The cannulae are then removed and hemostasis is secured. Pacing wires and a mediastinal drain are placed and, in the majority of cases, the sternum is closed. If there is any concern over myocardial function or hemorrhage, the sternum is left open and a PTFE patch is secured to the skin edges.

Depending on the cardiac anatomy, the operative technique is occasionally altered. In cases of transposition of the great vessels or if the aorta is large compared to the pulmonary artery, it may be simpler to transect both great vessels proximally. The aorta and pulmonary artery are then connected side-to-side along the adjacent edge followed by anastomosis to the augmented aortic arch. This technique avoids potential twisting of the reconstructed arch and decreases the likelihood of an excessively large patch compressing the posteriorly located pulmonary bifurcation.

A recent modification supported by Brawn, Mee, and others minimizes the use of prosthetic material by directly connecting the proximal pulmonary artery to the undersurface of the aortic arch. If this technique is used, extensive mobilization of the arch vessels is required so that the arch can come down to the pulmonary artery anastomosis without tension. Also, care must be taken to avoid kinking the diminutive ascending aorta, which serves as a common coronary artery. Because of problems with coronary inflow using this method, some centers now advocate dividing the ascending aorta and reimplanting it directly onto the antero-lateral aspect of the pulmonary artery. If there is significant aortic coarctation distal to the subclavian artery, the distal aorta also can be transected with excision of all ductal tissue followed by posterior reanastomosis to the arch prior to the connection with the proximal pulmonary artery.

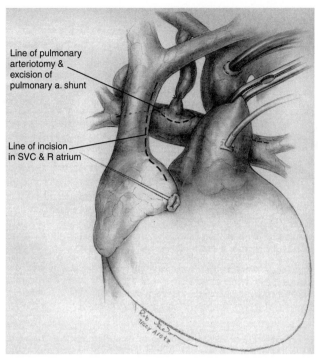

Figure 5
Initial dissection for the hemi-Fontan procedure. (*Reprinted from Fenestrated Fontan for hypoplastic left heart syndrome. In Spray T, editor:* Operative techniques in cardiac and thoracic surgery, *vol 2. Philadelphia, 1997, p 239, WB Saunders.*)

aorta), the shunt is encircled with a heavy ligature and purse-string sutures are placed in the neoaorta and right atrial appendage (Figure 5). Final dissection of the pulmonary artery behind the neoaorta may be left until after the patient is on cardiopulmonary bypass or during circulatory arrest if the adhesions are particularly dense; however, it should extend far enough to the left behind the neoaorta to allow the patch to span any branch pulmonary artery stenosis. The patient is heparinized, cannulae are placed, and cardiopulmonary bypass is initiated. The shunt is then ligated and the patient is cooled to a nasopharyngeal temperature of 18°C. The aorta is then cross-clamped, circulatory arrest is established, and cardioplegia is given into the root. The venous cannula is removed and the modified Blalock-Taussig shunt is divided adjacent to the pulmonary artery anastomosis. This anastomotic site is resected and a longitudinal incision is created extending from the right pulmonary hilum to the left. The azygos vein is ligated and an incision is placed in the medial aspect of the SVC extending onto the right atrial appendage (Figure 6). The posterior wall of the SVC and the right atrium are then sutured to the right pulmonary artery as shown in Figure 7. A large triangular patch of pulmonary homograft material is then used to augment the pulmonary artery beginning at the left hilum and extending to the previous suture line connecting the SVC to the right pulmonary artery. The inferior suture line is carried across the posterior cavoatrial junction, creating a dam between the SVC and the right atrium. Finally, the

Yet another modification of the technique involves minimizing the use of circulatory arrest. This method can be used either by creating the proximal modified Blalock-Taussig shunt (see Figure 4) without cardiopulmonary bypass or by cannulating the proximal pulmonary artery as described above followed by a brief period of circulatory arrest while the arterial cannula is moved to the shunt. It is often difficult to create the proximal shunt anastomosis without distorting the ascending aorta and thus causing myocardial dysfunction, so the use of bypass support during this maneuver is generally preferable. Once the aortic cannula has been secured to the distal shunt, the snares are tightened on the proximal innominate, left carotid, and left subclavian arteries and a vascular clamp is placed on the descending aorta beyond the planned reconstruction. Bypass flow is maintained at approximately 30% of normal and right radial artery pressures are monitored to maintain appropriate cerebral perfusion pressures. Using this technique cerebral perfusion is provided via the right carotid while some distal perfusion may occur via collaterals. Venous return is evacuated from the atrium either with the venous cannula or a sump suction placed in the atrium. Once the arch reconstruction is completed, the arterial cannula is replaced in the proximal neoaorta. The distal shunt anastomosis is performed during rewarming.

Stage 2

Following resternotomy and dissection of cardiac structures (superior vena cava [SVC], branch pulmonary arteries, and

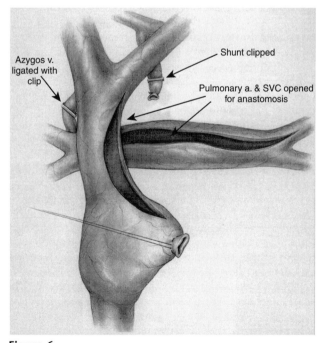

Figure 6
Hemi-Fontan procedure. The superior vena cava is incised with the incision extending onto the right atrial appendage. The pulmonary artery is incised, typically from hilum to hilum. The azygos vein is clipped. (*Reprinted from Fenestrated Fontan for hypoplastic left heart syndrome. In Spray T, editor:* Operative techniques in cardiac and thoracic surgery, *vol 2. Philadelphia, 1997, p 239, WB Saunders.*)

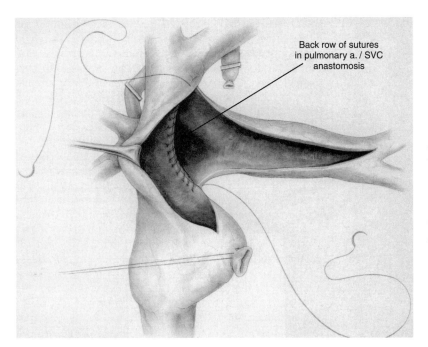

Back row of sutures
in pulmonary a. / SVC
anastomosis

Figure 7
Hemi-Fontan procedure. The posterior aspect of the superior vena cava is anastomosed to the right pulmonary artery using a running monofilament suture. (*Reprinted from Fenestrated Fontan for hypoplastic left heart syndrome. In Spray T, editor:* Operative techniques in cardiac and thoracic surgery, *vol 2. Philadelphia, 1997, p 239, WB Saunders.*)

homograft is folded down on itself as the anterior portion of the atrial suture line is completed to extend the dam up into the atrial appendage, thus preparing for a wide atriopulmonary connection at the third stage (Figure 8). Care must be taken to completely incorporate the doubled flap of homograft material along the right lateral portion of the suture line to prevent any baffle leaks between the SVC/pulmonary artery portion of the circulation and the atrium.

The atrium is then filled with saline prior to replacement of the venous cannula and reinstitution of cardiopulmonary bypass. The patient is rewarmed to 37°C and transthoracic monitoring lines are placed in both the pulmonary and atrial chambers (Figure 9). As with the first-stage procedure, modified ultrafiltration is typically used after weaning from bypass. Postoperatively, the patients are weaned from positive pressure ventilation as quickly as possible to improve hemodynamics across the pulmonary vasculature.

Stage 3

After resternotomy, limited dissection of the cardiac structures is required. The neoaorta must be sufficiently mobilized to allow placement of a cross-clamp and the lateral aspect of the right atrium must be dissected out. The patient is heparinized and cannulae are placed in the neoaorta and right atrial appendage. The patient is cooled to a nasopharyngeal temperature of 18°C, the aorta is clamped, circulatory arrest is initiated, and cardioplegia is given. The venous cannula is removed and an atriotomy is made along the lateral wall of the right atrium up to the level of the hemi-Fontan baffle (Figure 10). Under direct vision the baffle is excised leaving a circumferential rim of tissue to which the intraatrial baffle can later be attached (Figure 11). A segment of 10-mm-diameter PTFE graft is opened longitudinally and trimmed to appropriate length. A 4-mm punch hole is made in the lower end of the graft (Figure 12). The graft is then sewn to

the right atrium beginning with the posterior rim, which is secured to the lateral atrial wall anterior to the right pulmonary veins. This suture line is carried inferiorly to the eustachian valve where the graft is sutured medial to the inferior vena cava up the inferior end of the atriotomy incision. The other end of the posterior suture line is carried superiorly to the level of the excised hemi-Fontan baffle, which is included medially up to the superior end of the atriotomy. The graft can be trimmed at this point if it is too wide and the suture line is then continued so as to incorporate the anterior edge of the graft between the anterior and posterior edges of the atriotomy, creating a "PTFE sandwich" (Figure 13). After completion of the suture line, the atrium is filled with saline, the venous cannula is replaced, and cardiopulmonary bypass is reinstituted. Transthoracic monitoring lines are placed on either side of the baffle so as to measure pulmonary and atrial pressures. The patient is rewarmed to 37°C, weaned from bypass, and modified ultrafiltration is performed. As with the second stage, the patient is weaned from positive pressure ventilation as soon as possible so as to optimize the hemodynamics.

■ OUTCOMES

Survival after the first-stage operation has progressively improved since the 1980s. Currently, operative survival following the first-stage procedure is approximately 80%, with low risk patients (>2.5 kg and with no associated genetic syndromes) exceeding 90% operative survival. Analysis of long-term results reveals that after the second-stage procedure at 3 to 6 months, the intermediate-term survival is excellent with low mortality out to 15 years. The operative mortality for the second- and third-stage procedures has significantly improved so that current mortality is less than 1% for each of these procedures. While patients with HLHS have

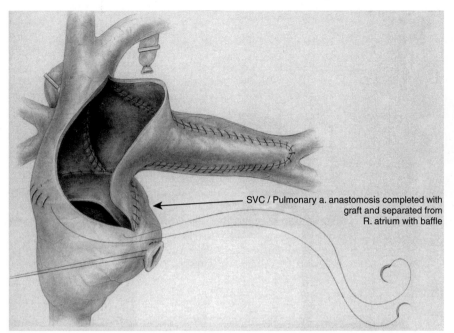

SVC / Pulmonary a. anastomosis completed with
graph and separated from
R. atrium with baffle

Figure 8
Hemi-Fontan procedure. Closure of the cavopulmonary anastomosis and creation of right atrial baffle. (*Reprinted from Fenestrated Fontan for hypoplastic left heart syndrome. In Spray T, editor: Operative techniques in cardiac and thoracic surgery, vol 2. Philadelphia, 1997, p 239, WB Saunders.*)

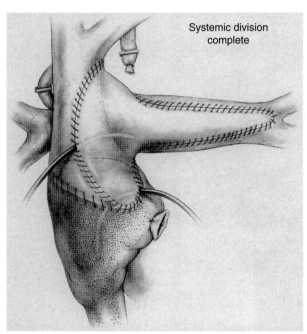

Systemic division complete

Figure 9
Hemi-Fontan procedure. Completion of systemic division and placement of transthoracic pressure monitoring lines in the pulmonary artery and common atrium directly through the suture lines. (*Reprinted from Fenestrated Fontan for hypoplastic left heart syndrome. In Spray T, editor: Operative techniques in cardiac and thoracic surgery, vol 2. Philadelphia, 1997, p 239, WB Saunders.*)

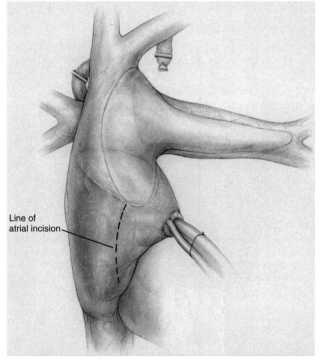

Line of atrial incision

Figure 10
Fenestrated lateral tunnel Fontan procedure. Initial dissection and a lateral right atriotomy up to the base of the previously placed hemi-Fontan baffle. (*Reprinted from Fenestrated Fontan for hypoplastic left heart syndrome. In Spray T, editor: Operative techniques in cardiac and thoracic surgery, vol 2. Philadelphia, 1997, p 239, WB Saunders.*)

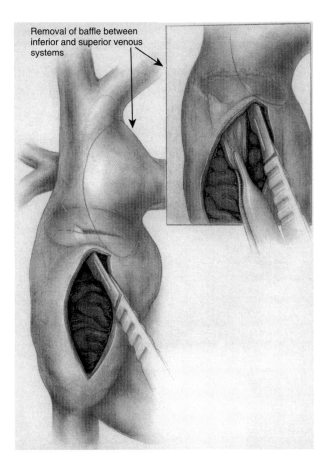

Removal of baffle between inferior and superior venous systems

Figure 11
Fenestrated lateral tunnel Fontan procedure. The dam of homograft between the atrium and the superior vena cava is excised, creating an opening that should be larger than the inferior vena caval orifice. (*Reprinted from Fenestrated Fontan for hypoplastic left heart syndrome. In Spray T, editor:* Operative techniques in cardiac and thoracic surgery, *vol 2. Philadelphia, 1997, p 239, WB Saunders.*)

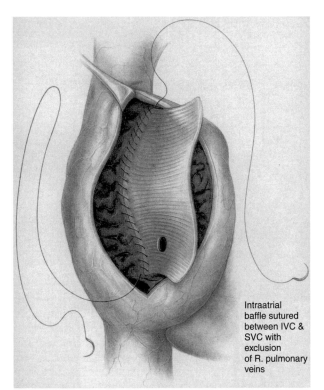

Intraatrial baffle sutured between IVC & SVC with exclusion of R. pulmonary veins

Figure 12
Fenestrated lateral tunnel Fontan procedure. Creation of lateral tunnel intraatrial baffle with PTFE graft. (*Reprinted from Fenestrated Fontan for hypoplastic left heart syndrome. In Spray T, editor:* Operative techniques in cardiac and thoracic surgery, *vol 2. Philadelphia, 1997, p 239, WB Saunders.*)

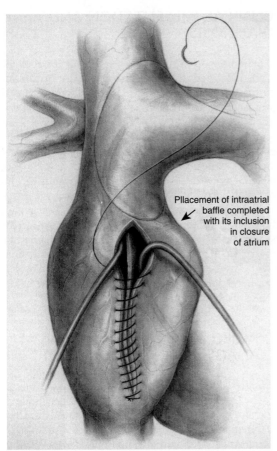

Pllacement of intraatrial baffle completed with its inclusion in closure of atrium

Figure 13
Fenestrated lateral tunnel Fontan procedure. Closure of atriotomy incorporating PTFE graft. (*Reprinted from Fenestrated Fontan for hypoplastic left heart syndrome. In Spray T, editor: Operative techniques in cardiac and thoracic surgery, vol 2. Philadelphia, 1997, p 239, WB Saunders.*)

been shown to score significantly lower than the normal population on scales of infant development and intelligence quotient testing, the majority of these patients remain within the normal range. Continued improvements in long-term outcomes can be expected as preoperative and postoperative management strategies are optimized and operative methods designed to minimize circulatory arrest while maximizing postoperative systemic perfusion are evaluated and used.

SUGGESTED READING

Cohen MI, et al: Modifications to the cavopulmonary anastomosis do not eliminate early sinus node dysfunction, *J Thorac Cardiovasc Surg* 120:891, 2000.

Gaynor JW, et al: Risk factors for mortality after the Norwood procedure, *Eur J Cardiothorac Surg* 2002.

Norwood WI, et al: Physiologic repair of aortic atresia: hypoplastic left heart syndrome, *N Engl J Med* 308:23, 1983.

Redo SF, et al: Atresia of the mitral valve, *Arch Surg* 82:678, 1961.

AORTIC ARCH INTERRUPTION

Luca A. Vricella
Duke E. Cameron

Interruption of the aortic arch is defined as the complete loss of continuity between contiguous segments of the aortic arch. Aortic luminal atresia with fibrous connection between aortic arch segments may also be included in this group of lesions that result in supravalvular left ventricular outflow tract obstruction.

The earliest description of aortic arch interruption was published in 1778, followed by several case reports over the ensuing decades; the first series of patients with interrupted aortic arch (IAA) and the original classification scheme based on location of the interruption were reported by Celeoria and Patton in 1959.

In normal morphogenesis, the proximal aortic arch (between innominate and left common carotid arteries) originates from the left horn of the aortic sac; the transverse or distal aortic arch (between left common carotid and left subclavian arteries) from the left fourth aortic arch. The third possible site of interruption (the isthmus, between left subclavian artery and ductus arteriosus) derives embryologically from the confluence of the dorsal aorta and the left sixth aortic arch.

The site of interruption therefore corresponds to specific segmental perturbation in the complex development of the aortic arch during embryogenesis. Aortic arch interruption accounts for 1% to 3% of all forms of congenital heart disease and has a prevalence of 0.005 in 1000 live births.

■ MORPHOLOGY

Aortic arch interruption has been categorized as three morphologic types, according to the location of aortic arch discontinuity (Figure 1). Isthmic interruption beyond the subclavian artery with ductus-dependent perfusion to the lower body is defined as Celeoria and Patton IAA type A. In type B, the atretic or absent portion of aorta is located between left common carotid and left subclavian arteries. This particular variant of IAA is the most common, occurring in over half of the cases and characteristically associated with thymic agenesis (DiGeorge syndrome) and 22q11 chromosomal microdeletion. Interruption between right brachiocephalic (innominate) and left common carotid arteries defines type C, the rarest of the three morphologic variants.

A large patent ductus arteriosus is always associated with aortic arch interruption. The ascending aorta is typically vertically oriented and, in comparison to the pulmonary trunk, of smaller caliber. In up to half of patients, the aortic valve is bicuspid. Other types of left ventricular outflow tract obstruction may also be present. In particular, a ventricular septal defect (VSD) with posterior deviation of the outlet septum can create a muscular ridge (the so-called muscle of Moulaert) that protrudes in the subaortic region, causing a subvalvular gradient. A large, nonrestrictive conoventricular VSD is typically associated with aortic arch interruption. Other lesions, such as common arterial trunk, transposition of the great arteries or aortopulmonary window, may coexist. A variety of aortic arch vessel anomalies may be present as well; the most common are aberrant retroesophageal right subclavian artery (associated most frequently with type B aortic arch interruption) and anomalous origin of the right pulmonary artery from the ascending aorta. A right-sided descending aorta is a rare associated finding.

■ CLINICAL PRESENTATION AND DIAGNOSIS

Most patients with aortic arch interruption present in the early postnatal period at the time of closure of the ductus arteriosus. Congestive heart failure secondary to left-to-right shunting across the VSD is worsened by the increase in impedance to left ventricular ejection that follows natural obliteration of the arterial duct. Hypoperfusion of the ductus-dependent systemic perfusion results in metabolic acidosis, splanchnic hypoperfusion, prerenal azotemia and, if untreated, circulatory collapse. Pediatric patients diagnosed in the neonatal period or early infancy may present with diminished pulses in the lower extremities, as well as electrocardiographic evidence of left ventricular hypertrophy. Physical examination is significant for a nonspecific systolic murmur auscultated over the precordium and, occasionally, differential cyanosis at the time of ductal closure. The pattern of peripheral pulses varies accordingly to the morphology of arch interruption.

■ DIAGNOSIS AND INITIAL MEDICAL MANAGEMENT

If untreated, IAA has a high neonatal mortality rate; nearly 75% of patients succumb within the first month of life. Only those children with isolated interruption and adequate collateral circulation survive untreated beyond the first year.

Diagnosis of aortic arch interruption with duct-dependent perfusion of the lower body should be considered in the differential diagnosis of newborns who present with circulatory collapse, unequal peripheral pulses, and a precordial murmur. Improvement of the clinical condition by prostaglandin infusion further supports the initial clinical suspicion. Chest radiographs typically show plethoric lung fields, while electrocardiogram is nonspecific. In the current era, echocardiography is the only diagnostic tool necessary before proceeding to surgical intervention. At the time of transthoracic echocardiogram, site of aortic arch interruption and presence/location of the VSD are noted, as well as left ventricular outflow tract obstruction or coexisting intracardiac anomalies.

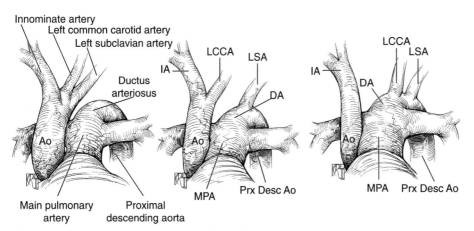

Figure 1
Classic morphologic classification of aortic arch interruption (Celeoria and Patton, 1959). Details are given in the text. *(Reproduced with permission from Jonas RA: Interrupted aortic arch. In Mavroudis C, Backer CL, editors:* Pediatric cardiac surgery, *ed 3. St Louis, 2003, Mosby, p 274.)*

In these often ill neonates and infants, there is currently almost no role for preoperative cardiac catheterization; magnetic resonance imaging is mostly of academic interest, although it can be substituted for angiography in cases with ambiguous anatomy.

Initial medical management is aimed at reversing metabolic acidosis, improving peripheral perfusion by reinstituting ductal patency, and improving cardiac performance. In infants diagnosed prenatally or presenting early in the postnatal period with hemodynamic collapse, infusion of prostaglandin E_1 and inotropic support are started immediately. Preoperative endotracheal intubation and pharmacologic paralysis facilitate manipulation of pulmonary and systemic vascular resistances to optimize perfusion. Calcium balance should also be closely monitored, as nearly one third of patients also have DiGeorge syndrome. For this specific reason, blood products should be irradiated until the syndrome is ruled out, and a fluorescence in situ hybridization (FISH) test should be obtained to rule out 22q11 chromosomal microdeletion. Once stabilized, the patient should proceed to operative correction, as the diagnosis of IAA per se constitutes an indication for surgical intervention.

■ SURGICAL TREATMENT

The first successful repair of type A aortic arch interruption by direct anastomosis via a left thoracotomy was reported by Samson in 1955. Alfred Blalock approached the same anatomic variant by turning down and anastomosing the distal left subclavian artery to the proximal descending aorta beyond the arterial duct (Blalock-Park procedure). In the early 1960s, synthetic interposition grafts were introduced. In 1970, Barratt-Boyes performed the first concomitant repair of aortic arch interruption and VSD closure, eliminating pulmonary artery banding as the initial palliative mean to avoid pulmonary overcirculation from the nonrestrictive interventricular communication. The procedure (under profound hypothermic circulatory arrest) was performed by first anastomosing a synthetic conduit via left thoracotomy to bypass the interruption and then performing VSD closure through a median sternotomy. Simultaneous VSD and IAA repair via an anterior approach without use of a prosthetic graft was reported by Trusler in 1975. During the past two decades, improvement in cardiopulmonary bypass techniques and the recent introduction of selective antegrade cerebral perfusion have allowed single-stage repair with direct anastomosis and without circulatory arrest, with excellent results in most congenital cardiac surgery units treating neonates and infants.

Staged palliation with initial pulmonary arterial banding and IAA repair (via median sternotomy or left thoracotomy depending on the site of interruption) followed by delayed VSD closure is rarely performed in the current era. Left thoracotomy is mainly used for primary repair of type A IAA without VSD, by directly anastomosing the proximal descending aorta to the underside of the distal aortic arch. More proximal interruptions are best dealt with through a median sternotomy. For neonates undergoing one-stage repair, an invasive arterial monitoring line should be placed in the right radial artery. This allows perfusion pressure monitoring when selective antegrade cerebral perfusion techniques are employed during aortic arch reconstruction. An umbilical artery or a femoral artery catheter should also be used to assess adequacy of distal perfusion during cooling and after repair. Single venous or bicaval cannulation is used, and the arterial perfusion line is split with a Y-connector to perfuse both the aortic arch proximal to the obstruction and the descending aorta. The latter limb of the arterial cannula is inserted into the pulmonary artery trunk and advanced toward the arterial duct (Figure 2A). The site of cannulation of the ascending aorta must be carefully chosen: the cannula should be placed so as to allow cerebral and myocardial perfusion (if needed) during arch repair and for perfusion of the descending aorta after completion of the arch anastomosis.

On initiation of cardiopulmonary bypass, snares are tightened around the branch pulmonary arteries, and prostaglandin infusion is discontinued. While cooling, extensive mobilization of the aorta and its branches is carried out to permit a tension-free anastomosis; for this reason, some authors have advocated routine sacrifice of the left subclavian artery. Cooling is continued for at least 20 minutes to allow homogeneous cerebral cooling. When profound hypothermia is reached (between 16° and 18°C core temperature), the descending aortic perfusion cannula is removed, the distal aorta is clamped, and, after ligation of the arterial duct at its origin from the pulmonary artery, all ductal tissue is excised. During this phase, cerebral and cardiac perfusion can be maintained at 50 ml/kg/min while monitoring right arm blood pressure. A direct end-to-side anastomosis is performed between the descending aorta and an aortotomy along the posterior aspect of the vertically oriented ascending aorta (Figure 2B). When there is also hypoplasia of other aortic arch segments, consideration should be given to patch augmentation of the aorta with a homograft.

While maintaining distal perfusion and after infusion of cold blood cardioplegia into the aortic root, the ascending aorta can be clamped and VSD and patent foramen ovale (PFO) closure is performed. If a single venous cannula is used, VSD closure and arch repair are performed during a period of circulatory arrest (with or without selective antegrade cerebral perfusion) or under low flow "suction bypass". Separation from cardiopulmonary bypass is followed by modified ultrafiltration; left atrial and pulmonary artery monitoring lines, as well as a peritoneal dialysis catheter, are routinely placed to guide early postoperative management.

Concomitant anomalies (VSD, transposition of the great arteries, and common arterial trunk among others) should be addressed at the time of aortic arch repair. Severe left ventricular outflow tract obstruction from posterior displacement of the outlet septum can be addressed by subaortic resection or, if the subaortic stenosis is severe, by a Damus-Kaye-Stansel aortopulmonary anastomosis. In the latter approach, the pulmonary artery is transected and the proximal end is anastomosed to the ascending aorta. The VSD is baffled to the pulmonary artery, and a conduit is interposed between the right ventriculotomy and the branch pulmonary arterial confluence.

■ OUTCOMES

Hospital mortality rate for single-stage IAA and VSD repair is below 10% in the current era. Specifically, mortality rates

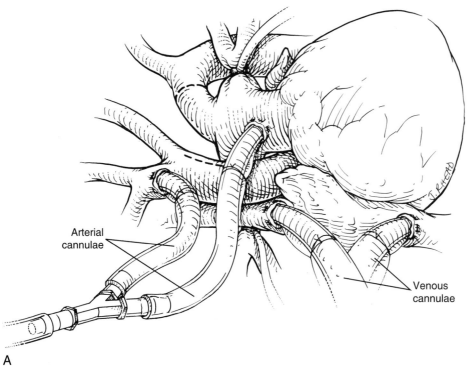

Arterial
cannulae

Venous
cannulae

A

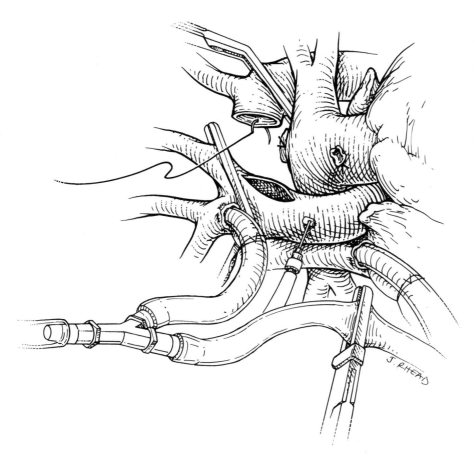

B

Figure 2
(A) Operative approach to aortic arch interruption (type B). The aortic return cannula is split with a Y-connector, allowing perfusion proximal and distal to the site of interruption during systemic cooling. Loops encircling the pulmonary arteries are snared. **(B)** Operative approach to aortic arch interruption (type B). While selectively perfusing the innominate and left common carotid arteries, continuity of the aortic arch is restored with an end-to-side anastomosis between the vertically oriented ascending aorta and the distal aortic arch. *(Reproduced with permission from Coarctation of the aorta and interrupted aortic arch. In Kouchoukos NT, editors: Kirklin/Barratt-Boyes cardiac surgery, ed 3. Philadelphia, 2003, Churchill Livingstone, pp 1358-1359.)*

as low as 4% have been reported with repair of type A interruption, and 11% with type B. Highest survival rates are obtained in patients with isolated type A interruption without VSD (essentially critical condition repaired via left thoracotomy). The lowest survival rates occur in the rare type C IAA. Incomplete preoperative resuscitation is indicated by low preprocedural pH. Severe left ventricular outflow tract obstruction (hypoplastic ascending aorta and aortic root) are predictive of early mortality. It is very difficult to predict which neonates will develop left ventricular outflow tract obstruction soon after repair and should therefore benefit from root enlargement or a Damus-Kaye-Stansel procedure at the time of aortic arch repair. In addition to persistent left ventricular outflow tract obstruction, left recurrent laryngeal and phrenic nerve injury are other procedure-related early complications and result from the magnitude of the surgical dissection. Furthermore, obstruction of the left main stem bronchus may result from compression by the downwardly displaced reconstructed aortic arch.

Long-term outcomes are influenced by the persistence or recurrence of a transaortic gradient, akin to that observed in neonates and infants undergoing resection and extended end-to-end anastomosis for coarctation. Similarly, percutaneous intervention is first-line therapy for late postoperative aortic obstruction in symptomatic children or for asymptomatic children when peak gradient exceeds 30 mm Hg. Actuarial freedom from reintervention for neonates after direct aortic anastomosis has been as high as 86% at 3-year follow-up.

Subaortic obstruction may also complicate late outcomes. Freedom from reintervention for subvalvular stenosis at 3 years is nearly 80%; the lesion may be persistent or recurrent. After complete intracardiac repair, 5-year survival now exceeds 70%.

SUGGESTED READING

Asou T, et al: Selective cerebral perfusion technique during aortic arch repair in neonates, *Ann Thorac Surg* 61:1546, 1996.

Bove EL, et al: The management of severe subaortic stenosis, ventricular septal defect and aortic arch obstruction in the neonate, *J Thorac Cardiovasc Surg* 105:289, 1993.

Jonas RA, et al: Outcomes in patients with interrupted aortic arch and ventricular septal defect. A multi-institutional study. Congenital Heart Surgeons Society, *J Thorac Cardiovasc Surg* 107:1099, 1994.

Mainwaring RD, Lamberti JJ: Mid-to long-term results of the two-stage approach to interrupted aortic arch and ventricular septal defect, *Ann Thorac Surg* 64:1782, 1997.

Serraf A, et al: Repair of interrupted aortic arch: a ten-year experience, *J Thorac Cardiovasc Surg* 223:1150, 1996.

PULMONARY ATRESIA WITH INTACT VENTRICULAR SEPTUM

Gary K. Lofland

Pulmonary atresia with intact ventricular septum (PA/IVS) is characterized by morphologic heterogeneity of right-sided cardiac structures—specifically, the tricuspid valve, the right ventricle, and the main pulmonary artery. It is the adequacy of these right-sided structures that determines the type of repair these patients may undergo: either single-ventricle palliation, one and one-half–ventricle palliation, or biventricular correction.

PA/IVS is a congenital cardiac lesion characterized by complete obstruction of the right ventricular outflow tract occurring at the level of the atretic pulmonary valve, an IVS with no ventricular septal defect, varying degrees of right ventricular and tricuspid valve hypoplasia, and variable coronary anatomy. The pulmonary valve, across which there is no forward flow, usually exists as a tough imperforate membrane. Because of relatively unimpeded inflow and totally obstructed outflow, the right ventricle is frequently markedly hypertrophic and may exhibit fibrosis and endocardial fibroelastosis. The right ventricle may be large and tripartite, but it is more frequently small because of hypoplasia or absence of the trabecular portion, the infundibular portion, or both. The tricuspid valve is usually proportionate to the size of the right ventricle and may exhibit varying degrees of incompetence. Right atrial enlargement and some form of interatrial communication are always present. Although they may sometimes be small, the pulmonary arteries are frequently normal or nearly normal in size, receiving blood flow through a patent ductus arteriosus.

■ INITIAL MEDICAL MANAGEMENT

PA/IVS is a ductus-dependent lesion. The sole source of pulmonary blood flow is the patent ductus arteriosus and every effort must be made to maintain patency of the ductus. Consequently, as soon as the diagnosis is established echocardiographically in the newborn, prostaglandin E_1 (PGE$_1$) infusion is initiated to both establish and maintain ductus patency, increase pulmonary blood flow, and relieve hypoxemia and acidosis. PGE₁ is typically infused at a dosage of 0.01 to 0.2 µg/kg/min and is adjusted according to systemic oxygen saturations. High doses of PGE₁ may cause mild hyperthermia and apnea, and one must be ready to intubate and mechanically ventilate the neonate if respiratory depression occurs. More severely hypoxic or acidotic neonates may also require endotracheal intubation and mechanical ventilation, coupled with reversal of acidosis with sodium bicarbonate, until ductus dependency can be clearly established and maintained. In addition to establishing the diagnosis of PA with ductus-dependent pulmonary blood flow, echocardiography is also used to define intracardiac structures, determine the adequacy of the atrial septal defect, and determine the presence or absence of coronary artery sinusoids and right ventricular dependent coronary circulation.

Once the patient is stabilized and resuscitated, cardiac catheterization with cineangiography is then expeditiously performed and may be both diagnostic and therapeutic. At the time of cardiac catheterization, balloon atrial septostomy may be performed to ensure unobstructed blood flow at the level of the atrial septum. If no coronary sinusoids with right ventricular dependent coronary circulation are found, the right ventricular outflow tract may be opened using radiofrequency perforation and balloon dilation of the atretic pulmonary valve (RFP/BPV) (Figure 1). If extensive coronary sinusoids are found, the decision to proceed down a single-ventricle pathway may be made in the neonatal period. Radiofrequency perforation with balloon valvotomy of the pulmonary valve has largely displaced open pulmonary valvotomy at our institution. It has the advantage of being able to decompress the right ventricle without

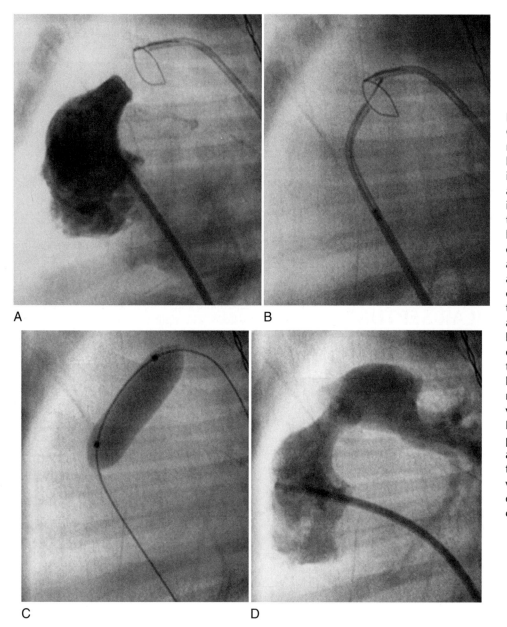

A   B   C   D

Figure 1
Cardiac catheterization with radiofrequency perforation and balloon pulmonary valvotomy in a patient with pulmonary atresia. An injection is made into the right ventricle. Note the well-developed infundibulum ending blindly **(A)**. The catheter is in the patient's aorta and has traversed the ductus arteriosus, with the tip of the catheter and snare lying in the proximal main pulmonary artery. A second catheter has been placed via right heart catheterization **(B)**. The tip of the catheter is in the infundibulum, and radiofrequency perforation of the atretic pulmonary valve has been accomplished. Balloon dilation of the atretic pulmonary valve has been accomplished **(C)**. Right ventricular injection post balloon valvotomy shows adequate opening of the right ventricular outflow tract **(D)**.

subjecting the patient to an open surgical procedure. If balloon valvotomy can be performed after RFP, the patient can then be slowly weaned off prostaglandins over several days. However, if oxygen saturations can be maintained, additional palliation with a systemic-to-pulmonary arterial shunt may be required. It should be noted that if RFP/BPV is attempted, the cardiac surgical team should be notified and be on standby, because perforation of the right ventricular outflow tract and pericardial tamponade can occur.

■ INITIAL SURGICAL MANAGEMENT

Initial surgical management is palliative and has two distinct goals. Goal 1 is to establish a reliable source of pulmonary blood flow through the creation of a systemic-to-pulmonary arterial shunt. Goal 2 is to decompress the right ventricle by opening the atretic pulmonary valve. If RFP/BPV is not available in an institution, open pulmonary valvotomy can be performed at the time the systemic-to-pulmonary arterial shunt is created. If there are extensive coronary sinusoids and right ventricular dependent coronary circulation, no attempt should be made to open the right ventricular outflow tract, because acute myocardial infarction can occur in that setting.

Most patients require a systemic-to-pulmonary arterial shunt, even if the right ventricular outflow tract is successfully opened. Although the shunt size is dictated to some extent by the patient's weight in some congenital cardiac lesions, all patients with PA/IVS in our series received a right modified Blalock-Taussig shunt using a 4-mm tube graft of expanded polytetrafluoroethylene.

Subsequent surgical procedures depend on the growth of the patient's right-sided cardiac structures. Patients who, in the first year of life, fail to achieve growth of the right ventricle will proceed down a single-ventricle (Fontan) pathway. Likewise, patients who have extensive coronary sinusoids and a right ventricular dependent coronary circulation will proceed down a single-ventricle pathway. Patients who achieve excellent growth of the right ventricle may require additional enlargement of the right ventricular outflow tract, takedown of the modified Blalock-Taussig shunt, closure of the atrial septal defect, or some combination of these procedures. Within this spectrum lies a group of patients in whom the right ventricle is still too small to handle the entire systemic venous drainage and pulmonary circulation but who still have good flow through the right ventricle. These patients may be candidates for additional augmentation of the right ventricular outflow tract, complete or partial closure of the atrial septal defect, and diversion of one third of their systemic venous drainage directly into the pulmonary circulation through a bidirectional Glenn shunt. This therapeutic strategy has sometimes been called a "one and one-half–ventricle correction."

Initial surgical palliation is accomplished in the first few days to 1 week of life. The need for, timing of, and type of subsequent surgical procedures involve careful follow-up and periodic reassessment using echocardiography and even cardiac catheterization in the first 2 years or so of the patient's life. It must always be kept in mind that considerable growth of even a small right ventricle can occur during this time.

■ LARGE RIGHT VENTRICLE

Patients with a large right ventricle constitute a small subgroup of PA/IVS (<10%). Our treatment strategy in this group is to perform RFP/BPV. In the past several years, we have not had to resort to open pulmonary valvotomy. After the catheter procedure, the patient can be observed in the neonatal intensive care unit while PGE_1 is tapered and discontinued. Oxygen saturations are carefully monitored while the ductus closes, allowing prostaglandins to be reinstituted if a fall in oxygen saturation occurs. This is usually the case, as significant infundibular obstruction is almost invariably present. At our institution, we then perform a right modified Blalock-Taussig shunt, through either right thoracotomy or median sternotomy. At our institution, more than 75 neonates with PA/IVS have been treated since 1998. Only two have not required a Blalock-Taussig shunt.

If RFP/BPV is unavailable, transventricular perforation and dilation using Hegar dilators, with or without cardiopulmonary bypass, or open pulmonary valvotomy with cardiopulmonary bypass may be performed.

Subsequent management includes hemodynamic reassessment by repeat cardiac catheterization at 12 to 18 months of age. This is followed by augmentation of the right ventricular outflow tract, usually with transannular patching with resection of infundibular muscle bundles and closure of the atrial septal defect using cardiopulmonary bypass.

■ HYPOPLASTIC RIGHT VENTRICLE

All patients in this subgroup require a systemic-to-pulmonary arterial shunt in the neonatal period. The indication for decompression of the right ventricle depends entirely on the presence or absence of the outlet or infundibular portion of the right ventricle. Patients with a completely absent infundibulum (5% to 10%) proceed down a single-ventricle pathway, as the small, nondecompressed right ventricle has no growth potential. Consequently, we create a right modified Blalock-Taussig shunt using a 4-mm tube graft of expanded polytetrafluoroethylene. This is performed through a right thoracotomy incision via the fourth intercostal space. The azygos vein is ligated and divided to mobilize the superior vena cava, thereby allowing the shunt to be placed more proximally on the right pulmonary artery, avoiding the branch vessels, especially the right upper lobe branch.

At 5 to 6 months of age, the infant then undergoes repeat cardiac catheterization to assess pulmonary artery morphology, and specifically to examine the right pulmonary artery for distortion. This is followed by takedown of the Blalock-Taussig shunt and creation of a bidirectional Glenn shunt. If there is distortion or scarring of the proximal right pulmonary artery, we perform a patch angioplasty of the proximal right pulmonary artery using an onlay patch of cryopreserved pulmonary artery allograft material.

At 2 to 3 years of age, the patient then undergoes repeat cardiac catheterization to determine suitability for completion Fontan, followed by surgical completion of the Fontan circulation, if appropriate.

Patients in whom a right ventricular infundibulum is present should receive a systemic-to-pulmonary arterial shunt in combination with RFP/BPV. Alternatively, transventricular valvotomy or open pulmonary valvotomy may be used. All three methods of opening the right ventricular outflow tract aim to decompress the right ventricle, thereby allowing for growth. Our policy is to open the right ventricular outflow tract at the time of cardiac catheterization, followed by the creation of a right modified Blalock-Taussig shunt soon after the catheterization once the patient has been stabilized.

Subsequent management includes repeat cardiac catheterization at about 12 months of age to determine growth of the right ventricle and tricuspid valve. If right ventricular and tricuspid valve growth has been satisfactory, complete correction can be performed. This consists of transannular patch enlargement of the right ventricular outflow tract, closure of the atrial septal defect, and takedown of the Blalock-Taussig shunt, performed using cardiopulmonary bypass.

If right ventricular growth has been marginal, further growth can be encouraged by transannular patch enlargement of the right ventricular outflow tract and resection of muscle bundles, leaving an interatrial communication. It is our policy to reduce the size of the atrial septal defect by taking a circular patch of expanded polytetrafluoroethylene, creating a 4- to 5-mm central defect using an aortic punch, placing small titanium vascular clips at several locations around the punched hole (to serve as markers during subsequent cardiac catheterizations), and then suturing the patch

to the rim of the atrial septal defect. The Blalock-Taussig shunt may be left open. At subsequent cardiac catheterizations, test closure of both the shunt and atrial septal defect can be performed, followed by device closure of both if hemodynamics are suitable.

Small coronary sinusoids involving the hypoplastic right ventricle may be found in many patients; as long as they are quite small, they usually close spontaneously. Patients with very large coronary sinusoids and a right ventricular dependent coronary circulation, however, are an especially high-risk group, as these patients are prone to sudden death from acute myocardial infarction in the neonatal period (Figures 2 and 3). No attempt whatsoever should be made to open the right ventricular outflow tract in these patients, as decompression of the right ventricle can lead to flow reversal in the coronary circulation and acute myocardial infarction. These patients should undergo balloon atrial septostomy followed by creation of a systemic-to-pulmonary arterial shunt (in our institution, a right modified Blalock-Taussig shunt). Careful monitoring in the intensive care unit for at least several days postoperatively is mandatory in these patients, as they are at risk for sudden death from acute myocardial infarction if coronary sinusoids are large. These patients should proceed down a single-ventricle pathway, with takedown of the Blalock-Taussig shunt and creation of a bidirectional Glenn shunt at 5 to 6 months of age, followed by completion Fontan using an extracardiac conduit at 2 to 3 years of age.

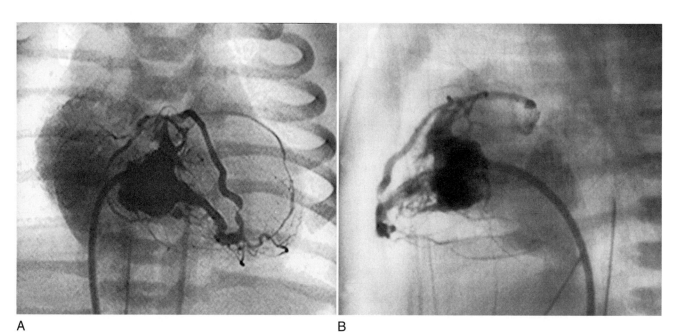

A   B

Figure 2
Cardiac catheterization and cineangiography in a newborn with pulmonary atresia and intact ventricular septum, anteroposterior and lateral projections. The tip of the catheter is in the markedly hypoplastic right ventricle. Note the absence of the infundibulum, the multiple coronary sinusoids, and retrograde filling of the coronary circulation. After uneventfully undergoing a right modified Blalock-Taussig shunt, this patient had daily episodes of ST-segment changes followed by ventricular tachycardia and fibrillation for the first 7 days postoperatively.

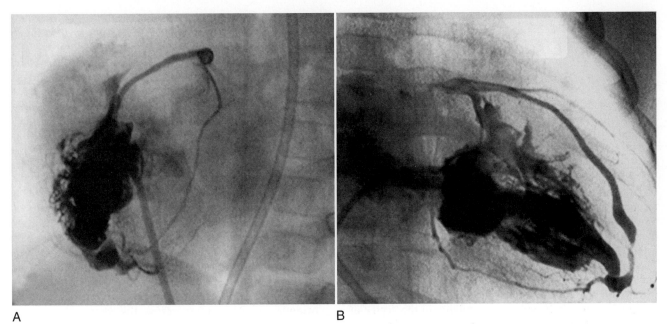

Figure 3
Cardiac catheterization and cineangiography at 9 months of age, anteroposterior and lateral projections. These cineangiograms were obtained on the same patient illustrated in Figure 2, before undergoing uneventful takedown of her right modified Blalock-Taussig shunt and creation of a bidirectional Glenn shunt. In Figure 2, multiple small branches emerged from her posterior descending coronary artery. In the cineangiograms obtained at 9 months of age, most of these vessels are gone. Spontaneous closure of these vessels undoubtedly caused the ST-segment changes and electrophysiologic instability this patient experienced during the neonatal period.

■ RESULTS

PA/IVS continues to present major medical and surgical challenges. In an earlier era, operative mortality rates exceeding 50% were reported by numerous groups. In recent years, these results have improved but PA/IVS continues to be a high-risk lesion.

The largest single study of neonates with PA/IVS was conducted between 1987 and 1997 by The Congenital Heart Surgeons Society. Thirty-three institutions were involved. Competing risk analysis was used to demonstrate prevalence of six end states.

Overall survival in this study was 77% at 1 month, 70% at 6 months, 60% at 5 years, and 58% at 15 years. Prevalence of end states 15 years after entry were two-ventricle repair, 33%; Fontan, 20%; one and one-half–ventricle repair, 5%; heart transplant, 2%; death before reaching definitive repair, 38%, and alive without definitive repair, 2%.

Patient-related factors discriminating among end states primarily included adequacy of right-sided heart structures, degree of aberration of coronary circulation, low birth weight, and tricuspid valve regurgitation.

SUGGESTED READING

Ashburn DA, et al: Determinants of mortality and type of repair in neonates with pulmonary atresia and intact ventricular septum, *J Thorac Cardiovasc Surg* (in press).

Cobanoglu A, et al: Valvulotomy for pulmonary atresia with intact ventricular septum, *J Thorac Cardiovasc Surg* 89:482, 1985.

deLeval M, et al: Pulmonary atresia and intact ventricular septum: surgical management based on a revised classification, *Circulation* 66:272, 1982.

Daubeney PE, et al: Pulmonary atresia with intact ventricular septum: range of morphology in a population-based study, *J Am Coll Cardiol* 39:1670, 2002.

COMPLETE ATRIOVENTRICULAR CANAL

Charles B. Huddleston

Atrioventricular (AV) canal is one of the more common forms of "complex" congenital heart anomalies. The association with trisomy 21 is well established: Approximately 70% of children with AV canal have this chromosomal defect. Conversely, 30% of children with trisomy 21 have AV canal. This anomaly is characterized by absence of the ventricular and atrial septa at the point where they normally are adjoined; this is also the confluence of the right and left AV valves (Figure 1). There is considerable variability in the degree of deficiency of the atrial and ventricular septa. In addition, there is variability in the formation and function of the AV valves. There can be imbalance in the positioning of the AV valves such that inlet into one of the ventricles is compromised, leading to varying degrees of hypoplasia of that ventricle. The specifics of surgical therapy and timing of intervention depend on these factors, which usually can be sorted out by a careful two-dimensional echocardiogram. There are a few instances in which cardiac catheterization should be performed, including when there is uncertainty about the systemic or pulmonary veins and when the patient's clinical status does not fit the echocardiographic findings. This chapter focuses on typical complete AV canal defects.

For the "garden variety" AV canal, most authors agree that palliative procedures, such as pulmonary artery banding, seldom are indicated, but they may be appropriate for infants with other severe congenital anomalies, multiple ventricular septal defects (VSDs), or significantly unbalanced ventricles. Most children with AV canal develop significant heart failure within the first 2 months of life. The response to medical therapy (digoxin, afterload reduction, and diuretics) is variable, but patients who respond can wait a few months for growth before surgical repair. If the response to medical therapy is poor, however, there is little benefit to delaying repair, even in an infant less than 3 kg. The risk of irreversible pulmonary hypertension increases as the age approaches 1 year and may be significant at age 6 months, particularly in children with trisomy 21. Our policy has been to offer repair before age 6 months, regardless of symptoms. In infants who do not respond to medical therapy, there may be other mitigating factors, such as pulmonary venoocclusive disease, a stenotic left-sided AV valve orifice, and a small left ventricular outflow tract (LVOT).

A debate has persisted for years as to whether the one-patch technique or two-patch technique is preferred. Both are satisfactory in experienced hands, and there is no substantial difference in operative survival or late outcome, including the competence of the left AV valve. More recently, there has been interest in closure of the ventricular and atrial components without use of patch material. For small defects, this approach seems feasible, but the advantages of avoiding patch material are not so great as to suggest this as a preferred approach, particularly if it results in distortion of the left or right AV valve.

Cardiopulmonary bypass is initiated using bicaval and aortic cannulation. Single venous cannulation and circulatory arrest are seldom necessary. After cardioplegic arrest, the right atrium is opened to provide exposure of the ventricular and atrial septa (Figure 2). The AV valve complex is inspected carefully to ascertain the relationship of formed commissures with the plane of the crest of the ventricular septum. This allows one to determine the degree of bridging of the superior and inferior leaflets of the common AV valve and to classify the defect according to the system described by Rastelli, which categorizes the defect according to the degree of bridging of the superior leaflet. The AV valve leaflets are floated into position by instillation of cold saline into the ventricles (Figure 3). The point of coaptation of the superior and inferior bridging leaflets over the midportion of the crest of the ventricular septum is identified and marked with a polypropylene stitch. If there is complete bridging of the leaflets across the ventricular septum (Rastelli type C), the leaflets are divided in a line parallel to and over the right side of the crest of the ventricular septum. This division allows excellent exposure for the closure of the VSD. If there is a well-formed commissure for the superior or inferior leaflet over the crest of the septum (Rastelli type A),

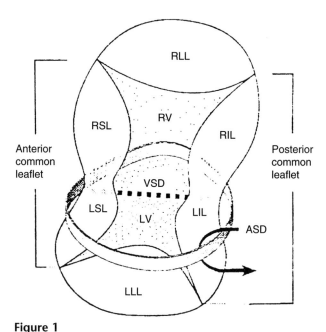

Figure 1

Schematic drawing of a complete AV canal defect. There is "sharing" of the anterior and posterior common leaflets between the right and left sides of the heart. The atrial septal defect (ASD) and ventricular septal defect (VSD) are actually one large defect with atrial and ventricular components. RLL, right lateral leaflet; RSL, right superior leaflet; RIL, right inferior leaflet; LSL, left superior leaflet; LIL, left inferior leaflet; LLL, left lateral leaflet; RV, right ventricle; LV, ventricle. (*From Backer CL et al: Repair of complete atrioventricular canal defects: results with two-patch technique,* Ann Thorac Surg *60:530, 1995. Reprinted with permission from the Society of Thoracic Surgeons.*)

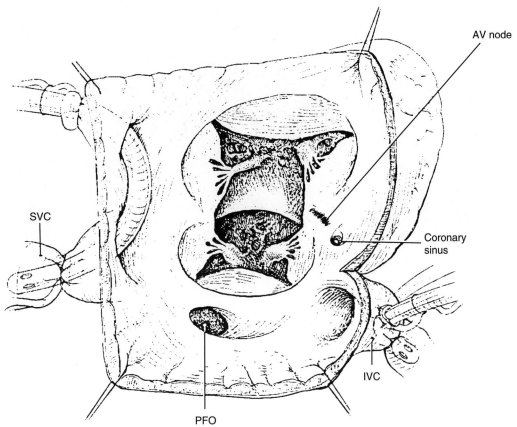

Figure 2
Appearance of a complete AV canal as viewed from a surgeon's perspective. Note relationship between the AV node and the edge of the defect and the coronary sinus. SVC, superior vena cava; IVC, inferior vena cava; PFO, patent foramen ovale. (*From Backer CL et al: Repair of complete atrioventricular canal defects: results with two-patch technique,* Ann Thorac Surg *60:530, 1995. Reprinted with permission from the Society of Thoracic Surgeons.*)

no division of the leaflet is necessary. Some secondary chordae from the right side of the AV valve complex may obstruct the view of the VSD; these may be divided because that portion of the AV valve is supported by the VSD patch. The patch is cut to the appropriate size and shape (Figure 4).

I prefer the two-patch technique, using synthetic material for the ventricular component and pericardium for the atrial side. The VSD patch usually is shaped like a half circle. Although some authors prefer closing the ventricular component of the defect with interrupted sutures, I find that the visualization of the defect is satisfactory for the quicker, continuous suture technique. The curved portion of the patch is sewn to the crest of the ventricular septum, starting at the midportion and proceeding inferiorly first, then superiorly. As one approaches the posterior AV valve annulus, care must be taken to avoid the conduction tissue located near the rim of the VSD. The suture line should veer away from the crest of the septum onto the body of the right ventricle a few millimeters. The stitch is brought up through the annulus of the AV valve complex. The other limb of the suture is sewn continuously and superiorly to the AV valve annulus.

At this point, the VSD closure is completed by attaching the divided components of the AV valve complex to the top margin of the synthetic patch. It is crucial that the AV valve leaflets be placed at the appropriate level to maintain competence of the AV valves, keeping in mind the preoperative echocardiographic appearance of the AV valves and the intraoperative evaluation when the common AV is floated into position. The amount of AV valve tissue taken up with each stitch should be the minimum necessary to hold the stitch without tearing. When this is completed, the surgeon should close the "cleft" in the "anterior leaflet of the mitral valve." This is not a true cleft in a true anterior leaflet or a true mitral valve. When bringing the edges of the superior and inferior bridging leaflets together, it is important to appose the so-called kissing edges of the leaflets—the portion where the leaflets coapt and not the free edge itself, which usually is attached to the chordal elements and folded under the kissing edge. I use horizontal mattress, interrupted, polypropylene suture to close the cleft. The degree of cleft closure necessary varies from patient to patient depending on the anatomy of the mitral valve orifice. In some cases, complete closure of the cleft may result in an orifice that is stenotic, whereas incomplete closure may result in postrepair mitral regurgitation.

I recommend careful assessment of the orifice based on the leaflet anatomy after closure of the VSD. In general, most patients have a satisfactory mitral valve orifice with nearly

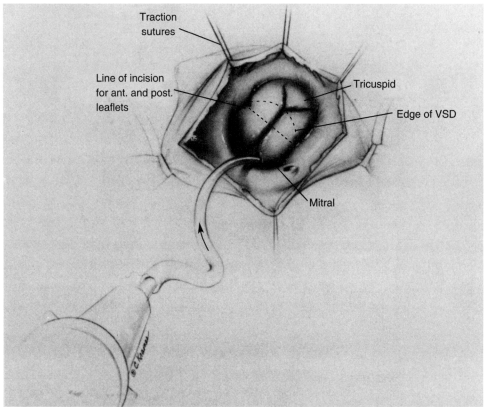

Figure 3
The AV valve leaflets are floated into position by instilling cold saline into the ventricles. The alignment of the AV valves with the ventricular septum is noted so that the inferior and superior bridging leaflets can by divided accordingly, and the point of coaptation of the inferior and superior bridging leaflets over the ventricular septum can be marked with a polypropylene stitch. (*From Santos A et al: Repair of atrioventricular septal defects in infancy,* J Thorac Cardiovasc Surg *91:505, 1986.*)

complete cleft closure. The stitches should be placed and tied down, and the competency of the mitral valve should be tested with infusion of cold saline into the left ventricle. If there is obvious regurgitation through the mitral valve, potential reasons are (1) failure of complete cleft closure, (2) inaccurate suspension of the leaflets on the VSD patch, (3) distortion of the mitral leaflets by cleft closure or VSD closure, and (4) inadequate residual mitral valve tissue remaining. If the leak is central, placing one or two stitches in the area of a commissure in the mitral valve to reduce the annulus may be sufficient. Occasionally, taking out one of the cleft closure stitches may reduce the regurgitation. Rarely, taking down the attachment of the AV valve to the VSD patch is appropriate; one must be careful with this, however, because the AV valve leaflet tissue is extremely thin and may be damaged in the process. It may not hold stitches as well the second time around.

The final step in repair is closing the atrial component. In the two-patch technique, a segment of pericardium appropriate to the size of the defect is harvested. Similar to the VSD patch, it is generally a half circle. It is sewn in place beginning with the attachment to the AV valve–VSD patch complex. Either interrupted stitches are placed

through the AV valve–VSD patch complex and then into the pericardium, or a running suture technique may be used. Care must be taken to incorporate the same AV valve tissue as was used in suspending the AV valve tissue to the top of the VSD patch. As one approaches the inferior/posterior portion of the AV valve–VSD patch complex, the conduction tissue is in proximity. Three approaches have been used for this part of the repair. One approach is to veer anteriorly and laterally around the coronary sinus, leaving it on the left atrial side of the atrial septal defect patch. The second is to take the suture line inferolaterally to the lateral edge of the coronary sinus, then proceed posteriorly within that. The third (my preference) is to follow the left AV valve annulus a short distance, then proceed onto the edge of the atrial septum when one is well away from the conduction tissue (Figure 5). I use the coronary sinus as a landmark for establishing a safe point at which the stitches might be placed into the edge of the atrial defect itself. The superior aspect of the atrial repair is a relatively safe area with the exception of the first few millimeters of the edge of the atrial septum. The aortic valve annulus is close to this portion and mandates that stitches not be placed too deeply at this spot. A secundum atrial defect frequently accompanies the AV canal

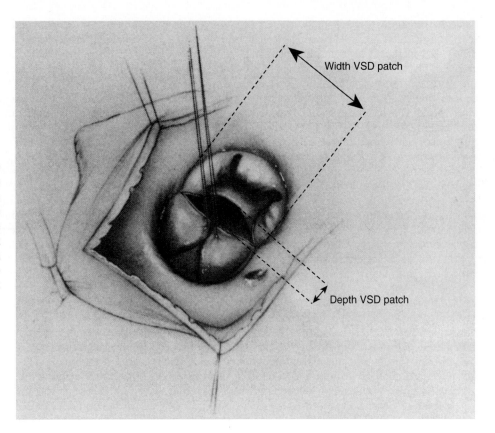

Figure 4
With the superior and inferior bridging leaflets divided, the ventricular septal defect (VSD) is easily seen. The stitch between the bridging leaflets helps to define the depth of the ventricular component of the AV canal. (*From Santos A et al: Repair of atrioventricular septal defects in infancy,* J Thorac Cardiovasc Surg *91:505, 1986.*)

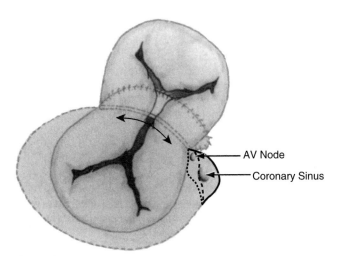

Figure 5
The inferolateral attachment of the patch for the atrial component of the AV canal may be placed in one of three positions—to the right and laterally *(dark solid line)*, to the right and posteriorly on the edge of the coronary sinus *(heavy dashed black line)*, or along the left AV valve annulus a short distance then posterolaterally to the edge of the atrial defect beyond the coronary sinus orifice *(black dotted line)*.

defect and should be closed separately or included in the closure of the primum atrial septal defect.

■ SPECIAL ISSUES

Double Orifice Left AV Valve
A so-called double orifice left AV valve occurs in approximately 5% of patients with AV canal. The best approach is to leave this part of the left-sided AV valve alone. This so-called minor orifice is usually competent and has its own chordal support system. Closure of the cleft must be done judiciously because of concerns regarding the resultant orifice size. Usually the cleft should be closed, however, as with a more typical AV canal defect.

Conotruncal Anomalies
Extension of the VSD anteriorly into the outlet septum with malalignment of the conal septum occurs with complete AV canal in approximately 5% of patients. This malalignment may vary from tetralogy of Fallot anatomy to double outlet right ventricle. The balance of the circulation varies with the degree of right ventricular outflow tract obstruction. The pulmonary valve itself may or may not be abnormal. Correction of this anomaly combines components of AV canal repair with those of tetralogy of Fallot. Exposure of the defect is through the right atrium initially. Although division of the superior bridging leaflet facilitates exposure of the anterosuperior portion of the VSD, usually the top of the

defect is seen better through an incision in the right ventricular outflow tract. The VSD patch is cut in a shape to fit this defect and appears like a comma. The VSD ordinarily is closed in part through the right atrium and in part through the ventriculotomy. The goals of correction are complete closure of the ventricular defect, complete closure of the atrial defect, relief of the right ventricular outflow tract obstruction, and competence of the AV valves. Ideally the pulmonary valve should remain competent, but when a transannular patch is necessary to relieve the right ventricular outflow tract obstruction, the pulmonary valve becomes regurgitant. The physiologic impact of this regurgitation is made worse when one or both AV valves leak. Generally, patients with either moderate left AV valve regurgitation or severe pulmonary valve regurgitation struggle postoperatively. Some surgeons advocate using a homograft conduit in the right ventricular outflow tract when repair of this lesion violates the pulmonary valve annulus.

Left AV Valve Regurgitation

Most surgeons use intraoperative transesophageal echocardiography to assess the status of the left AV valve after repair. When there is significant regurgitation, one should return to cardiopulmonary bypass to modify the repair. Strategies at this point include more complete closure of the cleft, annuloplasty stitches, and chordal shortening. The preferred repair technique may be inferred by the echocardiographic appearance of the left AV valve leaflets. When to revise the repair for left AV valve regurgitation (LAVVR) is influenced by the surgeon's estimate of likely improvement, how difficult the initial repair was, and the overall hemodynamic status of the patient. The experience of the cardiologist interpreting the echocardiogram also is a factor. Whenever there is moderate regurgitation or more, the likelihood of later reoperation is high. However, the correlation of intraoperative transesophageal echocardiography with late transthoracic echocardiography assessment of LAVVR is not as close as one would like. In addition to assessment of the regurgitation, the left AV valve should be interrogated for inflow stenosis. This stenosis can occur when the bridging leaflets compose more than 70% of the orifice of the left AV valve. Closing the cleft completely in this situation leaves an asymmetric, small orifice.

The incidence of reoperation for LAVVR varies from 2% to 20%. Possible factors contributing to development of LAVVR include preoperative LAVVR, early age at initial repair, single-patch versus double-patch technique, and failure to close the cleft in the left AV valve. None of these are conclusively demonstrated risk factors for late LAVVR, however. Most congenital heart surgeons believe that the incidence of late mitral regurgitation is higher without a closed cleft—whether left open at the original operation or open due to suture dehiscence. This opinion is supported by the observation that late LAVVR often can be repaired satisfactorily by merely closing the residual cleft. Several highly respected surgeons do not close this so-called cleft, however. Simple cleft closure is sufficient at reoperation for at least half of the patients who present with LAVVR late after repair of AV canal. For the other patients, the repair may require annuloplasty stitches, chordal shortening procedures, leaflet augmentation, or creation of a double orifice left AV valve.

Freedom from a second reoperation on the left AV valve is generally good—80% at 10 years. About 10% of patients require mitral valve replacement because of severe pathology of the left AV valve or failure of attempted repair. The incidence of complete heart block with this operation is high (25% to 40%). The operative mortality in young children also is relatively high but is less when valve replacement is performed after 1 year of age.

Subaortic Stenosis

The LVOT in patients with complete AV canal is narrowed and elongated as manifest by the so-called goose neck deformity seen angiographically. This deformity is related to the separation of the aorta and left AV valve and the deficient or "scooped out" septal crest. Subaortic stenosis is rare before repair but has an incidence of approximately 3% to 5% after repairs. This may be due to a discrete fibrous membrane, diffuse tunnel stenosis, accessory left AV valve tissue, aneurysmal AV valve tissue, asymmetric ventricular hypertrophy, and abnormal left-sided papillary muscle. It is seen more commonly after repair of "partial" AV canal or primum atrial septal defect, but also may present late after repair of complete AV canal. It seems to be more common in Rastelli type A than in Rastelli type C complete AV canal anatomy. The attachment of the superior bridging leaflet to the ventricular septal crest would seem to be a contributing factor. The technique of placement of the VSD patch also is thought to contribute to the development of subaortic stenosis. As noted earlier, there is some enthusiasm now for direct closure of small VSDs in patients with AV canal defects. When the VSD is anterior, this binds the AV valve leaflets to the deficient ventricular septum, however, and may narrow the LVOT. Providing a generous bit of VSD patch anteriorly may lessen the tendency toward subaortic stenosis.

Treatment of subaortic obstruction after repair of AV canal is challenging. If the underlying pathology is a fibrous connection between the LVOT and the left AV valve, simple resection of the tissue and septal myectomy may be performed, but the incidence of recurrence is 30% to 40%. Techniques to address the pathology directly include augmentation of the superior bridging leaflet of the left AV valve, detachment of the left AV valve with closure of the created VSD and resuspension of the left AV valve to the VSD patch, and the modified Konno procedure. The modified Konno procedure indirectly addresses the anatomic deformity by enlarging the LVOT in another direction. The risk inherent with augmentation or detachment with resuspension of left AV valve leaflet is valve regurgitation. One must realign the left AV valve tissue precisely and use patch material that neither shrinks nor stretches. This technique addresses the issue directly, however, and may provide the best anatomic solution.

■ SUMMARY

The treatment of AV canal defects represents much of what has transpired in pediatric cardiology and congenital heart surgery overall. There is a more thorough understanding of the natural history and the consequences of delayed surgery. Early surgical failures showed the need for thorough understanding of the anatomy of the defect and the conduction system.

With experience and refinement of surgical technique, operative repair of this anomaly now has a low mortality—1% to 2% in most centers—with few late deaths and overall good long-term results.

SUGGESTED READING

Bando K, et al: Surgical management of complete atrioventricular septal defects: a twenty-year experience, *J Thorac Cardiovasc Surg* 110:1543, 1995.

Chang C-I, Becker AE: Surgical anatomy of left ventricular outflow tract obstruction in complete atrioventricular septal defect: a concept for operative repair, *J Thorac Cardiovasc Surg* 94:897, 1987.

Gunther T, et al: Long-term results after repair of complete atrioventricular septal defects: analysis of risk factors, *Ann Thorac Surg* 65:754, 1998.

Rastelli GC, et al: Anatomic observations on complete form of persistent common atrioventricular canal with special reference to atrioventricular valves, *Mayo Clin Proc* 41:296, 1966.

Wilcox BR, et al: Anatomically sound, simplified approach to repair of "complete" atrioventricular septal defect, *Ann Thorac Surg* 64:487, 1997.

DOUBLE OUTLET RIGHT VENTRICLE

Piya Samankatiwat
Luca A. Vricella

Double outlet right ventricle (DORV) encompasses a spectrum of defects characterized by a wide spectrum of morphologic and pathophysiologic features. Recent advances in immunohistochemical techniques have settled some of the debate that surrounds the embryologic origin of this malformation, currently regarded as a primitive form of ventriculoarterial misconnection. As a consequence of both such extensive anatomic variability and the often associated malformations, DORV is considered by many to be one of the most challenging congenital anomalies that come to surgical attention.

■ DEFINITION AND MORPHOLOGY

DORV is a relatively uncommon congenital cardiac defect, with a reported incidence of 0.09 per 1000 live births. The anomaly is defined by the origin of both great arterial trunks (and the majority of both semilunar valves) from the morphologically right ventricle (RV). Although controversy still exists among cardiac morphologists as to some of the anatomic features observed in DORV, the definition can somewhat be simplified for surgical purposes. Most clinicians will accept the "50% rule" as definition of DORV: more than half of both great vessels arise from the ventricle associated with coarse trabeculations and a tricuspid atrioventricular valve. Another characteristic often seen in DORV is the presence of both subaortic and subpulmonary *infundibula*. A muscular

ridge supports the aortic and pulmonary valves, with absence of aortomitral continuity. This holds true in particular as the aortic valve is offset anterior to the pulmonary artery (PA), much like hearts with transposition of the great arteries.

The most used classification scheme of DORV was introduced in 1972 by Lev et al. It is based on the relationship between the interventricular communication and the great arteries (Figure 1). The ventricular septal defect (VSD) can be *subaortic* (60% to 70% of patients), *doubly committed* (located beneath both semilunar valves, 15% to 20%), *noncommitted* (remote from the great arteries, 3% to 8%), or *subpulmonic* (Taussig-Bing anomaly, 20% to 25%). A VSD is nearly always present and is restrictive in less than 10% of cases. Pulmonary stenosis (PS) is present in approximately 40% of DORV patients and can be either infundibular (more frequent) or valvular.

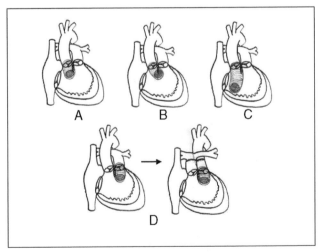

Figure 1

Anatomic variants of DORV and relative intracardiac baffle repair, based on relationship between ventricular septal defect and aortic valve. **A,** subaortic; **B,** doubly committed; **C,** noncommitted; **D,** subpulmonic/transposition-type.

■ PATHOPHYSIOLOGY AND CLINICAL PRESENTATION

The hemodynamic features and clinical implications of DORV depend on several anatomic factors: location of the interventricular communication, degree of restriction of the VSD, relationship between great arteries, and degree of right ventricular outflow tract obstruction (RVOTO). The combination of these anatomic characteristics results in varied clinical presentations, ranging from pulmonary overcirculation and congestive heart failure to cyanosis.

The pathophysiology of different forms of DORV can lead to three possible clinical scenarios, resembling nonrestrictive VSD, tetralogy of Fallot, and transposition of the great arteries. The presentation of DORV with subaortic interventricular communication resembles that of a large VSD, with high Q_p/Q_s and the development of pulmonary hypertension over time. When the VSD is doubly or noncommitted, similar pathophysiology will be observed. Should valvar or infundibular PS be associated with DORV, right-to-left shunting and varying degrees of cyanosis will be the most prominent features of the clinical presentation. In neonates and infants with the Taussig-Bing anomaly, oxygenated blood is ejected directly from the left ventricle (LV) into the PA, while systemic venous return is routed preferentially towards the ascending aorta. A transposition-type circulation with parallel circuits will result. The amount of PS and mixing will determine the degree of cyanosis in these neonates.

Median age at diagnosis of DORV is less than 2 months. The natural history of patients with uncorrected DORV is very poor and is determined primarily by the location of the VSD, the PS, and other anomalies. Growth retardation is typical of infants born with DORV and is associated with congestive heart failure and early development of pulmonary vascular obstructive disease. Severe pulmonary congestion and early vascular changes are typically accelerated in patients with large unobstructed VSD or the Taussig-Bing anomaly without PS. Complications similar to other cyanotic cardiac anomalies, such as cerebrovascular accident, clubbing, and polycythemia, may develop when DORV is associated with PS. Spontaneous closure of the restrictive VSD has been reported and is typically a lethal event. If DORV is left untreated, associated anomalies (and aortic coarctation in particular) further aggravate the already grim outlook.

■ DIAGNOSIS

The diagnosis of DORV is suggested by history, physical examination, chest radiography, and electrocardiography. Failure to thrive, tachypnea, signs of pulmonary overcirculation, or cyanosis are typical findings on physical examination. Radiographic and electrocardiographic findings are not specific. Chest radiographs will demonstrate cardiomegaly, with either plethoric or oligemic lung fields. Electrocardiography usually discloses signs of right atrial enlargement, RV hypertrophy, and right-axis deviation. Right bundle-branch block and first-degree atrioventricular block are frequently detected in the Fallot-type DORV with PS.

Transthoracic echocardiography is diagnostic (>95% accuracy) and delineates the origin of both arterial trunks from the RV, the absence of a left ventricular outflow tract (LVOT), the loss of aortomitral fibrous continuity, and bilateral subarterial *infundibula*. Location of the VSD and its size relative to the aorta are also accurately defined. Cardiac catheterization is not essential for the diagnosis of DORV; nevertheless, it is still valuable in the evaluation of infants who present late and when cardiac and coronary anatomy require further delineation.

■ TREATMENT

Several therapeutic options are available for the many morphologic variants of DORV. The most common palliative and corrective strategies are summarized in Table 1.

General Medical Supportive Measures
In neonates with DORV and duct-dependent pulmonary circulation, medical support with prostaglandin E_1 is still essential to ensure ductal patency. Medical therapy of congestive heart failure with diuretics, angiotensin-converting enzyme inhibitors, and digitalis is helpful in patients with pulmonary overcirculation.

Palliative Surgery
Although therapeutic trends have evolved toward complete intracardiac repair in the neonatal period or during early infancy, palliation for DORV remains an important option in selected cases. Palliative strategies include systemic-to-pulmonary shunts, pulmonary artery banding (PAB), and atrial septostomy or septectomy. Initial palliation may be followed by biventricular repair or by a Fontan-type staged palliation for neonates with unbalanced ventricles or severe atrioventricular valve straddling. Diagnosis and management of patients with single-ventricle physiology are discussed elsewhere in this textbook.

Systemic-to-pulmonary shunts are usually constructed as a thin polytetrafluoroethylene (PTFE) conduit between subclavian or innominate artery and the branch PA, through either a thoracotomy or a median sternotomy. This approach is indicated in deeply cyanotic newborns with DORV and critical PS in the setting of prematurity, very low birth weight, or associated malformations.

PAB is considered in patients with similar comorbidities and low birth weight in the setting of severe pulmonary overcirculation from a large unrestrictive VSD. Aortic coarctation and position of the VSD requiring a complex intracardiac conduit may also indicate banding as part of the initial procedure.

Percutaneous balloon atrial septostomy under fluoroscopic or echocardiographic guidance is performed in neonates with the Taussig-Bing anomaly, inadequate mixing, and/or a restrictive interatrial communication. An open or a closed (Blalock-Hanlon) atrial septectomy is rarely performed today.

Intracardiac Repair
In 1957, Kirklin and associates first reported successful repair of a Fallot-type DORV. The ultimate aim of complete

Table 1 Surgical Options Used in the Different Variants of Double Outlet Right Ventricle (DORV)

MORPHOLOGIC VARIANT	PALLIATIVE PROCEDURES	DEFINITIVE REPAIR
DORV with subaortic VSD		
Without RVOTO	PA banding for CHF	Intraventricular tunnel (LV to aorta)
With RVOTO	Systemic-pulmonary shunt	Intraventricular tunnel (LV to aorta) *plus*
		Infundibular resection or
		Transannular RVOT patch or
		RV-to-PA conduit
DORV with doubly committed VSD		
Without RVOTO	PA banding	Same as subaortic
With RVOTO	Systemic-to-pulmonary shunt	Same as subaortic
DORV with noncommitted VSD		
Without RVOTO	PA banding	Same as subaortic*
With RVOTO	Systemic-to-pulmonary shunt	Same as subaortic*
Unsuitable for repair	Systemic-to-pulmonary shunt or	Staged Fontan palliation
	PA banding	* Consider multiple patches and VSD
		enlargement or ASO with LV-to-PA baffle
DORV with subpulmonary VSD	PA banding (rarely performed)	"Side-by-side" great vessels:
	Balloon atrial septostomy or septectomy	Intracardiac baffle and RVOT reconstruction or REV
		ASO (LV-to-PA baffle)
		Offset great vessels (anteroposterior relationship)
		ASO (LV-to-PA baffle)
		Subaortic stenosis, nonreparable
		Damus-Kaye-Stansel reconstruction

Ao, aorta; AS, arterial switch operation; CHF, congestive heart failure; LV, left ventricle; PA, pulmonary artery; REV, reparation a l'etage ventriculaire; RVOTO, right ventricular outflow tract obstruction; VSD, ventricular septal defect.

intracardiac repair of DORV is to accomplish biventricular repair with unobstructed RVOT and LVOT. The morphologic variability of DORV derives from the different spatial relationship that may occur between great arteries, VSD and aorta, pulmonary and tricuspid valves, and the often-present RVOT obstruction; several surgical techniques are therefore used to address this variability. We will first discuss the surgical options that address the position of the VSD in relation to the great vessels (see Figure 1) and then briefly focus on the often-associated RVOTO.

The main principle of complete repair of DORV is to reroute blood flow from the LV to the aortic valve via the interventricular communication. This is now typically performed in infancy, with earlier intervention indicated by either severe symptoms or by the presence of transposition-type physiology.

DORV with Subaortic VSD
This group includes the majority of patients with DORV, and its correction is in many ways similar to that of a VSD with pronounced aortic overriding (Figure 1A). The VSD is usually nonrestrictive and becomes the future LVOT. A Dacron, pericardial, or PTFE baffle is used to create an intraventricular tunnel, which reroutes blood flow from the LV toward the aorta via the VSD. Some authors advocate the use of a Dacron conduit to take advantage of the geometric characteristics of a convex tunnel within the RV cavity. Repair can be accomplished through either a right atrial or an RV incision. A transatrial approach is favored by most surgeons to correct this anomaly. The diameter of the intraventricular baffle should be at least as large as that of the

aortic valve. Should the VSD be restrictive, it should be enlarged at the time of surgical correction; this is accomplished by excising a margin of the septum along the superoanterior aspect of the VSD, avoiding the conduction system.

DORV with Doubly Committed VSD
This uncommon type of DORV can be managed with an approach similar to that for DORV with subaortic VSD, through an infundibular incision (Figure 1B). The VSD observed in this subtype of DORV is usually large, and flow can be directed into the aorta without difficulty.

DORV with Noncommitted (Remote) VSD
This anatomic variant can be very challenging, as the feasibility and complexity of the repair largely depend on the relationship between the aortic valve and VSD (Figure 1C). The most common type of VSD encountered in this subgroup is an inlet-type defect. The conventional method of surgical repair of this variant is similar to that used for repairing the subaortic and doubly committed forms of DORV, but it can be far more complex because of the distance between VSD and the aorta and because of the difficulty in placing the conduit beneath the subvalvular tricuspid apparatus. Enlargement of the VSD anteriorly and inferiorly can improve exposure and facilitate creation of an unobstructed conduit. In these cases, a true conduit may be used rather than a baffle. As opposed to a long baffle, a conduit will limit the length of the suture line to the VSD and to the subaortic conus. On the other hand, a conduit may be more bulky and cause obstruction to PA inflow. This is particularly true if multiple patches or long conduits are used,

and often an RV-to-PA conduit is often required as a solution to this problem. Other structures at risk during correction of this subtype of DORV are the LVOT and the tricuspid valve. Exposure for conduit placement can be achieved via a combination of right atriotomy, right ventriculotomy, or through the aortic valve. Tunnelization of the VSD to the aorta carries the risk of long-term obstruction because of somatic growth of the patient relative to the LVOT size. If technically more convenient, the LV outflow can alternatively be rerouted toward the PA and followed by the arterial switch operation (ASO). When the RV cavity is small, when there is need for excessively complex rerouting, or when there are straddling atrioventricular valves or multiple VSDs, opting for single-ventricle palliation is both reasonable and safe. In this case, VSD enlargement and PAB should be considered at the time of initial intervention.

DORV with Subpulmonary VSD (Taussig-Bing Anomaly)

This is the most complex form of DORV, and the *repertoire* of surgical techniques includes several options (Figure 1D). Closure of the VSD with atrial inversion by Senning or Mustard procedures has been largely abandoned and replaced with the ASO. The latter procedure is indicated in patients with this anomaly and no evidence of subpulmonary stenosis. Should significant PS be present, an intracardiac conduit (LV to aorta) is performed in conjunction with oversewing of the proximal PA, resection of the subaortic *conus*, and creation of either an RV-to-PA conduit (Kawashima repair) or a direct anastomosis between the PA and RV (reparation a l'etage ventriculaire, or REV procedure).

The relationship between the great vessels can influence the surgical approach. If the great vessels are side by side, a classic ASO with a Lecompte maneuver (anterior translocation of the PA) may distort the left main coronary artery, resulting in myocardial ischemia. In this case, the Lecompte maneuver can be omitted altogether or, if performed, the neopulmonary arterial anastomosis can be positioned rightward along the right main PA. Alternatively, the arterial inversion strategy can be abandoned in favor of an intracardiac baffle between PA and aorta in conjunction with a Rastelli-type RV-to-PA conduit. If the great vessels relationship is offset with the aortic root anterior to the PA, performance of an ASO is more straightforward. The VSD is baffled in these cases toward the PA, with exposure achieved through the right atrium and the transected pulmonary root. Presence of a bicuspid aortic valve does not contraindicate arterial inversion.

In cases of critical subaortic stenosis not amenable to correction, a Damus-Kaye-Stansel procedure (aortopulmonary side-by-side anastomosis) is used. An ASO in this setting will result in unacceptable subpulmonary stenosis; a baffle is therefore used to direct LV outflow into the PA, which is transected and anastomosed to the ascending aorta. RV-to-PA continuity is subsequently restored with a conduit. This approach may also be considered for those neonates in whom coronary arterial anatomy precludes successful coronary button transfer.

Concomitant aortic coarctation or aortic arch hypoplasia poses an additional degree of complexity to an already difficult problem. Many, as opposed to initial palliation by means of PAB and coarctation repair, currently advocate simultaneous correction of both anomalies with circulatory arrest or selective antegrade low-flow cerebral perfusion.

■ RIGHT VENTRICULAR OUTFLOW TRACT OBSTRUCTION

RVOTO may present in several different forms of DORV or be acquired after repair if the intracardiac baffle obstructs inflow into the PA. These issues must be dealt with at the time of operative correction. In forms close to tetralogy, resection of the subpulmonary *conus*, division of parietal bands, and transannular patching will often suffice. The ventriculotomy must be carefully planned to avoid transection of anomalous coronaries or significant conal branches. Should RVOTO be associated with severe pulmonary arterial or branch stenosis, pulmonary hypertension, or anomalous coronary anatomy, a valved conduit is necessary to restore RV-to-PA continuity. Similarly, when an intracardiac baffle creates RVOT or LVOT obstruction, the RVOT is bypassed altogether. In this case, the PA is oversewn and a xenograft or homograft conduit is used to direct flow into the PA. Alternatively, the REV procedure can be used to establish RV-to-PA continuity.

■ POSTOPERATIVE MANAGEMENT

Postoperative management of neonates and infants with DORV is similar to that for patients with other forms of complex congenital heart disease. Optimally, residual defects should be identified and corrected before leaving the operating room. For this purpose, transesophageal or epicardial echocardiography is complementary to measured oxygen saturations and intraoperative shunt calculation. Direct measure of pressure gradients between RV and PA and between LV and aorta will detect RVOTO or LVOTO. Ventricular outflow tract obstruction and any residual shunt with Q_p/Q_s greater than 1.5:1 needs to be addressed immediately.

Aggressive treatment of pulmonary hypertension and RV diastolic dysfunction may be required in the early postoperative period. Among lesion-specific risks, atrioventricular conduction system injury is for obvious reasons more frequent in those cases in which complex intraventricular baffles are required for repair. Postoperative tachyarrhythmias, and junctional ectopic tachycardia in particular, can be associated with extensive infundibular resection, as typically performed for the tetralogy-type DORV.

■ RESULTS

Operative, short- and intermediate-term outcomes have greatly improved during recent years, regardless of the variability that is intrinsic to this particular pathology. In a large series of 154 patients with median follow-up of 52 months, Belli et al reported operative mortality of 9% and 10-year actuarial survival of 86%. Actuarial freedom from reintervention was 62% at the same interval, with higher incidence of reoperation observed for those patients who required

VSD enlargement as part of the initial procedure. Higher mortality has been observed in complex cases with noncommitted VSD, multiple VSDs, straddling atrioventricular valves, and unbalanced ventricles. In this particular group, single-ventricle palliation appears to outperform attempts at biventricular repair. When anatomically feasible, initial palliation does not offer survival advantage over complete neonatal repair. In particular, in patients with Taussig-Bing anomaly and aortic arch hypoplasia or interruption have better operative intermediate-term mortality and late functional class when total correction is performed early.

■ SUMMARY

DORV is characterized by variable morphology, clinical presentation, and surgical treatment. The natural history of patients with untreated DORV is poor, and complete intracardiac repair is advocated in the newborn period or early infancy. Various techniques of complete repair have been developed to achieve biventricular repair with unobstructed RVOT or LVOT. Ventricular septal defect closure techniques range in complexity from creation of a simple intracardiac baffle to ASO with concomitant aortic arch reconstruction. Despite the significant challenge posed by this heterogeneous cardiac anomaly, operative outcomes, late survival, functional class, and freedom from reintervention are now comparable to those of other less complex forms of congenital heart disease.

■ SUGGESTED READING

Anderson RH, et al: Double outlet right ventricle, *Cardiol Young* 11:329, 2001.

Lev M, et al: A concept of double-outlet right ventricle, *J Thorac Cardiovasc Surg* 64:271, 1972.

Black MD, et al: Direct neonatal ventriculo-arterial connections (REV): early results and future implications, *Ann Thorac Surg* 67:1137, 1999.

Belli E, et al: Biventricular repair for double-outlet right ventricle. Results and long-term follow-up, *Circulation* 98(Suppl II):II-360, 1998.

Kleinert S, et al: Anatomic features and surgical strategies in double-outlet right ventricle, *Circulation* 96:1233, 1997.

EBSTEIN'S ANOMALY

Renzo Pessotto
Vaughn A. Starnes

Ebstein's anomaly is a rare malformation of the tricuspid valve and right ventricle that accounts for less than 1% of all congenital heart disease. It is defined by the abnormal downward displacement of the septal and posterior leaflets of the tricuspid valve into the inlet portion of the right ventricle. The leaflets are abnormally formed and adherent to the underlying myocardium. The anterior leaflet normally is attached at the annulus but is redundant (sail-like) and in various degrees tethered to the ventricular wall, sometimes causing right ventricular outflow tract (RVOT) obstruction. The portion of the right ventricle between the true annulus and the displaced attachments of the posterior and septal leaflets is defined as the atrialized portion and presents various degrees of dilation. The right atrioventricular junction also is dilated. These anatomic and functional abnormalities cause tricuspid regurgitation with subsequent right atrial and ventricular dilation responsible for atrial and ventricular arrhythmias. In addition, 14% of the patients have accessory conduction pathways with Wolff-Parkinson-White syndrome.

■ CLINICAL PRESENTATION

The clinical presentation of Ebstein's anomaly is related strictly to the anatomic severity of the disease and the presence of associated malformations. In the most severe forms, neonatal heart failure or fetal hydrops and intrauterine death may occur. At the other end of the spectrum, patients with a mildly deformed tricuspid valve may remain asymptomatic for life.

Symptomatic neonates usually are critically ill with severe congestive heart failure, cyanosis, and metabolic acidosis. Although they require aggressive resuscitation with prostaglandin E_1, mechanical ventilation, and inotropic support, death ensues without surgical intervention. In some infants presenting with cyanosis and moderate congestive heart failure, symptoms improve early in life as pulmonary vascular resistance falls.

After the first year of life, many patients remain asymptomatic or have mild symptoms for several years. Symptomatic patients usually complain of fatigue, exertional dyspnea, and cyanosis. Episodes of paroxysmal supraventricular tachycardia occur in 25% of patients.

■ INDICATIONS FOR SURGERY

Symptomatic neonates require urgent surgical intervention after aggressive resuscitation. Patients who survive beyond early childhood usually can expect few limitations. Diagnosis alone should not be an automatic indication to proceed to surgery. For this reason, most patients in New York Heart Association (NYHA) functional class I and II can be managed medically, and there is a reasonable probability that they will have relatively normal biventricular function for many years.

The presence of progressive cyanosis, paradoxical emboli, or significant RVOT obstruction mandate earlier operation. Atrial arrhythmias related to accessory conduction pathways and the observation of progressive cardiomegaly are relative indications for operation. Surgery is indicated in all severely symptomatic patients (NYHA class III and IV) with severe tricuspid regurgitation. In borderline situations, precise definition of the tricuspid valve and right ventricular anatomy by echocardiography predicts the possibility of tricuspid valve repair and guides the indication to proceed with operation.

■ PREOPERATIVE EVALUATION

Two-dimensional and Doppler echocardiography is essential to provide the anatomic details of the malformation and measure the degree of tricuspid regurgitation. Points of interest include the size of the right atrium and tricuspid annulus, the degree of atrialization of the right ventricle, the fixation of the anterior leaflet of the tricuspid valve, and the presence of associated anomalies. Cardiac catheterization generally is not necessary in patients with Ebstein's anomaly. A preoperative electrophysiologic study is indicated in all patients with a history of recurrent supraventricular tachycardia, undefined wide-complex tachycardia, or syncope. If a reentry circuit is identified, radiofrequency ablation of the anomalous pathway is performed in the electrophysiology laboratory.

■ SURGICAL TECHNIQUES

Neonatal Repair

Treatment of symptomatic neonates with Ebstein's anomaly remains a surgical challenge. Severe congestive heart failure, marked cardiomegaly, need for mechanical ventilation, and dependence on prostaglandin E_1 are associated with a risk of 75% mortality. Two-dimensional echocardiography shows severe tricuspid regurgitation with marked right ventricular dysplasia. Various degrees of RVOT obstruction also are present. In neonates with mild RVOT obstruction from leaflet tissue rather than at the valve level, successful palliation has been obtained by conversion to univentricular physiology.

Cardiopulmonary bypass is established with aortic and bicaval cannulation. Under deep hypothermia (20°C) and continuous low-flow perfusion, the aorta is cross-clamped, and myocardial protection is achieved by direct injection in the ascending aorta of 15 ml/kg of cold blood cardioplegia. After snaring both cavae, the right atrium is entered through an oblique atriotomy. The septum primum is excised completely to create a large atrial septal defect to ensure unobstructed mixing at the atrial level. The tricuspid valve is closed using a patch of autologous pericardium secured with

continuous 6-0 polypropylene suture, leaving the ostium of the coronary sinus on the right ventricular side to minimize the risk of heart block (Figure 1). The right atrium is reduced in size by removing a portion of the right atrial free wall before closing the atriotomy. To provide pulmonary blood flow, a modified Blalock-Taussig shunt (3.5 or 4 mm in diameter) is constructed between the right innominate artery and the right pulmonary artery. In these patients, coronary sinus flow and thebesian vein flow still must be ejected from the right ventricle, and a patent RVOT is necessary.

Neonates with Ebstein's anomaly and severe pulmonary stenosis or atresia are not candidates for the aforementioned procedure. In the presence of severe RVOT obstruction, the right ventricle, distended by the venous return through the thebesian system, displaces the interventricular septum leftward, impairing left ventricular function. Heart transplantation may be the only appropriate therapy in this difficult subgroup of patients.

Repair after the Neonatal Period

After the neonatal period, the operative management of patients with Ebstein's anomaly consists of (1) reconstruction of the tricuspid valve when feasible or valve replacement; (2) plication of the atrialized portion of the right ventricle; (3) correction of associated anomalies, such as closure of atrial septal defect or relief of pulmonary stenosis; and (4) excision of redundant right atrial wall (right reduction atrioplasty).

The operation is performed through a standard median sternotomy. The ascending aorta and both venae cavae are cannulated. Under moderate hypothermia (32°C), the aorta is cross-clamped, and myocardial protection is achieved with

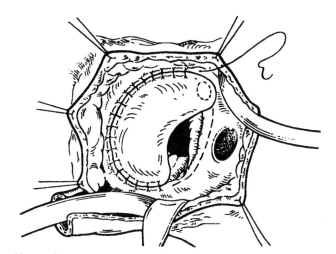

Figure 1
Conversion of neonatal Ebstein's anomaly to univentricular physiology. The right atrium is entered through an oblique atriotomy. The atrial septal defect is enlarged (*dark opening*) by resecting the septum primum. The tricuspid valve is closed using a patch of autologous pericardium secured with running 6-0 polypropylene suture. The ostium of the coronary sinus (*dotted circle*) is left on the right ventricular side to minimize the risk of heart block.

antegrade cold blood cardioplegia. Caval tourniquets are applied, and the right atrium is entered with an incision parallel to the atrioventricular groove.

When a secundum atrial septal defect or a patent foramen ovale is present, all the attenuated septum primum should be excised from the fossa ovalis, and the resulting defect should be closed using a patch of autologous pericardium treated in glutaraldehyde. Primary closure of the interatrial defect should be avoided because the high right atrial pressure may reopen the defect as a result of sutures pulling through the septal tissue. Among the various techniques proposed to reconstruct the tricuspid valve, two have been applied more extensively and have offered good results.

Danielson Technique

In 1972, Danielson developed a repair technique that consists of plicating the atrialized portion of the right ventricle, posterior tricuspid annuloplasty, and use of the anterior leaflet of the tricuspid valve to create a monocusp valve. A series of mattress pledgeted sutures is used to plicate the atrialized portion of the right ventricle. These sutures are passed through the base of the posterior and septal leaflets, then through the atrialized ventricle, and finally through the true annulus (Figure 2A and B). When these sutures are tied, the displaced leaflets come to lie at a more appropriate level relative to the rest of the tricuspid annulus (Figure 2C). The epicardial arteries are inspected after placement of each suture, and the suture is removed if an artery has been injured. A pledgeted mattress suture is used to perform a posterior annuloplasty with the purpose of completely obliterating the posterior part of the annulus (Figure 2D). Tying of this suture reduces the tricuspid annulus so that the large anterior leaflet can function as a monocusp valve. The competency of the repaired valve is tested by injecting saline into the ventricle and observing the valve for leaks.

Because this repair is based on the presence of a satisfactory anterior leaflet, significant abnormalities of the leaflet may compromise the result. In particular, the presence of a linear or hyphenated attachment of the free edge of the anterior leaflet to the right ventricular endocardium, a condition associated with absence of the papillary muscles and chordae, has been identified as a risk factor for recurrent severe tricuspid regurgitation.

Carpentier Technique

The Carpentier technique, introduced in 1980, differs from that described by Danielson in two important factors. First, a functionally bileaflet tricuspid valve is created instead of a monocusp valve. Second, the atrialized portion of the right ventricle is plicated longitudinally to restore the height of the ventricular cavity. The anterior leaflet except for its attachment at the anterior commissure and the adjacent portion of the posterior leaflet are detached as a single piece from the annulus (Figure 3A and B). Mobilization of the detached leaflets is obtained through this approach by cutting all the muscular trabeculations and cords restricting the leaflet motion. The anterior papillary muscle also is mobilized from the ventricular wall, leaving only the most distal attachments as an implant on the ventricle.

The atrialized right ventricle is longitudinally plicated with continuous 4-0 polypropylene, starting from the apex of the atrialized portion of the right ventricle to the ostium of the coronary sinus and including the attachments of the septal and posterior leaflets (Figure 3C). To avoid damage to the posterior descending coronary artery, the plicating suture has to be placed partial thickness. The anterior leaflet and the adjacent portion of the posterior leaflet are rotated clockwise to fill the circumference of the valve orifice, then are reattached to the tricuspid annulus (Figure 3D). A prosthetic annuloplasty ring can be used in adult patients to stabilize the annulus (Figure 3E).

Tricuspid Valve Replacement

Tricuspid valve replacement usually is necessary in patients with severe tricuspid regurgitation and a markedly abnormal anterior leaflet. When valve replacement is planned, the tricuspid valve leaflets are excised, and before placement of the valve sutures, deairing is completed, and the aortic clamp is removed to allow the heart to regain sinus rhythm. In this way, the rhythm can be monitored while pledgeted mattress sutures are placed around the tricuspid annulus from the ventricular to the atrial side. To avoid damage to the conduction system, the valve sutures are placed posterior (on the atrial side) to the ostium of the coronary sinus and the membranous septum. Anteriorly the valve stitches are placed directly through the tricuspid valve annulus.

A stented porcine bioprosthesis is the valve of choice. The large size of prosthesis that can be implanted and the low right ventricular pressures reduce the turbulence and stress on the bioprosthesis, allowing good long-term results. A mechanical valve also is a reasonable alternative in adult patients, especially patients with chronic atrial fibrillation requiring warfarin anticoagulation. After completion of valve repair or replacement, a portion of the wall of the right atrium is excised by an elliptical excision on each side of the oblique atriotomy. This reduction atrioplasty reduces the size of the dilated right atrium and may reduce the incidence of atrial fibrillation or flutter.

■ SURGICAL RESULTS

Neonates requiring palliative conversion to single-ventricle physiology usually have a difficult postoperative course requiring prolonged inotropic support and aggressive reduction of pulmonary vascular resistance with nitric oxide, sedation, and appropriate ventilation. Reported mortality is around 50%.

After the neonatal period, because of the known late problems with prosthetic valve replacement, current surgical efforts are directed toward valve repair rather than replacement. In the Mayo Clinic experience, valve repair was possible in almost 60% of the patients with a 7.3% mortality and a low incidence of reoperation. In the experience reported by Carpentier et al, valve repair was possible in 97% of the patients with a 10% operative mortality and 87.5% ± 7% freedom from reoperation at 14 years. Reported mortality for tricuspid valve replacement is 5.7%, and the 10-year freedom from tricuspid bioprosthesis degeneration, in patients older than age 18 years, is 94.4% ± 5.4%.

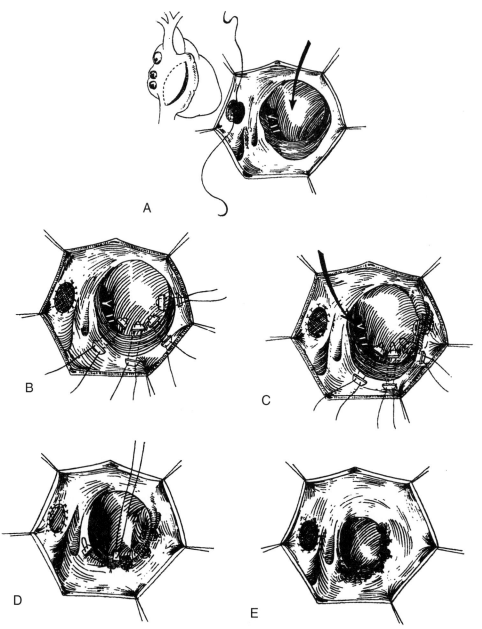

Figure 2
Repair of tricuspid valve in Ebstein's anomaly (Danielson technique). **A,** The right atrium is incised from the atrial appendage to the inferior vena cava (*left, inset*). Part of the redundant portion of the right atrium is excised (*dotted line*). Patch closure of the atrial septal defect (*right*). The large anterior leaflet of the tricuspid valve is indicated by the arrow. The posterior leaflet is displaced down from the annulus, and the septal leaflet is hypoplastic (not visible). **B,** Mattress sutures passed through pledgets of polytetrafluoroethylene (Teflon) felt are used to pull the tricuspid annulus and the valve together. Sutures are placed in the atrialized portion of the right ventricle as shown so that when they subsequently are tied, the atrialized ventricle is plicated, and the aneurysmal cavity is obliterated. **C,** Sutures are tied down sequentially. The hypoplastic, markedly displaced septal leaflet is now visible (*arrow*). **D,** The posterior annuloplasty is performed to narrow the annulus diameter. The ostium of the coronary sinus marks the posterior extent of the annuloplasty. To render the valve totally competent, one or more additional sutures may be required to obliterate the posterior aspect of the annuloplasty repair. The tricuspid valve annulus at this time admits two or more fingers in the adult. **E,** Completed repair, which allows the anterior leaflet to function as a monocusp valve.

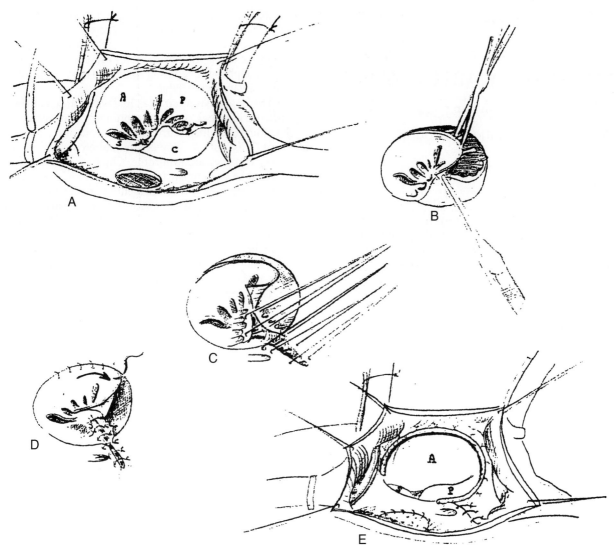

Figure 3
Repair of tricuspid valve in Ebstein's anomaly (Carpentier technique). **A,** Operative view.
B, The anterior leaflet and the adjacent portion of the posterior leaflet are detached from
the annulus. Leaflet mobilization requires cutting of the fibrous bands that connect the
leaflets to the ventricular wall. The intercordal spaces are fenestrated if obliterated. **C,** The
longitudinal plication of the right ventricle is obtained by simple sutures passed through
the remnants of the displaced septal and posterior leaflets. The tricuspid annulus and the
right atrium are plicated as well. **D,** The anterior and posterior leaflets are sutured to the
tricuspid annulus after clockwise rotation (*arrow*) to cover the entire orifice area. **E,** A prosthetic ring is inserted to remodel the orifice and to reinforce the repair. The atrial septal
defect is closed with a patch. A, anterior leaflet; C, atrialized chamber; P, posterior leaflet;
S, septal leaflet.

SUGGESTED READING

Carpentier A, et al: A new reconstructive operation for Ebstein's anomaly of
the tricuspid valve, *J Thorac Cardiovasc Surg* 96:92, 1988.

Danielson GK, et al: Operative treatment of Ebstein's anomaly, *J Thorac
Cardiovasc Surg* 104:1195, 1992.

Kiziltan HT, et al: Late results of bioprosthetic tricuspid valve replacement
in Ebstein's anomaly, *Ann Thorac Surg* 66:1539, 1998.

Starnes VA, et al: Ebstein's anomaly appearing in the neonate, *J Thorac
Cardiovasc Surg* 101:1082, 1991.

VASCULAR RINGS AND PULMONARY ARTERY SLING

Carl Lewis Backer
Constantine Mavroudis

The term *vascular ring* first was used by Gross in his report describing the first successful division of a double aortic arch in 1945. Since then, *vascular ring* has been used to refer to a collection of congenital vascular anomalies that encircle and compress the esophagus and trachea. In his original report, Gross described the two classic vascular rings: right aortic arch with left ligamentum and divided aortic arch (now called *double aortic arch*). In 1948, Gross reported successful suspension of the innominate artery to the sternum for innominate artery compression syndrome in a 4-month-old infant with wheezing and respiratory distress. In 1954, Potts and Holinger coined the term *pulmonary artery sling* when they reported the first successful repair of this anomaly in a 5-month-old infant with wheezing and intermittent attacks of dyspnea and cyanosis. Although innominate artery compression syndrome and pulmonary artery sling are not complete anatomic "rings," they are classified with the classic vascular rings because of the similarities in patient presentation, diagnosis, and surgical therapy. Tracheal stenosis secondary to complete cartilage tracheal rings occurs in 50% of patients with pulmonary artery sling—hence their inclusion with vascular rings. The most recent historic milestone in vascular ring surgery occurred in 1982 when Idriss reported the first successful use of pericardium to open the stenotic trachea of a child with complete tracheal rings.

■ EMBRYOLOGY

Vascular rings are a group of congenital anomalies caused by varying regressions and involutions from the normal embryonic aortic arch system. In the embryonic aortic arch system, the ventral and dorsal aorta are connected by six primitive aortic arches. The first, second, and fifth arches involute to form Edwards' classic double aortic arch. If the arch development arrests here, the patient has a double aortic arch. If the right fourth arch involutes, a normal left arch is formed. If the left fourth arch involutes, a right aortic arch is formed.

■ CLINICAL PRESENTATION AND DIAGNOSIS

In the 54 years between 1947 and 2001, 341 children underwent surgical repair of vascular rings, pulmonary artery sling, or complete tracheal rings at Chicago's Children's Memorial Hospital. Although there have been several different classification schemes proposed for vascular rings, we have preferred simply to call each vascular ring by its anatomic description rather than using a complex numbering or alphabetic lettering system. These diagnostic categories are shown in Table 1.

The classic symptom of a child with a vascular ring is the "seal-bark" cough. Other symptoms include stridor (noisy breathing), asthma, recurrent pneumonia, and cyanotic spells. Apnea is a common symptom in children with the innominate artery compression syndrome. Children with a pulmonary artery sling or complete tracheal rings often have severe respiratory distress requiring emergent intubation and ventilation. Dysphagia tends to occur as a symptom only in older children taking solid foods. Examinations that may lead to the correct diagnosis include chest radiograph, barium esophagogram, bronchoscopy, echocardiogram, computed tomography, magnetic resonance imaging, and angiography. The most cost-effective test is the barium esophagogram.

The chest radiograph usually can establish the location of the aortic arch—normal left, right, or indeterminate (likely a double aortic arch). The barium esophagogram is the most important and reliable technique for making the diagnosis of a vascular ring. It also is relatively inexpensive in the current era of heightened cost awareness. If the child has classic symptoms and a barium swallow that shows typical bilateral compression of the esophagus, we proceed to surgical intervention without further studies. Pulmonary artery sling is the only vascular ring that causes anterior compression of the esophagus with no posterior component. Bronchoscopic examination in a child with a vascular ring shows extrinsic (often pulsatile) "teardrop" compression of the trachea. Bronchoscopy is the diagnostic procedure of choice for infants with complete tracheal rings and innominate artery compression syndrome.

Echocardiography is useful for making the diagnosis of pulmonary artery sling, but is less useful for evaluating other vascular rings because segments without a lumen cannot be visualized. It should be used, however, to rule out a congenital heart lesion in a child with cyanotic episodes. In a child who has a classic vascular ring diagnosed by barium swallow, with no murmur or other cardiac symptoms, echocardiography is not necessary.

Computed tomography and magnetic resonance imaging are useful in that they identify the vascular structures and

Table 1 Types of Vascular Rings Undergoing Surgical Repair at Children's Memorial Hospital, 1947-2001

ANOMALY	NO. CHILDREN
Double aortic arch	105
Right aortic arch, left ligamentum	87
Right aortic arch, right ligamentum (absent LPA)	1
Innominate artery compression syndrome	84
Pulmonary artery sling	10
Complete tracheal rings	33
Ring-sling complex	21
Total	*341*

LPA, left pulmonary artery.

the tracheobronchial anatomy. In our practice, these studies chiefly have been employed if the diagnosis is not clear from the chest x-ray, barium swallow, and bronchoscopy. In patients with either a double aortic arch or a right aortic arch with a left ligamentum, there are four separate brachiocephalic vessels (instead of the normal three) in the superior mediastinum grouped around the trachea. This is called the *four vessel* sign. Angiography rarely is needed for the diagnosis of a vascular ring, but in unusual cases it can offer information not available from any other studies.

■ SURGICAL TECHNIQUE

Surgical intervention is indicated in all patients with clinical symptoms and a diagnosis of a vascular ring. Early and appropriate repair helps avoid serious complications that can occur from hypoxic or apneic episodes. Other reported complications from unrepaired vascular rings include aortic dissection, aortic aneurysm, and catastrophic bleeding from erosion of an indwelling endotracheal tube or nasogastric tube into the ring.

Double Aortic Arch

Infants with a double aortic arch typically present early in life (newborn to 6 weeks) and often have severe symptoms with the classic "barky" cough. Most patients can be diagnosed with a chest x-ray and a barium swallow. The surgical approach to a double aortic arch is through a left thoracotomy with a muscle-sparing technique. The chest is entered through the fourth intercostal space. The pleura overlying the vascular ring should be opened and careful dissection performed to identify clearly all the pertinent vascular structures. The most common form of double aortic arch is that in which the right (posterior) arch is dominant (75% of patients with a double aortic arch) (Figure 1A). The left (anterior) arch is dominant in 20% of these patients, and the arches are of equal size in 5% of patients. A portion of the smaller arch is atretic in one third of patients. This area of atresia commonly occurs where the lesser arch inserts into the descending thoracic aorta. Rare patients have been reported to have a coarctation of one or both arches.

The goal of surgical therapy is to divide the smaller of the two arches at a site that does not compromise the blood flow to the head vessels. Before dividing the arch, it should be occluded temporarily while the anesthesiologist checks right and left radial and carotid pulses. Arch division always should be done between vascular clamps by oversewing the divided stumps with polypropylene suture (Figure 1B and C). Simple ligation and division has been associated with ligature slippage and subsequent catastrophic hemorrhage. The divided stumps typically separate by 1.5 to 2 cm and often disappear into the posterior mediastinum, making precise hemostasis crucial. Thoracoscopic division of vascular rings using hemoclips has been reported in small series. There is a risk of hemorrhage, however, should a clip slip off when the vessel retracts. The operative repair is completed by freeing up all adhesive bands surrounding the esophagus in the area of the divided ring. The thoracotomy incision is closed without a chest tube by evacuating air from the

pleural space with a small suction catheter. Most children are extubated in the operating room, monitored in the hospital for 24 to 48 hours, then discharged home. It may take 1 year for the child's noisy breathing to disappear as the tracheobronchomalacia caused by the ring resolves.

Right Aortic Arch

Children with a right aortic arch and left ligamentum frequently present later in life (3 to 9 months old) because the ring is "looser," being formed partially by the low-pressure pulmonary artery and the ligamentum arteriosum. Similar to patients with a double aortic arch, most patients can be referred for surgery after a chest x-ray and barium swallow. In patients with a right aortic arch, there are two primary branching patterns: (1) retroesophageal left subclavian artery and (2) mirror image branching (Figure 2). Patients with a retroesophageal left subclavian artery have a vascular ring formed by the right arch, pulmonary artery, and ligamentum. When mirror image branching is present, the ligamentum usually arises anteriorly from the innominate artery, and a ring is not formed. Patients with a right aortic arch and left ligamentum can develop an aneurysm at the origin of the left subclavian artery. This is called a *Kommerell's diverticulum*, a remnant of the left fourth arch.

The surgical approach to a right aortic arch is via a muscle-sparing left thoracotomy through the fourth intercostal space. The vascular ring is addressed by dividing the ligamentum arteriosum. This is done using two vascular clamps and staged division after which the stumps of the ligamentum are oversewn. If there is an associated Kommerell's diverticulum, it is either resected and oversewn or (if small) fixed to the fascia of the vertebral column. This prevents compression of the trachea or esophagus from the diverticulum itself. Adhesive bands crossing the esophagus are divided. Some patients present with recurrent symptoms of Kommerell's diverticulum if it was not addressed at the first operation or subsequently enlarges. These patients respond to reoperation and diverticulum resection.

Innominate Artery Compression Syndrome

The innominate artery compression syndrome can cause stridor, cyanosis, apnea, and respiratory arrest. Frequently, apnea is associated with swallowing a bolus of food. The diagnosis of innominate artery compression syndrome is made by bronchoscopy. Because mild to moderate innominate artery compression can be found in infants who have no respiratory symptoms, we have used a criterion of 75% narrowing before considering patients for surgical intervention. Bronchoscopy shows a right anterolateral compression of the trachea that gives the lumen a classic triangular shape. Lifting the bronchoscope anteriorly against the compression causes obliteration of the right radial pulse.

We have treated innominate artery compression syndrome by suspending the innominate artery from the posterior aspect of the sternum through a small right anterolateral thoracotomy. Three separate pledgeted sutures are passed through the adventitia of the innominate artery, the ascending aorta, and the junction between the two. The sutures are tied to the posterior table of the sternum. This elevates the anterior tracheal wall and enlarges the tracheal lumen. The child is discharged the following day.

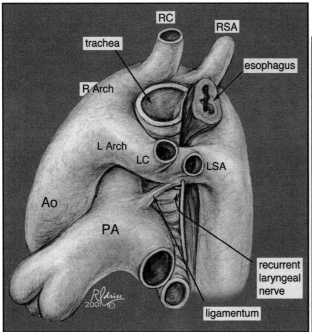

A

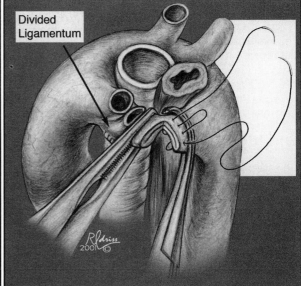

B

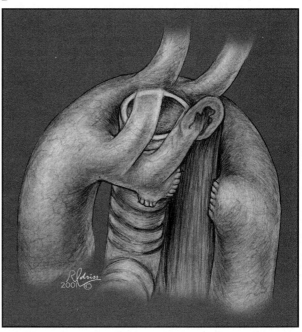

C

Figure 1
A, Double aortic arch, right arch dominant. Ao, aorta; LC, left carotid artery; RC, right carotid artery; R Arch, right arch; L Arch, left arch; PA, pulmonary artery; LSA, left subclavian artery; RSA, right subclavian artery. **B,** Dividing left aortic arch between two vascular clamps. Polypropylene suture is used to close the divided arches. **C,** Left arch divided; trachea and esophagus now are free.

Pulmonary Artery Sling

A pulmonary artery sling is formed when the left pulmonary artery originates from the right pulmonary artery and encircles the distal trachea, coursing between the trachea and esophagus to reach the hilum of the left lung (Figure 3A). The left pulmonary artery acts as a "sling" that applies pressure on the right main bronchus and right lower trachea. This anomaly first was reported in 1897 as an autopsy finding in a 7-month-old infant who died of severe respiratory distress. Bronchoscopy is performed in all infants diagnosed to have pulmonary artery sling to rule out associated

congenital tracheal stenosis with complete tracheal rings. In our experience, 50% of patients with pulmonary artery sling also have complete tracheal rings. This has been referred to as the *ring-sling complex.*

Surgical repair of pulmonary artery sling is undertaken urgently as soon as the diagnosis is made because of the usual tenuous nature of the respiratory status of the child. The mean age at the time of surgery in our series is 4 months. Pulmonary artery sling is repaired with a median sternotomy approach and the use of cardiopulmonary bypass. The left pulmonary artery is transected at its origin

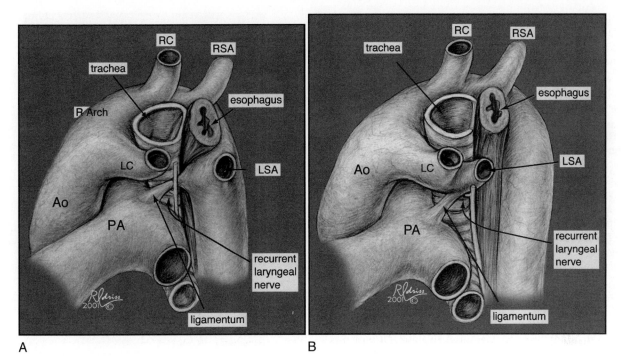

A   B

Figure 2
A, Right aortic arch, retroesophageal left subclavian artery, a vascular ring is formed. Ao, aorta; LC, left carotid artery; RC, right carotid artery; R Arch, right arch; L Arch, left arch; PA, pulmonary artery; LSA, left subclavian artery; RSA, right subclavian artery. **B,** Right aortic arch, mirror image branching, no vascular ring.

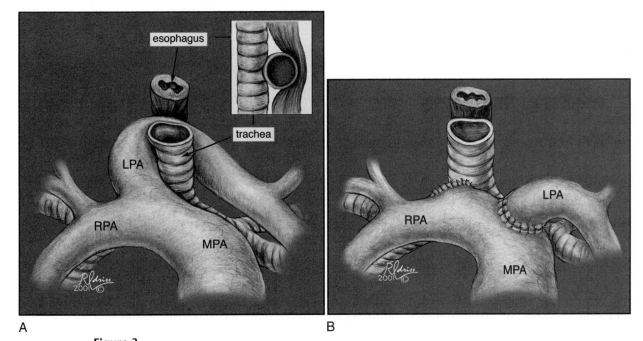

A   B

Figure 3
A, Pulmonary artery sling. RPA, right pulmonary artery; LPA, left pulmonary artery; MPA, main pulmonary artery. Inset shows anterior compression of esophagus. **B,** Repaired pulmonary artery sling. Left pulmonary artery has been anastomosed to main pulmonary artery anterior to trachea.

from the right pulmonary artery and is passed through the mediastinum posterior to the trachea. The left pulmonary artery is anastomosed to the main pulmonary artery anterior to the trachea (Figure 3B). In our series, the patency of the left pulmonary artery using a median sternotomy and cardiopulmonary bypass is 100%, with the mean blood flow to the left lung by nuclear scan being 35%.

Complete Tracheal Rings

Complete cartilage tracheal rings occur when there is congenital absence of the posterior membranous trachea. This causes tracheal stenosis that often leads to respiratory distress in infancy. Medical management of this lesion is associated with a 40% mortality rate. Many patients are referred when even the smallest endotracheal tube cannot be passed far below the vocal cords because of the stenosis. The diagnosis is confirmed by rigid bronchoscopy. In many patients, the bronchoscope itself cannot be passed, only the fine telescope. In patients diagnosed with complete tracheal rings, pulmonary artery sling is present in 35% of the patients and intracardiac defects in 22%; these anomalies should be ruled out with echocardiography.

A total of 54 patients have undergone repair of complete tracheal rings at Children's Memorial Hospital. Of patients, 28 have had pericardial tracheoplasty, 9 have had resection with end-to-end anastomosis, 2 have had slide tracheoplasty, and 15 have had a new technique developed at Children's Memorial Hospital—a free tracheal autograft. Other surgeons have reported good results with rib cartilage graft for the tracheal repair. Jacobs reported the successful application of cryopreserved tracheal homograft for infants with recurrent tracheal stenosis after repair of complete tracheal rings and pulmonary artery sling.

The pericardial patch tracheoplasty is performed through a median sternotomy with the use of cardiopulmonary bypass for respiratory support. The trachea is opened anteriorly the entire extent of the stenosis, then patched open with autologous pericardium (Figure 4). The patch is stented with an endotracheal tube for 10 to 14 days, at which time the child is extubated. Bronchoscopy is performed before extubation to remove secretions and granulation tissue and to perform dilation if necessary. Despite the low operative mortality of pericardial tracheoplasty, many patients had prolonged hospitalizations secondary to granulation tissue and scar tissue, and 6 of 28 patients required reoperation and surgical revision. Four patients required placement of balloon expandable metallic stents for collapsing tracheal or bronchial segments.

In an effort to improve the outcome of these patients, we developed the tracheal autograft technique. Using a median sternotomy and cardiopulmonary bypass, the trachea is incised anteriorly throughout the length of the stenosis. Approximately six to eight tracheal rings or 15 to 20 mm of trachea is harvested from the midportion of the trachea (Figure 5A). The trachea is reanastomosed posteriorly, and the autograft is used as an anterior patch (Figure 5B). In children with a shorter segment of tracheal stenosis, the autograft completes the patch. In patients with a longer stenosis, the autograft has been augmented superiorly with pericardium. This technique has been performed in 15 patients with one early and one late death. Of the nine patients who had a tracheal resection, there was one late death (awaiting liver transplant). Of the two patients who

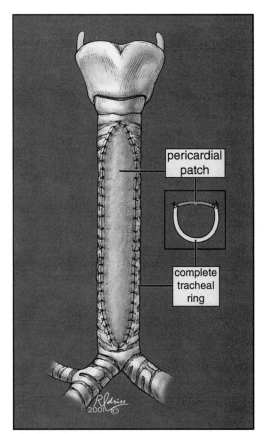

Figure 4
Pericardial patch tracheoplasty.

had a slide tracheoplasty, there was one late death from aortic valve endocarditis.

■ RESULTS AND CONCLUSIONS

There has been no operative mortality from an isolated vascular ring or pulmonary artery sling at Children's Memorial Hospital since 1959. The survival rate of infants with complete tracheal rings using the autograft technique is 87%. Of infants who undergo vascular ring repair, 92% are free of respiratory symptoms 1 year postoperatively.

Vascular rings are rare congenital anomalies that cause compression of the trachea and esophagus. Infants present with stridor, barky cough, respiratory distress, cyanosis, and apnea. Diagnosis is established best by barium esophagogram for double aortic arch and right aortic arch with left ligamentum. Bronchoscopy is used to diagnose innominate artery compression syndrome and complete tracheal rings. Echocardiogram is the diagnostic procedure of choice for pulmonary artery sling.

The surgical approaches to vascular rings include a left thoracotomy for double aortic arch and right aortic arch with ligamentum, right thoracotomy for innominate artery suspension, and median sternotomy with cardiopulmonary bypass for pulmonary artery sling and complete tracheal rings. Close cooperation between the cardiothoracic and otolaryngologic surgeons is essential to provide the optimal care for these children.

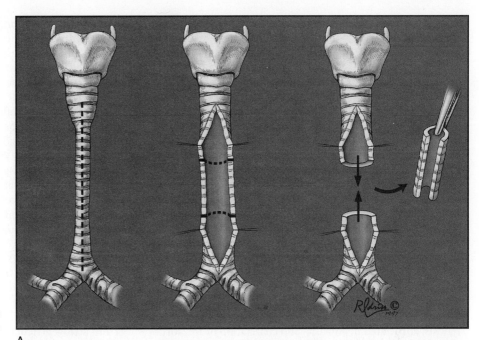

A

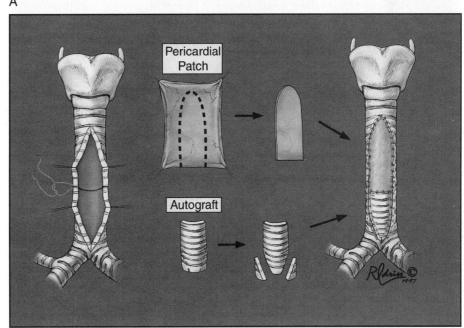

B

Figure 5
A, Tracheal autograft procedure. The trachea has been opened anteriorly and the autograft resected. **B**, The trachea is reanastomosed posteriorly, and the autograft is used as an anterior patch. A pericardial patch augments the repair superi-

SUGGESTED READING

Backer CL, et al: Vascular anomalies causing tracheoesophageal compression: review of experience in children, *J Thorac Cardiovasc Surg* 97:725, 1989.

Backer CL, et al: Repair of congenital tracheal stenosis with a free tracheal autograft, *J Thorac Cardiovasc Surg* 115:869, 1998.

Backer CL, et al: Pulmonary artery sling: results with median sternotomy, cardiopulmonary bypass, and reimplantation, *Ann Thorac Surg* 67:1738, 1999.

Gross RE: Surgical relief for tracheal obstruction from a vascular ring, *N Engl J Med* 233:586, 1945.

Potts WJ, et al: Anomalous left pulmonary artery causing obstruction to right main bronchus: report of a case, *JAMA* 155:1409, 1954.

PEDIATRIC MITRAL VALVE DISEASE

Jan Quaegebeur

Congenital malformations of the mitral valve are developmental lesions involving one and commonly multiple different components of the mitral valve apparatus. These lesions result in stenosis, incompetence, or sometimes both. Congenital mitral valve disease is rare and notoriously difficult to treat surgically, especially when this is necessary in small children. Often there are coexisting cardiac anomalies, particularly other elements of the left-sided cardiac structures, such as small or hypoplastic left ventricle, valvar or subaortic stenosis, aortic arch hypoplasia, and coarctation of the aorta (Shone's complex). Mitral valve anomalies may also be part of more complex malformations, such as univentricular heart, transposition of the great arteries, double outlet right ventricle, atrioventricular discordance, straddling atrioventricular valves, and, rarely, tetralogy of Fallot. Mitral incompetence may be associated with myxomatous degeneration (Marfan syndrome), cardiomyopathy, and anomalous left coronary artery. The mitral valve in the setting of atrioventricular septal defects is an entity in itself. This discussion here is limited to the congenital lesions of the mitral valve itself and do not extend to the difficult decision-making process in children with left ventricular hypoplasia and other complex associations.

■ CONGENITAL MITRAL VALVE LESIONS CAUSING OBSTRUCTION

Pure mitral stenosis is rare (0.6% of autopsy series) and may involve any component of the mitral valve, but usually the entire valve apparatus is affected.

Supravalvar Mitral Ring
A more or less circumferential ring is intimately attached to the left atrial side of the leaflets and may extend across the annulus. It can be very subtle and often best recognized by echocardiography. Rarely, a supravalvar ring is found at a distance from the mitral valve leaflets. It causes restriction of leaflet motion, particularly when the fibrous tissue covers the commissures. It can be isolated or associated with other mitral valve anomalies or left ventricular outflow tract obstruction.

Surgical treatment consists of finding a dissecting plane between the ring and the leaflets and then "peeling" it off the leaflets by blunt dissection, especially from the commissural areas. Once the ring is completely removed, the rest of the mitral valve must be inspected as well.

Mitral Annulus and Leaflets
Annular hypoplasia is almost always a coincident part of ventricular hypoplasia. Aortic coarctation can be associated

with a small mitral annulus. Surgical treatment of hypoplastic mitral annulus by itself has not been reported. Congenital absence of one or both commissures as an isolated lesion is rare and usually coexists with the presence of thickened chordae and papillary muscles. Fused commissures can be opened using a No. 11 blade. The line of incision can be found by gently pulling the leaflets in the opposite direction of the commissure. In small children, a commissurotomy of a few millimeters on both sides can result in a significant increase in effective valve area. Very often, thick chordae and papillary muscles must be incised as well to optimize leaflet motion. A double orifice mitral valve is formed by the presence of a band of leaflet tissue connecting the two leaflets. This cannot be resected without causing incompetence. Instead, opening one or both commissures should be attempted.

Chordae and Papillary Muscles
Embryologically, the mitral valve is formed from the inner layers of the myocardium of the left ventricular inlet portion. A process of "undermining" the myocardium results in the formation of papillary muscles, whereas the invagination of the atrioventricular sulcus provides the necessary tissue for the fibrous parts of the valve. Disruption of this myocardial maturation may lead to a group of mitral valve defects involving its tensor apparatus. These malformations are mostly stenotic and are characterized by the presence of thick and short chordae, absent chordae, and direct insertion of bulky papillary muscles directly on the valve leaflets and commissures, absent interchordal space, and decreased (or absent) interpapillary space. The location of these papillary muscles becomes more posterior, and sometimes they fuse with each other. This results in restricted motion of the valve leaflets during ventricular diastole. The mitral valve presents a typical "funnel shape," best seen on echocardiography, with the central opening being much smaller than the annulus size.

All of these defects share the same morphogenesis, but different names have been used to describe their specific pathology, from double orifice mitral valve, parachute mitral valve, hammock valve, or mitral arcade, to congenital stenosis with hypertrophied papillary muscles, and so on.

Surgical repair of these types of malformation is notoriously difficult. The aim is to improve diastolic leaflet opening by creating more interchordal space and interpapillary distance. These techniques include resection of secondary chordae, chordal fenestration, papillary muscle splitting, and resection of muscular attachments, often associated with commissurotomy. Even if the results of these maneuvers are suboptimal, the improvement in valve opening, especially in infants, may be significant and postpone valve replacement for several years.

■ CONGENITAL MITRAL VALVE LESIONS CAUSING INCOMPETENCE

Mitral valve incompetence may be associated with any of the obstructive lesions described previously.

Annular Dilation
Primary isolated annular dilation is very rare and involves mostly the posterior leaflet or a commissural area. In these

cases, the dilation is eccentric. Usually annular dilation is secondary to left ventricular dilation caused by cardiomyopathy, anomalous left coronary artery, or coronary fistula. It has been described with atrial and ventricular septal defects.

Different forms of annuloplasty have been described and are usually effective both in short- and long-term follow-up. The annuloplasty is centered around the area of maximum dilation (usually posterior). Interrupted, pericardium pledgeted mattress sutures, placed at the desired location, are very effective. If the commissures are involved, eccentric commissuroplasty (Wooler type) has provided excellent results. The use of fixed annuloplasty rings should be avoided because they impede annular growth.

Deficient Leaflet Tissue

Abnormal fenestration or localized agenesis of leaflet tissue may be encountered. Especially in the posterior leaflet, a sliding plasty supported by a localized annuloplasty is often possible.

Leaflet Prolapse

This is usually caused by chordal and/or papillary muscle elongation. Chordal elongation involves one or more chordae attached to one papillary muscle. It is seen in Barlow's syndrome and Marfan's syndrome. Chordal shortening, as described by Carpentier, is usually effective. Chordal transfer from the posterior to the anterior leaflet may occasionally be used, especially in older children.

Absence of chordae along a portion of the free edge of the leaflet is treated by resection of that portion and primary reconstruction. Papillary muscle elongation is usually secondary to myocardial ischemia (severe aortic stenosis, anomalous origin of left coronary artery). The papillary muscle is thin and fibrotic and can be shortened by burying its base within a trench made in the ventricular wall. A variety of these techniques have been described by Carpentier.

Cleft Leaflets

The best-known cleft in the anterior leaflet is associated with atrioventricular septal defects. It is usually located in the middle of the leaflet and is oriented toward the middle of the inlet septum. Of different embryologic origin is the isolated cleft in the anterior leaflet, which is usually eccentric and points toward the aortic valve. Rarely, clefts are observed in the posterior leaflet.

Clefts may or may not be incompetent (especially in atrioventricular septal defects). Incompetence usually results from absence of supporting chordae on the free rim of the cleft. In older children, that rim may be fibrotic and thickened secondary to a long-standing jet. Closing the unsupported area of the cleft, in association with an annuloplasty, offers excellent results. It is better to create an apposition zone by placing the sutures at a slight distance from the free edge, rather than simply closing the free edges of the cleft themselves. Closing the entire cleft (including the zone supported by chordae) may result in mitral stenosis.

■ MITRAL VALVE REPAIR VERSUS REPLACEMENT

For obvious reasons, it is preferable in children to repair the mitral valve rather than replace it. However, in some cases valve replacement might be the only option to obtain a satisfactory hemodynamic result. Between 1990 and 2000, 74 children with primary mitral valve lesions were operated on in our center. Obstructive lesions were encountered in 41 patients (55%). Repair was possible in 36 patients, and 5 needed valve replacement (12%). Shone's syndrome was found in 41.5%. Half of the patients were infants. Primary mitral incompetence was seen in 33 patients, of whom only 2 (6%) required valve replacement. The children were usually older, and only 2 had Shone's syndrome. Three infants (7%) with mitral stenosis died; all were younger than 3 months.

During the same period of time, 33 patients underwent mitral valve replacement with a hospital mortality rate of 6% (both infants). All patients received a bileaflet mechanical valve and were anticoagulated with warfarin. There was one late death. In small patients (nine were <2 years old), the 16- or 18-mm CarboMedics valve (Austin, TX) was the prosthesis of choice.

Of 67 patients who underwent successful mitral valve repair, 8 (12%) required subsequent valve replacement. Their initial disease was usually mitral stenosis. Additional procedures that were necessary during mitral valve replacement included aortic valve or root replacement, Rastelli procedure, Glenn shunt, arterial switch, and tetralogy repair.

■ SUMMARY

Although this section focuses on the mitral valve anomalies themselves, it is clear that congenital mitral valve disease is complex and often associated with other cardiac abnormalities. With this in mind, approximately 80% of these patients undergo successful mitral valve repair. Valve repair should always be attempted, but if it fails, valve replacement offers an acceptable solution and should be performed before significant cardiac failure or hypertension occurs. The use of a small prosthesis can be lifesaving in infants and small children. Furthermore, when children outgrow their prostheses, sometimes up to 10 years later, a significantly larger valve can always be implanted.

SUGGESTED READING

Carpentier A: Congenital malformations of the mitral valve. In Stark J, de Leval M, editors: *Surgery for congenital heart defects*, ed 2. Philadelphia, 1996, WB Saunders, p 588.

Embray RP, Behrendt D: Congenital abnormalities of the mitral valve. In Baue AE, et al, editors: *Glenn's Thoracic and cardiovascular surgery*, ed 6. Appleton and Lange, 1996, p 1463.

Wenink AC, et al: Developmental considerations of mitral valve anomalies, *Int J Cardiol* 11:85, 1986.

PEDIATRIC CARDIAC TRANSPLANTATION

Harry Zemon

David D. Yuh

■ HISTORY

Cardiac transplantation has become the procedure of choice for children with end-stage congenital and acquired heart disease. In 1968, Kantrowitz attempted the first heart transplantation in an infant; however, it was not until 1984 that Yacoub et al performed the first successful pediatric heart transplant. The field of pediatric heart transplantation has since made tremendous strides. Long-term survival is now comparable to that of adult heart transplantation, and 4500 pediatric heart transplantations have been performed worldwide since 1982.

■ INDICATIONS AND CONTRAINDICATIONS

Cardiac transplantation is now considered the most effective therapy for end-stage heart disease and is the procedure of choice for managing both acquired cardiomyopathy and congenital heart disease. The most common indications for heart transplantation differ among the pediatric age groups (Table 1). Congenital heart disease is the most common indication for heart transplantation in the neonatal and infant age group (<1 year) comprising 75% of the heart transplants performed in that age group. In contrast, congenital heart disease represents only 25% in the 11- to 17-year-old age

Table 1 Indications and Survival for Pediatric Cardiac Transplantation Based on Ages

	<1 YEAR OLD	1 TO 10 YEARS OLD	11 TO 17 YEARS OLD
Indication			
Congenital	76%	37%	25%
Myopathy	20%	53%	66%
Other	3%	5%	6%
Retransplant	1%	5%	3%
Survival			
30-Day	87%	90%	91%
1-Year	80%	85%	88%
3-Years	74%	78%	80%
5-Years	63%	70%	67%

Adapted from the International Society of Heart and Lung Transplantation Registry and United Network of Organ Sharing Registry 2001.

group, which is similar to the adult heart transplantation population. Children aged 1 to 10 years and 11 to 17 years who have various types of cardiomyopathy represent the majority of pediatric cardiac transplant recipients (53% and 66%, respectively). Symptomatic congestive heart failure, recurrent uncontrolled arrhythmia and limitation of activity in conjunction with cardiac disease are indications for transplantation.

An estimated 2500 to 3000 infants are born each year in the United States with congenital heart disease not amenable to palliative surgical repair. Hypoplastic left heart syndrome is the most common diagnosis in these patients. Transplantation offers greater survival over palliative repair of this congenital defect.

The major contraindication to transplantation is fixed pulmonary hypertension greater than 8 Wood units, unresponsive to pulmonary vasodilators. High pulmonary vascular resistance is a risk factor for right ventricular failure and early death after heart transplantation. Other relative contraindications include active, untreated malignancy, multisystem organ failure, and multiple congenital anomalies. In addition, socioeconomic factors that could lead to noncompliance with drug regimens and postoperative follow-up should also be considered relative contraindications.

■ TIMING

Often, the greatest challenge facing cardiac transplant surgeons is the timing of transplantation. Surgeons must weigh the likelihood of successful outcome for each patient in the context of maximizing pediatric organ utilization. Timing also plays an essential role in the long-term success of the patient. Perioperative mortality and morbidity are reduced when transplantation is performed before circulatory collapse and multisystem organ failure develop. A poor prognosis is associated with an elevated left ventricular end-diastolic pressure greater than 25 mm Hg, poor ejection fraction, and a family history of cardiomyopathy; therefore, these factors should be taken into consideration prior to transplantation. Ultimately, the decision to proceed with transplantation is multifactorial and resides with the transplant center, surgeon, patient, and family.

Pediatric and particularly neonatal heart transplantation is extremely limited by the supply of available hearts. Mortality while on the waiting list is reported as 12% to 39%. As the popularity and expanded indications of heart transplantation increase, recipient waiting times and resulting morbidity have increased. A strategy to sustain severely ill children while waiting for a suitable donor is essential. Options for mechanical support in the neonatal heart are limited, with historically poor outcomes using univentricular assist devices. However, extracorporeal membrane oxygenation (ECMO) has become a useful modality as a bridge to transplantation in infants when an organ becomes available within a relatively short time period. Several studies show survival rates ranging from 45% to 73% for using ECMO as a bridge to cardiac transplantation. Conversely, intermediate-sized children and adolescents have excellent survival using long-term ventricular assist devices (VADs) as a bridge to transplantation. Both ECMO and VADs have successfully reduced overall mortality during the waiting list period without negatively affecting the outcome of cardiac transplantation. Early listing for transplantation allows a greater window for the surgeon and patient to optimize the timing of transplantation. Placing patients on the transplant list carries little disadvantage to the potential recipient as the critical decision comes only when a donor is available. In addition, early listing has been associated with a decrease in morbidity while awaiting transplantation.

■ TECHNIQUE

The standard biatrial technique for cardiac transplantation developed by Lower and Shumway in 1967 has stood the test of time (Figure 1A). However, the bicaval modification of this operation is currently the most common technique for orthotopic heart transplantation. In a worldwide survey, it was found that more than half of the existing cardiac transplant centers predominately use the bicaval technique, whereas only 22% predominately use the standard biatrial technique. The standard technique creates oversized atria whereby the recipient's atrial cuff is anastomosed to the donor's atria. The standard biatrial technique is favored by some centers in cases of dilated cardiomyopathy because the large pericardial sac accommodates the extra atrial tissue. However, subsequent distortion of the right atrial geometry may lead to atrioventricular valvular insufficiency, arrhythmias, and bradycardia. The bicaval technique preserves the atrial morphology (Figure 1B) by completely excluding the native right atria and anastomosing the intact donor right atria via the superior and inferior vena cava. The left atrial

cuff of the recipient incorporating the native pulmonary veins is anastomosed to the left atrial cuff of the donor heart. Children with prior cardiac surgery who receive oversized donor hearts often cannot accommodate extraatrial tissue and are more suitable for the bicaval technique. The complete atrioventricular technique or "total anastomotic" technique was developed to keep both the right and the left atria intact with separate anastomoses to the cavae and pulmonary veins (Figure 1C). This technique was introduced by the Harefield and Carpentier groups in 1989. Potential complications from this modification include bleeding from inaccessible suture lines in the posterior pericardial space; reduced patency of the pulmonary veins caused by twisting or narrowing of the graft; and size discrepancies that lead to difficult pulmonary venous anastomoses. Benefits of both modified techniques compared with the standard biatrial technique have been reported in several studies.

Heterotopic transplantation can be a useful option for infants and children with elevated pulmonary vascular resistance or who can only receive an undersized donor heart. The donor heart acts as an accessory pump and is attached to and assists the recipient's left-sided heart. A possible benefit of this procedure is that it allows recovery of the recipient's native heart function. Disadvantages of this method include pulmonary dysfunction from compression by the heterotopic donor heart; emboli from thrombus in a weakly contracting native heart; continued angina from ischemic heart muscle; and ongoing deterioration of the recipient's native heart. Operative mortality is high, and the 5-year survival of heterotopic transplantation is approximately 71%.

Improvement in donor organ preservation techniques has prolonged acceptable ischemic times and facilitates

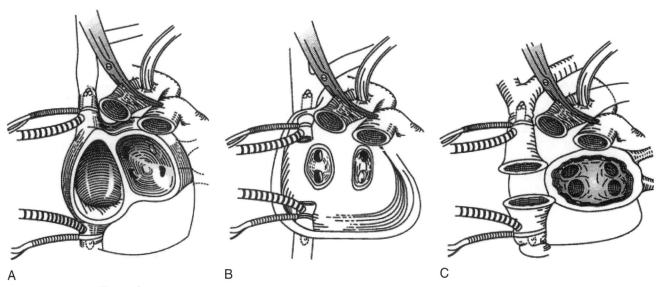

A   B   C

Figure 1
Preparation of the recipient's mediastinum prior to heart transplantation. The main differences in the methods of recipient heart explantation are displayed. **(A)** Standard: the main bulk of right and left atria are preserved. **(B)** Total: left and right pulmonary veins cuffs are prepared for total atrioventricular transplantation. **(C)** Bicaval: the donor left atrium is anastomosed to small recipient's left atrial cuff, which includes the pulmonary veins. (*Reprinted with permission from Wythenshawe Hospital Cardiac Transplant Unit.*)

better allocation to recipients in greatest need. In 1998, an International Society for Heart and Lung Transplantation (ISHLT) study reported a correlation between prolonged ischemic times and first-year mortality for orthotopic heart transplants, especially when ischemic times were greater than 6 hours. In response, transplant centers have set standardized maximum ischemic times of approximately 4 hours. Recently, the use of cardioplegia solution during transport and portable hypothermic perfusion systems have increased acceptable ischemic times to 8 to 16 hours with good results. Currently, U.S. and European centers accept ischemic times between 5 and 6 hours and 20% of transplant centers accept donor hearts with ischemic times of up to 7 hours.

■ RESULTS

Five-year survival for the 11- to 17-year-old age group compares favorably to the adult population, whereas the <1-year-old age group has the poorest survival (see Table 1). The infant age group has a high mortality rate from early graft failure in the first month posttransplant. Interestingly, ongoing mortality for infants who survive past the first month posttransplant is similar to the older children and adult age group. Strategies for improving early donor heart function for the infant age group are currently under investigation.

Donor-recipient matching for age and size has significant impact on 5-year survival. A donor heart relatively larger than the recipient is associated with improved outcomes. Recently, a UNOS allocation algorithm was revised to allocate adolescent donor hearts to adolescent recipients before being offered to an adult. This change was mandated due to a higher incidence of transplant coronary artery disease (TCAD) when the donor is of advanced age. In addition to TCAD, statistically significant differences in survival exist between children who receive advanced aged donors' hearts and those who receive hearts from age-appropriate donors. As such, advanced age donors' hearts are not placed into pediatric patients except for the critically ill who are unable to wait for a suitably aged heart.

The majority of long-term survivors enjoy the achievement of normal developmental milestones, normal growth, and integration into mainstream society. Most children exhibit "catch up" growth following transplantation; however, various studies differ as to whether patients attain target heights. Growth parameters at the time of transplant and cardiac pathology are a major determinant of final achieved height.

■ COMPLICATIONS

Rejection and infection are the most common complications associated with heart transplantation. Other problems that develop include hypertension, seizures, renal dysfunction, hematologic abnormalities, and hepatic dysfunction. Reduction in renal function is common and associated with immunosuppression drugs; however, dialysis dependence is rare. Late complications such as chronic rejection, transplant coronary artery disease, and posttransplant lymphoproliferative disease (PTLD) ultimately lead to graft failure and death. Ventricular dysfunction, infection, TCAD, graft failure, and rejection are the leading causes of death among cardiac transplant recipients.

Transplant Coronary Artery Disease

TCAD is emerging as a significant problem and contributes to a large percentage of late morbidity and mortality in pediatric cardiac transplantation. Early estimates of TCAD prevalence range between 10% to 15%. Introduction of intracoronary ultrasound as an adjunct screening modality for TCAD suggests a prevalence of 74%. A very strong correlation between TCAD and rejection has emerged, and TCAD is sometimes considered synonymous with chronic rejection. Children with multiple rejection episodes should be approached with a high index of suspicion for TCAD. Upward adjustments in immunosuppression and salvage therapy are recommended on initial diagnosis of TCAD. Retransplantation is currently the only primary therapy for TCAD. Listing for retransplantation is highly recommended on making the diagnosis of severe coronary artery disease, as early cardiac events are imminent. Medical therapy for TCAD is under investigation with preliminary survival results exceeding retransplantation survival. However, long-term graft durability with medical therapy needs further investigation.

Posttransplant Lymphoproliferative Disease

Current data show a strong relationship between PTLD and EBV. In addition, higher prevalence of EBV in children correlates with the higher incidence of PTLD, especially when compared with adults. The incidence is reported to be 10%, and mortality is reported to be 60% to 70%. Levels of immunosuppression are an important risk factor for the development of PTLD and therefore the incidence varies widely between the different pediatric transplant groups. Reduction in immunosuppressants, acyclovir, and chemotherapy are the current treatments for PTLD.

Rejection

Despite improvements in immunosuppressive therapy, rejection is the most common cause of death among transplant recipients accounting for a 29% overall mortality and 25% of the deaths during the first year posttransplant. Acute rejection leads to graft dysfunction, heart failure, and death. Twenty-five percent of pediatric transplant recipients will experience recurrent episodes of acute rejection or refractory acute rejection. The incidence of acute rejection in pediatric recipients is higher than that in the adult population and likely related to the wide age range and varied doses and responses to immunosuppressive therapy. Rejection in the first year is a predictor for subsequent complications and late mortality. A 25% reduction in QRS voltages, irritability, and morphologic changes on echocardiogram are warning signs for rejection and should be investigated thoroughly. Interestingly, the incidence of rejection in the infant population is much lower, probably due in part to a relatively naïve immune system.

Rejection with hemodynamic compromise is a serious complication that occurs in approximately 11% of the pediatric heart recipients compared with 5% in the adult.

Associated mortality is extremely high at 40%. Risk factors associated with this type of rejection are non-white race and older recipient age, with 10 to 18 year olds twice as likely to experience hemodynamic compromise compared with infants. Close surveillance and aggressive treatment may aid in reducing mortality.

Endomyocardial biopsy is considered the gold standard for rejection surveillance and considered safe for pediatric heart recipients of all ages. Close surveillance permits early diagnosis and treatment. Advocates of endomyocardial biopsy recommend surveillance biopsies during the first 5 years with additional biopsies after changes in immunosuppression or after acute rejection episodes.

Immune Suppression

Choices of immunosuppressive drug regimens take on greater significance in terms of side effects to a growing child. Triple-drug therapy with cyclosporine or tacrolimus, azathioprine, and steroids are the primary immunosuppressive agents used in cardiac transplantation. Corticosteroids are associated with long-term morbidity and as such are used primarily for induction and then tapered quickly.

The wide age range of pediatric transplant recipients parallels the wide range of responses to immunosuppressive therapy, making selection of a proper combination difficult. Those patients receiving induction therapy with cytolytic agents may experience graft rejection because of milder immunosuppressive regimens compared with adults. Long-term steroid use is associated with a myriad of complications including growth retardation, hypertension, hyperlipidemia, peptic ulcer disease, osteoporosis, and obesity. Several studies support the use of tacrolimus in the pediatric population as a primary immunosuppression agent and in conversion therapy for episodes of acute rejection. However, recent studies do not show a survival advantage over cyclosporine. As with any immunosuppressive agent, lower doses lead to subtherapeutic levels and acute rejection, whereas higher doses are associated with renal and neurologic toxicity. Early acute rejection and toxicity may be avoided by frequent monitoring of serum drug levels. Induction therapy in the pediatric population is not well studied; however, some preliminary results show efficacy in reducing late mortality in the less than 6-month-old infant population.

Retransplantation

Indications for retransplantation include irreversible rejection, graft vasculopathy, and primary organ failure. Roughly 4% of all pediatric heart transplants are performed for retransplantation. The merits of retransplantation are often in question, given the limitation of available donors and historically poor survival. Again, the surgeon must weigh timing and the probability of success in the decision to allocate a second heart to one patient. Nevertheless, early and intermediate-term survival results for the pediatric population are now comparable to primary transplantation. Therefore, elective retransplantation is considered a viable therapeutic option.

■ FUTURE DIRECTION

The future holds great promise for continued success and advancements in pediatric heart transplant surgery. The prospects for organ-specific immune tolerance will likely drive organ transplantation into a new era. Xenotransplantation offers the potential of an unlimited organ supply and is currently being investigated. In the interim, pediatric cardiac transplantation is faced with a paucity of donors and charged with developing strategies to maximize allocation of this limited resource. Despite the challenges and obstacles ahead, pediatric heart transplant continues to provide excellent outcomes with improved quality of life and is an effective and long-lasting therapy for the pediatric population.

SUGGESTED READING

Fricker FJ, et al: Heart transplantation in children: indications, *Pediatr Transplant* 3:333, 1999.

Hosenpud JD, et al: The Registry of the International Society for Heart and Lung Transplantation: eighteenth official report 2001, *J Heart Lung Transplant* 20:805, 2001.

Kantrowitz A, et al: Transplantation of the heart in an infant and an adult, *Am J Cardiol* 22(6):782. 1968.

Laks H, et al: Heart transplantation in the young and elderly, *Heart Fail Rev* 6:221, 2001.

Renlund DG, et al: New UNOS rules: historical background and implications for transplantation management, *J Heart Lung Transplant* 18:1065, 1999.

Index

Note: Page numbers followed by f refer to figures; page numbers followed by t refer to tables.

A

Abdominal accessory lobe, 108t, 110
Abscess
  amebic, 231, 231t
  lung, 225–226
Achalasia, 428–429, 463–464
  Chagas', 444, 446f, 447–448, 447f
Acid burns, esophageal, 98–101, 99f, 100t
Acquired immunodeficiency syndrome. *See* Human
    immunodeficiency virus (HIV) infection.
Actinomycosis, 217–218
Adenoid cystic carcinoma, 157
Adenoma, bronchial, 152–155, 154f, 156–157
Adenovirus infection, after lung transplantation, 266
Adrenal glands, metastatic cancer of, 167
Adult respiratory distress syndrome, extracorporeal life
    support in, 569–572, 570t, 571t
AIDS. *See* Human immunodeficiency virus (HIV) infection.
Air
  mediastinal. *See* Pneumomediastinum.
  thoracic. *See* Pneumothorax.
Air embolism
  in hemothorax, 60–61
  with pacemaker implantation, 512
Air leak
  after tube thoracostomy, 292
  after video-assisted thoracic surgery, 470
Air trapping, in emphysema, 26
Airway. *See also* Larynx; Trachea.
  acute obstruction of, 74–75
  debulking of, 37
  difficult, 27–31. *See also* Difficult airway.
  esophagectomy-related injury to, 391
  in non–small cell lung cancer, 168
  rupture of, with single-lung ventilation, 23
  stenting of, 37–38, 37f, 138–141, 139t
    imaging in, 139, 139f
    indications for, 138–139, 139t
    metal stents for, 139, 140
    Montgomery T-tube for, 140, 140f
    silicone stents for, 139–140, 139f
    Y-stents for, 140
  trauma to, 56–59
    complications of, 58–59
    evaluation of, 56–57
    in children, 111–112
    mechanisms of, 56
    treatment of, 57–58
  tumors of, 111
Airway obstruction
  acute, 74–75
  congenital, 111
  in non–small cell lung cancer, 168
Alkali burns, esophageal, 98–101, 99f, 100t
Amebiasis, 230–231, 231t
ε-Aminocaproic acid, in cardiovascular surgery, 484,
    499, 500
Analgesia, 9–10, 32–34. *See also* Anesthesia.
  intercostal nerve cryoablation for, 33
  interpleural anesthesia for, 33–34
  local anesthetics for, 34
  neuraxial opioids for, 34

  regional anesthetic techniques for, 33–34
  systemic, 32–33
Anastomotic leaks, after esophagectomy, 391–392
Anesthesia, 21–35
  difficult airway and, 27–31, 28f, 29f, 29t. *See also*
    Difficult airway.
  epidural, 24
  for airway obstruction, 75
  for bronchoscopy, 24
  for cardiovascular surgery, 481–483
  for esophagectomy, 25–26
  for esophagogastrectomy, 25–26
  for Ivor Lewis esophagectomy, 370
  for left thoracoabdominal esophagogastrectomy, 377–378
  for lung volume reduction, 26
  for mediastinoscopy, 24
  for mediastinotomy, 24–25
  for pain control, 24, 33–34
  for thoracoscopy, 25
  for thoracotomy, 25
  for thymectomy, 26
  for tracheal resection, 25
  in pulmonary trauma, 68
  intercostal nerve block for, 24
  intrapleural, 24
  intrathecal, 24
  monitoring of, 21–22
  premedication for, 21
  preoperative evaluation for, 21
  selection of, 23–24
  single-lung ventilation and, 22–23
Aneurysm
  aortic, 4, 578–586, 580f, 581t, 583t, 651
  cerebral, 641
  coronary artery, 728, 730f, 731
  venous, pulmonary, 332
  ventricular, 527, 675–677, 676f
Angiocentric lymphoma, pulmonary, 213
Angiography
  aortic, 651
  coronary, 645–650. *See also* Coronary angiography.
  left ventricular, 650–651, 651f
Angioplasty
  in congenital heart disease, 698–699
  in superior vena cava syndrome, 183
Anomalous circumflex coronary artery, from right aortic
    sinus of Valsalva, 727
Anomalous left coronary artery, from pulmonary artery,
    726, 726f
Antegrade cerebral perfusion, in cardiac surgery, 594–595
Antibiotics
  in actinomycosis, 218
  in esophageal injury, 64
  in lung abscess, 225
  in nocardiosis, 220
  preoperative, 7
  prophylactic
    in endocarditis, 643, 643t
    in traumatic hemothorax, 59–60
Anticoagulation
  during pediatric extracorporeal membrane
    oxygenation, 715